FAMILY PRACTICE GUIDELINES

Jill C. Cash, MSN, APRN, FNP-BC, a family nurse practitioner (FNP) for over 24 years, currently practices at Vanderbilt University Medical Center for the Vanderbilt Medical Group at Westhaven Family Practice in Franklin, Tennessee. She is a faculty member for the School of Nursing at Vanderbilt University. She has been a clinical preceptor for NP students for a variety of programs over the past several years. She also serves as a clinical preceptor for the Vanderbilt Program in Interprofessional Learning, which includes students from other disciplines, including the Vanderbilt Medical School, Nurse Practitioner, Pharmacy, and Social Work programs. Her previous experience includes high-risk obstetrics as a clinical nurse specialist in maternal–fetal medicine, as well as practicing as an NP in women's health, family practice, and rheumatology. In 2017, Ms. Cash was awarded the 2017 American Association of Nurse Practitioners State Award for Excellence in Illinois. Ms. Cash has authored several chapters in a variety of nursing and NP textbooks. She is the coauthor of *Family Practice Guidelines* (first, second, third, fourth, and fifth editions), *Adult-Gerontology Practice Guidelines* (first and second editions), and the first edition of *Canadian Family Practice Guidelines*. Ms. Cash is an active member of the American Association of Nurse Practitioners and Sigma Theta Tau International Honor Society.

Cheryl A. Glass, MSN, APRN, WHNP, RN-BC, a women's health nurse practitioner (NP) for over 22 years, currently practices as a clinical research specialist for KEPRO in TennCare's Medical Solutions Unit in Nashville, Tennessee. She is also an adjunct faculty at Vanderbilt University School of Nursing. Previously, Ms. Glass was a clinical trainer and trainer manager for Healthways. Her previous NP practice was as clinical research coordinator on pharmaceutical clinical trials at Nashville Clinical Research. She also worked in a Collaborative Clinical OB Practice with the director and assistant directors of maternal–fetal medicine at Vanderbilt University Medical Center Department of Obstetrics-Gynecology. Ms. Glass is the coauthor of *Family Practice Guidelines* (first, second, third, fourth, and fifth editions), *Adult-Gerontology Practice Guidelines* (first and second editions), and the first edition of *Canadian Family Practice Guidelines*. She has published five refereed journal articles. In 1999, Ms. Glass was named Nurse of the Year by the Tennessee chapter of the Association of Women's Health, Obstetric, and Neonatal Nurses. Ms. Glass is an active member of the American Association of Nurse Practitioners and Nurse Practitioners in Women's Health.

Jenny Mullen, DNP, MSN, FNP-BC, ACHPN, has been a practicing family nurse practitioner (FNP) for over 25 years in internal medicine. Currently Dr. Mullen is with Advanced Care Group in Nashville, Tennessee, where she is dedicated to serving families and geriatric populations through hospice/palliative care. Additional experience includes Director of Medical Services with Wellness Solutions Geriatrics, supervising medical healthcare providers in LTC facilities in southern state regions; endocrinology practice at Frist Clinic in Nashville, Tennessee; family practice and behavior health with United Neighborhood Health Services, primarily reaching the uninsured; and family/palliative practice with Holston Medical Group in Kingsport, Tennessee. In addition, she has been a clinical preceptor for NP/physician assistant (PA) students from Tennessee State University, Vanderbilt University, Trevecca Nazarene University, and Belmont University. Dr. Mullen is an adult-geriatric consultant for *Adult-Gerontology Practice Guidelines* (second edition) and is a peer reviewer for the *Journal of Doctoral Nursing Practice*. She is an active member of Tennessee Nurses Association/American Nurses Association, American Association of Nurse Practitioners, Hospice & Palliative Nurses Association, and Sigma Theta Tau International Honor Society.

FAMILY PRACTICE GUIDELINES

FIFTH EDITION

Jill C. Cash, MSN, APRN, FNP-BC

Cheryl A. Glass, MSN, APRN, WHNP, RN-BC

Jenny Mullen, DNP, MSN, FNP-BC, ACHPN

EDITORS

SPRINGER PUBLISHING COMPANY

Springer Publishing Company, LLC
11 West 42nd Street
New York, NY 10036
www.springerpub.com

Acquisitions Editor: Adrianne Brigido
Compositor: diacriTech

ISBN: 978-0-8261-3583-4
ebook ISBN: 978-0-8261-3584-1
DOI: 10.1891/9780826135841

A Procedures Supplement and Editable Client Teaching Guides may be accessed at connect.springerpub.com/book/978-0-8261-3584-1

20 21 22 23 24 / 5 4 3

The author and the publisher of this Work have made every effort to use sources believed to be reliable to provide information that is accurate and compatible with the standards generally accepted at the time of publication. Because medical science is continually advancing, our knowledge base continues to expand. Therefore, as new information becomes available, changes in procedures become necessary. We recommend that the reader always consult current research and specific institutional policies before performing any clinical procedure or delivering any medication. The author and publisher shall not be liable for any special, consequential, or exemplary damages resulting, in whole or in part, from the readers' use of, or reliance on, the information contained in this book. The publisher has no responsibility for the persistence or accuracy of URLs for external or third-party Internet websites referred to in this publication and does not guarantee that any content on such websites is, or will remain, accurate or appropriate.

Library of Congress Control Number: 2020937424

Contact us to receive discount rates on bulk purchases.
We can also customize our books to meet your needs.
For more information please contact: sales@springerpub.com

To my kids, Kaitlin and Carsen—
thank you for always being there and for being you!

*"Sometimes you will never know the value of a moment,
until it becomes a memory."* — Dr. Seuss

Jill C. Cash

To my beloved Ed, I miss you.

*"She watched the gap between ship and shore grow to a huge gulf like dying.
Perhaps this was a little like dying, the departed no longer visible to the others,
yet both still existed, only in different worlds."* — Susan Wiggs

Cheryl A. Glass

This is dedicated to my husband, Jeff Nelson, and to all my family who have given me much love,
patience, and support. I'm so very grateful for each of you in my life.

*"Wholeness and meaning in life are not the products of what you have or don't have,
what you've done or haven't done. You are already a whole person and possess a life of infinite
meaning and purpose because of who you are—a child of God."* — Neil T. Anderson

Jenny Mullen

Contents

I. Guidelines

1. Health Maintenance Guidelines

2. Public Health Guidelines

3. Pain Management Guidelines

4. Dermatology Guidelines

5. Eye Guidelines

13. Obstetrics Guidelines

14. Gynecological Guidelines

15. Sexually Transmitted Infections Guidelines

16. Infectious Disease Guidelines

17. Systemic Disorders Guidelines

18. Musculoskeletal Guidelines

IV. Appendices

Contributors

Julie Adkins, DNP, APN, FNP-BC, FAANP
Certified Family Nurse Practitioner
Adkins Family Practice
West Frankford, Illinois

Rhonda Arthur, DNP, CMN, WHNP-BC, FNP-BC, CNE
Associate Professor
Department of Family Nursing
Frontier Nursing University
Hyden, Kentucky

Jill C. Cash, MSN, APRN, FNP-BC
Nurse Practitioner
The Vanderbilt Medical Group
Westhaven Family Practice
Vanderbilt University Medical Center
Nashville, Tennessee

Kala Christopherson, DNP, RN, FNP-C
Family Nurse Practitioner Program Co-Coordinator
Assistant Professor of Clinical Nursing
Department of Graduate Studies
University of Texas Health Science Center
    Houston-Cizik School of Nursing
Houston, TX

Michelle Collins, Ph.D., CNM, RN-CEFM, FACNM, FAAN, FNAP
Associate Dean of Academic Affairs, Professor,
Women's, Children, and Family Nursing
Rush University College of Nursing
Chicago, IL

Moya Cook, APN, CNP
Nurse Practitioner
Marion VA Medical Center
Marion, Illinois

Susan B Drummond RN MSN C-EFM
Senior Associate in Obstetrics
OBGYN
Vanderbilt University Medical Center
Nashville, TN

Doncy Joji Eapen, PhD, MSN, APRN, FNP-BC
Assistant Professor, Clinical Nursing
Department of Undergraduate Studies
UTHealth Cizik School of Nursing
Houston, Texas

Cheryl A. Glass, MSN, APRN, WHNP-BC
Clinical Research Specialist
KEPRO Peer Review
Medical Solutions Unit
Paducah, Kentucky

Debbie A. Gunter MSN, APRN, FNP-BC, ACHPN
Family and Palliative Care Nurse Practitioner
Cognitive Neurology
Emory Healthcare
Atlanta, Georgia

Mellisa A. Hall, DNP, AGPCNP-BC, FNP-BC
Graduate Nursing Chair
Nursing
University of Southern Indiana
Evansville, Indiana

Dana Hughes, MSN, MPH
Nurse Practitioner
Infectious Disease
Vanderbilt University Medical Center
Nashville, Tennessee

Carole Mackavey, DNP, MSN, APRN, FNP-C
Assistant Professor/FNP Program Coordinator
Cizik School of Nursing, The University of Texas
    Health Science Center
Houston, Texas

Jenny Mullen, DNP, MSN, FNP-BC, ACHPN
Palliative Care Services
The Advanced Care Group/Advanced Care
Nashville, Tennessee

Robertson Nash, Ph.D., ACNP-BC
Assistant in Medicine
Department of Medicine
Vanderbilt University Medical Center
Nashville, Tennessee

Merita O'Sullivan, MSN, RN, CNM
Director of Midlevel Providers in OB/GYN and
    Reproductive Sciences
University of Texas Health Science Center at
    Houston
Houston, Texas

Laura A. Petty, MSN, GNP-BC
Gerontological Nurse Practitioner
Self-Employed/ Contractor
Belmont University (BSN) & Vanderbilt University
    (MSN)
Lebanon, Tennessee

Christina C. Reed, WHNP
Women's Health Nurse Practitioner
The University of Texas Health Science Center at
    Houston
Houston, Texas

Kathleen Siders DNP, APRN, FNP-C
Assistant Professor
Graduate Studies
Cizik School of Nursing at The University of Texas
    Health Science Center at Houston (UTHealth)
Houston, Texas

**Mariya Tankimovich, DNP, MSN, RN, APRN,
    FNP-C, CNE**
Assistant Professor-Clinical
UTHealth Cizik School of Nursing
Department of Graduate Studies
Family Nurse Practitioner Track
Houston, Texas

Sarah Hendershott Taylor, APRN, MSN, FNP
Otolaryngology Nurse Practitioner
Vanderbilt University Medical Center
Nashville, Tennessee

Nancy Pesta Walsh, DNP, MSN, FNP
Family Nurse Practitioner
Hutchinson Health and Frontier School of
    Midwifery and Family Nursing
Hyden, Kentucky

Kimberly D. Waltrip, Ph.D, APRN-BC
Instructor of Nursing
College of Health Professions
Western Governors University
Salt Lake City, Utah

Kenneth E. Watford, DNP
Nurse practitioner/Assistant professor
Otolaryngology, Head and Neck Surgery
Vanderbilt University Medical Center
Nashville, Tennessee

Jamie G. Wiggleton, ANP-BC
Nurse Practitioner
Otolaryngology, Head and Neck Surgery
Vanderbilt University Medical Center
Nashville, Tennessee

Alyson Wolz, DNP, APRN, PMHCNS, BC, CBIS
NeuroRestoritive
Carbondale, Illinois

Preface

We are excited to collaborate on this new fifth edition of *Family Practice Guidelines*. The guidelines have been written and updated by experienced nurse practitioners. This valuable resource is designed to assist nurse practitioners in organizing and using the content in a quick-reference format. Emphasis is placed on history taking, physical examination, and key elements of the diagnosis. Useful website links have also been incorporated, along with updated client teaching guides.

This book is organized into chapters using a body-system format. The disorders included within each chapter are organized in alphabetical sequence for easy access. Disorders that are more commonly seen in the primary care setting are included. Client teaching guides are also available for many topics, and clinical pearls and bold and italic text alert the practitioner to key information.

Organization

The book is organized into three major sections:

- *Section I: Guidelines* – Chapters containing the individual disorder guidelines.
- *Section II: Procedures* – Procedures that are commonly conducted within the office or clinic setting.
- *Section III: Client Teaching Guides* – Written information that is easy to distribute to patients as a take-home teaching guide. The teaching guides are arranged in alphabetical order for ease of reference and the pages are perforated for easy pull-out and photocopying.

Notable Updates

- The most up-to-date Centers for Disease Control and Prevention (CDC) guidelines on health maintenance and immunization schedules for adults and children.
- An entire chapter is dedicated to the sports pre-participation examination.
- The Dermatology Guidelines include the newest guidelines for Wound Care Management. The Dermatology Guidelines also include color photos of skin rashes and skin disorders, along with the latest standard of care for treatment.
- The Respiratory Guidelines include the updated treatment guidelines for Chronic Obstructive Pulmonary Disease (COPD) and Pneumonia.
- The Cardiovascular Guidelines include the newest guidelines for Heart Failure and Hypertension.
- The Genitourinary Guidelines include an updated subchapter on Erectile Dysfunction and a new subchapter on Premature Ejaculation.
- The Obstetric Guidelines include a new section on the overview of prenatal care from the initial prenatal visit through the overview of postpartum care.
- The Neurologic Guidelines include an updated subchapter on Stroke.
- The Rheumatological Guidelines chapter includes the most common rheumatic conditions encountered in primary care, including Fibromyalgia, Psoriatic Arthritis, Gout, and many others.
- The Infectious Diseases Guidelines chapter includes guidelines for the diagnosis and management of coronavirus disease 2019 (COVID-19).
- The Psychiatric Guidelines include the newest treatment recommendations in psychiatric conditions, including the subchapters Bipolar Disorder, Depression, Sleep Disorders, and so forth.
- Diet Recommendations have been updated with a new section on the Fermentable Oligosaccharides, Disaccharides, Monosaccharides, and Polyols (FODMAP) Diet.

We hope you find this fifth edition of *Family Practice Guidelines* easy to access and a valuable resource during your clinical practice. We appreciate your support for our first four editions and hope you find the fifth edition as rewarding as the others.

Jill C. Cash
Cheryl A. Glass
Jenny Mullen

FAMILY PRACTICE
GUIDELINES

I

GUIDELINES

1

Health Maintenance Guidelines

Jill Cash and Mariya Tankimovich

This chapter provides an overview and resources for a successful health promotion and disease prevention visit for populations across the life span. Current world population presents many challenges, including cultural and genetic ones. This chapter helps a provider understand the needs of different socio-cultural groups and best practices for providing care accepted by each individual.

Cultural Diversity and Sensitivity

Angelito Tacderas and Mariya Tankimovich

Each office visit is an opportunity to gain more knowledge about a client's health beliefs and practices. Cultural sensitivity is the responsibility of all healthcare providers. Inadequate awareness of the client's health beliefs and practices influenced by culture may lead to mistrust. This may result in barriers, including inappropriate delivery of care, increased cost, noncompliance, and seeking care elsewhere. Thus, this may eventually lead to even more barriers to healthcare access, resulting in unfavorable healthcare outcomes. Title VI of the Civil Rights Act is very specific about providing services that are less than the existing standard of care to anyone based on race, age, sex, or financial status. According to this document, "No person in the United States shall, on the grounds of race, color or national origin be excluded in the participation in, be denied the benefits of, or be discriminated under any programs or activity receiving federal financing assistance" (U.S. Department of Justice [USDJ], 2017).

Culture is more than nationality or race. Culture influences a person's reasoning, decisions, and actions. It is the accumulation of learned beliefs, values, habits, and practices. Culture influences decision-making, thoughts, what is approved or disapproved, what is normal or not, which are all acquired from close personal relations (family/members of society) over time.

Cultural diversity exists when groups from different cultures must coexist within an environmental area (family, neighborhood, township, city, or country). Knowing that there are differences in cultures, and not assigning values among different cultures, reflects cultural sensitivity. However, significant differences may exist in the way healthcare is perceived and practiced because of the differing values and beliefs regarding health and illness inherent among people of varying cultural backgrounds.

Factors Contributing to Cultural Diversity

- Fewer White non-Hispanic children
- Increase in immigration
- Efficiency in transportation and travel
- Increase in the homeless and the poor populations
- Increase in divorce rate
- Increase in single parenting
- Grandparents raising grandchildren
- Substance abuse
- Violence
- Transgender sex changes
- Homosexual acceptance
- Information explosion/high technology
- Illiteracy
- Increase in non-English-proficient healthcare providers
- Federal regulations

Thoughtful Consideration

Providing care without being sensitive to the cultural needs of a client may suggest that the healthcare provider's values and beliefs are superior to those of the client and may lead to disparity of care. The limited patient involvement in care may result in noncompliance, placing patients at greater risk of health-related complications. The delay in provision of healthcare can result in life-threatening complications.

Numerous cultural resources are available throughout the literature and the Internet. Preference as to which educational/assessment tools to use is the healthcare provider's prerogative.

The following are guidelines for promoting cultural sensitivity in the clinical setting:

A. Provide a cultural diversity self-assessment/practice organization.

   1. Consult online Internet self-assessment tools; for example, on the Centers for Disease Control and Prevention (CDC, 2015) website.

   2. Download self-assessment tools from public sites. **Resettlement Assistance Program, Cultural**

Competence, provides a validated tool (http://rapworkers.com/resources/cultural-competence).

3. Use existing self-assessment tools and make necessary changes to fit the need of your community.

B. Identify the need of the population served.

1. Understand the community and its health status.

2. Evaluate resources, attitudes, and barriers inside the community and practice location.

    a. Access to resources

    b. Notification of assistance

    c. Range of assistance options:

        i. Transportation

        ii. Communication; consider an interpreter (personal vs. automated).

           1) Identify bilingual staff.

           2) Use family members or personal acquaintances as interpreters (adults only).

           3) Provide multilingual written materials.

        iii. Education (meaningful/multilingual)

           1) User friendly

           2) Friendly technology

C. Educate staff to cultural diversities.

1. Assessments should include the patient's health values and beliefs.

2. Communication should be meaningful.

    a. Be precise and clear.

    b. Maintain eye contact when speaking.

    c. Use plain language.

    d. Observe facial expressions and body language.

    e. Use short sentences to explain lengthy information.

    f. Avoid medical jargon.

    g. Use repetition for emphasis.

    h. Ask questions to confirm understanding.

D. Schedule longer appointments if needed.

E. Healthcare providers should clarify the limitations of a healthcare provider's role.

(Spector, 2017; Pigozi & Jones Bartoli, 2016; Muronda, 2016; Andrews & Boyle, 2015; Douglas, et al., 2014)

Bibliography

Andrews, M. M., & Boyle, J. S. (2015). *Transcultural concepts in nursing care* (7th ed.). Philadelphia, PA: Lippincott Williams & Wilkins.

Centers for Disease Control and Prevention. (2015, March 11). Cultural competence. Retrieved from https://npin.cdc.gov/pages/cultural-competence

Douglas, M. K., Rosenkoetter, M., Pacquiao, D. F., Callister, L. C., Hattar-Pollara, M., Lauderdale, J., … Purnell, L. (2014). Guidelines for implementing culturally competent nursing care. *Journal of Transcultural Nursing: Official Journal of the Transcultural Nursing Society/Transcultural Nursing Society*, 25(2), 109–121. doi:10.1177/1043659614520998

Muronda, V. (2016). The culturally diverse nursing student: A review of the literature. *Journal of Transcultural Nursing*, 4, 400–412. doi:10.1177/1043659615595867

Ontario Council of Agencies Serving Immigrants (OCASI). (2019). Cultural competence. Retrieved from http://rapworkers.com/resources/cultural-competence

Pigozi, P. L., & Jones Bartoli, A. J.(2016). School nurses' experiences in dealing with bullying situations among students. *Journal of School Nursing*, 32(3), 177–185. doi:10.1177/1059840515613140

Spector, R. E. (2017). *Cultural diversity in health and illness* (9th ed.). Upper Saddle River, NJ: Prentice-Hall.

U.S. Department of Justice. (2017). Retrieved from https://www.justice.gov/crt/fcs/T6manual1

Health Maintenance During the Life Span

Jill C. Cash, Debbie Gunter, and Mariya Tankimovich

Health maintenance involves identifying individuals who are at risk for health problems and encouraging these individuals to develop behaviors that reduce these risks. An important aspect of health maintenance is patient education, including teaching individuals about risk factors for a disease and ways to modify their behaviors to reduce risks of comorbidities. This book contains Client Teaching Guides that the practitioner may use for patient education; these forms are found in Section III: Client Teaching Guides. They may be photocopied by the practitioner, filled in according to the patient's evaluation and needs, and given to the patient.

Family history is an important component of any patient visit. Health maintenance visits allow more time for a more thorough collection of the detailed family history. Advances in genetic sciences contribute to increased value to understanding detailed family history in medical practice. The American Medical Association includes information and guides for understanding and collecting family and genetic history in the website accessed through https://www.ama-assn.org/delivering-care/precision-medicine/collecting-family-history.

This chapter describes tools that the practitioner can use in preventive healthcare assessment, which include websites, screening guidelines, and suggestions for patient education and counseling.

Pediatric Well-Child Evaluation

The 2019 Recommendations for Preventative Pediatric Health Care provided by American Academy of Pediatrics (AAP) are available in a chart on the AAP website (https://www.aap.org/en-us/documents/periodicity_schedule.pdf). It is designed for use starting with prenatal care visits and throughout adolescence, ending at 21 years of age. A detailed documentation from each visit is required and is documented either in Electronic Health/Medical Record (HER or EMR) or on paper. One of the documentation formats used arranges information under Subjective, Objective, Assessment, and Plan (SOAP). The American Academy of Family Physicians provides a website with several forms for different types of visits. These forms can be used for when either paper charting is unavoidable or when choosing a new EHR/EMR program for the practice. These forms are accessible through the following link: https://www.aafp.org/fpm/toolBox/viewToolBox.htm

The growth charts for children are available in imperial and metric systems as well as in multiple languages. They can be found on the Centers for Disease Control and Prevention (CDC) website www.cdc.gov/growthcharts. Immunization schedules for children and adults are accessible through the CDC website as well (https://www.cdc.gov/vaccines/schedules/index.html). Most of the states have online record systems for easy tracking of immunizations administered. They could be accessed through the CDC Immunization Information Systems (IIS) website found at: https://www.cdc.gov/vaccines/programs/iis/contacts-locate-records.html. IIS is helpful in cases of school transfer and lost paper records. Paper records are available on numerous on-line sites. Below are two examples for children/teens and adults:

- Vaccine Administration Record for Children and Teens (available at http://immunize.org/catg.d/p2022.pdf)
- Vaccine Administration Record for Adults (available at http://immunize.org/catg.d/p2023.pdf)

Many cases of rejection of immunization have been reported. It is important to realize that parents and adults have a right to refuse immunizations for their children or themselves. However, it is essential to educate population about latest research and implication of declining immunizations.

Anticipatory Guidance by Age
The anticipatory guidance outline and resources for motivational interviewing are provided by AAP (2019a) and Bright Futures and are found at: https://brightfutures.aap.org/search/Pages/default.aspx?k=motivational%20interviewing. It provides a quick reference for the practitioner conducting either the child's initial visit or an adult's annual visit. A more detailed resource called, Promoting Healthy Development, focuses on intricate details of quickly-growing and changing children. It can be found at https://brightfutures.aap.org/Bright%20Futures%20Documents/BF4_HealthyDevelopment.pdf. This resource lists topics that the practitioner should discuss with the caregiver. Information discussed during the visit should be supplemented with booklets, teaching guides, and brochures for the caregiver. Additional tools for health promotion and more information for effective health promotion visits are found on the Bright Futures website: https://brightfutures.aap.org/materials-and-tools/guidelines-and-pocket-guide/Pages/default.aspx.

Nutrition
Proper nutrition is an essential part of maintaining health and preventing diseases. Providers should promote well-balanced diets for all patients with an emphasis on the prevention of obesity. Diet modification is an important part of disease or disorder management. The U.S. Department of Agriculture (USDA) provides a variety of interactive educational tools on nutrition, weight management, and physical activity. It is recommended that patients use these tools for family education on healthy diet and lifestyle. Diet information is found in Appendix B: Diet Recommendations. The Mayo Clinic provides an excellent on-line resource for healthy diets for children. It can be accessed through https://www.mayo-clinic.org/healthy-lifestyle/childrens-health/in-depth/nutrition-for-kids/art-20049335. The USDA produces a food pyramid guide at https://www.cnpp.usda.gov/sites/default/files/archived_projects/FGPPamphlet.pdf, and one of the easiest guides for determining servings is at https://www.choosemyplate.gov/grains-group-food-gallery. More detailed serving size recommendations are available on the website by the Government of Canada through

https://www.canada.ca/en/health-canada/services/canada-food-guide/about/history-food-guide/eating-well-with-canada-food-guide-2007.html.

The obesity epidemic is affecting global population health. It is the responsibility of all healthcare providers to alert and educate families about healthy nutrition. Each office visit is an opportunity to evaluate the patient's weight and to discuss exercise programs. As pain assessment becomes the "fifth vital sign" in the hospital setting, the body mass index (BMI) becomes the fifth vital sign in the outpatient setting.

Teaching parents the correct serving sizes for children will help guide their children's eating habits for life. The American Academy of Pediatrics-sponsored healthychildren.org, (2015) recommends that portion sizes for fruits and vegetables are one-quarter cup cooked, one-half piece fresh, or one-quarter cup of juice for children aged 1 to 6 years. Serving sizes for older children and adults are based on the food pyramids. Use the food pyramid to teach and reinforce proper nutrition. Some helpful websites about nutrition are as follows:
A. The USDA resources for nutrition and health are located at www.choosemyplate.gov.
B. My Plate kids' place is located at https://www.choosemyplate.gov/kids.
C. The Childhood Nutrition website is located at www.nourishinteractive.com. This informative website gives helpful information such as:
    1. Controlling portion sizes
    2. Parent tips tool
    3. Interactive nutrition tools
    4. A fun area for children with interactive nutrition games
    5. Healthy living tips ready to print
D. The Harvard Medical School on-line publication provides a good resourse for vitamins found in foods. It can be accessed through https://www.health.harvard.edu/staying-healthy/the-best-foods-for-vitamins-and-minerals
E. The American Heart Association (AHA) is another valuable resource for education about nutrition. The website provides information about serving size for each group at: https://www.heart.org/en/healthy-living/healthy-eating/eat-smart/nutrition-basics/suggested-servings-from-each-food-group

Height and weight are used to calculate BMI. The mathematical calculation is BMI = kg/m^2; however, the Internet provides easy-to-use BMI calculators.
A. The National Heart, Lung, and Blood Institute (NHLBI, 2019) includes a calculator in its Obesity Education Initiative: www.nhlbi.nih.gov/health/educational/lose_wt/BMI/bmicalc.htm. This support site also includes patient information on risk assessment, weight control, and helpful recipes.
B. The CDC provides an online source for the calculation of BMI for children and teens: https://www.cdc.gov/healthyweight/bmi/calculator.html. The CDC's website also provides information on weight loss, physical activity, and parental tips.

Malnutrition and vitamin and mineral deficiency are commonly seen in the elderly population. Vitamins B6,

B12, D, E, folic acid, zinc, calcium, and iron are often deficient in the elderly diet, along with protein and calorie deficiencies (Stepler, 2016). The National Institute on Aging provides an excellent resourse on vitamin needs for people over 50 years of age at the website: https://www.nia.nih.gov/health/vitamins-and-minerals

Using Zawada's (1996) acronym WEIGHT LOSS can help you easily identify common causes of weight loss in the elderly.

W: Wandering and not eating, because of forgetting to take time to eat

E: Emotional problems, including depression

I: Impecuniosity (finances do not meet the needs to buy food and other things)

G: Gut problems

H: Hyperthyroidism or other endocrine abnormalities

T: Tremor or neurologic problems that make eating and holding utensils difficult

L: Low-salt, low-cholesterol diets avoided, often because of disliking the taste of recommended diets

O: Oral problems: edentulous, poor dental care, dentures not fitting, mouth disorders such as oral ulcers

S: Swallowing problems, difficulty swallowing or chewing food because of stroke or other impairment

S: Shopping or food preparation barriers, inability to purchase or prepare food, and no resources for assistance

Identification of factors contributing to an elderly patient's malnutrition assists you, the patient, and the patient's family in resolving them. Utilize your state's Area Agencies on Aging (AAA) for information on elder care resources in your area. Local area agiencies could be located through the National Association of Area Agiencies on Aging at https://www.n4a.org/.

Exercise

Physical exercise is a vital component of health maintenance. Exercise provides cardiovascular fitness and weight control, prevents osteoporosis through weight-bearing exercise, and decreases lipids. Exercise is important for flexibility, strength, and coordination. Exercise can also be used for both weight control and reduction. The Mayo Clinic (2018), at the following site—https://www.mayoclinic.org/healthy-lifestyle/weight-loss/in-depth/calories/art-20048065—states that approximately 3,500 calories must be burned to lose 1 pound of fat. Therefore, along with exercise, caloric intake must remain the same or be decreased to result in weight loss.

Planning an Exercise Program

Exercise plans should be started after a health provider screens a patient because heavy physical exertion may trigger an acute myocardial infarction. Factors most likely to influence risk are age, medical conditions, hypertension,

and the intensity of the exercise planned. The medical history screening identifies individual and family history of problems such as coronary heart disease, hypertension, and diabetes. Review health habits such as previous exercise or sedentary lifestyle, diet, and smoking/tobacco use.

Providers need to evaluate the patient using screening tests before prescribing an exercise program. Consider the patient's age and all comorbidities for additional tests.

A. Complete blood count
B. Blood glucose
C. Cholesterol screening
D. EKG (in patients older than 40 years)
E. Holter monitoring for arrhythmias

Persons with a heart murmur or other abnormal physical finding should defer exercise until the full nature of the disorder is evaluated. The best measure of an exercise work capacity is the determination of oxygen consumption at maximal activity, which is measured with a stress test. Hypertension, elevated resting blood pressures, and chronic obstructive lung disease are other factors that require attention before participation in exercise. Persons with hypertension should undergo a thorough evaluation, have antihypertensive agent(s) prescribed, and be monitored periodically during their prescribed graded exercise program.

Physical exercise should be strictly monitored in the following conditions and may need to be curtailed, or even stopped, based on the condition:

A. Congestive heart failure
B. Uncontrolled hypertension
C. Uncontrolled epilepsy
D. Uncontrolled diabetes
E. Atrioventricular (AV) heart block
F. Aneurysms
G. Ventricular instability
H. Aortic valve disease

Measurement of the heart rate during exercise is an easy and inexpensive method to evaluate cardiovascular fitness. Target heart rates vary by physical condition and a person's age. The Mayo Clinic (2019b) provides a formula to calculate target heart/aerobic activity level zone range at the following website: https://www.mayoclinic.org/healthy-lifestyle/fitness/in-depth/exercise-intensity/art-20046887

Patient Education Before Exercise

All exercise program prescriptions should include frequency, duration, intensity, and time to abort the exercise. Persons should be educated on the signs and symptoms of heat exhaustion and should be advised when to seek first aid.

The AHA (2018) (at the following website—https://www.heart.org/en/healthy-living/fitness/fitness-basics/aha-recs-for-physical-activity-in-adults) provides recommendations for exercise activity for adults and children in accordance with guidelines made available by the Office of Disease Prevention and Health Promotion (ODPHP) through the following website: https://health.gov/paguidelines/second-edition. Both organizations recommend evenly spreadout weekly 150 minutes of moderate or 75 minutes of vigorous exercises or a combination of both for adults, and daily 60 minutes of vigorous activity for adolescents. It is recommended for children to be active throughout the day. Descriptions of different types of exercises could be accessed through the AHA website at https://www.heart.org/en/healthy-living/fitness/fitness-basics/aha-recs-for-physical-activity-in-adults. ODPHP website includes scientific report and information about Move Your Way Campaign. Both can be used to encourage patients to move more and are accessible through https://health.gov/paguidelines/second-edition/

The American College of Obstetricians and Gynecologists (ACOG, 2017) provides recommendations for continuing or starting excersise programs during pregnancy at the website https://www.acog.org/Patients/FAQs/Exercise-During-Pregnancy. ACOG's recommendation is to start prenatal visits early and to discuss exercise plans with a healthcare provider.

Swimming and cycling are considered to be low impact exercise types by the Arthritis Foundation (https://www.arthritis.org/living-with-arthritis/exercise/arthritis-friendly/lap-swimming.php) and Norwegian sports medicine and sciences researchers. It is recommended to include resistance training exercises for swimmers and cyclists (Andersen et al., 2018).

For exercise to benefit individuals, it must be continued lifelong. The healthcare provider should evaluate individual lifestyle and preferences in designing an exercise program. One exercise program can become boring over an extended period and probably will not be continued. A variety of activities, class participation, and positive reinforcement help to keep physical activity fun as an integral part of a health maintenance program. *See Section III: Client Teaching Guide for this chapter, "Exercise."*

Healthcare professionals who will be monitoring and prescribing exercise plans for large numbers of individuals are encouraged to seek special training and certification. The American College of Sports Medicine (ACSM) has a program that includes training for healthcare professionals and a book titled *ACSM's Guidelines for Exercise Testing and Prescription.*

Bibliography

American Academy of Family Physicians. (2019). FPM toolbox. Retrieved from www.asfp.org/fpm/toolBox/viewToolBox.htm

American Academy of Pediatrics. (2019a). Recommendations for preventive pediatric health care. *Bright Futures: American Academy of Pediatrics.* Retrieved from https://www.aap.org/en-us/documents/periodicity_schedule.pdf

American Academy of Pediatrics.(2019b). Engaging patients and families: Periodicity schedule. Retrieved from https://www.aap.org/en-us/professional-resources/practice-transformation/managing-patients/Pages/Periodicity-Schedule.asp

American College of Obstetricians and Gynecologists. (2017). Exercise during pregnancy. Retrieved from https://www.acog.org/Patients/FAQs/Exercise-During-Pregnancy

American College of Sports Medicine. (2018). *ACSM's Guidelines for Exercise Testing and Prescription* (10th ed.). Philadelphia, PA: Wolters Kluwer.

American Heart Association. (2018). American Heart Association recommendations for physical activity in adults and kids. Retrieved from https://www.heart.org/en/healthy-living/fitness/fitness-basics/aha-recs-for-physical-activity-in-adults

Andersen, O. K., Clarsen, B., Garthe, I., Morland, M., & Stensrud, T. (2018). Bone health in elite Norwegian endurance cyclists and runners: A cross sectional study. *BMJ Open Sport and Exercise Medicine, 4*(1), 1–7.

Arthritis Foundation. (2019). Lap swimming. Retrieved from www.arthritis.org/living-with-arthritis/exercise/arthritis-friendly/lap-swimming.php

Centers for Disease Control and Prevention. (2016a). CDC catch-up immunization schedule for persons aged 4 months through 18 years who start late or who are more than 1 month behind—United States 2016. Retrieved from https://www.cdc.gov/vaccines/schedules/hcp/imz/catchup.html

Centers for Disease Control and Prevention. (2016b). CDC recommended adult immunization schedule—United States 2016. Retrieved from https://www.cdc.gov/vaccines/schedules/hcp/adult.html

Centers for Disease Control and Prevention (CDC). (2016c). CDC recommended immunization schedule for persons aged 0 through 6 years—United States 2016. Retrieved from https://www.cdc.gov/vaccines/schedules/hcp/imz/child-adolescent.html

Centers for Disease Control and Prevention. (2016d). Information for travelers. Retrieved from www.cdc.gov/travel/page/traveler-information-center

Centers for Disease Control and Prevention. (2016e). Growth charts. Retrieved from https://www.cdc.gov/growthcharts

Centers for Disease Control and Prevention. (2019a). BMI percentile calculator for child and teen: English version. Retrieved from https://nccd.cdc.gov/dnpabmi/calculator.aspx

Centers for Disease Control and Prevention. (2019b). CDC Vaccine Schedules App for Health Care Providers. Retrieved from https://www.cdc.gov/vaccines/schedules/hcp/schedule-app.html

Centers for Disease Control and Prevention. (2019c). Immunization schedules. Retrieved from www.cdc.gov/vaccines/schedules/index.html

Childhood Nutrition. (n.d.). Serving sizes. Retrieved from http://www.nourishinteractive.com

ConsultGeri. (2019). The 2019 American Geriatrics Society Updated Beers Criteria® for potentially inappropriate medication use in older adults. Retrieved from https://consultgeri.org/try-this/general-assessment/issue-16

Healthy Children. (2015). Portions and serving sizes. *Healthychildren.org.* Retrieved from www.healthychildren.org/English/healthy-living/nutrition/Pages/Portions-and-Serving-Sizes.aspx

Mayo Clinic. (2019a). Healthy lifestyle: Children's health. Hutrition for kids: Guidelines for a healthy diet. Retrieved from https://www.mayoclinic.org/healthy-lifestyle/childrens-health/in-depth/nutrition-for-kids/art-20049335

Mayo Clinic. (2019b). Healthy lifestyle: Fitness. Exercise intensity: How to measure it. Retrieved from www.mayoclinic.org/healthy-lifestyle/fitness//in-depth/exercise-intensity/art-20046887

Mayo Clinic. (2018). Healthy lifestyle: Weight loss. Retrieved from www.mayoclinic.org/healthy-lifestyle/weight-loss/in-depth/calories/art-20048065

Mayo Foundation for Medical Education and Research. (2016, January). Nutrition for kids: Guidelines for a healthy diet. Retrieved from http://www.mayoclinic.com/health/nutrition-for-kids/NU00606

Miller, N., Reicks, M., Redden, J. P., Mann, T., Mykerezi, E., & Vickers, Z. (2015). Increasing portion sizes of fruits and vegetables in an elementary school lunch program can increase fruit and vegetable consumption. *Appetite, 91,* 426–30. doi:10.1016/j.appet.2015.04.081

National Heart Lung and Blood Institute. (2019). Obesity education initiative: BMI calculator. Retrieved from http://www.nhlbi.nih.gov/health/educational/lose_wt/BMI/bmicalc.htm

National Institutes of Health, Office of Dietary Supplements. (2015). Food sources for common vitamin and mineral deficiencies. Retrieved from https://ods.od.nih.gov/factsheets/Mvms-HealthProfessional/

Steinweg, D. L., & Worth, H. (1993). Alcoholism: The keys to the CAGE. *The American Journal of Medicine 94,* 520–523. DOI: 10.1016/0002-9343(93)90088-7

Stepler, R. (2016). World's centenarian population projected to grow eightfold by 2050. Washington, DC: Pew Research Center. Retrieved from http://www.pewresearch.org/fact-tank/2016/04/21/worlds-centenarian-population-projected-to-grow-eightfold-by-2050

U.S. Census. (n.d.). Quickfacts. Retrieved from https://quickfacts.census.gov/qfd/staes/oooo.html

U.S. Department of Agriculture. (n.d.). Food pyramid. Retrieved from https//www.choosemyplate.gov

U.S. Department of Agriculture. (n.d.). *My Plate kids' place.* Retrieved from https://www.choosemyplate.gov/kids

Zawada, E. (1996). Malnutrition in the elderly: Is it simply a matter of not eating enough? *Postgraduate Medicine, 100*(1), 208.

Other Collaborating Providers

Jill C. Cash, Debbie Gunter, and Mariya Tankimovich

The role of the primary care provider is to ensure that the patient becomes a partner in preventive health measures to avoid disease, disease complications, and comorbidities. The practitioner should refer the patient to other healthcare providers to continue health maintenance according to specialty. The primary care provider functions as the main point of care coordination.

A. Dental care:
   1. Dental care should be routinely discussed.
   2. Once teeth emerge, brushing should begin with a small, soft brush.
   3. In children, dental care should begin with soft, rubber brushes for gum care.
   4. Encourage the child to brush teeth twice daily to promote healthy habits.
   5. Refer the patient to a dentist at 3 years, unless problems arise earlier.
   6. Older children should be encouraged to use mouth guards with contact sports.
   7. Encourage flossing when the child has the cognitive and developmental dexterity to use dental floss.
B. Vision care:
   1. Begin initial vision screening for children at 3 years of age using the age-appropriate eye chart.
   2. School screening should include a vision-screening component.
   3. Refer patients to an optometrist for routine evaluation.

Adult Risk Assessment Form

Jill C. Cash, Debbie Gunter, and Mariya Tankimovich

The Adult Risk Assessment Form (Exhibit 1.1) should be used for all adult patients. It is used to evaluate a patient's risk for particular diseases. The practitioner should interview the patient, assessing for the risk factors listed on the Risk Assessment Form. The family history of first-degree relatives (parents, siblings, and children) should also be discussed, as many diseases are related to genetic factors. Use provided form to guide HER/EMR upgrades. For paper charts, keep a copy of the Risk Assessment Form in the front of the patient's chart, and update yearly or as needed. When complete, this tool can guide the practitioner in determining the assessment needs of each patient.

EXHIBIT 1.1 Adult Risk Assessment Form

Name _____ DOB _____ Chart # _____

Allergies _____

Occupation _____

Assess the patient for the following risk factors:

Family History	
First-degree relatives with remarkable diseases (e.g., asthma, allergies, hypertension, diabetes mellitus, coronary artery disease [CAD], cancer, and thyroid disease)	
1.	6.
2.	7.
3.	8.
4.	9.
5.	10.

A. Coronary heart disease
   1. High-fat/high-cholesterol diet
   2. Obese
   3. Elevated cholesterol level
   4. Stroke
   5. Hypertension
   6. Tobacco use
B. Lung cancer
   1. High-fat/high-cholesterol diet
   2. Tobacco use
   3. Smoking

C. Cervical cancer
   1. Early age of first intercourse
   2. Multiple sexual partners
   3. HPV Immunization series
D. Breast cancer
   1. Nulliparous
   2. Primigravida after age 35 years
   3. High-fat diet
   4. Family history at early age
E. Colon cancer
   1. History of polyps
   2. High-fat diet
F. Osteoporosis
   1. Less than 1 g of calcium per day
   2. History of tobacco or alcohol use
   3. Sedentary lifestyle
   4. Thin, Caucasian
   5. Female gender
G. Glaucoma/visual impairment
   1. Family history of glaucoma
   2. Diabetes mellitus
H. Sexually transmitted infections (STIs)/HIV
   1. Alcohol and drug use or abuse
   2. Multiple sexual partners
   3. Homosexual or bisexual partner
   4. History of intravenous drug use
   5. History of blood transfusion
   6. Exposed to or past history of STI
I. Substance abuse
   1. Alcohol or drug use history
   2. Family history of substance abuse

(continued)

EXHIBIT 1.1 Adult Risk Assessment Form *(continued)*

3. Stress or poor coping mechanisms
4. Administer the *CAGE* assessment (Steinweg & Worth, 1993),
   Have you ever tried to **C**ut down on your alcohol/drug use?
   Do you get **A**nnoyed if someone mentions your use is a problem?
   Do you ever feel **G**uilty about your use?
   Do you ever have an "**E**ye-opener" first thing in the morning after you have been drinking or using the night before?

J. Accidents and suicide
   1. Family history of suicide
   2. Alcohol or tobacco use
   3. History of depression
   4. High-stress or "hot-reactor" personality

5. Male gender
6. Alcohol use
7. Previous suicide attempt
8. Poor coping mechanisms or stress

K. Safety
   1. Does not use seat belt or car seat
   2. Drinks and drives
   3. Drives over the speed limit
   4. Does not wear safety helmet if driving motorcycle
   5. Inadequate number of smoke detectors or none in the home
   6. Firearms in the home
   7. Feels safe at home/at risk for domestic violence

Bibliography

Steinweg, D. L., & Worth, H. (1993). Alcoholism: The keys to the CAGE. *The American Journal of Medicine 94*, 520–523. DOI: 10.1016/0002-9343(93)90088-7

Adult Preventive Healthcare

Jill C. Cash, Debbie Gunter, and Mariya Tankimovich

The flow sheet given in Exhibit 1.2 helps the practitioner identify changes in the adult patient's risk factor status, make recommendations for health maintenance (e.g., immunizations, laboratory work, physical examinations), and educate patients in prevention (Exhibit 1.3). Screening guidelines for each of these can be found in the associated chapters in this book, according to the national association recommendations (e.g., screening recommendations for mammograms were obtained from the American Cancer Society). The Adult Health Maintenance Guide in Exhibit 1.3 can be used as a quick reference for the practitioner to evaluate the patient's adherence to preventive measures. Keep a copy of this flow sheet and guide in the front of the patient's chart where they can be reviewed routinely and updated as necessary. If using electronic medical records, a special section should be identified as routine health maintenance.

EXHIBIT 1.2 Adult Preventive Healthcare Flow Sheet

Immunization Schedule				
Immunization	**Date**	**Date**	**Date**	**Date**
Tetanus/diphtheria or tetanus/diphtheria/ pertussis				
Measles, mumps, rubella (MMR)				
Tuberculosis (TB; yearly)				
Hepatitis A				
Hepatitis B				
Influenza (yearly)				
Prevnar 13 and Pneumovax 23				
Zoster				

Assess patients for the following behaviors:

Risk Assessment				
Examination	**Date**	**Date**	**Date**	**Date**
Tobacco, amount				
Alcohol, amount				
Substance use				

(continued)

EXHIBIT 1.2 Adult Preventive Healthcare Flow Sheet (*continued*)

Risk Assessment				
Examination	Date	Date	Date	Date
Domestic violence				
Depression screening				

Patients should be educated about any behavior modifications that can reduce their risk factors for health problems. The practitioner should note the date as well as the type of counseling given to a patient.

Patient Education				
Behavior Modification	Date	Date	Date	Date
Diet/exercise				
Tobacco/alcohol/ vaping				
Injury prevention				
Skin protection				
Hormone replacement therapy				
Sexual practices				
Occupational hazards				
Self-examination: Breast/testicular				

EXHIBIT 1.3 Adult Health Maintenance Guide

Name _____ DOB _____ Chart # _____

Allergies _____ Occupation _____

The following tests should be performed according to the individual patient's risk factors, as part of preventive healthcare. The practitioner should fill in the date and result of each test and highlight any remarkable results. This list is not exhaustive and special populations may need additional screenings. www.uspreventiveservicestaskforce.org/BrowseRec/Index/browse-recommendations

Test	Date	Result	Date	Result	Date	Result	Date	Result
Height								
Weight								
Body mass index (BMI)								
Blood pressure (BP)								
Skin examination								
Oral cavity examination								
EKG								
Thyroid-stimulating hormone (TSH)								
Lipid profile								
Urinalysis								
Rectal examination								
Hemoccult								
Chest x-ray (lung cancer screening)								
Colonoscopy								
Prostate-specific antigen (PSA)								
Testicular examination								

(*continued*)

EXHIBIT 1.3 Adult Health Maintenance Guide (*continued*)

Test	Date	Result	Date	Result	Date	Result	Date	Result
Pelvic examination/Pap smear								
Breast examination								
Mammogram								
Bone mineral density								
Sexually transmitted disease (STD)/HIV								
Additionally, the practitioner should ensure that the patient receives other healthcare as needed. Assess the patient's adherence to other preventive healthcare examinations:								
Dental examination								
Vision/glaucoma examination								

Immunizations

The CDC is the primary source for the current immunization schedules. Consult the CDC's website for pocket-sized schedules, printable versions, and versions for mobile devices. The download information for your smartphone is available on the CDC website at https://www.cdc.gov/vaccines/schedules/hcp/index.html

Immunizations for Travel

The CDC recommends certain vaccines to protect travelers from illnesses present in other parts of the world and to protect others on return to the United States. The CDC's Travelers' Health website is located at https://wwwnc.cdc.gov/travel. It is an interactive website to individualize the needs of travelers to their specific destination. Vaccinations required are dependent on area of travel and other optional factors (cite https://wwwnc.cdc.gov/travel):

A. Travel destination
B. Travel season
C. Age
D. Pregnancy or breastfeeding
E. Traveling with infants or children
F. Immune-compromized
G. Chronic disease
H. Extended stay
I. Visiting friends and family

The CDC also has a Health Education sheet for travelers at: https://wwwnc.cdc.gov/travel/page/traveler-information-center

Medications

Evaluating medications for safety is an important part of every healthcare visit for patients at any age. Young and old people are particularly vulnerable to harmful effects of medications. Always check appropriateness of medications and dosage during healthcare maintenance visits. The American Geriatrics Society (AGS) Beers Criteria for Potentially Inappropriate Medication Use in Older Adults is available on AGS's website for purchase and for members at https://geriatricscareonline.org/ProductAbstract/american-geriatrics-society-updated-beers-criteria/CL001.

Bibliography

Centers for Disease Control and Prevention. (2016a). CDC recommended adult immunization schedule—United States 2016. Retrieved from https://www.cdc.gov/vaccines/schedules/hcp/adult.html

Centers for Disease Control and Prevention. (2016b). Information for travelers. Retrieved from www.cdc.gov/travel/page/traveler-information-center

Centers for Disease Control and Prevention. (2019). Immunization schedules. Retrieved from www.cdc.gov/vaccines/schedules/index.html

ConsultGeri. (2019). The 2019 American Geriatrics Society Updated Beers Criteria® for potentially inappropriate medication use in older adults. Retrieved from https://consultgeri.org/try-this/general-assessment/issue-16

2 Public Health Guidelines

Homelessness

Robertson Nash and Cheryl A. Glass

Overview

Homelessness is a multifaceted structural problem that has a syndemic effect on people. The term *syndemic* refers to situations in which the net effect of multiple physical and social comorbidities is worse than the sum of the individual effects (Merrill, 2009). There is no specific time limit on homelessness. Due to the extremely limited incomes of most families, experiencing homelessness can sometimes last an extended period of time. In the case of people experiencing homelessness, consider all of the possible interactions among unmanaged chronic diseases (diabetes mellitus type 2, hypertension, hyperlipidemia), multiple caries and gingival abscesses, chronic soft tissue infections, and untreated depression and anxiety. For people without the support of stable housing and nutrition, these interactions can be overwhelming. Data show that, on average, people who are chronically homeless live approximately 20 years less than their housed peers.

Definition (Federal)

A. The U.S. Department of Housing and Urban Development (HUD) is responsible for defining the criteria by which an individual's housing status is assessed. The required criteria for the determination of homelessness include the following (HUD, 2012):

1. People who are living in a place not meant for human habitation, in emergency shelter, in transitional housing, or are exiting an institution where they temporarily resided if they were in shelter or a place not meant for human habitation before entering the institution. People will be considered homeless if they are exiting an institution where they resided for up to 90 days and were homeless immediately prior to entering that institution.
2. People who are losing their primary nighttime residence, which may include a motel or hotel or a doubled-up situation, within 14 days and lack resources or support networks to remain in housing

3. Families with children or unaccompanied youth who are unstably housed and likely to continue in that state. This is a new category of homelessness, and it applies to families with children or unaccompanied youth (up to age 24) who have not had a lease or ownership interest in a housing unit in the past 60 or more days, who have had two or more moves in the past 60 days, and who are likely to continue to be unstably housed because of disability or multiple barriers to employment.
4. People who are fleeing or attempting to flee domestic violence, dating violence, sexual assault, stalking, or other dangerous or life-threatening situations related to violence; have no other residence; and lack the resources or support networks to obtain other permanent housing

Incidence

A. Statistics from the U.S. Department of HUD Office of Community Planning and Development's 2018 Annual Homeless Assessment Report to Congress (AHAR) Point-in-Times (PIT) estimates offer a snapshot of homelessness—both sheltered and unsheltered—on a single night. The one-night counts are conducted during the last 10 days of January each year.

1. On a single night in 2018, roughly 553,000 people were experiencing homelessness in the United States.
   a. About two-thirds (65%) were staying in sheltered locations—emergency shelters or transitional housing programs; about one-third (35%) were in unsheltered locations, such as on the street, in abandoned buildings, or in other places not suitable for human habitation.
   b. About 36,000 people were experiencing homelessness as unaccompanied youth—that is, people under the age of 25 experiencing homelessness on their own. Most unaccompanied youth (89%) were between the ages of 18 and 24.
   c. Two in three people experiencing homelessness (67%) were adults in households without children. The remaining 33% of people experiencing homelessness did so as part of a family.

d. Seven in 10 people experiencing homelessness as individuals identified as men. The remaining 30% identified as women, transgender, or gender nonconforming.

B. In the United States, relates the Interagency Council on Homelessness in its report Homelessness in America: Focus on Chronic Homelessness Among People with Disabilities (2018), more than two-thirds (69%) of individuals with disabilities who experience chronic homelessness were staying in unsheltered locations, such as on sidewalks or in doorways, parks or encampments, under bridges, in cars, buses, or abandoned buildings rather in emergency shelters at the time of the January PIT count.

Pathogenesis

A. Homelessness is a catastrophic experience at the individual level and family level. However, most of the factors that contribute to homelessness are structural in nature and are beyond the control of any one client or provider. For example, cities with an inadequate supply of Section 8 housing will not be able to provide people experiencing homelessness with a place to live. Furthermore, the disparity between federal and state minimum wages and the living wage translates to mean that the people who work 40 or more hours a week are often unable to secure housing.

Predisposing Factors

A. Chronic illnesses: People who are homeless suffer from chronic illnesses at rates that exceed those in the general population. In many cases, overlapping and negatively interacting manifestations of illness exacerbate each other, leading to several complicated comorbidities whose management may tax the resources available to both client and provider.

Common Complaints

A. Refer to chapter-specific conditions, complaints, and treatments
B. Chronic illnesses:
   1. Hypertension
   2. Diabetes
   3. Coronary artery disease
   4. Congestive heart failure
   5. Peripheral vascular disease
   6. Hypercholesterolemia
C. Respiratory:
   1. Bronchitis
   2. Pneumonia
   3. Tuberculosis
   4. Influenza
   5. Asthma
   6. COPD
   7. Cough
D. Infections:
   1. HIV/AIDS
   2. Sexually transmitted infections
   3. Hepatitis A, B, and C
   4. Wound and skin infections
   5. Tetanus
E. Dental abscesses, gingivitis, tooth loss

F. Problems being outdoors:
   1. Sleep deprivation
   2. Animal bites
   3. Food insecurity/poor nutrition
   4. Dehydration
G. Weather-related illnesses:
   1. Heat-related illnesses:
      a. Cramps
      b. Heat exhaustion
      c. Heat stroke
   2. Cold-related illnesses:
      a. Frostbite
      b. Hypothermia
H. Skin and foot problems:
   1. Lice
   2. Scabies
   3. Abrasions, abscesses, corn calluses, onychomycosis, tinea pedis
   4. Ulcerations and cellulitis from edema and venous stasis
   5. Immersion foot
I. Mental health-related complaints:
   1. Physical violence/sexual abuse
   2. Anger
   3. Major depression
   4. Schizophrenia
   5. Bipolar disorders
   6. Posttraumatic stress
   7. Suicide
   8. Substance abuse problems:
      a. Opioid-related overdose and death
      b. Alcoholism
J. Unintended pregnancies
K. Children-related issues:
   1. Lead poisoning
   2. Behavioral problems (e.g., anxiety, depression, withdrawal, aggression, hostility)
   3. Delayed development
   4. Growth delays
   5. Learning disabilities
   6. Separation from family

Other Signs and Symptoms

A. Does the client smell of smoke, as if he or she has been sleeping outdoors by a fire? If so, this would trigger a chest x-ray and detailed pulmonary examination.
B. Does the client smell of urine, suggesting a possible urinary tract infection? If so, this would trigger a genitourinary skin examination, urinalysis, and social work consult regarding access to clean clothing.
C. Unilateral lower extremity pitting edema, pain, and tenderness suggest the presence of a deep vein thrombosis (DVT), which is considered a medical emergency.
D. Bilateral lower extremity pitting edema may be a sign of heart failure. This finding would trigger a thorough clinical examination for the following: S3, S4 heart sounds, jugular venous pulse, and jugular venous distension.
E. Brawny edema and venous stasis ulcerations would trigger a thorough peripheral vascular examination and a sensory examination of the plantar surfaces of both feet.

F. Itchiness suggests pest infestation, needs treatment, shower, wash cloth, new clothes, and contact shelter to treat the environment.

G. Unusual behavior, for example, hallucination, visible depression, intoxication, and so on, refer to mental health.

Subjective Data: Factors to Consider When Evaluating People Experiencing Homelessness

A. Where did the client sleep last? Does the client have a safe place to sleep tonight?

B. When was the last time the client was able to bathe?

C. When was the last time the client ate?

D. Is the client able to find bathrooms when needed?

E. Are symptoms of depression and anxiety interfering with survival?

F. Is the client being physically, sexually, or emotionally abused?

G. Is the client being forced to engage in behaviors against his or her will in exchange for food and shelter?

H. Does the client have a safe way to manage medications on the street, such as insulin or inhalers?

I. Assess/discuss current substance abuse (refer to Substance and Use Disorders in this section).

▶ *See Section III: Client Teaching Guide for this chapter, "Alcohol and Drug Dependence."*

Physical Examination

Providers should be aware that, due to past trauma, many people experiencing homelessness are reluctant to touch. Take your time with the physical examination, ask permission for each step of the physical examination, and explain what you are doing and why.

A. Check temperature (as indicated), pulse, respirations, blood pressure, height and weight to calculate BMI.

B. Inspect:
  1. Scalp—assess for nits.
  2. Oral cavity—assess for caries or active oral abscesses.
  3. Assess skin for burns, abrasions, trauma, and evidence of accidental or intentional injury. Visualize both feet for infection and trauma.

C. Palpate the abdomen for tenderness or masses. Perform pelvic examination as appropriate. This may not be possible on the first examination. For some females, intentionally poor hygiene is viewed as protection against male assault.

D. Auscultate heart, lungs, and abdomen.

E. Neurologic examination:
  1. Assess for neuropathy in feet.
  2. Assess hearing and vision, as these faculties are central to survival when living on the street

F. Mental health examination:
  1. Perform depression/anxiety screening. See depression/anxiety in Chapter 22: Psychiatric Guidelines, for screening.
  2. Evaluate suicidal ideation. See Chapter 22: Psychiatric Guidelines, for assessment/screening.
  3. Assess for active audio/visual hallucinations
  4. Assess for paranoia

Diagnostic Tests

A. Complete blood count (CBC)

B. Comprehensive metabolic panel (CMP)

C. B12/folate

D. Urine: urinalysis for protein/glucose and *Neisseria gonorrhea*/chlamydia

E. Rapid plasma reagin (RPR)

F. HIV

G. HAV/HBV profile, hepatitis C virus antibody

H. Glycosylated hemoglobin A1c

I. Purified protein derivative (PPD)/T-SPOT

Differential Diagnoses

A. Substance use/abuse

B. Depression

C. Malnutrition

D. Schizophrenia

Plan

A. General interventions:
  1. There are no disease-based standards of care that specifically address people who are homeless. Rather, providers must be creative and resourceful, working with clients toward higher levels of self-efficacy within the resource bounds imposed on the situation by society at large.
  2. Community-based care: No single provider or ancillary service organization (ASO) can provide all of the care needed by people experiencing homelessness. In order to maximize care, providers should make an effort to identify and be in communication with their local ASOs before a crisis so that resources can be coordinated and maximized when acute issues arise.
  3. Identifying and assisting the client with current health needs is imperative. In addition to homelessness, the client may have other acute and chronic health conditions that should be addressed and treated as appropriate.
  4. Immunize according to standard guidelines for flu, pneumonia, hepatitis A and B, tetanus, so on.

B. Client teaching:
  1. Lifestyle modifications, focusing on diet, exercise, and smoking cessation, form the cornerstone of APRN client teaching for chronic disease management. The following principles should be used to guide the teaching of these principles in the homeless population:
    a. People experiencing homelessness rarely have access to exercise facilities. In addition, they often lack a safe place to store their belongings while they exercise.
    b. People experiencing homelessness have little to no control over their food selection. Dependence on volunteer-driven, charity-led food banks and meal programs is a significant impediment to healthy eating as many of these programs assume that a high-carbohydrate, calorie-dense meal, such as spaghetti and bread, is what people experiencing homelessness like and want to eat.

c. The prevalence of poor dentition among the homeless greatly exceeds that of the stably housed, employed population. Accordingly, people experiencing homelessness may not be able to eat fresh fruits and vegetables.

d. The rates of substance abuse among the chronically homeless exceed those in the general population. Some people may be successfully clean and sober from alcohol yet continue to smoke tobacco. Although this situation is not ideal, focus on client strengths, praise sobriety, and acknowledge that smoking cessation is perceived as being more difficult than sobriety from alcohol and may need to have a lower priority in a client's overall plan of care.

e. Blanket dietary and exercise recommendations developed around stably housed, fully employed people will likely not translate well to people experiencing homelessness. Failure to account for the unique challenges of people experiencing homelessness will exacerbate feelings of depression, low self-worth, and decreased self-efficacy.

f. Caring for individuals experiencing homelessness requires a team approach. Successful teams include clinicians, social workers, behavioral health providers, psychiatric providers, and nursing staff. No one provider or discipline can address all of the needs of people experiencing homelessness. It is critical that the care team work well together and prioritize the work of building rapport with the client, whose life experiences have likely reinforced his/her distrust of the systems that we all depend on to deliver care.

Follow-Up

A. One of the primary challenges facing providers of those experiencing homelessness is the deep-seated lack of trust that homeless people have in the healthcare system within which most providers operate. In order to encourage people to return to the clinic for appropriate follow-up care, every effort must be made during the first visit to establish a true therapeutic relationship with the client. Providers should attempt to work with clients to identify and address concerns that are important to the client. Providers should remember that topics such as smoking cessation and sobriety from alcohol may best be deferred during an initial visit. All clinic staff should be trained to treat all clients with a professional, welcoming, and empathetic manner.

Consultation/Referral

A. Referring clients to specialists is an everyday part of primary care, and advanced practice nurses serve important screening and gatekeeper functions in this role. However, the insurance-based system that we rely on for care is not available to most people experiencing homelessness, as they lack health insurance. Should insurance be available, then providers must still identify specialists willing to take specific insurances and work with people experiencing homelessness. Effective providers will identify specialists in their local communities and seek to build relationships that will facilitate referrals. Given the lack of access to transportation in this population, it is important to set an expectation that a missed appointment does not mean that the client does not want or need care and that specialists may need to be flexible regarding missed appointments with people in this population.

Individual Considerations

A. Pediatrics/minors:
1. The National Runaway Safeline estimates that on any given night there are approximately 1.3 million homeless youth living unsupervised on the streets, in abandoned buildings, with friends (couch surfing), or with strangers. Homeless youth are at a higher risk for physical abuse, sexual exploitation, mental health disabilities, substance abuse, and death. It is estimated that 5,000 unaccompanied youth die each year as a result of assault, illness, or suicide.
2. The National Alliance to End Homelessness (2019) notes youth homelessness is often rooted in family conflict. Other contributing factors include economic circumstances like poverty and housing insecurity, racial disparities, and mental health and substance use disorders (SUDs). Young people who have had involvement with child welfare and juvenile justice systems are also more likely to become homeless. Many homeless youth and young adults have experienced significant trauma before and after becoming homeless and are particularly vulnerable to sexual trafficking and exploitation. Youth who identify as LGBTQ, pregnant and parenting youth, youth with special needs or disabilities, and youth of color, particularly African American and Native American youth, are also more likely to become homeless.
3. Homeless children and youth report that school is a home to them—a place they see the same faces, sit in the same seat, and receive meals.
4. A lot of young people don't seek out services because of fear that they will be turned into the child welfare or juvenile justice system or refused services. The more information they have about what they can directly access, the more likely they are going to seek the services again. Providers should make contact with their community YMCA/YWCA resources to develop a referral plan should a homeless minor present for care.

B. Pregnancy: All pregnant women who are experiencing homeless and present for care should be seen by a social worker before leaving the site. In cases where abuse is suspected, law enforcement must be notified.

C. Elderly: All people older than 60 years of age who are experiencing homelessness and present for care should be seen by a social worker before leaving the site. In cases where abuse is suspected, law enforcement must be notified.

Resources

Federal

HUD Exchange: Homelessness Assistance: www.hudex -change.info

National Coalition to End Homelessness: www.national -homeless.org

National Health Care for the Homeless Council: www .nhchc.org

National Conference of State Legislatures: www.ncsl .org

United States Interagency Council on Homelessness: https://www.usich.gov/

State

Providers should use the Internet search engine of choice to locate emergency shelters and care for people experiencing homelessness in their locale. There is no centralized database of state/local shelters. Many larger shelters will have a list of local places for people to find food and community assistance, and this information can be invaluable for providers to keep on hand.

Homeless Shelter Directory: https://www.home lessshelterdirectory.org/

Bibliography

FYSB Family & Youth Services Bureau. (n.d.). *About runaway and homeless youth. RHYi National clearinghouse on homeless youth & families.* Retrieved from https://rhyclearinghouse.acf.hhs.gov/about-runaway -and-homeless-youth

Maness, D. L., & Khan, M. (2014, April 15). Care of the homeless: An overview. *American Family Physician, 89*(8), 634–640.

National Alliance to End Homelessness. (2012, January 4). *Changes in the HUD definition of "homeless."* Retrieved from http://endhomelessness.org/wp-content/uploads/2012/01/changes-in-hud-definition-homeless.pdf

National Alliance to End Homelessness. (2019). *Youth and young adults.* Retrieved from https://endhomelessness.org/homelessness-in-america/who-experiences-homelessness/youth/

National Conference of State Legislatures. (2016, April 14). *Homeless and runaway youth.* Retrieved from http://www.ncsl.org/research/human -services/homeless-and-runaway-youth.aspx

Santos, M. (2017, October). *The most frequently asked questions on the educational rights of children & youth in homeless situations.* Retrieved from https://naehcy.org/wp-content/uploads/2018/02/2017-10-16_NAEHCY-FAQs.pdf

U.S Department of Housing and Urban Development Office of Community Planning and Development. (2018, December). *The 2018 annual homeless assessment report (AHAR) to congress, Part 1: Point-in-time estimates of homelessness.* Retrieved from https://www.wpr.org/sites/default/files/2018-ahar-part-1-compressed.pdf

United States Interagency Council on Homelessness. (2018, August). *HOMELESSNESS IN AMERICA: Focus on chronic homelessness among people with disabilities.* Retrieved from https://www.usich.gov/resources/uploads/asset_library/Homelessness-in-America-Focus-on-chronic.pdf

Obesity

Cheryl A. Glass, Angelito Tacderas, and Bunny Pounds

Definition

A. Obesity is a multifactorial disease with physical, psychological, and social consequences. The body mass index (BMI) is a standard measuring tool. BMI is the most commonly used approach to determine if adults are overweight or obese and is also the recommended measure to determine if children are overweight. The BMI is calculated by using the formula weight in kilograms divided by height in meters squared (weight [kg]/height [m]^2). In adults, obesity is defined as a BMI >30 kg/m^2.

B. The BMI for children is calculated the same way as for adults, but is interpreted using age- and gender-specific percentages (BMI-for-age) clinical charts (see Tables 2.1 and 2.2). The Centers for Disease Control and Prevention (CDC) defines childhood obesity by percentiles. The CDC recommends that healthcare providers use World Health Organization (WHO) growth charts to monitor growth for infants and children ages 0 to 2 years in the United States and recommend the use of the CDC growth charts to monitor growth for children 2 years and older in the United States. CDC charts for children are available on the CDC website at www.cdc.gov/growthcharts/clinical_charts.htm. The BMI percentile calculator for children and teens is available at www.cdc.gov/healthyweight/bmi/calculator.html. WHO growth charts are available at www.cdc.gov/growthcharts/who_charts.htm. The adult BMI calculator is available at www.cdc.gov/healthyweight/assessing/bmi/adult_BMI/english_bmi_calculator/bmi_calculator.html.

Incidence

Obesity now affects 1 in 5 children and adolescents in the United States. Data from the 2015–2016 National Health and Nutrition Examination Survey (NHANES) notes the prevalence of obesity is 39.8% in adults and

TABLE 2.1   CHILDHOOD OBESITY BY PERCENTILES

Childhood Obesity Category	BMI Definitions by Percentiles
Underweight	<5th percentile
Healthy weight	5th to <85th percentile
Overweight	85th to <95th percentile
Obese	≥95th percentile

BMI, body mass index.

TABLE 2.2   ADULT OBESITY BY BMI FOR ADULTS 20 YEARS OLD AND OLDER

Classification of Adult Obesity by BMI	BMI (kg/m²)
Underweight	<18.5
Normal	18.5–24.9
Overweight (pre-obese)	25.0–29.9
Obesity	Level I: 30.0–34.9 Level II: 35–39.9 Level III: 40.0–49.9
Super morbidly obese	>50.0
Super-super morbidly obese (SSO)	≥60.0

BMI, body mass index.

18.5% in youth. The prevalence of obesity was higher among middle-aged adults (42.8%) than among younger adults (35.7%). The prevalence of obesity was higher among youth aged 6 to 11 years (18.4%) and adolescents aged 12 to 19 years (20.6%) compared with children aged 2 to 5 years (13.9%). Obesity rates cross all groups in society, regardless of age, sex, race, ethnicity, socioeconomic status, educational level, or geographic group. Hispanics and non-Hispanic blacks have the highest age-adjusted prevalence of obesity, followed by non-Hispanic whites and non-Hispanic Asians.

Pathogenesis
Numerous factors contribute to the development of obesity, including biological, genetic, behavioral, social, cultural, and environmental influences.
A. Imbalance between energy intake and energy output
B. Genetics (e.g., Prader–Willi syndrome)
C. Medical conditions (e.g., Cushing's syndrome, polycystic ovary syndrome [PCOS])
D. Age
E. Pregnancy
F. Environmental factors
G. Drug-induced obesity:
   1. Antidepressants (amitriptyline, doxepin, imipramine, mirtazapine, nortriptyline, paroxetine, phenelzine)
   2. Antihistamines (cyproheptadine)
   3. Antipsychotics (clozapine, haloperidol, olanzapine, quetiapine, risperidone, thioridazine)
   4. Antidiabetics (insulin, sulfonylureas, thiazolidinediones)
   5. Anticonvulsants (sodium valproate, carbamazepine, gabapentin)
   6. Steroids (contraceptives, glucocorticoids, progestational steroids)
   7. Beta- or alpha-adrenergic blockers (propranolol, doxazosin)
   8. Glucocorticoid steroids
H. Sleep disturbance–induced obesity
I. Quitting smoking

Predisposing Factors
A. Consuming too many calories/high-fat diet
B. Poor dietary choices
C. Readily available food sources, especially fast foods
D. Lack of exercise/sedentary lifestyle
E. Decreased/eliminated physical education requirements in public schools
F. Television, computer, hand-held electronic devices, video game use more than a total of 3 hours a day
G. Increased leisure time
H. Lack of funding and planning for community parks and recreation areas
I. Ethnic background: African American, Hispanic
J. Family history of obesity
K. Poverty
L. Insomnia, difficulty staying asleep and frequent wakefulness

Common Complaints
A. Difficulties with activities of daily living (ADLs) or functional impairment
B. Lack of interest/inability to tolerate exercise
C. Shortness of breath and/or asthma exacerbations
D. Difficulty with personal hygiene
E. Urinary incontinence
F. Lack of desire to lose weight
G. Decreased quality of life (e.g., depression, disability, shame and guilt, social isolation)

Other Signs and Symptoms
A. Obstructive sleep apnea (OSA)
B. Increased asthma symptoms
C. Infertility/PCOS
D. Symptoms associated with cholelithiasis
E. Hypertension
F. Gynecologic problems (e.g., irregular periods, early sexual maturity in girls)
G. Joint pain (OA)—cartilage and joint breakdown of lower extremities
H. Other complications: type 2 diabetes, gallbladder disease, depression/anxiety, dyslipidemia, stroke, coronary artery disease, metabolic syndrome, cancer (colon, endometrial, lung cancer), erectile dysfunction, nonalcoholic fatty liver disease (NASH)

Subjective Data
A. Review the onset of weight gain and duration of obesity. Identify when the client first noticed the weight gain.
B. Ask the client about other symptoms secondary to obesity.
C. Review full medical history.
D. Review medications, including over-the-counter (OTC) herbals and diet products.
E. Review the client's previous history of weight-loss attempts.
F. Assess ADLs and functional limitations and the presence of exercise intolerance.
G. Elicit history of sleep disorders (i.e., snoring and obstruction, sleep apnea).
H. Review 24-hour dietary recall. Review the client's normal average meals per day, including snacks and portion sizes.
I. Review consumption of high-calorie drinks and alcohol intake.
J. Review frequency of fast food consumption.
K. Assess for history of binge eating, purging, night eating syndrome, lack of satiety, food-seeking behaviors, and other abnormal feeding habits.
L. Assess for depression.
M. Assess for readiness and commitment for weight loss. People who voluntarily enroll in a weight-loss program generally lose weight.
N. Ask the client to describe his or her activity level, exercise routine, and daily activity (work activity).
O. Ask about screen time.
P. Ask about family history of obesity.

Q. Ask about possible biopsychosocial and behavioral risk factors for weight gain such as starting a new medication, change in occupation or marital status, recent illness, pregnancy, menopause, stressful events, or smoking cessation.

Physical Examination

A. Check pulse, respirations, and blood pressure supine, sitting, and standing.
B. Measurements:
 1. Determine height and weight to calculate BMI.
 2. Measure waist and hip circumferences to calculate the waist-to-hip circumference ratio. The waist-to-hip ratio is the strongest anthropometric measure that is associated with myocardial infarction risk and is a better predictor than BMI. A waist-to-hip ratio that is >0.8% usually has some form of premetabolic syndrome or insulin resistance.
 3. Measure neck circumference to evaluate risk factor of OSA.
C. Inspect:
 1. Observe the overall appearance and note body fat distribution.
 2. Examine the skin.
 3. Mouth and teeth: assess dental enamel for signs of purging.
D. Auscultate:
 1. Heart
 2. Lungs
 3. Carotid arteries
 4. Abdomen
E. Palpate:
 1. Neck and thyroid
 2. Extremities—noting edema
 3. Abdomen for masses, tenderness, rebound tenderness

Diagnostic Tests

A. Thyroid function
B. Lipid panel
C. Liver enzymes
D. CBC
E. 25-hydroxy vitamin D test
F. Pregnancy test
G. Fasting blood sugar/3-hour glucose tolerance test (GTT)
H. Consider fasting insulin level
I. Sleep study (if indicated)
J. Consider genetic testing
K. Nocturnal hypoxemia study

Differential Diagnoses

A. Pseudo tumor cerebri
B. Binge eating
C. Genetic syndrome (e.g., Prader–Willi syndrome)
D. Cushing's syndrome
E. Diabetes mellitus
F. Insulin resistance syndrome
G. Primary pulmonary hypertension

Plan

Manage obesity as a chronic relapsing disease, including the comanagement of other diseases secondary to obesity (i.e., diabetes, hypertension).
A. General interventions:
 1. Treat any underlying cause of obesity.
 2. Reinforce the positive impact that weight-loss measures (diet, exercise) can have and the overall health benefits of weight loss. Weight loss of even 5% to 15% can provide a significant reduction in obesity-related complications.
 3. Identify and monitor any cardiovascular complications.
 4. Behavior modification: Intensive behavior therapy has been shown to lead to better success with weight loss and sustainable weight loss for longer periods of time. Behavior therapy includes weekly meetings with healthcare professionals for at least 6 to 8 weeks.
  a. Dietary plan:
   i. Consume 500 to 1,000 fewer calories per day for 1- to 2-pound-per-week weight loss.
   ii. Most diets have good short-term efficacy but limited sustainability.
   iii. Diets shown to be effective include portion control, low-fat, Mediterranean, low-carbohydrate, low glycemic index, and commercial weight-loss diets.
   iv. Increase water intake, particularly drinking 500 mL of water before meals.
   v. Protein-dense and high-fiber foods increase satiety with fewer calories.
  b. Exercise: children:
   i. Sixty minutes or more of moderate-to-vigorous physical activity daily is recommended for children and adolescents ages 6 to 17.
    a) Within the 60 minutes of daily physical activity, children and adolescents should engage in muscle-strengthening, bone strengthening, and vigorous intensity physical activities at least 3 days per week.
  c. Exercise: adults:
   i. Single episodes of physical activity promote acute improvements in executive function for a period of time. Physical activity also improves other components of cognition, including memory, processing speed, attention, and academic performance.
   ii. Approximately 150 minutes (2½ hours) of moderate intensity exercise aerobic physical activity is recommended per week for adults; 155 to 180 minutes per week for children.
   iii. Multiple short sessions (four 10-minute sessions per day, 5 days per week) may have the same benefit as fewer longer sessions (one 40-minute session, 5 days per week). At least two times a week strength exercises (push-ups, sit-ups, lifting weights) are also recommended.

iv. Walking 30 minutes per day has been shown to prevent weight gain; higher amounts of exercise promote weight loss.

v. The combination of exercise and diet is more effective than either alone.

d. Wide range of benefits of exercise and weight loss:

i. Helps lower blood pressure

ii. Improves cholesterol count

iii. Helps lower hemoglobin A1c in diabetes

iv. Helps strengthen bones

v. Promotes weight loss

vi. Improves depression (reduces depressive symptoms among people both with and without clinical depression)

vii. Boosts immune system

viii. Reduces stress

ix. Reduces symptoms of anxiety, both chronic levels of anxiety and acute feelings

x. Improves sense of well-being

xi. Believed to be a major driving force in lifestyle change

xii. Improves joint pain

xiii. Improves the quality of sleep

xiv. Improves the ability to more easily accomplish the tasks of daily living, such as climbing stairs or carrying groceries

xv. Reduces risk of falls and fall-related injuries

xvi. Single episodes of physical activity promote acute improvements in executive function for a period of time. Physical activity also improves other components of cognition, including memory, processing speed, attention, and academic performance.

xvii. For children ages 5 through 13, the evidence indicates that both acute bouts and regular moderate-to-vigorous physical activity improve cognition, including memory, processing speed, attention, and academic performance.

xviii. Among older children and youth through high school age, the evidence continues to demonstrate that moderate-to-vigorous physical activity improves cardiovascular and muscular fitness, bone health, weight status, and cardiometabolic risk factor status.

e. Obtain counseling on stimulus control, goal setting, self-monitoring, and contracts that reward behaviors.

f. Pre-exercise medical evaluation:

i. Before beginning a sport or vigorous exercise program, children and adults should undergo screening (i.e., a history and physical examination), with emphasis on detecting cardiovascular risks.

g. Contraindication to exercise: There are several contraindications for beginning exercise:

i. Individuals with recent myocardial infarction (2 weeks)

ii. Unstable angina

iii. Severe aortic stenosis

iv. Decompensated congestive heart failure (low ejection fraction)

v. Left ventricular outflow obstruction

vi. Uncontrolled dysrhythmias

vii. Uncontrolled diabetes or diabetic complications

viii. Uncontrolled hypertension

ix. Uncontrolled respiratory conditions such as asthma and COPD

h. Key guidelines for safe physical activity:

i. Understand the risks and yet be confident that physical activity is safe for almost everyone.

ii. Choose to do types of physical activity that are appropriate for the client's current fitness level and health goals, because some activities are safer than others.

iii. The risk of injury is directly related to the rate of progression or change in volume of physical activity. Increase physical activity gradually over time whenever more activity is necessary to meet guidelines or health goals. Inactive people should "start low and go slow" by gradually increasing how often and how long activities are done.

iv. Tell client to protect self by using appropriate gear and sports equipment, looking for safe environments, following rules and policies, and making sensible choices about when, where, and how to be active.

v. People with disabilities should try to get the same amount of physical activities

B. Client teaching on obesity treatment modalities:

1. Advise the client to keep a food diary to identify food triggers and for accountability. Clients who maintain a food diary have been shown to have as much as 90% more weight loss than those who do not keep a diary.

2. Counsel clients about pharmaceutical therapy drug side effects and the lack of long-term safety data. Stress to the client the temporary nature of weight-loss medication. Typical weight loss is modest, <5 kg (10–11 lb) at 1 year.

3. Teach clients how to read food labels.

C. Pharmaceutical therapy:

1. After an adequate trial (minimum of 6 months) of diet and exercise therapy, consider adding pharmaceutical therapy. Pharmacological intervention is not covered by some health plans. State statutes should be considered before prescribing weight-control products.

2. Studies lack evidence to support whether one drug is more efficacious than another; the literature does not support the use of combination therapy for increased weight loss.

3. The choice of a pharmaceutical agent depends on the side-effects profile of the drug and tolerance of the side effects.

4. There are no OTC appetite suppressant drugs that have been approved by the Food and Drug Administration (FDA). The FDA has approved two medications, Qsymia (phentermine and topiramate extended release [ER]) and Belviq (lorcasern), for adults at least 18 years of age with a BMI of 30 or greater or the client's BMI is 27 or greater and has at least one other weight-related condition. Qsymia and Belviq are considered lifelong therapies in clients who respond to and tolerate them when used in conjunction with a balanced diet and exercise. Other appetite suppressants that are FDA approved for weight-loss medications for use up to 2 years in adults include the following:

 a. Phentermine, diethylpropion, benzphetamine, and phendimetrazine are approved for short-term (12 weeks) use.

 b. Sibutramine (Meridia, Reductil) is FDA approved for 1-year use.

 c. Orlistat (Xenical) is FDA approved for 2-year use.

5. Appetite suppressants:

 a. Qsymia (phentermine and topiramate ER). Start with 3.75/23 mg ER per day for initial BMI >30 kg/m^2, or BMI >27 kg/m^2 in the presence of risk factors. May gradually increase dose to 15/92 mg:

  i. Avoid evening dose

  ii. Not to be taken by adolescents younger than 18 years of age

  iii. Avoid in pregnancy. Weight loss offers no potential benefit to a pregnant woman. Qsymia carries a risk for birth defects (cleft lip with or without cleft palate) in infants exposed during the first trimester.

  iv. Monitor for hypersensitivity to phentermine and topamax.

  v. These drugs are not recommended in the presence of hypertension, hyperthyroidism, cardiovascular disease, drug or alcohol abuse, or history of kidney stones (topamax).

  vi. Do not use if a history of glaucoma or hyperthyroidism is present, or within 14 days of use of monoamine oxidase inhibitors (MAOIs).

 b. Lorcasern (Belviq), 10 mg twice a day for initial BMI >30 kg/m^2, or BMI >27 kg/m^2 in the presence of risk factors:

  i. Discontinue if 5% weight loss is not achieved by week 12.

  ii. Not to be taken by pediatric below the age of 18 years

  iii. Avoid in pregnancy. Weight loss offers no potential benefit to a pregnant woman. Qsymia carries a risk for birth defects (category X drug classification).

  iv. Do not use if a history of valvular heart disease, type 2 diabetes with hypoglycemia that requires the assistance of another person, or within 14 days of use of MAOIs or antipsychotics

  v. Discontinue in clients who experience suicidal thoughts or behaviors.

 c. Phentermine (Adipex-P) 37.5 mg orally once daily before or 1 to 2 hours after breakfast, or 18.75 mg one to two times per day for initial BMI >30 kg/m^2, or BMI >27 kg/m^2 in the presence of risk factors such as controlled elevated blood pressure, diabetes, and high cholesterol:

  i. Avoid late-evening dosing

  ii. Not recommended for children younger than 16 years

  iii. Not recommended in the presence of hypertension, hyperthyroidism, cardiovascular disease, and drug or alcohol abuse

  iv. Do not prescribe during or within 14 days of MAOIs.

 d. Benzphetamine (Didrex) 25 to 50 mg orally, initially in the midmorning or midafternoon. Increase if needed to 25 to 50 mg one to three times a day:

  i. Not recommended in children or adolescents

  ii. Not recommended in the presence of hypertension, hyperthyroidism, cardiovascular disease, and drug or alcohol abuse

  iii. Not to be prescribed during or within 14 days of MAOIs

  iv. Pregnancy category X: known to cause fetal abnormalities or toxicity in animal and human studies

 e. Diethylpropion (Tenuate) 25 mg one tablet every 8 hours, 1 hour before meals. May add one additional dose for night hunger. Half-life of 4 to 6 hours:

  i. Avoid late-evening dosing

  ii. Not recommended for children younger than 16 years

  iii. Not recommended in the presence of hypertension, hyperthyroidism, cardiovascular disease, and drug or alcohol abuse

  iv. Do not prescribe during or within 14 days of MAOIs.

 f. Phendimetrazine (Bontril PDM) 35 mg orally two or three times daily 1 hour before meals. May reduce to 17.5 mg/dose. Maximum dose 210 mg/d in three evenly divided doses. Also available in slow-release 105 mg taken in the morning 30 to 60 minutes before breakfast:

  i. Not recommended in children or adolescents

  ii. Not recommended in the presence of hypertension, hyperthyroidism, cardiovascular disease, and drug or alcohol abuse

  iii. Not to be prescribed during or within 14 days of MAOIs

6. Lipase inhibitor:
a. Orlistat (Xenical) for use with a low-fat diet. Recommend 30% of calories spread over three main meals:
   i. Take one 120-mg capsule orally during or up to 1 hour after main meals up to three times per day.
   ii. If a meal is missed or had no fat, skip dosage.
   iii. May decrease absorption of fat-soluble vitamins and beta carotene
   iv. Orlistat carries an FDA warning regarding safety and efficacy for use in clients younger than 12 years and in pregnancy and lactation as it interferes with the absorption of fat-soluble vitamins.
   v. Supplement diet with a multivitamin.
   vi. FDA approved for up to 2 years' use in adults
   vii. Gastrointestinal side effects include fatty/oily stools, oily spotting, flatus with discharge, fecal urgency, and fecal incontinence
   viii. Contraindicated in chronic malabsorption syndrome and cholestasis
   ix. May affect doses for antidiabetic medications
   x. Monitor warfarin and cyclosporine levels
b. Alli, a lipase inhibitor, is the only FDA-approved OTC weight-loss product.
7. Glucagon-like peptide-1 (GLP-1) receptor agonist:
a. Liraglutide (Saxenda) subcutaneous was FDA approved for chronic weight management as an adjunct to a reduced-calorie diet and increased physical exercise in December of 2014 for use in adults with BMI of 30 kg/m² or greater or 27 kg/m² or greater with at least one weight-related comorbidity:
   i. Start with 0.6 mg once daily for a week; may increase by 0.6 mg daily at weekly intervals up to 3 mg once daily.
   ii. Delay dose increase if tolerance is an issue.
   iii. If 3 mg once daily is not tolerated, discontinue drug. Efficacy has not been established for lower doses.
   iv. Evaluate at 16 weeks of therapy; discontinue if at least 4% of baseline body weight loss has not been achieved.
   v. Pregnancy category X; contraindicated in clients with multiple endocrine neoplasia syndrome type 2 (MEN2).
8. Off-label medications used for obesity: These medications are not FDA approved for weight loss. The client should be counseled regarding off-label medications and use at discretion.
a. Metformin (Glucophage) is used to decrease central adiposity in weight loss, lower insulin levels, and slow down the process of gluconeogenesis.
   i. Start Metformin 500 mg at the evening meal. The dosage can be increased by 500 mg/wk in divided doses up to the maximum of 2,000 mg/d.
   ii. Titrate slowly because of the gastrointestinal side effects.
   iii. Check a metabolic panel before and every 3 to 6 months to evaluate for lactic acidosis.
   iv. Metformin is contraindicated in clients with renal impairment; assess renal function before instituting metformin and monitor regularly.
   v. Metformin must be stopped before any procedure with radiographic dye.
   vi. May be used in children with central adiposity, especially those with signs of premetabolic syndrome
   vii. May be used on a client with a waist-to-hip ratio >0.8%
b. Topiramate (Topamax) is used to treat seizures and several types of headache. In small doses, it can be used alone or as adjunct with phentermine to suppress appetite longer. Be familiar with the risks associated with the use of Topamax.
   i. If used alone, the drug may start at 25 mg daily in the morning. Increase up to two or three times a day. Topamax has a long half-life of 19 to 25 hours.
   ii. May be used as adjunct with phentermine. Start client at 18.75 mg of phentermine and 12.5 mg of Topamax. Gradually increase the dose to 37.5 mg of phentermine and 25 mg of Topamax.
   iii. Always give the phentermine in the morning, preferably 30 minutes before meals. Topamax should be dosed in the afternoon or evening.
   iv. Phentermine (Adipex-P) 37.5 mg orally once daily before or 1 to 2 hours after breakfast, or 18.75 mg one to two times per day for initial BMI >30 kg/m² or BMI >27 kg/m² in the presence of risk factors such as controlled elevated blood pressure, diabetes, or high cholesterol.
   v. Avoid late-evening dosing
   vi. Not recommended for children younger than 16 years
   vii. Not recommended in the presence of hypertension, hyperthyroidism, cardiovascular disease, drug or alcohol abuse, or history of kidney stones
   viii. Do not prescribe during or within 14 days of MAOIs.

Follow-Up

A. Re-evaluate the client every week for 6 to 8 weeks, and then monthly if pharmaceutical therapy is used until goal is achieved.
B. Maintain the recommended schedule for comorbid conditions.
C. If the client is a candidate for bariatric surgery, follow recommended pretreatment/reauthorization guidelines required by the payer and bariatric center.

Consultation/Referral

A. Refer to a nutritionist/registered dietitian for consultation.

B. Consider a referral to a bariatric center/surgical consultation and evaluation of bariatric surgery.

C. Consider a psychology consultation (may be required before bariatric surgery).

D. If the family is eligible, refer to the Women, Infant, and Children (WIC) program. Referral to some commercial weight-loss programs may be beneficial. See www.fns.usda.gov/wic/women-infants-and-children-wic.

Individual Considerations

A. Pregnancy:

1. Category X drugs: phentermine and topiramate ER (Qsymia), lorcasern (Belviq), and benzphetamine (Didrex). Avoid use during pregnancy.

2. Weight loss should never be a goal during pregnancy.

3. Counsel clients regarding appropriate weight gain and healthy eating habits during pregnancy.

B. Pediatrics:

1. The cornerstone for management of obesity in children is modification of dietary and exercise habits.

2. The first step for overweight children older than 2 years is maintenance of baseline weight if there is no secondary complication of obesity (i.e., diabetes and hypertension). Any dietary modification must ensure adequate nutrients for the growing child (My Plate kids' place is located at https://www.choosemyplate.gov/kids).

3. The weight-loss goal should be approximately 1 pound per month for a BMI below the 85th percentile.

4. Decrease sedentary behaviors (i.e., watching TV, use of handheld electronic devices, surfing the Internet, and playing video games more than a total of 3 hours a day).

5. Increase physical activity and incorporate exercise into family time.

6. Long-term safety and effectiveness of low-carbohydrate, high-protein diets, such as the Atkins diet, have not been adequately studied in children.

7. Use of pharmacotherapies in children and adolescents requires further research, unless previously noted under drug therapies.

C. Geriatrics:

1. All adults should avoid inactivity. Some exercise is better than none. Any dietary modification must ensure adequate nutrients for the aging adult (The USDA resources for nutrition and health are located at www.choosemyplate.gov).

Resources

American Heart Association: www.heart.org

American Heart Association Go Red for Women: https://www.goredforwomen.org

Centers for Disease Control and Prevention (CDC). *Overweight and obesity*: www.cdc.gov/obesity/index.html

National Institute on Aging. *Exercise: A guide:* www.nia.nih.gov/HealthInformation/Publications/Exercise Guide

President's Council on Fitness, Sports & Nutrition: www.fitness.gov

The Obesity Society: www.obesity.org/home

SHAPE America, Society for Health and Physical Educators: www.shapeamerica.org/

Bibliography

2018 Physical Activity Guidelines Advisory Committee. (2018, February). *2018 physical activity guidelines advisory committee scientific report.* Washington, DC: U.S. Department of Health and Human Services. Retrieved from https://health.gov/paguidelines/second-edition/report/pdf/PAG_Advisory_Committee_Report.pdf

Arena Pharmaceuticals. (2014, December). *Highlights of prescribing information: Belviq.* Retrieved from https://www.accessdata.fda.gov/drugsatfda_docs/label/2014/022529s003lbl.pdf

Centers for Disease Control and Prevention. (2015). *Overweight & obesity.* Retrieved from https://www.cdc.gov/obesity/index.html.

Centers for Disease Control and Prevention. (2018a, August 13). *Adult obesity facts.* Retrieved from https://www.cdc.gov/obesity/data/adult.html.

Centers for Disease Control and Prevention. (2018b, September 11). *Childhood overweight and obesity.* Retrieved from https://www.cdc.gov/obesity/childhood/index.html

Centers for Disease Control and Prevention, National Center for Health Statistics. (2010, September 9). *WHO growth standards are recommended for use in the U.S. for infants and children 0 to 2 years of age.* Retrieved from https://www.cdc.gov/growthcharts/who_charts.htm

Centers for Disease Control and Prevention, National Center for Health Statistics. (2016, December 7). *Growth charts.* Retrieved from https://www.cdc.gov/growthcharts/cdc_charts.htm

DynaMed Plus. (2018, November 30). *Obesity in adults.* Ipswich, MA: EBSCO Information Services. Retrieved from https://www.dynamed.com/topics/dmp~AN~T115009/Obesity-in-adults.

FRAC: Food Research & Action Center. (2019). *Factors contributing to obesity.* Retrieved from http://frac.org/obesity-health/factors-contributing-obesity

Hales, C. M., Carroll, M. D., Fryar, C. D., & Ogden, C. (2017, October). *NCHS data brief No. 288. Prevalence of obesity among adults and youth: United states, 2015-2016.* Retrieved from https://www.cdc.gov/nchs/data/databriefs/db288.pdf

Jensen, M. D., Ryan, D. H., Donato, K. A., Apovian, C. M., Ard, J. D., Comuzzie, A. G., & Yanovski, S. Z. (2014). Special issue: Guidelines for managing overweight and obesity in adults. *Obesity, 22*(S2), 1–16. S1–S410. doi:10.1002/oby.20818

MacMillan, A. (n.d.). *What is obesity? WebMD.* Retrieved from https://www.webmd.com/diet/obesity/features/am-i-obese#1

Mayo Clinic. (n.d.). *Obesity.* Retrieved from https://www.mayoclinic.org/diseases-conditions/obesity/symptoms-causes/syc-20375742

Michalsky, M., Reichard, K., Inge, T., Pratt, J., & Lenders, C. (2012). ASMBS pediatric committee best practice guidelines. *Surgery for Obesity and Related Diseases, 8*, 1–7. doi:10.1016/j.soard.2011.09.009. Retrieved from https://asmbs.org/app/uploads/2011/09/Pediatric BestPracticeGuidelines-January2012.pdf

U.S. Food and Drug Administration. (n.d.). *Medications target long-term weight control.* Retrieved from https://www.fda.gov/consumers/consumer-updates/medications-target-long-term-weight-control

WebMD. (2018). *Appetite suppressants: What you should know.* Retrieved from https://www.webmd.com/diet/appetite-suppressants#1

Post-Bariatric Surgery Long-Term Follow-Up

Cheryl A. Glass and Bunny Pounds

Definition

A. The number of obese people in the United States has more than doubled in the past 50 years, with severe obesity increasing more rapidly than nonsevere obesity. The traditional management of obesity, a combination of diet, exercise, and behavioral modification, often results in moderate success with limited sustainability. Increasing prevalence of obesity combined with improvements in surgical weight-loss procedures and improved insurance coverage has resulted in exponential growth of the number of people opting for surgical management. Clients who undergo surgical weight-loss procedures have unique healthcare needs and require lifelong follow-up. Although the bariatric treatment team is the ideal source of follow-up and monitoring, primary care providers can play a critical role and need to be cognizant of the unique needs of this population.

B. The primary mechanism of action for surgical weight-loss procedures is either restriction or a combination of restriction and malabsorption (see Table 2.3). All procedures have some form of restriction that reduces the volume of food that can be ingested. Restriction can occur by means of a physical barrier such as a laparoscopic adjustable gastric band (LAGB; see Figure 2.1), or an intragastric balloon (see Figure 2.2), or by removing a portion of the digestive tract such as with the gastric sleeve (GS; see Figure 2.3). Malabsorptive procedures cause weight loss by changing the way nutrients are absorbed, which is accomplished by removing portions of the stomach and/or small intestine and sometimes by rerouting the digestive tract (Roux-en-Y; see Figure 2.4). The success of surgical weight loss is defined by initial weight loss, maintenance of weight loss, and prevention of complications. Success is directly related to the aftercare a person receives.

Incidence

A. The CDC notes that obesity now affects one in five children and adolescents in the United States. According to the 2015–2016 NHANES, the prevalence of obesity is 39%; among adults aged 40–59 years, the prevalence is higher (42.8%).

FIGURE 2.1 Laparoscopic adjustable gastric band (LAGB).

Source: Reproduced from Cash, J. C., & Glass, C. A. (2019). *Adult-gerontology practice guidelines* (2nd ed.). New York, NY: Springer Publishing Company.

TABLE 2.3	SURGICAL WEIGHT-LOSS PROCEDURES AND MECHANISM OF ACTION		
Procedure	**Mechanism of Action**	**Advantages**	**Disadvantages**
LAGB; Figure 2.1	Restriction	No cutting or rerouting of digestive tract Reversible and adjustable Lowest risk of nutritional deficiencies	Slower (more gradual) weight loss Greater chance of failure to lose 50% of excess weight Foreign device in body; slippage and erosion possible Highest rate of reoperation
Intragastric balloons; Figure 2.2	Restriction	Approved for BMI 30–40. Placed endoscopically under conscious sedation or general sedation. Can be adjunctive therapy to achieve weight-loss reduction prior to bariatric surgery	Designed to remain implanted for 6 months and allow adjustments in fluid volume to address client symptoms and weight-loss plateaus
GS; Figure 2.3	Restriction and some malabsorption	No rerouting Hormonal hunger suppression, appetite reduction, and increased satiety	Not reversible Potential for nutrient deficiencies Higher complication rate than LAGB
RYGB; Figure 2.4	Restriction and malabsorption	Reduces appetite, enhances satiety Better initial and long-term weight loss compared with LAGB	Long-term nutritional deficiency risk Lifelong adherence to diet and supplementation required Higher complication rate compared with LAGB and GS
BPD/DS	Malabsorption and some restriction	Greatest weight loss overall Reduces appetite, improves satiety Most effective for treatment of diabetes mellitus	Greatest risk of nutritional deficiencies Strict lifetime adherence to diet and supplements Highest complication rate

BPD/DS, biliopancreatic diversion with duodenal switch; GS, gastric sleeve; LAGB, laparoscopic adjustable gastric band; RYGB, Roux-en-Y gastric bypass.

FIGURE 2.2 Intragastric balloon.

Source: Reproduced from Cash, J. C., & Glass, C. A. (2019). *Adult-gerontology practice guidelines* (2nd ed.). New York, NY: Springer Publishing Company.

A

B

FIGURE 2.4 Roux-en-Y gastric bypass (RYGB).

Source: Reproduced from Cash, J. C., & Glass, C. A. (2019). *Adult-gerontology practice guidelines* (2nd ed.). New York, NY: Springer Publishing Company.

FIGURE 2.3 Sleeve bypass procedure with stomach resection.

Source: Reproduced from Cash, J. C., & Glass, C. A. (2019). *Adult-gerontology practice guidelines* (2nd ed.). New York, NY: Springer Publishing Company.

B. The American Society for Metabolic and Bariatric Surgery (ASMBS) reports an estimated 208,000 weight-loss operations were performed in 2017. About 90% of surgical weight-loss procedures are performed laparoscopically now. The most common procedures performed today are gastric bypass, GS, adjustable gastric band, and biliopancreatic diversion with duodenal switch (BPD/DS). The intragastric balloons were FDA approved in 2015; only about 2.75% were done in 2017.

C. The ASMBS pediatric committee best practice guidelines recommend the selection criteria for adolescents being considered for a bariatric procedure should include a BMI of ≥35 kg/m² with major comorbidities (i.e., type 2 diabetes mellitus, moderate to severe sleep apnea [apnea-hypopnea index >15], pseudotumor cerebri, or severe NASH) or a BMI of ≥40 kg/m² with other comorbidities (e.g., hypertension, insulin resistance, glucose intolerance, substantially impaired quality of life or ADLs, dyslipidemia, sleep apnea with apnea–hypopnea

index >5). The associated risk/benefit analysis should also include the consideration of the potential long-term health risks of untreated or inadequately treated obesity for the individual candidate.

Pathogenesis

A. The pathogenesis of obesity is reviewed under "Obesity" in this chapter. Significant improvements in the safety of surgical weight-loss procedures in recent years result from improved surgical techniques, accreditation, and the use of laparoscopy. The overall mortality rate is about 0.5%. The incidences of complications vary by surgical procedure. Postoperative complications may occur immediately or may occur many years after surgery. Nutritional deficiencies are by far the most common long-term complication.

Predisposing Factors

A. Higher BMI
B. Noncompliance with bariatric diet and exercise
C. Lack of follow-up with healthcare professionals
D. Obesity-related health problems:
   1. OSA
   2. Diabetes

3. Arthritis
4. Hypertension
5. GERD
6. Nonalcoholic fatty liver disease and nonalcoholic steatohepatitis
7. Pseudotumor cerebri
8. Depression
E. Complexity and type of surgery

Common Complaints
Functional and Nutritional
A. Dumping syndrome usually occurs within 30 minutes of eating high-fat/high-sugar foods and involves flushing, sweating, lightheadedness, tachycardia, palpitations, nausea, diarrhea, and cramping.
B. Hypoglycemia occurs 1 to 3 hours after eating high-carb meals and involves shakiness, anxiety, sweating, chills, clamminess, confusion, rapid heart rate, dizziness, hunger, and nausea.
C. New or exacerbated reflux is more common with a GS.
D. Vitamin deficiencies or toxicities. Refer to Table 2.4.
   1. Most common:
     a. Iron deficiency—fatigue, lethargy, pica, food cravings
     b. Iron toxicity—gastrointestinal irritation, nausea, vomiting, indigestion, constipation, diarrhea

TABLE 2.4 MOST COMMON NUTRIENT DEFICIENCIES

Nutrient	Protein	Iron	Folate	Calcium	Vitamin B12	Vitamin D
Assay	Serum albumin <3.5 mg/dL May need prealbumin and serum creatinine levels also	Iron saturation <10% Serum ferritin <10 ng/mL or iron saturation <7% regardless of ferritin value	Serum folic acid	Total and ionized calcium Phosphorus 24-hr urinary calcium excretion Intact serum parathyroid hormone Bone density	Serum B12 level May need methylmalonic acid level also	25 (OH)D3 <30 ng/mL
Incidence	18%–25% after malabsorptive procedures	6%–50%	1%–10%	10%–25%	5%–25%	Up to 63%
Complications and symptoms	Anemia Edema Alopecia Asthenia (weakness, decreased muscle mass, brittle hair, generalized edema)	Microcytic, hypochromic anemia (pallor, fatigue, poor capillary refill, palpitations, pica, brittle hair)	Megaloblastic or macrocytic anemia (palpitations; fatigue; diarrhea; smooth, sore tongue) Neural tube defects May aggravate B12 deficiency	Secondary hyperparathyroidism Enhanced bone loss Metabolic bone disease (tetany, tingling, cramping)	Megaloblastic anemia with macrocytosis Neuropathy Cognitive dysfunction (glossitis, constipation, diarrhea, neurologic changes, depression, dementia)	Myopathy Secondary hypocalcemia
Recommended daily amount for prevention	1.1–1.5 g/kg ideal body weight/day 10%–35% of total energy intake should be from protein	45–60 mg/d from multivitamins and iron supplements for malabsorptive procedures Menstruating women may need more	400 mcg/d	1,200–1,500 mg/d of calcium citrate from food and supplements	500 mcg/d oral for band 1,000 mcg/d oral for malabsorptive procedures; may need 500–1,000 mcg/mo intramuscular	At least 3,000 IU of oral D3 daily, better to titrate to therapeutic level
Treatment dosing	If previous options are not effective, may need parenteral nutrition	150–200 mg of elemental iron twice daily, preferably with vitamin C	1,000 mcg/d for 3 months	2,000 mg/d with adequate vitamin D supplementation	Depends on the level of deficiency Recheck levels after 3–6 months of repletion	6,000–10,000 IU/d or 50,000 IU/wk up to 50,000 IU/d Recheck level every 3 months

Sources: Data from Becker, Balcer, & Galetta (2012); Handzlik-Orlik, Holecki, Orlik, Wylezol, & Dulawa (2015); and Kerner (2014).

c. Protein deficiency—weakness, decreased muscle mass, brittle hair, generalized edema

d. Folate deficiency—fatigue, palpitations, sore tongue, diarrhea, restless legs

e. Calcium deficiency—usually silent, hyperparathyroidism

f. Calcium toxicity—constipation, nausea, vomiting, dry mouth, loss of appetite

g. Vitamin D deficiency—spasms/twitching of eyes, burning in mouth, sweating, weakness

h. Vitamin B12 deficiency—fatigue, burning lips/mouth, rapid heart rate, palpitations, sore tongue, weakness, mood changes, neurologic changes

2. Less common:

a. Thiamine (B1) deficiency—usually in first 3 months postop, often a result of vomiting, blurred or double vision, difficulty swallowing, rapid heart rate, fatigue, confusion, memory loss, burning feet, leg weakness, amnesia

b. Zinc deficiency—loss of smell, diminished sense of taste, poor wound healing, skin rashes or roughness, hair loss, poor appetite, lethargy, grooved or deformed nails, canker sores

c. Magnesium deficiency—hyperexcitability, cramps, tremors, fasciculation, spasms, fatigue, loss of appetite, apathy, confusion, insomnia, irritability, poor memory

d. Selenium deficiency (very rare)—signs of hypothyroidism (selenium is necessary for conversion of thyroxine into its active form, triiodothyronine)

e. Selenium toxicity (rare)—hair loss, abnormal nails, dermatitis, peripheral neuropathy, nausea, diarrhea, fatigue, irritability, garlic odor of breath

E. Surgical complications:

1. Short term:

a. Anastomotic leak—<1% to 3% with Roux-en-Y gastric bypass (RYGB)

b. Gastrointestinal hemorrhage, bleeding—0.5% to 2%

c. Wound infection—more common with open approach

d. Thromboembolism—DVT <1%

e. Anastomotic strictures—typically within first 3 months, nausea and/or vomiting

f. Acute distention of the distal stomach

g. Respiratory insufficiency, pneumonia

2. Long term:

a. Band slippage—abdominal pain, acid reflux, regurgitation, or dysphagia

b. Band erosion—may be asymptomatic, abdominal pain, gastrointestinal bleeding, weight loss, abdominal sepsis

c. Intestinal obstruction—caused by internal hernias, adhesions, and anastomotic stenosis—colicky central abdominal pain, nausea, vomiting, abdominal distention, absolute constipation

d. Hepatobiliary complications—rapid weight loss associated with gallstone formation

e. Gastrointestinal bleeding—rare and usually caused by ulceration

f. Marginal ulcers—abdominal pain, vomiting, bleeding, or anemia

g. Micronutrient deficiencies

Other Signs and Symptoms

A. Expected weight loss:

1. LAGB—initial loss of 40% to 50% of excess body weight in 3 to 5 years. Expected maintenance <50%

2. GS—initial loss of >50% of excess body weight in 3 to 5 years. Expected maintenance >50%

3. RYGB—initial loss of 60% to 80% of excess body weight in 1 year. Expected maintenance >50%

4. BPD/DS—initial loss of 60% to 70% of excess body weight in 1 year. Expected maintenance of 60% to 70%

5. Intragastric balloons—loss of about 10% to 15% of body weight is typical during the 6 months following intragastric balloon placement. Expected maintenance: the gastric balloon is only placed for 6 months then removed.

B. Weight regain of up to 20 pounds is common after 2 years.

C. Constipation and/or diarrhea may occur, depending on the procedure

D. Weight loss of <25% of excess body weight is considered a surgical failure and may be revised.

E. Even if weight loss is adequate, clients may express disappointment and/or depression related to rate or amount of weight lost.

F. Nausea and vomiting after LAGB may indicate need for band adjustment.

Subjective Data

A. Review onset and duration of symptoms.

B. Elicit the date of surgery, type of surgery, and any reoperations or complications.

C. Review previous highest weight and amount of excess weight lost since surgery.

D. Evaluate the location and level of pain/discomfort.

E. Evaluate the overall psychosocial changes since surgery

F. Review a 24-hour food recall, choices of healthy foods, skipping meals, food aversion (e.g., red meat), serving size, and intolerance.

G. Review medications and supplement use.

Physical Examination

A. Check height, weight, waist, and hip circumference. Calculate BMI, waist/hip ratio, pulse, respirations, and blood pressure. Check temperature if infection is suspected.

B. Inspect:

1. Examine the skin, evaluate surgical site(s), evaluate redness and tenderness.

2. Oral/dental examination

3. Evaluate for dehydration

4. Eye examination: evaluate eye movement (thiamine deficiency).

5. Evaluate gait.
6. General overview of personal presence and affect
C. Auscultate:
1. Auscultate the heart and lungs.
2. Auscultate the abdomen for bowel sounds.
D. Palpate abdomen:
1. Evaluate for the presence of tenderness.
2. Evaluate for masses.
E. Neurologic examination:
1. Perform neurologic examination, including checking deep tendon reflexes (DTRs), sense of smell, and Babinski reflex (vitamin B12 deficiency).

Diagnostic Tests

A. Laboratory testing is recommended annually for all procedures. Refer to Table 2.5.
1. CBC with differential
2. Liver function tests
3. Glucose
4. Creatinine
5. Electrolytes
B. Annual laboratory testing suggested for LAGB; recommended for all other procedures:
1. Iron/ferritin
2. Vitamin B12
3. Folate
4. Calcium
5. Intact parathyroid hormone (PTH)
6. 25-hydroxy vitamin D
7. Albumin/prealbumin

C. Optional labs that may be required based on symptoms:
1. Zinc
2. Copper
3. Vitamin B1
4. Vitamin B6
5. Vitamin A
D. Other labs as appropriate for condition and prevention:
1. Monitor HgA1c and blood glucose closely in clients with diabetes. Diabetes has resolved after bariatric surgery in some clients.
2. Lipid profile
E. Abdominal ultrasound
F. CT scan abdomen
G. Doppler ultrasound of limb for suspected DVT
H. Pulmonary ventilation/perfusion scan for suspected pulmonary embolus
I. Bone mineral density (dual-energy x-ray absorptiometry [DEXA]) scan: recommended annually until stable after malabsorptive procedures
J. Endoscopy as needed for abdominal complaints

Differential Diagnoses

A. Postoperative surgical complication(s)
B. Infection
C. Abdominal pain
D. Fascial dehiscence
E. DVT
F. Bowel obstruction
G. Band slippage
H. Anastomosis leakage

TABLE 2.5   RECOMMENDED ANNUAL LABORATORY MONITORING FOR BYPASS CLIENTS

	Gastric Band	Gastric Sleeve	Gastric Bypass	BPD/DS
Complete blood count	X	X	X	X
Liver function tests	X	X	X	X
Glucose	X	X	X	X
Creatinine	X	X	X	X
Electrolytes	X	X	X	X
Iron/ferritin	Suggested	X	X	X
Vitamin B12	Suggested	X	X	X
Folate	Suggested	X	X	X
Calcium	Suggested	X	X	X
Intact PTH	Suggested	X	X	X
Vitamin D 25-OH	Suggested	X	X	X
Albumin/prealbumin	Suggested	X	X	X
Bone mineral density		X	X	X
Zinc		Optional	Optional	Optional
Vitamin B1		Optional	Optional	Optional
Vitamin A		Optional 24 months and beyond	Optional 24 months and beyond	Optional 24 months and beyond

BPD/DS, biliopancreatic diversion with duodenal switch; PTH, parathyroid hormone.

Source: Adapted from Heber, D., Greenway, F. L., Kaplan, L. M., Livingston, E., Salvador, J., Still, C., … Endocrine Society. (2010). Endocrine and nutritional management of the post-bariatric surgery client: An Endocrine Society clinical practice guideline. *Endocrine Society, 95*(11), 4823–4843. doi:10.1210/jc.2009-2128.

I. Stomal stenosis/stricture
J. Cholecystitis
K. Dumping syndrome
L. Food intolerance
M. Gastric ulcer
N. Gastroenteritis
O. Vitamin deficiency
P. Malnutrition/protein deficiency
Q. Incisional hernia
R. Osteoporosis

Plan
A. General interventions:
1. Lifelong follow-up is required after bariatric surgery. Ideally, clients should follow up with their surgical group, but many do not. Primary care providers are well positioned to capture those lost to follow-up. Continuous reinforcement of good nutritional habits is important.
B. Client teaching: Many complications can be prevented by adhering to diet and lifestyle recommendations.
1. Supplements are required lifelong; strict adherence will prevent deficiencies.
2. Dumping syndrome can be prevented by avoiding foods that trigger it, such as high-sugar and/or high-fat foods. Clients can keep food diaries to identify triggers.
3. Hypoglycemia can usually be prevented by careful monitoring of carbohydrate intake.
4. Surgery does not replace the need for a balanced diet or exercise. Approximately 150 minutes of moderate activity each week is recommended, though safety and tolerance differ, so exercise recommendations should be individualized. Any activity is better than none.
5. Food should be chewed thoroughly and consumed slowly. Liquids should be avoided 30 minutes before and after meals. Avoid eating and drinking liquids simultaneously.
6. Protein is important for maintaining muscle mass during rapid weight loss and avoiding hunger during maintenance. Between 60 and 100 g of protein daily is recommended. Limit carbohydrate intake to 50 g per day or less. Limiting carbohydrate intake reduces risk of weight regain by preventing rebound hunger.
7. To prevent dehydration as well as reduce the risk of kidney stones and constipation, encourage clients drink 64 ounces of fluids daily.
8. Stress, boredom, and emotions often affect eating habits. Identifying problems and seeking help early are important.
9. Support groups can be a vital source of education and social support, both of which are key to weight loss and maintenance.
10. Weight plateaus are common and normal. They are the body's way of trying to establish a new set point. Do not be discouraged by plateaus. Consistency is key to overcoming them.
11. Adequate sleep and successful stress management are also key to successful weight loss and maintenance.
C. Pharmaceutical therapy:
1. Medication absorption can be altered after bariatric surgery. Evaluate need for adjustments of medication dosing, especially diabetic, psychiatric, and antihypertensive medications as well as any medication with a narrow therapeutic window.

> Drugs with a small therapeutic window such as digoxin, carbamazepine, theophylline, and phenytoin should not be crushed due to the increase in toxicity.

2. Clients may require alternate formulations of medications, including crushed, chewable, liquid, patches, intramuscular (IM), or subcutaneous. Long-acting (LA), ER, or enteric coated medications may not be absorbed as well and may need to be switched to immediate release. Medications designed to release slowly should not be crushed or chewed since the full dose will be released faster than expected.
3. Recommended supplementations:
   a. Multivitamin plus mineral supplements containing iron, folic acid, zinc, copper, selenium, and thiamin (200% of RDA):
      i. LAGB: One daily
      ii. All other procedures: two daily
   b. Calcium: (all procedures) 1,200 to 1,500 mg daily from food and calcium citrate in divided doses
   c. Vitamin D: (all procedures):
      i. 3,000 IU daily [as ergocalciferol (vitamin D_2), or cholecalciferol (vitamin D_3)], titrate to reach normal concentrations of 30 ng/mL
      ii. Treatment for deficiency: 50,000 IU vitamin D_2 or D_3 one time per week for 8 weeks, followed by maintenance therapy of 1500–2000 IU/d to achieve normal concentrations
   d. Iron:
      i. LAGB: not usually necessary unless iron intake from food is insufficient
      ii. All other procedures: 45 to 60 mg elemental daily from multivitamin plus additional supplementation
      iii. Treatment for deficiency: 150–200 mg elemental supplement/d
   e. Vitamin B12 (cobalamin):
      i. LAGB: not usually necessary
      ii. All other procedures: 250–350 mcg/d or 1000 mcg/month IM, or 3000 mcg every 6 months IM after RYGB and BPD
      iii. Treatment for deficiency: 1000–2000 mcg/d sublingual
   f. Thiamin (all procedures):
      i. Should be included in the routine multivitamin supplement

ii.   Treatment for deficiency: 500 mg thiamin/d intravenous (IV) for 3 to 5 days, then 250 mg/d for 3 to 5 days or until the symptoms disappear, and then further treatment by oral administration of 100 mg/d as needed

g. Folate (folic acid) (all procedures):

i.   400 mcg/d should be included in the routine multivitamin; pregnant women or those planning to conceive should take 800–1000 mcg folic acid/d included in a multivitamin supplement or separately.

ii.   Treatment for deficiency: 1000 mcg folic acid/d

h. Fat-soluble vitamins (A, K, and E):

i.   6000 IU vitamin A should be included in the routine multivitamin; for pregnant women or those planning to conceive, the beta carotene form of vitamin A is preferred over retinol

ii.   After BPD: 10,000 IU vitamin A/d, 300 mcg vitamin K/d, and 400 IU vitamin E/d (included in a multivitamin or separately):

1)   Treatment for deficiency when changes in the cornea appear: 50,000–100,000 IU IM for 3 days followed by 50,000 IU/d for 2 weeks IM is recommended

iii.   Treatment for deficiency:

1)   Vitamin A deficiency without corneal changes: 10,000–25,000 IU/d orally to achieve clinical improvement

2)   Vitamin E deficiency: 800–1200 IU/d to reach normal serum concentrations

3)   Vitamin K deficiency: 10 mg IM or submuscular, followed by 1–2 mg/wk parenterally or orally

i. Zinc (Zn):

i.   The routine daily multivitamin should contain 15 mg/d.

ii.   Treatment of deficiency: 60 mg Zn two times per day

j. Copper (Cu):

i.   The routine daily multivitamin should contain 2 mg Cu.

ii.   Severe deficiency requires 2–4 mg Cu/day IV for 6 days.

k. Vitamin C:

i.   The routine daily multivitamin should follow the RDA recommendation for vitamin C.

ii.   Treatment: 100 mg vitamin C three times per day or 500 mg/d for 1 month

4. Long-term anticoagulation may be needed for DVT/pulmonary embolism (PE) prophylaxis.

5. Nonsteroidal anti-inflammatory drugs (NSAIDs) and corticosteroids should be avoided to reduce the risk of marginal ulcers.

D. Psychosocial changes: Bariatric surgery often results in dramatic lifestyle and body changes and may require significant psychosocial adjustments for the client as well as his or her friends and family.

1. Monitor for depression/anxiety, body image concerns, and social support.

2. Alcoholism can be a concern after bariatric surgery. Less alcohol is needed to elevate blood alcohol levels and blood alcohol levels are sustained longer after bariatric surgery.

Follow-Up

A. Bariatric surgery requires lifelong follow-up, ideally by a multidisciplinary team of healthcare providers. Initial follow-up schedules are set by the surgeon. Long-term follow-up (after the first 2 years) is usually provided for by the bariatric surgery program, but research has shown that follow-up is often poor, which leads to poor outcomes and substandard client care.

B. Laboratory and diagnostic testing is required as listed in Table 2.5. Early recognition of nutritional deficiencies can prevent permanent damage and even death.

C. Chronic disease management (particularly diabetes, lipids, and bone disease) can be simpler or more complex after bariatric surgery, depending on the client's adherence to lifestyle and nutritional recommendations.

Consultation/Referral

A. Bariatric surgeon for surgical complications, revisions

B. Surgeon for cholecystectomy (preferably bariatric surgeon or general/GI surgeon experienced in the care of bariatric clients)

C. Gastroenterology consult

D. Nutrition consultation and/or counseling

E. Psychologist consultation

F. Physical therapy/exercise specialist

G. Support group

Individual Considerations

A. Women:

a. All women of childbearing age should receive adequate folate supplementation and be given contraception and preconception counseling.

b. Oral contraceptives (OCPs) may not be as effective after bariatric surgery because of changes in absorption.

B. Pregnancy:

a. Pregnancy should be delayed for 12 to 18 months after bariatric surgery or however long it takes for weight loss to stabilize.

b. Bariatric surgeon consult may be required.

c. Increased folic acid may be needed preconception to reduce risk of neural tube defects.

d. Increased vitamin supplementation may be necessary during pregnancy. Vitamin A should be limited to 5,000 IU daily.

e. Gastric band may need to be adjusted during pregnancy.

f. Serial ultrasounds may need to be done to follow fetal growth.

Bibliography

Ali, M., Moustarah, F., & Kim, J. (2015). *American society for metabolic and bariatric surgery position statement on intra-gastric balloon therapy, Draft.* Retrieved from https://asmbs.org/app/uploads/2015/10/IntraGastricBalloon_Statement_DRAFT.pdf

American Society for Metabolic and Bariatric Surgery. (n.d.). *Life after bariatric surgery.* Retrieved from https://asmbs.org/patients/life-after-bariatric-surgery

American Society for Metabolic and Bariatric Surgery. (2016, March). *Endorsed procedures and devices.* Retrieved from https://asmbs.org/resources/endorsed-procedures-and-devices?/resources/approved-procedures

American Society for Metabolic and Bariatric Surgery. (2018, June). *Estimates of bariatric surgery numbers, 2011–2017.* Retrieved from https://asmbs.org/resources/estimate-of-bariatric-surgery-numbers

Becker, D. A., Balcer, L. J., & Galetta, S. L. (2012). The neurological complications of nutritional deficiency following bariatric surgery. *Journal of Obesity, 2012.* doi:10.1155/2012/608534

Dagan, S. S., Goldenshluger, A., Globus, I., Schweiger, C., Kessler, Y., Sandbank, G. K., ... Sinai, T. (2017). Nutritional recommendations for adult bariatric surgery patients: Clinical practice. *Advances in Nutrition, 8*(2), 382–394. doi:10-3945/an.116.014258

Handzlik-Orlik, G., Holecki, M., Orlik, B., Wylezol, M., & Dulawa, J. (2015). Nutrition management of the post-bariatric surgery client. *Nutrition in Clinical Practice: Official Publication of the American Society for Parenteral and Enteral Nutrition, 30*(3), 383–392. doi:10.1177/0884533614564995

Hamdan, K., Somers, S., & Chand, M. (2011). Management of late post-operative complications of bariatric surgery. *British Journal of Surgery, 98*(10), 1345–1355. doi:10.1002/bjs.7568

Heber, D., Greenway, F. L., Kaplan, L. M., Livingston, E., Salvador, J., Still, C., ... Endocrine Society. (2010). Endocrine and nutritional management of the post-bariatric surgery client: An Endocrine Society clinical practice guideline. *Endocrine Society, 95*(11), 4823–4843. doi:10.1210/jc.2009-2128

Iannelli, A., Dainese, R., Piche, T., facchiano, E., & Gugenhein, J. (2008). Laparoscopic sleep gastrectomy for morbid obesity. *World Journal of Gastroenterology, 14,* 821–827. doi:10.3748/wjg.14.821

Parrott, J., Frank, L., Rabena, R., Craggs-Dino, L., Isom, K. A., & Greiman, L. (2017). American Society for Metabolic and Bariatric Surgery integrated health nutritional guidelines for the surgical weight loss patient 2016 update: Micronutrients. *Surgery for Obesity and Related Diseases, 13*(5), 727–741. doi:10.1016/j.soard.2016.12.018

Pounds, B. P. (2015). *Improving primary care provider knowledge regarding malabsorptive nutritional deficiencies after bariatric surgery.* Hyden, KY: Frontier Nursing University. Unpublished manuscript.

University of California, San Francisco, UCSF Health. (n.d.). *Dietary guidelines after bariatric surgery.* Retrieved from https://www.ucsfhealth.org/education/dietary_guidelines_after_gastric_bypass/index.html

Substance Use Disorders

Cheryl A. Glass, Karen M. Kress, Moya Cook, and Robertson Nash

Definition

A. Alcoholism and drug dependence and addiction, known as substance use disorders (SUDs), are complex problems. Most scientists and medical researchers now consider dependence on alcohol or drugs to be a long-term illness, like asthma, hypertension (high blood pressure), or diabetes. Most people who drink alcohol drink very little, and many people can stop taking drugs without a struggle. However, some people develop an SUD—use of alcohol or drugs that is compulsive or dangerous (or both).

B. The National Survey on Drug Use and Health (NSDUH) states misuse of prescription drugs is defined as use in any way not directed by a doctor, including use without a prescription of one's own; use in greater amounts, more often, or longer than told to take a drug; or use in any other way not directed by a doctor:

  1. The National Institute on Drug Abuse (NIDA) notes many misused drugs can alter a person's thinking and judgment, leading to health risks, including addiction, drugged driving, infectious disease, and potential harm to babies with prenatal exposure. Table 2.6 is the NIDA's list of commonly abused substances. Table 2.7 is a list of commonly abused prescription medications.

TABLE 2.6   NATIONAL INSTITUTE ON DRUG ABUSE LIST OF COMMONLY ABUSED DRUGS

Substances: Category and Name	Examples of Commercial and Street Names	DEA Schedule[a]/How Administered[b]	Acute Effects/Health Risks
Tobacco			Increased blood pressure and heart rate/chronic lung disease; cardiovascular disease; stroke; cancers of the mouth, pharynx, larynx, esophagus, stomach, pancreas, cervix, kidney, bladder, and acute myeloid leukemia; adverse pregnancy outcomes; addiction
Nicotine	Found in cigarettes, cigars, bidis, hookahs, and smokeless tobacco (snuff, spit tobacco, chew)	Not scheduled/smoked, snorted, chewed, and vaporized	
Alcohol			In low doses, euphoria, mild stimulation, relaxation, lowered inhibitions; in higher doses, drowsiness, slurred speech, nausea, emotional volatility, loss of coordination, visual distortions, impaired memory, sexual dysfunction, loss of consciousness/increased risk of injuries, violence, fetal damage (in pregnant women); depression; neurologic deficits; hypertension; liver and heart disease; addiction; fatal overdose
Alcohol (ethyl alcohol)	Found in liquor, beer, and wine	Not scheduled/swallowed	

(*continued*)

TABLE 2.6   NATIONAL INSTITUTE ON DRUG ABUSE LIST OF COMMONLY ABUSED DRUGS (*continued*)

Substances: Category and Name	Examples of Commercial and Street Names	DEA Schedule[a]/How Administered[b]	Acute Effects/Health Risks
Cannabinoids			Euphoria; relaxation; slowed reaction time; distorted sensory perception; impaired balance and coordination; increased heart rate and appetite; impaired learning, memory; anxiety; panic attacks; psychosis/cough; frequent respiratory infections; possible mental health decline; addiction
Marijuana	Blunt, dope, ganja, grass, herb, joint, bud, Mary Jane, pot, reefer, green, trees, smoke, sinsemilla, skunk, weed	I/smoked, swallowed	
Hashish	Boom, gangster, hash, hash oil, hemp	I/smoked, swallowed	
Opioids			Euphoria; drowsiness; impaired coordination; dizziness; confusion; nausea; sedation; feeling of heaviness in the body; slowed or arrested breathing; constipation; endocarditis; hepatitis; HIV; addiction; fatal overdose
Heroin	Diacetylmorphine: smack, horse, brown sugar, dope, H, junk, skag, skunk, white horse, China white, cheese (with OTC cold medicine and antihistamine)	I/injected, smoked, snorted	
Opium	Laudanum, paregoric: big O, black stuff, block, gum, hop	II, III, V/swallowed, smoked	
Stimulants			Increased heart rate, blood pressure, body temperature, metabolism; feelings of exhilaration; increased energy, mental alertness; tremors; reduced appetite; weight loss; irritability; anxiety; panic; paranoia; violent behavior; psychosis; insomnia; cardiac or cardiovascular complications; stroke; seizures; addiction Also, for cocaine—nasal damage from snorting Also, for methamphetamine—severe dental problems
Cocaine	Cocaine hydrochloride: blow, bump, C, candy, Charlie, coke, crack, flake, rock, snow, toot	II/snorted, smoked, injected	
Amphetamine	Biphetamine, dexedrine: bennies, black beauties, crosses, hearts, LA turnaround speed, truck drivers, uppers	II/swallowed, snorted, smoked, injected	
Methamphetamine	Desoxyn: meth, ice, crank, chalk, crystal, fire, glass, go fast, speed	II/swallowed, snorted, smoked, injected	
Club Drugs			MDMA—mild hallucinogenic effects; increased tactile sensitivity, empathic feelings; lowered inhibition; anxiety; chills; sweating; teeth clenching; muscle cramping/sleep disturbances; depression; impaired memory; hyperthermia; addiction Flunitrazepam—sedation; muscle relaxation; confusion; memory loss; dizziness; impaired coordination/addiction GHB—drowsiness; nausea; headache; disorientation; loss of coordination; memory loss/unconsciousness; seizures; coma
MDMA	Ecstasy, Adam, clarity, Eve, lover's speed, peace, uppers	I/swallowed, snorted, injected	
Flunitrazepam	Rohypnol: forget-me pill, Mexican Valium, R2, roach, Roche, roofies, roofinol, rope, rophies	IV/swallowed, snorted	
GHB[c]	Gamma-hydroxybutyrate: G, Georgia home boy, grievous bodily harm, liquid ecstasy, soap, scoop, goop, liquid X	I/swallowed	
Dissociative Drugs			Feelings of being separate from one's body and environment, impaired motor function/anxiety, tremors, numbness, memory loss, nausea Also for ketamine—analgesia, impaired memory, delirium, respiratory depression and arrest, death Also for PCP and analogs—analgesia, psychosis, aggression, violence, slurred speech, loss of coordination, hallucinations Also for DXM—euphoria, slurred speech, confusion, dizziness, distorted visual perceptions
Ketamine	Ketalar SV: cat Valium, K, special K, vitamin K	III/injected, snorted, smoked	
PCP and analogs	Phencyclidine: angel dust, boat, hog, love boat, peace pill	I, II/swallowed, smoked, injected	
Salvia divinorum	Salvia, shepherdess's herb, Maria Pastora, magic mint, Sally-D	Not scheduled/chewed, swallowed, smoked	
Dextromethorphan (DXM)	Found in some cough and cold medications: Robotripping, Robo, Triple C	Not scheduled/ swallowed	

(*continued*)

TABLE 2.6   NATIONAL INSTITUTE ON DRUG ABUSE LIST OF COMMONLY ABUSED DRUGS (*continued*)

Substances: Category and Name	Examples of Commercial and Street Names	DEA Schedule[a]/How Administered[b]	Acute Effects/Health Risks
Hallucinogens			Altered states of perception and feeling; hallucinations; nausea Also for LSD and mescaline—increased body temperature, heart rate, blood pressure; loss of appetite; sweating; sleeplessness; numbness; dizziness; weakness; tremors; impulsive behavior; rapid shifts in emotion Also for LSD—flashbacks, hallucinogen persisting perception disorder Also for psilocybin—nervousness; paranoia; panic
LSD	LSD: acid, blotter, cubes, microdot, yellow sunshine, blue heaven	I/swallowed, absorbed through mouth tissues	
Mescaline	Buttons, cactus, mesc, peyote	I/swallowed, smoked	
Psilocybin	Magic mushrooms, purple passion, shrooms, little smoke	I/swallowed	
Other Compounds			Steroids—no intoxicating effects; blood clotting and cholesterol changes; liver cysts; hostility and aggression; acne; in adolescents—premature stoppage of growth; in males—prostate cancer, reduced sperm production, shrunken testicles, breast enlargement; in females—menstrual irregularities, development of beard and other masculine characteristics Inhalants (varies by chemical)—stimulation; loss of inhibition; headache; nausea or vomiting; slurred speech; loss of motor coordination; wheezing/cramps; muscle weakness; depression; memory impairment; damage to cardiovascular and nervous systems; unconsciousness; sudden death
Anabolic steroids	Anadrol, Oxandrin, Durabolin, Depo-Testosterone, Equipoise, roids, juice, gym candy, pumpers	III/injected, swallowed, applied to skin	
Inhalants	Solvents (paint thinners, gasoline, glues); gases (butane, propane, aerosol propellants, nitrous oxide); nitrites (isoamyl, isobutyl, cyclohexyl): laughing gas, poppers, snappers, whippets	Not scheduled/inhaled through nose or mouth	
Prescription Medications			
CNS depressants	For more information on prescription medications, please visit www.nida.nih.gov/DrugPages/ PrescripDrugsChart.html		
Stimulants			
Opioid pain relievers			

CNS, central nervous system; DEA, Drug Enforcement Administration; GHB, gamma-hydroxybutyric acid; LSD, lysergic acid diethylamide; MDMA, methylenedioxymethamphetamine; OTC, over the counter; PCP, phenylcyclidine.

[a]Schedule I and II drugs have a high potential for abuse. They require greater storage security and have a quota on manufacturing, among other restrictions. Schedule I drugs are available for research only and have no approved medical use; Schedule II drugs are available only by prescription (unrefillable) and require a form for ordering. Schedule III and IV drugs are available by prescription, may have five refills in 6 months, and may be ordered orally. Some Schedule V drugs are available OTC.

[b]Some of the health risks are directly related to the route of drug administration. For example, injection drug use can increase the risk of infection through needle contamination with staphylococci, HIV, hepatitis, and other organisms.

[c]Associated with sexual assaults.

Sources: National Institute on Drug Abuse (NIDA): Visit NIDA at www.drugabuse.gov; National Institutes of Health (NIH); U.S. Department of Health and Human Services; The NIH: Turning Discovery Into Health.

2. Rates of opioid overdose deaths doubled from 2010 to 2016, with the sharpest increase in deaths related to illicitly made fentanyl and fentanyl analogs (synthetic opioids). In response to the opioid crisis, the U.S. Surgeon General released a public health advisory to urge more individuals, including family, friends, and those who are personally at risk for an opioid overdose, to keep the drug naloxone, an opioid antagonist, on hand as a potentially lifesaving medication that can reverse the effects of an opioid overdose.

C. NSDUH defines binge drinking for males as drinking five or more drinks on an occasion on at least 1 day in the past 30 days and for females as drinking four or more drinks on an occasion on at least 1 day in that period. Heavy alcohol use is defined as binge drinking on 5 or more days in the past 30 days. Any alcohol use, binge drinking, and heavy drinking are not mutually exclusive categories of use: heavy use is included in estimates of binge and current use, and binge use is included in estimates of current use.

Incidence

A. Statistics indicate that the most commonly used legal substances are caffeine, alcohol, and nicotine. According to the NIDA, tobacco use is the leading preventable cause of disease, disability, and death in the United States.

TABLE 2.7 NATIONAL INSTITUTE ON DRUG ABUSE LIST OF COMMONLY ABUSED PRESCRIPTION DRUGS

Substances: Category and Name	Examples of Commercial and Street Names	DEA Schedule[a]/How Administered	Intoxication Effects/Health Risks
Depressants			Sedation/drowsiness; reduced anxiety; feelings of well-being; lowered inhibitions; slurred speech; poor concentration; confusion; dizziness; impaired coordination and memory/slowed pulse; lowered blood pressure; slowed breathing; tolerance; withdrawal; addiction; increased risk of respiratory distress and death when combined with alcohol For barbiturates—euphoria; unusual excitement; fever; irritability/life-threatening withdrawal in chronic users
Barbiturates	*Amytal, Nembutal, Seconal, Phenobarbital:* barbs, reds, red birds, phennies, tooies, yellows, yellow jackets	II, III, IV/injected, swallowed	
Benzodiazepines	*Ativan, Halcion, Librium, Valium, Xanax, Klonopin:* candy, downers, sleeping pills, tranks	IV/swallowed	
Sleep medications	*Ambien (zolpidem), Sonata (zaleplon), Lunesta (eszopiclone)*	IV/swallowed	
Opioids and Morphine Derivatives[b]			Pain relief; euphoria; drowsiness; sedation; weakness; dizziness; nausea; impaired coordination; confusion; dry mouth; itching; sweating; clammy skin; constipation/slowed or arrested breathing; lowered pulse and blood pressure; tolerance; addiction; unconsciousness; coma; death. Risk of death increased when combined with alcohol or other CNS depressants For fentanyl—80 to 100 times more potent analgesic than morphine For oxycodone—muscle relaxation/twice as potent analgesic as morphine; high abuse potential For codeine—less analgesia, sedation, and respiratory depression than morphine For methadone—used to treat opioid addiction and pain; significant overdose risk when used improperly
Codeine	*Empirin with Codeine, Fiorinal with Codeine, Robitussin A-C, Tylenol with Codeine:* Captain Cody, Cody, schoolboy; (with glutethimide: doors and fours, loads, pancakes and syrup)	II, III, IV/injected, swallowed	
Morphine	*Roxanol, Duramorph:* M, Miss Emma, monkey, white stuff	II, III/injected, swallowed, smoked	
Methadone	*Methadone, Dolophine:* fizzies, amidone (with MDMA: chocolate chip cookies)	II/swallowed, injected	
Fentanyl and analogs	*Actiq, Duragesic, Sublimaze:* Apache, China girl, dance fever, friend, good-fella, jackpot, murder 8, TNT, Tango and Cash	II/injected, smoked, snorted	
Other opioid pain relievers: Oxycodone HCL, hydrocodone bitartrate, hydromorphone, oxymorphone, meperidine, propoxyphene	*Tylox, Oxycontin, Percodan, Percocet:* oxy, O.C., oxycontin, oxycet, hillbilly heroin, percs; *Vicodin, Lortab, Lorcet:* vike, Watson-387; *Dilaudid:* juice, smack, D, footballs, dillies; *Opana, Numorphan, Numorphone:* biscuits, blue heaven, blues, Mrs. O, octagons, stop signs, O bomb; *Demerol, meperidine hydrochloride:* demmies, pain killer; *Darvon, Darvocet*	II, III, IV/chewed, swallowed, snorted, injected, suppositories	
Stimulants			Feelings of exhilaration; increased energy; mental alertness/increased heart rate, blood pressure, and metabolism; reduced appetite; weight loss; nervousness; insomnia; seizures; heart attack; stroke For amphetamines—rapid breathing; tremor, loss of coordination; irritability; anxiousness; restlessness/delirium; panic; paranoia; hallucinations; impulsive behavior; aggressiveness; tolerance; addiction For methylphenidate—increase or decrease in blood pressure; digestive problems; loss of appetite; weight loss
Amphetamines	*Biphetamine, Dexedrine, Adderall:* bennies, black beauties, crosses, hearts, LA turnaround, speed, truck drivers, uppers	II/injected, swallowed, smoked, snorted	
Methylphenidate	*Concerta, Ritalin:* JIF, MPH, R-ball, skippy, the smart drug, vitamin R	II/injected, swallowed, snorted	

(continued)

TABLE 2.7   NATIONAL INSTITUTE ON DRUG ABUSE LIST OF COMMONLY ABUSED PRESCRIPTION DRUGS *(continued)*

Substances: Category and Name	Examples of Commercial and Street Names	DEA Schedule[a]/How Administered	Intoxication Effects/Health Risks
Other Compounds			Euphoria; slurred speech/increased heart rate and blood pressure; dizziness; nausea; vomiting; confusion; paranoia; distorted visual perceptions; impaired motor function
DXM	Found in some cough and cold medications: robotripping, robo, triple C	Not scheduled/ swallowed	

CNS, central nervous system; DEA, Drug Enforcement Administration; DXM, dextromethorphan; HCl, hydrochloride; MDMA, methylenedioxymethamphetamine.

[a]Schedule I and II drugs have a high potential for abuse. They require greater storage security and have a quota on manufacturing, among other restrictions. Schedule I drugs are available for research only and have no approved medical use. Schedule II drugs are available only by prescription and require a new prescription for each refill. Schedule III and IV drugs are available by prescription, may have five refills in 6 months, and may be ordered orally. Most Schedule V drugs are available OTC.

[b]Taking drugs by injection can increase the risk of infection through needle contamination with staphylococci, HIV, hepatitis, and other organisms. Injection is a more common practice for opioids, but risks apply to any medication taken by injection.

Source: National Institute on Drug Abuse (NIDA): Visit NIDA at www.drugabuse.gov; National Institutes of Health (NIH); U.S. Department of Health and Human Services; The NIH: Turning Discovery Into Health.

1. According to the CDC, approximately one in five premature deaths in the United States every year is the result of cigarette smoking. On average, smokers die 10 years earlier than nonsmokers. In 2017 14.0% of all adults age 18 years or older were current cigarette smokers.

2. According to the E-Cigarette Use Among Youth and Young Adults 2016 Report of the Surgeon General, e-cigarettes are now the most commonly used tobacco product among youth in the United States:

   a. These products are now the most commonly used form of tobacco among youth in the United States, surpassing conventional tobacco products, including cigarettes, cigars, chewing tobacco, and hookahs.

   b. E-cigarette use is strongly associated with the use of other tobacco products among youth and young adults, including combustible tobacco products.

   c. These devices are referred to, by the companies themselves and by consumers, as "e-cigarettes," "e-cigs," "cigalikes," "e-hookahs," "mods," "vape pens," "vapes," and "tank systems."

   d. Ingestion of e-cigarette liquids containing nicotine can cause acute toxicity and possibly death if the contents of refill cartridges or bottles containing nicotine are consumed.

B. Research suggests that sexual minorities (e.g., people who identify as lesbian, gay, or bisexual) are at greater risk for substance use and mental health issues compared with the sexual majority population that identifies as being heterosexual. Although sexual orientation is not a new construct, many federally funded surveys have only recently begun to identify sexual minorities in their data collections. In 2015, NSDUH added two questions on sexual orientation, one for sexual identity and one for sexual attraction, making it the first nationally representative, comprehensive source of federally collected information on substance use and mental health issues among sexual minority adults. Sexual minority adults identified as being lesbian, gay, or bisexual. Sexual majority adults identified as being heterosexual or straight.

The 2015 NSDUH obtains information on 10 categories of illicit drugs: marijuana; cocaine in any form, including crack; heroin; hallucinogens; inhalants; methamphetamine; and the misuse of prescription pain relievers, tranquilizers, stimulants, and sedatives. The survey noted sexual minority adults were more likely than sexual majority adults to have engaged in the following:

   a. Cocaine use (5.1% vs. 1.8%)

   b. Heroin use (0.9% vs. 0.3%)

   c. Use of hallucinogens (5.0% vs. 1.6%), including use of lysergic acid diethylamide (LSD) (1.7% vs. 0.5%) and Ecstasy (3.2% vs. 0.9%)

   d. Use of inhalants (3.7% vs. 0.3%)

   e. Methamphetamine use (2.3% vs. 0.6%)

   f. Misuse of prescription tranquilizers (5.9% vs. 2.2%)

   g. Misuse of prescription stimulants (4.2% vs. 1.9%)

   h. Misuse of prescription sedatives (1.2% vs. 0.6%)

C. NSDUH asks respondents about their alcohol use in the 30 days before the interview (i.e., current use). Sexual minority adults aged 18 or older were more likely than sexual majority adults to be current alcohol drinkers or binge drinkers in the past month. However, similar percentages of sexual minority and sexual majority adults were heavy alcohol users in the past month. Among sexual minority adults, 63.6% were current alcohol drinkers and 36.1% were binge alcohol drinkers.

> A substance abuse problem is recognized in as few as one in 20 substance-abusing clients seeking medical attention.

Pathogenesis

A. No single gene has been identified as the culprit in the predisposition to substance dependence. Certain biological features seem to be inherited by first-degree relatives (particularly males) of alcoholics, for example, a resistance to intoxication, a subnormal cortisol rise after drinking, and a subnormal epinephrine release following stress.

B. Some theories postulate alterations in metabolism of alcohol and drugs in people who are dependent. Studies pertaining to alcohol have included research into genetic heritability, flawed metabolism of alcohol by alcoholics, insensitivity to alcohol inherited by alcoholics (thus tending to increase tolerance or ability to know when to stop), and alterations in brain waves in alcoholics.

C. Although much of the research is specific to only one drug, much of what is known about the research can be applied to other drugs.

D. According to the NIDA, people begin taking drugs for a variety of reasons, including:
1. To feel good/pleasure of "high"
2. To feel better, for example, relieve stress, pain, sleep
3. To do better/improve performance
4. Curiosity/boredom
5. Peer pressure

E. According to the E-Cigarette Use Among Youth and Young Adults 2016 Report of the Surgeon General, the most commonly cited reasons for using e-cigarettes among both youth and young adults are:
1. Curiosity
2. Flavor/taste
3. Low perceived harm
4. Aid to quit conventional cigarettes

Predisposing Factors

Factors vary among individuals, and no one factor can account entirely for the risk of substance abuse. Studies indicate a high correlation between substance use and the presence of psychiatric disorders, especially anxiety disorders, depression, schizophrenia, and, in women, eating disorders.

A. Genetic
B. Familial
C. Environmental
D. Occupational
E. Socioeconomic
F. Cultural
G. Personality
H. Life stress
I. Psychiatric comorbidity
J. Biological
K. Social learning and behavioral conditioning
L. Sexual minority adults identified as being lesbian, gay, or bisexual

Common Complaints

Clients' complaints will be focused on the symptoms of the problem rather than the substance dependence. The problem itself will be avoided through the use of denial, minimization, blaming, and projection (all signs of the disease of substance dependence).

A. Chronic anxiety and tension
B. Insomnia
C. Chronic depression
D. Headaches and/or back pain
E. Blackouts
F. Gastrointestinal problems
G. Tachycardia/palpitations
H. Frequent falls or minor injuries
I. Problems with a loved one, problems at work, or with friends

> An estimated 20% of clients presenting to physician offices with noncancer pain symptoms or pain-related diagnoses (including acute and chronic pain) have received an opioid prescription. Consider clients who present frequently with somatic complaints, such as back pain or headache, as "drug seeking," especially when the client knows what drugs work best or asks for specific narcotic analgesics.

> Substance abuse should be suspected in all clients who present with accidents or signs of repeated trauma, especially to the head.

Other Signs and Symptoms

A. Defensiveness about alcohol/drug use or vagueness with answers
B. History of problems with family life, marital relationships, work, finances, and physical health
C. Change in spiritual beliefs (stops attending religious services)
D. Unexplained job changes and multiple traffic accidents
E. History of impulsive behavior, fighting, or unexplained falls
F. Arrest for public drunkenness, driving under the influence, or illegal activity when alcohol/drugs were involved
G. Tremors (shakes)
H. Delirium tremens (DTs)
I. Seizures related to drugs
J. Hallucinations
K. History of chronic family chaos and instability
L. Physical indications of chronic alcohol/drug use include spider angiomas, ruddy nose and face, nasal lesions, bruxism, swollen features, bruises, needle marks/tracks, cutaneous abscesses, malnourishment, anemia, jaundice, and severe dental problems such as "meth mouth"
M. Active withdrawal symptoms include nausea and vomiting, malaise, weakness, tachycardia, diaphoresis, tremors, lightheadedness or dizziness, insomnia, irritability, confusion, perceptual abnormalities or hallucinations (auditory, visual, or tactile), paresthesia, blurred vision, diarrhea, anorexia, abdominal cramps, severe depression, severe anxiety, piloerection, fasciculation (muscle twitching), rhinorrhea, fever, elevated blood pressure and pulse, tinnitus, nystagmus, delirium, or seizures
N. Overdose symptoms related to drug(s) include seizures, cardiovascular depression/collapse, and respiratory depression/collapse. Be prepared to provide cardiovascular and respiratory support and supportive care until transport

Subjective Data

A. Review the onset, duration, and course of presenting complaints.

B. Question the client regarding relatives with a history of alcohol, tobacco, or drug use or problems pertaining to use.

C. When questioning the client, assume some use. Start with the least invasive questions first, for example, "At what age did you first start drinking?" Then ask about tobacco products, e-cigarettes, OTC medications, prescription medications, marijuana, stimulants, opiates, sedatives, hypnotics, benzodiazepines, barbiturates, hallucinogens, inhalants, steroids, and other drugs.

D. Review use of the following drugs concerning quantity and type (if cigarettes, brand smoked, e-cigarettes; if alcohol, type of alcohol: beer, wine, hard liquor) and age at initiation. Query regarding previous attempts to stop use.

E. Start with the past and proceed to the present with use; include first use of the mood-altering substance, amounts, and the last use of the particular substance and amount

F. Choose evidence-based screening tools and assessments. The NIDA website has links to multiple tools specific to alcohol and/or drugs, client age, and indicates if the tool is self-administered or clinician-administered. The website is https://www.drugabuse.gov/nidamed-medical-health-professionals/screening-tools-resources/chart-screening-tools.

　1. Assess using the CAGE test. The **CAGE** (two out of four) is highly predictive of addiction.

　　a. Have you ever tried to **cut** down on your alcohol/drug use?

　　b. Do you get **annoyed** if someone mentions your use is a problem?

　　c. Do you ever feel **guilty** about your use?

　　d. Do you ever have an **"eye-opener"** first thing in the morning after you've been drinking or using the night before?

　2. Assess the client's pain and function regularly using a validated instrument such as the three-item PEG Assessment Scale. A 30% improvement in pain and function is considered clinically meaningful. If your client does not have a 30% improvement in pain and function, consider reducing dose or tapering and discontinuing opioids. Ask client:

　　a. What number best describes your pain on average in the past week? (from 0 = no pain to 10 = pain as bad as you can imagine)

　　b. What number best describes how, during the past week, pain has interfered with your enjoyment of life? (from 0 = does not interfere to 10 = completely interferes)

　　c. What number best describes how, during the past week, pain has interfered with your general activity? (from 0 = does not interfere to 10 = completely interferes)

　3. Assess for depression using the Patient Health Questionnaires (PHQ). The PHQ-9 has been validated for use in primary care settings and can be used to make a tentative diagnosis of depression and to monitor depression severity and response to treatments in the past 2 weeks. The PHQ-9 is available at https://d14rmgtrwzf5a.cloudfront.net/sites/default/files/files/PatientHealthQuestionnaire9.pdf.

　4. NIDA has two brief online validated adolescent substance use screening tools to assess for SUD risk among adolescents 12–17 years old. The Brief Screener for Tobacco, Alcohol, and other Drugs (BSTAD) and the Screening to Brief Intervention (S2BI) ask clients about frequency of past year use and triage them into one of three levels of SUD risk: no reported use, lower risk, and higher risk.

　　a. The BSATD online tool is located at https://www.drugabuse.gov/ast/bstad/#/.

　　b. The S2BI online tool is located at https://www.drugabuse.gov/ast/s2bi/#/.

G. If client admits drinking or drug use, ascertain specific amounts and last use of each substance. Has the client ever needed the use of naloxone for overdose or been hospitalized?

H. Determine whether client experiences suicidal ideation and whether there is a history of past attempts (see Chapter 22, Psychiatric Guidelines, Suicide).

Physical Examination

A. Check temperature (if indicated), pulse, respirations, blood pressure, height and weight to calculate BMI.

B. Inspect:

　1. Observe general appearance, dress, grooming, breath odor, wasted appearance, attitude, sad affect, psychomotor retardation, or tremors.

　2. Conduct a dermal examination for spider angiomas, bruises, track marks, color, pallor, rash, jaundice, petechiae, and gynecomastia in men (hallucinogens).

　3. Examine the eyes for sclera color and features, pupil size, and reactivity.

　4. Inspect the nasal mucosa for erythema, edema, spider telangiectasis, and discharge; look for septal lesions or perforation, deviation, and polyps.

　5. Inspect the mouth/pharynx: Oral lesions, poor dental hygiene, erythema, and teeth for uneven surfaces, tooth decay, and gum erosion.

C. Palpate:

　1. Palpate the neck and thyroid.

　2. Palpate the axilla and groin for lymphadenopathy.

　3. Palpate the abdomen; note hepatomegaly/tenderness.

D. Percuss:

　1. Percuss the chest; note pulmonary consolidation.

　2. Percuss the abdomen for hepatosplenomegaly.

E. Auscultate:

　1. Auscultate the heart for murmur, new S4 gallop, single S2, and arrhythmias.

　2. Auscultate the lungs for rales, effusion, and consolidation.

F. Perform neurologic examination/mental status.

Diagnostic Tests

A. Blood alcohol level

B. Cotinine level (nicotine; where available)

C. Urine drug screen

D. CBC with differential

E. Platelet count
F. HIV or hepatitis

> IV drug use contributes strongly to the spread of AIDS, hepatitis B and hepatitis C, and other infectious diseases. Consider evaluation for sexually transmitted infections.

G. Antinuclear antibody, erythrocyte sedimentation rate, and rheumatoid factor
H. Electrolytes
I. Liver panel:
1. Elevated liver enzymes can also be attributed to overuse of acetaminophen (Tylenol), found in combination with opiates.
J. Blood cultures (fever)
K. Bone density studies:
1. Clients who have been drinking for years should have bone density studies done because alcohol increases the risk for osteoporosis.

Differential Diagnoses
A. Chronic pain syndrome
B. Anxiety
C. Depression

Plan
A. General interventions:
1. Discuss your concerns about alcohol, nicotine, or drug use and discuss addiction treatment with the client.
2. Principles of Drug Addiction Treatment:
a. Everyone entering treatment receives a clinical assessment. A complete assessment of an individual is needed to help treatment professionals offer the type of treatment that best suits the client. The assessment also helps program counselors work with the person to design an effective treatment plan. Although clinical assessment continues throughout a person's treatment, it starts at or just before a person's admission to a treatment program. The assessment includes:
i. Cultural issues around use of alcohol or drugs
ii. Effects of drug or alcohol use on the person's life
iii. Medical history
iv. Current medical problems or needs
v. Current medications (including pain medication)
vi. Mental health issues or behavioral problems
vii. Family and social issues and needs
viii. Legal or financial problems
ix. Educational background and needs
x. Current living situation and environment
xi. Employment history, stability, problems, and needs
xii. School performance, problems, and needs, if relevant
xiii. Previous treatment experiences or attempts to quit drug or alcohol use

b. More than three decades of scientific research show that treatment can help drug-addicted individuals stop drug use, avoid relapse, and successfully recover their lives. Based on this research, 13 fundamental principles that characterize effective drug abuse treatment have been developed. These principles are detailed in NIDA's *Principles of Drug Addiction Treatment: A Research-Based Guide*. The guide also describes different types of science-based treatments and provides answers to commonly asked questions.
i. **Addiction is a complex but treatable disease that affects brain function and behavior.** Drugs alter the brain's structure and how it functions, resulting in changes that persist long after drug use has ceased. This may help explain why abusers are at risk of relapse even after long periods of abstinence.
ii. **No single treatment is appropriate for everyone.** Matching treatment settings, interventions, and services to an individual's particular problems and needs is critical to his or her ultimate success.
iii. **Treatment needs to be readily available.** Because drug-addicted individuals may be uncertain about entering treatment, taking advantage of available services the moment people are ready for treatment is critical. Potential clients can be lost if treatment is not immediately available or readily accessible.
iv. **Effective treatment attends to multiple needs of the individual, not just his or her drug abuse.** To be effective, treatment must address the individual's drug abuse and any associated medical, psychological, social, vocational, and legal problems.
v. **Remaining in treatment for an adequate period of time is critical.** The appropriate duration for an individual depends on the type and degree of his or her problems and needs. Research indicates that most addicted individuals need at least 3 months in treatment to significantly reduce or stop their drug use and that the best outcomes occur with longer durations of treatment.
vi. **Counseling—individual and/or group—and other behavioral therapies are the most commonly used forms of drug abuse treatment.** Behavioral therapies vary in their focus and may involve addressing a client's motivations to change, building skills to resist drug use, replacing drug-using activities with constructive and rewarding activities, improving problem-solving skills, and facilitating better interpersonal relationships.
vii. **Medications are an important element of treatment for many clients, especially when combined with counseling and**

other behavioral therapies. For example, methadone and buprenorphine are effective in helping individuals addicted to heroin or other opioids stabilize their lives and reduce their illicit drug use. Also, for persons addicted to nicotine, a nicotine replacement product (nicotine patches or gum) or an oral medication (bupropion or varenicline) can be an effective component of treatment when part of a comprehensive behavioral treatment program.

viii. **An individual's treatment and services plan must be assessed continually and modified as necessary to ensure it meets his or her changing needs.** A client may require varying combinations of services and treatment components during the course of treatment and recovery. In addition to counseling or psychotherapy, a client may require medication, medical services, family therapy, parenting instruction, vocational rehabilitation, and/or social and legal services. For many clients, a continuing care approach provides the best results, with treatment intensity varying according to a person's changing needs.

ix. **Many drug-addicted individuals also have other mental disorders.** Because drug abuse and addiction—both of which are mental disorders—often co-occur with other mental illnesses, clients presenting with one condition should be assessed for the other(s). And when these problems co-occur, treatment should address both (or all), including the use of medications as appropriate.

x. **Medically assisted detoxification is only the first stage of addiction treatment and by itself does little to change long-term drug abuse.** Although medically assisted detoxification can safely manage the acute physical symptoms of withdrawal, detoxification alone is rarely sufficient to help addicted individuals achieve long-term abstinence. Thus, clients should be encouraged to continue drug treatment following detoxification.

xi. **Treatment does not need to be voluntary to be effective.** Sanctions or enticements from family, employment settings, and/or the criminal justice system can significantly increase treatment entry, retention rates, and the ultimate success of drug treatment interventions.

xii. **Drug use during treatment must be monitored continuously, as lapses during treatment do occur.** Knowing their drug use is being monitored can be a powerful incentive for clients and can help them withstand urges to use drugs. Monitoring also provides an early indication of a return to drug use, signaling a possible need to adjust an individual's treatment plan to better meet his or her needs.

xiii. **Treatment programs should assess clients for the presence of HIV/AIDS, hepatitis B and C, tuberculosis, and other infectious diseases, as well as provide targeted risk-reduction counseling to help clients modify or change behaviors that place them at risk of contracting or spreading infectious diseases.** Targeted counseling specifically focused on reducing infectious disease risk can help clients further reduce or avoid substance-related and other high-risk behaviors. Treatment providers should encourage and support HIV screening and inform clients in whom highly active antiretroviral therapy (HAART) has proven effective in combating HIV, including among drug-abusing populations.

c. At each office visit, provide support to help prevent relapse. If relapse occurs, encourage the client to try again immediately.

d. Consider signing a contract with the client to stop smoking, drinking, or using drugs.

e. Verify abstinence by urine drug screen and pill counts at each visit.

f. Assess potential for suicide with every office visit.

g. If possible, obtain confirmation of the client's abstinence from a family member.

h. Stress the importance of 12-step meetings such as Alcoholics Anonymous (AA), Cocaine Anonymous (CA), and Narcotics Anonymous (NA).

i. Have the client sign a written release of information so that you can speak with a rehabilitation counselor. If the client is willing, refer to an alcohol and drug treatment facility or smoking-cessation program, after initial assessment and differential diagnosis is made.

j. Treat physical/laboratory findings as indicated.

k. Identify potential withdrawal symptoms from the cessation of stimulants, such as caffeine intake reduction, alcohol, and drug use.

l. If malnourished, discuss dietary needs and treatment.

B. Client teaching: *See Section III: Client Teaching Guide for this chapter, "Alcohol and Drug Dependence."*

1. Educate the client about the impact of alcohol, tobacco, and drugs on physical/emotional health. Provide information for the client to read at home.

2. Educate the client about safe disposal of medications:

a. Many communities have drug take-back programs; some pharmacies have mail-back programs and disposal kiosks for unused/expired medicines.

b. Almost all medicines, except those on the FDA flush list, can be thrown into household trash, including prescription and OTC drugs in pills, liquids, drops, patches, creams, and inhalers.

i. Mix medications with an unappealing substance such as dirt or kitty litter, place in a sealed container such as a zip-locking bag, and dispose in the household trash.

ii. Mark out or scratch out personal information on used prescription bottles before placing them in the household trash.

iii. The fentanyl adhesive patch, even after used, contains a lot of medication, therefore flushing the patch is recommended for disposal.

C. Pharmaceutical therapy:

1. The CDC Guideline for Prescribing Opioids for chronic pain recommends optimization of nonopioid pharmacotherapy and nonpharmacological therapy, rather than a trial of opioids. The principles of chronic pain treatment using nonopioid treatments is noted in Exhibit 2.1.

2. The CDC's Guideline for Prescribing Opioids for Chronic Pain was published March 2016 and is located at https://www.cdc.gov/mmwr/volumes/65/rr/rr6501e1.htm. The guideline provides 12 recommendations about the appropriate prescribing of prescription opioids and other treatment options to improve pain management and client safety. The guideline is not intended for clients who are in active cancer treatment, palliative care, or end-of-life care.

a. Nonpharmacologic therapy and nonopioid pharmacologic therapy are preferred for chronic pain. Clinicians should consider opioid therapy only if expected benefits for both pain and function are anticipated to outweigh risks to the client. If opioids are used, they should be combined with nonpharmacologic therapy and nonopioid pharmacologic therapy, as appropriate.

b. Before starting opioid therapy for chronic pain, clinicians should establish treatment goals with all clients, including realistic goals for pain and function, and should consider how opioid therapy will be discontinued if benefits do not outweigh risks. Clinicians should continue opioid therapy only if there is clinically meaningful improvement in pain and function that outweighs risks to client safety.

c. Before starting and periodically during opioid therapy, clinicians should discuss with clients known risks and realistic benefits of opioid therapy and client and clinician responsibilities for managing therapy.

d. When starting opioid therapy for chronic pain, clinicians should prescribe immediate-release opioids instead of ER/LA opioids (ER/LA opioids include methadone, transdermal fentanyl, and ER versions of opioids).

e. When opioids are started, clinicians should prescribe the lowest effective dosage. Clinicians should use caution when prescribing opioids at any dosage, should carefully reassess evidence of individual benefits and risks when considering increasing dosage to ≥50 morphine milligram equivalents (MME)/day, and should avoid increasing dosage to ≥90 MME/day or carefully justify a decision to titrate dosage to ≥90 MME/day.

f. Long-term opioid use often begins with treatment of acute pain. When opioids are used for acute pain, clinicians should prescribe the lowest effective dose of immediate-release opioids and should prescribe no greater quantity than needed for the expected duration of pain severe enough to require opioids. Three days or less will often be sufficient; more than 7 days will rarely be needed.

g. Clinicians should evaluate benefits and harms with clients within 1 to 4 weeks of starting opioid therapy for chronic pain or of dose escalation. Clinicians should evaluate benefits and harms of continued therapy with clients every 3 months or more frequently. If benefits do not outweigh harms of continued opioid therapy, clinicians should optimize other therapies and work with clients to taper opioids to lower dosages or to taper and discontinue opioids.

h. Before starting and periodically during continuation of opioid therapy, clinicians should evaluate risk factors for opioid-related harms. Clinicians should incorporate into the management plan strategies to mitigate risk, including considering offering naloxone when factors that increase risk for opioid overdose, such as history of overdose, history of SUD, higher opioid dosages (≥50 MME/day), or concurrent benzodiazepine use, are present.

i. Clinicians should review the client's history of controlled substance prescriptions using state prescription drug monitoring program (PDMP) data to determine whether the client is receiving opioid dosages or dangerous combinations that put him or her at high risk for overdose. Clinicians should review PDMP data when starting opioid therapy for chronic pain and periodically during opioid therapy for chronic pain, ranging from every prescription to every 3 months.

j. When prescribing opioids for chronic pain, clinicians should use urine drug testing before starting opioid therapy and consider urine drug testing at least annually to assess for prescribed medications as well as other controlled prescription drugs and illicit drugs.

k. Clinicians should avoid prescribing opioid pain medication and benzodiazepines concurrently whenever possible.

l. Clinicians should offer or arrange evidence-based treatment (usually medication-assisted treatment with buprenorphine or methadone in combination with behavioral therapies) for clients with opioid use disorder.

3. Opioid antagonist: Depending on the state, friends, family members, and others in the community may give naloxone to someone that has overdosed. Some states require a prescription; in other states, pharmacies may distribute naloxone in an outpatient setting without a prescription. There are three FDA-approved formulations of naloxone:

a. IV injectable: professional training required for administration

b. Autoinjectable Evzio: prefilled autoinject device that makes it easy for families or emergency

EXHIBIT 2.1 Nonopioid Therapy

NONOPIOID TREATMENTS FOR CHRONIC PAIN

PRINCIPLES OF CHRONIC PAIN TREATMENT

Patients with pain should receive treatment that provides the greatest benefit. Opioids are not the first-line therapy for chronic pain outside of active cancer treatment, palliative care, and end-of-life care. Evidence suggests that nonopioid treatments, including nonopioid medications and nonpharmacological therapies can provide relief to those suffering from chronic pain, and are safer. Effective approaches to chronic pain should:

Use nonopioid therapies to the extent possible

Identify and address co-existing mental health conditions (e.g., depression, anxiety, PTSD)

Focus on functional goals and improvement, engaging patients actively in their pain management

Use disease-specific treatments when available (e.g., triptans for migraines, gabapentin/pregabalin/duloxetine for neuropathic pain)

Use first-line medication options preferentially

Consider interventional therapies (e.g., corticosteroid injections) in patients who fail standard non-invasive therapies

Use multimodal approaches, including interdisciplinary rehabilitation for patients who have failed standard treatments, have severe functional deficits, or psychosocial risk factors

NONOPIOID MEDICATIONS

MEDICATION	MAGNITUDE OF BENEFITS	HARMS	COMMENTS
Acetaminophen	Small	Hepatotoxic, particularly at higher doses	First-line analgesic, probably less effective than NSAIDs
NSAIDs	Small-moderate	Cardiac, GI, renal	First-line analgesic, COX-2 selective NSAIDs less GI toxicity
Gabapentin/pregabalin	Small-moderate	Sedation, dizziness, ataxia	First-line agent for neuropathic pain; pregabalin approved for fibromyalgia
Tricyclic antidepressants and serotonin/norephinephrine reuptake inhibitors	Small-moderate	TCAs have anticholinergic and cardiac toxicities; SNRIs safer and better tolerated	First-line for neuropathic pain; TCAs and SNRIs for fibromyalgia, TCAs for headaches
Topical agents (lidocaine, capsaicin, NSAIDs)	Small-moderate	Capsaicin initial flare/burning, irritation of mucus membranes	Consider as alternative first-line, thought to be safer than systemic medications. Lidocaine for neuropathic pain, topical NSAIDs for localized osteoarthritis, topical capsaicin for musculoskeletal and neuropathic pain

U.S. Department of Health and Human Services
Centers for Disease
Control and Prevention

LEARN MORE | www.cdc.gov/drugoverdose/prescribing/guideline.html

CS263451   April 27, 2016

RECOMMENDED TREATMENTS FOR COMMON CHRONIC PAIN CONDITIONS

Low back pain

Self-care and education in all patients; advise patients to remain active and limit bedrest

Nonpharmacological treatments: Exercise, cognitive behavioral therapy, interdisciplinary rehabilitation

Medications

- First-line: acetaminophen, non-steroidal anti inflammatory drugs (NSAIDs)
- Second-line: Serotonin and norepinephrine reuptake inhibitors (SNRIs)/tricyclic antidepressants (TCAs)

Migraine

Preventive treatments

- Beta-blockers
- TCAs
- Antiseizure medications
- Calcium channel blockers
- Non-pharmacological treatments (Cognitive behavioral therapy, relaxation, biofeedback, exercise therapy)
- Avoid migraine triggers

Acute treatments

- Aspirin, acetaminophen, NSAIDs (may be combined with caffeine)
- Antinausea medication
- Triptans-migraine-specific

Neuropathic pain

Medications: TCAs, SNRIs, gabapentin/pregabalin, topical lidocaine

Osteoarthritis

Nonpharmacological treatments: Exercise, weight loss, patient education

Medications

- First-line: Acetamionphen, oral NSAIDs, topical NSAIDs
- Second-line: Intra-articular hyaluronic acid, capsaicin (limited number of intra-articular glucocorticoid injections if acetaminophen and NSAIDs insufficient)

Fibromyalgia

Patient education: Address diagnosis, treatment, and the patient's role in treatment

Nonpharmacological treatments: Low-impact aerobic exercise (e.g., brisk walking, swimming, water aerobics, or bicycling), cognitive behavioral therapy, biofeedback, interdisciplinary rehabilitation

Medications

- FDA-approved: Pregabalin, duloxetine, milnacipran
- Other options: TCAs, gabapentin

personnel to inject naloxone quickly into the outer thigh. Once activated, the device provides verbal instructions to the user describing how to deliver the medication, similar to automated defibrillators.

Caregivers and family members should practice administration technique using the trainer injector that is supplied with the product before naloxone is needed.

---

c. Narcan nasal spray: prefilled, needle-free device that requires no assembly and is sprayed into one nostril while the client lies on back

d. Dosing:

i. **Adults**

0.4 to 2 mg IV, IM, or subcutaneously, up to a total dose of 10 mg; doses may be repeated every 2 to 3 minutes, as needed. In emergency settings, clinical practice guidelines recommend 0.4 to 2 mg IV; alternatively, 0.4 to 0.8 mg may be given by IM or subcutaneous injection if systemic perfusion is adequate. Repeat doses as needed to attain desired response.

ii. **Children and adolescents 5 to 17 years or weighing more than 20 kg**

2 mg IV or IO is recommended for total reversal of narcotic effect (PALS recommendation); may require repeated doses to prevent recurrent apnea. The FDA-approved labeling recommends an initial dose of 0.01 mg/kg IV, IM, or subcutaneously; may repeat dose every 2 to 3 minutes until sufficient response.

iii. **Infants and children younger than 5 years or weighing 20 kg or less**

0.1 mg/kg/dose IV or IO is recommended for total reversal of narcotic effect (PALS recommendation); may require repeated doses to prevent recurrent apnea. The FDA-approved labeling recommends an initial dose of 0.01 mg/kg/dose IV, IM, or subcutaneously; may repeat dose every 2 to 3 minutes until sufficient response.

iv. **Neonates**

0.1 mg/kg/dose IV is recommended by clinical practice guidelines and may require repeated doses to prevent recurrent apnea. If IV access is not available, IM administration is acceptable. The FDA-approved labeling recommends 0.01 mg/kg/dose IV, IM, or subcutaneously every 2 to 3 minutes until the desired response is obtained.

v. **Intranasal dosage (Narcan nasal spray)**

NOTE: Restrict use of the 2 mg nasal spray to opioid-dependent clients expected to be at risk for severe opioid withdrawal in situations where there is a low risk for accidental or intentional opioid exposure by household contacts

1) **Adults, adolescents, children, infants, and neonates**

Spray, which delivers 2 mg or 4 mg of naloxone, by intranasal administration. Seek immediate medical attention after administration of the first dose. If additional doses are available, may repeat dose in alternate nostrils every 2 to 3 minutes as needed if the desired response is not attained or if the client relapses into respiratory depression. Each device contains a single dose. Family or caregiver should monitor the client closely until emergency medical personal arrive. Pediatric clients should continue to be monitored for at least 24 hours after administration.

4. Nicotine replacement:

a. Consider nicotine replacement for those who smoke more than one pack of cigarettes per day or who smoke their first cigarette within 30 minutes of waking. Stress that there is *no smoking* while using the nicotine patch.

b. Nicotine patch—Nicoderm (dosing based on more than 10 cigarettes/d habit):

i. 21 mg/qD for 6 weeks (14 mg qD × 6 weeks for <10 cigarettes/d) *then*

ii. 14 mg/qD for 2 weeks (7 mg qD × 6 weeks for <10 cigarettes/d) *then*

iii. 7 mg/qD for 2 weeks (only for more than 10 cigarettes/d habit)

c. Nicotine gum:

2 to 4 mg of nicotine gum per hour with maximum of 24 pieces/d for up to 12 weeks

d. Nicotine lozenges:

i. 2–4 mg every 1–2 hours for 6 weeks

ii. 2 mg every 2–4 hours for 3 weeks

iii. 2 mg every 4–8 hours for 3 weeks

5. Nonnicotine therapy: adults—bupropion (Zyban, Wellbutrin) 150 ER mg daily for 3 days, then increase to 150 mg ER twice daily. Treat for 7 to 12 weeks. The client may continue to smoke during the first 2 weeks of starting medication. This medication should not be given to clients with seizure disorders.

6. Varenicline (Chantix): start at 0.5 mg/d for the first 3 days, then for the next 4 days, 0.5 mg twice daily. After the first 7 days the dose is 1 mg twice daily × 11 weeks:

a. Encourage the client to choose a stop date for smoking and start the Chantix 1 to 2 weeks before this stop date.

b. Clients should be encouraged to quit even if they have relapses.

c. Instruct clients that the most common side effects of Chantix are insomnia, vivid or strange dreams, and nausea. Advise that side effects are usually transient.

d. Warn the client regarding potential side effects of mood swings, aggression, homicidal thoughts, psychosis, anxiety, and panic disorder, which may occur on rare occasions.

e. See package inserts or the *Physicians' Desk Reference* for detailed instructions.

7. Detoxification and methadone maintenance: should be performed by specially licensed and trained professionals

8. Disulfiram (Antabuse) therapy is not recommended. Clients who consume alcohol after taking Antabuse can become extremely ill.

9. Refer the client to a physician or specialist if the client is experiencing withdrawal; consider admission to rehabilitation center for detoxification and treatment.

Follow-Up

A. Make a follow-up appointment weekly. Make contact with the referral source (smoking cessation program, alcohol/drug rehabilitation program) before the next follow-up visit to check on the client's progress. At the weekly visit, question the client regarding compliance.

B. Order blood alcohol, urine drug screen, or nicotine level (as appropriate) with every office visit while in outpatient treatment and throughout the year following treatment.

C. Once positive change is seen, the client can be seen monthly. Discuss changes the client has made, past relapses, circumstances under which they occurred, and any special concerns.

D. Refer to the medical diagnosis for other applicable follow-up recommendations.

Consultation/Referral

A. Refer clients with drug and/or alcohol dependence to a community mental health center that has an outpatient alcohol/drug rehabilitation program or to a specialist in the community who deals frequently with substance abuse/dependence.

1. Substance Abuse and Mental Health Services Administration (SAMHSA): search for alcohol, drug, or mental health treatment facilities around the country, confidentially and anonymously located in your area.

2. National Helpline 1-800-662-HELP (4357) for treatment referral and information 24/7

3. Behavioral Health Treatment Locator https://findtreatment.samhsa.gov/

4. Medication-Assisted Treatment (MAT) for Substance Use Disorders, SAMHSA Opioid Treatment Program Directory: https://dpt2.samhsa.gov/treatment/

5. Buprenorphine Practitioners Locator: https://www.samhsa.gov/medication-assisted-treatment/practitioner-program-data/treatment-practitioner-locator

B. Planning a family intervention to confront the client is best done with the help of an experienced mental health professional.

C. Have referral numbers close at hand so that the client's moment of motivation is not lost.

Individual Considerations

A. Pregnancy:

1. Substance-dependent pregnant women frequently avoid early prenatal care for fear of identification and reprisal.

2. Cocaine use is associated with abruptio placenta and preterm labor. Consider drug screen for emergent admissions for clients in preterm labor and abruption.

3. Notify the hospital nursery personnel/neonatologist before delivery to closely monitor the newborn for neonatal abstinence syndrome.

4. Nicotine/smoking use is associated with intrauterine growth restriction, preterm delivery, and bleeding in pregnancy.

5. Nicotine-dependent pregnant women should be encouraged to stop smoking without pharmacological treatment. The nicotine patch should be used during pregnancy only if the increased likelihood of smoking cessation, with its potential benefits, outweighs the risk of nicotine replacement and potential concomitant smoking. Similar factors should be considered in lactating women.

6. Pregnant women who use alcohol, tobacco, or drugs should always be classified as substance dependent rather than substance abusive.

B. Pediatrics:

1. Infants of smokers have increased risk of sudden infant death syndrome (SIDS).

2. The diagnosis of substance dependence is more difficult to make in children younger than 18 years. If there is any indication of substance dependence, children should be referred to a pediatrician who deals specifically with this problem.

3. Consider drug use when alienation of friends and family, falling grades, and isolation occur

4. "Huffing" is common with gasoline, glues, aerosol sprays, and spray paints.

5. The use of synthetic cannabinoid products is on the rise in the adolescent population. K2, Spice, and bath salts and others are available in tobacco stores, gas stations, over the Internet, and in other small shops. These products can be very harmful. They are not detected on routine toxicology drug screens. Be aware of illicit drug use if clients present with change in behavior, depression, paranoid delusion, and aggressive behaviors. Educate the client and family regarding the toxic use of these OTC substances. Stress to the client that these are abusive substances that can potentially be fatal. Stress cessation of use and refer to specialist.

C. Adults:

1. Alcohol:

a. With women, tolerance can be established by asking the question, "How many drinks does it take to make you high?" More than two drinks indicates some tolerance.

b. In considering a diagnosis of alcohol dependence, consider the following diagnostic findings: hypertension; nonspecific EKG changes; cardiomyopathy; palpitations; increased mean cell volume; decreased red blood cell count; low platelet count; increased alanine aminotransferase (ALT), aspartate aminotransferase (AST), lactic dehydrogenase, gamma-glutamyl transpeptidase, alkaline phosphatase; type IV hyperlipoprotein-emia; gout; and adult-onset diabetes mellitus.

D. Geriatrics:

1. In this population, consumption of as little as 1 oz/d can indicate a problem.

2. Pain medications and benzodiazepines, along with multiple medications for health problems, may create a substance abuse problem.

E. Partners/family members:

1. For fear of retribution, the family may remain silent about the problem, even if accompanying the client to the healthcare visit.

2. Some studies by corporate business show that, per capita, business spends more money on the care of family members of substance-dependent clients than on the employee.

3. Refer family members of alcoholics/drug addicts to Al-Anon, Nar-Anon, Co-dependents Anonymous, or Adult Children of Alcoholics (ACOA) meetings.

4. Discuss availability and administration of Narcan.

Resources

Adult Children of Alcoholics: 562-595-7830; https://www.adultchildren.org

Al-Anon Family Group Headquarters, Inc. (Al-Anon and Alateen): 888-4AL-ANON (meeting information line); Spanish website: www.al-anon.alateen.org/inicio

Alcoholics Anonymous: 212-870-3400; www.aa.org

Cocaine Anonymous World Services (CAWSO): 800-347-8998; https://www.ca.org

Co-Dependents Anonymous (CoDA®): 888-444-2359; www.coda.org

Drug-Free Workplace: 1-800-WORKPLACE (967-5752)

Dual Recovery Anonymous (DRA) Central Service Office: 913-991-2703; www.draonline.org

Marijuana Anonymous World Services: 800-766-6779; www.marijuana-anonymous.org

National Association for Children of Alcoholics (NACoA): 888-554-COAS; https://www.nacoa.org

National Families in Action (NFIA): 404-248-9676; www.nationalfamilies.org

National Institute on Drug Abuse (NIDA): https://www.drugabuse.gov

NIDA for Teens: https://teens.drugabuse.gov

National Suicide Prevention Lifeline: 1-800-273-TALK (8255)

Nicotine Anonymous: 877-879-6422; www.nicotine-anonymous.org

Parents, Families and Friends of Lesbians and Gays (PFLAG): 202-467-8180; https://www.pflag.org

Substance Abuse and Mental Health Services Administration (SAMHSA): https://www. samhsa.gov

Veteran's Crisis Line: 1-800-273-TALK (8255)

Women for Sobriety, Inc.: 215-536-8026; https://www.womenforsobriety.org

Bibliography

Busse, J. (Ed.). (2017). *National pain center. The 2017 Canadian guideline for opioids for chronic non-cancer pain*. Retrieved from http://nationalpaincentre.mcmaster.ca/documents/Opioid%20GL%20for%20CMAJ_01may2017.pdf

Centers for Disease Control and Prevention. (n.d.). *Assessing benefits and harms of opioid therapy*. Retrieved from https://www.cdc.gov/drugoverdose/pdf/Assessing_Benefits_Harms_of_Opioid_Therapy-a.pdf

Centers for Disease Control and Prevention. (2016, April). *Nonopioid treatments for chronic pain, principles of chronic pain treatment*. Retrieved from https://www.cdc.gov/drugoverdose/pdf/nonopioid_treatments-a.pdf

Centers for Disease Control and Prevention, Office on Smoking and Health, National Center for Chronic Disease Prevention and Health Promotion. (2019, February 6). *Smoking & tobacco use, fast facts*. Retrieved from https://www.cdc.gov/tobacco/data_statistics/fact_sheets/fast_facts/index.htm

Dowell, D., Haegerich, T. M., & Chou, R. (2016). CDC guideline for prescribing opioids for chronic pain—United States, 2016. *MMWR Recommendations Reports, 65*(No. RR-1), 1–49. doi:10.15585/mmwr.rr6501e1

Ewing, J. A. (1984). Detecting alcoholism. The CAGE questionnaire. *Journal of the American Medical Association, 252*(14), 1905–1907. doi:10.1001/jama.1984.03350140051025

Hardy, S. (2013). Prevention and management of depression in primary care. *Nursing Standard (Royal College of Nursing (Great Britain): 1987), 27*(26), 51–56; quiz 58. doi:10.7748/ns2013.02.27.26.51.e7240. Retrieved from https://rcni.com/nursing-standard/evidence-and-practice/clinical

National Institute on Drug Abuse. (2018a, June). *Commonly abused drugs*. Retrieved from https://www.drugabuse.gov/drugs-abuse/commonly-abused-drugs-charts

National Institute on Drug Abuse. (2018b, June). *Commonly abused prescription drugs chart*. Retrieved from www.drugabuse.gov/drugs-abuse/commonly-abused-drugs-charts

National Institute on Drug Abuse. (2018c, April). Opioid overdose reversal with naloxone (Narcan, Evzio). Retrieved from https://www.drugabuse.gov/related-topics/opioid-overdose-reversal-naloxone-narcan-evzio

National Institute on Drug Abuse. (2018d, June). *Screening and assessment tools chart*. Retrieved from https://www.drugabuse.gov/nidamed-medical-health-professionals/screening-tools-resources/chart-screening-tools

National Institute on Drug Abuse. (2019, May). *Screening tools for adolescent substance use*. Retrieved from https://www.drugabuse.gov/nidamed-medical-health-professionals/screening-tools-resources/screening-tools-for-adolescent-substance-use

Novo Nordisk. (2018, October). *Highlights of prescribing information, Saxenda (liraglutide)*. Retrieved from https://www.novo-pi.com/saxenda.pdf

O'Malley, P. A. (2012). Baby boomers and substance abuse: The curse of youth again in old age: Implications for the clinical nurse specialist. *Clinical Nurse Specialist, 26*(6), 305–307. doi:10.1097/NUR.0b013e318272f7a6

PDR | Prescriber's Digital Reference. (2019). *Naloxone hydrochloride injection (0.4mg/mL) drug information*. Retrieved from https://www.pdr.net/drug-summary/Naloxone-Hydrochloride-Injection--0-4-mg-mL--naloxone-hydrochloride-777

Saha, S., Wilson Deanne, J., & Adger, R. J. (2012). K2, spice, and bath salts drugs of abuse commercially available. *Contemporary Pediatrics, 29*(10), 22–28. Retrieved from http://www.contemporarypediatrics.com/.

SAMHSA. (2014). *What is substance abuse treatment? A booklet for families. HHS publications No. (SMA) 14-4126*. Retrieved from https://store.samhsa.gov/system/files/sma14-4126.pdf

SAMHSA: Medley, G., Lipari, R. N., Bose, J., RTI International: Cribb, D. S., Kroutil, L. A., & McHenery, G., (2016, October). *Sexual orientation and estimates of adult substance use and mental health: Results from the 2015 national survey on drug use and health. National survey on drug use and health NSDUH data review*. Retrieved from https://www.samhsa.gov/data/sites/default/files/NSDUH-SexualOrientation-2015/NSDUH-SexualOrientation-2015/NSDUH-SexualOrientation-2015.htm

U.S. Department of Health and Human Services. (2016). *E-cigarette use among youth and young adults: A report of the surgeon general*. Retrieved from https://e-cigarettes.surgeongeneral.gov/documents/2016_SGR_Full_Report_non-508.pdf

U.S. Department of Health and Human Services. (2019, February). *Office of the surgeon general opioid overdose prevention.* Retrieved from https://www.hhs.gov/surgeongeneral/priorities/opioids-and-addiction/opioids-overdose-prevention/index.html

U.S. Food and Drug Administration. (2019, May 30). *Disposal of unused medicines: What you should know.* Retrieved from https://www.fda.gov/drugs/safe-disposal-medicines/disposal-unused-medicines-what-you-should-know#Medicines_recommended

Wendell, A. D. (2013). Overview and epidemiology of substance abuse in pregnancy. *Clinical Obstetrics and Gynecology, 56*(1), 91–96. doi:10.1097/GRF.0b013e31827feeb9

Violence: Children

Cheryl A. Glass, Moya Cook, and Robertson Nash

Definition

The definitions of *sexual abuse, childhood abuse,* and the age of children included in statistics changes with each state in the United States. Any family member, friend, or stranger can perpetrate abuse; however, fathers, mothers' boyfriends, female babysitters, and mothers are the most common perpetrators of abuse. Nonaccidental injury/abuse may result in serious physical or emotional harm and may result in failure to thrive (FTT), delayed developmental progress, or death.

A. Physical abuse: infliction of pain/harm producing injuries, including skeletal fractures, skin (i.e., burns), and CNS injuries (i.e., abusive head trauma [AHT] and shaken baby syndrome [SBS]/shaking-impact syndrome)

B. Sexual abuse: inappropriate exposure; fondling; sexual stimulation; coercion; oral, genital, buttock, breast contact; anal or vaginal penetration; foreign-body insertion; sharing obscene images and making use of child pornography photos or videos

C. Emotional abuse: rejection, lack of affection or stimulation, ignoring, dominating, intimidating, describing the child negatively, blaming the child, and verbal abuse (belittle, yell, threats of severe punishment) resulting in impaired psychological growth and development

D. Child neglect: isolation; starvation; lack of medical care; inadequate supervision; failure to provide love, affection, and emotional support; and failure to enroll/attend school

Incidence

A. Childhood abuse occurs worldwide; the exact incidence is not known. It occurs across all cultures and at all racial, socioeconomic, and educational levels.

B. Approximately 3.6 million referrals are made to child protective agencies (CPS), involving more than 6.6 million children (a referral can include multiple children), for child abuse and/or neglect reported annually.

C. Sexual abuse is underreported, underrecognized, and undertreated.

D. Approximately one in six boys is sexually abused before the age of 16 years.

E. More than 15 million children live with families in which partner violence occurs at least once a year. Seven million children live in families in which severe partner violence occurs. Witnessing domestic violence is associated with experiencing physical abuse and witnessing physical abuse of a sibling.

Pathogenesis

A. Society, lack of parenting skills, the home environment, substance abuse, and untreated mental illness are all factors that contribute to abuse.

Predisposing Factors

A. Children:
1. Minority children
2. Disabled or medically fragile children:
   a. Congenital anomalies
   b. Mental retardation
   c. Handicapped
   d. Chronic medical illness
   e. Hyperactive
   f. Adopted children/stepchildren
   g. Poor bonding
3. Age of children (physical abuse):
   a. Younger than 1 year
   b. Children younger than 3 years

B. Parental factors:
1. Young or single parents
2. Distant or absent extended family
3. Low educational level of parents
4. Parent's lack of understanding of children's needs, child development, and parenting skills
5. Nonbiological, transient caregivers in the home (e.g., mother's male partner)
6. Acute or chronic instability and stress in the family:
   a. Loss of employment
   b. Divorce/death
   c. Drug/alcohol abuse
   d. Parents with a history of abuse/neglect as a child (learned behavior)
   e. Presence of psychiatric illness
   f. Poverty
   g. Criminal history
   h. Parental thoughts and emotions that tend to support or justify maltreatment behaviors

C. Sexual abuse risk factors:
1. Male:
   a. Younger than 13 years
   b. Non-white
   c. Low socioeconomic status
   d. Not living with the biological father
   e. Disabled
2. Female:
   a. Young age between 7 and 14 years
   b. Absence of a parent
   c. Appearance of isolation, depression, or loneliness

Common Complaints

A. Oral/facial injuries:
1. Oropharyngeal sexually transmitted infections: sexual abuse
2. Black eyes
3. Nasal perforation/septal deviation
4. Skull fracture
5. Traumatic alopecia
6. Retinal hemorrhage
7. Hearing loss/tympanic injury

B. Burns (6%–20% of injuries):
1. Cigarette burns (pathognomonic for child abuse)
2. Scalding/immersion
3. Caustic exposure
4. Branding
5. Microwave burns
6. Stun-gun burns
C. Fractures (second most common injury)
D. Bruises (most common type of injury)
E. Lacerations
F. Bites
G. Force-feeding/"bottle jamming"/forced ingestion (water, salt, pepper, poisons)
H. Starvation
I. Sexual abuse:
1. Difficulty with bowel movements
2. Urinary tract infections
3. Vaginal infections, itching, or discharge
4. Complains of stomachaches
5. Headaches
6. Vaginal or rectal bleeding
7. Difficulty walking or sitting
J. Behavioral signs:
1. Loss of appetite/eating disorder
2. Clinging, withdrawn, or aggressive
3. Nightmares, disturbed sleep pattern, and fear of the dark
4. Regression (i.e., bedwetting, thumb sucking, crying)
5. Poor grades/school attendance
6. Expression of interest or affection inappropriate for the child's age
7. Intercourse or masturbation or other sexual acting out
8. Self-injurious behavior (i.e., cutting, biting, pulling out hair)

Other Signs and Symptoms

A. A caregiver's refusal to allow an interview of the child alone in the examination room is considered a "red flag" for abuse.
B. The history is inconsistent, changes with repeated questioning, conflicts with other family members/caregivers who are interviewed, is implausible, or there is a total lack of history (i.e., "I don't know how it happened").
C. History is inconsistent with the child's developmental ability/stage.
D. Caregiver behaviors that may indicate abuse include delay in seeking care, argumentativeness, lack of emotional response, inappropriateness, or violence.
E. Radiographs should be obtained for a history of "soft," easily broken bones.
F. The child exhibits inappropriate behavior for his or her developmental age.

Subjective Data

A. Use open-ended questions during the history to evaluate how injuries were sustained. As the interview continues, ask specific questions related to responses. If the child can talk, direct questions to him or her before the caregiver.
B. If this is the first clinic visit, ask whether the child had routine healthcare, including immunizations.

Physical Examination

The physical examination should be performed with the child totally unclothed; however, clothing can be removed as the physical progresses from head to toe (i.e., upper body, torso, lower body, lastly perineum/rectum). Detailed documentation of history is essential.
A. Check blood pressure, pulse, and respirations, height and weight to calculate BMI and plot on growth charts.
B. A forensic examination requires thorough documentation of injuries:
1. Use color photographs before any treatment is started.
2. Photograph damaged clothing.
3. Take at least one full-body photograph and a facial photograph.
4. Take close-up photographs of all injuries.
5. Use a ruler to identify/document the size of injuries.
6. Document on the back of the photographs the client's name, date, photographer's name, as well as any witnesses to the examination. The photographer should also sign each photograph.
C. General observation:
1. Observe the interactions between the caregiver and the child. Is the child fearful or reluctant to have the examination? Are there signs of discomfort during the examination with movement such as range of motion (ROM)?
2. Evaluate the child's overall appearance. Is the child clean and are his or her clothes appropriate for the season? Observe for poor hygiene, body odor, malnourishment, dehydration, depression, violence, withdrawnness, behavioral compliance even during a painful examination of the rectum/genitalia, and level of consciousness.
3. Dermal examination: evaluate from head to toe, including the palms, soles of the feet, and between toes; observe for injuries in different stages of healing and new trauma, including burns, lesions, swelling, bruises, and signs of pinching. Evaluate the corner of the mouth for signs of being gagged. Examine the head for alopecia from hair pulling. Evaluate bruises and burns for the characteristics of shapes (i.e., iron, handprints, long belt marks, loops, bite marks, ligature marks).
4. Eye examination: observe for retinal hemorrhages, black eyes, periorbital edema, and papilledema (indicates increased intracranial pressure).
5. Ear examination: evaluate hearing, hemotympanum or possible laceration to the external canal, and insertion of foreign objects.
6. Nasal examination: evaluate the presence of blood, swelling, and foreign objects.
7. Mouth and throat: evaluate the presence of caustic ingestion; observe for ligature marks and cry/voice quality.
D. Auscultate:
1. Heart
2. Lungs
3. Abdomen in all four quadrants

4. Over the globes of the eyes if warranted (bruit may indicate traumatic carotid cavernous fistula)

5. The carotid arteries bilaterally if warranted (bruit may indicate carotid dissection)

E. Palpate:

1. Examine for facial fractures; palpate for instability of the facial bones, including the zygomatic arch.

2. Palpate abdomen in all four quadrants for guarding, tenderness, and masses (hematoma).

3. Examine for any trauma to the spine.

F. Neurologic examination:

1. Assess mental status and memory: determine whether the client is awake, alert, cooperative, and oriented (to person, place, time, and situation). Temporary impairment of memory is one of the most common deficits after a head injury.

2. Assess cranial nerve function:

   a. Opthalmoscopic/visual examination (cranial nerve II)

   b. Pupillary response (cranial nerve III)

   c. Extraocular movements (cranial nerves III, IV, VI)

   d. Facial sensation and muscles of mastication (cranial nerve V)

   e. Facial expression and taste (cranial nerve VII)

3. Perform a motor examination on all four extremities.

4. Perform a sensory examination on all four extremities.

G. Genital/rectal examination:

1. Evaluate genitals/anal area for redness, swelling, bruising, hematomas, abrasions, or lacerations.

2. Evaluate for evidence of sperm.

3. Evaluate for presence of condyloma.

4. Evaluate for presence of foreign bodies.

Diagnostic Tests

Diagnostic tests and x-rays are ordered dependent on the type of presenting complaints and physical examination.

A. CBC with differential and peripheral smear; bleeding evaluation, including prothrombin time/partial thromboplastin time (PT/PTT), alanine aminotransferase (ALT), and aspartate aminotransferase (AST), to evaluate injury to the liver, serum amylase, or lipase to rule out pancreatic injury

B. Urinalysis

C. Drug screen/toxicology (urine and serum)

D. Obtain forensic DNA samples from the skin, under nails, vagina, rectum, and saliva from bite marks using sterile cotton-tipped applicators that have been moistened with sterile saline. These should be sent to a crime laboratory as soon as possible.

E. Test for sexually transmitted infections/HIV

F. Pregnancy test (age appropriate)

G. Radiographs for facial injury, anteroposterior (AP) and lateral radiograph for any areas of bone tenderness, swelling, deformity, or limited ROM

H. Neuroimaging CT/MRI for any suspected nonaccidental head injury (i.e., head trauma, history of shaking, and scalp hematoma)

Differential Diagnoses

A. Congenital syphilis

B. Rickets

C. Osteogenesis imperfecta (OI)

D. Mongolian spots

E. Impetigo

F. Dermatitis herpetiformis

G. Folk-healing practices

H. Immune thrombocytopenia (ITP)

I. Malignancy

J. Meningitis: neurologic signs

Plan

A. General interventions:

1. Each state may have a requirement for parental permission before taking any photographs.

B. Safety planning is the first priority.

C. Increase public awareness.

D. Failure to report a suspected case of sexual abuse may incur criminal charges.

Client Teaching

A. Reinforce that abuse/neglect is not the client's fault.

B. Help is available.

Pharmaceutical Therapy

A. Prescribe antibiotics to treat sexually transmitted infections or wounds.

B. Antidepressant therapy may be appropriate.

Follow-Up

A. Each state mandates reporting of child abuse. Refer to your state requirements or laws. CPS is responsible for inves-tigations. Depending on your locality, police involvement may be mandatory. The Child Abuse Prevention Services (CAPS) website lists individual state abuse hotlines at www.capsli.org/reporting-abuse/individual-state-hotlines.

B. Hospitalization may be required, depending on physical findings, child safety, and parental observation.

C. Abused and neglected children are at high risk of depression, anxiety, eating disorders, discipline problems, drug/alcohol use, runaway tendencies, and low self-esteem. Therapy and follow-up vary for each individual child. Family participation in a recommended treatment program is helpful. The goal of treatment is to help the child regain his or her prior state of mental and psychological health. Neglect is the major reason that children are removed from a home, especially when the parents have drug/alcohol problems.

Consultation/Referral

A. Consult with other healthcare providers who have greater experience with abuse (i.e., CPS, physician, psychiatrist or psychologist, social worker).

B. Refer for a nurse in-home assessment if available/indicated.

C. Specialty consultations:

1. Genetic consultation: OI

2. Orthopedic consultation

3. Plastic surgeon

4. Child psychiatrist
5. Ophthalmology

Resources

Childhelp Prevention and Treatment of Child Abuse: www.childhelp.org

Childhelp National Child Abuse Hotline: 1-800-422-4453

Rape, Abuse & Incest National Network (RAINN): 1-800-656-HOPE

Stop It Now: 1-888-PREVENT (1-888-773-8368)

Bibliography

American Society for the Positive Care of Children. (2018). *Physical child abuse*. Retrieved from https://americanspcc.org/physical-child-abuse/

Centers for Disease Control and Prevention. (2019, February 26). *Violence prevention, risk and protective factors*. Retrieved from https://www.cdc.gov/violenceprevention/childabuseandneglect/riskprotectivefactors.html

Childhelp. (n.d.). *Child abuse statistics & facts*. Retrieved from https://www.childhelp.org/child-abuse-statistics/

Futures Without Violence, Formerly Family Violence Prevention Fund. (n.d.). *The facts on children's exposure to intimate partner violence*. Retrieved from https://www.futureswithoutviolence.org/the-facts-on-childrens-exposure-to-intimate-partner-violence

Giardino, A. P. (2017, April 24). *Physical child abuse. Medscape*. Retrieved from http://emedicine.medscape.com/article/915664-overview

HelpGuide.org. (n.d.). *Child abuse and neglect: Recognizing, preventing, and reporting child abuse*. Retrieved from https://helpguide.org/articles/abuse/child-abuse-and-neglect.htm/

Prevent Child Abuse America. (2016a, February). *Fact sheet: Emotional child abuse*. Retrieved from www.preventchildabuse.org/images/docs/emotionalchildabuse.pdf.

Prevent Child Abuse America. (2016b, February). *Fact sheet: Maltreatment of children with disabilities*. Retrieved from http://www.preventchildabuse.org/images/docs/maltreatmentofchildrenwithdisabilities.pdf.

Prevent Child Abuse America. (2016c, February). *Recognizing child abuse: What parents should know*. Retrieved from www.preventchildabuse.org/images/docs/recognizingchildabuse-whatparentsshouldknow.pdf.

Rape, Abuse & Incest National Network. (n.d.[a]). *State resources*. Retrieved from https://www.rainn.org/state-resources

Rape, Abuse & Incest National Network. (n.d.[b]). *Victims of sexual violence: Statistics*. Retrieved from http://www.rainn.org

U.S. Department of Defense. (2019, April 30). *Sexual assault accountability and investigation task force*. Retrieved from https://media.defense.gov/2019/May/02/2002127159/-1/-1/1/SAAITF_REPORT.PDF

Violence: Intimate Partner

Definition

A. Intimate partner violence (IPV) is defined as intentional power and control or victimization of a person with whom the abuser has had or is currently in an intimate, romantic, or spousal relationship. Domestic IPV crosses all cultures and economic boundaries; it encompasses violence between both genders, including gay and lesbian relationships. Abusive behaviors can occur in a single event, sporadically, or continually. The Duluth Model Power and Control Wheel from the Domestic Abuse Intervention Project illustrates the abuser's power and control over the client (see Figure 2.5). The following is

FIGURE 2.5 The Duluth Model Power and Control Wheel from the domestic abuse intervention project.

Source: Reproduced with permission from Domestic Abuse Intervention Programs. Retrieved from https://www.theduluthmodel.org/wheel-gallery/

a list of the many forms through which IPV may manifest itself.

B. Physical abuse, sexual assault, coercion, social isolation, emotional abuse, economic control, and deprivation are associated with IPV. There is no typical abuser, although all abusers tend to be violent in the home setting and their behavior at work is normal.

C. Forms of physical violence include threatening or assaulting with weapons, pushing, shoving, slapping, punching, choking, kicking, holding, throwing objects, and binding.

D. Psychological abuse includes threats of physical harm to the client or others, humiliations, intimidation, degradation, ridicule, false accusation, isolation, and deprivation of food, economic coercion, access to healthcare, and transportation.

E. Psychological abuse in LGBT relationships includes the threat to "out" their partner as well as threats related to custody of coparent children.

F. Digital abuse is use of technologies and/or social media networking to intimidate, harass, or threaten. Intimate partner stalking can occur during a relationship or after the relationship ends.

1. Monitoring cell phone activity
2. Demanding passwords
3. Cyberbullying
4. Nonconsensual sexting
5. Posting photographs or other types of humiliation on social media
6. Threatening texts or stalking on social media

G. Sexual abuse is nonconsensual (unwanted kissing or touching) or painful sexual acts.

H. Reproductive coercion is another form of IPV.

1. Partner sabotage of safe-sex practices (i.e., refusal to use condoms, exposing the client to sexually transmitted infections)
2. Refusal/control of contraception
3. Forcing the woman to have an abortion, or utilizing physical violence to endanger a pregnancy
4. Controlling access to healthcare

Incidence

> The exact incidence of IPV is unknown because of the lack of reporting. The United Nations estimates that more than 603 million women live in countries where domestic violence is not considered a crime. The most significant reason for missing the diagnosis of IPV is failure to ask the client.

A. Domestic violence is the leading cause of homicide in women globally.

B. Up to 75% of domestic assaults occur after separation; women are most likely to be murdered when reporting abuse or attempting to leave an abusive relationship.

C. Stalking is often linked to both IPV and sexual assault. Examples of stalking includes the perpetrator approaching the client or showing up at places the client frequents; threatening physical harm; damaging personal property; making unwanted online contact (via email, instant message, or social media) or unwanted telephone calls; leaving

unwanted gifts or strange items; and sneaking into the client's car/home.

D. An estimated 4% to 15% of women presenting in emergency departments have situations related to domestic violence.

E. Women who separate have a risk of violence approximately three times that of divorced women.

1. More than half of the children who witness domestic violence intervene in some way, including yelling to the abuser to stop, calling for help, and trying to get away.

F. The incidence of abused men is estimated as one in three. Men are also clients of attempted or complete rape, at approximately 7% during their lifetime.

G. Pregnancy and the postpartum period have an increased incidence of violence.

1. One in five young women and 35% of women overall have experienced pregnancy coercion.
2. 53% of young women have experienced birth control sabotage.
3. It is estimated that 324,000 of intimate partner abuse occurs against pregnant women.
   a. The American College of Obstetricians and Gynecologists (ACOG) recommends screening for IPV at the first prenatal visit, at least once per trimester, and at the postpartum checkup.

H. Sexual violence, rape, physical assault, or stalking by an intimate partner occurs in 11% of lesbians and in 15% of men with male partners.

I. Among college women, 20% to 30% report violence during a date.

J. Physical, emotional, or verbal abuse is estimated in one in three adolescent girls from a dating partner in the United States.

1. The tween population (ages 11 to 14 years) reports that half of their friends have experienced dating violence.
2. The tween population reports that their friends are victims of verbal abuse.
3. Teen clients are more likely to smoke, use drugs, and have other risky behaviors.

K. Women and men in the military are recognized as a vulnerable population susceptible to abuse because of geographical location away from family and friends and the social isolation within the military culture.

1. Men are far more likely to consider sexual assault as hazing, bullying, physical abuse, or an act with the intent to humiliate rather than sexual harassment or sexual assault, thus contributing to the low reporting rate by men.
2. In 2018, the Department of Defense (DoD) estimated that in the U.S. military approximately 30% instances of unwanted sexual contact were reported.
3. Most sexual assault incidents in the military involve individuals who know each other. In reported cases, the parties often agree sexual activity took place but contest matters of consent.
4. Most criminal investigations conducted today involve the need to analyze computers, laptops, cell phones, Internet-connected home assistants, digital

data stored in vehicles, so on. Digital devices almost always contain relevant evidence (e.g., emails, texts, photographs, Internet search logs, geo-location data, social media uploads/downloads) particularly helpful in sexual assault case–associated crimes (e.g., stalking).

Pathogenesis

Intrapartner violence is not associated with an underlying medical condition. The cycle of abuse has three phases.

A. Tension building, in which the client tries to avoid violence and is described as "walking on eggs," unsure what will trigger an abusive incident

B. Explosion and acute battering occur

C. "Honeymoon phase," noted for the absence of tension and reconciliation

D. Clients stay with their partners for multiple reasons, including fear, shame, denial, religious reasons, lack of resources, custody issues and other legal issues, fear of being "outed," and family pressures.

Predisposing Factors

A. Gender: Clients are predominantly female.

B. Race: African Americans, American Indians, Hispanic women, and Alaskan Natives

C. Higher incidence in interracial couples

D. Pregnancy

E. History of violence:
   1. Violence present in family of origin
   2. Abuse as a child: 50% report abuse as an adult

F. History of drug use

G. Posttraumatic stress disorder (PTSD)

H. Lack of social support systems

I. Impulse control disorders

J. Poor economic status

K. LGBT

Common Complaints

A. Vague complaints

B. Sexual problems

C. Depression

D. Chronic pain inconsistent with organic disease

E. Chronic headaches/migraines

F. Stress:
   1. Anxiety
   2. Panic attacks

G. Alcohol or drug abuse (the batterer, client, or both)

H. Current or past self-mutilation

I. Gynecologic and obstetric complaints:
   1. Dyspareunia
   2. Frequent vaginal or urinary tract infections
   3. Pelvic pain/infection
   4. Recurrent sexually transmitted infections
   5. Unintended pregnancy
   6. Late prenatal care
   7. Miscarriage
   8. Preterm bleeding/delivery

J. Complaints of falls and other recurrent accidents

K. Eating disorders

L. Gastrointestinal complaints/irritable bowel syndrome

M. Musculoskeletal complaints

Other Signs and Symptoms

A. Multiple prior visits to the emergency department for traumatic and nontraumatic complaints

B. A delay between injury and office visits (may result from lack of transportation or the inability to leave the house)

C. Noncompliance with the treatment or missed appointments (lack of access to money or telephones)

D. Suicide attempt (25% higher in women with IPV)

E. A partner who accompanies the client at all visits

Subjective Data

The "gold standard" research method to document the prevalence of women's exposure to violence includes conducting the interview one on one, in private, and asking specific direct questions.

A. The batterer often refuses to leave the client alone and may answer questions for the client. Translators should not be a member of the client's or suspected abuser's family.

B. Use direct questions: Women-validated Partner Violence Screen (PVS):
   1. Have you been hit, punched, kicked, or otherwise hurt by someone in the past year? If yes, by whom and were you injured?
   2. Do you feel safe in your current relationship?
   3. Is a partner from a previous relationship making you feel unsafe now?
   4. Are you here today because of injuries from a partner?
   5. Are you here today because of illness or stress related to threats, violent behavior, or fears of a partner?

C. Assess whether the client has ever told family or friends, called hotlines, or attempted to leave the abuser.

D. Has the client sought help with law enforcement or legal help, that is, filed a criminal complaint or got an order of protection?

E. Are there any weapons in the home?
   1. Has the abuser ever threatened or tried to kill you?
   2. Are you thinking of suicide? Have you ever considered or attempted to commit suicide because of problems in your relationship?
   3. Have you ever considered or attempted killing your batterer?
   4. Do you have a plan?

Physical Examination

A. Enforce the need to interview and conduct physical examinations in private. Do a full-body examination, including the head/scalp:
   1. Most injuries are to the central (breast, chest, and abdomen) area, which is easily concealed by clothing.
   2. Other frequent sites of injury include the head, face, throat, and genitals.
   3. Explain the physical examination and touch with permission.
   4. Forensic examinations need thorough documentation of injuries:
      a. Take color photographs before any treatment is started.
      b. Photograph damaged clothing.

c. Take at least one full-body photograph and a facial photograph.

d. Take close-up photographs of all injuries.

e. Use a ruler to identify/document the size of injuries.

f. Document on the back of the photographs the client's name, date, and photographer's name, as well as any witnesses to the examination. The photographer should also sign each photograph.

g. Use direct quotes of the client's history of the violence.

B. Check blood pressure, pulse, and respirations.

C. General observation: observe for depression/withdrawnness or flat affect, anxiousness, fearfulness, evasiveness, poor eye contact, and wearing heavy makeup or clothing to conceal signs of abuse. Evaluate voice changes: dysphonia and aphonia. Observe for difficulty breathing

D. Inspect:

1. Dermal examination for the presence of cigarette burns, impression marks, rope burns, welts, abrasions, scratch marks, claw marks, bite marks, ligature marks, petechiae, and contusions at multiple sites (e.g., back, legs, buttocks).

2. Eye examination:

a. Observe subconjunctival hemorrhages from strangulation/struggle.

b. Perform a funduscopic examination (if indicated secondary to trauma).

3. Evaluate the genitals for lacerations and hematomas of the vagina or labia.

E. Auscultate:

1. All lung fields

2. The bowel sounds in all four quadrants of the abdomen

F. Palpate:

1. Evaluate skull/facial trauma to the maxillofacial area, eye orbits, mandible, and nasal bones. Facial injuries are reported in 94% of clients.

2. Evaluate for dislocations, fractures (including spiral fractures), sprains, and contusions to the wrists and forearms, and shoulders.

G. Percuss abdomen, chest, and areas of injury (if indicated secondary to trauma).

H. Perform a neurologic examination (if indicated secondary to trauma).

I. Genital/rectal examination:

1. Evaluate genitals/anus area for redness, swelling, bruising, hematomas, abrasions, or lacerations.

2. Perform bimanual examination (females).

3. Order an anoscopy (if indicated).

4. Evaluate for evidence of sperm (recto/vaginal).

5. Evaluate for the presence of condyloma (perineum, rectum, vagina).

6. Evaluate for the presence of foreign bodies (recto/vaginal).

Diagnostic Tests

Diagnostic tests and x-rays are ordered dependent on the type of presenting complaints and physical examination.

A. Administer a domestic abuse assessment screening tool and have the client mark a body map of injuries (see Exhibit 2.2).

B. CBC with differential and peripheral smear, bleeding evaluation, including PT/PTT, ALT, and AST, to evaluate injury to the liver, serum amylase, or lipase to rule out pancreatic injury

C. Urinalysis

D. Drug/toxicology screen (urine and blood)

E. Obtain forensic DNA samples from the skin, under nails, vagina, rectum, and saliva from bite marks using sterile cotton-tipped applicators that have been moistened with sterile saline. These should be sent to a crime laboratory as soon as possible.

F. Test for sexually transmitted infections/HIV.

G. Pregnancy test (if indicated)

H. Radiographs for facial injury, AP, and lateral radiograph for any areas of bone tenderness, swelling, deformity, or limited ROM

I. Ultrasounds as indicated

J. Neuroimaging CT/MRI may be used for any suspected nonaccidental head injury (i.e., head trauma, or scalp hematoma).

Differential Diagnoses

A. Rape

B. Other: related to presenting symptoms

Plan

A. Provide a safe environment. Assess for immediate danger.

B. Clearly document the history, physical findings, and interventions.

C. Determine the risk to the client and any children.

D. Evaluate the need for emergency department/hospital admission.

E. Battery is a crime; assess the client's readiness for police intervention and need for a court order of protection.

F. Help develop a safety plan:

1. Plan a safe place to go in advance, choose a place where the client will be able to alert authorities that her or his partner does not know about. Make up a code word to alert family and friends that the client in danger.

2. Ask the client to inform his or her school or place of work so that a safety plan can be implemented with their support.

3. Memorize important phone numbers in case the cell phone is taken away.

4. Keep an extra set of house and car keys in a safe, hidden place, or with someone that can be trusted.

5. Keep extra money available.

6. Encourage changing email addresses, cell phone number, and other contact information on social network sites.

G. Assess readiness to leave: Signs include collection of important papers (e.g., birth certificates, custody papers, divorce papers, and legal agreements, address book, copies of restraining orders), access to money/credit cards, and telling family and friends.

EXHIBIT 2.2 Abuse Assessment Screening Tool with Body Map

ABUSE ASSESSMENT SCREEN

1. Have you ever been emotionally or physically abused by your partner or someone important to you?
   Yes ☐   No ☐
   If yes, by whom? _____
   Total number of times _____

2. Within the last year, have you been hit, slapped, kicked, or otherwise physically hurt by someone?
   Yes ☐   No ☐
   If yes, by whom? _____
   Total number of times _____

3. Since you've been pregnant, have you been hit, slapped, kicked, or otherwise physically hurt by someone?
   Yes ☐   No ☐
   If yes, by whom? _____
   Total number of times _____

4. Within the last year, has anyone forced you to engage in sexual activity?
   Yes ☐   No ☐
   If yes, by whom? _____
   Total number of times _____

5. Are you afraid of your partner or anyone you listed previously?
   Yes ☐   No ☐

MARK THE AREA OF INJURY ON A BODY MAP AND SCORE EACH INCIDENT ACCORDING TO THE FOLLOWING SCALE

If any of the descriptions for the higher number apply, use the higher number.

1 = Threats of abuse, including use of a weapon
2 = Slapping, pushing; no injury and/or lasting pain
3 = Punching, kicking, bruises, cuts, and/or continuing pain
4 = Beating up, severe contusions, burns, broken bones
5 = Head injury, internal injury, permanent injury
6 = Use of weapon; wound from weapon

Source: Reprinted with permission from Parker, B., McFarlane, J., Soeken, K., Torres, S., & Campbell, D. (1993). Physical and emotional abuse in pregnancy: A comparison of adult and teenage women. *Nursing Research*, 42(3), 173–178. doi:10.1097/00006199-199305000-00009

H. Provide contact numbers for shelters. Have the client hide information in her shoes.
I. Counsel that violence may escalate.

Client Teaching
A. Reinforce that the violence is not the client's fault. IPV is very common and the clients do not deserve to be abused. Discuss the cycle of abuse.
B. Violence increases in frequency and severity.
C. Help is available.

Pharmaceutical Therapy
A. Prescriptions are related to physical injuries.
B. Treatment may be offered for sexually transmitted infections in the oral anal genital areas.
C. Tranquilizers may impair the client's ability to flee or defend herself/himself and should not be prescribed.

Follow-Up
A. Develop a follow-up plan:
   1. What type of help does the client want?
   2. Does the client have a plan for returning? Is the batterer home? Do they think it is safe?
   3. Does she have a place to stay with family or friends, or does she want to go to a shelter?
   4. Give the telephone numbers for shelters and crises hotlines.
B. Screen the client for abuse at all subsequent visits.
C. Mandatory reporting:
   1. States require reporting when domestic violence involves a child younger than 18 years and abuse or neglect of the child is suspected.
   2. Abuse of a disabled person must be reported to the Disabled Persons Protection Commission.

3. Reporting elder abuse may be mandatory in your state.

D. Your state may mandate reporting and intervention with law enforcement. Refer to the Domestic Violence, Sexual Assault, and Stalking Data Resource Center at www.jrsa.org/dvsa-drc/st-summary.shtml.

E. The 2013 National Protocol for Sexual Assault Medical Forensic Examination for Adults and Adolescents is available at https://ncjrs.gov/pdffiles1/ovw/241903.pdf.

Consultation/Referral

A. Facilitate referrals to a shelter, counseling, and legal services.

B. Contact a Sexual Assault Nurse Examiner (SANE)– qualified healthcare provider if indicated.

C. Refer to community or private support groups and agencies.

D. Refer for a consultation with a psychiatrist if the client is homicidal or suicidal.

E. Refer for a neurologic or neurosurgical consultation for intracranial injuries or focal neurologic findings.

F. Refer for an orthopedic consultation for fractures.

Individual Considerations

A. Pregnancy is a known period of increased risk of violence:

1. The genitals, breast, and abdomen are common sites targeted for trauma.

2. Women may present with a miscarriage or premature labor.

3. Blunt trauma is a common injury in pregnancy.

4. Perform universal screening at each trimester and postpartum as abuse often begins during pregnancy.

Resources

Dating Abuse Stops Here: www.datingabusestopshere.com

Domestic Violence, Sexual Assault and Stalking Data Resource Center: www.jrsa.org

Futures Without Violence (*Formerly Family Violence Prevention Fund*): www.futureswithoutviolence.org

National Domestic Violence Hotline: 1-800-799-7233

National TEEN Dating Abuse Helpline: 1-866-311-9474

Rape, Abuse & Incest National Network (RAINN) Hotline: 1-800-656-4673; www.domesticviolence.org

Bibliography

American College of Obstetricians and Gynecologists. (2019). *Domestic violence during pregnancy*. Retrieved from https://www.acog.org/ About-ACOG/ACOG-Departments/Violence-Against-Women/ Domestic-Violence-During-Pregnancy?IsMobileSet=false

American College of Obstetricians and Gynecologists. (2012, February). Intimate partner violence. *Committee Opinion, 518*, 1–5. Retrieved from https://www.acog.org/Clinical-Guidance-and-Publications/Committee -Opinions/Committee-on-Health-Care-for-Underserved-Women/ Intimate-Partner-Violence?IsMobileSet=false

Break the Cycle. (2014). *Learning about dating abuse*. Retrieved from http:// www.breakthecycle.org/learn-about-dating-abuse

Dating Abuse Stops Here. (n.d.). *Warning signs in depth*. Retrieved from www.datingabusestopshere.com/warning-signs/warning-signs-indepth

Dating Abuse Stops Here. (2019). *Create a safety plan*. Retrieved from www .datingabusestopshere.com/create-a-safety-plan/

Devries, K. M., Mak, J. Y. T., Garcia-Moreno, C., Petzold, M., Child, J. C., Falder, G., … Watts, C. H. (2013, June 30). *The global prevalence of intimate partner violence against women. Sciencexpress*. Retrieved from http://www.sciencemag.org/content/early/recent

Futures Without Violence, Formerly Family Violence Prevention Fund. (n.d.). *The facts on children's exposure to intimate partner violence*. Retrieved from https://www.futureswithoutviolence.org/the-facts-on-childrens -exposure-to-intimate-partner-violence

HelpGuide.org. (n.d.[a]). *Domestic violence and abuse: Signs of abuse and abusive relationships*. Retrieved from https://www.helpguide.org/articles/ abuse/getting-out-of-an-abusive-relationship.htm?pdf=12327

HelpGuide.org. (n.d.[b]). *Help for abused men: Escaping domestic violence by women or domestic partners*. Retrieved from https://www.helpguide.org/ articles/abuse/help-for-med-who-are-being-abused.htm

Office for Victims of Crime. (2018). *Stalking*. Retrieved from https://ovc .ncjrs.gov/ncvrw2018/info_flyers/fact_sheets/2018NCVRW_ Stalking_508_QC_v2.pdf

Parker, B., McFarlane, J., Soeken, K., Torres, S., & Campbell, D. (1993). Physical and emotional abuse in pregnancy: A comparison of adult and teenage women. *Nursing Research, 42*(3), 173–178. doi:10.1097/00006199- 199305000-00009

Rape, Abuse & Incest National Network. (n.d.[a]). *State resources*. Retrieved from https://www.rainn.org/state-resources

Rape, Abuse & Incest National Network. (n.d.[b]). *Victims of sexual violence: Statistics*. Retrieved from http://www.rainn.org

Ross, R., Roller, C., Rusk, T., Martsolf, D., & Draucker, C. (2009). The SATELLITE sexual violence assessment and care guide for perinatal clients. *Women's Health Care: A Practical Journal for Nurse Practitioners, 8*(11), 25–31. Retrieved from https://www.ncbi.nlm.nih.gov/pmc/articles/ PMC3324818/pdf/nihms316342.pdf.

United Nations Development Programme. (2013, November 25). *Violence against women is not acceptable and can be prevented*. Retrieved from https://www.undp.org/content/undp/en/home/presscenter/pressre -leases/2013/11/25/violence-against-women-is-not-acceptable-and-can -be-prevented.html

U.S. Army SHARP: Sexual Harassment/Assault Response & Prevention. (n.d.). *What we know about sexual assault of military men*. Retrieved from https://www.sexualassault.army.mil/whatweknow_militarymen .aspx

U.S. Department of Defense. (2019, April 30). *Sexual assault accountability and investigation task force*. Retrieved from https://media.defense .gov/2019/May/02/2002127159/-1/-1/1/SAAITF_REPORT.PDF

U.S. Department of Justice, Office on Violence Against Women. (2013). *A national protocol for sexual assault medical forensic examinations: Adults/ adolescents* (2nd ed.). Washington, DC: Author. Retrieved from https:// www.ncjrs.gov/pdffiles1/ovw/241903.pdf

World Health Organization. (2011). *Intimate partner violence during pregnancy*. Retrieved from https://apps.who.int/iris/bitstream/ 10665/70764/1/WHO_RHR_11.35_eng.pdf

Violence: Older Adults

Definition

Abuse in older individuals, defined as older than age 65, is associated with loss of functional capacity, depression, cognitive impairment, and increased morbidity and mortality. Perpetrators include partners and family members (of all ages), as well as strangers. There are several types of maltreatment in this population.

A. Physical abuse: willful unnecessary restraint, the infliction of physical pain, or injury

B. Sexual abuse: nonconsensual sexual contact

C. Psychological abuse: infliction of emotional harm, bullying, ridicule, verbal abuse, terrorizing, and threating to place in a long-term facility until the elder submits

D. Neglect: failing to provide for needs and protection of a vulnerable adult

E. Self-neglect (subset of neglect): malnutrition, dehydration, lack of personal hygiene, listlessness, hoarding

F. Abandonment: desertion

G. Financial exploitation: misappropriation of resources, utilities turned off for nonpayment, essential purchases including food or medicine not made, discrepancies in personal bookkeeping including unexplained credit card activities, recent change in property titles, deeds, and refinancing mortgages

H. Healthcare fraud and abuse: not providing care but charging for services, overmedicating or undermedicating

I. Confinement: restraining or isolating an older adult other than for medical reasons

Incidence

A. The U.S. Census Bureau's 2017 National Population Projections, based on the 2010 Census, estimates by 2030 all baby boomers will be older than age 65, meaning that one in every five residents will be in retirement age.

B. The incidence of elder abuse, neglect, exploitation, and self-neglect is approximately one in 10 Americans aged 60 years and older. The incidence is underreported because of the reluctance to report abuse, fear of implicating family members, and fear of being removed from the home.

C. Abuse is not uncommon in the institutional setting.

D. The highest rate of abuse is among elderly women older than age 80, with the abuser being the spouse or adult child. In the case of cognitive impairment, the client may not remember or recognize abuse.

Pathogenesis

Maltreatment of vulnerable adults occurs by people who have an ongoing relationship with the older person when there is an expectation of responsibility: sons/daughters, spouses/intimate partners, other family members such as grandchildren, and others, including paid and unpaid caregivers. There are several identifying psychopathologies in the abusers.

A. Physical frailty and mental impairment of the client play an indirect role. The client may have a decreased ability to defend or escape.

B. Caregiver stressors from caring for the elderly client, including the client's physical and verbal demands, contribute. Psychosocial factors of the caregiver, mental illness, and alcohol or drug abuse also contribute.

C. The child who was once abused may continue the cycle of violence transferred to the parent.

Predisposing Factors

A. Age: 65 years and older

B. Institutionalized

C. Cognitive impairment/diminished capacity

D. Decreased capacity for performing ADLs:
   1. Difficulty feeding self
   2. Difficulty bathing and dressing self
   3. Difficulty going to the toilet and performing personal hygiene

E. Decreased capacity performing instrumental activities of daily living (IADLs):
   1. Ability to prepare meals
   2. Ability to do household chores
   3. Ability to use the telephone
   4. Ability to manage personal finances

F. Females have a higher incidence of physical/sexual abuse.

G. Male gender is associated with self-neglect associated with impaired ADLs and IADLs.

H. Family stressors involving the caretaker

Common Complaints

A. Depression

B. Falls

C. History of hip fracture

D. Pressure ulcers

E. Bruises, lacerations, and burns

Other Signs and Symptoms

A. Indications of healing spiral fractures on x-ray

B. Poor nutrition: lack of resources/transportation to obtain food; caregiver not providing adequate nutrition/withholding food

C. Multiple hospitalizations

D. Recurrent urinary tract infections

E. Noncompliance: may not be able to pay for medications; medications may be withheld, or even given in excess by the caregiver

F. Complaints of sexual abuse:
   1. Pain or soreness in the genital area
   2. Bruises or lacerations on the perineum/rectum
   3. Vaginal or rectal bleeding

G. Traumatic tooth and/or hair loss

H. Sedation from overmedicating

I. Changes in personality

Subjective Data

A. The caregiver often refuses to leave the client alone and may answer questions for the client.

B. The caregiver has a different explanation of the injury.

C. Ask the client directly about abuse, neglect, or exploitation:
   1. Has anyone at home threatened or ever hurt you?
   2. Are you afraid of anyone at home?
   3. Are you left alone for long periods of time?
   4. Who cooks your meals? How often and what amounts of food do you eat?
   5. Who handles your financial business? Have you signed any documents that you did not understand?

D. Assess the client's living arrangements. Has the client ever told family or friends of his or her concerns, called hotlines, or attempted to leave the caregiver?

Physical Examination

A. Assessment:
   1. Observation: If abuse is suspected, enforce the need to do the physical examination in private. Do a full-body examination.
      a. Forensic examinations need thorough documentation of injuries.
         i. Take color photographs before any treatment is started
         ii. Take at least one full-body photograph and a facial photograph.

iii. Take close-up photographs of all injuries.

iv. Use a ruler to identify/document the size of the injuries.

v. Document the back of the photographs the client's name, date, and photographer's name, as well as any witness to the examination. The photographer should also sign each photograph.

vi. Use direct quotes of the client's history.

2. Check blood pressure, pulse, respirations, height and weight to calculate BMI.

3. General observation: observe for depression, withdrawal demeanor, flat affect, fearfulness, poor eye contact, inappropriate dress, and signs of malnutrition.

4. Observe for poor hygiene, presence of urine and feces, matted or lice-infected hair, odors, dirty nails and skin, and soiled clothing.

5. Assess cognitive abilities, depression, and functional ability of ADLs and IADLs

B. Inspect:

1. Dermal examination for signs of burns, tears, lacerations, impression marks, and bruises in different stages of healing. Frequent areas of the body involved are the neck, arms, and/or legs. Evaluate for the presence of decubitus/pressure ulcers. Signs of dehydration include dry fragile skin, dry sore mouth, and mental confusion.

2. Oral examination for poor oral hygiene, absence of dentures, and dry mucous membranes.

3. Evaluate breasts and genitals for lacerations and hematomas of the vagina or labia.

C. Auscultate:

1. All lung fields

2. Bowel sounds in all four quadrants of the abdomen

D. Palpate: evaluate for dislocation, fractures, sprains, and contusions to the wrists, forearms, and shoulders.

E. Percuss abdomen and chest (if indicated).

F. Genital/rectal examination:

1. Evaluate genitals/anus for redness, swelling, bruising, hematomas, abrasions, or lacerations.

2. Evaluate for evidence of sperm.

3. Evaluate for the presence of foreign bodies.

Diagnostic Tests

A. Diagnostic tests and x-rays are ordered dependent on the type of presenting complaints.

B. Obtain a CT for evaluation of injuries to the head and assault to the face, neck, or head. A CT or Doppler ultrasound may be ordered for abdominal injuries.

C. Order laboratory testing to evaluate dehydration, malnutrition, electrolyte imbalance, and medication/substance abuse:

1. CBC

2. Chemistry-7

3. Urinalysis

4. Calcium, magnesium, and phosphorus

5. Drug/alcohol screen

6. Serum levels for relevant medications

D. Obtain DNA samples if sexual abuse is present.

Differential Diagnoses

A. Depression

B. Abdominal trauma

C. Sexual assault

D. Gait disturbance/fall

E. Pathologic fracture

F. Epidural/subdural hematoma

Plan

A. Provide a safe environment.

B. Clearly document the history, physical findings, and interventions.

C. Determine the perpetrator(s).

D. Evaluate the need for emergency department/hospital admission.

Client Teaching

A. Reinforce that abuse/neglect is not the client's fault. Elder abuse is very common.

B. Help is available.

Pharmaceutical Therapy

A. Ensure prescriptions are related to physical injuries.

B. Recommend treatment for sexually transmitted infections in the oral anal genital areas.

Follow-Up

The Department of Health and Human Services National Center on Elder Abuse Administration on Aging maintains a State-by-State Resource site that includes directories, helplines, hotlines, referral sources, state government agencies and laws, and regulations related to elder abuse; it is located at ncea.acl.gov/Resources/State.aspx.

A. Develop a follow-up plan. All states have legislation protecting against abuse, neglect, and exploitation of the older population.

B. Know whether your state has mandatory requirements to report any suspicion of elder mistreatment.

C. Abuse of a disabled person must be reported to the Disabled Person Protection Commission.

D. Know whether your state has additional regulations related to self-neglect. Contact adult protective services or law enforcement agencies.

E. At the present time, there is no recommendation for universal screening of all older adult clients except in nursing facilities.

Consultation/Referral

A. Schedule a social work consultation to coordinate an in-home geriatric assessment visit.

B. Facilitate referrals to a shelter, counseling, and legal services.

C. Contact a SANE-qualified healthcare provider if indicated.

D. Refer to the community Area Agency on Aging for assistance.

E. Refer for a psychiatric consultation if indicated.

F. Refer for a neurologic or neurosurgical consultation for intracranial injuries or focal neurologic findings.

G. Refer for an orthopedic consultation for fractures.

Resources

The AARP: www.aarp.org

Clearinghouse on Abuse and Neglect of the Elderly (CANE): www.elderabusecenter.org

Help hotline for suspected elder abuse, neglect, or exploitation: 1-800-677-1116

National Adult Protective Services Association (NAPSA): www.napsa-now.org

National Center on Elder Abuse Administration on Aging (NCEA): www.ncea.acl.gov

Bibliography

HelpGuide.org. (n.d.). *Elder abuse and neglect: Warning signs, risk factors, prevention, help*. Retrieved from https://www.helpguide.org/articles/abuse/elder-abuse-and-neglect.htm

National Center on Elder Abuse. (n.d.). *State resources*. Retrieved from https://ncea.acl.gov/Resources/State.aspx

National Council on Aging. (n.d.). *Elder abuse facts*. Retrieved from https://www.ncoa.org/public-policy-action/elder-justice/elder-abuse-facts/

3 Pain Management Guidelines

Moya Cook and Kala Christopherson

Definition
A. The American Academy of Pain Medicine defined *acute pain* as the "physiologic response and experience to noxious stimuli that can become pathologic, is normally sudden in onset, time limited, and motivates behaviors to avoid actual or potential tissue injuries." Acute pain can last up to 7 days but, depending on its etiology, may last up to 30 days, which can assist in differentiating acute pain from subacute and chronic pain. Pain can be categorized as somatic (involving skin, muscles, or joints), visceral, or neuropathic (involving the nervous system).

Incidence
A. Acute pain is the most common reason for self-medication and presentation for treatment in the healthcare system. Acute pain is very individual, and if not treated properly it can have devastating physiological and psychological effects. Because pain is very subjective, the client care plan needs to be individualized to meet the client's needs. Proper management of acute pain could prevent the transition to chronic pain.

Pathogenesis
A. Acute pain is usually the result of stimulation of the sympathetic nervous system. Noxious stimuli activate the nociceptors (pain-producing sensors) to the thalamus and into the somatosensory cortex. Serotonin, norepinephrine, and neuropeptides are neurotransmitters utilized in pain transmission.

Predisposing Factors
A. Recent trauma/injury
B. Recent surgery
C. Stress
D. Illness
E. Compromised immune system
F. Chronic conditions that affect immune system (diabetes, etc.)
G. Age (children/elderly)

Common Complaints
A. Pain at a specific site
B. Increased heart rate
C. Increased respiratory rate
D. Elevated blood pressure (BP)
E. Sweating
F. Nausea

Other Signs and Symptoms
A. Urinary retention
B. Dilated pupils
C. Pallor

Subjective Data
A. Onset: Determine cause or mechanism of injury or etiology of pain.
B. Location/distribution/radiation of pain
C. Duration and pattern/timing
D. Characteristic of pain—quality
E. Precipitating/aggravating factors
F. Alleviating factors
G. Severity by utilizing a pain scale (0–10, with 0 indicating no pain and 10 being the worst pain imaginable) and by noting the effects of pain on activities of daily living (ADLs)
H. Associated symptoms related to pain

> Adaptations need to be made when assessing special populations who are not able to express pain adequately. These include the very young, cognitively impaired, and potentially the elderly. There are other scales and tools available to evaluate pain in these populations.

Physical Examination
In client presenting with acute pain, the physical examination is based on the location and etiology of pain. A general guide can be altered based on the type/location/cause of pain.
A. Check temperature, pulse, respiration, and BP.
B. Inspect:
   1. Observe overall appearance.
   2. Note affect and ability to express self and pain.

3. Note facial grimaces with movement.
4. Note gait, stance, and movements.
5. Inspect area at pain site.
C. Auscultate:
1. Auscultate heart and lungs.
2. Auscultate neck and abdomen.
D. Palpate:
1. Palpate affected area of pain.
E. Percuss (if applicable):
1. Percuss chest.
2. Percuss abdomen.
F. Perform abdominal examination (if applicable).
G. Perform musculoskeletal examination.

> When performing a musculoskeletal examination, identify the location of pain, presence of trigger points, evidence of injury or trauma, edema, erythema, warmth, lesions, petechiae, tenderness, decreased range of motion, pain with movement, crepitus, laxity of ligaments or cords, spasms, or guarding.

1. Perform a complete musculoskeletal examination, concentrating on the area of pain.
2. Assess deep tendon reflexes (DTRs).
H. Neurologic examination:
1. Perform a complete neurologic examination.
2. Identify changes in gait, sensory function, skin tenderness, weakness, muscle atrophy, and/or loss of DTRs.

Diagnostic Tests

A. No diagnostic testing is required unless clearly indicated to rule out organic cause of pain. If organic disease is suspected, diagnostic testing may include:
1. CT imaging
2. MRI
3. Blood chemistries
4. Radiographic x-ray
5. Lumbar puncture
6. Ultrasound
7. EKG/echocardiogram

Differential Diagnoses

The common differential diagnoses are organized by location of the acute pain.
A. Head:
1. Migraine
2. Cluster headache/migraine headache
3. Temporal arteritis
4. Intracranial bleeding or stroke
5. Sinusitis
6. Dental abscess
B. Neck:
1. Meningitis
2. Muscle strain/sprain
3. Whiplash injury
4. Thyroiditis
C. Chest:
1. Pulmonary emboli
2. Myocardial infarction
3. Pneumonia

4. Costochondritis
5. Angina
6. Gastroesophageal reflux disease/esophagitis
D. Abdomen:
1. Peritonitis
2. Appendicitis
3. Ectopic pregnancy/uterine pregnancy
4. Endometriosis
5. Pelvic inflammatory disease
6. Peptic ulcer
7. Cholelithiasis
8. Colitis/diverticulitis
9. Constipation
10. Gastroenteritis
11. Irritable bowel syndrome
12. Urinary tract infection, kidney stone, pyelonephritis
13. Prostatitis
14. Malignancies
E. Musculoskeletal:
1. Muscle sprain/strain/tear
2. Skeletal fracture
3. Viral infection
4. Gout
5. Vitamin D deficiency

Plan

A. General interventions:
1. Acute pain is a symptom, not a diagnosis.
2. Analgesic treatment should be provided as soon as possible and not be delayed by diagnostics.
3. Identify the cause or source of the acute pain depending on the location. If the pain is organic in nature, make the appropriate referral.
4. The overall goal is to treat the acute pain appropriately.
B. Client teaching:
1. The pain management plan must include client and family education regarding preventing and controlling pain, potential medication side effects, and how to prevent side effects.
2. Nonsteroidal anti-inflammatory drugs (NSAIDs) are often equally or more effective in pain management of some acute pain etiologies.
3. The newest (2016) recommendation from the Centers for Disease Control and Prevention (CDC) is the lowest possible dose of narcotics for pain for no longer than 3 to 5 days before reevaluation.
4. Opioid addiction education should be discussed. Explain that risk of addiction is low when medication is used as directed for a short duration. Explain that complete pain relief may not be achievable initially, but the overall goal is to decrease the pain, thus allowing some daily activities at home to begin recovery.
C. Pharmaceutical therapy:
1. *Visceral pain*: Treatment of choice is corticosteroids, intraspinal local anesthetics, NSAIDs, and opioids. Extended- or sustained-release opioids should not be prescribed for acute pain.

2. *Somatic pain*: Acetaminophen, cold packs, corticosteroids, localized anesthetics, NSAIDs, aspirin, and opioids. Extended- or sustained-release opioids should not be prescribed for acute pain.

3. *Neuropathic pain*: Tricyclic antidepressants (TCAs), using amitriptyline, are the first-line treatment for neuropathic pain. Anticonvulsants like carbamazepine (Tegretol), phenytoin (Dilantin), and valproic acid (Depakene) can be useful in treating neuropathic pain. Gabapentin is also prescribed and is the first oral treatment approved by the Food and Drug Administration (FDA) for postherpetic neuralgia. Other treatments include local anesthetics, tramadol (Ultram), and glucocorticoids.

D. Nonpharmaceutical treatment

Nonpharmacological treatment can be used in conjunction with analgesics during acute pain. Treatment should be chosen based on etiology and severity.

1. Application of heat or ice
2. Immobilization or exercise, which can include physical therapy treatment
3. Massage, compression, spinal manipulation, tactile stimulation, transcutaneous electrical nerve stimulation (TENS), or acupuncture

> Know each medication's mechanism of action, potential adverse side effects, half-life, and drug–drug interaction potential. Always document that you have advised on the potential for sedation, suggested no driving/machinery use, and indicated no alcohol should be consumed while taking medication with these potential adverse side effects. The FDA advises extreme caution when using nonsteroidal anti-inflammatory drugs (NSAIDs) with clients with cardiovascular disease due to the increased risk of heart attack and stroke.

Follow-Up
A. Once an organic cause of pain has been ruled out, initial follow-up is 48 to 72 hours after onset.
B. Ensure that the client has consistent access to care.

Consultation/Referral
If the acute pain is organic, make the appropriate referral to a specialist.

Individual Considerations
A. Geriatrics:
1. Physiologic changes that occur in the elderly, such as decreased body mass, hepatic dysfunction, and renal dysfunction may cause increased serum drug concentrations of pain medication. Use caution when prescribing pain medication to this population.
2. Anti-inflammatories are not recommended for the elderly as a general rule due to the effects of the medication on the kidneys and cardiovascular system.

Bibliography
American Society for Pain Management Nursing. (2010). *Optimizing the treatment of pain in patients with acute presentations*. Retrieved from http://aspmn.org/Documents/OptimizingPositionPaper.pdf

Centers for Disease Control and Prevention. (2016a, March 15). CDC guidelines for prescribing opioids for chronic pain—United States, 2016. *Morbidity and Mortality Weekly Reports*. Retrieved from https://www.cdc.gov/mmwr/volumes/65/rr/rr6501e1.htm

Centers for Disease Control and Prevention. (2016b, March 22). Checklist for prescribing opioids for chronic pain. Retrieved from https://www.cdc.gov/drugoverdose/pdf/PDO_Checklist-a.pdf

Kasper, D., Fauci, A., Hauser, S., Longo, D., Jameson, J., & Loscalzo, J. (2016). *Harrison's manual of medicine* (19th ed.). New York, NY: McGraw-Hill Education.

Kent, M. L., Tighe, P. J, Belfer, I., Brennan, T., Bruehl, S., Brummett, C., … Terman, G. (2017). The ACTION-APS-AAPM Pain Taxonomy (AAAPT) multidimensional approach to classifying acute pain conditions. *Journal of Pain*, 18(5), 479–489. doi:10.1016/j.jpain.2017.02.421

Mundkur, M., Franklin, J., Adbia, Y., Huybrechts, K., Patorno, E., Gagne, J., … Bateman, B (2019, February 15). Days' Supply of Initial Opioid Analgesic Prescriptions and Additional Fills for Acute Pain Conditions Treated in the Primary Care Setting - United States, 2014. *Morbidity and Mortality Weekly Report*, 68(6), 140–143. Retrieved from https://www.cdc.gov/mmwr/volumes/68/wr/mm6806a3.htm

National Pharmaceutical Council. (n.d.). Pain: Current understanding of assessment, management, and treatments. American Pain Society. Retrieved from http://americanpainsociety.org/uploads/education/section_4.pdf

Sridhar, S. B., Shariff, A., Dallah, L., Anas, D., Ayman, M., & Rao, P. G. (2018). Assessment of nature, reasons, and consequences of self-medication practice among general population of Ras Al-Khaimah, UAE. *International Journal of Applied & Basic Medical Research*, 8(1), 3–8. Retrieved from https://www.ncbi.nlm.nih.gov/pubmed/29552527

Tighe, P., Buckenmaier, C. C. 3rd, Boezaart, A. P., Carr, D. B., Clark, L. L., Herring, A. A., … Reisfield, G. (2015). Acute pain medicine in the United States: A status report. *Pain Medicine [APM Shared Interest Group of the American Academy of Pain Medicine]*, 16(9), 1806–1826. doi:10.1111/pme.12760

Chronic Pain

Kathleen Siders and Moya Cook

Definition
A. The International Association for the Study of Pain defined *general pain* as an "unpleasant sensory and emotional experience associated with actual or potential tissue damage or described in terms of such damage."
B. Many definitions of *chronic pain* exist, but the general consensus describes chronic pain as lasting 3 months or longer than the normal tissue healing time. Chronic pain may be continuous or recurrent and of sufficient duration and intensity to interfere with a person's ability to function with normal daily activities as well as decrease a person's quality of life.
C. The CDC distinguishes *high-impact chronic pain* as that which "frequently limits life or work activities."

Incidence
Pain syndromes are commonly seen in clinical practice. Chronic pain costs the American people about $635 billion yearly in healthcare expenses, disability costs, and lost productivity. The CDC estimates 20.4% of U.S. adults (50.0 million) experience chronic pain and 8.0% of U.S adults (19.6 million) experience high-impact chronic pain. The prevalence increases with advancing age. As the U.S. population continues to age, primary care providers will care for increasing numbers of clients with chronic diseases including chronic pain. Pain prevalence is higher in women than in men. Onset can begin at any age but

usually occurs in the fourth, fifth, or sixth decades and is often associated with marked functional disability.

Pathogenesis

A. *Skeletal muscle pain* occurs in the soft tissue involving the neck, shoulders, trunk, arms, low back, hips, and lower extremities. *Myofascial pain syndrome* relates to the fascia surrounding the muscle tissue.

B. *Inflammatory pain* arises from complex relationships between the immune system and injured tissue leading to the stimulation of the pain receptors (nociceptors). Multiple chemical mediators are involved in the expression of pain. Examples include arthritis, infection, tissue injury, skeletal muscle pain, and postoperative pain.

C. *Neuropathic pain* is caused by a lesion or disease of the central or peripheral somatosensory system. The most common types include diabetic neuropathy, sciatica from nerve root compression, trigeminal neuralgia, and postherpetic neuralgia.

D. The *nociceptive system* involves neurons that detect noxious stimuli, including mechanical, thermal, and chemical. Nociceptors are found in all tissues except the central nervous system and generally produce pain sensation proportionate to the injury. Somatic pain is generally described as dull and aching, whereas visceral pain additionally is described as pressure-like and vague. They both respond well to opioids, with the exception of arthritis.

Predisposing Factors

A. Younger adults
B. Female gender
C. History of seeking multiple healthcare providers for the purpose of obtaining multiple prescriptions for pain management
D. Occupational exposures
E. Depression; lack of social support
F. Behavior health disorders, including moods, fears, expectations, and dysfunctional coping efforts
G. History of childhood trauma
H. Pre- and post-surgery
I. Job dissatisfaction, low work status
J. Effects of a developing chronic disease

Common Complaints

A. Specific to site of pain
B. Emotional distress related to fear, maladaptive or inadequate support systems, and other coping resources
C. Treatment-induced complications
D. Overuse of drugs
E. Inability to work
F. Financial complications
G. Disruption of usual activities
H. Sleep disturbances
I. Pain becomes primary life focus.

Other Signs and Symptoms

A. Pain lasts longer than 6 months.
B. There may be anger and loss of faith or trust in the healthcare system. This type of client frequently takes too many medications, spends a great deal of time in bed, sees many physicians, and experiences little joy in either work or play.

Subjective Data

A. Elicit a clear description of the onset, location, quality, intensity, and time course of pain, and any factors that aggravate or relieve it.
   1. Use the acronym OLD CARTS-U: O = onset, L = location, D = duration, C = characteristics, A = aggravating triggers, R = relieving triggers, T = timing, S = severity, U = YOU. What do YOU think is going on? What have YOU done to relieve it?
   2. Or use the acronym PQRST: P = provokes, palliate; Q = quality, quantity; R = radiation; S = severity; T = timing, temporal.
   3. For clients on opioid analgesics, ask:
      a. Analgesia: Effectiveness of medications
      b. Activity: Can they do more?
      c. Adverse reactions: Constipation and other side effects
      d. Aberrant behaviors: Other drug use including ethyl alcohol (ETOH), self-escalating doses
      e. Affect: Changes in mood?

B. *Self-reporting pain assessment tools* should be used early in the process of client evaluation. Use the tool at each office visit to see progression or regression. Lack of pain assessment is a barrier to good pain control. Consider the age of the client; his or her physical, emotional, and cognitive status; and preference when choosing the self-reporting pain assessment tool.
   1. Numeric rating scales (NRS) rate pain intensity from 0 to 10. They are client friendly and quick to complete.
   2. Verbal rating scales rate pain as mild (1–3 NRS), moderate (4–6 NRS), or severe (7–10 NRS).
   3. The Faces scale is useful for pediatric and cognitively impaired clients. Multicultural translations may be downloaded at www.wongbakerfaces.org.

C. Determine the extent to which the client is suffering, disabled, and unable to enjoy usual activity. It is important to inquire about ADLs and functional limitations.

D. Obtain a complete review of systems, including nausea, numbness, weakness, insomnia, loss of appetite, dysphoria, malaise, fatigue, or depression signs and symptoms.

E. Obtain a complete family and social history. Address spiritual and cultural issues. History of chemical dependency is of interest in this client population.

F. Inquire about childhood trauma or abuse, including sexual abuse.

G. Obtain the client's medical history relevant to the pain, including diagnosis, testing, treatments, and outcomes.

H. Obtain a pain history to identify the client's attitudes, beliefs, level of knowledge, and previous experiences with pain. Are previously used methods for pain control helpful? What is the client's attitude toward the use of certain pain medications? Often, the client discusses certain adverse side effects or allergies from undesired pain medication.

Physical Examination
A. Check temperature, pulse, respirations, and BP.
B. Inspect:
  1. Observe overall appearance.
  2. Note affect and ability to express self and pain.
  3. Note facial grimaces with movement.
  4. Note gait, stance, and movements.
  5. Inspect area at pain site.
C. Auscultate:
  1. Heart and lungs
  2. Neck and abdomen
D. Palpate the affected area of pain.
E. Percuss:
  1. Chest
  2. Abdomen
F. Perform musculoskeletal examination.

> When performing the musculoskeletal examination, identify the location of pain, presence of trigger points, evidence of injury or trauma, edema, erythema, warmth, heat, lesions, petechiae, tenderness, decreased range of motion, pain with movement, crepitus, laxity of ligaments or cords, spasms, or guarding.

  1. Perform a complete musculoskeletal examination, concentrating on the area of pain.
  2. Note limitations in range of motion.
G. Neurologic examination:
  1. Perform a complete neurologic examination.
  2. Note the client's affect and mood. Is the client cooperative during examination?
  3. Identify abnormal sensory function such as allodynia (painful sensation to non-noxious stimuli) or hyperpathia (pain sensation that lingers after non-noxious stimuli are extinguished).
  4. Measure muscle strength, noting any weakness and/or muscle atrophy.
  5. Grade DTRs and presence of clonus or other signs of spasticity.
H. Functional assessment:
  1. A baseline functional assessment provides objective measurable data on a client's physical abilities and limitations. This assessment can be useful in evaluating the validity and reliability of the client's efforts and complaints.
  2. The information may be used to identify areas of impairment, establish specific functional goals, and measure the effectiveness of treatment interventions.
  3. These objective data may be used in worker compensation cases, returning-to-work status, federal disability, and motor vehicle accident lawsuits.
  4. Know the resources in your area prepared to perform functional assessments.

Diagnostic Tests
A. None required unless clearly indicated to establish an organic cause of pain:
  1. Remember that pain previously diagnosed as chronic pain syndrome can be organic, and vice versa. Organic causes must always be evaluated and excluded.
  2. Plain radiography should be ordered first for muscle, inflammatory, or skeletal pain. Plain radiography will diagnose a fracture. Additional studies may be recommended by the radiologist if a lesion/abnormality is seen on plain radiography.
  3. MRI and CT are ordered if the plain radiograph is negative and the client continues to complain of pain.
  4. Electromyography and nerve conduction studies are used to evaluate neuropathic pain. Numerous serum and urine studies should also be considered if the neuropathic pain is undiagnosed.
B. Depression screening tool: Consider using a depression assessment tool such as the Beck Depression Inventory or Patient Health Questionnaire 9 (PHQ9). These tools can be administered at a subsequent appointment to follow the client's symptoms.

Differential Diagnoses
A. Pain disorder
B. Pain related to a disease with no cure/malignancy
C. Somatization disorder
D. Conversion disorder
E. Hypochondriasis
F. Depression
G. Chemical dependency

Plan
A. General interventions:
  1. Treatment is multidimensional and should not focus on pharmacological treatment alone.
  2. Offer hope and potential for improvement of pain control, but *not* a cure.
  3. Identify realistic functional physical goals for clients and reassess at each visit. The client discussion needs to include the idea that the goal may be decreasing pain intensity, not eliminating pain.
  4. The pain is real to the client, and acceptance of the problem must occur before a mutually agreed-on treatment plan can be initiated.
  5. Depression and anxiety are common emotional disturbances in clients with chronic pain and are treatable
  6. Identify specific and realistic ADL goals for therapy, such as having a good night's sleep, going shopping, yardwork, cooking, or returning to work.
  7. Carefully assess the level of pain using available tools such as a daily pain diary or other pain assessment scales.
  8. Avoid pain reinforcement such as sympathy and attention to pain. Provide a positive response to productive activities. Improving activity tolerance assists in desensitizing the client to pain.
  9. Shift the focus from the pain to accomplishing daily assigned self-help tasks. The accomplishment of these tasks functions as positive reinforcement.
B. Client teaching: *See Section III: Client Teaching Guide for this chapter, "Chronic Pain."*

C. Pharmaceutical interventions:

1. Skeletal muscle pain: Treatment should focus on physical rehabilitation and behavioral management. TCAs and muscle relaxants (cyclobenzaprine) may be used. Research is lacking regarding the effectiveness of opioids. All muscle relaxers are on the Beers list and should be carefully prescribed in the elderly population. In children and adults, some muscle relaxers can cause a dangerous withdrawal syndrome if suddenly discontinued.

2. Inflammatory pain: NSAIDs and corticosteroids are first-line pharmaceutical interventions. Topical creams and solutions have been used in treating arthritis and other somatic sources of pain.

3. Mechanical/compressive pain: Opioids may be used to manage these symptoms while other measures are being taken.

4. Neuropathic pain:

   a. Gabapentin (Neurontin) and pregabalin (Lyrica) have become first-choice treatments in recent years for diabetic neuropathy, fibromyalgia, neuropathic pain associated with spinal cord injury, and postherpetic neuralgia.

   b. TCAs are extremely useful. Clients who are not depressed obtain excellent pain relief with TCAs such as amitriptyline and doxepin.

   c. Selective serotonin reuptake inhibitors (SSRIs) are also effective for chronic pain control. Duloxetine (Cymbalta) has been approved for chronic pain as monotherapy or in conjunction with TCAs.

   d. Anticonvulsants are useful in controlling some neuropathic pain: carbamazepine (Tegretol), phenytoin (Dilantin), and valproic acid (Depakene). Clients need to be monitored monthly for hepatic dysfunction and hematopoietic suppression.

   e. Topical agents: Capsaicin applied three to four times per day can reduce pain without significant systemic effects. Topical lidocaine 5% patches are approved for postherpetic neuralgia but are used off-label for other topical pain.

   f. Carbamazepine is used as the first-line treatment for trigeminal neuralgia.

   g. Opioids: Tramadol is considered to be a good choice if an opioid is indicated. In addition to pain control, tramadol causes serotonin reuptake inhibition similar to that seen with the TCAs. Peak plasma levels occur approximately 1.5 hours after ingestion and elimination; the half-life of tramadol is approximately 5 to 6 hours. Risk for seizures and serotonin syndrome increases even at recommended doses with coadministration of other SSRIs, alcohol, TCAs, and antipsychotics. Know the Drug Enforcement Administration's (DEA) and the state's rules and regulations within the Prescription Drug Monitoring Programs (PDMP) database systems for opioid prescribing.

5. All therapies need a 2- to 3-week trial period to adequately evaluate therapy. Some medications take longer than that to evaluate.

6. NSAIDs should be used for flare-ups of mild to moderate inflammatory or non-neuropathic pain.

7. Opioids require careful client selection, titration, and monitoring. Explain to the client starting on an opioid that this will be a trial to see if the opioid is effective. The goal is to improve function and quality of life more than to reduce the pain scale. Have an exit plan when starting an opioid if the opioid is ineffective or not well tolerated. Avoid long-term, daily treatment with short-acting opioids (Vicodin, Norco, and Percocet). For as-needed use, prescribe small quantities.

8. Benzodiazepines and barbiturates are not advised for treatment of chronic pain due to the high risk of substance abuse.

9. Mitigate risks when considering opioids. A checklist for prescribing opioids can be found at www.cdc.gov/drugoverdose/pdf/PDO_Checklist-a.pdf.

   a. Check your state's PDMP before prescribing controlled substances, as needed, and at least annually. PDMPs are state-run electronic databases that track dispensing of controlled substances. PDMPs provide clinicians with critical information about client narcotic prescription history and identify drug-seeking behavior patterns. For more details regarding PDMPs and your state's information, visit www.cdc.gov/drugoverdose/pdmp/states.html.

   b. Contact the client's pharmacy for a list of current medications. Currently, the PDMP access time is less than 5 minutes real time, and all active client prescriptions are available from the pharmacy.

   c. Perform urine drug screens before prescribing controlled substances initially, as needed, and annually. National guidelines recommend the enzyme immunoassay (EIA) and gas chromatography/mass spectroscopy urine drug test. Depending on the results of urine drug screening, the provider may seek additional consultation, change medication therapy, refer for substance abuse, or discharge the client.

   d. A written controlled substance treatment agreement among the client, provider, and clinic is recommended. Include expectations of the client: No other controlled substances will be prescribed by any other provider. One pharmacy only should be used. Medications must be taken as prescribed. Prescriptions of controlled substances will not be filled early. The client must agree to random drug tests and may be called to report to the clinic for random drug screening and/or pill counts. Both analgesic goals and functional goals should be defined and realistic expectations established. Potential risks including common opioid side effects, abuse/addiction risks, respiratory depression, overdose, and death should be discussed with the client. The client should be informed of alternative treatments plans that do not include opioids. All of these risks should be addressed in follow-up appointments as well.

   e. Utilize tools such as the Screener and Opioid Assessment for Patients with Pain (SOAPP) and/or the Opioid Risk Tool (ORT).

   f. Red flags for misuse, abuse, addiction, and diversion with opioids include:

      i. Psychiatric illness

      ii. Personal history of alcohol or drug abuse

      iii. Family history of alcohol or drug abuse

      iv. Younger age

      v. Male gender

      vi. Preadolescent

      vii. Psychiatric comorbidities

      viii. Psychotropic medication use

      ix. Sleep-disordered breathing

D. Alternative interventions:

1. Psychological interventions: Cognitive behavioral therapy is most commonly used and is currently being adopted more widely as an effective method of treatment to decrease pain and improve function. Examples include problem-solving, guided imagery, controlled breathing exercises, attention diversion, meditation, and yoga exercises; progressive muscle relaxation (PMR) to help relax major muscle groups; Acceptance Commitment Therapy; biofeedback; and mindfulness.

2. Exercise: Examples of exercise include yoga exercises and PMR. Research indicates that yoga decreases a large degree of bothersome pain after 12 weeks of regular exercise. The benefits of yoga exercise include improved strength, balance, coordination, range of motion, and reduced anxiety. Yoga instruction by a qualified teacher is a low-cost intervention. Yoga is an effective form of self-care and is an affordable way to alleviate pain. Always advise clients to start slowly and be prepared for an approach to pain management that may take several weeks of therapy.

3. Alternative therapies: Randomized controlled trials showed significant reduction in pain with alternative interventions such as music, relaxation, distraction, acupuncture, myofascial release treatments, and massage use.

4. Occupational therapy

5. Vocational therapy

6. Physical therapy such as noninvasive techniques, transcutaneous electrical nerve stimulation, hot or cold therapy, hydrotherapy, traction, massage, bracing, and exercise

7. Individual and family therapy or counseling

8. Aesthetic or neurosurgical procedures

9. Clients may inquire about the use of herbal products to treat chronic pain. Advise clients that these products are not regulated by the FDA. Advise them that these herbal products may interact with current medications and cause complications. Advise them to research all herbal products on reputable medically based websites, not blogs or chat rooms. Caution clients regarding devil's claw, feverfew, willow bark, glucosamine, and chondroitin. Discourage any use of dimethylsulfoxide.

10. Acupuncture and acupressure may be considered

11. Neuromodulation with spinal cord stimulators and/or intrathecal pumps can be explored with a board-certified pain management physician.

Follow-Up

A. See clients every 4 to 6 weeks for evaluation.

B. Ensure that the client has access to care on a regular schedule.

C. These brief visits should be consistent so that care is not perceived to be dependent on escalation of symptoms.

Consultation/Referral

A. Consider client referral to a pain management clinic if pain control is not adequate. Interventions commonly performed at the specialty clinic include facet joint injections, percutaneous radiofrequency neurotomy, epidural corticosteroid injections, transforaminal epidural injections, and sacroiliac joint injections.

B. Consult with the full interdisciplinary team and/or an addictionologist for suspected substance abuse and/or addiction.

C. Refer to a certified pain specialist physician if the client is taking high doses of opioids and detoxification is indicated. Buprenorphine (Suboxone) is the most common medication prescribed by a certified pain specialist physician.

D. Consider a rheumatology consult if indicated.

Bibliography

Centers for Disease Control and Prevention. (2016a, March 15). CDC guidelines for prescribing opioids for chronic pain—United States, 2016. *Morbidity and Mortality Weekly Reports*. Retrieved from https://www.cdc.gov/mmwr/volumes/65/rr/rr6501e1.htm

Centers for Disease Control and Prevention. (2016b, March 22). Checklist for prescribing opioids for chronic pain. Retrieved from https://www.cdc.gov/drugoverdose/pdf/PDO_Checklist-a.pdf

Centers for Disease and Prevention. (2019). What states need to know about PDMPs. *CDC: Opioid. State Information*. Retrieved from https://www.cdc.gov/drugoverdose/pdmp/states.html

Dahlhamer, J., Lucas J., Zelaya, C., Nahin, R., DeBar, L., Kerns, R., … Helmick, C. (2018). Prevalence of chronic pain and high-impact chronic pain among adults—United States 2016. *Morbidity and Mortality Weekly Report, 67*(36), 1001–1006. doi:10.15585/mmwr.mm6736a2

Donaldson, M. (2018). Resilient to pain: A model of how yoga may decrease interference among people experiencing chronic pain. *Explore.* doi:10.1016/j.explore.2018.11.002

International Association for the Study of Pain Terminology. (2017). IASP terminology. Retrieved from https://www.iasp-pain.org/Education/Content.aspx?ItemNumber=1698#Pain

Kasper, D., Fauci, A., Hauser, S., Longo, D., Jameson, J., & Loscalzo, J. (2016). *Harrison's manual of medicine* (19th ed.). New York, NY: McGraw-Hill Education.

Murphy, K. R., Han, J. L., Yang, S., Hussaini, S. M. Q., Elsamadicy, A. A., Parente, B., … Lad, S. P. (2017). Prevalence of specific types of pain diagnoses in a sample of United States adults. *Pain Physician, 20*, E257–E268. Retrieved from https://www.painphysicianjournal.com/current/pdf?article=NDExNQ%3D%3D&journal=102

Lower Back Pain

Kathleen Siders and Moya Cook

Definition

Painful conditions of the lower back may be categorized as follows:

A. Potentially serious disorders: Acute fracture, tumor, progressive neurologic deficit, nerve root compression, and cauda equina syndrome

B. Degenerative disorders: Aging or repetitive use, degenerative disease, and osteoarthritis

C. Nonspecific disorders: Benign and self-limiting with unclear etiology

Incidence

A. Lower back pain is commonly seen in clients from ages 20 to 40 years.

B. Approximately 70% to 80% of people experience back pain at one point in their lifetime.

Pathogenesis

A. Pain arises from fracture, tumor, nerve root compression, degenerative disc, osteoarthritis, and strain of the ligaments and musculature of the lumbosacral area.

Predisposing Factors

A. Trauma causing ligament tearing; stretching of vertebra, muscles, tendons, ligaments, or fascia

B. Repetitive mechanical stress

C. Tumor

D. Exaggerated lumbar lordosis

E. Abnormal, forward-tipped pelvis

F. Uneven leg length

G. Chronic poor posture due to inadequate conditioning of muscle strength and flexibility, improper lifting techniques causing excessive strain, and poor body mechanics

H. Inadequate rest

I. Emotional depression

Common Complaints

A. Pain in the lower back area may range from discomfort to severe back pain, with or without radiation

Other Signs and Symptoms

A. Ambulating with a limp

B. Limited range of motion

C. Posture normal to guarded

Subjective Data

A. Ask the client to discuss the origin of pain. How has the pain progressed or changed since the initial injury?

B. Ask the client to point to an area where pain is felt.

C. Have the client describe the pain. Is it radiating, with sharp, shooting pain down to the lower leg and feet?

D. Ask: What makes the pain worse or better? Does activity make the pain worse or better? Have the client list current medications or therapies used for pain, noting results of treatment.

E. Investigate occurrence of systemic symptoms such as fever and weight loss.

F. Explore the client's past medical history. Note previous trauma or overuse, tuberculosis, arthritis, cancer, and osteoporosis.

G. Inquire about symptoms such as dysuria, bowel or bladder incontinence, muscle weakness, paresthesia, and loss of sensation. Bowel or bladder dysfunction, bilateral sciatica, and saddle distribution of dysesthesias may be symptoms of severe compression of the cauda equina that necessitate an urgent workup and referral. Other red flags include fever, history of cancer, history of intravenous (IV) drug use, immunosuppression, steroid use, history of osteoporosis, and worsening symptoms.

H. Ask the client about precipitating factors such as athletics, heavy lifting, driving, yardwork, occupation, sleep habits, any new activity, or systemic disease.

I. Use a pain scale to describe the worst pain and the best pain levels.

Physical Examination

A. Check temperature, pulse, BP, and respiration.

B. Inspect:

1. Observe general appearance; note discomfort and grimacing on movement and/or examination.

2. Distraction may distinguish pain behavior from actual pathology.

3. Note evidence of trauma with bruises, cuts, and fractures.

4. Note posture and gait.

C. Palpate:

1. Palpate spine and paravertebral structures, noting point tenderness and muscle spasm. Palpation elicits paravertebral tenderness and generalized tenderness over the lower back to upper buttocks.

2. Examine abdomen for masses and presence of aortic aneurysm, which can present as back pain.

3. Extremities: Palpate peripheral pulses.

D. Perform neurologic examination:

1. Identify sensation and pain distribution.

2. Determine motor strength and evaluate whether muscle strength is symmetrical: Upper extremity resistance is equal bilaterally.

3. Test DTRs, check for clonus, and assess strength of dorsiflexion of the big toes.

E. Check sensation of perineum to rule out cauda equina syndrome.

F. Perform traction tests: Straight leg raises, crossed leg raises, Yeoman Guying, and Patrick's test. Musculoskeletal findings include the following:

1. Straight leg raising and dorsiflexion of foot on the affected side may reduce lower back discomfort

2. Elevate each leg passively with flexion at the hip and extension of the knee. Positive straight leg raise produces radicular pain when the leg is raised to 30 degrees to 60 degrees.

3. Crossed leg raises: Test is positive when pain occurs in the leg not being raised.

4. Yeoman Guying: Unilateral hyperextension in prone position identifies lumbosacral mechanical disorder

5. Patrick's test: Place heel on opposite knee and apply lateral force; check for hip or sacroiliac disease

6. Range of motion: Increased pain with extension often indicates osteoarthritis. Increased pain with flexion often indicates strain or injured disc.

G. Pelvic examination: Consider pelvic and rectal examination, if indicated. If the client has fallen on the coccyx, a rectal examination is needed to check for stability.

Diagnostic Tests

A. Laboratory: Complete blood count, erythrocyte sedimentation rate, serum calcium, alkaline phosphatase, urinalysis, and serum immunoelectrophoresis when inflammatory, neoplastic, diffuse bone disease, or renal disease is suspected

B. Radiography of spine

1. In the absence of red flags, do not perform an x-ray unless pain persists past 6 weeks. When possible, begin with plain radiographs with at least two views.

2. If radiographs and/or persistent symptoms indicate, consider MRI to rule out disc disease and tumors

3. Consider a bone scan to rule out cancer.

Differential Diagnoses

A. Back pain secondary to musculoskeletal pain
B. Herniated intervertebral disease
C. Sciatica
D. Fracture (compression or pars)
E. Ankylosing spondylitis
F. Malignancy/tumor
G. Abdominal aneurysm
H. Pyelonephritis
I. Metabolic bone disease
J. Gynecologic disease
K. Peripheral neuropathy
L. Depression
M. Prostatitis
N. Spinal stenosis
O. Osteoarthritis
P. Osteoporosis
Q. Abdominal aortic aneurysm

Plan

A. General interventions:

1. The client should continue physical activity as tolerated. Total bed rest is not recommended.

2. For acute muscle strain, have the client apply local cold packs 20 to 30 minutes several times a day for the first 24 hours. Heat packs are recommended after the initial 24 hours of injury.

3. Chronic or recurrent pain may be treated with either ice or heat applications, whichever gives relief.

B. Client teaching:

1. Give accurate information on the prognosis for quick recovery such as continuing light physical activity, performing back-strengthening exercises, and avoiding overuse of medications.

2. Improvement occurs in most cases in a few weeks, although mild symptoms may persist.

3. Joint guidelines by the American College of Physicians and the American Pain Society recommend rehabilitative therapies for clients who do not improve after medications and self-care recommendations. Rehabilitative therapies include exercise therapy, acupuncture, massage therapy, spinal manipulation, cognitive behavioral therapy, and yoga.

4. Provide educational handouts on back exercises; *see Section III: Client Teaching Guide for this chapter,* ◄ *"Back Stretches."*

5. After intense pain abates, the client may perform low-back exercises for range of motion and strengthening, and isometric tightening exercises of abdominal and gluteal muscles.

6. Teach client knee–chest exercises. Recommend to the client to place the back against the wall and contract the abdominal and gluteal muscles, with 5 to 10 repetitions performed four to six times per day.

7. Research indicates that yoga is beneficial for many types of back pain. Types of back pain benefited by yoga include musculoskeletal injury, herniated disc, spinal stenosis, spondylolisthesis, piriformis syndrome, arthritis, and sacroiliac joint derangement.

8. Encourage the client to perform walking, swimming, or pool exercise daily.

9. Teach relaxation techniques.

10. Encourage the client to modify work hours and job tasks.

11. Refer the client for therapeutic massage or physical therapy as needed.

12. Obesity is often related to decreased exercise and poor physical fitness with reduced trunk muscle strength and endurance. Obese clients may experience back pain with normal activity.

13. Protective factors:

  a. Moderate physical activity
  b. Controlling weight
  c. Avoiding injuries
  d. Adequate preoperative and postoperative analgesia
  e. Resilience and positive affect

C. Pharmaceutical therapy:

1. Analgesics: Acetaminophen 350 to 650 mg every 4 to 6 hours. Maximum dose is 4,000 mg per day. Inquire about use of any other current medications and/or over-the-counter preparations containing acetaminophen.

2. NSAIDs: Unless contraindicated due to gastrointestinal symptoms or cardiovascular disease:

  a. Aspirin: 325 to 650 mg every 4 to 6 hours
  b. Ibuprofen: 200 to 800 mg every 6 to 8 hours; maximum dose is 3.2 g per day under the care of the provider, otherwise 1.2 g per day

c. Naproxen: 500 mg initially, followed by 250 mg every 6 to 8 hours

d. Piroxicam (Feldene): 20 mg every day

e. Meloxicam (Mobic): 7.5 to 15 mg daily

f. Celebrex: 100 to 200 mg twice a day

3. Muscle relaxants:

a. Cyclobenzaprine HCl (Flexeril): 10 mg three times daily

b. Carisoprodol (Soma): 350 mg three times daily; avoid use due to risk of addiction.

c. Methocarbamol (Robaxin): 500 to 750 mg three to four times a day

d. Orphenadrine citrate (Norflex): 100 mg twice a day

e. Metaxalone (Skelaxin): 800 mg three to four times a day

f. Tizanidine (Zanaflex): 2 to 6 mg TID

Follow-Up

A. If pain is severe or unimproved, follow up in 24 hours.

B. If pain is moderate, reevaluate the client in 7 to 10 days.

C. See the client in 2 to 4 weeks to reevaluate his or her condition and behavioral changes.

D. Recurrences are not uncommon but do not indicate a chronic or worsening case.

Consultation/Referral

A. Consult with a physician when considering red flag diagnoses such as cauda equina syndrome, herniated disc, widespread neurologic involvement, carcinoma, or significant trauma.

B. Referral to a physician is needed for clients who note significant morning stiffness with a gradual onset prior to age 40 years, with continuing spinal movements in all directions, and involving some peripheral joints, iritis, and skin rashes indicating inflammatory disorders such as ankylosing spondylitis and related disorders.

Individual Considerations

A. Pregnancy: Pregnancy is often associated with low-back discomfort. This is due to the redistribution of body weight. As weight increases in the abdominal area with the growing fetus, clients tend to compensate by changing posture and tilting the spine back.

B. Adults:

1. For clients older than 50 years presenting with no prior history of backache, consider a differential diagnosis of neoplasm. The most common metastasis seen is secondary to the primary site of breast cancer, prostate cancer, or multiple myeloma. Pain most prominent in a recumbent position rarely radiates into the buttock or leg.

2. Men and women in their early adulthood (ages 20–45 years) who present with chronic back pain that improves with activity should be further evaluated for ankylosing spondylitis.

Bibliography

American Society for Pain Management Nursing. (2010). Optimizing the treatment of pain in patients with acute presentations. Retrieved from http://aspmn.org/Documents/OptimizingPositionPaper.pdf

Centers for Disease Control and Prevention. (2016a, March 15). CDC guidelines for prescribing opioids for chronic pain—United States, 2016. Morbidity and Mortality Weekly Reports. Retrieved from https://www.cdc.gov/mmwr/volumes/65/rr/rr6501e1.htm

Centers for Disease Control and Prevention. (2016b, March 22). Checklist for prescribing opioids for chronic pain. Retrieved from https://www.cdc.gov/drugoverdose/pdf/PDO_Checklist-a.pdf

Dahlhamer, J., Lucas J., Zelaya, C., Nahin, R., DeBar, L., Kerns, R., … Helmick, C. (2018). Prevalence of chronic pain and high-impact chronic pain among adults—United States 2016. Morbidity and Mortality Weekly Report, 67(36), 1001–1006. doi:10.15585/mmwr.mm6736a2

Donaldson, M. (2018). Resilient to pain: A model of how yoga may decrease interference among people experiencing chronic pain. Explore, 15, 230–238. doi:10.1016/j.explore.2018.11.002

Institute of Medicine. (2011). Relieving pain in America: A blueprint for transforming prevention, care, education, and research. Washington, DC: National Academies Press.

International Association for the Study of Pain Terminology. (2017). IASP terminology. Retrieved from https://www.iasp-pain.org/Education/Content.aspx?ItemNumber=1698#Pain

Kasper, D., Fauci, A., Hauser, S., Longo, D., Jameson, J., & Loscalzo, J. (2016). Harrison's manual of medicine (19th ed.). New York, NY: McGraw-Hill Education.

Kent, M. L., Tighe, P. J, Belfer, I., Brennan, T., Bruehl, S., Brummett, C., … Terman, G. (2017). The ACTION-APS-AAPM Pain Taxonomy (AAAPT) multidimensional approach to classifying acute pain conditions. Journal of Pain, 18(5), 479–489. doi:10.1016/j.jpain.2017.02.421

Mundkur, M., Franklin, J., Adbia, Y., Huybrechts, K., Patorno, E., Gagne, J., … Bateman, B (2019, February 15). Days' supply of initial opioid analgesic prescriptions and additional fills for acute pain conditions treated in the primary care setting—United States, 2014. Morbidity and Mortality Weekly Report, 68(6), 140–143. Retrieved from https://www.cdc.gov/mmwr/volumes/68/wr/mm6806a3.htm

Murphy, K. R., Han, J. L., Yang, S., Hussaini, S. M. Q., Elsamadicy, A. A., Parente, B., … Lad, S. P. (2017). Prevalence of specific types of pain diagnoses in a sample of United States adults. Pain Physician, 20, E257–E268. Retrieved from https://www.painphysicianjournal.com/current/pdf?article=NDExNQ%3D%3D&journal=102

National Pharmaceutical Council. (n.d.). Pain: Current understanding of assessment, management, and treatments. American Pain Society. Retrieved from http://americanpainsociety.org/uploads/education/section_4.pdf

Ronchetti, S., Migliorati, G., & Delfin, D. V. (2017). Association of inflammatory mediators with pain perception. Biomedicine & Pharmacotherapy, 96, 1445–1452. doi:10.1016/j.biopha.2017.12.001

Tighe, P., Buckenmaier, C. C. 3rd, Boezaart, A. P., Carr, D. B., Clark, L. L., Herring, A. A., … Reisfield, G. M. (2015). Acute pain medicine in the United States: A status report. Pain Medicine [APM Shared Interest Group of the American Academy of Pain Medicine], 16(9), 1806–1826. doi:10.1111/pme.12760

4 Dermatology Guidelines

Acne Rosacea

Jill C. Cash and Amy C. Bruggemann

Definition

A. A multifactorial vascular skin disorder, acne rosacea, is characterized by chronic inflammatory processes in which flushing and dilation of the blood vessels occur primarily on the face (Figure 4.1). It is manifested in four stages of pathologic events.

Incidence

A. Acne rosacea affects approximately 13 million people in the United States. It occurs in all ethnic backgrounds but is frequently observed in people with fair pigmented skin. Prevalence ranges from 1% to 10% of fair-skinned people. Women over the age of 30 years also tend to have a higher incidence of rosacea. Rosacea can occur in adolescence; however, it is rarely seen in children.

Pathogenesis

A. Rosacea is a functional vascular anomaly with a tendency toward recurrent dilation and flushing of the face. Inflammatory mediator release to cutaneous microorganisms, extravasation of inflammatory cells of the immune system, exposure to UV light, and heightened activity of the vascular system are the factors that are believed to cause the symptoms of rosacea. Ocular involvement may also include the eyelid and conjunctiva.

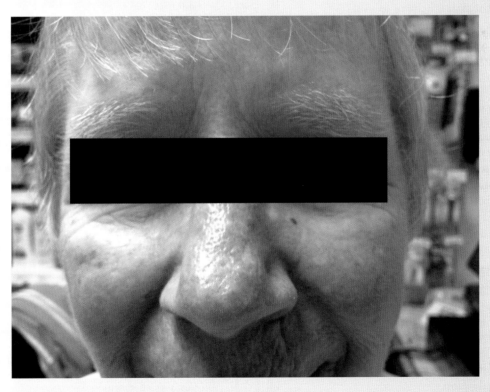

FIGURE 4.1 Acne rosacea.

Source: Reproduced from Lyons, F., & Ousley, L. (2015). *Dermatology for the advanced practice nurse*. New York, NY: Springer Publishing Company, Figure III.47.

Predisposing Factors
A. Tendency to flush frequently
B. Exposure to heat, cold, or sunlight
C. Consumption of hot or spicy foods and alcoholic beverages
D. Some topical medications, astringents, or toners
E. Psychological stress
F. Menopause hot flashes

Common Complaints
A. **Papules, pustules, and nodules. Hallmarks for diagnosis are the small papules and papulopustules. Many presenting erythematous papules have a tiny pustule at the crest. No comedones are present.**
B. Periodic reddening or flushing of face, primarily the nose and medial cheeks
C. Increase in skin temperature of face
D. Face flushing in response to heat stimuli (hot liquids) in mouth

Other Signs and Symptoms
A. Periorbital erythema
B. Telangiectasia, paranasally and on cheeks
C. Rhinophyma
D. Blepharoconjunctivitis with erythematous eyelid margins
E. Conjunctivitis: Diffuse hyperemic type or nodular
F. Keratitis: Lower portion of cornea, associated with pain, photophobia, and foreign-body sensation

Subjective Data
A. Ask the client to describe the location and the onset. Was the onset sudden or gradual? How have the symptoms continued to develop?
B. Assess if the skin is itchy or painful.
C. Assess for any associated discharge (blood or pus).
D. Complete a drug history. Has the client recently taken any antibiotics or other medications?
E. Determine whether the client has used any topical medications, astringents, toners, or new skin-care products.
F. Rule out any possible exposure to industrial or domestic toxins, insect bites, and possible contact with venereal disease or HIV.
G. Ask the client about close contact with others with skin disorders.
H. Identify whether exposure to heat, cold, or sunlight provokes the symptoms.
I. Ask whether eating or drinking hot or spicy foods or consumption of alcoholic beverages provokes the symptoms.

Physical Examination
A. Check temperature, pulse, and blood pressure.
B. Inspect:
  1. Skin, focusing on face and scalp
  2. Nose and paranasal structures
  3. Eyes, eyelids, conjunctiva, and cornea. **An ocular manifestation, rosacea keratitis, may cause corneal ulcers to develop.**

Diagnostic Tests
Consider skin biopsy to rule out lupus, sarcoidosis, or other possible causes if history and physical examinations warrant further testing.

Differential Diagnoses
A. Acne rosacea
B. Acne vulgaris
C. Steroid-induced acne
D. Perioral dermatitis
E. Seborrheic dermatitis
F. Lupus erythematosus
G. Cutaneous sarcoidosis

Plan
A. General interventions: Identify any causative or provocative factors—heat, cold, hot or spicy foods, alcoholic beverages, sunlight, so forth.
  1. Advise washing face with a mild cleanser such as Cetaphil or Cerave in the morning and at night.
  2. Avoid direct sunlight exposure by wearing protective clothing/hats when outdoors. Suggest using a sunscreen of sun protection factor (SPF)-30 when exposed to sunlight.
B. Client teaching: *See Section III: Client Teaching Guide* ◀ *for this chapter, "Acne Rosacea."*
C. Pharmaceutical therapy:
  1. Topical treatment:
    a. Metronidazole 0.75%: apply twice daily after cleansing skin. Cheapest and best used for facial sensitivity
    b. Sodium sulfacetamide may be used as an alternative.
    c. Azelaic acid: This is dicarboxylic acid that decreases swelling and redness, kills bacteria, and reduces the production of keratin. Apply gel to skin twice a day.
    d. Ivermectin: This is an antiparasitic agent that targets parasites and inflammation on the skin.
  2. Oral treatment
    a. Drug of choice: Tetracycline 500 to 1,000 mg twice to four times daily for 2 to 4 weeks
    b. Others: Doxycycline 100 mg daily until clear
    c. Minocycline (Minocin) 50 to 200 mg daily which is divided into two doses
  3. **Steroids:** Do not use topical steroids. Topical steroids may worsen irritation.
  4. Isotretinoin: Oral isotretinoin is used to treat severe acne and refractory cases. Must be closely monitored and suggested to the dermatologist for treatment

Follow-Up
A. Follow up in 2 weeks to evaluate therapy.
B. See clients monthly for evaluation until maintenance is reached.
C. Relapses are common following discontinuance of antibiotics; repeat treatment.

Consultation/Referral
A. Consult or refer the client to a dermatologist if there is no improvement or if the client is unable to reach maintenance.
B. Provide an immediate referral to an ophthalmologist for treatment and follow up for ocular involvement.

Individual Considerations
A. Adults: Tinted sulfacetamide (Sulfacet-R) lotion may be used to cover erythema in fair-skinned clients

Bibliography
Acmaz, G., Cınar, L., Acmaz, B., Aksoy, H., Kafadar, Y. T., Madendag, Y., … Muderris, I. (2019). The effects of oral isotretinoin in women with acne and polycystic ovary syndrome. *BioMed Research International, 2019*, 1–5. doi:10.1155/2019/2513067

Brackenbury, J. (2016). Recommended topical treatments for managing adult acne in women. *Nurse Prescribing, 14*(3), 126–129. doi:10.12968/npre.2016.14.3.126

dall'Oglio, F., Lacarrubba, F., Luca, M., Boscaglia, S., & Micali, G. (2018). Clinical and erythema-directed instrumental evaluation of papulopustular rosacea treated with topical ivermectin. *Journal of the American Academy of Dermatology, 79*(3), AB75. doi:10.1016/j.jaad.2018.05.335

Gold, L. S., Lain, E. L., & Harvey, A. (2018). The anti-inflammatory properties of ivermectin and brimonidine in the treatment of papulopustular rosacea. *Journal of the American Academy of Dermatology, 79*(3), AB281. doi:10.1016/j.jaad.2018.05.1115

Oge, L. K., Muncie, L. H., & Phillips, A. R. (2015). Rosacea: Diagnosis and treatment. *American Family Physician, 92*(3), 187–196.

Palmer, W. J. (2019). New therapies in development to manage acne, rosacea. *Dermatology Times, 40*(4), 1–20.

Radley, K. (2015). The management and treatment of acnes. *Primary Health Care, 25*(4), 34–41. doi:10.7748/phc.25.4.34.e996

Acne Vulgaris

Jill C. Cash and Amy C. Bruggemann

Definition
A. Acne vulgaris is a disorder of the sebaceous glands and there are numerous hair follicles on the face, back, and chest (Figure 4.2). The sebaceous glands become inflamed and form papules, pustules, cysts, open or closed comedones, and/or nodules on an erythema base. In severe cases, scarring can result.

Incidence
A. Acne vulgaris is the most common skin disorder in the United States, affecting 40 to 50 million persons of all ages and races. Nearly 80% to 90% of all adults experience

FIGURE 4.2   Acne vulgaris.

Source: StatPearls Publishing. (2019). Retrieved from https://www.ncbi.nlm.nih.gov/books/NBK459173/

acne during their lifetime. Acne vulgaris, commonly seen in adolescence, may even extend into the third or fourth decade of life.

Pathogenesis
A. Sebum is overproduced and collected in the sebaceous gland. Sebum and keratinized cells are collected in the hair follicle. With the presence of *Propionibacterium acnes*, the duct becomes clogged, and lesions (noninflammatory and/or inflammatory) evolve.

Predisposing Factors
A. Age (adolescence)
B. External irritants to skin (makeup, oils, equipment contact on skin)
C. Hormones (oral contraceptives with high progestin content)
D. Medications (lithium, halides, hydantoin derivatives, rifampin)
E. Hot, humid weather

Common Complaints
A. Outbreak of pimples on face, chest, shoulders, and back that do not resolve with over-the-counter (OTC) treatment
B. Acne rosacea: Presence of Telangiectasia, flushing, and rhinophyma

Other Signs and Symptoms
A. Mild: Open comedones (blackhead) and closed comedones (whitehead)
B. Moderate: Comedones with papules and pustules
C. Severe: Nodules, cysts, and scars

Subjective Data
A. Elicit the age of onset of outbreak, duration, and course of symptoms.
B. Determine what makes the lesions worse or better.
C. Ask whether there are certain times of the month or year when lesions are better or worse.
D. Identify the client's current method of cleanser or moisturizer treatment.
E. Ask if the client has ever been treated by a provider for this problem. If so, determine the treatment and results of the treatment.
F. Assess whether other family members have the same problem.
G. Ask the client for a description of his or her environment and occupation.
H. Explore with the client any current stress factors in his or her life.

Physical Examination
A. Inspect:
   1. Observe skin for location and severity of lesions.
   2. Rate severity of lesions as mild, moderate, or severe:
      a. Mild: Few papules/pustules, no nodules
      b. Moderate: Several papules/pustules, rare nodules
      c. Severe: Many papules/pustules with many nodules
   3. Take a picture of areas of affected skin for chart and document date. Use this for future appointments as a reference to compare results for follow-up visits.

Diagnostic Tests

A. No tests are generally required

B. Culture lesions to rule out gram-negative folliculitis with clients on antibiotics

C. Consider hormone testing if other primary causes of acne are taken into account (follicle-stimulating hormone, luteinizing hormone, testosterone levels)

Differential Diagnoses

A. Acne vulgaris

B. Acne rosacea

C. Steroid rosacea

D. Folliculitis

E. Perioral acne

F. Drug-induced acne

Plan

A. General interventions:

1. Document location and severity of lesions. Assess quality of improvement at each office visit.

2. The primary goal of treatment is prevention of scarring. Good control of lesions during puberty and early adulthood is required for best results. Anticipate ups and downs during the normal course of treatment.

B. Client teaching:

▶ 1. *See Section III: Client Teaching Guide for this chapter: "Acne Vulgaris."*

2. Instruct the client on proper cleansing routine. The client should wash affected areas with a mild soap (Purpose, Cetaphil) twice a day and apply medications as directed.

3. Warn the client that washing the face more than two to three times a day can decrease oil production and cause drying.

4. Discuss current stressors in the client's life and discuss treatment options.

5. Recommend an exercise routine 3 to 5 days a week.

6. Recommend oil-free sunscreens.

C. Pharmaceutical therapy: **It may take 1 to 3 months before results are visible when using these medications**.

1. Mild: Treatment of choice is topical. Use one of the following:

a. Benzoyl peroxide, 2.5%, 5%, 10%; begin with 2.5% at bedtime; may graduate to 5% or 10% twice daily, if needed, as tolerated

b. T-Stat: Apply to dried areas twice daily. Avoid eyes, nose, and mouth creases.

c. Topical tretinoin 0.1% (Retin-A Micro); use at bedtime.

i. With Retin-A use, the client may see rapid turnover of keratin plugs

ii. Instruct the client to avoid abrasive soaps

iii. Warn the client regarding photosensitivity

iv. Warn the client regarding increased dryness. May apply a moisturizer such as Cerave or Cetaphil if needed.

d. Desquam E: Use at bedtime. Wash face with soap and then apply Desquam E.

2. Moderate: Use one of the aforementioned topical medications in addition to one of the following oral medications for 3 to 4 months.

a. Tetracycline 500 mg twice daily for 3 to 6 weeks, for adolescents older than 14 years. As condition improves, begin tapering medication to 250 mg twice daily for 6 weeks, then to daily or to every other day.

i. Instruct the client to take tetracycline on an empty stomach and to avoid dairy products, antacids, and iron.

ii. Warn the client about photosensitivity. This medication may be used as a maintenance dose at 250 mg daily or every other day for those clients who break out after discontinuing antibiotic therapy. No drug resistance is seen with tetracycline.

b. Erythromycin 250 mg four times per day after meals or topical erythromycin 2%, solution or gel, twice daily, or clindamycin (Cleocin T) solution, pads, or gel, twice daily. Erythromycin resistance has been seen.

c. Minocycline 100 mg twice daily. When this is effective, taper to 50 mg twice daily.

i. Have the client drink plenty of fluids.

ii. Central nervous system (CNS) side effects (headaches) have been seen.

d. Bactrim single strength twice daily if the aforementioned regimens do not work well. Bactrim works well if others fail because it is effective for gram-negative folliculitis

e. Doxycycline 100 mg twice daily. Re-evaluate every 4 to 6 months.

f. Oral contraceptives with higher doses of estrogen have also been effective for girls. There are three oral contraceptives approved by the FDA to be used for acne. These three contraceptives are:

i. Estradiol 20/30/35 mcg/norethindrone 1 mg (Estrostep)

ii. Ethinyl estradiol 35 mcg/norgestimate 180/215/2,501 mcg (Ortho Tri-Cyclen)

iii. Ethinyl estradiol 20 mcg/drospirenone 3 mg (Yaz)

g. Spironolactone may be used for women who fail topical and oral antibiotics and contraceptives. Spironolactone 50 to 100 mg/d, split into two divided doses. Medical history should be evaluated for comorbidities such as heart disease, renal disease, and other medications/risks of causing hyperkalemia since spironolactone is a potassium-sparing drug. Levels may be checked prior to starting medication and periodically while on the medication.

3. Severe: Medications such as isotretinoin should be prescribed by the dermatologist.

4. Underlying disorders: Women with hyperandrogenism should be evaluated and treated for underlying endocrine disorders. Mild cases can be treated with hormone therapy (oral contraceptive agents).

Follow-Up

See clients every 6 to 8 weeks for evaluation.

A. Mild: Adjust dose depending on local irritation.

B. Moderate (oral and topical medications):

1. Adjust dose according to irritation.

2. Taper oral antibiotics with discretion and/or continue topical medications.

3. Oral antibiotics may be tapered and discontinued when inflammatory lesions have resolved.

C. Severe: Recommend referral to dermatology and follow-up with the specialty.

D. A minimum of 3 to 6 months should be trialed before switching to another alternative.

Consultation/Referral

A. Consult with a physician if treatment is unsuccessful after 10 to 12 weeks of therapy or if acne is severe.

B. The client may need dermatology consultation.

Individual Considerations

A. Pregnancy:

1. Acne may flare up or improve during pregnancy.

2. Medications preferred during pregnancy are topical retinoids.

3. **Teratogens include tretinoin, tetracycline, and minocycline.**

a. **When using teratogenic medications, contraception must be practiced to avoid pregnancy to prevent severe fetal malformations.**

b. **Begin contraception 1 month before starting the medication and continue contraception 1 month after finishing the medication.**

c. Safe antibiotics to use during pregnancy include oral /topical erythromycin, topical clindamycin, or azelaic acid.

B. Teens/adults:

1. Review risk factors prior to using oral contraceptives for treatment for acne. Avoid in clients who may have an increased risk of deep vein thrombosis (DVT).

2. Contraceptives with progestin only and/or high androgenic properties should be avoided due to worsening acne for these clients.

Bibliography

Acmaz, G., Cınar, L., Acmaz, B., Aksoy, H., Kafadar, Y. T., Madendag, Y., … Muderris, I. (2019). The effects of oral isotretinoin in women with acne and polycystic ovary syndrome. *BioMed Research International, 2019*, 1–5. doi:10.1155/2019/2513067

Brackenbury, J. (2016). Recommended topical treatments for managing adult acne in women. *Nurse Prescribing, 14*(3), 126–129. doi:10.12968/npre.2016.14.3.126

Graber, E. (2019) Treatment of acne vulgaris. *UpToDate*. Retrieved from https://www.uptodate-com.ckmproxy.vumc.org/contents/treatment-of-acne-vulgaris?search=acne%20vulgaris&sectionRank=3&usage_type=default&anchor=H40&source=machineLearning&selectedTitle=1-150&display_rank=1#H40

Kang, A., Lyons, A., Herrmann, J., & Moy, R. (2019). Treatment of moderate-to-severe facial acne vulgaris with solid-state fractional 589/1, 319-nm laser. *Journal of Clinical & Aesthetic Dermatology, 12*(3), 28–31.

Radley, K. (2015). The management and treatment of acnes. *Primary Health Care, 25*(4), 34–41. doi:10.7748/phc.25.4.34.e996

Zito, P. M., & Murgia, R. D., III. (2019). Complementary alternative therapies: Green tea flavonoids in acne vulgaris. *Journal of the Dermatology Nurses' Association, 11*(2), 91–92. doi:10.1097/JDN.0000000000000453

Animal Bites, Mammalian

Jill C. Cash and Amy C. Bruggemann

Definition

A. Bites of any mammalian animal to the human can be potentially dangerous. Human bites are included.

Incidence

A. There are approximately 4.5 million animal bites in the United States each year. Ninety percent of those are dog bites and 20% of those bites become infected.

B. There are approximately 400,000 cat bites per year in the United States, accounting for 10% of total animal bites and up to 50% of those bites become infected.

C. Human bites account for 250,000 bites annually and 10% of those bites become infected.

D. Children and the elderly are more prone to bites.

Pathogenesis

A. Mechanical trauma and break in skin and/or underlying structures

B. Infection from transmission of bacteria:

1. *Pasteurella multocida* is primarily associated with cat bites but may also be associated with dog bites.

2. *Staphylococcus aureus*, *Staphylococcus epidermis*, and *Enterobacter* species can be transmitted by dog and cat bites.

3. *Streptobacillus moniliformis* can be transmitted by rat and mouse bites.

4. *Streptococcus, Staphylococcus*, and *Eikenella* can be transmitted by human bites.

5. Human bites can transmit diseases such as actinomycosis, syphilis, tuberculosis, hepatitis B, and potentially HIV.

C. Rabies, an acute viral infection, may be transmitted by means of infected saliva or by an infected animal licking mucosa of an open wound. It is rarely contracted by means of airborne transmission, but this has been reported to occur in bat-infested caves.

Predisposing Factors

A. Entering an animal's territorial space and/or surprising an animal

Common Complaints

A. Bitten

B. Pain

C. Redness

D. Swelling

Other Signs and Symptoms

A. Normal: Mild redness and swelling, sero-sanguinous oozing, discomfort

B. Abnormal: Erythema, fever, pus, red streaks, pain, loss of sensation

Subjective Data

A. What person or type of animal bit the client?

B. Was this a provoked or an unprovoked attack?

C. Did the client identify and contact the owner of the animal?

D. What was the behavior of the animal: Unusual, strange, or ill appearing?

E. How much time elapsed from being bitten to seeking treatment?

F. Did the client start any self-treatment?

G. What is the client's tetanus immunization status?

H. Review history for any prior rabies immunizations

I. Does the client know if the animal was a domestic animal? Is the animal's vaccination status known?

J. If the bite is of human origin, determine if it is a closed-fist injury or plain bite.

Physical Examination

A. Check blood pressure, pulse, and respirations, and observe overall respiratory status.

B. See Table 4.1.

Diagnostic Tests

A. Refer to Table 4.1.

Differential Diagnoses

A. Animal bite: Dog, cat, human, and so forth:

1. Cat bites more frequently become infected.

2. Bites on the hand have the highest infection rates. Bites on the face have the lowest infection rates.

B. Cellulitis and abscesses

C. High-risk potential for rabies from the following:

1. Skunks, foxes, raccoons, and bats are primary carriers.

2. Rabbits, squirrels, chipmunks, rats, and mice are seldom infective for rabies.

3. Properly vaccinated animals seldom are infective.

Plan

A. General interventions:

1. Control bleeding.

2. Perform wound care:

   a. Immediately wash wound copiously with soap and water.

   b. Irrigate wound with saline using a 20-gauge or larger catheter.

   c. Use 150 to 1,000 mL of solution.

   d. Direct saline stream on the entire wound surface.

   e. Scrub entire surrounding area.

   f. Debride all wounds.

   g. Trim any jagged edges to prevent cosmetic and/or functional complications.

   h. Cover with dry dressing.

3. Do not suture wounds with high risk of infection:

   a. Hand bites, closed-fist injuries

   b. Bites older than 12 hours (greater than 24 hours on the face)

   c. Deep, crush, or puncture wounds

   d. Bites with extensive injury of surface or underlying structures

4. Rabies control measures:

   a. Consult with the local health department regarding the risk of rabies in the area.

   b. The domestic animal should be identified, caught, and confined for 10 days of observation. If the animal develops any signs of rabies, it should be destroyed and its brain tissue should be

---

TABLE 4.1   EXAMINATION AND TESTING FOR BITES

Animal	Signs and Symptoms	Physical Examination: Check Client Temperature for All Animal Bites	Diagnostic Tests
Dog	Crush injury, lacerations, and abrasions	Inspect site; underlying structures; and distal neurovascular, motor, and sensory functions. Palpate area. If wound is more than 24 hours old, check for any signs of cellulitis or lymphangitis	If infected—Laboratory: CBC, culture, and sensitivity for anaerobes and aerobes
Cat	Puncture wounds, may be deep	Determine depth and extent of wound. Check for foreign bodies. If wound is more than 24 hours old, check for any signs of cellulitis or lymphangitis	If sepsis suspected— Laboratory: CBC, culture, and sensitivity of abscess/ tissue site
Rat and squirrel	Laceration, abrasions; more superficial in nature	Check for signs of infection if wound is more than 24 hours old. Check for any signs of cellulitis or lymphangitis.	
Human	Crush injury, laceration; wound of hand (closed-fist wound)	Check for signs of infection if wound is more than 24 hours old. Check for any signs of cellulitis or lymphangitis. Also, examine for fractures, air in the joint, subchondral bone defects, and osteomyelitis. Examine for full range of interphalangeal and metacarpophalangeal joints.	If infected—Laboratory: CBC, culture, and sensitivity Also, take an X-ray film of structures underlying the bite.

analyzed. No treatment is necessary if results are negative.

c. The wild animal should be caught and destroyed for brain tissue analysis. No treatment is necessary if results are negative.

d. If the bat or wild carnivore cannot be found, rabies prophylaxis is instituted.

B. Client teaching:

1. Stress the importance of keeping the site free from infection. Instruct the client on how to keep the site free from infection such as teaching cleaning techniques, good handwashing, and using medications as prescribed.

2. Discuss symptoms to report to the provider if signs of infection begin (erythema, swelling, drainage, and tenderness).

C. Pharmaceutical therapy:

1. Antibiotic prophylaxis is controversial, but it is generally recommended for wounds involving subcutaneous tissues and deeper structures. Prophylaxis may be prescribed 3 to 5 days and antibiotic treatment for established infection is 5 to 14 days.

a. Amoxicillin/clavulanic acid (Augmentin) 875 mg every 12 hours; for children, prescribe 25 to 45 mg/kg/dose in two divided doses for 3 to 7 days. Available as 200 mg/5 mL and 400 mg/ 5 mL liquid

b. **For adults allergic to penicillin**, prescribe doxycycline 100 mg twice per day for 3 to 7 days; TMP-SMX 1 tab twice a day , or fluroquinolone (ciprofloxacin 500–750 bid or levofloxacin 750 mg daily) PLUS metronidazole 500 mg three times per day or clindamycin 300 to 450 mg three times per day OR moxifloxacin 400 mg daily monotherapy

c. For children allergic to penicillin, prescribe clindamycin 7.5 to 10 mg per kg divided every 6 to 8 hours PLUS trimethoprim/sulfamethoxazole 4 to 6 mg per kg (trimethoprim component) divided every 12 hours for 3 to 7 days

2. Tetanus prophylaxis: Tetanus-toxoid-containing vaccine should be given for any wound (minor or major) if vaccination status is unknown or less than three doses have been received in the past. For major wounds: Human tetanus immune globulin should also be given to anyone of unknown status or has received less than three doses in the past. Tetanus-toxoid-containing vaccine should be given to anyone who has received more than three doses in the past if the last dose is more than 10 years for clean/ minor wounds and more than 5 years for all other major wounds. Human tetanus immunoglobulin is not recommended for anyone who has received more than three previous doses of tetanus toxoid.

3. Rabies prophylaxis:

a. Active immunization: Human diploid cell vaccine (HDCV), 1 mL, is given intramuscularly (IM) on the first day of treatment, and repeat doses are administered on days 3, 7, 14, and 28.

b. Passive immunization: Rabies immunoglobulin (RIG); (human) should be used simultaneously with the first dose of HDCV; the recommended dose of RIG is 20 IU/kg. Approximately one half of RIG is infiltrated into the wound, and the remainder is given IM.

Follow-Up

A. Evaluate wound and change dressing in 24 to 48 hours.

B. Reevaluate as indicated. If the client is on immunoprophylaxis and has no signs of infection, see the client in 1 week.

C. Instruct the client to return immediately in case of any signs of infection.

Consultation/Referral

A. Refer all clients with bites in the ears, face, genitalia, hands, and feet.

B. Consult with a doctor if suspicion of rabies is involved.

C. Contact the local health department.

D. Wounds involving tendon, joint, or bone require hospitalization and surgical consultation.

Individual Considerations

A. Pregnancy: Use appropriate antibiotic management.

B. Pediatrics: Children are more prone to animal bites.

C. Geriatrics: The elderly population is more prone to animal bites.

Bibliography

Aziz, H., Rhee, P., Pandit, V., Tang, A., Gries, L., & Joseph, B. (2015). The current concepts in management of animal (dog, cat, snake, scorpion) and human bite wounds. *Journal of Trauma and Acute Care Surgery, 78*(3), 641–648. doi:10.1097/TA.0000000000000531

Bula-Rudas, F. J., & Olcott, J. L. (2018). Human and Animal Bites. *Pediatrics in Review, 39*(10), 490–500. doi:10.1542/pir.2017-0212

Benign Skin Lesions

Jill C. Cash and Amy C. Bruggemann

Definition

A benign skin lesion is a cutaneous growth with no harmful effects to the body. Benign lesions must be distinguished from the following:

A. Basal cell carcinoma (BCC): Nodular tumor with pearly surface, telangiectasia on surface, and depressed center or rolled edge

B. Squamous cell carcinoma (SCC): Irregular papule, with scaly, friable, bleeding surface

C. Malignant melanoma: Asymmetric papule, with irregular border, of two or more colors, and size varies

Incidence

A. Benign lesions are common to all races, and they are seen primarily in the adult and elderly populations.

Pathogenesis

A. The course varies, depending on the specific type of lesion.

Predisposing Factors
A. Sun exposure in the adult and elderly populations
B. Dermatosis papulosa nigra: Common in African Americans and Asians

Common Complaints
New lesion of the skin

Other Signs and Symptoms
A. Actinic keratosis (Figure 4.3): Rough, scaly patch on your skin that develops from years of exposure to the sun. They are most commonly found on your face, lips, ears, back of your hands, forearms, scalp, or neck. These areas should be monitored closely as they can become cancerous.
B. Dermatosis papulosa nigra: Hyperpigmented mole located on face or neck; a pedunculated papule that is symmetric, 1 to 3 mm in diameter
C. Cherry angioma: Vascular papule, red to purple, located on trunk in adults; begins in early adulthood; 1- to 3-mm diameter papules that do not blanch
D. Solar lentigines (liver spots): Tan maculae on sun-exposed areas in elders, especially on face and hands; border is irregular, and the size varies
E. Sebaceous hyperplasia: Enlarged sebaceous glands that appear as yellow papules on sun-exposed areas, especially on the face in elders; papules have central umbilication, and their size varies

FIGURE 4.3 Example of actinic keratosis.

Source: Reproduced from Lyons, F., & Ousley, L. (2015). *Dermatology for the advanced practice nurse.* New York, NY: Springer Publishing Company, Figure III.48.

F. Seborrheic keratosis: Waxy papules with a stuck-on appearance are seen in adults; they appear symmetric, 0.2 to 3.0 cm in size, with a well-demarcated border and a variety of colors (tan, black, and brown)

Subjective Data
A. Identify when the client first discovered the lesion.
B. Determine whether the lesion has changed in size, shape, or color.
C. Ask if the client has discovered more lesions.
D. Elicit information regarding a family history of skin lesions or cancer.

Physical Examination
A. Inspect:
    1. Observe skin; note all lesions and evaluate each for asymmetry, border, color, diameter, evolving changes, and/or elevation change.
    2. Note the client's skin type.

Diagnostic Tests
A. Benign lesions do not require any tests.
B. If unsure regarding possible malignancy, a biopsy is recommended.

Differential Diagnoses
A. Benign skin lesion:
    1. Seborrheic keratosis
    2. Dermatosis papulosa nigra
    3. Cherry angioma
    4. Solar lentigines
    5. Senile sebaceous hyperplasia
    6. Keratoacanthoma

Plan
A. General interventions:
    1. Reassure the client that lesions are benign. No treatment is required unless the client chooses to have the lesion removed for cosmetic purposes.
    2. Benign skin lesions may be removed using cryotherapy if they are bothersome for the client.
B. Client teaching: *See Section III: Client Teaching Guide for this chapter, "Skin Care Assessment."* ◄
C. Pharmaceutical therapy:
    1. Medications are not recommended for treatment.

Follow-Up
A. Routine skin examinations should be performed yearly

Consultation/Referral
A. Immediately refer the client to a dermatologist if malignancy is suspected or confirmed by biopsy.

Individual Considerations
A. Adults: Skin lesions begin to appear in early adulthood. Encourage clients to monitor lesions over time.
B. Geriatrics: Benign lesions are commonly seen in the elderly population.

Bibliography
Boer, F. L., ten Eikelder, M. L. G., Kapiteijn, E. H., Creutzberg, C. L., Galaal, K., & van Poelgeest, M. I. E. (2019). Vulvar malignant melanoma: Pathogenesis, clinical behaviour and management: Review of

the literature. *Cancer Treatment Reviews*, *73*, 91–103. doi:10.1016/j.ctrv.2018.12.005

Broccolo, F., Drago, F., Ciccarese, G., Genoni, A., Porro, A., Parodi, A., … Toniolo, A. (2019). Possible long-term sequelae in hand, foot, and mouth disease caused by Coxsackievirus A6. *Journal of the American Academy of Dermatology*, *80*(3), 804–806. doi:10.1016/j.jaad.2018.08.034

Candidiasis

Jill C. Cash and Amy C. Bruggemann

Definition

A. A fungal infection of the mucous membranes and/or skin, candidiasis is caused by the *Candida albicans* fungus (Figure 4.4).

Incidence

A. It occurs frequently in women, children, and the elderly population.

Pathogenesis

An overgrowth of *C. albicans* occurs when mucous membranes and/or skin are exposed to moisture, warmth, and an alteration in the membrane barrier.

Predisposing Factors

A. Immunosuppression
B. Use of antibiotics
C. Hyperglycemia
D. Chronic use of steroid
E. Frequent douching by women
F. Adults wearing dentures

Common Complaints

A. Oral: A persistent white patch on the tongue or roof of mouth may be slightly reddened with or without crevices on the tongue.
B. Vaginal: Thick, white, "cottage-cheese-like" vaginal discharge with or without vaginal itching.

FIGURE 4.4 Candidiasis (diaper rash on female newborn).

Source: Reproduced from Kifer, Z. A. (2012). *Fast facts for wound care nursing: Practical wound management in a nutshell* (p. 264). New York, NY: Springer Publishing Company.

C. Genital: Bright red rash with well-demarcated satellite lesions advancing to pustules or erosions in genital or diaper area.
D. Males: Erythemic rash that may advance to erosions seen on male genitalia; scrotum is perhaps involved.

Subjective Data

A. Question the client about onset, duration, and location of lesions.
B. Determine whether the client has a history of previous infections.
C. Inquire into medical history and current medications.
D. Rule out the presence of any other current medical conditions.

Physical Examination

A. Inspect:
    1. Assess skin and mucous membranes for discharge and lesions.
    2. Observe location and severity of lesions.
B. Palpate
    1. Palpate lymph nodes in neck and groin.

Diagnostic Tests

A. Vaginal and genital infections need to be evaluated for sexually transmitted infections (STIs), especially if the client is sexually active with multiple partners. Vaginal/genital culture specimen should be sent for gonorrhea/chlamydia testing.
B. Other specimens to consider include wet prep/potassium hydroxide (KOH) 10% solution, Gram stain vaginal culture for *Candida*.

Differential Diagnoses

A. Oral candidiasis:
    1. Leukoplakia
    2. Stomatitis
    3. Formula (for newborns)
B. Diaper area:
    1. Candidiasis
    2. Contact dermatitis
    3. Bacterial infection
C. Genital area:
    1. Candidiasis
    2. Bacterial infection
    3. Bacterial vaginosis
    4. Chlamydia
    5. Gonorrhea
    6. Trichomoniasis

Plan

A. General interventions:
    1. Treatment can be successful with good hygiene and medications.
    2. Stress to the client to keep the affected area cool and dry. Frequent changes of clothing may be necessary to keep the area cool and dry to avoid damp conditions.
    3. Diaper area will need to be changed more frequently; suggest using cloth diapers and allowing skin to be exposed to air for short periods.

B. Client teaching:
1. Use medication on the skin to help with symptoms.
2. Do not scratch. Keep fingernails short.
C. Pharmaceutical therapy: Choose *one* of the following pharmaceutical therapies:
1. Oral:
a. Nystatin (Mycostatin) oral suspension 100,000 U/mL, 2 mL for infants and 4 to 6 mL for older children and adults, four times daily for 7 to 10 days
b. Gentian violet aqueous solution, 1% for infants and 2% for adults, one to two times per day
c. Lotrimin buccal troches, five times per day for 2 weeks, only for adults
2. Diaper:
a. Nystatin cream, three to four times per day for 7 to 10 days
b. Mycolog II; apply sparingly to skin twice daily until resolved
3. Vaginal:
a. Clotrimazole 1% cream, 5 g intravaginally for 7 to 14 days
b. Miconazole 2% cream, 5 g intravaginally for 7 days (over the counter [OTC])
c. Terconazole 0.8% cream, 5 g intravaginally for 3 days
d. Terconazole 80 mg vaginal suppository, at bedtime for 3 days
e. Fluconazole (Diflucan) 150 mg, oral tablet one time
f. Other preparations available in stronger or weaker doses

Follow-Up
A. None indicated unless not resolved or complications arise

Consultation/Referral
A. Consult a physician if not resolved within 2 weeks.

Individual Considerations
A. Pregnancy:
1. Most effective medications for pregnant women are clotrimazole, miconazole, and terconazole
2. Recommend a full 7-day course of treatment during pregnancy
B. Adults:
1. Consider immunosuppression in all adults with oral candidiasis (HIV, diabetes, chemotherapy, leukemia)
2. Adults with oral lesions need to be assessed for leukoplakia, especially if the client has a history of smoking or chewing tobacco

Bibliography
Hillier, S., Gould, V., Beamer, M., Kaiser, J., & Juul, J. (2019). Diagnostic accuracy of clinical criteria for bacterial vaginosis, vulvovaginal candidiasis and BV/VVC co-infections. *American Journal of Obstetrics & Gynecology*, *221*(6), 671–672. https://doi-org.proxy.library.vanderbilt.edu/10.1016/j.ajog.2019.10.085

Latti, P., Ramanarayanan, S., & Prashant, G. M. (2019). Antifungal efficacy of spice extracts against Candida albicans: An in vitro study. *Indian Journal of Community Medicine*, *44*, S77–S80. https://doi-org.proxy.library.vanderbilt.edu/10.4103/ijcm.IJCM_140_19

Contact Dermatitis

Jill C. Cash and Amy C. Bruggemann

Definition
A. Contact dermatitis is a cutaneous response to direct exposure of the skin to irritants (irritant contact dermatitis) or allergens (allergic contact dermatitis). See Figure 4.5 for examples of contact dermatitis.
1. Irritant contact dermatitis is a nonimmunologic response of the epidermis.
2. Allergic contact dermatitis is an immunologic response after one or more exposures to a particular agent.

Incidence
A. Occurs in all ages. People who work with chemicals daily and wash their hands numerous times a day have a higher incidence of irritant dermatitis. Irritant contact dermatitis is seen in the elderly because of dry skin.

Pathogenesis
A. Irritant contact dermatitis is caused by an alteration of the outer layer of the dermis caused by exposure to chemicals; lotions; cold, dry air; soaps; detergents; or organic solvents.
B. Allergic contact dermatitis is caused by an alteration in the epidermis when, after exposure to an allergen, the immune system responds by producing inflammation of the cutaneous tissue. Common allergens include poison ivy, poison oak, sumac, nickel jewelry, hair dye, rubber and leather chemicals (latex gloves), cleaning supplies, harsh soaps, detergents, and topical medicines.

Predisposing Factors
A. Occupation (hairdresser, nurse, housecleaner, etc.)
B. Jewelry
C. Activities in yard or woods

Common Complaints
A. Irritation of the skin, ranging from redness to pruritic inflammation, with possible progression of blisters:
1. Poison oak, ivy, and sumac induce classic presentation: Lesions (vesicles) and papules on an erythemic base presenting in a linear fashion with sharp margins
2. Diffuse pattern with erythema may be seen when oleoresin is contacted with pets or smoke from burning fire.
B. Exposure to some type of irritant known to the client. Round or annular lesions may have an internal cause such as a drug reaction.

Other Signs and Symptoms
A. Chronic:
1. Erythema with thickening
2. Scaling
3. Fissures
4. Inflammation; with chronic dermatitis, lichenification may occur with scales and fissures
B. Diaper dermatitis: Prominent red, shiny rash on buttocks and genitalia

FIGURE 4.5 (ABC) Examples of contact dermatitis and (D) facial contact dermatitis.

Source: Reproduced from Lyons, F., & Ousley, L. (2015). *Dermatology for the advanced practice nurse.* New York, NY: Springer Publishing Company, Figures III.15, III.16.

C. Candidiasis diaper rash:
  1. Bright red rash with satellite lesions at margins
  2. Inflammation and excoriations present
  3. Creases may be involved

Subjective Data

A. Ask the client when irritation began and how it has progressed.

B. Elicit history of exposure to allergens.

C. Question the client regarding activity and skin contact with irritants before outbreak (cleaning agents, walking in woods, hobbies, change in soap/laundry detergent, shaving cream, lotions, etc.).

D. List occupation and family history of allergens.

E. Review medication list, including prescription, OTC, and herbal medicines, to evaluate an interaction.

F. List medications used to relieve symptoms and results.

Physical Examination

A. Check temperature (if indicated).

B. Inspect:
  1. Inspect skin, noting types of lesions and location of lesions. **Note the pattern of inflammation. The shape of irritation may mimic the shape of the irritant, such as the skin under a ring or watch, for example.**

  2. Determine progression of lesions.
  3. Differentiate between primary and secondary lesions.

Diagnostic Tests

A. Consider none if source is known.

B. Wet mount (potassium hydroxide [KOH], saline) to rule out fungal infection if candida is suspected

C. Culture/sensitivity of pustules

D. Patch test to rule out allergic contact dermatitis

Differential Diagnoses

A. Irritant contact dermatitis

B. Allergic contact dermatitis

C. Diaper dermatitis

D. Candida

E. Tinea pedis, corporis, cruris

F. Drug reactions

G. Pityriasis rosea

H. Scabies

Plan

A. General interventions:
  1. Irritant contact dermatitis: Removal of irritating agent:
     a. Use topical soaks with saline or Burow's solution (1:40 dilution) for weeping areas.

b. Suggest lukewarm baths (not hot); or oatmeal (Aveeno) baths, as needed.

c. For dry erythematous skin, recommend Eucerin or Aquaphor ointments to rehydrate skin.

d. Remind the client to avoid scratching skin and to keep nails short.

e. Suggest use of mild soaps and cleansers.

2. Allergic contact dermatitis:

a. Instruct the client to avoid contact with the causative agent.

b. Have the client wash the affected area with cool water immediately after exposure.

c. Recommend lukewarm baths with oatmeal (Aveeno) three to four times per day.

d. Tell the client to apply calamine lotion after baths.

3. Diaper dermatitis:

a. Instruct the caretaker to change the client's diaper frequently, cleaning with water only, and allow skin to air dry 15 to 30 minutes four times a day. Tell the parent not to use lotions or powders, but to apply zinc oxide (Desitin ointment or powder, or Happy Hiney) with each diaper change.

b. If candidiasis diaper rash presents, for treatment refer to the "Candidiasis" section in this chapter.

▶ B. Client teaching: *See Section III: Client Teaching Guide for this chapter, "Dermatitis."*

C. Pharmaceutical therapy:

1. Irritant contact dermatitis: Hydrocortisone 2.5% ointment three to four times per day for 2 weeks

2. Allergic contact dermatitis:

a. Low-dose topical steroids: Hydrocortisone 2.5% ointment three to four times per day for 1 to 2 weeks after blistering stage. Triamcinolone acetonide 0.025% (Kenalog) ointment/cream twice daily

b. Intermediate-dose topical steroids: Triamcinolone acetonide 0.1% (Kenalog) cream twice daily. Cream/ointment should not be used longer than 2 weeks at a time.

c. High-potent topical steroids: Fluocinonide 0.05% (Lidex) ointment three to four times per day; not to be used on face or skin folds. Cream/ointment should not be used longer than 2 weeks at a time.

d. Hydroxyzine 25 to 50 mg four times daily, diphenhydramine Hcl (Benadryl) 25 to 50 mg four times daily. For children, 0.5 mg/kg/dose three times daily as needed

e. If the rash is severe (face, eyes, genitalia, mucous membranes), consider prednisone 60 to 80 mg/d to start and taper over 10 to 14 days.

f. Triamcinolone acetonide (Kenalog) 40 to 60 mg by IM injection

3. Secondary bacterial infections: Erythromycin 250 mg four times daily or amoxicillin/clavulanic acid (Augmentin) 875 mg twice daily for 10 days

4. Candidiasis:

a. Use miconazole nitrate 2% cream, miconazole powder, or nystatin cream.

b. Use clotrimazole (Lotrimin) or ketoconazole (Nizoral) cream three to four times per day for 10 days.

c. If inflammation is present along with yeast, use Mycolog II.

d. If secondary bacterial infection is present, use mupirocin (Bactroban) ointment three times daily for 7 to 10 days.

Follow-Up

A. None required if case is mild.

B. See the client again in 2 to 3 days for severe cases, or phone to assess progress.

Consultation/Referral

A. Consult with a physician when steroid treatment is necessary or if worsening symptoms develop despite adequate therapy.

Individual Considerations

A. Pregnancy: If medications are necessary during pregnancy, consider the gestational age of the fetus and category of medication.

B. Pediatrics: For infants and children, consider hydroxyzine (Atarax) 0.5 mg/kg/dose three times daily as needed for severe pruritus.

C. Elderly: Clients may only exhibit scaling as the prominent irritation rather than erythema and inflammation. Topical medications (neomycin, vitamin E, lanolin) and acrylate adhesives are common causes of contact dermatitis.

Bibliography

Schadler, E. D., & Kamat, D. (2019). Common annular lesions in the pediatric population: Part 2. *Pediatric Annals, 48*(3), e135–e138. doi:10.3928/19382359-20190222-01

Trayes, K. P., Savage, K., & Studdiford, J. S. (2018). Annular lesions: Diagnosis and treatment. *American Family Physician, 98*(5), 283–291.

Eczema or Atopic Dermatitis

Jill C. Cash and Amy C. Bruggemann

Definition

A. This pattern of skin inflammation has clinical features of erythema, itching, scaling, lichenification, papules, and vesicles in various combinations. Currently, the term *eczema* is used interchangeably with *dermatitis*. Most common variants are atopic dermatitis (Figure 4.6) and atopic eczema. Classification is done by cause, either endogenous or exogenous.

Incidence

A. Overall prevalence of all forms of eczema is about 18 in 1,000 in the United States.

FIGURE 4.6 Atopic dermatitis.

Source: Reproduced from Kifer, Z. A. (2012). *Fast facts for wound care nursing: Practical wound management in a nutshell* (p. 264). New York, NY: Springer Publishing Company.

B. With atopic dermatitis, 60% of those affected become afflicted between infancy and 12 years of age. It is more common in boys. Approximately 20% of children and 3% of adults are affected.

Pathogenesis

A. Eczema is characterized by a lymphohistiocytic infiltration around the upper dermal vessels. Epidermal spongiosis or intercellular epidermal edema and inflammation are seen.

Predisposing Factors

A. Family history of atopic triad: Dermatitis, asthma, and allergic rhinitis
B. Exposure to allergens:
   1. Common foods: Cow's milk, nuts, wheat, soy, and fish
   2. Common environmental allergens: Dust, mold, cat dander, and low humidity (dry air)
C. Exposure to topical medications, most commonly neomycin, lanolin, and topical anesthetics like benzocaine
D. Skin irritants: Harsh soaps, skin-care products with perfumes, chemicals and alcohol, fabrics containing wool, tight clothing
E. Stress

Common Complaints

A. Skin changes:
   1. Itching, impossible to relieve
   2. Dryness
   3. Discoloration, lichenification, and scaling
   4. Skin thickening
   5. Associated bleeding and oozing skin

Other Signs and Symptoms

A. Primary lesions, papules, and pustules that may lead to excoriation
B. Lesions commonly seen on trunk, face, and antecubital and popliteal fossae of children. Adults will have lesions on the face, trunk, neck, and genital area.
C. Other common features include infraorbital fold (Dennie sign), increased palmar creases, facial erythema, and scaling.

Subjective Data

A. Determine whether the onset was sudden or gradual.
B. Ask the client if the skin is itchy or painful.
C. Assess if there is any associated discharge (blood or pus).
D. Ask if the client has recently taken any antibiotics, other oral drugs, or topical medications.
E. Ask the client about use of soaps, creams, or lotions.
F. Assess for any preceding systemic symptoms (fever, sore throat, anorexia, vaginal discharge).
G. Ask the client about recent travel abroad.
H. Rule out insect bites.
I. Rule out any possible exposure to industrial or domestic toxins.
J. Elicit what precipitates itching.
K. Evaluate for increased stress level at home, work, in relationships, and so forth.

Physical Examination

A. Check temperature (if indicated).
B. Inspect:
   1. Inspect skin for lesions.
   2. Recognize bacteria-infected eczema; *S. aureus* is the most common pathogen. It appears with acute weeping dermatitis; crusted, and small, superficial pustules.

Diagnostic Tests

A. Culture skin lesions to determine viral, bacterial, or fungal etiology.
B. Blood work: Serum immunoglobulin E (IgE) is elevated with atopic dermatitis.

Differential Diagnoses

A. Atopic dermatitis, acute or chronic
B. Contact dermatitis, acute or chronic
C. Seborrheic dermatitis
D. Ichthyosis vulgaris
E. Bacterial/fungal infections
F. Neoplastic disease
G. Immunologic and metabolic disorders

Plan

A. General interventions:
   1. Frequently treat the dry skin with emollients (Aquaphor, Eucerin).
   2. Pat, do not rub skin.
   3. Children: Only bathe every two to three nights. Avoid excessive use of soap and water when bathing. Use gentle cleansers such as Cetaphil or Cerave when bathing.
   4. Avoid wool products and lanolin preparations.

5. Keep fingernails cut short to prevent scratching/scarring skin.

6. May need to treat secondary bacterial infections as appropriate.

7. Eliminate trigger foods one at a time for 1 month at a time to see improvement. Begin with eliminating cow's milk products. Consider soy-based foods instead.

8. Allergy testing may be considered if symptoms continue.

9. Ointments are usually recommended over creams for moisturizing.

▶ B. Client teaching: *See Section III: Client Teaching Guide for this chapter, "Eczema."*

C. Pharmaceutical therapy:

1. Atopic: Acute, adult:
   a. Wet dressings with Burow's solution and change every 2 to 3 hours.
   b. Potent topical corticosteroid: Betamethasone valerate 0.1% two to three times daily for up to 2 to 3 weeks
   c. Antihistamine of choice: Cetirizine Hcl (Zyrtec) or diphenhydramine Hcl (Benadryl)
   d. Severe cases: Oral steroid: Prednisone 1 mg/kg (40–60 mg/d) tapered over 2 to 3 weeks

2. Atopic: Acute; occurs in infants and children:
   a. Hydrocortisone: Infants and children—2.5% ointment twice daily; 1% on face and intertriginous areas
   b. Adolescents: Triamcinolone acetonide 0.1% (Aristocort) ointment; apply thinly twice daily for 2 to 3 weeks. **Precautions should be given regarding possibility of hypopigmentation of skin even with short-term use of steroids on skin.**
   c. Antihistamines for itching:
      i. Infants and children: Hydroxyzine (Atarax) 0.5 mg/kg/dose three times daily as needed or diphenhydramine Hcl (Benadryl); for those 2 to 6 years: 6.25 mg every 4 to 6 hours; for those 6 to 12 years: 12.5 to 25 mg every 4 to 6 hours
      ii. Adolescents: Hydroxyzine 25 to 50 mg/dose every 4 to 6 hours or diphenhydramine Hcl (Benadryl)
      iii. Atopic: Chronic, adult—short course of potent topical corticosteroid betamethasone dipropionate (Diprolene) or clobetasol propionate (temovate) twice daily for 7 days
   d. Alternative therapies:
      i. Probiotics have limited benefit.
      ii. Melatonin has been studied and shown to be useful for children 6 to 12 years of age, in addition to the usual treatment of topical corticosteroids and emollients.

3. Antibacterial treatments for secondary bacterial infections: *S. aureus.*
   a. Adults:
      i. Augmentin 875 mg by mouth twice a day for 10 to 14 days
      ii. Keflex 500 mg by mouth four times a day for 10 to 14 days
      iii. Erythromycin 500 mg by mouth four times a day for 10 to 14 days *or*
      iv. Dicloxacillin 250 mg every 6 hours for 10 days
   b. Children:
      i. Augmentin 25 to 45 mg/kg/d by mouth in two divided doses for 10 days
      ii. Erythromycin 30 to 50 mg/kg/d by mouth in two, three, or four evenly divided doses for 10 days
      iii. Omnicef (cefdinir): Not recommended for children younger than 6 months; 6 to 12 months: 7 mg/kg every 12 hours for 10 days

Follow-Up

A. See client in office in 1 to 2 weeks and then every month until condition is stabilized.

B. Monitor the client for superimposed staphylococcal infection; may use oral erythromycin or dicloxacillin.

C. Client may be seen every 3 to 6 months thereafter for client education updates.

Consultation/Referral

A. Eczema herpeticum (herpes simplex type 1) may progress rapidly. Refer the client to a dermatologist.

B. Refer the client to a dermatologist if skin eruptions are severe or fail to respond to conservative treatment.

Individual Considerations

A. Pregnancy: Avoid oral steroids.

B. Children: Teach clients to apply emollients when they have an itch rather than scratching. The goal is to control the rash and symptoms.

C. Young adults and elderly: Nummular eczema is commonly seen, characterized by coin-shaped vesicles and papules seen on extremities and/or trunk.

Bibliography

Nutten, S. (2015). Atopic dermatitis: Global epidemiology and risk factors. *Annals of Nutrition & Metabolism, 66*(Suppl. 1), 8–16. doi:10.1159/000370220

Shi, K., & Lio, P. A. (2019). Alternative treatments for atopic dermatitis: An update. *American Journal of Clinical Dermatology, 20*(2), 251–266. doi:10.1007/s40257-018-0412-3

Tanei, R., & Hasegawa, Y. (2016). Atopic dermatitis in older adults: A viewpoint from geriatric dermatology. *Geriatrics & Gerontology International, 16*(1), 75–86. doi:10.1111/ggi.12771

Trayes, K. P., Savage, K., & Studdiford, J. S. (2018). Annular lesions: Diagnosis and treatment. *American Family Physician, 98*(5), 283–291.

Vandiver, A., & Cohe, B. A. (2016). Vesicular rash in an infant with eczema. *Contemporary Pediatrics, 33*(6), 38–40.

Voelker, R. (2019). Older adults may fuel an upturn in eczema cases. *JAMA: Journal of the American Medical Association, 321*(11), 1038–1039. doi:10.1001/jama.2019.0384

Erythema Multiforme

Jill C. Cash and Amy C. Bruggemann

Definition

A. This dermal and epidermal inflammatory process is characterized by symmetric eruption of erythematous, iris-shaped papules ("target" lesions), and vesiculobullous lesions (Figure 4.7).

FIGURE 4.7 Erythema multiforme.

Source: Reproduced from Kifer, Z. A. (2012). *Fast facts for wound care nursing: Practical wound management in a nutshell* (p. 262). New York, NY: Springer Publishing Company.

Incidence

A. Erythema multiforme accounts for up to 1% of dermatology outpatient visits.
B. Children younger than 3 years and adults older than 50 years are rarely affected.
C. It may occur in seasonal epidemics.
D. Approximately 90% of cases of erythema multiforme minor follow a recent outbreak of herpes simplex virus (HSV)-1 or mycoplasma infection.

Pathogenesis

A. The disorder is thought to be an immunologic reaction in the skin, possibly triggered by circulating immune complexes

Predisposing Factors

A. Infections: Recurrent HSV, mycoplasmal infections, and adenoviral infections
B. Drugs: Sulfonamides, phenytoin, barbiturates, phenylbutazone, penicillin
C. Idiopathic: Greater than 50%; consider occult malignancy

Common Complaints

A. Rash with intense pruritus
B. Nonspecific upper respiratory infection followed by rash
C. General malaise, body aches, and joint pain
D. Fever

Other Signs and Symptoms

A. Primary: Macules, papules, and plaques
B. Secondary: Erythema, dull red target-like lesions blanch to pressure; distribution is symmetric, primarily on flexor surfaces. **Classic target lesions develop abruptly and symmetrically and are heaviest peripherally; they often involve palms and soles.**
C. Swelling of hands and feet
D. Painful oral lesions

E. Eye discomfort (redness, itching, burning, pain, visual changes)

Subjective Data

A. Ask if the client has ever been diagnosed with erythema multiforme.
B. Determine whether the onset of symptoms was sudden or gradual.
C. Assess for any associated discharge (blood or pus).
D. Identify the location of the symptoms.
E. Complete a drug history. Has the client recently taken any antibiotics or other drugs? Question the client regarding use of any topical medications.
F. Determine the presence of any preceding systemic symptoms (fever, sore throat, anorexia, or vaginal discharge).
G. Rule out any possible exposure to industrial or domestic toxins.
H. Question the client concerning any possible contact with venereal disease.
I. Ask the client about any close physical contact with others with skin disorders.
J. Elicit information concerning any possible exposure to HIV.
K. Rule out sources of chronic infection, neoplasia, or connective tissue disease.

Physical Examination

A. Check temperature, pulse, respirations, and blood pressure.
B. Inspect:
   1. Skin for lesions
   2. Mouth and mucous membranes for lesions
C. Palpate abdomen for masses and tenderness.
D. Auscultate heart, lungs, and abdomen.
E. Neurologic examination

Diagnostic Tests

A. Punch biopsy of skin
B. Complete blood count (CBC)
C. Urinalysis

Differential Diagnoses

A. Erythema multiforme:
   1. Erythema multiforme minor: Pruritus, swelling of hands and feet, painful oral lesions
   2. Erythema multiforme major: Fever, arthralgias, myalgias, cough, oral erosions with severe pain
B. Urticaria
C. Viral exanthems
D. Stevens–Johnson syndrome (SJS): **SJS is a severe, life-threatening, systemic reaction with fever, malaise, cough, sore throat, chest pain, vomiting, diarrhea, myalgia, arthralgia, and severe skin manifestations with painful bullous lesions on mucous membranes (Figure 4.8).**
E. Pemphigus vulgaris
F. Bullous pemphigoid
G. Other bullous diseases
H. Staphylococcal scalded skin syndrome
I. Vasculitis

FIGURE 4.8   Stevens–Johnson syndrome.

Source: Reproduced from Kifer, Z. A. (2012). *Fast facts for wound care nursing: Practical wound management in a nutshell* (p. 253). New York, NY: Springer Publishing Company.

Plan

A. General interventions:
1. Identify and treat precipitating causes or triggers.
2. Burow's solution or warm compresses may be used for mild cases as needed.
3. Oral lesions may be treated with saline solution, warm salt water, and/or Mary's mouthwash (Benadryl, lidocaine, and Kaopectate).
4. Discontinue any medications suspected of precipitating symptoms.
5. Provide adequate pain relief if skin or oral lesions are painful. Lesions remain fixed at least 7 days.
6. Maintain nutrition and fluid replacement for this hypercatabolic state.
7. Consider chronic viral suppression therapy for recurrent herpes simplex viral infections.
► B. Client teaching: *See Section III: Client Teaching Guide for this chapter, "Erythema Multiforme."*
C. Pharmaceutical therapy:
1. Antihistamines, such as Benadryl or Claritin, may be used for itching.
2. Acetaminophen may be used to reduce fever and for general discomfort/pain.
3. Potent topical corticosteroids: Betamethasone dipropionate 0.05% or clobetasol propionate 0.05% twice daily for up to 2 weeks. Avoid use on face and groin.
4. Open lesions should be treated like open burn wounds. Stop offending medications that may cause blistering of wounds and treat with steroids.
5. Oral antibiotics may be needed to control secondary bacterial skin infection.
6. Oral steroids may be used for severe oral mucosal lesions, oral prednisone 40 to 60 mg/d tapering over 2 to 4 weeks.
7. Hospitalization for severe cases. Intravenous immunoglobulins may be needed.

Follow-Up

A. See the client in the office in 1 to 2 days to evaluate initial treatment.

Consultation/Referral

A. If the client has recurrent or chronic infection, refer him or her to a physician.
B. Immediate consultation and/or hospital admission is critical if SJS is suspected.

Individual Considerations

A. Pediatrics: Systemic corticosteroids may increase the risk of infection and prolong healing. Use low- to mid-potency topical corticosteroids.
B. Adults/Pediatrics: Eye involvement can lead to keratitis, scarring or vision loss. Referral to ophthalmologist is recommended.

Bibliography

dall'Oglio, F., Lacarrubba, F., Luca, M., Boscaglia, S., & Micali, G. (2018). Clinical and erythema-directed instrumental evaluation of papulopustular rosacea treated with topical ivermectin. *Journal of the American Academy of Dermatology*, *79*, AB75. doi:10.1016/j.jaad.2018.05.335

Hashemi, D. A., Carlos, C., & Rosenbach, M. (2019). Herpes-associated erythema multiforme. *JAMA Dermatology*, *155*(1), 108. doi:10.1001/jamadermatol.2018.3973

Kaplan, D. L. (2018). What is the cause of these papules? *Consultant (00107069)*, *58*(7), 1–4.

Trayes, K. P., Savage, K., & Studdiford, J. S. (2018). Annular lesions: Diagnosis and treatment. *American Family Physician*, *98*(5), 283–291.

Folliculitis

Jill C. Cash and Amy C. Bruggemann

Definition

A. Folliculitis is a bacterial infection of the hair follicle.
B. Malassezia folliculitis, also known as pityrosporum, is an inflammatory skin disorder of the hair follicle triggered by yeast (Figure 4.9). This is often confused with acne vulgaris; the defining difference is itch.

Incidence

A. A very common disorder, folliculitis occurs in all ages and is seen more frequently in males.
B. Malassezia folliculitis is commonly seen in clients with immunosuppression, diabetes, and antibiotic use.

Pathogenesis

A. Bacterial organisms (most commonly *S. aureus*) invade the follicle wall and cause an infectious process.
B. For malassezia folliculitis, fungal organisms invade the follicle walls and cause a fungal infection that causes a pruritic rash.

Predisposing Factors

A. Break in the skin tissue
B. Use of razors on skin
C. Poor hygiene
D. Diabetes

Common Complaint

A. Outbreak of pustules on the face, scalp, or extremities that do not resolve despite proper hygiene and care

FIGURE 4.9 Folliculitis.

Source: Reproduced from Kifer, Z. A. (2012). *Fast facts for wound care nursing: Practical wound management in a nutshell* (p. 260). New York, NY: Springer Publishing Company.

Other Signs and Symptoms

A. Tenderness and itching at the site
B. Furuncle (abscess): A deep pustule, tender, firm or fluctuant, found in groin, axilla, waistline, or buttocks
C. Carbuncle: A group of follicles coalescing into one larger, painful, infected area; fever and chills possible
D. Excoriated folliculitis: Chronic thickened, excoriated papules or nodules

Subjective Data

A. Elicit the initial outbreak of lesions and onset and progression of lesions.
B. Identify what makes the lesions better or worse.
C. Ask the client what medications, soaps, or lotions have been used on the lesions.
D. Complete a medical history. Ask if the client has had an outbreak similar to this before.
E. Describe systemic symptoms if they have occurred (fever, chills, etc.).
F. Does the client have a beard, shave his face, or use a razor frequently?
G. Is there a recent history of use of a hot tub? (Commonly seen 1–4 days after use of hot tub, whirlpool, or swimming pool)
H. Does the client wear tight pants/jeans or use oils that clog pores in the groin area?
I. Is the client currently being treated with antibiotics for acne? (May see flare of gram-negative folliculitis with chronic use of antibiotics)

Physical Examination

A. Check temperature, pulse, respirations, and blood pressure.
B. Inspect: Assess skin for lesions and describe.
C. Palpate: Palpate lesions and associated lymph nodes.

Diagnostic Tests

A. Culture and sensitivity to verify appropriate antibiotic coverage
B. Gram stain
C. Potassium hydroxide (KOH)/wet prep
D. Fungal culture hair if fungi suspected (tinea of scalp)
E. Skin biopsy for the diagnosis of malassezia folliculitis

Differential Diagnoses

A. Folliculitis
B. Acne vulgaris
C. Ingrown hair follicle
D. Keratosis pilaris
E. Contact dermatitis

Plan

A. General interventions:
    1. Apply warm, moist compresses to site for comfort.
B. Client teaching:
    1. *See Section III: Client Teaching Guide for this chapter, "Folliculitis."*
    2. If razors are used on the area, have the client use clean, sharp razors, throw old razors away, and not share razors. Avoid use of irritating creams or lotions on affected area.
    3. Encourage proper hygiene, with frequent washing of hands and skin with an antibacterial soap.
    4. Warm compresses three to four times a day are encouraged at the site for 15 to 20 minutes.
    5. Bleach bath (0.5–1 cup of bleach to 20 L water) reduces spread of *Staphylococcus* infection.
C. Pharmaceutical therapy:
    1. Mild cases: Topical antibiotics are recommended before oral antibiotics. Apply mupirocin (Bactroban) ointment to affected area three times daily until resolved.
    2. *S. aureus:*
        a. Dicloxacillin (Dynapen) 250 mg by mouth four times daily for 10 to 14 days
        b. Erythromycin 250 mg by mouth four times daily for 10 to 14 days
        c. Cephalexin (Keflex) 500 mg by mouth for 10 to 14 days
    3. *Pseudomonas aeruginosa:*
        a. Ciprofloxacin (Cipro) 500 mg by mouth twice daily for 10 days
        b. Ofloxacin 400 mg by mouth twice daily for 10 days
    4. Antistaphylococcal antibiotics:
        a. Cephalexin 250 to 500 mg four times a day (children: 25–50 mg/kg/d given in two divided doses)
        b. Clindamycin 150 to 300 mg four times a day (children: 8–16 mg/kg/d in three to four doses per day)
        c. Dicloxacillin 125 to 500 mg four times a day (children: 12.5 mg/kg/d four times a day)
        d. Erythromycin 250 to 500 mg four times a day (children: 30–50 mg/kg/d four times a day)
    5. Bacterial infections caused by organisms other than *Staphylococcus* may be treated for an extended period, 4 to 8 weeks. These areas may include axilla, chest, back, beard, and groin.

6. Methicillin-resistant *S. aureus* (MRSA):
   a. Bactrim DS 160/800 twice a day (children: 8–10 mg/kg/d divide and give q12h)
   b. Doxycycline 100 mg twice daily for 1 day and then once a day for the remainder of the duration (children: 2.2 mg/kg twice daily for 1 day and then for the remainder of the duration once a day)
7. Severe cases may be treated with oral antibiotics with topical permethrin every 12 hours every other night for a 6-week period or itraconazole 400 mg daily, isotretinoin 0.5 mg/kg/d for up to 4 to 5 months with ultraviolet B (UVB) light therapy. Consider dermatology referral for severe cases.
8. Treatment for malessezia folliculitis is as follows:
   a. Antifungal treatment: Oral antifungal medications (itraconazole, fluconazole, or ketoconazole) should be prescribed for at least 4 weeks for treatment

Follow-Up

A. If not resolved in 2 weeks, further evaluation is needed.
B. Severe cases, in which carbuncles are not improved with antibiotic therapy, warrant incision and drainage and referral to dermatology.
C. Continue to follow every 2 weeks until resolved.
D. Test for diabetes mellitus in severe cases.

Consultation/Referral

A. Refer the client to a physician for testing for immunodeficiency if severe cases occur or if resistance is seen.
B. Dermatology referral

Bibliography

Rambhia, P. H., Conic, R. R. Z., Murad, A., Atanaskova-Mesinkovska, N., Piliang, M., & Bergfeld, W. (2019). Updates in therapeutics for folliculitis decalvans: A systematic review with evidence-based analysis. *Journal of the American Academy of Dermatology*, *80*(3), 794. doi:10.1016/j.jaad.2018.07.050

Hand, Foot, and Mouth Syndrome

Jill C. Cash and Amy C. Bruggemann

Definition

A. This is a viral infection caused by coxsackievirus A16, with vesicular lesions present on the hands, feet, and oral mucosa (Figure 4.10).

Incidence

A. Hand, foot, and mouth syndrome is most commonly seen in preschool children.

Pathogenesis

A. Enteroviruses invade the intestinal tract of humans and are spread to others by fecal–oral and/or oral–oral (respiratory) routes. The incubation period is approximately 4 to 6 days.

Predisposing Factors

A. Childhood
B. Confined households or day-care centers, camps
C. Seasonal: Summer and fall most common

FIGURE 4.10 Hand, foot, and mouth syndrome.

Source: Reproduced from Kifer, Z. A. (2012). *Fast facts for wound care nursing: Practical wound management in a nutshell* (p. 252). New York, NY: Springer Publishing Company.

Common Complaints

A. Generalized rash, with lesions on the tongue, gums, and roof of the mouth
B. Lesions (vesicles) also present on the hands, feet, and buttocks

Other Signs and Symptoms

A. Fever
B. Sore throat
C. Some enteroviruses have been associated with severe consequences such as meningitis, encephalitis, and others. The family should monitor symptoms carefully.

Subjective Data

A. Question the client regarding onset, duration, and progression of symptoms and lesions.
B. Determine whether any family member or other contact person had similar symptoms.
C. Identify areas where the child comes in contact with numerous children (child care facility, nurseries at church, school, etc.).
D. If not noted in the presenting symptoms, ask the client about his or her upper respiratory symptoms (sore throat, fever, headache, runny nose, cough, etc.).

Physical Examination

A. Check temperature, pulse, respirations, and blood pressure.
B. Inspect skin, ears, nose, and oral cavity for lesions.
C. Palpate:
   1. Palpate abdomen and lymph nodes in neck.
   2. Assess for meningism.
D. Auscultate lungs and heart.

Diagnostic Tests

A. Usually none; consider cultures of oral lesions if secondary bacterial infection is suspected.

Differential Diagnoses

A. Hand, foot, and mouth syndrome
B. Pharyngitis
C. Pneumonia

D. Meningitis

E. Meningococcemia: Exanthem, petechial rash

Plan

A. General interventions:

1. Supportive treatment—warm saline gargles, acetaminophen (Tylenol) as needed for discomfort, and increased fluids. Popsicles are useful to soothe oral lesions, especially for small children.

B. Client teaching:

1. Reinforce good oral and body hygiene. The virus may be harbored in the gastrointestinal tract for long periods.

C. Pharmaceutical therapy:

1. None is recommended.

2. Acetaminophen (Tylenol) as needed for fever and malaise

Follow-Up

A. None is recommended unless symptoms worsen or do not resolve in 7 to 10 days.

Consultation/Referral

A. Refer to physician for any symptoms related to meningitis or encephalitis.

Individual Considerations

A. Pediatrics: Seen primarily in the pediatric population.

Bibliography

Bian, L., Gao, F., Mao, Q., Sun, S., Wu, X., Liu, S., … Liang, Z. (2019). Hand, foot, and mouth disease associated with coxsackievirus A10: More serious than it seems. *Expert Review of Anti-Infective Therapy*, *17*(4), 233–242. doi:10.1080/14787210.2019.1585242

Broccolo, F., Drago, F., Ciccarese, G., Genoni, A., Porro, A., Parodi, A., … Toniolo, A. (2019). Possible long-term sequelae in hand, foot, and mouth disease caused by Coxsackievirus A6. *Journal of the American Academy of Dermatology*, *80*(3), 804–806.

Shayegan, L. H., Antonov, N. K., Morel, K. D., & Garzon, M. C. (2019). Casting new light on hand-foot-and-mouth disease. *Journal of Pediatrics*, *207*, 259. doi:10.1016/j.jpeds.2018.11.032

Herpes Simplex Virus Type 1

Jill C. Cash and Amy C. Bruggemann

Definition

Herpes simplex virus type 1 (HSV-1) viral infection of the cutaneous tissue manifests itself by vesicular lesions on the mucous membranes and skin. HSV-1 is most often associated with oral lesions (mouth and lips; Figure 4.11), and HSV-2 is associated with genital lesions. The virus appears in three stages:

A. Primary

B. Latent

C. Recurrent infections

Incidence

A. HSV-1 is seen in clients of all ages and in equal numbers of males and females.

B. There are approximately 776,000 new cases of herpes diagnosed annually in the United States.

FIGURE 4.11 Herpes simplex virus type 1.

Source: Reproduced from Kifer, Z. A. (2012). *Fast facts for wound care nursing: Practical wound management in a nutshell* (p. 259). New York, NY: Springer Publishing Company.

Pathogenesis

A. Viral infection can be transmitted from a vesicular lesion or fluid (saliva) containing the virus to the skin or mucosa of another person by direct contact, with an incubation period of 2 to 14 days. Trigeminal ganglia are the host of the oral virus. The virus can be reactivated, whereupon it travels along the affected nerve route and produces recurrent lesions. Common sites of infection are the lips, face, buccal mucosa, and throat.

Predisposing Factors

A. Immunocompromised clients

B. Prior HSV infections

C. Exposure to virus

Common Complaints

A. Painful lips, gums, and oral mucosa

Other Signs and Symptoms

A. Primary lesion: Fever, blisters on lips, malaise, and tender gums

B. Recurrent episodes: Fever blisters with prodrome of itching, burning, and tingling sensation at the site before vesicles appear

Subjective Data

A. Ask questions regarding location, onset, and duration of lesions.

B. Elicit description of prodromal symptoms.

C. Ask the client if systemic symptoms occur with vesicular outbreak.

D. Determine when the initial outbreak of lesions occurred (commonly seen in childhood).

E. Inquire whether the client has been exposed to anyone with similar lesions.

F. If the lesion(s) is recurrent, ask the client if stress, skin trauma, or sun exposure stimulates an outbreak of fever blisters.

Physical Examination

A. Inspect the skin and note location, appearance, and stage of vesicles.

B. Palpate lymph nodes for lymphadenopathy.

Diagnostic Tests

A. Viral cultures

Differential Diagnoses

A. Impetigo: Appears as amber-colored vesicular lesions with crusting

B. Stomatitis: Appears as erythemic or erosion lesions in the mouth and lips

C. Herpes zoster: Causes vesicles that run along a single dermatome

D. Stevens–Johnson syndrome (SJS)

E. Herpangina: Vesicles can be noted on the soft palate, tonsillary area, and uvula area; usually caused by the coxsackievirus

Plan

A. General interventions:

1. Comfort measures. Ice may be used to reduce swelling as needed.

2. Vaseline or other lip ointments may be applied as needed and lip ointment with SPF-30 or greater may be applied when exposed to sunlight.

B. Client teaching:

1. Educate the client regarding the disease process of HSV-1.

2. Instruct the client to wash hands frequently.

3. Suggest proper care of lips to prevent drying and to reduce pain.

4. Educate regarding transmission of virus to others.

5. Teach the client to expect recurrences at variable times.

C. Pharmaceutical therapy:

1. Precautions should be used when administering medication to clients who are immunocompromised and who have a history of renal insufficiency:

a. Lidocaine 2% as needed for comfort

b. Diphenhydramine (Benadryl) elixir may be used to rinse mouth as needed.

c. Acetaminophen (Tylenol) as needed for pain

d. Campho-Phenique application as needed

e. Initial episode: Acyclovir 200 mg by mouth five times per day for 7 to 10 days or until resolved

f. Recurrent episodes: Begin one of the following when prodrome begins or within 2 days of onset of lesions to get maximum effect:

i. Acyclovir 200 mg by mouth five times per day for 5 days

ii. Acyclovir 800 mg by mouth twice daily for 5 days

iii. Other alternative antivirals: Dosage depends on renal function:

1) Famciclovir (Famvir)

2) Valacyclovir (Valtrex)

g. Suppressive therapy:

i. Acyclovir 200 mg by mouth two to five times per day for 1 year

ii. Acyclovir 400 mg by mouth twice daily for 1 year

Follow-Up

A. None needed if resolved without complications

Consultation/Referral

A. Refer the client to a physician if treatment is unsuccessful or further complications arise.

Individual Considerations

A. Pediatrics:

1. Initial outbreak commonly occurs in childhood.

B. Adolescents/adults:

1. HSV-1 can also be transmitted sexually when having oral sex. Educate teens/adults regarding transmitting the virus during sexual contact. Transmission is possible if having sexual relations with partners; avoid contact when lesions are present.

2. Advise using a dental dam during oral sex to prevent transmission.

3. Avoid sharing toothbrushes and eating utensils.

Bibliography

Centers for Disease Control and Prevention. (2019). Genital herpes—CDC fact sheet. Retrieved from https://www.cdc.gov/std/herpes/STDFact-Herpes.htm

Herpes Zoster or Shingles

Jill C. Cash and Amy C. Bruggemann

Definition

Herpes zoster is a viral infection manifested by painful, vesicular lesions on the skin, limited to one side of the body, following one body dermatome (Figure 4.12).

Incidence

A. Infection may occur at any age; however, it is more common in older adults and the elderly. It occurs in 10% to 20% of the U.S. population.

FIGURE 4.12 Varicella zoster.

Source: Reproduced from Kifer, Z. A. (2012). *Fast facts for wound care nursing: Practical wound management in a nutshell* (p. 259). New York, NY: Springer Publishing Company.

Pathogenesis

A. After the primary episode of chickenpox (varicella zoster), the virus remains dormant in the body. Herpes zoster occurs when the varicella virus has been stimulated and reactivated in the dorsal root ganglia, producing the clinical manifestations of herpes zoster as discussed in the following. Duration of infection usually lasts 14 to 21 days, but may be longer in elderly or debilitated clients.

Predisposing Factors

A. Adulthood
B. Immunocompromised clients
C. Spinal cord trauma or injury

Common Complaints

A. Prodrome: Itching, burning, tingling, or painful sensation at lesion sites
B. Active: Malaise, fever, headache, or pruritic rash on the skin

Other Signs and Symptoms

A. Lesions: Clusters of vesicles on an erythemic base that burst and produce crusted lesions. These are most commonly found on the chest and back area, but they may also occur on the head and neck area or extremities. Distribution of lesions typically appears along a single dermatome.
B. Motor weakness (may be seen in approximately 5% of clients)

Subjective Data

A. Determine onset, location, and progression of rash
B. Ask the client about prodromal symptoms: Burning, itching, tingling, or painful sensation at the site before lesions break out
C. Evaluate client status regarding immunosuppressive agents, diseases, and so forth

Physical Examination

A. Check temperature, pulse, respiration, and blood pressure
B. Inspect
   1. Observe skin for lesions, noting characteristics and distribution
   2. Inspect ears, nose, and throat
C. Auscultate heart and lungs

Diagnostic Tests

A. Usually none
B. Culture vesicular lesions
C. Consider Tzanck smear
D. Young clients with herpes zoster: Consider test for HIV

Differential Diagnoses

A. Herpes zoster
B. Varicella
C. Poison ivy
D. HSV
E. Contact dermatitis
F. Coxsackievirus
G. Postherpetic neuralgia

Plan

A. General interventions:
   1. Comfort measures. Instruct the client to apply wet dressings (Burow's solution) on the site for 30 to 60 minutes at least four times a day. Calamine lotions may be used as needed; oatmeal (Aveeno) bath may be used for comfort; acetaminophen (Tylenol) is taken as needed for malaise, temperature, and comfort.
B. Client teaching:
   1. *See Section III: Client Teaching Guide for this chapter, "Herpes Zoster, or Shingles."*
   2. Tell the client that the rash usually lasts approximately 2 to 3 weeks.
   3. Instruct the client to monitor for signs/symptoms of postherpetic neuralgia.
   4. Instruct the client to call if symptoms worsen or do not improve, or signs of bacterial infection occur.
   5. Emphasize to the client that the virus is easily transmitted to vulnerable persons.
C. Pharmaceutical therapy:
   1. Antiviral medications should be initiated within 24 to 48 hours after outbreak.
      a. Acyclovir (Zovirax) 800 mg every 4 hours while awake for 7 to 10 days
      b. Famciclovir (Famvir) 500 to 750 mg by mouth three times daily for 7 days
      c. Valacyclovir (Valtrex) 1,000 mg by mouth three times daily for 7 days
   2. Acetaminophen (Tylenol) or ibuprofen as needed for pain or discomfort
   3. Narcotics may be used for severe pain as needed.
   4. Postherpetic neuralgia:
      a. Postherpetic neuralgia may be treated with narcotics or other pain-relieving medications.
      b. Long-term medications may be needed for control of pain:
         i. Gabapentin 100 to 600 mg three times daily
         ii. Amitriptyline 25 mg every bedtime or other low-dose tricyclic antidepressants
   5. If secondary bacterial infection of the skin occurs, apply silver sulfadiazine (Silvadene) topically to the site until resolved.
   6. Use of steroids is controversial. Corticosteroids may be used with caution. May increase risk of dissemination.

Follow-Up

A. As needed for complications
B. Monitor the client for complications: Postherpetic neuralgia, Guillain–Barré syndrome, motor weakness, secondary infection, meningoencephalitis, ophthalmic and facial palsy, corneal ulceration, and so forth.

Consultation/Referral

A. Ramsay Hunt syndrome occurs when a shingles outbreak affects the facial nerve near one of the ears. This can cause facial paralysis and hearing loss in the affected ear. Consult a physician.

B. Hutchinson's sign refers to vesicles in the peri-orbital region. These clients require an ophthamologist referral.
C. Consult with a physician if secondary infection occurs or if secondary complications arise.

Individual Considerations

A. Pregnancy:

1. Acyclovir falls under category C drug classification. The safety and efficacy of the use of the antiviral medications during pregnancy need to be considered.
2. Pregnant women whom are not immune to the virus need to take precautions to prevent contact with the virus while pregnant. Complications during pregnancy may include congenital varicella for the fetus and varicella pneumonia for the mother.

B. Pediatrics: Shingles is rarely seen in children.

C. Elderly:

1. Postherpetic neuralgia occurs in approximately 15% of clients. It is commonly seen in elderly clients.
2. The Centers for Disease Control and Prevention (CDC) recommends the shingles vaccine for all clients 50 years of age and older, irrespective of whether they have had the chickenpox or shingles infection in the past. There are two types available: the CDC recommends the recombinant vaccine (Shingrix) over the live vaccine unless contraindicated. For those who have had a recent shingles outbreak, it is recommended that resolution of the rash be complete before administering the vaccination.

    a. Shingrix—recombinant zoster vaccine guidelines:

      i. Administration dosing:

- Two doses administered IM: first dose given on day 0, and, the second dose should be administered 2 to 6 months after the first.

      ii. Indications:

- Immunocompetent clients older than 50 years
- Clients who previously received the varicella vaccine and the (live) zoster vaccine. The CDC recommends waiting 2 months to administer the Shingrix vaccine if Zostavax was previously administered.
- Clients with comorbid conditions

      iii. Contraindications:

- Clients with known allergy to components of the vaccine

3. The virus is contagious for those who have not had chickenpox.

Bibliography

Centers for Disease Control and Prevention. (2017, October 2017). Shingles (herpes zoster). Retrieved from https://www.cdc.gov/shingles

Chu, L., Daganzo, S., & Aronowitz, P. (2019). Chickenpox in a Vaccinated Adult. *JGIM: Journal of General Internal Medicine, 34*(3), 479–480. doi:10.1007/s11606-018-4816-9

Jones, G., & Whittle, N. (2019). Understanding the health risks of varicella zoster virus in pregnancy. *Primary Health Care, 29*(2), 45–50. doi:10.7748/phc.2019.e1522

Shafran, S. D. (2019). Prevention of shingles: Better protection and better value with recombinant vaccine. *Annals of Internal Medicine, 170*(6), 416–417. doi:10.7326/M19-0141

Impetigo

Jill C. Cash and Amy C. Bruggemann

Definition

A. Impetigo is a bacterial infection of the skin, most commonly caused by *S. aureus* or *Streptococcus pyogenes*, or both (Figure 4.13).

Incidence

A. It occurs equally in males and females and is most commonly seen in children, especially those 2 to 5 years of age.

Pathogenesis

A. An alteration in the skin integrity allows bacterial invasion into the epidermis, causing an infection. Small, moist vesicles ranging from red macules to honey-colored crusts or erosions occur singly or grouped together. Most common organisms are *S. aureus* and Group A beta-hemolytic *S. pyogenes*.

Predisposing Factors

A. Poor hygiene
B. Warm climate
C. Break in the skin

Common Complaint

A. Tender sores around the mouth and nose area in which the lesions continue to spread and worsen, despite OTC medication treatment

Subjective Data

A. Elicit onset, progression, duration, and location of lesions.
B. Ask the client whether he or she has had contact with any other child or person with similar lesions.
C. Assess whether the client exhibits any other symptoms, especially systemic symptoms (fever, malaise, etc.).
D. Elicit what treatment has been tried, if any.

FIGURE 4.13 Impetigo.

Source: Reproduced from Kifer, Z. A. (2012). *Fast facts for wound care nursing: Practical wound management in a nutshell* (p. 255). New York, NY: Springer Publishing Company.

Physical Examination
A. Check temperature.
B. Inspect:
   1. Examine skin, noting types of lesions and skin involvement.
   2. Examine ears, nose, mouth, and throat.
C. Auscultate lungs and heart.

Diagnostic Tests
A. None required
B. May perform culture if recurrent or resistant to treatment

Differential Diagnoses
A. Impetigo
B. Varicella
C. Folliculitis
D. Erysipelas
E. Herpes simplex
F. Second-degree burns
G. Pharyngitis or tonsillitis: Throat erythema, with tonsillary hypertrophy and exudate present; lymph nodes: Adenopathy of anterior cervical chain
H. Ecthyma: Severe case of impetigo with lymphadenitis
I. Insect bites
J. Necrotizing fasciitis
K. Contact dermatitis
L. Scabies

Plan
A. General interventions:
   1. Crusted lesions may be removed with thorough, gentle washing with mild soap three to four times daily.
   2. Impetigo must be adequately treated and resolved to prevent postinfection complications such as the following: Poststreptococcal acute glomerulonephritis, cellulitis, ecthyma, and bacteremia.

B. Client teaching: Encourage good handwashing and hygiene to reduce spreading infection.
C. Pharmaceutical therapy:
   1. If few lesions are noted without involvement of cellulitis: Topical mupirocin (Bactroban) ointment—to site three times daily for 5 days. Alternative topical ointment: retapamulin applied to site twice a day for 5 days.
   2. Systemic antibiotics are recommended for several lesions. Oral treatment recommended for 7 days (Refer to Table 4.2).

Follow-Up
Schedule appointment in 10 to 14 days to determine resolution of infection

Consultation/Referral
A. Consult a physician if complications arise or if resolution is not complete with antibiotic therapy.

Bibliography

Galli, L., Venturini, E., Bassi, A., Gattinara, G. C., Chiappini, E., Defilippi, C., … Villani, A. (2019). Common Community-acquired Bacterial Skin and Soft-tissue Infections in Children: An Intersociety Consensus on Impetigo, Abscess, and Cellulitis Treatment. *Clinical Therapeutics*, *41*(3), 532. doi:10.1016/j.clinthera.2019.01.010

Madden, J., Buck, S., Beachkofsky, T., & Xia, Y. (2018). Diffuse facial rash in a former collegiate wrestler: The patient described a history of "recurrent impetigo," which led to an uncommon diagnosis. *Journal of Family Practice*, *67*(12), 783–785.

May, P. J., Tong, S. Y. C., Steer, A. C., Currie, B. J., Andrews, R. M., Carapetis, J. R., & Bowen, A. C. (2019). Treatment, prevention and public health management of impetigo, scabies, crusted scabies and fungal skin infections in endemic populations: A systematic review. *Tropical Medicine & International Health*, *24*(3), 280–293. doi:10.1111/tmi.13198

Rosen, T., Albareda, N., Rosenberg, N., Roth, S., Zsolt, I., & Hebert, A. A. (2018). Efficacy and safety of ozenoxacin 1% cream, a novel antibiotic for the topical treatment of impetigo in children and adults. *Journal of the American Academy of Dermatology*, *79*(3), AB121. doi:10.1016/j.jaad.2018.05.509

TABLE 4.2   RECOMMENDED ANTIBIOTICS FOR IMPETIGO

	Adults	Children
Cephalexin	250–500 mg 4 times a day	25–50 mg/kg/d in 3–4 divided doses
Dicloxacillin	250–500 mg 4 times a day	25–50 mg/kg/d in 4 divided doses
Alternative for allergy to penicillin and cephalosporin:		
Erythromycin	base 250 mg 4 times a day	40 mg/kg/d in 3–4 divided doses
Clarithromycin	250 mg twice a day	15 mg/kg/d in 2 divided doses
Methicillin-resistant S. aureus (MRSA) suspected or confirmed:		
Clindamycin	300–450 mg 4 times a day	20 mg/kg/d in 3 divided doses
OR		
Trimethoprim–sulfamethoxazole	1–2 double strength tabs twice a day	8–12 mg/kg/d in 2 divided doses
OR		
Doxycycline	100 mg twice a day	2–4 mg/kg/d in 2 divided doses

Insect Bites and Stings

Jill C. Cash and Amy C. Bruggemann

Definition

A. Bites and/or stings on the skin come from commonly encountered insects: Bees, hornets, wasps, mosquitoes, chiggers, ticks, fleas, fire ants, and bedbugs.

Incidence

A. Bites are seen in all age groups, more common in summer months.

Pathogenesis

A. Some bites elicit local tissue inflammation and destruction because of proteins and enzymes in the poison or venom of the insect.

B. Immunoglobulin E (IgE)-mediated allergic reactions (immediate or delayed) may occur.

C. Serum-sickness reaction may appear 10 to 14 days after a sting with venom. Toxic reactions can also occur from multiple stings yielding large inoculation of poison or venom.

D. With tick bites, exposure to Rocky Mountain spotted fever, Lyme disease, ehrlichiosis, and babesiosis disease may occur.

Predisposing Factors

A. Exposure to areas of heavy insect infestations

B. Warm-weather months

C. Outdoor exposure with barefeet, bright clothes

D. Use of perfumes and/or colognes

E. Previous sensitization

Common Complaints

A. Local reaction: Pain, swelling, and redness at the site after insect bite

B. Toxic reaction: Local reaction plus headache, vertigo, gastrointestinal symptoms (nausea, vomiting, diarrhea), syncope, convulsions, and/or fever

Subjective Data

A. Did the client see what bit or stung him or her?

B. If the client felt the bite or sting, was he or she bitten or stung once or multiple times?

C. How long ago did it occur?

D. Where was the client when the injury occurred (environment)?

E. Has the client ever been bitten or stung before? If so, did he or she have any reaction then? If so, what was the treatment?

Physical Examination

A. Check temperature, pulse, respiration, and blood pressure. Observe overall respiratory status.

B. Inspect:
   1. Inspect site of injury for local reaction; note erythema, rash, or edema.
   2. Perform ear, nose, and throat examination.

C. Auscultate: Assess heart and lungs.

D. Palpate:
   1. Palpate injured site.
   2. Assess nodes for lymphadenopathy.
   3. Perform abdominal examination, if appropriate.

Diagnostic Tests

A. None is required.

B. Consider taking skin scrapings to evaluate under a microscope.

C. Consider culture if infection is suspected.

Differential Diagnoses

A. Insect bite:
   1. Bees, hornets, wasps, bedbugs: Local pain, redness, pruritus, and swelling occur at the site. Red papules and wheals appear, enlarge, and then subside within hours. Delayed hypersensitivity occurs within 7 days with enlarged, local reaction, with fever, malaise, headache, arthralgias, and lymphadenopathy. Toxicity can occur. Anaphylaxis may be seen with generalized warmth and urticaria, erythema, angioedema, intestinal cramping, bronchospasm, laryngospasm, shock, and collapse.
   2. Ticks: Local redness, swelling, itching; enlarged area of redness and swelling may occur.
   3. Mosquitoes and chiggers: Local redness, swelling, and itching occur. Delayed reaction can include edema and burning sensation.
   4. Fleas: Local redness, swelling, and itching occur. Usually papules noted in a zigzag pattern, especially on legs and waist. Note hemorrhagic puncta surrounded by erythematous and urticarial patches. Flea bites can transmit diseases.
   5. Body lice: Small noninflammatory red spots, intensely pruritic, are found on waist, shoulders, axilla, and neck. Note linear scratch marks. Note secondary infection.
   6. Scabies: Pruritus is the dominant symptom. Note inflammation and burrows in skin with papules and vesicles, especially in the webs of the hands and feet.
   7. Fire ants: Papules appear and turn to pustules within 6 to 24 hours after bite. Watch for localized necrosis with scarring. Urticaria and angioedema can occur (see Figure 4.14).

B. Allergic reaction

Plan

A. General interventions. Anaphylaxis: Activate emergency medical services (EMS) immediately.
   1. With all bites and stings, treat anaphylaxis first.
   2. Local reactions: Treat with analgesic of choice. Apply ice packs to the site for approximately 10 minutes. Elevate affected extremities.
   3. Delayed reactions: Administer antihistamines as needed. Consider corticosteroid use.
   4. Routine wound care: Cleanse wound. Remove stinger. If it is a painful sting, apply a cotton ball soaked in meat tenderizer or sodium bicarbonate paste.
   5. Debride as necessary.

FIGURE 4.14 Pustules resulting from fire ant bites.

6. For embedded insects, apply petroleum jelly, nail polish, or alcohol over site for 30 minutes and wait for insect or tick to withdraw.

7. Referral to allergist-immunologist is recommended for clients with a severe systemic reaction for skin testing and to evaluate for candidacy of venom immunotherapy treatment.

8. Hospitalize the client for severe reactions.

▶ B. *See Section III: Client Teaching Guide for this chapter, "Insect Bites and Stings."*

C. Pharmaceutical therapy:
   1. Antihistamines:
      a. Children:
         i. Younger child: 2 to 6 years: Diphenhydramine 6.25 mg every 4 to 6 hours
         ii. Older child: 6 to 12 years: Diphenhydramine 12.5 to 25 mg every 4 to 6 hours
      b. Adult: Diphenhydramine (Benadryl) 50 mg every 6 hours as needed
   2. Mild anaphylaxis:
      a. Epinephrine 1:1,000 (aqueous) administered subcutaneously. Usual dose is as follows:
         i. Children: 0.01 mg/kg; may repeat in 4 hours if needed
         ii. Adults: 0.3 mg IM; may repeat if needed
   3. Oral antihistamines for next 24 hours (Atarax):
      a. Children: Hydroxyzine hydrochloride (Atarax) 2 to 4 mg/kg/d divided into three doses
      b. Adults: Hydroxyzine hydrochloride (Atarax) 10 to 25 mg four times daily
   4. Severe anaphylaxis:
      a. Epinephrine 1:1,000 (aqueous), given subcutaneously (see mild anaphylaxis, mentioned earlier)
      b. Oxygen 2 to 4 L as needed
      c. Albuterol (Ventolin) 5 mg/mL per dose by nebulizer:
         i. Children: 0.1 to 0.15 mg/kg in 2 mL of saline
         ii. Adults: 2.5 mg (0.5 mL of 0.5% solution) in 2 mL saline

   5. Self-treatment for anaphylaxis (emergency treatment kits):
      a. Ana-Kit contains a preloaded syringe.
      b. Epipen and Epipen Junior Auto-Injectors are spring-loaded automatic injectors. Children: 0.01 mg/kg IM in thigh. Adults: 0.3 mg IM in thigh

Follow-Up
A. Follow up in 2 weeks to evaluate effectiveness of treatment. If symptoms worsen before this, reevaluation is needed.

Consultation/Referral
A. Consult with a physician when anaphylaxis occurs.

Individual Considerations
A. Pediatrics:
   1. Children are at a higher risk than adults for complications of a reaction.
B. Geriatrics:
   1. Elderly adults are at high risk for complications of reactions.

Bibliography
Abrams, E., & Chan, E. (2018). Stinging insect hypersensitivity: Evaluation and management in children and youth. *Paediatrics & Child Health (1205–7088), 23*(8), 557. doi:10.1093/pch/pxy140

Schub, T., & Cabrera, G. (2018). Bites: Head lice. *CINAHL Nursing Guide.*

Lice (Pediculosis)

Jill C. Cash and Amy C. Bruggemann

Definition
Pediculosis (lice) is an infestation of the louse on human beings in one of three areas:
A. Head (Pediculosis capitis)
B. Pubic area (Pthirus pubis)
C. Body (Pediculosis corporis)

Incidence
A. Pediculosis capitis is most common in children. It is estimated that head lice infestations occur in the school systems anywhere from 10% to 40% of the time.
B. They are more commonly found in girls than boys.
C. Phthirus pubis infestation is more common in adults.
D. Lice affect all demographics; all social, racial, and economic groups get lice.

Pathogenesis
A. Head and body lice are transmitted by direct contact from person to person, that is, through sharing hats, combs, brushes, and so forth. The parasite hatches from an egg, or nit. Once hatched, the lice live on humans by sucking blood through the skin. The average adult louse lives 9 to 10 days. The nits appear as small white eggs on the hair shaft. Nits are very difficult to remove and survive up to 3 weeks after removal from the host. Body lice lay nits in the seams of clothing.

B. Pubic lice are found at the base of the hair shaft, where they lay nits. Pubic lice are transmitted through sexual contact.

Predisposing Factors
A. Head and body lice: Exposure to crowded public areas, such as schools; inability to clean and launder clothing, bed linens, and so forth
B. Pubic lice: Sexual contact with infected people
C. Poor hygiene

Common Complaints
A. Head lice: Severe itching and scratching of the head, neck area, and commonly behind the ears
B. Body lice: Severe itching on the body, which may lead to secondary infections of the skin
C. Pubic lice: Severe itching of genital area

Other Signs and Symptoms
A. Excoriated skin from intense scratching
B. Visible lice or nits in hair, body, or clothing
C. Papules with an erythemic base may develop on the genital area, axilla, chest, beard, or eyelashes.
D. *Phthirus pubis* or nits or lice are found on eyelashes of children.

Subjective Data
A. Inquire as to exposure to anyone known to have lice.
B. Identify whether the client attends a crowded environment such as school, day care, and so forth.
C. Ask if lice and nits have been seen by the client or guardian.
D. Determine onset, duration, and course of symptoms. Ask: When were lice or nits first discovered?
E. Assess whether the client has been symptomatic (itching, scratching).
F. Inquire about social habits of cleaning, laundry, and so forth.

Physical Examination
A. Check temperature to rule out any secondary infection.
B. Inspect:
   1. Inspect hair, body, pubic area, and clothing seams for nits or lice.
   2. Note excoriation of skin.
   3. Examine eyelashes of children.
   4. Examine skin for secondary bacterial infection.

Diagnostic Tests
A. None
B. Culture excoriated area if secondary bacterial infection suspected.

Differential Diagnoses
A. Lice
B. Scabies

Plan
A. General interventions:
   1. Treat immediately with appropriate pediculicides (see Pharmaceutical therapy, in the following).

   2. After treatment, it is imperative to remove each nit and louse; use fine-tooth comb for nit removal.
   3. Evaluate entire family for lice.
   4. Treat secondary bacterial infection as needed.
B. Client teaching:
   1. *See Section III: Client Teaching Guide for this chapter, "Lice (Pediculosis."* ◀
   2. Specific instructions need to be given to clients on how to get rid of lice and nits.
   3. Reinforce good hygiene; teach children not to share combs, brushes, hats, and hair accessories.
C. Pharmaceutical therapy:
   1. Malathion lotion 0.5% (Ovide): Pediculicidal and partially ovicidal
   2. Permethrin lotion 1% (Nix): Pediculicidal only. Available OTC for treatment.
   3. Synergized pyrethrins (Rid 0.3%; Available OTC)
   4. Apply, repeat in 24 hours, and then again in 1 week.
   5. Do not use a shampoo/conditioner or conditioner before using head lice treatments. Do not wash hair for 1 to 2 days after using lice treatment regimen.
   6. Pthirus pubis: Lindane (Kwell) or permethrin (Nix); apply to pubic area as directed.
   7. **Lindane (Kwell) toxicity may occur from ingestion or overuse and is exhibited by headaches, dizziness, and convulsions.**
   8. Eyelash manifestation: After removing nits, apply petroleum jelly to lashes three to four times a day for 8 to 10 days. **Eyelashes should never be treated with pediculicides.**

Follow-Up
A. None recommended
B. Some schools and institutions require follow-up to evaluate whether infestation is resolved before admitting the child back into the classroom.

Consultation/Referral
A. If lice are a repeated problem, contact social services or the health department to have a visiting nurse or aide visit the home to evaluate home conditions and to teach the family how to prevent infestations.

Individual Considerations
A. Pregnancy:
   1. Lindane (Kwell) is contraindicated during pregnancy
B. Pediatrics:
   1. Head lice is commonly seen in school-aged children
   2. Lindane (Kwell) should not be used in infants. The American Academy of Pediatrics does not recommend lindane as a first-line treatment for head lice for children secondary to the toxic effects of the brain and CNS.
C. Geriatrics:
   1. For adult/elderly clients with the diagnosis of lice, consider self-neglect, unsuitable living conditions, cognitive/psychiatric impairments, and/or abuse/neglect of the elderly.
   2. Consider a home visit for evaluation of the client.

Bibliography

Sanchezruiz, W. L., Nuzum, D. S., & Kouzi, S. A. (2018). Oral ivermectin for the treatment of head lice infestation. *American Journal of Health-System Pharmacy, 75*(13), 937–943. doi:10.2146/ajhp170464

Schub, T., & Cabrera, G. (2018). Bites: Head lice. *CINAHL Nursing Guide.*

Lichen Planus

Jill C. Cash and Amy C. Bruggemann

Definition
A. Lichen planus is a relatively common acute or chronic inflammatory dermatosis. It affects skin and mucous membranes with characteristic flat-topped, shiny, violaceous (purplish color) pruritic papules with lacy lines on the skin, and milky-white papules in the mouth.

Incidence
A. Lichen planus accounts for 0.1% to 1.2% of office visits to dermatologists.
B. It exhibits no racial preference.

Pathogenesis
A. Etiology is unknown, although it is possibly a cell-mediated immune response. Most cases remit within 7 years. Lesions may heal with significant postinflammatory hyperpigmentation.

Predisposing Factors
A. Severe emotional stress
B. Drugs may induce lichenoid plaques.

Common Complaints
A. Rash with or without pruritus
B. Primary lesions: Small, flat-topped papules that are polygonal, lightly scaly, and violaceous
C. Secondary lesions: Erythema, scales, and erosions

Other Signs and Symptoms
A. Distribution: Volar aspect of wrists, ankles, mouth, genitalia, and lumbar region
B. Wickham's striae (white, lacelike pattern on surface)
C. Scalp: Atrophic skin with alopecia
D. Nails: Destruction of nail fold and bed, especially in the large toe
E. Men: Lesions of glans penis
F. Women: Erosive lesions of labia and vulva

Subjective Data
A. Determine whether the onset was sudden or gradual.
B. Ask the client to describe if the skin is itchy or painful.
C. Assess lesions for any associated discharge (blood or pus).
D. Identify the location(s) of the problem.
E. Complete a drug history. Ask the client if he or she has recently taken any antibiotics or other drugs. Ask if he or she has used any topical medications, lotions, or other creams.
F. Determine the presence of any preceding systemic symptoms (fever, sore throat, anorexia, or vaginal discharge).
G. Rule out insect bites.
H. Identify any possible exposure to industrial toxins, domestic toxins, or color-film-developing chemicals.
I. Ask if the client has had any possible sexual contact with persons with HIV or STIs.
J. Ask if the client has had close physical contact with others with skin disorders.

Physical Examination
A. Inspect:
1. Inspect skin and note lesion distribution.
2. Inspect mucous membranes: Buccal mucosa, tongue, and lips.
3. Examine hair and nails.
4. Observe genitalia.

Diagnostic Tests
A. A drop of mineral oil accentuates the papule.
B. If necessary to confirm diagnosis, deep shave or punch biopsy of developed lesions
C. HIV or STI testing if indicated
D. Hepatitis testing should be completed to assess for hepatitis C as lichen planus has been shown to have a correlation.

Differential Diagnoses
A. Lichenoid drug eruptions
B. Leukoplakia
C. Chronic graft-versus-host disease
D. Candidiasis (thrush)
E. Lupus erythematosus
F. Contact dermatitis
G. Bite trauma
H. Secondary syphilis

Plan
A. General interventions: Discontinue any suspected drug agent.
B. Client teaching: *See Section III: Client Teaching Guide for this chapter, "Lichen Planus."*
1. Instruct clients that the disease may be chronic; most cases resolve spontaneously.
2. Encourage the client to avoid severe emotional stress.
3. Encourage the client to avoid scratching and prevent secondary infection.
4. Reassure the client that lichen planus is not contagious.
C. Pharmaceutical therapy:
1. Oral antihistamines: Hydroxyzine hydrochloride 10 to 50 mg four times daily as needed for pruritus, or cetirizine Hcl (Zyrtec) 10 mg daily
2. Medium- to high-potency topical corticosteroids:
a. Mouth lesions: Fluocinonide 0.05%, ointment or gel, two or three times daily
b. Body lesions: Betamethasone dipropionate (Diprolene) 0.05%, triamcinolone (Kenalog), clobetasol (Temovate, Cormax) 0.05%, or other

class 1 cream or ointment, two times daily for 2 to 3 weeks and then stop use. **Caution clients about steroid atrophy.**

   c. Genital lesions: Desonide cream 0.05% twice daily initially, although higher potency creams may be necessary. Topical corticosteroids should be used on genitalia in short bursts only.

   d. Hypertrophic lesions: Intralesional injections, such as injecting triamcinolone 5 to 10 mg/mL, 0.5 to 1 mL per 2-cm lesion, are helpful for pruritus relief. Use cautiously in dark-skinned clients because of risk of hypopigmentation.

  3. Oral prednisone is rarely used, but if necessary use with a short course only and taper

Follow-Up
A. See the client in 1 week for evaluation of treatment.

Consultation/Referral
A. Refer the client to a dermatologist if there is no response to initial treatment.

Individual Considerations
A. Pregnancy:
  1. Use caution with medications prescribed.
B. Pediatrics:
  1. For severe itching, consider oral antihistamine.
C. Geriatrics:
  1. Avoid first-generation anticholinergics because of risk of confusion, dry mouth, constipation, and other anticholinergic effects or toxicity.

Bibliography
Leung, A. K. C., Barankin, B., & Leong, K. F. (2018). What is the cause of this boy's asymptomatic papular rash? *Consultant (00107069)*, *58*(1), 1–7.

Plensdorf, S., Livieratos, M., & Dada, N. (2017). Pigmentation disorders: Diagnosis and management. *American Family Physician*, *96*(12), 797–804.

Trayes, K. P., Savage, K., & Studdiford, J. S. (2018). Annular lesions: Diagnosis and treatment. *American Family Physician*, *98*(5), 283–291.

Pityriasis Rosea

Jill C. Cash and Amy C. Bruggemann

Definition
A. Pityriasis rosea is an acute, self-limiting, benign skin eruption characterized by a preceding "herald patch" that is followed by widespread papulosquamous lesions (Figure 4.15).

Incidence
A. Pityriasis rosea is relatively common, with more than 75% of cases in individuals from 10 to 35 years of age.
B. Incidence is slightly higher in women than in men.
C. Incidence is higher during the spring and autumn.

Pathogenesis
A. Disease is idiopathic; some evidence exists to support a viral origin or autoimmune disorder.

FIGURE 4.15   Pityriasis rosea.

Source: Centers for Disease Control and Prevention.

Predisposing Factor
A. Recent acute infection

Common Complaints
A. Rash: Salmon, pink, or tawny-colored lesions generally are concentrated in the trunk, but may develop on arms, legs, and rarely on the face
B. Mild pruritus

Other Signs and Symptoms
A. Earliest lesions may be papular but may progress to 1- to 2-cm oval plaques.
B. Long axes of oval lesions run parallel to each other, hence the term "Christmas tree distribution."
C. Preceding herald patch (2–10 cm with central clearing) closely resembles ringworm; usually appears abruptly a few days to several weeks before the generalized eruptive phase.

Subjective Data
A. Elicit information about occurrence of initial, single, 2- to 10-cm round to oval lesion.
B. Question the client as to known contact with similar symptoms. Small epidemics have been identified in fraternity houses and military bases.

Physical Examination
A. Check temperature to rule out any infection.
B. Inspect:
  1. Examine all body surfaces with client unclothed.
  2. Look for characteristic lesions and distribution.
  3. Check the mucous surfaces, palms, and soles, which are usually spared by pityriasis rosea.

Diagnostic Tests
A. Generally none required; however, potassium hydroxide (KOH) wet preparation may be useful to distinguish a herald patch from tinea corporis.
B. Serology to rule out syphilis, if applicable.
C. If unable to identify herald patch, a serologic test for syphilis should be ordered because syphilis may be clinically indistinguishable from pityriasis rosea.
D. White blood count (WBC) normal; no specific laboratory markers for pityriasis rosea.

Differential Diagnoses

A. Pityriasis rosea
B. Nummular eczema
C. Tinea corporis
D. Tinea versicolor
E. Viral exanthems
F. Drug eruptions:
   1. Captopril
   2. Bismuth
   3. Barbiturates
   4. Clonidine
   5. Metronidazole
G. Secondary syphilis
H. Lichen planus

Plan

A. General interventions:
   1. Direct sunlight to the point of minimal erythema hastens the disappearance of lesions and decreases itching. UVB light in five consecutive daily exposures can decrease pruritus and shorten rash, particularly if administered within the first week of eruption.
   2. Not proven to be contagious and relatively harmless, so isolation is not required
B. Client teaching:
   1. *See Section III: Client Teaching Guide for this chapter, "Pityriasis Rosea."*
   2. Advise clients that the disease is self-limiting and clears spontaneously in 1 to 3 months.
C. Pharmaceutical therapy:
   1. Generally none is required, but for itching the following recommendations exist: Group V topical steroids and oral antihistamines as per usual dosing
   2. Prednisone 20 mg twice daily for 1 to 2 weeks in rare cases of intense itching

Follow-Up

A. None is required unless secondary infection (impetigo) develops. Disease may recur in approximately 2% of clients.

Consultation/Referral

A. Consult or refer the client to a physician when disease persists beyond 3 months.

Individual Considerations

A. Pregnancy:
   1. Disease has not been shown to affect fetus.
B. Pediatrics:
   1. Rash more frequently affects face and distal extremities.
   2. Impetigo may result from scratching or poor hygiene.
C. Geriatrics: Disease is rarely seen in geriatric clients. Strongly consider other differential diagnoses, particularly drug reactions.
   1. Avoid first-generation anticholinergics because of risk of confusion, dry mouth, constipation, and other anticholinergic effects or toxicity.

Bibliography

Kim, H. S., Kim, H., & Lee, J. D. (2017). An annular plaque on the back. *American Family Physician, 96*(4), 255–256.
Trayes, K. P., Savage, K., & Studdiford, J. S. (2018). Annular lesions: Diagnosis and treatment. *American Family Physician, 98*(5), 283–291.
Villalon-Gomez, J. M. (2018). Pityriasis rosea: Diagnosis and treatment. *American Family Physician, 97*(1), 38–44.

Precancerous or Cancerous Skin Lesions

Jill C. Cash and Amy C. Bruggemann

Definition

A. Skin cell changes that occur in the body that may be precancerous or cancerous

Incidence

A. Actinic keratosis is the most common precancerous skin disorder that occurs in approximately 58 million Americans, which is an estimate because it is not commonly reported and/or often occurs without diagnosis.
B. Basal cell carcinoma (BCC) is the most common form of skin cancer, with approximately 400,000 new cases per year in the United States (Figure 4.16). It is often seen in the sixth or seventh decade of life. It is commonly seen in Caucasians and noted to be 30% higher in men than women. The occurrence of BCC is greater in people living in the states that are closer to the equator than those in the Midwest, thought to be related to increased exposure to UV light.
C. Squamous cell carcinoma (SCC) is the second leading type of skin cancer and accounts for 20% of all skin cancers. It is most often seen in the middle-aged and elderly populations.
D. Malignant melanoma is the fifth leading cause of cancer in men and women and accounts for less than 5% of all skin cancers (Figure 4.17). The median age at diagnosis is 61 years of age.

Pathogenesis

A. Actinic keratosis: A precancerous skin lesion commonly caused by damage to the skin that is the result of exposure to UV rays or tanning beds. If not treated, these skin lesions may turn into a form of skin cancer, such as SCC.
B. BCC: Abnormal cells of the basal layer of the epidermis expand. The surrounding stroma supports the basal cell growth. UV rays (sunlight) are the major contributor to BCC. BCC is a slow-growing tumor that rarely metastasizes.
C. SCC: Abnormal cells of the epidermis penetrate the basement membrane of the epidermis and move into the dermis, producing SCC. This often begins as actinic keratosis that undergoes malignant change.
D. Malignant melanoma: Abnormal cells proliferate from the melanocyte system. Initially, the cells grow superficially and laterally into the epidermis and papillary dermis. After a period, the cells begin growing up into the reticular dermis and subcutaneous fat. Malignant tumors occur because of the inability of the damaged cells to protect themselves from the long-term exposure of the UV rays.

FIGURE 4.16 Basal cell carcinoma.

Source: Reproduced from Kifer, Z. A. (2012). *Fast facts for wound care nursing: Practical wound management in a nutshell* (p. 252). New York, NY: Springer Publishing Company.

Predisposing Factors

A. Advanced age (older than age 50 years)
B. Median age of 40 years for malignant melanoma
C. Exposure to UV light (sun exposure)
D. Fair complexion
E. Smokers (damaged lips)
F. Skin damaged by burns and/or chronic inflammation
G. History of blistering sunburns before 18 years of age increases risk

Common Complaints

A. New lesions found on the skin
B. Ulcer that does not heal

Other Signs and Symptoms

A. Actinic keratosis (solar keratosis): Scaly, crusted lesions commonly found on sun-exposed skin areas such as the face, ears, scalp, lips, and hands that are usually rough in texture and appearance
B. BCC: Tumors arising from the basal cell layer of the epidermis. Tumors may be seen on face and neck; may appear as an open sore, pink growth, or nodule that is greater than 1 cm that appears shiny, pearly in color with telangiectasia; center may cave in.
C. SCC: Skin lesions seen in sun-exposed areas of the skin, or skin damaged by burns or chronic inflammation; lower lip lesions common; firm, irregular papules with scaly, bleeding, friable surface like sandpaper; grows rapidly
D. Malignant melanoma: Asymmetrical tumor of skin with irregular border, variation in color, greater than 6 mm in diameter; can metastasize to any organ
E. Bowen's disease (SCC in situ): Chronic, nonhealing erythemic patch with sharp, irregular borders; occurs on skin and/or the mucocutaneous tissue; resembles eczema but does not respond to steroids

Subjective Data

A. Have the client identify when lesion was first noted.
B. Ask the client to describe any changes in size, color, or shape of the lesion.

FIGURE 4.17 Example of malignant melanoma.

Source: National Cancer Institute.

C. Determine whether the client has noted any new lesions
D. Ascertain any family history of malignant melanoma.
E. Determine the client's history of skin exposure to the sun or any other UV rays.
F. Ask the client about smoking history. If the client smokes, ask how many packs per day.

Physical Examination

A. Inspect:
   1. Perform full body exam of the skin for lesions.
   2. Note surface, size, shape, border, color, and diameter of lesion.
   3. Examine scalp and ears for lesions.

Diagnostic Test

A. Biopsy suspicious lesions.

Differential Diagnoses

A. Actinic keratosis
B. BCC
C. SCC
D. Malignant melanoma
E. Solar lentigo
F. Seborrheic keratosis
G. Common nevus
H. Leukoplakia

Plan

A. General interventions:
   1. Monitor progress/change of lesions detected.
   2. Biopsy any suspicious lesions. Excise lesion with narrow margins, making sure to include all margins. If biopsy results of specimen are inadequate for accurate histologic diagnosis or staging, repeat biopsy. Include all clinical history information on the pathology report with the specimen when sending to pathology.
B. Client teaching:
   1. *See Section III: Client Teaching Guide for this chapter, "Skin Care Assessment."*
   2. Educate clients regarding importance of early identification of lesions and monthly assessment of skin. The U.S. Preventive Services Task Force

(USPSTF) recommends counseling adolescents and young adults less than 24 years of age regarding reducing the amount of UV radiation exposure, especially between the hours of 10 a.m. and 3 p.m. In adults older than 24 years of age, the USPSTF did not find sufficient evidence to determine the effects of counseling these clients regarding the use of sun protection.

3. Instruct clients on monthly skin evaluation. Teach the "ABCD" method of exam for changes in lesions: **A**symmetry, **B**order, **C**olor, and **D**iameter. A body map may be used to mark skin changes and monitor progress. Mark the site of the lesion on the body map, including measurements and date found. A body map may be found at www.skincancer.org/skin-cancer-information/early-detection/body-map.

C. Pharmaceutical therapy: None indicated

Follow-Up
A. When a diagnosis is made, follow up according to diagnosis. Differentiate between benign skin lesions and malignant melanoma. Follow-up/treatment depends on diagnosis (nonsurgical versus surgical removal for diagnosis). Surgical removal recommended for recurrent and suspicious lesions.

Consultation/Referral
A. Refer all clients to the dermatologist if skin cancer is suspected.

Individual Considerations
A. Pediatrics:
1. Teach parents to use SPF-30 or greater on pediatric clients exposed to the sun.
B. Geriatrics:
1. The elderly is at higher risk for skin cancer because of their decreased immune system as they age, as well as their cumulative chronic disease risk factors. Educate these clients regarding their risk factors and teach them how to assess the skin for lesions. Encourage frequent skin assessment and early diagnosis for improved outcomes.

Bibliography
Jansen, M. H. E., Kessels, J. P. H. M., Nelemans, P. J., Kouloubis, N., Arits, A. H. M. M., van Pelt, H. P. A., ... Mosterd, K. (2019). Randomized trial of four treatment approaches for actinic keratosis. *New England Journal of Medicine*, 380(10), 935–946. doi:10.1056/NEJMoa1811850

Wei, E. X., Li, X., & Nan, H. (2019). Extremity nevus count is an independent risk factor for basal cell carcinoma and melanoma, but not squamous cell carcinoma. *Journal of the American Academy of Dermatology*, 80(4), 970–978. doi:10.1016/j.jaad.2018.09.044

Psoriasis

Jill C. Cash and Amy C. Bruggemann

Definition
A. A common benign, chronic, inflammatory skin disorder, psoriasis is characterized by whitish scaly patches commonly seen on the scalp, knees, and elbows (see Figure 4.18).

FIGURE 4.18 Psoriasis.

Source: Reproduced from Kifer, Z. A. (2012). *Fast facts for wound care nursing: Practical wound management in a nutshell* (p. 252). New York, NY: Springer Publishing Company.

Incidence
A. Disease occurs in about 1% to 3% of the world population.
B. Psoriasis affects 7.5 million people in the United States. Approximately 80% of those clients have plaque psoriasis.
C. It occurs at any age:
1. Peak of onset seen in adolescence.
2. Seen in young adult (16–22 years old)
3. Occurs in adults 50 to 60 years old

Pathogenesis
A. Etiology is unknown; this is a multifactorial disease with a definite genetic component. Hyperproliferation of the epidermis and inflammation of the epidermis and dermis are seen, with epidermal transit time rapidly increased (six- to ninefold). A T-lymphocyte-mediated dermal immune response may occur because of microbial antigen or autoimmune process.

Predisposing Factors
A. Family history
B. Drugs that exacerbate condition:
1. Lithium
2. Beta-blockers
3. Nonsteroidal antiinflammatory drugs (NSAIDs)
4. Antimalarial
5. Sudden withdrawal of systemic or potent topical corticosteroids
C. Stress (common triggering factor)
D. Local trauma or irritation
E. Recent streptococcal infection
F. Alcohol use
G. Tobacco use
H. HIV association; suspected if onset is abrupt

Common Complaint
A. Dry scaly rash

Other Signs and Symptoms
A. Pruritic and/or painful lesions

B. Silvery scales on discrete erythematous plaques:
 1. Onset commonly occurs as a guttate form with small, scattered, teardrop-shaped papules and plaques after a streptococcal infection in a child or young adult.
 2. Larger, chronic plaques occur later in life.
C. Lesions commonly seen on the scalp, elbows, and knees, but may involve any area of the body
D. Glossitis or geographic tongue: Small pits or yellow-brown spots (oil spots)
E. Positive Auspitz sign: Punctate bleeding points with removal of scale
F. Onycholysis
G. Stippled nails and pitting; approximately 50% of clients have nail involvement
H. Periarticular swelling of small joints of fingers and toes. **Joint pain and involvement signals psoriatic arthritis.**
I. Pustular variant with predominant involvement of hands and/or feet, including nails

Subjective Data

A. Question the client regarding any predisposing factors listed earlier to identify risk factors.
B. Ask the client if there have been changes in the course of symptoms.
C. Ascertain whether the symptoms worsen in winter and improve in summer.
D. Determine the site of the lesion and whether the onset is sudden and/or painful.
E. Ask the client to describe the skin, whether it is itchy or painful.
F. Assess lesions for any associated discharge (blood or pus)
G. Ask if the client is using any new soaps, creams, or lotions
H. Rule out any exposure to industrial or domestic toxins
I. Ask the client about any possible contact with venereal disease (sexually transmitted diseases [STDs])
J. Review whether there has been any close physical contact with others with skin disorders
K. Elicit information regarding any preceding systemic symptoms (fever, sore throat, and anorexia)

Physical Examination

A. Check temperature (if indicated).
B. Inspect:
 1. Inspect skin; note type of lesion and distribution. Assess oral mucosa, nails, and nail beds.
 2. Assess joints for erythema and/or synovitis (inflammation of the synovial membrane).
C. Palpate joints for tenderness and synovitis.

Diagnostic Tests

A. None is indicated unless HIV infection is suspected; if so, order HIV test.
B. If joint inflammation is present, consider rheumatoid factor, erythrocyte sedimentation rate, and uric acid.
C. If there is a history of streptococcal infection, order antistreptolysin O titer.

Differential Diagnoses

A. Psoriasis
B. Scalp: Seborrheic dermatitis
C. Body folds: Candidiasis
D. Trunk: Pityriasis rosea, tinea corporis
E. Hand dermatitis
F. SCC
G. Cutaneous lupus erythematosus
H. Eczema

Plan

A. General interventions:
 1. This is a chronic disorder that requires long-term treatment, a high degree of client involvement, and therapy that is simple and inexpensive.
 2. Aim of treatment is control, not cure.
 3. Exposure to sunlight may be beneficial. However, symptoms worsen in a small percentage of clients with exposure to sunlight.
 4. Sequence of agents for involvement of less than 20% body surface is as follows:
  a. Emollients (Eucerin cream or Aquaphor cream)
  b. Keratolytic agents (salicylic acid gel or ointment)
  c. Topical corticosteroids: Use lowest potency to control disease.
  d. Calcipotriene ointment: Vitamin D analogue (calcipotriene ointment 0.005%)
  e. Anthralin: Use as short-contact therapy 1% to 3%
  f. Coal tar (Estar, PsoriGel): Use in conjunction with topical steroids or anthralin. May apply at bedtime or in the morning for 15 minutes and then shower off.
  g. Medicated shampoos: Useful for scalp psoriasis, in conjunction with topical steroids and other treatments
B. Client teaching:
 1. *See Section III: Client Teaching Guide for this chapter, "Psoriasis."* ◄
 2. Help the client understand the chronic nature of this disease characterized by flares and remission. Teach stress monitoring and control. Assist with coping techniques.
 3. A trial of a gluten-free diet may be tried to help symptoms. See Appendix B: "Gluten-Free Diet."
 4. Encourage the client to reach out to the National Psoriasis Foundation for education and resources for the client and family.
C. Pharmaceutical therapy: If the disease is not controlled with the first agent, then an alternative agent may be tried.
 1. Mild to moderate disease: Topical steroids as first-line therapy
 2. Emollients to start treatment (e.g., Eucerin Plus lotion or cream, Lubriderm Moisture Plus, Moisturel)
 3. Scalp: Use coal tar shampoo (Zetar, T/Gel, Pentrax) in place of regular shampoo two times per week.
  a. Apply lather to scalp, allow to soak for 5 minutes, and then rinse.

b. If plaques are very thick, use P and S Liquid (OTC). Massage in at night and wash out in the morning.

4. For additional treatment as needed, apply triamcinolone acetonide 0.1% (Kenalog 0.1%) lotion or equivalent to scaly, stubborn areas once or twice daily until controlled. **Avoid face.**

5. Dovonex scalp solution: Apply on dry scalp as directed.

6. Face and skin folds: Hydrocortisone cream 1%, apply sparingly up to 4 weeks, preferably no more than 2 weeks. If lesions are unresponsive, consider increasing to 2.5% and taper quickly with improvement.

7. Body, arms, and legs: Use triamcinolone acetonide 0.025% (Aristocort A) cream twice daily up to 2 weeks. **Avoid normal skin.**

8. For thick plaques, try Keralyt gel (6% salicylic acid), then corticosteroids

9. Use coal tar (Estar gel) once or twice daily in combination with corticosteroids.

10. Anthralin (Dritho-Creme) is beneficial as an alternate to steroid lotion for scalp psoriasis. **Avoid sunlight.**

11. Vitamin D₃ analogue: (Calcipotriol), twice daily up to 8 weeks, is comparable to midpotency corticosteroids. **Avoid face and skin folds.**

12. **Systemic agents for moderate to severe psoriasis may be used if other measures fail. Systemic agents should be prescribed by a dermatology specialist; these medications include retinoids, methotrexate, cyclosporine, and apremilast. These medications should be monitored closely for liver/kidney function changes.**

Follow-Up

A. See clients in 2 to 3 weeks to evaluate treatment.

B. Follow up in 2 months to monitor side effects.

C. Follow-up must be individualized for each client.

Consultation/Referral

A. Medical management: For involvement greater than 20% of body, refer the client to a dermatologist for the following:

    1. Light therapy with ultraviolet A (UVA) or UVB. UVB light therapy is often used in conjunction with keratolytic agents.

    2. Synthetic retinoids: Etretinate or acitretin are options.

    3. Low-dose cyclosporine or Azulfidine can be effective.

B. Refer clients with extensive disease, psoriatic arthritis, or inflammatory disease to a rheumatologist. Medications are used to suppress the immune system's response, which include adalimumab (Humira), etanercept (Enbrel), infliximab (Remicade), and ustekinuman (Stelara).

C. Cases of generalized pustular psoriasis of exfoliative erythroderma should be referred immediately to a dermatologist.

D. All systemic therapies should be given under supervision of a dermatologist or rheumatologist.

Individual Considerations

A. Geriatrics:

    1. First-line therapy for mild to moderate psoriasis in the elderly population is topical treatments. Systemic steroid therapies place geriatrics at a higher risk for adverse effects including atrophy, rebound phenomenon, tachyphylaxis, secondary skin infections, telangiectasia, and purpura.

    2. If topical treatment is not effective, before considering other treatments, do an assessment for client adherence and physical function abilities. Verify the client is using the medication correctly and consistently.

    3. If the medication is being implemented appropriately, then consider second-line treatments of systemic medications or UVB phototherapy. Second-line therapies must have a thorough review of comorbidities, any client needs for assistance, and an evaluation of functional status before initiating the systemic/phototherapy.

Bibliography

Frampton, J. E. (2019). Tildrakizumab: A review in moderate-to-severe plaque psoriasis. *American Journal of Clinical Dermatology*, *20*(2), 295–306. doi:10.1007/s40257-019-00435-9

Menter, A., Strober, B. E., Kaplan, D. H., Kivelevitch, D., Prater, E. F., Stoff, B., ... Leonardi, C. L. (2019). Joint AAD-NPF guidelines of care for the management and treatment of psoriasis with biologics. *Journal of the American Academy of Dermatology*, *80*(4), 1029–1072. doi:10.1016/j.jaad.2018.11.057

Sparks, J. A., Lesperance, T., Accortt, N. A., & Solomon, D. H. (2019). Subsequent cardiovascular events among patients with rheumatoid arthritis, psoriatic arthritis, or psoriasis: Patterns of disease-modifying antirheumatic drug treatment. *Arthritis Care & Research*, *71*(4), 512–520. doi:10.1002/acr.23609

Trayes, K. P., Savage, K., & Studdiford, J. S. (2018). Annular lesions: Diagnosis and treatment. *American Family Physician*, *98*(5), 283–291.

Scabies

Jill C. Cash and Amy C. Bruggemann

Definition

A. Scabies is a contagious skin infestation by the mite *Sarcoptes scabiei* (Figure 4.19).

Incidence

A. Scabies occurs mainly in individuals in close contact with many other individuals such as schoolchildren or nursing-home residents. It is rare among African Americans.

FIGURE 4.19 Scabies.

Source: Reproduced from Kifer, Z. A. (2012). *Fast facts for wound care nursing: Practical wound management in a nutshell* (p. 255). New York, NY: Springer Publishing Company.

Pathogenesis

A. Scabies is transmitted through close contact with an individual who is infested with the mite *S. scabiei*. Transmission may occur through sexual contact or contact with mite-infested clothing or sheets. The fertilized female mite burrows into the stratum corneum of a host and deposits eggs and fecal pellets. Larvae hatch, mature, and repeat the cycle.

B. A hypersensitivity reaction is responsible for the intense pruritus.

Predisposing Factors

A. Close contact with large numbers of individuals
B. Institutionalized
C. Poverty
D. Sexual promiscuity

Common Complaints

A. Intense itching, worse at night
B. Skin excoriation
C. Generalized pruritus
D. Rash

Other Signs and Symptoms

A. Mites burrow in finger webs, at wrists, in the sides of hands and feet, at the axilla buttocks, and in the penis and scrotum in males
B. Discrete vesicles and papules, distributed in linear fashion
C. Erythema
D. Secondary infections caused by scratching or infection (pustules and pinpoint erosions)
E. Nodules in covered areas (buttocks, groin, scrotum, penis, and axilla), which may have slightly eroded surfaces that persist for months after mites have been eradicated
F. Diffuse eruption that spares the face

Subjective Data

A. Elicit information regarding housing conditions, close contact, or sexual contact with potentially infected individuals.
B. Question the client regarding onset, duration, and location of itching.

Physical Examination

A. Check temperature.
B. Inspect:
    1. Examine all body surfaces with client unclothed.
    2. Use a magnifying lens to identify characteristic burrows in finger webs, wrists, and penis.
    3. Inspect adult pubic area for lesions.

Diagnostic Tests

A. Three findings are diagnostic of scabies:
    1. Microscopic identification of *S. scabiei* mites
    2. Eggs
    3. Fecal pellets (scybala)
B. Burrow identification: Ink the suspected area with a blue or black felt-tipped pen, then wipe with an alcohol swab. The burrow absorbs the ink, while the surface ink is wiped clean.

C. A tiny black dot may be seen at the end of a burrow, which represents the mite, ova, or feces, and can be transferred by means of a 25-gauge hypodermic needle to immersion oil on a slide for microscopic identification.
D. Place a drop of mineral oil on a suspected lesion, scrape the lesion with a #15 blade, and transfer the shaved material to a microscope slide for direct examination of the mite under low power.

Differential Diagnoses

A. Atopic dermatitis
B. Insect bites
C. Pityriasis rosea
D. Eczema
E. Seborrheic dermatitis
F. Syphilis
G. Pediculosis
H. Allergic or irritant contact dermatitis

Plan

A. General interventions:
    1. Implement comfort measures to reduce pruritus.
    2. Treat secondary infection(s) with antibiotics
    3. Household members should be treated simultaneously as a prophylactic measure and to reduce the chance of reinfection.
    4. The client should be advised that pruritus may continue for up to a week even with a successful treatment because of local irritation.
B. Client teaching: *See Section III: Client Teaching Guide* ◄ *for this chapter, "Scabies."*
C. Pharmaceutical therapy:
    1. First line of therapy, because of its low toxicity, is 5% permethrin (Elimite cream) applied to all body areas from the neck down and washed off in 8 to 14 hours. One application is highly effective, but some dermatologists recommend retreatment in 1 week.
    2. Alternative therapy is lindane (Kwell) cream, applied to all skin surfaces from the neck down and washed off in 8 to 12 hours. Some dermatologists retreat in 1 week.
    3. An oral dose of the anthelmintic agent ivermectin (200 mcg/kg) followed by a repeat dose in 1 to 2 weeks has been shown to be effective and to rapidly control pruritus in healthy clients and HIV clients
    4. Diphenhydramine (Benadryl) 25 to 50 mg may be given by mouth every 4 to 6 hours if indicated for pruritus. Other nonsedating antihistamines may be used. Toxicity is usually a result of client overtreatment (failure to follow prescribed regimen). Advise the client of this danger.

Follow-Up

A. Follow up in 2 weeks to assess treatment response.

Consultation/Referral

A. Consult or refer the client to the physician if, at 2-week follow-up, pharmaceutical therapy has been ineffective.

Individual Considerations

A. Pregnancy:
1. Permethrin is preferred to lindane in pregnant and/or lactating women because of decreased toxicity.
2. Client should be warned of its potential to cause neurotoxicity and convulsions with overuse (more than two treatments).

B. Pediatrics:
1. Infants and toddlers often have more widespread involvement that can include the face and scalp.
2. Vesicular lesions on palms and soles are more commonly seen.
3. Drug of choice is permethrin 5% cream; apply over the head, neck, and body, avoiding the eyes. The cream should be removed by bathing within 8 to 14 hours.
4. Lindane should not be used in infants and toddlers.
5. Infants and children with underlying cutaneous disease, malnutrition, prematurity, or a history of seizure disorders should be treated with special caution because of their increased risk of toxicity.

C. Partners:
1. All intimate contacts within the past month and close household and family members should be treated.

D. Geriatrics:
1. The elderly tend to have more severe pruritus despite fewer lesions.
2. They are at risk of extensive infections because of age-related decline in immunity.
3. The excoriations may become severe and may be complicated by cellulitis.
4. Avoid first-generation anticholinergics because of risk of confusion, dry mouth, constipation and other anticholinergic effects or toxicity.
5. Geriatric clients that have dementia or declining functional abilities need a thorough home environment assessment and an evaluation for any issues of neglect or abuse.

Bibliography

May, P. J., Tong, S. Y. C., Steer, A. C., Currie, B. J., Andrews, R. M., Carapetis, J. R., & Bowen, A. C. (2019). Treatment, prevention and public health management of impetigo, scabies, crusted scabies and fungal skin infections in endemic populations: A systematic review. *Tropical Medicine & International Health, 24*(3), 280–293. doi:10.1111/tmi.13198

Seborrheic Dermatitis

Jill C. Cash and Amy C. Bruggemann

Definition

A. A common chronic, erythematous, scaling dermatosis, seborrheic dermatitis occurs in areas of the most active sebaceous glands such as the face and scalp, body folds, and presternal region (see Figure 4.20).

Incidence

A. Seborrheic dermatitis is very common, affecting approximately 1% to 5% of the general population.
B. Incidence is higher in HIV-infected individuals, ranging from 34% to 83%.

Pathogenesis

A. Etiology is unknown. There is a possibility that it is hormonally dependent, has a fungal (*Pityrosporum ovale* or *C. albicans*) component, is neurogenic, or may reflect a nutritional deficiency.
B. Currently, it is identified as an inflammatory disorder that most probably results from a dysfunction of sebaceous glands.

Predisposing Factors

A. Possible link between infantile and adult forms
B. Possible familial trend
C. High association with HIV-infected individuals

Common Complaints

A. Infants: "Cradle cap"
B. Adults: "Dandruff," dry flaky scalp
C. Rash with "sticky flakes"

> Often no presenting complaints are found on a routine physical examination.

Other Signs and Symptoms

A. Variable pruritus, often increasing with perspiration and in winter
B. Oily, flaking skin on erythemic base around ears, nose, eyebrows, and eyelids
C. Red, cracking skin in body folds; axilla; groin; or anogenital, submammary, or umbilical areas
D. Primary lesions: Plaques
E. Secondary lesions: Erythema, scales, fissures, exudate, and symmetric eyelid involvement
F. Lesions with drainage or crusting may indicate secondary bacterial infection
G. Distribution pattern in infants: Scalp and diaper area
H. Distribution area in adults: Scalp, eyebrows, paranasal area, nasolabial fold, chin, behind ears, chest, and groin
I. Secondary impetigo in children

FIGURE 4.20 Infantile seborrheic dermatitis.

Subjective Data

A. Identify location, onset, and progression of symptoms.

B. Ask the client to describe symptoms. Ask if the skin is itchy or painful.

C. Assess lesions for any associated discharge (blood or pus)

D. Elicit information regarding use of topical medications, soaps, creams, or lotions. Quiz the client regarding any oral medications being taken.

E. Determine whether there were any preceding systemic symptoms (fever, sore throat, anorexia, or vaginal discharge).

F. Rule out any possible exposure to industrial or domestic toxins.

G. Ask the client to identify what improves or worsens this condition.

Physical Examination

A. Inspect:
1. Inspect skin; note areas of lesions and distribution.
2. Assess eyes for blepharitis.
3. Inspect ears and nose.

B. Palpate:
1. Skin, noting texture and moisture.

Diagnostic Tests

A. None required

B. Consider fungal culture in children and adolescents to rule out a fungal infection.

C. Consider possible skin biopsy to rule out other conditions.

Differential Diagnoses

A. Seborrheic dermatitis
B. Atopic dermatitis
C. Candidiasis
D. Dermatophytosis
E. Histiocytosis X
F. Psoriasis vulgaris
G. Rosacea
H. Systemic lupus erythematosus
I. Tinea capitis
J. Tinea versicolor
K. Vitamin deficiency
L. Impetigo
M. Eczema
N. Secondary syphilis

Plan

A. General interventions:
1. Shampooing is the foundation of treatment.
   a. Infants: Rub petroleum jelly into scalp to soften crusts 20 to 30 minutes before shampooing.
   b. Shampoo daily with baby shampoo using a soft brush.
   c. Toddlers or adolescents: Shampoo every other day with antiseborrheic shampoo (Selsun Blue, Exsel, or Nizoral).
2. If skin does not clear after 1 to 2 weeks of treatment, it is appropriate to use ketoconazole 2% cream.

3. Seborrheic blepharitis:
   a. Hot compresses plus gentle debridement with cotton-tipped applicator and baby shampoo twice a day
   b. For secondary bacterial infection, sulfacetamide sodium 10% (ophthalmic Sodium Sulamyd)
4. Continue treatment for several days after lesions disappear.

B. Client teaching: *See Section III: Client Teaching Guide for this chapter, "Seborrheic Dermatitis."*

C. Pharmaceutical therapy:
1. Most shampoos should be used two times per week. Those with coal tar can be used three times per week.
2. Medicated shampoos:
   a. Coal tar (Denorex, T/Gel, Pentrax, Tegrin) shampoo, apply as directed
   b. Salicylic acid (Ionil Plus, P and S) shampoo, apply as directed
   c. Selenium sulfide (Exsel, Selsun Blue) shampoo, use daily
   d. Ketoconazole 2% (Nizoral) cream, apply to affected area twice daily for 4 to 6 weeks
   e. Combination shampoos: Coal tar and salicylic acid (T/Sal); salicylic acid and sulfur (Sebulex). These shampoos may be used one to two times a week, alternating with other shampoos during the week. Always apply corticosteroids in a thin layer only; avoid the eyes.
3. Topical corticosteroid lotions or solutions: Use in combination with medicated shampoo if 2 to 3 weeks of treatment with shampoo alone fails.
4. Adults: Scalp:
   a. Start with medium potency, for example, betamethasone valerate 0.1% lotion 20 to 60 mL twice daily
   b. If treatment is not effective in 2 weeks, increase potency, for example, fluocinonide 0.05% solution 20 to 60 mL twice daily, or fluocinolone acetonide 0.01% oil 120 mL nightly with shower cap
   c. As dermatitis is controlled, decrease to mild potency, for example, hydrocortisone 1% to 2.5% lotion 20 to 60 mL once or twice daily
5. Adults: Face or groin:
   a. Low-potency agents, for example, hydrocortisone 1% cream or desonide 0.05% cream once or twice daily
   b. Consider lotion for eyebrows for easier application.
   c. Metronidazole 1% gel on face once or twice daily
6. Recalcitrant disease:
   a. Add ketoconazole 2% cream (15, 30, or 60 g) every day.
   b. Use sulfacetamide sodium 10%, with sulfur 5%, lotion 25 g once or twice daily.

Follow-Up

A. Advise the client to call the office in 5 to 6 days to report progress.

B. The client should return to the office if no improvement is seen.

Consultation/Referral

A. Refer the client to a dermatologist if the condition does not clear in 10 to 14 days.

Individual Considerations

A. Pregnancy:
   1. Ketoconazole is not recommended.
B. Pediatrics:
   1. Avoid using tar preparations on infants.
   2. Use baby shampoo only.
   3. If lesions are inflammatory, use topical steroids no stronger than hydrocortisone 0.5% to 1.0% twice daily.
   4. Betamethasone valerate (Valisone) lotion may be used daily for scalp only if other treatments fail.
   5. Be aware of potential for emotional distress in adolescents
   6. Treat with antiseborrheic shampoo every other day for adolescents.
C. Geriatrics:
   1. Seborrheic dermatitis is one of the most common inflammatory skin disorders with the elderly population. Clients with light dry skin have the greater risk of an occurrence, especially during the winter.

Bibliography

Barak-Shinar, D., & Green, L. J. (2018). Scalp seborrheic dermatitis and dandruff therapy using a herbal and zinc pyrithione-based therapy of shampoo and scalp lotion. *Journal of Clinical & Aesthetic Dermatology*, *11*(1), 26–31. Retrieved from http://search.ebscohost.com.proxy.library.vanderbilt.edu/login.aspx?direct=true&AuthType=ip,uid,cpid&custid=s9007717&db=ccm&AN=127294010&site=ehost-live

Friedmann, D. P., Mishra, V., & Batty, T. (2018). Progressive facial papules in an African-American patient: An atypical presentation of seborrheic dermatitis. *Journal of Clinical & Aesthetic Dermatology*, *11*(7), 44–45. Retrieved from http://search.ebscohost.com.proxy.library.vanderbilt.edu/login.aspx?direct=true&AuthType=ip,uid,cpid&custid=s9007717&db=ccm&AN=130845905&site=ehost-live

Tinea Corporis (Ringworm)

Jill C. Cash and Amy C. Bruggemann

Definition

A. Tinea corporis (ringworm) is a fungal infection of the skin tissue (keratin) commonly seen on the face, trunk, and extremities (Figure 4.21).
B. Tinea capitis is a fungal infection of scalp hair.
C. Tinea cruris is a fungal infection of the groin.
D. Tinea pedis is a fungal infection of the foot.
E. Tinea unguium (dermatophyte onychomycosis) is a fungal infection of the nail.

Incidence

A. Ringworm is a fairly common fungal infection seen in adults and children.

Pathogenesis

A. The causative fungal species varies, depending on the location of the infection. Three common organisms are *Epidermophyton, Microsporum,* and *Trichophyton.*
B. The infection can be obtained from other people, animals (puppies, kittens), and the soil.

Predisposing Factors

A. Exposure to person or facilities (e.g., locker rooms) infected with the fungus
B. Poor nutrition
C. Poor health
D. Poor hygiene
E. Warm climates
F. Immunosuppression

Common Complaints

A. Scaly, itchy patch of skin
B. When circular in shape, usually tinea corporis (ringworm)
C. When nails are thickened and yellow usually tinea unguium

Other Signs and Symptoms

A. Tinea capitis: Erythema, scaling of scalp, with hair loss at site asymptomatic
B. Tinea corporis: Circular, erythematous, well-demarcated lesion on the skin with hypopigmentation in center of lesion; usually pruritic
C. Tinea cruris: Well-demarcated scaling lesions on groin (not scrotum) or thigh; usually pruritic
D. Tinea pedis: Scaly, erythemic vesicles on feet, between toes, and in arch, with extreme pruritus

FIGURE 4.21 Tinea corporis.

Source: Reproduced from Kifer, Z. A. (2012). *Fast facts for wound care nursing: Practical wound management in a nutshell* (p. 258). New York, NY: Springer Publishing Company.

E. Tinea unguium (onychomycosis): Thickening and yellowing of toenail or fingernail, often with other fungal infection or alone

Subjective Data

A. Ask the client about onset, duration, and progression of the patch or rash on the skin.
B. Assess the client about other areas of skin involvement.
C. Ask if the lesion is pruritic.
D. Inquire as to the client's exposure to anyone with similar symptoms.
E. Determine whether the client has a history of similar lesions.
F. Query the client regarding predisposing factors.
G. Review with the client what remedies were used and with what results.

Physical Examination

A. Check temperature (if indicated).
B. Inspect:
   1. Examine all areas of skin.
   2. Note type of lesions present.

Diagnostic Tests

A. Obtain scrapings of the border of the lesion for evaluation:
   1. Potassium hydroxide (KOH)
   2. Wet prep
   3. Fungal cultures

Differential Diagnoses

A. Tinea corporis
B. Dermatitis
C. Alopecia areata
D. Psoriasis
E. Contact dermatitis
F. Atopic eczema
G. Subacute cutaneous lupus erythematous
H. Pityriasis rosea

Plan

A. General interventions:
   1. Identify type of lesion.
   2. Identify other infected family members or sexual partners for treatment.
B. Client teaching:
   1. *See Section III: Client Teaching Guide for this chapter, "Ringworm Tinea."*
   2. Reinforce medication regimen for 4- to 8-week period for resolution.
C. Pharmaceutical therapy:
   1. Tinea capitis:
      a. Adults: Griseofulvin 500 mg by mouth per day for 4 to 8 weeks.
      b. Children: Griseofulvin 10 to 20 mg/kg/d for 4 to 8 weeks. **Griseofulvin is best absorbed with high-fat foods.**
      c. Ketoconazole (Nizoral) may also be used.

   2. Tinea corporis, pedis, and cruris:
      a. Use wet dressings with Burow's solution along with one of the following:
         i. Clotrimazole 1% (Lotrimin) cream, or econazole nitrate 1% cream, twice daily for 14 to 28 days
         ii. Terbinafine 1% cream (Lamisil), topical, apply once or twice daily for 1 to 4 weeks. Not recommended for children
   3. Onychomycosis: Successful treatment is difficult.
      a. Itraconazole (Sporanox) 100 mg, two tablets by mouth twice daily for 7 days. Repeat in 1 month, then repeat again in 1 more month.

Monitor liver function tests (LFTs) at 6 weeks after starting medication.

---

      b. Terbinafine 1% cream (Lamisil)
         i. Fingernail: 250 mg once daily for 6 weeks
         ii. Toenail: 250 mg daily for 12 weeks
      c. Home cure: Apply Vicks VapoRub on toenail bed and cover with a sock every night at bedtime for approximately 4 to 6 months or until resolved. This treatment offers a safe, cost-effective alternative to oral medications.

Follow-Up

A. A 2- to 4-week follow-up is recommended to evaluate progress.
B. When using Sporonox, monitor LFTs at 6 weeks. If the medication is continued, monitoring LFTs every 6 to 8 weeks is recommended.

Consultation/Referral

A. Consult a physician if the infection has not improved.

Individual Considerations

A. Pregnancy: Oral antifungal medications are not recommended during pregnancy.
B. Pediatrics:
   1. Tinea capitis is common in children 2 to 10 years old. When hair has been lost, regrowth takes time.
   2. Tinea pedis is common in adolescents.
   3. Tinea unguium is common in adolescents, but rare in children.
C. Adults:
   1. Tinea capitis is rare in adults.
   2. Tinea cruris is more common in obese males, but rare in females.
   3. Tinea pedis is common in adults.
   4. Tinea unguium is seen in adults.
   5. Transient and/or permanent hearing loss has been documented in some clients with the use of itraconazole. These cases were reported when itraconazole was used with quinidine, which is contraindicated.

D. Elderly:
1. Itraconazole should be used cautiously in the elderly client.
2. Recommendation for tinea treatment with the elderly population is Terbinafine because of its decreased risk for cardiac complications and drug interactions.

Bibliography

Hudson, A., Sturgeon, A., & Peiris, A. (2018). Tinea versicolor. *JAMA: Journal of the American Medical Association, 320*(13), 1396. doi:10.1001/jama.2018.12429

May, P. J., Tong, S. Y. C., Steer, A. C., Currie, B. J., Andrews, R. M., Carapetis, J. R., & Bowen, A. C. (2019). Treatment, prevention and public health management of impetigo, scabies, crusted scabies and fungal skin infections in endemic populations: A systematic review. *Tropical Medicine & International Health, 24*(3), 280–293. doi:10.1111/tmi.13198

Shear, N. H., Gupta, A. K., Piguet, V., Versteeg, S. G., Tosti, A., & Piraccini, B. M. (2019). A practical guide to curing onychomycosis: How to maximize cure at the patient, organism, treatment, and environmental level. *American Journal of Clinical Dermatology, 20*(1), 123–133. doi:10.1007/s40257-018-0403-4

Trayes, K. P., Savage, K., & Studdiford, J. S. (2018). Annular lesions: Diagnosis and treatment. *American Family Physician, 98*(5), 283–291.

Tinea Versicolor

Jill C. Cash and Amy C. Bruggemann

Definition
A. Tinea versicolor is a fungal infection of the skin, which may be chronic in nature (Figure 4.22). It is most commonly seen on the upper trunk; however, it may spread to extremities.

Incidence
A. Tinea versicolor is seen most frequently in adolescents and young adults.

Pathogenesis
A. Tinea versicolor is a fungal infection of the skin caused by an overgrowth of *Pityrosporum orbiculare*, part of the normal skin flora.
B. Discoloration of the skin is seen, forming round or oval maculae, which may become confluent.

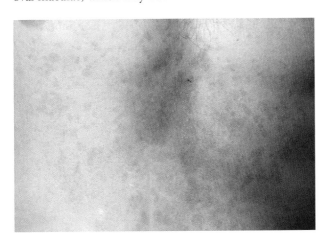

FIGURE 4.22 Examples of tinea versicolor.

Source: Reproduced from Lyons, F., & Ousley, L. (2015). *Dermatology for the advanced practice nurse.* New York, NY: Springer Publishing Company, Figure III.55.

C. Maculae range from 1 cm to very large, greater than 30 cm.

Predisposing Factors
A. Immunosuppressive therapy
B. Pregnancy
C. Warm temperatures
D. Corticosteroid therapy

Common Complaint
A. Scaly rash on the upper trunk with occasional mild itching

Other Signs and Symptoms
A. Annular maculae with mild scaling
B. Asymptomatic or pruritic
C. Pink-, white-, or brown-colored rash

Subjective Data
A. Ascertain when and where the rash began.
B. Have the client describe how the rash has changed.
C. Assess the client for any associated symptoms with the rash such as itching and burning.
D. Identify what products the client has used on the skin to treat rash and with what results.
E. Elicit information regarding a history of similar rashes.
F. Query the client regarding current medications.
G. Review any medical history for comorbid conditions.

Physical Examination
A. Inspect:
1. Inspect skin and note type of lesion.
2. Examine other areas of skin for similar lesions.

Diagnostic Tests
A. Wet prep/potassium hydroxide (KOH)
B. Wood's lamp: Wood's lamp is useful in examining skin to determine the extent of infection. Inspection of fine scales with Wood's lamp reveals scales with a pale yellow-green fluorescence that contains the fungus.
C. Culture lesion: When obtaining a sample scraping, obtain the sample from the edge of the lesion for the best sample of hyphae. (Hyphae and spores have a "spaghetti and meatball" appearance.)

Differential Diagnoses
A. Tinea versicolor
B. Tinea corporis
C. Pityriasis alba
D. Pityriasis rosea: Herald patch is clue to diagnosis.
E. Seborrheic dermatitis
F. Vitiligo

Plan
A. General interventions:
1. Apply medication as directed.
B. Client teaching:
1. *See Section III: Client Teaching Guide for this chapter, "Tinea Versicolor."*

2. These causative species are a normal inhabitant of skin flora; recurrence is possible.

3. Skin pigmentation returns after infection is cleared up. This may take several months to resolve.

C. Pharmaceutical therapy:

1. Selenium sulfide 2.5% (Selsun Blue)

a. Advise client to shower at bedtime. Then apply selenium sulfide 2.5% cream to skin, covering entire body from chin down to toes. Leave treatment on skin for 8 to 10 hours. Shower off in the morning.

b. A second treatment option includes applying the selenium sulfide 2.5% cream to skin lesions daily for 12 days. Leave treatment on skin for 30 minutes, then shower off.

c. Treatment may be needed monthly until desired results are obtained. Encourage use of Selsun Blue on entire body surface except for face and head.

2. Other medications used:

a. Clotrimazole 1% cream twice daily for 4 weeks

b. Ketoconazole (Nizoral) cream daily for 14 days

c. Fluconazole 300 mg once weekly for 2 weeks. When using fluconazole as treatment, caution the client regarding liver damage with toxicity.

Follow-Up

A. None is required if resolution occurs.

B. Monitor LFTs every 6 weeks if client is on ketoconazole.

Consultation/Referral

A. Consult with a physician if current treatment is unsuccessful.

Individual Considerations

A. Pediatrics:

1. Commonly seen in adolescents

B. Adults:

1. Commonly seen in young adults

Bibliography

Lipner, S. R., & Scher, R. K. (2019). Onychomycosis: Clinical overview and diagnosis. *Journal of the American Academy of Dermatology, 80*(4), 835–851. doi:10.1016/j.jaad.2018.03.062

May, P. J., Tong, S. Y. C., Steer, A. C., Currie, B. J., Andrews, R. M., Carapetis, J. R., & Bowen, A. C. (2019). Treatment, prevention and public health management of impetigo, scabies, crusted scabies and fungal skin infections in endemic populations: A systematic review. *Tropical Medicine & International Health, 24*(3), 280–293. doi:10.1111/tmi.13198

Plensdorf, S., Livieratos, M., & Dada, N. (2017). Pigmentation disorders: Diagnosis and management. *American Family Physician, 96*(12), 797–804.

Shear, N. H., Gupta, A. K., Piguet, V., Versteeg, S. G., Tosti, A., & Piraccini, B. M. (2019). A practical guide to curing onychomycosis: How to maximize cure at the patient, organism, treatment, and environmental level. *American Journal of Clinical Dermatology, 20*(1), 123–133. doi:10.1007/s40257-018-0403-4

Warts

Jill C. Cash and Amy C. Bruggemann

Definition

A. A wart is an elevation of the epidermal layer of the skin (skin tumor). Warts are caused by the papillomavirus.

Incidence

A. Warts occur in people of all ages, more common in children and during early adulthood.

B. By adulthood, 90% of all people have positive antibodies to the virus.

C. Warts are seen more frequently in females than in males.

Pathogenesis

A. A circumscribed mass develops on the skin that is limited to the epidermal layer. The virus, papillomavirus, is located within the nucleus of the cell.

B. The virus may be transmitted by touch and is commonly seen on the hands and feet.

C. Most warts resolve without treatment within 12 to 24 months.

Predisposing Factors

A. Skin trauma

B. Immunosuppression

C. Exposure to public showers, pools, locker rooms, and so forth

Common Complaints

A. Bump on the skin or specific area of the body (hands, feet, arms, and legs)

B. Usually painless unless present on the bottom of the foot

Other Signs and Symptoms

A. Common wart (verruca vulgaris): Flesh-colored, irregular lesion with rough surface; black dots in center of lesion occasionally seen, which is thrombosed capillaries; can occur on any body part

B. Filiform wart (verruca filiformis): Thin, threadlike, projected papule on face, lips, nose, or eyelids

C. Flat wart (verruca plana): Flat-topped, flesh-colored papule, 1 to 3 mm in diameter, with smooth surface; seen in clusters or in a line, on face and extremities

D. Plantar wart (verruca plantaris): Firm papula, 2 to 3 cm in diameter, indented into skin with verrucous surface; painful with ambulation, when placed on ball or heel of foot

E. Genital warts: See Chapter 15: Sexually Transmitted Infections Guidelines.

Subjective Data

A. Determine onset, location, and duration of tumor.

B. Elicit information regarding a history of previous warts.

C. Identify with the client what treatment has been used in the past and what the results were. Question the client regarding length of time OTC medications were used, and how aggressive he or she was with the treatment.

FIGURE 4.23 Molluscum contagiosum.

Source: Reproduced from Kifer, Z. A. (2012). *Fast facts for wound care nursing: Practical wound management in a nutshell* (p. 250). New York, NY: Springer Publishing Company.

Physical Examination

A. Inspect:
1. Assess skin for lesions, noting location, appearance, size, and surface texture of tumor.
2. Examine the entire body for other lesions.

Diagnostic Test

A. None indicated

Differential Diagnoses

A. Wart:
1. Verruca vulgaris
2. Verruca filiformis
3. Verruca plana
4. Verruca plantaris
B. Seborrheic keratosis
C. Callus
D. Molluscum contagiosum: Flesh-colored group of firm papules found on the face, trunk, and/or extremities (Figure 4.23). A white core may be expressed from the lesion. Lesion may be successfully removed by curettage or cryotherapy.

Plan

A. General interventions:
1. Identify the type of wart.
2. Conservative treatment is recommended for children.
▶ B. Client teaching: *See Section III: Client Teaching Guide for this chapter, "Warts."*
C. Pharmaceutical therapy:
1. Common wart: After soaking and filing wart with a nail file, apply one of these:
   a. Salicylic acid 17% (Compound W) gel twice daily for up to 12 weeks, if needed. Keep site covered with adhesive.
   b. Apply duct tape to site after treatment. Repeat this treatment every night for up to 12 weeks or until resolved.
   c. Cryotherapy with liquid nitrogen to site. Repeat every 3 to 4 weeks until resolved. Apply adhesive tape over site and keep covered.
2. Flat wart:
   a. Retinoic acid: Apply to site twice daily for 4 to 6 weeks

b. Aldara (imiquimod) 5% cream may be applied by the client at home. Although the labeled use is for genital warts, the client may consider off-label use at bedtime and wash off after 6 to 8 hours every other day until resolved. Precautions should be stressed regarding the caustic nature of the cream to healthy skin.
3. Plantar wart: Salicylic acid 40% (Mediplast), apply over wart. Remove in 24 to 48 hours, and remove dead skin with a pumice stone or by scraping or using a nail file. Educate the client to throw away the emory board nail file after each use. If using a nail file, after each use, cleanse with alcohol. Repeat every 24 to 48 hours until wart is removed. May take up to 6 to 8 weeks.
4. Filiform wart:
   a. Cryotherapy with liquid nitrogen to site. Repeat every 3 to 4 weeks until resolved. Apply adhesive tape over the site and keep covered.
   b. Dermatologist referral for surgical removal

Follow-Up

A. Follow the client every 4 to 6 weeks until resolved.

Consultation/Referral

A. If diagnosis is unclear, refer the client to a dermatologist for surgical excision and biopsy.

Individual Considerations

A. Pediatrics:
1. Warts are commonly seen in young school-aged children.
B. Geriatrics.
1. Use caution if client elects cryotherapy to treat a wart secondary to thinness of aging skin. Always assess if the client is taking aspirin or anticoagulant therapy prior to incisional removal or cryotherapy.

Bibliography

Efficacy and safety of hydrogen peroxide topical solution, 45% (w/w) for treatment of common warts: 8-Week results from the phase 2 WART-203 trial. (2019). *Journal of the American Academy of Dermatology, 81*, AB53. https://doi-org.proxy.library.vanderbilt.edu/10.1016/j.jaad.2019.06.223

Long-term efficacy and safety of hydrogen peroxide topical solution, 45% (w/w) in patients with common warts: Posttreatment results from the phase 2 WART 203 trial. (2019). *Journal of the American Academy of Dermatology, 81*, AB89. https://doi-org.proxy.library.vanderbilt.edu/10.1016/j.jaad.2019.06.345

Wound Care: Lower Extremity Ulcer

Amy C. Bruggemann

Definition

A. Vascular ulcer:
1. Arterial/ischemic ulcer:
   a. Skin ulcers usually found on the medial or lateral foot or ankle; ulcers are nonhealing because of inadequate arterial flow
2. Venous ulcer:
   a. Chronic skin and subcutaneous lesions are usually found on the lower extremity between the

ankle and knee, thought to occur from intracellular edema or inflammatory processes

B. Diabetic foot ulcer:

1. Skin ulcers are usually found on the plantar surface of the foot, most commonly occurring from trauma or plantar pressure

Incidence

A. Diabetic foot ulcers precede more than 80% of lower extremity amputations in the United States.

B. The financial burden of venous ulcers is estimated to be $2 billion per year in the United States.

C. Up to 20% of lower extremity ulcers have been shown to have mixed etiology disease.

Pathogenesis

A. An ulcer that is found between the knees and toes constitutes a lower extremity ulcer, and guidelines are based according to the etiology. Many times lower extremity ulcers have more than one cause. The most common etiologies are venous insufficiency, arterial insufficiency, diabetic foot ulcer, and/or pressure.

Predisposing Factors

A. Arterial insufficiency

B. Congestive heart failure

C. Coronary artery disease

D. Diabetes

E. Edema

F. Hyperlipidemia

G. Obesity

H. Age: Older than 65 years

I. Venous insufficiency

J. Peripheral neuropathy

Common Complaints

A. Lower extremity or foot pain

B. Bleeding

C. Drainage

D. Hyperglycemia

Subjective Data

A. Ask the client to describe the location and onset. What does he or she think may have been the cause? Was the onset sudden or gradual? How have the symptoms continued to develop?

B. Assess if the area is pruritic or painful. Does the client note any change in sensation?

C. Assess for any associated drainage. Ask about the color and if any odor is noted.

D. Complete a drug history. Ask the client if he or she is taking any steroids or anticoagulants.

E. Has the client been treated in this location before? If so, describe.

F. Determine whether the client has attempted to treat this at home. If yes, inquire about treatments that have been performed.

G. Does the client have any numbness or tingling in the lower extremities? Does the client wake up at night with pain? Does he or she have any pain with ambulation? Does he or she have sensation in the feet?

H. Rule out any possible exposure to industrial or domestic toxins, or insect bites.

I. Assess for iodine and sulfa allergies before starting treatment.

Physical Examination

A. Check temperature, pulse, respiration, and blood pressure.

B. Inspect:

1. Assess the lower extremities, feet, and toes:

a. Color of the skin:

i. Assess skin; begin at the top of the legs, move down the legs to the toes looking for changes in color that may exhibit signs of ischemia.

ii. Hemosiderin staining may exhibit venous insufficiency.

2. Inspect the ulcer:

a. Measure length × width × depth:

i. Undermining: Measure and note location, using the face of a clock to document the site of undermining: 12 o'clock, 3 o'clock, 6 o'clock, or 9 o'clock

ii. Tunneling (destroyed tissue pathway that creates dead space underneath the skin): Measure and note the location, using the face of a clock to document the site of tunneling: 12 o'clock, 3 o'clock, 6 o'clock, or 9 o'clock

b. Describe the wound bed:

i. Tissue in the wound bed

1) Necrotic tissue, slough tissue, granulation tissue, or epithelial tissue. Percentage of each together should equal 100%.

ii. Color of the tissue (percentage to equal 100%, i.e., 80% pink, 20% yellow)

1) Red, pink, yellow, brown, tan, or black

iii. Drainage:

1) Amount:

a) None, scant, moderate, or copious

2) Color:

a) Serous, sanguineous, purulent, yellow, serosanguineous, or green

iv. Odor:

1) Odor present: Yes or no

v. Periwound:

1) Intact

2) Not intact:

a) Describe periwound: Note erythema, fever, induration, maceration, excoriation, calloused, or epiboly.

3. Palpate:

1. Note temperature of the skin.

2. Assess sensation of the skin.

3. Check capillary refill.

4. Assess pulses in bilateral extremities.

Diagnostic Tests

A. Ankle brachial index (ABI)
B. Arterial Doppler
C. Bone scan
D. CBC
E. Hemoglobin A1c (Hgb A1c)
F. MRI
G. Wound culture
H. Wound biopsy
I. Venous Doppler
J. X-ray

Differential Diagnoses

A. Vascular ulcer:
   1. Arterial/ischemic ulcer
   2. Venous ulcer
B. Diabetic foot ulcer
C. Abscess
D. Atypical ulcers
E. Dermatological disorder
F. Necrotizing fasciitis
G. Skin cancers
H. Pressure ulcer
I. Trauma
J. Pyoderma gangrenosum

Plan

A. General interventions
   1. Vascular ulcers:
      a. Arterial ulcer:
         i. Refer to vascular surgery for assessment to improve arterial flow.
         ii. Refer to wound care specialist.
      b. Venous ulcer:
         i. Establish arterial flow
            1) Refer to vascular surgeon if deficiency found.
         ii. For signs and symptoms of infection, treat the infection first with tissue culture and sensitivity. Treat per pharmaceutical recommendations. Treat with silver alginate to the site for moderate drainage and silver gel to the site for scant drainage.
         iii. Once arterial flow has been established as sufficient and infection has been ruled out, compression therapy is the mainstay of treatment for venous ulcers. Compression therapy recommendations:
            a) ABI: 0.8 to 1.0 full compression:
               ❍ Pro-fore
               ❍ Apply calcium alginate to ulcer, then wrap with an Unna Boot and cover with a coban wrap.
               ❍ Change in 3 days; if tolerating, then change weekly.
            b) ABI: 0.6 to 0.8 Light compression:
               ❍ Pro-fore lite

               ❍ Apply calcium alginate to ulcer, then wrap with a Unna Boot, and then cover with a coban wrap.
               ❍ Change in 3 days; if tolerating well, then change weekly.
   2. Diabetic foot ulcer:
      a. Establish arterial flow.
         i. Refer to a vascular surgeon if deficiency found.
      b. For signs and symptoms of infection, use a sterile culturette to obtain a tissue culture and sensitivity first to assess what organism is present and to determine sensitivities. Treat per pharmaceutical recommendations. Treat with silver alginate to the site for moderate drainage, and silver gel to the site for scant drainage.
      c. Initiate offloading to site:
         i. Refer to an orthotist for assessment if devices are required.
      d. Treatment options:
         i. To debride: Cleanse with normal saline (NS), apply Santyl, and change dressing daily and as needed.
         ii. To granulate an ulcer with scant drainage: Cleanse with NS, apply hydrogel, and change dressing daily and as needed.
         iii. To granulate an ulcer with moderate drainage: Cleanse with NS, apply calcium alginate, and change dressing daily as needed.
B. Client teaching:
   1. *See Section III: Client Teaching Guide for this chapter, "Wound Care: Lower Extremity Ulcers."* ◀
C. Pharmaceutical therapy:
   1. If culture and sensitivity are performed, antibiotics may be used as recommended per sensitivity.

Follow-Up

A. Follow up in 1 to 2 weeks to evaluate therapy.
B. See clients every 1 to 2 weeks until healing well; then client may reduce to 2- to 4-week evaluation until complete closure.

Consultation/Referral

A. Consult or refer the client to a wound care specialist when the client has:
   1. Extensive ulcer that you are not comfortable with:
      a. Visible bone, muscle, or tendon
   2. Multiple medical comorbidities (especially diabetes)
   3. Not responded to treatment of 2 to 4 weeks
   4. Ulcer showing decline on follow-up visit
   5. Infection present

Individual Considerations

A. Adults:
   1. Ischemic ulcers warrant immediate referral
   2. Complaints of severe pain, lack of pulse, cool digit, or new onset of purplish/bluish discolorations to the feet require immediate workup for arterial clot to lower extremity

Wound Care: Pressure Ulcers

Amy C. Bruggemann

Definition

A. "A pressure injury is localized damage to the skin and underlying soft tissue usually over a bony prominence or related to a medical or other device. The injury can present as intact skin or an open ulcer and may be painful. The injury occurs as a result of intense and/or prolonged pressure or pressure in combination with shear. The tolerance of soft tissue for pressure and shear may also be affected by microclimate, nutrition, perfusion, comorbidities and condition of the soft tissue" (National Pressure Ulcer Advisory Panel [NPUAP], 2016).

Incidence

A. Acute care: 0.4% to 38%
B. Long-term care: 2.2% to 23.9%
C. Home care: 0% to 17%

Pathogenesis

A. Pressure ulcers occur when an area of tissue remains in surface contact for a period of time. This contact causes occlusion of microvascular vessels, which leads to tissue hypoxia and eventually may cause ischemia. Over time, a pressure ulcer develops. The amount of time this takes is client dependent and can be altered by physical and/or environmental factors of time.

Predisposing Factors

A. Acute illness
B. Fecal/urinary incontinence
C. Malnutrition
D. Weight loss
E. Failure or inability to offload:
    1. For example, fracture, elevation of head of bed (HOB), lack of education, or noncompliance

Common Complaints

A. Pain
B. Bleeding
C. Drainage

Subjective Data

A. Ask the client to describe the location and onset. What did he or she think may have been the cause? Was the onset sudden or gradual? How have the symptoms continued to develop?
B. Assess if the area is itchy or painful.
C. Assess for any associated drainage. Ask about the color and if any odor is noted.
D. Complete a drug history. Ask the client if he or she is taking any steroids or anticoagulants.
E. Has the client been treated in this location before? If so, describe.
F. Determine whether the client has attempted to treat this problem at home. If yes, ask with what.
G. Rule out any possible exposure to industrial or domestic toxins, or insect bites.

H. Assess for iodine and sulfa allergies before starting treatment.

Physical Examination

A. Check temperature, pulse, respirations, and blood pressure.
B. Inspect:
    1. Measure pressure ulcer: length × width × depth.
        a. Undermining: Measure and note location, using the face of a clock to document the site of undermining: 12 o'clock, 3 o'clock, 6 o'clock, or 9 o'clock
        b. Tunneling: Measure and note location, using the face of a clock to document the site of tunneling: for example, 12 o'clock, 3 o'clock, 6 o'clock, or 9 o'clock
    2. Describe the wound bed:
        a. Tissue in the wound bed
            i. Necrotic tissue, slough tissue, granulation tissue, or epithelial tissue **(percentage of each should together equal 100%)**
        b. Drainage:
            i. Amount:
                1) None, scant, moderate, or copious
            ii. Color:
                1) Serous, sanguineous, purulent, yellow, serosanguineous, or green
        c. Odor
        d. Periwound
            i. Intact
            ii. Not intact:
                1) Erythema, fever, induration, maceration, excoriation, calloused, or epiboly

Diagnostic Tests

A. CBC
B. Wound culture
C. Wound biopsy
D. X-ray
E. MRI
F. Bone scan

Diagnosis: Staging Pressure Injuries/Ulcers

A. **Deep-tissue pressure injury (DTPI)**
    1. Intact or nonintact skin with persistent nonblanchable discoloration (purple, deep red, maroon) or epidermal separation revealing a blood-filled blister or darkened wound bed.
    2. Changes in pain/temperature may precede changes in skin color. Discoloration may be difficult to detect in highly pigmented skin.
    3. DTPI may be due to intense pressure and shear forces at the bone–muscle interface.
    4. The wound may resolve without tissue loss, or rapid evolution may occur to reveal extent of damage.
    5. If fascia, muscle, necrotic/subcutaneous/granulation tissue, or other underlying structures are visible, this is likely a full-thickness pressure injury (Stage 3, 4, or unstageable).
    6. Do not use DTPI staging to describe neuropathic, vascular, dermatologic, or traumatic conditions.

B. **Stage 1 pressure injury**
1. Intact skin with nonblanchable, localized erythema. Discoloration may be difficult to detect in highly pigmented skin.
2. Changes in sensation, temperature, or firmness may precede visual changes.
3. Do not use Stage 1 to describe purple, deep red, or maroon discoloration; these may indicate DTPI.

C. **Stage 2 pressure injury:**
1. Partial-thickness loss of skin with exposed dermis
2. The wound is moist, pink or red, viable, and may present as an intact or ruptured serum-filled blister.
3. Deeper tissues and adipose (fat) are not visible.
4. Eschar, slough, and granulation tissue is not present.
5. Stage 2 pressure injuries are the result of adverse microclimate or shear forces.
6. Do not use Stage 2 to describe the following:
    a. Skin tears, burns, or abrasions.
    b. Moisture-associated skin damage (MASD), including:
        i. Incontinence-associated dermatitis (IAD)
        ii. Intertriginous dermatitis (ITD)
        iii. Medical adhesive-related skin injury (MARSI)

D. **Stage 3 pressure injury**
1. Full-thickness loss of skin, with visible adipose
2. Granulation tissue and epibole (rolled wound edges) are present.
3. Eschar and slough are present.
4. The extent of tissue damage varies by anatomical location; deep wounds may develop in areas of significant adiposity.
5. Undermining/tunneling may occur.
6. Muscle, tendon, ligament, cartilage, fascia and/or bone are not exposed.
7. Do not use Stage 3 if eschar or slough obscures the depth of tissue loss; this indicates an Unstageable Pressure Injury.

E. **Stage 4 pressure injury:**
1. Full-thickness loss of skin and tissue
2. Muscle, tendon, ligament, cartilage, fascia, and/or bone are exposed or directly palpable
3. Epibole (rolled wound edges), undermining, and/or tunneling often occur.
4. The extent of tissue damage varies by anatomical location.
5. Eschar or slough may be present. If either or both obscure the depth of tissue loss, this indicates an Unstageable Pressure Injury.

F. **Unstageable pressure injury**
1. Full-thickness loss of skin and tissue
2. Eschar or slough obscures the extent of tissue loss; removing these will reveal a Stage 3 or 4 Pressure Injury.

3. Do not soften or remove stable eschar (dry, adherent, intact without erythema or fluctuance) on the heel or ischemic limb.

G. **Medical device–related pressure injury**
1. This is the result of using devices intended for diagnostic or therapeutic purposes.
2. The pressure injury generally conforms to the shape or pattern of the device.
3. The injury should be staged using the staging system.

H. **Mucosal membrane pressure injury**
1. Found on mucous membranes with a history of medical device use at the injury's location
2. These ulcers cannot be staged due to the anatomy of the tissue

Differential Diagnoses
A. Pressure ulcer
B. Abscess
C. Trauma
D. Skin cancer
E. Vascular ulcer
F. Diabetic foot ulcers
G. Dermatological disorder

Plan
A. General interventions:
1. Identify the cause of pressure and alleviate.
2. To debride: NS cleanse, apply santyl and dressing change daily and as needed throughout.
3. To granulate an ulcer with scant drainage: NS cleanse, apply hydrogel and dressing change daily as needed.
4. To granulate an ulcer with moderate drainage: NS cleanse, apply calcium alginate and dressing change daily as needed.
B. Client teaching:
1. Educate client and family regarding stage of ulcer and treatment plan.
2. Wound nurse should be caring for wound and educating client and family of daily/weekly care.
C. Pharmaceutical therapy:
1. Treatment dependent on stage of ulcer

Follow-Up
A. Follow up in 1 to 2 weeks to evaluate therapy.
B. See clients every 1 to 2 weeks until healing well; then client may reduce to 2- to 4-week evaluation until complete closure.

Consultation/Referral
A. Consult or refer the client to a wound care specialist for the following:
1. Extensive ulcer that you are not comfortable treating
2. Client with multiple medical comorbidities (especially diabetes)
3. Client not responding to treatment of 2 to 4 weeks
4. Ulcer showing decline on follow-up visit
5. Infection present needing alternative treatment

Source: Adapted from National Pressure Ulcer Advisory Panel. (2016). NPUAP pressure injury stages. Retrieved from http://www.npuap.org/resources/educational-and -clinical-resources/npuap-pressure-injury-stages/

Individual Considerations

A. Adults:

    1. Clients at end of life may develop pressure ulcers related to the dying process, referred to as Kennedy terminal ulcers. These clients are treated for comfort.

B. Geriatrics:

    1. Research suggests that pressure ulcers in the elderly population (especially those suffering dementia) appear to accelerate health deterioration, which leads to lower survival and higher mortality rates.

    2. Educate the client and surrogates regarding good nutrition, fall prevention, skin care, and meticulous wound care techniques could help decrease pressure ulcer complications and increase survival time.

Wound Care: Wounds of the Skin

Jill C. Cash and Amy C. Bruggemann

Definition

Wounds are breaks in the external surface of the body

Pathogenesis

Wounds can be caused by any one of the innumerable objects that breach the skin. Lacerations and abrasions typically heal by a three-stage process of clotting, inflammation, and skin cell proliferation. The most common pathogens of wound infections are *S. aureus* and beta-hemolytic streptococcus.

Predisposing Factors

A. Exposure to accidental or intentional injury

B. Accident prevention failure

C. High-risk behaviors

D. Conditions that predispose to poor wound healing:

    1. Diabetes

    2. Corticosteroid therapy

    3. Immunodeficiency

    4. Advanced age

    5. Undernourishment

    6. Comorbidities

Common Complaints

A. Bleeding

B. Pain

C. "Cut" in the skin integrity

D. Drainage

Other Signs and Symptoms

A. Signs and symptoms of infection: Deep wounds and dirty wounds have increased risk for infection.

B. Soft-tissue damage: Wounds with tissue necrosis have increased risk for infection.

Subjective Data

A. Elicit the client's description of how the wound occurred, including where and when the injury was sustained.

B. Ascertain how much time elapsed until treatment. If 6 hours have elapsed, bacterial multiplication is likely.

C. Ask if the client is currently immunized for tetanus.

D. Complete a drug history; include any allergies to medications, anesthetics, or dressings.

E. Ask if the client is taking any medications, especially steroids, or anticoagulants.

F. Assess iodine and sulfa drug allergies before starting treatment.

G. Review with the client whether anything significant in the past medical history may interfere with the healing process (e.g., immunodeficiency).

Physical Examination

A. Check temperature, pulse, respirations, and blood pressure.

B. Inspect:

    1. Inspect wound.

    2. Measure wound for size: Length, width, and depth. Wounds with untidy edges may heal more slowly and with disfigurement.

    3. Assess underlying bony structures.

    4. Inspect for foreign objects.

C. Palpate:

    1. Palpate extremities for neurovascular function and sensation.

    2. Palpate tissue distal to wound.

    3. Palpate lymph nodes surrounding injured area.

D. Neurologic examination: Assess motor function distal to wound.

Diagnostic Tests

A. Culture wound site if suspicious of infection.

B. Take X-ray films for deep or crushing wounds.

Differential Diagnoses

A. Wound, minor

B. Nonaccidental self-inflicted injury

C. Self-inflicted injury

D. Domestic violence

E. Bite

Plan

A. General interventions:

    1. Wounds that require open-wound management:

        a. Abrasions and superficial lacerations

        b. Wounds with great amount of tissue damage

        c. Wounds more than 6 hours old

        d. Contaminated wounds

        e. Large area of superficial skin denudation

        f. Puncture wounds

    2. For wounds that do not require sutures:

        a. Cleanse wound well with NS; remove all dirt and foreign bodies.

        b. Forceful irrigation may be needed; use fine-pore sponge (Optipore) with a surfactant such as poloxamer 188 (Skin-Clens). If wound edges easily approximate, apply Steri-Strips.

        c. Dry, sterile dressings (Telfa, Duoderm, or Opsite) may be used.

3. If inflammation is present, soak and wash for 15 to 20 minutes three to four times per day. Cover with clean, dry dressing. **Do not use Steri-Strips.**

4. For wounds that require sutures:

a. Clean with warm water and soap. Irrigate with sterile saline solution.

b. Anesthetize with 1% to 2% lidocaine (Xylocaine). Do not use solution with epinephrine at fingertips, nose, or ears. Probe wound for any remaining foreign bodies. Approximate wound edges.

c. Suture with technique appropriate to site:

i. Skin sutures: Nonabsorbable material (e.g., nylon, Prolene, or silk)

ii. Subcutaneous and mucosal sutures: Absorbable material (e.g., Dexon, Vicryl, or plain or chromic gut)

iii. Extremities: 4-0 nylon

iv. Soles of feet: 2-0 nylon

d. Cover with clean, dry dressing; change after first 24 hours.

e. Suture removal is based on location:

i. Head and trunk: 5 to 7 days

ii. Extremities: 7 to 10 days

iii. Soles and palms: 7 to 10 days

iv. Distal extremities: 10 to 14 days

f. Tetanus prophylaxis (see Health Maintenance Guidelines)

▶ B. Client teaching: *See Section III: Client Teaching Guide for this chapter, "Wound Care: Pressure Ulcers."*

C. Pharmaceutical therapy:

1. Control pain with acetaminophen (Tylenol) as needed.

2. Topical antibiotic ointments: Bacitracin and mupirocin

3. Oral antibiotics for prophylaxis:

a. Amoxicillin, clavulanic acid (Augmentin) given for 7 to 10 days:

i. Adults: 875 mg oral twice daily

ii. Adolescents: 250 to 500 mg twice daily

iii. Children: 25 to 45 mg/kg/d twice daily for 7 to 10 days; available as 200 mg/5 mL or 400 mg/5 mL liquid

b. With penicillin allergy, use erythromycin given for 7 to 10 days:

i. Adults: 500 mg oral twice a day

ii. Adolescents: (E-Mycin) 250 mg four times daily for 7 to 10 days

iii. Children: (Eryped) 30 to 60 mg/kg/d four times daily for 7 to 10 days; available as 200 mg/5 mL or 400 mg/5 mL liquid

4. Other alternatives: Cephalexin (Keflex), cefadroxil (Duricef), ciprofloxacin

5. Tetanus toxoid 0.5 mL by IM) injection in deltoid, if no booster has been administered in the last 5 years

6. Wounds diagnosed with MRSA should be treated with the following oral antibiotics:

a. Trimethoprim sulfamethoxazole (Bactrim)

b. Minocycline or doxycycline

c. Clindamycin rifampin (should be used in combination with one of the previous antibiotics)

d. Linezolid.

7. Antibiotics not recommended because of high resistance include the following:

a. Beta lactams

b. Fluoroquinolones

c. Dicloxacillin

d. Cephalexin

8. Treating the nares with Bactroban ointment twice a day and having the client use hibiclens soap when showering will help to prevent recurrent infections.

9. For severe cases of infection, the client requires hospitalization for aggressive antibiotic treatment.

Follow-Up

A. Have the client return for evaluation and dressing change in 24 to 48 hours.

Consultation/Referral

Refer the client to a physician for wounds of the type listed here:

A. Facial wounds

B. Subcutaneous tissue penetration

C. Functional disturbance of tendons, ligaments, vessels, or nerves

D. Grossly contaminated wounds

E. Wounds requiring hospitalization or aggressive antimicrobial therapy for evidence of pyogenic abscess, cellulitis, and ascending lymphangitis

Individual Considerations

A. Adults:

1. Adults with chronic conditions such as diabetes or immune deficiency, or those with compromised immune systems should be monitored closely for infection and delayed wound healing.

B. Geriatrics:

1. Avoid use of NSAIDs in clients that have chronic kidney disease Stage IV or less (creatinine clearance <30 mL/min).

2. Medications commonly used in the elderly population are associated with poor wound healing: cytotoxic antineoplastic agents, corticosteroids, aspirin, NSAIDs, anticoagulants, bisphosphonates, and pain medications that contain morphine

Bibliography

Anrys, C., Van Tiggelen, H., Verhaeghe, S., Van Hecke, A., & Beeckman, D. (2019). Independent risk factors for pressure ulcer development in a high-risk nursing home population receiving evidence-based pressure ulcer prevention: Results from a study in 26 nursing homes in Belgium. *International Wound Journal*, 16(2), 325–333. doi:10.1111/iwj.13032

Au, Y., Holbrook, M., Skeens, A., Painter, J., McBurney, J., Cassata, A., & Wang, S. C. (2019). Improving the quality of pressure ulcer management in a skilled nursing facility. *International Wound Journal*, 16(2), 550–555. doi:10.1111/iwj.13112

Baranoski, S., & Ayello, E. (2015). *Wound care essentials: Practice principle*. Philadelphia, PA: Lippincott Williams, and Wilkins.

Furuya-Kanamori, L., Walker, R. M., Gillespie, B. M., Clark, J., Doi, S. A. R., & Thalib, L. (2019). Effectiveness of different topical treatments in the healing of pressure injuries: A network meta-analysis. *Journal of the American Medical Directors Association, 20*(4), 399–407. doi:10.1016/j.jamda.2018.10.010

Kennedy, K. (2016). *Understanding the Kennedy terminal ulcer.* Retrieved from http://www.kennedyterminalulcer.com

National Pressure Ulcer Advisory Panel. (2016, April 13). Pressure injury staging. Retrieved from http://www.npuap.org/resources/educational-and-clinical-resources/npuap-pressure-injury-stages

National Pressure Ulcer Advisory Panel and European Pressure Ulcer Advisory Panel. (2009). *Prevention and treatment of pressure ulcers; clinical practice guideline.* Washington, DC: Author.

Thakral, G., La Fontaine, J., Kim, P., Najafi, B., Nichols, A., & Lavery, L. A. (2015). Treatment options for venous leg ulcers: Effectiveness of vascular surgery, bioengineered tissue, and electrical stimulation. *Advances in Skin & Wound Care, 28*(4), 164–172. doi:10.1097/01.ASW.0000462328.60670.c3

Weller, C. D., Team, V., Ivory, J. D., Crawford, K., & Gethin, G. (2019). ABPI reporting and compression recommendations in global clinical practice guidelines on venous leg ulcer management: A scoping review. International Wound Journal, 16(2), 406–419. doi:10.1111/iwj.13048

Yapp, J. H., Raja Ahmad, R. M. K., Ahmad, S. A., Mahmud, R., Mohtarrudin, N., Mohamad Yusof, L., … Abu Bakar, M. Z. (2019). Determining weight-bearing tissue condition using peak reactive hyperemia response trend and ultrasonographic features: Implications for pressure ulcer prevention. *Wound Repair & Regeneration, 27*(3), 225–234. doi:10.1111/wrr.12698

Wound Healing: High-Protein Nutrition

Cheryl A. Glass

A. Nutrition is an essential component in the healing of any wounds. Protein, carbohydrates, fats, vitamins, minerals, and amino acid needs are increased for tissue repair. Table 4.3 summarizes the recommended amount of protein intake needed under different circumstances for tissue repair:
1. Consult with a dietitian for medical nutrition therapy (MNT).
2. Evaluate protein intake.
3. Evaluate the client's weight:
   a. Serial weights—use same scales
   b. Diet diary or 24-hour recall
   c. The dietary and weight history is used to determine additional needs.
   d. Excessive protein potentially leads to dehydration.
4. Lab testing:
   a. CBC
   b. Basic metabolic panel (BMP)
   c. Protein: Albumin, total protein
   d. Renal: Blood urea nitrogen (BUN) and creatinine

5. Evaluate wound stage/healing.
6. Supplemental protein supplement may be required:
   a. Sources of protein:
      i. Whole eggs are considered the "gold standard" protein.
      ii. Meat: Red and white meat
      iii. Fish
      iv. Liver
      v. Dairy: Milk, cheese, yogurt
      vi. Soybeans
      vii. Legumes
      viii. Seeds
      ix. Nuts
      x. Grains
   b. Encourage meals and snacking, double portions of meat and eggs, commercial supplements, and fluids:
      i. Eat five to six smaller meals throughout the day.
      ii. Keep ready-to-eat meals and snacks.
      iii. Drink shake-type beverages that contain protein, vitamins, and minerals.
      iv. Add protein powder to drinks.
   c. Consider appetite stimulants.
   d. Enteral nutrition should be considered if oral food and fluid intake is not adequate.

Other Considerations

A. The elderly have multiple risk factors for intake of insufficient protein for wound healing:
1. Financial:
   a. Expense of high-protein foods
   b. Expense of oral supplemental nutrition drinks
2. Difficulty chewing:
   a. Dental problems
   b. Loose-fitting dentures
   c. Edentulous
3. Assistive needs:
   a. Inability to prepare foods
   b. Need to have a caregiver feed the elderly person
   c. Given inadequate time to consume food if being fed
4. Dysphagia
5. Anorexia
6. Fatigue
7. Psychosocial:
   a. Depression
   b. Loneliness

TABLE 4.3	RECOMMENDED PROTEIN NEEDS PER DAY FOR WOUND HEALING
Elderly: Baseline protein needs	1.0–1.2 g/kg body weight/d
Healthy adults	0.8–1.0 g/kg body weight/d
Large burns	1.5–3.0 g/kg body weight/d (varies by extent of the burn)
Postsurgery	1.0–1.5 g/kg body weight/d (varies by extent of the surgery)
Pressure ulcers	1.0–2.0 g/kg body weight/d

B. Consultation with a dietitian for MNT, wound care specialist, social worker, occupational therapist, and behavioral health evaluations is advised

Bibliography

Au, Y., Holbrook, M., Skeens, A., Painter, J., McBurney, J., Cassata, A., & Wang, S. C. (2019). Improving the quality of pressure ulcer management in a skilled nursing facility. *International Wound Journal, 16*(2), 550–555.

Baranoski, S., & Ayello, E. (2015). *Wound care essentials: Practice principle.* Philadelphia, PA: Lippincott Williams, and Wilkins.

Xerosis (Winter Itch)

Jill C. Cash and Amy C. Bruggemann

Definition
A. Xerosis, often called "winter itch," is dry skin.

Incidence
A. Xerosis occurs in 48% to 98% of clients with atopic dermatitis.
B. It occurs more frequently in elderly clients.

Pathogenesis
A. Dry skin may fissure, appear shiny and cracked, and leave subsequent inflammatory changes.

Predisposing Factors
A. Frequent bathing with hot water and harsh soaps
B. Cold air
C. Low humidity
D. Central heating or cooling
E. Alcohol use
F. Poor nutrition
G. Cholesterol-lowering drugs
H. Systemic disease manifested by thyroid, renal, or hepatic disease; anemia; diabetes; or malignancy

Common Complaints
A. Dry, rough skin, especially on legs

Other Signs and Symptoms
A. Pruritic, scaling skin, particularly on legs, with cracks and/or fissures
B. Pruritus may be associated with systematic disorders or other infections. Itching of scabies is particularly intense at night.
C. Plaques 2 to 5 cm in diameter
D. Erythema
E. Wheal-and-flare response typical of urticaria

Subjective Data
A. Obtain the client's description of the onset of symptoms and whether it was sudden or gradual.
B. Ask the client to identify any discomfort. Ask if the skin is itchy or painful.
C. Assess lesions for any associated discharge (blood or pus).
D. Determine whether the client has recently ingested any new medicines (antibiotics, cholesterol-lowering medications, or other drugs), alcohol, or new foods.
E. Ask the client about use of any topical medications.
F. Identify any preceding systemic symptoms (fever, sore throat, anorexia, or vaginal discharge).
G. Ask the client about bathing in hot water and if client is bathing regularly.
H. Review the client's full medication history for comorbid conditions.

Physical Examination
A. Inspect:
    1. Inspect skin for lesions, noting texture of skin.
B. Palpate:
    1. Palpate abdomen for masses and hepatosplenomegaly.
    2. Palpate lymph nodes.

Diagnostic Tests
A. There are no diagnostic tests for xerosis.

Differential Diagnoses
A. Scabies
B. Atopic dermatitis

Plan
A. General interventions:
    1. Hydrate and lubricate the skin.
    2. Assess for and treat secondary infection.
B. Client teaching:
    1. *See Section III: Client Teaching Guide for this chapter, "Xerosis (Winter Itch)."*
    2. Avoid alkaline soaps: Use Dove, Basis, mild soap, or soap substitute such as Cetaphil or Aquaphor.
C. Pharmaceutical therapy:
    1. Apply emollient cream or lotion (Sarna, Lac-Hydrin, or Eucerin).
    2. Use OTC skin lubricants (petroleum jelly, mineral oil, or cold cream).
    3. Topical corticosteroid.
        a. Triamcinolone 0.025% two to four times daily or 0.1% two to three times daily; apply sparingly
        b. Hydrocortisone 1% or 2.5% two to four times daily; apply thin film, avoid face
    4. Systemic antihistamine is used to control pruritus, such as diphenhydramine (Benadryl) 25 to 50 mg every 4 to 6 hours as needed

Follow-Up
A. Follow up as indicated until resolved.

Consultation/Referral
A. Consult or refer the client to a dermatologist if no improvement is seen.

Individual Considerations
A. Pediatrics:
    1. Avoid corticosteroid preparation or use low-potency corticosteroid only.
B. Geriatrics:
    1. Monitor the client for possible skin breakdown and/or ulceration.

2. Xerosis is common among elderly population. Several nonpharmacological treatments to consider before using topical hydrocortisone would include increasing home environment humidity, avoiding excessive bathing and bath oils, encouraging oatmeal baths, and using emollient ointment (e.g., Aquaphor or Eucerin) and ceramide lotions (e.g., AmLactin) to smooth cracked rough skin and decrease pruritus.

Bibliography

Anderson de Oliveira Cruz, R., Palhano, D. B., & Costa, M. M. L. (2019). Nursing care for skin xerosis in elderly. *Journal of Nursing UFPE/Revista de Enfermagem UFPE, 13*(3), 875–878. https://doi-org.proxy.library.vanderbilt.edu/10.5205/1981-8963-v13i03a237348p875-878-2019

Mekić, S., Jacobs, L. C., Gunn, D. A., Mayes, A. E., Ikram, M. A., Pardo, L. M., & Nijsten, T. (2019). Prevalence and determinants for xerosis cutis in the middle-aged and elderly population: A cross-sectional study. *Journal of the American Academy of Dermatology, 81*(4), 963. https://doi-org.proxy.library.vanderbilt.edu/10.1016/j.jaad.2018.12.038

5 Eye Guidelines

Amblyopia

Jill C. Cash, Nancy Pesta Walsh, and Jenny Mullen

Definition
A. Amblyopia is a decrease in the visual acuity of one eye. It is commonly diagnosed in younger adults and children, and often referred to as "lazy eye."
B. It cannot be corrected with either glasses or contact lenses.

Incidence
A. Amblyopia is most commonly diagnosed in children and occurs in approximately 3% of the population.
B. Effective return of vision occurs with approximately 75% of children that experienced occlusion therapy. Fifty percent of those children had mild visual acuity loss over time, which emphasizes the importance of referring clients early in life.
C. Most common cause of childhood vision loss

Pathogenesis
Amblyopia has numerous causes, including:
A. Congenital defect
B. Develops from a corneal scar or cataract
C. Occurs from an uncorrected high refractive error, which causes visual blurring
D. Develops when each eye has a different refractive error that leads to blurred vision
E. Strabismic amblyopia may also occur due to the loss of vision in the eye that turns inward or outward.

Predisposing Factors
A. One parent with amblyopia
B. Prematurity
C. Small for gestational dates
D. Maternal smoking or alcohol use

Common Complaints
A. Decreased vision—complains of sitting close to the TV, sitting in the front row of a classroom, having trouble seeing the ball in sports, and so on
B. Vision that is not corrected with either glasses or contact lenses
C. Wandering eye and frequent eye squinting
D. Clients often describe vision as distorted or confused.

Other Signs and Symptoms
A. Frequent rubbing of the eyes
B. Tired eyes

Subjective Data
A. Elicit the onset of visual changes, noting course of symptoms and severity
B. Assess for pain or any new injury or trauma to the eye
C. Inquire about new events or changes in health history, including contact lenses, glasses, illnesses, and cataracts
D. Review client and family history of amblyopia

Physical Examination
A. Inspect eyes:
  1. Note extraocular movements (EOMs) of eyes.
  2. Examine sclera, pupil, iris, and fundus.
  3. Examine eyes for red reflex.
B. Assess vision based on age, using LEA SYMBOLS®, Sloan letters, Sloan numerals, Tumbling E, and the HOTV. The Kindergarten Eye Chart and the Snellen Chart are less preferred methods, as they do not meet the World Health Organization (WHO)/Committee on Vision Standards.
C. Visual fields may be assessed with a parent holding the child in his or her lap.

Diagnostic Test
A. None

Differential Diagnoses
A. Amblyopia
B. Organic brain lesion

Plan
A. General interventions:
  1. All children need to have a visual examination prior to starting school.
  2. Recommend examination by an ophthalmologist for children with strabismus and for those with a family history of amblyopia.
  3. Measures for refractive correction or patching of the stronger eye are usually performed to encourage the weak eye to develop.
  4. Surgery may be required for abnormal positioning of the eye.

Follow-Up
A. Follow-up with an ophthalmologist.

Consultation/Referral
A. Refer the client to an ophthalmologist for evaluation and treatment.

Individual Consideration
A. Pediatrics: Closely monitor children post-surgery to ensure they do not peek from under bandages. Establish a reward system to assist children adherence with eye patch.

Bibliography
Blair, K., Cibis, G., & Gulani, A. (2019). *Amblyopia.* StatPearls NCBI Resources, e1–e5. Retrieved from https://www.ncbi.nlm.nih.gov/books/NBK430890/

Blepharitis

Jill C. Cash, Nancy Pesta Walsh, and Jenny Mullen

Definition
A. Blepharitis is dryness and flaking of the eyelashes, resulting from an inflammatory response of the eyelid.

Incidence
A. A recent survey of the U.S. ophthalmologists and optometrists discovered up to 47% of clients had signs of blepharitis.
B. Blepharitis affects all age and ethnic groups. Current studies indicated the mean age of clients affected with blepharitis is 50 years, and clients with staphylococcal blepharitis were approximately 42 years old and primarily women.

Pathogenesis
A. Seborrheic: excessive shedding of skin cells and blockage of glands
B. *Staphylococcus:* most common bacteria found, responsible for bacterial infection of lid margin
C. Commonly seen with inadequate flow of oil and mucus into the tear duct

Predisposing Factors
A. Diabetes
B. Candida
C. Seborrheic dermatitis
D. Acne rosacea
E. Demodicosis (demodex mites)
F. Isotretinoin oral medication used to treat cystic acne
G. Clients who wear contact lens and have acquired giant papillary conjuctivitis

Common Complaints
A. Burning and itching
B. Lacrimal tearing
C. Photophobia
D. Recurrent eye infections, styes, or chalazions
E. Dry, flaky secretions on lid margins and eyelashes
F. Dry eyes

Other Signs and Symptoms
A. Seborrheic blepharitis: Lid margin swelling and erythema, flaking, nasolabial erythema, and scaling
B. *Staphylococcus aureus* blepharitis: Erythema/edema, scaling, burning, tearing, itching, and recurrent stye or chalazia
C. Meibomian gland dysfunction: prominent blood vessels crossing the mucocutaneous junction, frothy discharge along eyelid margin, thick discharge, and chalazion; may have rosacea or seborrheic dermatitis
D. May have dandruff of scalp and eyebrows

Subjective Data
A. Elicit onset and duration of signs and symptoms
B. Note sensations of itching, burning, or pain in the eye
C. Ask what makes signs and symptoms worse? What makes signs and symptoms better?
D. Any change in soaps, creams, lotions, or shampoos?
E. Has the client had similar signs and symptoms in the past?
F. Note any visual change or pain since the last eye examination
G. Note contributing factors involved if present

Physical Examination
A. Inspect:
    1. Inspect eyes, noting EOMs of eyes.
    2. Examine sclera, pupil, iris, and fundus.
    3. Examine eyes for red reflex.
    4. Note erythema or edema on lid margin; note dryness, scaling, and flakes.
    5. Assess vision based on age, using Snellen chart for children older than 3 years.
    6. Visual fields may be assessed with a parent holding the child in his or her lap.

Diagnostic Test
A. None; however, cultures of eyelid margins may be warranted if signs/symptoms indicate.

Differential Diagnoses
A. Blepharitis:
    1. *Staph. aureus*
    2. Seborrheic
    3. Meibomian gland dysfunction
B. Conjunctivitis
C. Squamous cell carcinoma
D. Stye
E. Upper respiratory infection
F. Sinusitis

Plan
A. General interventions:
    1. Assess client and rule out bacterial infection and vision changes.
    2. When examining a child, notify the parent of diagnosis and educate the parent regarding findings.
    3. Clients with recurrent blepharitis need further follow-up.
B. Client teaching:
    1. Wash eye with antibacterial soap and water. May use gentle baby shampoo

2. Apply warm compresses to the eye for comfort daily for approximately 10 to 20 minutes.
3. Stop use of contacts until the eye is healed.
4. Encourage good hygiene for prevention of recurrent episodes.
C. Pharmaceutical therapy:
1. Apply bacitracin or erythromycin ophthalmic ointment to the margin of the eye at bedtime, taking care not to contaminate the medication bottle.
2. Oral antibiotics: Tetracycline 250 mg by mouth, four times a day, or doxycycline 100 mg by mouth, twice a day, tapering after clinical improvement, for a total of 2 to 6 weeks. Alternative: Erythromycin 250 to 500 mg daily or azithromycin 250 to 500 mg one to three times a week for 3 weeks.
3. Consider long-term treatment with doxycycline if infections reoccur.

Follow-Up

A. Recommend follow-up with a primary provider in 1 to 2 weeks.
B. Consider referral to an eye specialist for recurrent episodes of blepharitis and for slit-lamp examination.

Individual Considerations

A. Pediatrics:
1. Tetracycline is not recommended for children younger than 8 years.
B. Pregnant or lactating women:
1. Tetracycline is not recommended.
2. Azithromycin may lead to abnormalities of heart electrical rhythm; use with caution in clients with a high risk of cardiovascular disease.

Bibliography

Amescua, G., Akpek, E. K., Farid, M., Garcia-Ferrer, F. J., Lin, A., Rhee, M. K., . . . Mah, F. S. (2019). Blepharitis preferred practice pattern. *Ophthalmology, 126*(1), 56–93. doi:10.1016/j.ophtha.2018.10.019
Tonk, R., & Hossain, K. (2019). Blepharitis: Disease entity. *American Academy of Ophthalmology*, pp. e1–e7. Retrieved from https://eyewiki.aao.org/Blepharitis

Cataracts

Jill C. Cash, Nancy Pesta Walsh, and Jenny Mullen

Definition

A. A cataract, opacity of the crystalline lens of the eye, causes progressive, painless loss of vision (functional impairment). Presenile and senile cataract formation is painless and progresses throughout months and years. Cataracts are frequently associated with intraocular inflammation and glaucoma.

Incidence

A. Cataracts are the most common cause of blindness and are responsible for >51% of vision loss in the world.
B. Ninety-five percent of people older than 60 years have cataracts without visual disturbance.
C. Fifty percent of people older than 40 years have significant visual loss due to cataracts.
D. Prevalent cases in the United States are 61% female and 39% male.
E. The National Institutes of Health projected that by year 2030 approximately 40 million U.S. citizens are expected to suffer from cataracts, and approximately 50 million people by 2050.

Pathogenesis

A. Age-related changes of the lens of the eye result from protein accumulation, which produces a fibrous thickened lens that obscures vision.

Predisposing Factors

A. Age
B. Trauma
C. Medications (e.g., topical or systemic steroids, major tranquilizers, or some diuretics)
D. Medical diseases (e.g., diabetes mellitus, Wilson's disease, hypoparathyroidism, glaucoma, congenital rubella syndrome, chronic anteri, or uveitis)
E. Chronic exposure to UV B light
F. Alcohol use
G. Family history
H. Prior intraocular surgery
I. Obesity
J. Smoking

Common Complaints

A. Decreased vision
B. Blurred or foggy vision, "ghost" images
C. Inability to drive at night

Other Signs and Symptoms

A. Initial visual event can be a shift toward nearsightedness.
B. Visual impairment can be more marked at distances, with abnormal visual acuity examinations.
C. Severe difficulty with glare can occur.
D. Altered color perception may be noticed.
E. Frequent falls or injuries may occur.

Subjective Data

A. Review the onset, course, and duration of visual changes, including altered day or night vision and nearsighted versus farsighted vision.
B. Assess whether involvement is in one or both eyes.
C. Determine what improves vision—use of glasses or use of extra light.
D. Review the client's medical history and current medications.
E. Review the client's history for traumatic injury.
F. Discuss the client's occupation and leisure activities to determine exposure to UV rays.

Physical Examination

A. Inspect:
1. Conduct a funduscopic examination:
a. Check red reflex and opacity:
i. A bright red reflex is seen in the normal eye.
ii. Cataract formation is seen by the disruption of the red reflex.

iii. Lens opacities appear as dark areas against the background of the red-orange reflex.
   b. Examine color of opacity. For brunescent cataracts, the nucleus acquires a yellow-brown coloration and becomes progressively more opaque.
   c. Check retinal abnormalities, hemorrhage, scarring, and drusen (small yellow deposits)

Diagnostic Tests
A. Perform visual acuity examination.
B. Perform peripheral vision examination.
C. Perform slit-lamp examination to determine the exact location and type of cataract
D. Dilated eye examination

Differential Diagnoses
A. Cataracts
B. Glaucoma
C. Age-related macular degeneration (macular degeneration causes vision loss that is symptomatically similar to cataracts)
D. Diabetic retinopathy
E. Temporal arteritis

Plan
A. General interventions:
   1. Monitor the client for increased interference of visual impairment on his or her lifestyle.
   2. Cataracts do not need to be removed unless there is impairment of normal, everyday activities.
   3. Surgery is the definitive treatment; however, modification of glasses may improve vision adequately to defer surgery. Contact lenses are optically superior to glasses.
B. Client teaching:
   1. Prevention is important. Teach the client to use protective eyewear to prevent trauma.
   2. Use sunglasses to prevent the penetration of UV B rays.
   3. Wear a hat with a visor to protect eyes when outdoors.

Follow-Up
A. Surgical removal is indicated if the visual disturbance is interfering with the client's life, such as causing falls or prohibiting reading.

Consultation/Referral
A. Refer client for ophthalmologic consultation
B. Clients should be followed by an ophthalmologist to monitor the cataract for increased size and progressive visual impairment.
C. Contact a social worker or community resources as needed

Individual Considerations
A. Adults:
   1. In light of advancing intraocular technologies and new surgical approaches, the American Academy of Ophthalmology advocates educating clients regarding

the long-standing standard of care in the U.S. for cataract surgery: small-incision phacoemulsification with foldable intraocular lens implantations
   2. Topical NSAID used to treat ocular inflammation and pain was FDA approved in 1988, however, it remains controversial for post cataract surgery. Current research indicates it may be used for clients with diabetic retinopathy and other high-risk comorbidities to prevent cystic macular edema.

Bibliography
National Institutes of Health. (2019). Cataracts. *Statistics and Data*, pp. e1–e4. Retrieved from https://nei.nih.gov/eyedata/cataract

Prall, F., Ciulla, T., Criswell, M., Harris, A., Talavera, F., Charles, S., Dahl, A., & Phillpotts, B. (2018). Exudative (wet) age-related macular degeneration (AMD). Macular degeneration: Ophthalmology. *MedScape*, pp. e1–e24. Retrieved from https://emedicine.medscape.com/article/1226030-overview

Chalazion

Jill C. Cash, Nancy Pesta Walsh, and Jenny Mullen

Definition
A. Chalazion is a chronic lipogranulomatous inflammation of a meibomian gland located in the eyelid margin. It differs from a hordeola because it is a result of gland obstruction rather than an infection. Inflammation occurs from occlusion of the ducts.

Incidence
A. Commonly seen, though the incidence is unknown
B. More prominent in adults aged 30 to 50 years than in children secondary to androgenic hormones influences sebaceous secretion and viscosity

Pathogenesis
A. Meibomian glands secrete the oil layer of the tear film that covers the eye. When the glands become blocked, the oil or lipid extrudes into the surrounding tissue, causing the formation of a nodule.

Predisposing Factor
A. Chalazion may occur as a secondary infection of the surrounding tissues.

Common Complaints
A. Swelling, nontender palpable nodule, usually pea-sized, inside lid margin or eye
B. Discomfort or irritation due to swelling

Other Signs and Symptoms
A. Tearing
B. Feeling of a foreign body in the eye
C. If infection is present, the entire lid becomes painfully swollen.

Subjective Data
A. Review the onset of symptoms, their course and duration, and any concurrent visual disturbance.
B. Question the client regarding possible foreign body or trauma to the eye.

C. Elicit the quality of pain or tenderness of the eyelid.

D. Review the past eye problems and the treatment received.

Physical Examination

A. Temperature

B. Inspect:

1. Inspect the eye, sclera, and conjunctiva for a foreign body.

2. Check for red- or gray-colored subconjunctival mass.

C. Palpate:

1. Palpate the eyelid for masses and tenderness. Usually a hard, nontender nodule is found on the middle portion of the tarsus, away from the lid border; it may develop on the lid margin if the opening of the duct is involved. Some chalazia continue to increase in size and can cause astigmatism by putting pressure on the eye globe.

2. Chalazia may become acutely tender; however, note the difference between the chalazia and the stye, which is found on the lid margin.

3. Check for preauricular adenopathy.

Diagnostic Test

A. Perform visual acuity examination.

Differential Diagnoses

A. Chronic dacryocystitis

B. Hordeolum (Stye)

C. Blepharitis

D. Xanthelasma

E. Cellulitis of the eyelid

Plan

A. General interventions:

1. Small chalazia, usually, do not require treatment.

B. Client teaching:

1. Instruct client regarding warm, moist compresses applied for 15 minutes four times a day.

2. Educate client regarding the importance of good handwashing to prevent spreading infection.

C. Pharmaceutical therapy:

1. Sulfacetamide sodium (Sulamyd) ophthalmic ointment 10%, four times daily, for 7 days for bacterial infection

2. Tobradex ophthalmic drops: 1 to 2 drops every 2 hours for first 24 to 48 hours, then every 4 to 6 hours. Reduce dose as the condition improves. Treat for 5 to 7 days as needed. Not recommended in children younger than 2 years

3. Intrachalazion corticosteroid injection is performed by an ophthalmologist.

Follow-Up

A. For large infected chalazia, follow up with client in 1 week and then evaluate the client every 2 to 4 weeks.

Consultation/Referral

A. If the chalazion does not resolve spontaneously, incision and curettage by an ophthalmologist may be necessary.

Individual Considerations

A. Pediatrics:

1. If a chalazion recurs in a child or young adult, evaluate further for viral conjunctivitis or Job syndrome (hyper-IgE).

B. Geriatrics:

1. If a chalazion recurs in an elderly client, then consider conditions that charade as a chalazion: sebaceous carcinoma, squamous cell, and other cancers.

Bibliography

Carlisle, R. T., & Digiovanni, J. (2015). Differential diagnosis of the swollen red eyelid. *American Family Physician, 15*(92), 106–112.

Deschênes, J., Fansler, J., Plouzinkoff, A., Talavera, F., Dahl, A., Brenner, B., … Talavera, F. (2018). Chalazion: Ophthalmology. *MedScape*, pp. e1–e17. Retrieved from https://emedicine.medscape.com/article/1212709-overview

Conjunctivitis

Jill C. Cash, Nancy Pesta Walsh, and Jenny Mullen

Definition

A. Conjunctivitis is inflammation of the conjunctiva.

Incidence

A. Viral conjunctivitis is the most common type; conjunctivitis occurs in 1% to 12% of newborns

B. Every year, approximately 135 bacterial conjunctivitis cases per 10,000 population occur in the United States and constitute 1% of primary care consultations. Internationally, isolated epidemics have reported newborn blinding infections, which have caused blindness in almost 8% of the affected region's population.

C. An estimated 6 million new cases of viral conjunctivitis occur in the United States annually, and often present as an epidemic in schools, offices, athletic teams, military organizations, shipyards, and residential communities.

D. Most common viral conjunctivitis affect: 20 to 40 years (*adenovirus*), young children and infants (*herpes simplex* and *varicella zoster*), young adults and children in lower socioeconomic regions (*picornavirus*), and all ages (*latent varicella zoster*).

Pathogenesis

Primarily three types of conjunctivitis are seen:

A. Bacterial (*Haemophilus influenzae, Streptococcus pneumoniae, Streptococcus aureus, Neisseria gonorrhoeae,* and *Chlamydia*). See Figure 5.1.

B. Viral (adenovirus, coxsackievirus, and enteric cytopathic human orphan [ECHO] viruses). See Figure 5.2.

C. Allergic (seasonal pollens or allergic exposure). See Figure 5.3.

Predisposing Factors

A. Contact with another person with the diagnosis of conjunctivitis

B. Exposure to sexually transmitted infection (STI)

C. Other atopic conditions (allergies)

FIGURE 5.1 Bacterial conjunctivitis.

Source: Image courtesy of Tanalai.

FIGURE 5.2 Viral conjunctivitis.

Source: Image courtesy of Joyhill09.

Common Complaints
A. Red eyes
B. Eye drainage
C. Itching (with allergic conjunctivitis)

Other Signs and Symptoms
A. Bacterial:
  1. Fast onset, 12 to 24 hours of copious purulent or mucopurulent discharge
  2. Burning, stinging, or gritty sensation in eyes
  3. Crusted eyelids upon awakening, with swelling of eyelid
  4. Usually starts out unilaterally; may progress to bacterial infection
  5. Bacterial conjunctivitis may present as beefy red conjunctiva.
B. Viral:
  1. Symptoms may begin in one eye and progress to both eyes.

FIGURE 5.3 Allergic conjunctivitis.

Source: Image courtesy of James Heilman, MD.

  2. Tearing of eyes
  3. Sensation of foreign body
  4. Systemic symptoms of upper respiratory infection (runny nose, sore throat, sneezing, fever)
  5. Preauricular or submandibular lymphadenopathy
  6. Photophobia, impaired vision
  7. Primary herpetic infection: vesicular skin lesion, corneal epithelial defect in form of dendrite, uveitis
C. Allergic:
  1. Itchy, watery eyes, bilateral
  2. Seasonal symptoms
  3. Edema of eyelids without visual change
  4. With allergic conjunctivitis, hyperemia of eyes is always bilateral and giant papillae on tarsal may be seen.
  5. May also see eczema, urticaria, and asthma flare

Subjective Data
A. Elicit the onset, duration, and course of symptoms.
B. Question client regarding the presence of discharge upon awakening.
C. Elicit changes in vision since symptoms began.
D. Determine whether there has been any injury or trauma to the eye.
E. Assess whether these symptoms have appeared before.
F. Rule out exposure to anyone with conjunctivitis.
G. Ask client about any new events, such as use of contact lenses or change in contact lenses or solutions.
H. Review client and family history of allergies.

Physical Examination
A. Check temperature.
B. Inspect:
  1. Observe eyes for color and foreign objects. Perform complete eye examination.
  2. Note lid edema.
  3. Assess pupillary reflexes.
  4. Examine skin.
  5. Inspect ears, nose, and throat.
C. Auscultate:
  1. Auscultate heart and lungs.

D. Palpate:
    1. Preauricular lymph nodes and anterior and posterior cervical chain lymph nodes.

Diagnostic Tests
A. Gram stain testing for discharge/exudate extracted from eyes if gonococcal infection is suspected and/or all neonates
B. Culture for *chlamydia*, if suspected
C. Perform fluorescein stain of eye if foreign body is suspected or corneal abrasion/ulceration is suspected
D. Test visual acuity with an age-appropriate visual acuity chart. Assess peripheral vision and EOMs

Differential Diagnoses
A. Corneal abrasion
B. Blepharitis
C. Drug-related conjunctivitis
D. Herpetic keratoconjunctivitis
E. Iritis
F. Gonococcal or chlamydial conjunctivitis

Plan
A. General interventions:
    1. Distinguish among bacterial, allergic, or viral infection.
    2. Consider other diagnoses if eye pain is noted.
▶ B. Client teaching: *See Section III: Client Teaching Guide for this chapter, "Eye Medication Administration."*
    1. Cool compresses to the affected eye should be applied several times a day.
    2. Clean eyes with warm, moist cloth from inner to outer canthus to prevent spreading infection.
    3. Encourage good handwashing technique with antibacterial soap.
    4. Instruct on the proper method of instilling medication into eye. Give client the teaching guide on how to administer eye medications.
    5. Instruct the female client to discard all eye makeup, including mascara, eyeliner, and eye shadow, worn at the time of the infection.
    6. Teach the client/parent the difference among bacterial, allergic, and viral infections. Educate according to appropriate diagnosis.
    7. If using aminoglycoside or neomycin ointments or drops, use caution and monitor closely for reactive keratoconjunctivitis.
    8. Bacterial conjunctivitis is contagious until 24 hours after beginning medication.
    9. Viral conjunctivitis is contagious for 48 to 72 hours, but it may last up to 2 weeks. This is typically self-limiting, and does not require antibiotic treatment.
C. Pharmaceutical therapy:
    1. Bacterial:
        a. Aminoglycosides: Gentamicin 0.3%: Severe infections: 2 gtts every hour on day 1, then 1 to 2 gtts every 4 hours for 5 to 7 days. Mild/moderate infections: 1 to 2 gtts every 4 hours for 5 to 7 days

        b. Tobramycin 0.3%; severe infections: 2 gtts every hour on day 1, then 1 to 2 gtts four times a day for 5 to 7 days. Mild-to-moderate infections: 1 to 2 gtts four times a day for 5 to 7 days
        c. Polymyxin B: trimethoprim/polymyxin B sulfate (Polytrim) ophthalmic ointment in each eye four times daily for 7 days. Polymyxin B/bacitracin (Polysporin) drops may also be used, 1 gtt every 3 hours for 7 to 10 days
        d. Macrolides: erythromycin (Ilotycin) ophthalmic ointment 0.5% in each eye four times daily for 7 days
        e. Fluoroquinolones: Ciprofloxacin 0.3%: 1 to 2 gtts every 2 hours for 2 days, then every 4 hours for 5 days. Moxifloxacin (Vigamox) 0.5% 1 gtt three times a day for 7 days
    2. Viral
        a. Antiviral medications
            i. Trifluridine 1% drops: 1 drop every 2 hours while awake; no more than 9 drops per day. May then alter to 1 drop every 4 hours for 7 days. Not recommended for children younger than 6 years.
            ii. Oral antiviral medications (trifluridine, valacyclovir) may be used for herpes simplex keratitis. Herpes zoster ophthalmicus is often treated with acyclovir, famciclovir, or valacyclovir and lessens symptoms if started within 72 hours of onset of symptoms.
    3. Allergic:
        a. Topical antihistamines/mast cell stabilizer:
            i. Azelastine HCl (Optivar): not recommended for those younger than 3 years. For those older than 3 years, 1 drop to the affected eye twice a day
            ii. Olopatadine HCl (Pataday) 0.2%: not recommended for those younger than 3 years. For those older than 3 years, 1 drop to the affected eye daily
            iii. Olopatadine HCl (Patanol) 0.1%: not recommended for those younger than 3 years. For those older than 3 years, 1 drop twice a day to the affected eye
        b. Mast cell stabilizer:
            i. Cromolyn sodium (Crolom) ophthalmic solution for children older than 4 years, 1 to 2 drops four to six times daily
        c. Topical nonsteroidal anti-inflammatory drug (NSAID):
            i. Ketorolac tromethamine (Acular) 0.5%: not for use in children younger than 3 years: 1 drop four times a day. This is used for severe symptoms of atopic keratoconjunctivitis.
        d. Artificial tears four to five times daily
        e. Oral antihistamines may be used in severe cases (loratadine or diphenhydramine HCl).
    4. Concurrent conjunctivitis and otitis media should be treated with a systemic antibiotic; no topical eye antibiotic is needed.

Follow-Up

A. If resolution occurs within 5 to 7 days after proper treatment, follow-up is not needed.

B. If client continues to have symptoms or if different symptoms appear, then follow-up with the primary provider is recommended.

Consultation/Referral

A. Consult or refer client to a physician if client is not responding to treatment.

B. Refer if client is suspected of having periorbital cellulitis.

C. Refer to eye specialist if client has vision change or eye pain, or is not responding to treatment.

Individual Considerations

A. Pediatrics:

   1. In neonates, consider gonococcal and chlamydial conjunctivitis. Perform culture if suspected.

B. Partners:

   1. Check partners for *gonorrhea* and *chlamydia* when adolescent or adult presents with gonococcal or chlamydial conjunctivitis.

C. Geriatrics:

   1. Avoid diphenhydramine secondary to risks of confusion, constipation, blurred vision, delirium, dry mouth, and other anticholinergic symptoms. May consider only for acute treatment of a severe allergic reaction

Bibliography

Channa, R., Zafar, S., Canner, J., Haring, S., Schneider, E., & Firedman, D. (2016). Epidemiology of eye-related emergency department visits. *JAMA Ophthalmology, 134*(3), 312–319. doi:10.1001/jamaophthalmol.2015. 5778

Maya, Y., Tashimo, A., & Mitsuhito, O. (2018). Persistent red and swollen eyelids. *The Lancet, 392*(10157), p 1552. doi: https://doi.org/10.1016/S0140-6736(18)32327-4. Retrieved from https://www.thelancet.com/article/S0140-6736(18)32327-4/fulltext

Varu, D.M., Rhee, M.K., Akpek, E.K., Amescua, G., Farid, F., Garcia-Ferrer, F. J., . . . Dunn, S. P. (2018). Conjunctivitis preferred practice pattern. *Ophthalmology, 126*(1), 94–169. doi:10.1016/j.ophtha.2018.10.020

Yeung, K., & Dahl, A. (2019). Bacterial conjunctivitis (pink eye). *MedScape*, pp. e1–e8. Retrieved from https://emedicine.medscape.com/article/1191730-overview#a6

Corneal Abrasion

Jill C. Cash, Nancy Pesta Walsh, and Jenny Mullen

Definition

A. A corneal abrasion is the loss of epithelial tissue, either superficial or deep, from trauma to the eye. See Figure 5.4.

Incidence

A. In the United States, approximately 2.4 million eye injuries occur annually.

B. Corneal abrasions account for approximately 10% of new admissions to eye emergency units. Eighty percent of those visits are for cornea abrasions or foreign bodies.

C. More males than females are treated for corneal abrasions; and automotive employees, 20–29 years old, have the highest incidence of these eye injuries.

FIGURE 5.4 Corneal abrasion with fluorescein staining.

Source: Image courtesy of James Heilman, MD.

Pathogenesis

1. Trauma occurs in the epithelial tissue of the cornea.

Predisposing Factors

A. Trauma in the eye are commonly caused from: a human fingernail, contact lens, animal paws, makeup applicators, UV light burns (from tanning beds and welding arcs), tree branches, wood particles, children's toys, and sports injuries.

B. A history of surgical trauma may cause globe weakening.

Common Complaints

A. Sudden onset of eye pain

B. Foreign-body sensation in the eye

C. Watery eye

D. Mild photophobia

E. Blurred vision

F. Headache

Other Signs and Symptoms

A. Change in vision

B. Redness, swelling, inability to open the eye

Subjective Data

A. Elicit the onset, duration, and course of symptoms; note any past history of similar symptoms.

B. Question the client regarding visual changes (blurred, double, or lost vision, or loss of a portion of the visual field).

C. Question the client regarding the mechanism of injury and how much time has elapsed since the injury (minutes, hours, or days). Ask what is his or her occupation, and what sports are involved? Were goggles being worn and are they routinely worn during the sport or activity?

D. Review the client's history of exposure to herpetic outbreaks.

E. Determine the degree of pain if any; headache; photophobia; redness; itching; or tearing.
F. Ascertain whether the client wears contact lenses or glasses and for what length of time.
G. Ask if the client has tried any treatments before presentation to the office. If so, what?
H. Rule out the presence of any other infections, such as sinus infection. Conjunctival discharge signifies an infectious etiology.

Physical Examination
A. Vital signs: temperature
B. Inspect:
  1. Observe *both* eyes.
  2. Test visual acuity and pupil reactivity and symmetry.
  3. Observe the corneal surface with direct illumination, noting any shadow on the surface of the iris.
  4. Perform funduscopic examination.
  5. Evert eyelids for cornea inspection.
  6. Inspect for foreign body and remove if indicated
  7. Fluorescein stain to visualize changes in epithelial lining. Cobalt blue light or Wood's lamp should be used for visualization.

Diagnostic Test
1. Perform fluorescein stain test: An epithelial defect that stains with fluorescein is the hallmark symptom.

Differential Diagnoses
A. Corneal foreign body
B. Acute-angle glaucoma
C. Herpetic infection (herpes simplex virus [HSV]): HSV is associated with decreased corneal sensation
D. Recurrent corneal ulceration
E. Ulcerative keratitis
F. Corneal erosion
G. Blepharitis

Plan
A. General interventions:
  1. Superficial corneal abrasions do not need patching.
  2. For deeper abrasions, apply a patch that prevents lid motion for 24 to 48 hours.
  3. Pressure patch is no longer recommended.
B. Client teaching:
  1. Discuss the use of protective eyewear and prevention of future ocular trauma for the client with a history of use of power tools or hammering.
  2. *See Section III: Client Teaching Guide for this chapter, "Eye Medication Administration."*
  3. Advise that the client should not use/wear contact lenses until the eye is completely healed.
C. Pharmaceutical therapy:
  1. Antibiotic drops or ointment. Ointments are suggested over drops as they provide lubrication for the eye. Never instill antibiotic ointment if there is a possibility of a perforation. Patch the eye and refer the client to a physician or ophthalmologist.
    a. Adults and children: sulfacetamide sodium ophthalmic solution 10% (Sulamyd), 1 to 2 drops instilled into the lower conjunctival sac every 2 to 3 hours during the day; may instill every 6 hours during the night × 5 to 7 days
    b. Sulfacetamide's sodium (Sulamyd) ophthalmic solution or ointment interacts with gentamicin. Avoid using them together.
    c. Para-aminobenzoic acid (PABA) derivatives decrease sulfacetamide's action. Wait 0.5 to 1 hour before instilling sulfacetamide.
    d. Sulfacetamide precipitates when used with silver preparations. Avoid using them together.
  2. Adults and children: polymyxin B sulfate (Polytrim) 10,000 U/g, bacitracin zinc 500 U/g ophthalmic ointment (Polysporin), a small ribbon of ointment applied into the conjunctival sac one or more times daily or as needed
  3. Adults and children: erythromycin ophthalmic ointment 0.5% (Ilotycin), 1-cm ribbon of ointment applied into the conjunctival sac up to four to six times daily, depending on the severity of infection
  4. Bacitracin 500 U/g ointment, 1/2-inch ribbon twice a day to four times a day for 7 days
  5. Contact lens wearers are often colonized with *Pseudomonas* and should be treated with either a fluoroquinolone or an aminoglycoside. Ciprofloxacin 0.3% solution, 1 to 2 drops four times a day, for 3 to 5 days; gentamycin 0.3% solution 1 to 2 drops, four times a day, for 3 to 5 days; or tobramycin (Tobrex) ointment or drops, four times a day for 3 to 5 days
  6. Analgesics: Topical analgesics should be used sparingly. Diclofenac (Voltaren) 0.1% solution to eye four times a day as needed, or ketorolac (Acular) 0.5% solution in eye four times a day as needed.
  There is moderate evidence that topical NSAID ointment/drops suggested a decreased need for oral analgesics 24-hours post-treatment for corneal abrasions.
  7. Avoid use of home prescriptions that will interfere with the healing process.
  8. Avoid the use of medications containing steroids. These products may increase the risk of superinfection and may slow down the healing process.

Follow-Up
A. Reevaluate the client within 24 hours. The cornea usually heals within 24 to 48 hours.
B. Ophthalmic ointment or drops should be continued for a minimum of 4 days after reepithelialization occurs to help in the healing process.
C. If the client is still symptomatic in 48 hours, consider referral to an ophthalmologist.
D. Recurrent erosion could become a lifetime challenge for clients that experienced moderate to severe cornea abrasions. Consider a nightly hyperosmotic ointment (sodium chloride 5%), and a daily hypertonic drop (such as Systane) for 7 to 8 weeks while monitoring the cornea tissue for healing.

Consultation/Referral

> Immediate referral to an ophthalmologist is required for large or central lesions, or deep or penetrating wounds.

Individual Considerations

A. Pregnancy:

1. Retinal detachment should be considered as a source of eye pain and visual loss, especially in a woman with severe pregnancy-induced hypertension.

B. Pediatrics:

1. The use of ointments is suggested over the use of eye drops due to the lubricating effect. Blurry vision may be experienced; therefore, apply the ointment at nap time and bedtime. Eye drops commonly burn/sting.

2. Pressure patches are not recommended for children. Children commonly pull patches off and this counteracts the purpose of the use of a pressure patch.

3. Preventive precautions include encouraging the use of protective eyewear for contact sports, including hockey, soccer, baseball, and basketball.

Bibliography

Channa, R., Zafar, S., Canner, J., Haring, S., Schneider, E., & Firedman, D. (2016). Epidemiology of eye-related emergency department visits. *JAMA Ophthalmology, 134*(3), 312–319. doi:10.1001/jamaophthalmol.2015.5778

Swaminathan, A., Otterness, K., Milne, K., & Rezaie, S. (2015). The safety of topical anesthetics in the treatment of corneal abrasions: A review. *Journal of Emergency Medicine, 49*(5), 810–815. doi:10.1016/j.jemermed.2015.06.069

Verma, A., Khan, F., Dahl, A., Gordon, K., Rapuano, C., & Talavera, F. (2019). Corneal abrasion: Ophthalmology. *MedScape*, pp. e1–e22. Retrieved from https://emedicine.medscape.com/article/1195402-overview

Waldman, N., Window, B., Denise, I., Gray, A, McMaster, S., Giddings, G. & Meanley, J. (2018). An observational study to determine whether routinely sending patients home with a 24-hour supply of topical tetracaine from the emergency department for simple corneal abrasion pain is potentially safe. *Annals of Emergency Medicine, 71*(6), 776–778. doi:10.1016/j.annemergmed.2017.02.016

West, J. R. (2019). Are topical non steroidal anti-inflammatory drugs useful for analgesia in patients with traumatic corneal abrasions? *Annals Emergency Medicine, 73*(2), 157–159. doi:10.1016/j.annemergmed.2018.08.420

Wipperman, J. L., & Dorsch, J. N. (2015). Evaluation and management of corneal abrasions. *American Family Physician, 87*(2), 114–120

Dacryocystitis

Jill C. Cash, Nancy Pesta Walsh, and Jenny Mullen

Definition

A. Infection or inflammation of the lacrimal sac, or dacryocystitis, can be acute or chronic.

B. Dacryocystitis is usually secondary to obstruction.

Incidence

A. Dacryocystitis occurs more often with infants and adults older than 40.

B. Females comprise 70% to 83% of cases with a peak age of 60 to 70 years.

C. Caucasians tend to be more affected than other races because the lacrimal canal is longer and is inclined to deviate.

Pathogenesis

A. Bacterial infection of the lacrimal sac usually is caused by *Staphylococcus* or *Streptococcus*.

Predisposing Factors

A. Nasal trauma

B. Deviated septum

C. Nasal polyps

D. Congenital dacryostenosis

E. Inferior turbinate hypertrophy

Common Complaints

A. Pain in the eye

B. Redness

C. Swelling

D. Fever

E. Tearing

Other Signs and Symptoms

A. Purulent exudate may be expressed from the lacrimal duct.

Subjective Data

A. Elicit the onset, course, and duration of symptoms. Are symptoms bilateral or unilateral?

B. Review the client's activity when the symptoms began to determine if etiology is chemical, traumatic, or infectious.

C. Review other presenting symptoms such as fever and discharge.

D. Review the client's history for previous episodes. Note treatments used in past.

E. Review history for a recent HSV or fever blister.

F. Review ophthalmologic history.

G. Review medications.

Physical Examination

A. Check temperature, pulse, and blood pressure.

B. Inspect:

1. Assess both eyes.

2. Check peripheral fields of vision, and sclera.

3. Evaluate conjunctiva for distribution of redness, ciliary flush, and foreign bodies.

4. Inspect lid margins: evaluate for crusting, ulceration, and masses.

C. Palpate:

1. Palpate lacrimal duct. Discharge can be expressed from the tear duct with the application of pressure.

Diagnostic Tests

A. Check visual acuity.

B. Culture discharge for *Neisseria* if suspected.

Differential Diagnoses

A. Chalazion

B. Blepharitis

C. Xanthoma

D. Bacterial conjunctivitis

E. Hordeolum

F. Foreign body

G. Cellulitis

H. Complications of sarcoidosis

Plan

A. General interventions:

   1. Apply warm, moist compresses at least four times per day.

   2. Instruct female clients to discard old makeup, including mascara, eyeliner, and eye shadow, used before infection.

B. Client teaching:

   1. Application of compresses, handwashing, and proper cleaning. *See Section III: Client Teaching Guide for this chapter, "Eye Medication Administration."* See Figure 5.5: How to instill eye drops into the eye.

C. Pharmaceutical therapy:

   1. Dicloxacillin 250 mg by mouth four times daily for 7 days

   2. Erythromycin 250 mg by mouth four times daily for 7 days

Follow-Up

A. Follow up in 2 weeks if symptoms are not resolved.

Consultation/Referral

A. Refer the client to an ophthalmologist for irrigation and probing if needed.

B. Lab studies are generally performed by an ophthalmologist.

FIGURE 5.5   How to instill eye drops into the eye.

Bibliography

Gilliland, G., Law, S., & Ing, E. (2018). Dacrocystitis: Ophthalmology. *MedScape*, pp. e1–e20. Retrieved from https://emedicine.medscape .com/article/1210688-overview

Dry Eyes

Jill C. Cash, Nancy Pesta Walsh, and Jenny Mullen

Definition

A. Insufficient lubrication of the eye, or dry eyes, is caused by a deficiency of any one of the major components of the tear film.

B. Defects in tear production are uncommon but may occur in conjunction with systemic disease. Presence of systemic disease should be evaluated.

Incidence

A. It is estimated that 6.8% (16.4 million people) of U.S. adult population has been diagnoses with dry eye disease.

B. Prevalence increased among young adults 18 to 34 years old.

C. The highest risk diagnosed were adults 45 to 54 years old and was higher among women than men.

D. The elderly population is vulnerable to dry eye disease due to decreased rate of lacrimal gland secretions.

Pathogenesis

A. Decreased production of one or more components of the tear film results in dry eyes. The tear film comprises three layers:

   1. An outermost lipid layer, excreted by the lid meibomian glands

   2. A middle aqueous layer, secreted by the main and accessory lacrimal glands

   3. An innermost mucinous layer, secreted by conjunctival goblet cells

B. A defect in the production of the aqueous phase by lacrimal glands causes dry eyes or keratoconjunctivitis sicca. The condition most often occurs as a physiological consequence of aging, and it is commonly exacerbated by dry environmental factors. It may also develop in clients with connective tissue disease.

C. In Sjögren's syndrome, the lacrimal glands become involved in immune-mediated inflammation.

D. Mucin production may decline with vitamin A deficiency.

E. Loss of goblet cells can occur secondary to chemical burns.

Predisposing Factors

A. History of severe conjunctivitis

B. Eyelid defects such as fifth or seventh cranial nerve palsy, incomplete blinking, exophthalmos, and lid movement hindered by scar formation

C. Drug-induced conditions, including the use of anticholinergic agents:

   1. Phenothiazine

   2. Tricyclic antidepressants

   3. Antihistamines

   4. Diuretics

   5. Isotretinoin (Accutane)

D. Systemic disease such as rheumatoid disease, Sjögren's syndrome, and neurologic disease

E. Environmental factors such as heat (wood, coal, and gas), air conditioners, winter air, and tobacco smoke

F. Use of contacts

G. Increasing age

H. Lipid abnormalities

Common Complaints

A. Ocular fatigue

B. Foreign-body sensation in the eye

C. Itching, burning, irritation, or dry sensation in the eye

D. Redness

E. Eye discharge

Other Signs and Symptoms

A. Photophobia

B. Cloudy, blurred vision

C. Rainbow of color around lights. Acute-angle-closure glaucoma can present with a red, painful eye; cloudy, blurred vision, and a rainbow of color around lights; dilatation of the pupil; nausea and vomiting

D. Bell's palsy, signs of stroke, or other conditions affect the blinking mechanism

Subjective Data

A. Elicit the onset, duration, and frequency of symptoms.

B. Note factors that worsen or alleviate symptoms.

C. Note medical history for systemic conditions and strokes.

D. List current medications, noting anticholinergic drugs and isotretinoin (Accutane) use.

E. Note whether the client wears contact lenses or glasses, and ask for what length of time.

F. Review occupational and home exposure to irritants and allergens.

G. Assess whether the client produces tears. Note eye drainage amount, color, and frequency.

H. Review history of any previous ocular disease, surgeries, and so forth.

Physical Examination

A. Check temperature, pulse, respirations, and blood pressure.

B. Inspect:

    1. Observe and evaluate *both* eyes.

    2. Conduct a detailed eye examination Check the eye, lid, and conjunctiva for masses and redness

    3. Check pupil reactivity and corneal clarity. The corneal reflex should be checked if there is concern about a neuroparalytic keratitis or facial nerve palsy.

    4. Complete a funduscopic examination. Check for completeness of lid closure as well as position of eyelashes.

    5. Examine mouth for dryness.

    6. Inspect skin for butterfly rash.

C. Palpate:

    1. Palpate lacrimal ducts for drainage.

    2. Invert upper lid and check for foreign body or chalazion.

    3. Check sinuses for tenderness.

    4. Palpate thyroid.

    5. Palpate joints for warmth and redness or inflammation.

Diagnostic Test

A. Perform Schirmer's test. Use Whatman no. 41 filter paper, 5 mm by 35 mm. A folded end of filter paper is hooked over the lower lid nasally, and the client is instructed to keep his or her eyes lightly closed during the test. Wetting is measured after 5 minutes; less than 5 mm is usually abnormal. More than 10 mm is normal.

Differential Diagnoses

A. Stevens–Johnson syndrome

B. Sjögren's syndrome: Chronic dry mouth, dry eyes, and arthritis triad suggest Sjögren's syndrome. Facial telangiectasias, parotid enlargement, Raynaud's phenomenon, and dental caries are associated features. Clients complain first of burning and a sandy, gritty, foreign-body sensation, particularly later in the day.

C. Systemic lupus erythematosus

D. Scleroderma

E. Ocular pterygium

F. Superficial pemphigoid

G. Vitamin A deficiency

Plan

A. General interventions:

    1. If no ocular disease is present, reduce environmental dryness by use of a room humidifier for a 2-week trial.

    2. Apply artificial tear substitutes and nonprescription drops.

    3. Consider stopping medications being used that may be contributing to the source of dry eye symptoms.

    4. Caution should be used when using over-the-counter (OTC) allergy medications, if allergy is a contributing cause. Topical antihistamines may exacerbate the condition over time.

B. Client teaching: *See Section III: Client Teaching Guide for this chapter, "Eye Medication Administration."*

C. Pharmaceutical therapy:

    1. Topical artificial tears 1 or 2 drops four times daily, preferably one without preservatives (i.e., Thera-tears, Dry Eye Therapy, Tears Naturale)

    2. Drops may be instilled as often as desired.

Follow-Up

A. Determined by the severity of the issue. Reevaluate the client in 2 weeks

Consultation/Referral

A. Refer the client to an ophthalmologist if symptoms are unrelieved at the 2-week follow-up.

B. Make an immediate referral for red eye, visual disturbance, or eye pain.

Individual Consideration

A. Geriatrics:

    1. The rate of lacrimal gland secretions diminishes with age; therefore, the elderly are at an increased risk for developing dry eye.

B. Adults:

    1. ACE inhibitors may reduce the risk of dry eye syndrome in some clients. Consider treatment with ACE inhibitors for hypertension as appropriate in clients.

C. Pediatrics:

    1. Current research indicated that children that used smartphones were strongly associated with dry eye disease. Grade-school children who had less outdoor activity and increased indoor smartphone usage

(schoolwork, study, and APP games) had greater risk for dry eyes.

2. Consider education regarding appropriate smartphone use with pediatrics (and all age groups) such as eye-rest, optic lubricants, and increase outdoor activity without using smartphone.

Bibliography

American Academy of Ophthalmology. (2018). Dry eye syndrome preferred practice guidelines. *Ophthalmology*, *126*(1), 286–334. doi:10.1016/j.ophtha.2018.10.023

Ferrand, K., Fridman, M., Stillman, I., & Schaumberg, D. (2017). Prevalence of diagnosed dry eye disease in the United States among adults aged 18 years and older. *American Journal of Ophthalmology*, *182*, 90–98. doi:10.1016/j.ajo.2017.06.033

Galor, A., Levitt, R., Felix, E., Martin, E., & Sarantopoulos, C. (2015). Neuropathic ocular pain: an important yet underevaluated feature of dry eye. *The Scientific Journal of Royal College of Ophthalmologists*, *29*(3), 301–312. doi:10.1038/eye2014.263

Maturi, R., Franklin, A., Law, S., Charles, S., Dahl, A., & Phillpotts, B. (2018). Nonexudative (dry) age-related macular degeneration (AMD). Macular degeneration: Ophthalmology. *MedScape*, pp. e1–e23. Retrieved from https://emedicine.medscape.com/article/1223154-overview

Moon, J., Kim, K., & Moon, N. (2016). Smartphone use is a risk for pediatric dry eye disease according to region and age: A case control study. *BioMed Central: BMC Ophthalmology*, *16*(188), e1–e14. doi:10.1186/s12886-016-0364-4

Excessive Tears

Jill C. Cash, Nancy Pesta Walsh, and Jenny Mullen

Definition

A. Excessive tears disorder is an overproduction of tears. Complaints vary from watery eyes to overflowing tears that run down the cheeks, a condition known as *epiphora*.

Incidence

A. The incidence is unknown. Previous research has reported the highest incidence of excessive tearing is in individuals between 50 and 70 years old, and more prevalent in women.

Pathogenesis

A. The most common cause is reflex overproduction of tears (as occurs in the elderly) due to a deficiency of the tear film.

B. Lacrimal pump failure and obstruction of the nasolacrimal outflow system are other causes of excessive tears.

C. Canalicular infections may be caused by *Actinomyces israelii* (Streptothrix) and *Candida*.

Predisposing Factors

A. Blepharitis (inflammation of the eyelid)

B. Allergic conjunctivitis (infectious or foreign body)

C. Exposure to cold, air conditioning, or dry environment

D. Lid problems: impaired pumping action of the lid motion due to seventh nerve palsy or conditions that stiffen the lids such as scars or scleroderma

E. Lid laxity from aging or ectropion (sagging of the lower lid)

F. Sinusitis

G. Atopy

H. Age: increased incidence in the elderly due to an overproduction of tears by the lacrimal gland

I. Congenital obstruction

Common Complaints

A. Watery eyes or tears running down cheeks are common complaints.

Other Signs and Symptoms

A. Unilateral tearing: obstructive etiology

B. Bilateral tearing: environmental irritants

Subjective Data

A. Inquire about onset, course, and duration of symptoms. Note frequency of excessive tearing.

B. Ascertain whether this is a new symptom or whether the client has a past history of similar complaints. Ask how it was treated, and what was the response to treatment(s).

C. Determine severity. Do the tears run down the cheek?

D. Ascertain whether tearing is unilateral or bilateral.

E. Review common environmental predisposing factors.

F. Question the client regarding vision changes.

G. Review medical history.

H. Review recent history for sinus infections or drainage, facial fractures, and surgery.

Physical Examination

A. Inspect:

1. Evaluate *both* eyes

2. Observe the lid structure and motion.

3. Conduct a dermal examination to rule out butterfly rash.

B. Palpate:

1. Apply gentle pressure over the lacrimal sac to check drainage.

2. Invert upper lid to check for foreign body.

3. Palpate face for sinus tenderness.

Diagnostic Test

A. Culture any drainage expressed from the lacrimal sacs.

Differential Diagnoses

A. Excessive tears

B. Dendritic ulcer: Early symptoms are tears running down cheeks associated with a foreign-body sensation.

C. Congenital glaucoma

D. Dacryocystitis (purulent discharge)

E. Reflex tearing caused by dry eye

F. Blepharitis

Plan

A. General interventions:

1. Eliminate identifiable irritants.

2. Treatment is mainly aimed at the underlying condition (i.e., ocular infection).

3. Dacryocystitis is treated with hot compresses at least four times a day and systemic antibiotics.

B. Client teaching:
1. Instruct the client on the application of compresses.
C. Pharmaceutical therapy:
1. None is required for diagnosis of excessive tears without infectious pathology.
2. Dacryocystitis:
    a. Erythromycin 250 mg four times daily for 7 days
    b. Dicloxacillin 250 mg four times daily for 7 days

Follow-Up

A. See client in 48 to 72 hours to evaluate symptoms, especially if antibiotic therapy was needed.

Consultation/Referral

A. Clients unresponsive to treatment should be promptly referred to an ophthalmologist.
B. Consider referral for lid malposition or nasolacrimal duct obstructions.

Individual Consideration

A. Pediatrics:
1. Nasolacrimal duct obstruction. Approximately 6% of newborns are diagnosed with a congenital obstruction within the first weeks of life. With moist heat and massage, many resolve spontaneously.

Bibliography

Worak, S., Bengzon, A., Law, S., Roy, H., Pelton, R., & Camara, J. (2018). Nasolacrimal duct obstruction and epiphora. Epiphora: Ophthalmology. *MedScape*, pp. e1–e17. Retrieved from https://emedicine.medscape.com/article/1210141-overview

Eye Pain

Jill C. Cash, Nancy Pesta Walsh, and Jenny Mullen

Definition

A. Sensation of pain may affect the eyelid, conjunctiva, or cornea.

Incidence

A. Unknown. Pain in the eye is most often produced by conditions that do not threaten vision.

Pathogenesis

A. The external ocular surfaces and the uveal tract are richly innervated with pain receptors. As a result, lesions or disease processes affecting these surfaces can be acutely painful.
B. Pathology confined to the vitreous, retina, or optic nerve is rarely a source of pain.

Predisposing Factors

A. Eyelids: inflammation such as hordeolum (stye), trichiasis (in-turned lash), and tarsal foreign bodies
B. Conjunctiva: viral and bacterial conjunctivitis or allergic conjunctivitis; toxic, chemical, and mechanical injuries
C. Cornea: keratitis (inflammation of the cornea) accompanying trauma, infection, exposure, vascular disease, or decreased lacrimation; microbial keratitis from contact use. If blood vessels invade the normally avascular corneal stroma, vision may become cloudy. Severe pain is a prominent symptom; movement of the lid typically exacerbates symptoms.

Common Complaints

A. Eye pain (sharp, dull, deep): The quality of the pain needs to be considered. Deep pain is suggestive of an intraocular problem. Inflammation and rapidly expanding mass lesions may cause deep pain. Displacement of the globe and diplopia may ensue.
B. Eye movement may cause sharp pain due to meningeal inflammation (the extraocular rectus muscles insert along the dura of the nerve sheath at the orbital apex). Most cases are idiopathic, but 10% to 15% are associated with multiple sclerosis.
C. Deep dull ache and discomfort associated with eyestrain, blurred vision, and sometimes headache with neck and shoulder pain. Research suggested that approximately 70% of people who work on computer screens, tablets, and cellphones have at least one symptom. This type of eye pain is referred to as digital eye strain or computer vision syndrome (CVS).
D. Eye pain behind the eyes associated with headache might be stemming from a sinus infection or allergy. If eye pain is behind one eye, then it suggests a possible migraine, especially if accompanied in another area on the same side of the cranium.

Other Signs and Symptoms

These symptoms may be unilateral or bilateral.
A. Eyelids:
1. Tenderness
2. Sensation of foreign body
3. Redness
4. Edema
B. Conjunctiva:
1. Mild burning
2. Sensation of foreign body
3. Itching (allergic)
C. Cornea:
1. Burning
2. Foreign-body sensation
3. Considerable discomfort
4. Reflex photophobic tearing
5. Blinking exacerbates pain
6. Pain relieved with pressure (i.e., holding the lid shut). With a foreign body or a corneal lesion, pain is exacerbated by lid movement and relieved by cessation of lid motion.
D. Sclera: redness
E. Uveal tract (uveitis or iritis):
1. Dull, deep-seated ache and photophobia
2. Profound ocular and orbital pain radiating to the frontal and temporal regions accompanying sudden elevation of pressure (acute-angle-closure glaucoma)

3. Vagal stimulation with high pressure may result in nausea and vomiting.

4. Usual history of mild intermittent episodes of blurred vision preceding onset of throbbing pain, nausea, vomiting, and decreased visual acuity

5. Halos around light

F. Orbit:

1. Deep pain with inflammation and rapidly expanding mass lesions

2. Eye movement causing sharp pain due to meningeal inflammation

G. Sinusitis: secondary orbital inflammation and tenderness on extremes of eye movement

Subjective Data

A. Review the onset, duration, and course of symptoms. Inquire regarding the quality of pain.

B. Review any predisposing factors such as trauma or a foreign object. Ask was the onset sudden or gradual?

C. Note reported changes in visual acuity or color vision

D. Note aggravating or alleviating factors.

E. Determine whether the eye pain is bilateral or unilateral.

F. Review history for herpes, infections, and toxic or chemical irritants.

G. Review history for glaucoma and previous eye surgeries or treatments.

H. Assess the client for any other symptoms such as migraine headache, sinusitis, or tooth abscess.

I. Inquire whether the client has lost a large amount of sleep.

J. Inquire whether he or she has been exposed to a large amount of UV light or sunlight (vacation, tanning beds).

K. Review history for any other medical problems such as lupus, sarcoidosis, or inflammatory bowel disease.

Physical Examination

A. Inspect:

1. Evaluate *both* eyes

2. Test visual acuity and color vision.

3. Observe for EOMs.

4. Check the eye, lid, and conjunctiva for masses and redness.

5. Check pupil reactivity and corneal clarity.

6. Conduct a funduscopic examination for disc abnormalities.

7. Perform ear, nose, and throat examination.

B. Palpate:

1. Palpate lacrimal ducts for drainage.

2. Palpate sinus for tenderness.

3. Invert upper lid and check for foreign body or chalazion.

Diagnostic Tests

A. Fluorescein stain

B. Measurement of intraocular pressure (IOP)

Differential Diagnoses

A. Hordeolum

B. Chalazion

C. Acute dacryocystitis

D. Irritant exposure

E. Conjunctival infection

F. Corneal abrasion

G. Foreign body

H. Ulcers

I. Ingrown lashes

J. Contact lens abuse

K. Scleritis

L. Acute-angle-closure glaucoma may present with fixed, midposition pupil, redness, and a hazy cornea

M. Uveitis

N. Referred pain from extraocular sources such as sinusitis, tooth abscess, tension headache, temporal arteritis, and prodrome of herpes zoster

Plan

A. General interventions:

1. The initial task is to be sure that there is no threat to vision.

2. Treatment modality depends on the underlying cause of eye pain.

B. Client teaching: *See Section III: Client Teaching Guide for this chapter, "Eye Medication Administration."* See Figure 5.5: How to instill eye drops into the eye.

C. Pharmaceutical therapy: Medication depends on the underlying cause.

D. Digital eye strain treatment

1. American Optometric Association's 20–20–20 rule is to take a 20-second break to view something 20-feet away every 20-minutes.

2. Keep blinking; that will naturally rinse eyes.

3. Correct lighting by keeping window light to the side, use blinds, use an anti-glare screen, and position computer screen to reduce reflections of overhead light and windows.

4. Station monitor 20 inches from eyes, with the center approximately 4 to 6 inches below eyes. Adjust the screen downward and choose settings that are comfortable (polarity, resolution, brightness, contrast, etc.).

5. Suggest computer glasses that an optometrist could prescribe and advise any purchased retail bluelight/UV eyeglasses be evaluated through the optometrist.

6. Encourage annual comprehensive eye exam with ophthalmologist to examine eye health and assess for any changes related to diabetes, hyperlipidemia, hypertension, glaucoma, and macular degeneration.

Follow-Up

A. Follow-up depends on the underlying cause.

Consultation/Referral

A. Any change in visual acuity or color vision requires an urgent ophthalmologic consultation.

Bibliography

America Academy of Ophthalmology. (2017b November). *Retina Summary Benchmarks 2018*. Retrieved from https://www.aao.org/summary-benchmark-detail/retina-summary-benchmarks-2018

American Optometric Association. (2019). *Computer vision syndrome*. Retrieved from https://www.aoa.org/patients-and-public/caring-for-your-vision/protecting-your-vision/computer-vision-syndrome

Brady, C. (2018). Eye pain. *Merck Manual: Professional Version*. Retrieved from https://www.merckmanuals.com/professional/eye-disorders/symptoms-of-ophthalmologic-disorders/eye-pain#

Lin, C., Yeh, F., Wu, B., & Yang, C. (2019). The effects of reflected glare and visual field lighting on computer vision syndrome. *Clinical and Experimental Optometry, 102*(2), 513–520. doi:10.1111/cxo.12878

Prall, F., Ciulla, T., Criswell, M., Harris, A., Talavera, F., Charles, S., Dahl, A., & Phillpotts, B. (2018). Exudative (wet) age-related macular degeneration (AMD). Macular degeneration: Ophthalmology. *MedScape*, pp. e1–e24. Retrieved from https://emedicine.medscape.com/article/1226030-overview

Sheppard, A., & Wolffsohn, J. S. (2018). Digital eye strain: Prevalence, measurement and amelioration. *British Medical Journal, 3*(1), e1–e10. doi:10.1136/bmjophth-2018-000146

Glaucoma

Jill C. Cash, Nancy Pesta Walsh, and Jenny Mullen

Definition

A. This ocular emergency is caused by elevations in IOP that damage the optic nerve, leading to loss of peripheral fields of vision; it can lead to loss of central vision and result in blindness.

Incidence

A. An estimation of more than 3 million Americans has glaucoma and only 50% know of their diagnosis. WHO reported it is the leading cause of blindness in the world (greater than 60 million) and may increase to 80 million by 2020. It accounts for 12% of all cases of blindness in the United States.

B. Open-angle glaucoma is the most common form of glaucoma and is diagnosed more often with African Americans than Caucasians. Currently, 2.7 million 40 years and older have open-angle glaucoma.

C. High-risk groups are people greater than 60 years old, diabetics, and people who are severely nearsighted.

D. Angle-Closure glaucoma is an urgent dramatic event that develops and peaks around the age of 60 years old and affects women 50% more than men. High-risk groups are people with smaller eyes that are often far-sighted, geriatrics, Asian and Indian ethnicity, and have a family history of angle-closure glaucoma.

Pathogenesis

A. The essential pathophysiologic feature of glaucoma is an IOP that is too high for the optic nerve. Increased IOP increases vascular resistance, causing decreased vascular perfusion of the optic nerve and ischemia. Light dilates the pupil, causing the iris to relax and bow forward. As the iris bows forward, it comes into contact with the trabecular meshwork and occludes the outflow of aqueous humor, resulting in increased IOP.

B. Basic differences between open-angle glaucoma and angle-closure glaucoma:

    1. Open-angle glaucoma: Most common of all glaucoma cases. Open-angle means there is an abnormally wide and open angle where the iris meets the cornea. It causes the drainage canals to become sluggish and build pressure. The symptoms are gradual and unnoticed.

    2. Angle-closure glaucoma is less common yet an emergent case. The acute closure angle describes the abnormally narrow angle between the iris and cornea closing. It develops quickly and suddenly blocks drainage canals that increases pressure. These symptoms are usually immediately noticed.

Predisposing Factors

A. Narrow anterior ocular chamber
B. Prolonged periods of darkness
C. Drugs that dilate the pupils (i.e., anticholinergics)
D. Advancing age: Greater than 60 years
E. African American heritage
F. Family history
G. Trauma
H. Neoplasm
I. Corticosteroid therapy
J. Neovascularization
K. Female sex

Common Complaints

A. Ocular pain
B. Blurred vision, decreased visual acuity, "cloudiness" of vision
C. "Halos" around lights at night
D. Neurologic complaints (headache, nausea, or vomiting)

Other Signs and Symptoms

A. Red eye with ciliary flush
B. "Silent blinder" causes extensive damage before the client is aware of visual field loss
C. Dilated pupil
D. Hard orbital globe
E. No pupillary response to light
F. Increase IOP (normal IOP is 10–20 mmHg).

Subjective Data

A. Review the onset, course, and duration of symptoms; note visual changes in one or both eyes.
B. Review medical history and medications.
C. Review family history of glaucoma.
D. Determine whether there has been any difficulty with peripheral vision, any headache photophobia, or any visual blurring.
E. In children, ask about rubbing of eyes, refusal to open eyes, and tearing.
F. Rule out presence of any chemical, trauma, or foreign bodies in the eye.
G. Review any recent history of herpes outbreak.
H. Ask the client whether this has ever occurred before, and if so, how it was treated.
I. The National Glaucoma Research recommends assessing the following medications that may develop or affect glaucoma, and to defer these clients to their ophthalmologist:

    1. COPD: Atrovent, Spiriva
    2. Bladder conditions: Detrol, Ditropan

3. Indigestion: Tagamet, Zantac
4. Muscle spasms: Norflex, Artane
5. Depression: Prozac, Paxil, Elavil , Tofranil
6. Allergies: Diphenhydramine
7. Nausea: Phenergan
8. Anxiety: Vistaril
9. Cold remedies: Ephedrine
10. Oral steroids: prednisone

Physical Examination
A. Blood pressure
B. Inspect:
1. Examine both eyes.
2. Rule out foreign body.
3. Inspect for redness, inflammation, and discharge.
4. Check pupillary response to light.
5. Redness noted around iris, pupil is dilated, and cornea appears cloudy.
6. Inspect anterior chamber of eye by holding penlight laterally and direct toward nasal area. Shallow chamber will cast a shadow on the nasal side of the iris.
C. Palpate: globe of the eye, which will feel firm on palpation
D. Funduscopic examination: This may reveal notching of the cup and a difference in cup-to-disc ratio between the two eyes.

Diagnostic Tests
A. Check visual acuity and peripheral fields of vision
B. Measure IOP with a tonometer. Normal level is 10 to 21 mmHg; acute-angle-closure glaucoma IOP is greater than 50 mmHg; open-angle glaucoma would be a noted rise in ocular pressures >21 mmHg in comparison to previous exams. Tonometer examination is not recommended if external infection is present.
C. Slit-lamp examination: edematous and/or cloudy cornea

Differential Diagnoses
A. Acute iritis
B. Acute bacterial conjunctivitis
C. Iridocyclitis
D. Corneal injury
E. Foreign body
F. Herpetic keratitis

Plan
A. General interventions:
1. Severe attacks of acute-angle-closure glaucoma can cause blindness in 2 to 3 days. Seek medical attention immediately to prevent permanent vision loss.
2. Frequency of attacks is unpredictable.
3. All pressure changes greater than 21 mmHg need further evaluation from an ophthalmologist.
▶ B. Client teaching: *See Section III: Client Teaching Guide for this chapter, "Eye Medication Administration."*

C. Pharmaceutical therapy: must be instituted by an ophthalmologist:
1. Acetazolamide (Diamox). For acute-angle-closure glaucoma: 500 mg PO/IV followed by 125 to 250 mg PO every 4 hours for 2 to 3 days or until ocular pressure stabilizes. For open-angle exacerbations: 250 mg to 1 g PO/IV followed by 250 to 500 mg PO every 6 or 12 hours until ocular pressure stabilizes
2. Pilocarpine (Pilocar). For acute-angle-closure glaucoma: 2% solution 1 drop in eye(s) every 15 to 60 minutes for 2 to 4 doses until ocular pressure stabilizes. For open-angle glaucoma: 1% to 4% solution, 1 to 2 drops three to four times a day until ocular pressure stabilizes
Common medications to treat chronic glaucoma:
Alpha adrenergic agonists: apraclonidine, epinephrine, brimonidine
Beta blockers: timolol, levobunolol, carteolol, betatoxolol
Carbonic anhydrase inhibitors: brinzolamide, acetazolamide
Prostaglandin analogs: latanoprost, travoprost
3. A new class of prostaglandin analogs is called rho kinase inhibitors: Rhopressa (netarsudil) 0.02% solution. This drug assists in lowering IOP, is dosed daily, and carries very few systemic safety concerns.
D. Surgical intervention:
1. Surgery is indicated if IOP is not maintained within normal limits with medications or if there is progressive visual field loss with optic nerve damage.
2. Surgical treatment of choice is peripheral iridectomy—excision of a small portion of the iris whereby the aqueous humor can bypass the pupil.

Follow-Up
A. Annual eye examinations by an ophthalmologist are necessary to monitor IOP and treatment efficacy.

Consultation/Referral
A. All clients should be referred to an ophthalmologist *immediately* for measurement of IOP, acute management, and possible surgical intervention (laser peripheral iridectomy).

Individual Considerations
A. Pediatrics
1. Congenital pediatric glaucoma is a rare and usually diagnosed in the first year of life. Symptoms in childhood include enlarged eyes, cornea cloudiness, excessive tearing (child constantly rubbing eyes), and photosensitivity. Refer immediately to pediatric ophthalmologist
2. In uncomplicated cases, surgery corrects structural defects. Inform parents that children often adapt and participate in their own ocular self-care.
B. Adults:
1. Women normally have slightly higher IOPs than men.
2. Asians may have higher IOPs than African Americans and Caucasians.

3. Individuals older than age 40 years should have their IOP measured periodically. Every 3 to 5 years is sufficient after a stable baseline is established for the client.

C. Geriatrics:

1. Incidence increases with age, usually in those older than 60 years.

Bibliography

American Academy of Ophthalmology. (2017, November). *Glaucoma summary benchmarks 2018*. Retrieved from https://www.aao.org/summary-benchmark-detail/glaucoma-summary-benchmarks-2018

BrightFocus Foundation. (2019). Glaucoma: Facts & figures. *BrightFocus*, pp. e1–e5. Retrieved from https://www.brightfocus.org/glaucoma/article/glaucoma-facts-figures

Glaucoma Research Foundation. (2017a). Childhood glaucoma. *Glaucoma Research Foundation*. Retrieved from https://www.glaucoma.org/glaucoma/childhood-glaucoma-1.php

Glaucoma Research Foundation. (2017b). Glaucoma facts and stats. *Glaucoma Research Foundation*. Retrieved from https://www.glaucoma.org/glaucoma/glaucoma-facts-and-stats.php

Glaucoma Research Foundation. (2017c). Types of glaucoma. *Glaucoma Research Foundation*. Retrieved from https://www.glaucoma.org/glaucoma/types-of-glaucoma.php

National Glaucoma Research. (2019). National glaucoma research report 2019. *Bright Focus Foundation Program*. Retrieved from https://www.brightfocus.org/sites/default/files/national-glaucoma-research-report-winter-2019.pdf

Hordeolum (Stye)

Jill C. Cash, Nancy Pesta Walsh, and Jenny Mullen

Definition

A. Hordeolum is an infection of the glands of the eyelids (follicle of an eyelash or the associated gland of Zeis [sebaceous] or Moll's gland [apocrine sweat gland]), usually caused by *Staph. aureus*. See Figure 5.6.

B. If swelling is under the conjunctival side of the eyelid, it is an internal hordeolum.

C. If swelling is under the skin of the eyelid, it is an external hordeolum.

Incidence

A. The incidence is unknown; it is more common in children and adolescents than in adults.

FIGURE 5.6   Stye of upper eyelid.

B. Clients with recurrent blepharitis, seborrheic dermatitis, rosacea, diabetes, and hyperlipidemia are have an increased risk for hordeola development.

Pathogenesis

A. Acute bacterial infection of the meibomian gland (internal hordeolum) or of the eyelash follicle (external hordeolum) is usually caused by *Staph. aureus*.

Predisposing Factor

A. Age: more common in the pediatric population

Common Complaints

A. Eye tenderness

B. Sudden onset of a purulent discharge

Other Signs and Symptoms

A. Redness and swelling of the eye

Subjective Data

A. Review the onset, course, and duration of symptoms.

B. Determine whether there is any visual disturbance.

C. Note whether this is the first occurrence. If not, ask how it was treated before.

D. Evaluate how much pain or discomfort the client is experiencing.

E. Review the client's history for chemical, foreign body, and/or trauma etiology.

F. Review the client's medical history and medications.

Physical Examination

A. Inspect:

1. Examine both eyes; note redness, site of swelling, and amount and color of discharge.

2. Evert the lid and check for pointing.

3. Assess sclera and conjunctivae for abnormalities.

4. Inspect ears, nose, and throat.

B. Palpate:

1. Palpate eye for hardness and expression of discharge.

2. Evaluate for preauricular adenopathy.

Diagnostic Tests

A. Test visual acuity.

B. Discharge can be cultured but is usually treated presumptively.

Differential Diagnoses

A. Chalazion: The main differential diagnosis is chalazia, which point on the conjunctival side of the eyelid and do not usually affect the margin of the eyelid.

B. Blepharitis

C. Xanthoma

D. Bacterial conjunctivitis

E. Foreign body

Plan

A. General interventions:

1. Contain the infecting pathogen. Crops occur when the infectious agent spreads from one hair follicle to another.

B. Client teaching:
1. *See Section III: Client Teaching Guide for this chapter, "Eye Medication Administration."* See Figure 5.5: How to instill eye drops into the eye.
2. Reinforce good handwashing.
3. Instruct on proper eyelid hygiene.
4. Clients should discard all eye makeup, including mascara, eyeliner, and eye shadow.
C. Pharmaceutical therapy:
1. Sulfacetamide sodium (Sulamyd) ophthalmic ointment 10%; 0.5 to 1.0 cm placed in the conjunctival sac four times daily for 7 days
2. Sulfacetamide sodium (Sulamyd) 10% ophthalmic drops; 2 drops instilled every 3 to 4 hours for 7 days
3. Polymyxin B sulfate and bacitracin zinc (Polysporin) ophthalmic ointment; 0.5 to 1.0 cm placed in the conjunctival sac four times daily for 7 days
4. If crops of styes occur, some clinicians recommend a course of tetracycline to stop recurrences (consult with a physician).

Follow-Up
A. Have client telephone or visit the office in 48 hours to check response
B. If crops occur, diabetes mellitus must be excluded. Perform blood glucose evaluation.

Consultation/Referral
A. Hordeolum may produce a diffuse superficial lid infection known as *preseptal cellulitis* that requires referral to an ophthalmologist.
B. If hordeolum does not respond to topical antimicrobial treatment, refer the client to an ophthalmologist.

Individual Consideration
A. Adults:
1. Address underlying conditions such as rosacea, frequent blepharitis, uncontrolled diabetes, and high cholesterol in order to prevent recurrent hordeolum in these clients.

Bibliography

Bragg, K., Le, J., & Le, P. (2020). Hordeolum. In *StatPearls NCBI Resources* (pp. e1–e4). Bethesda, MD: National Center for Biotechnology Information. Retrieved from https://www.ncbi.nlm.nih.gov/books/NBK441985/

Carlisle, R. T., & Digiovanni, J. (2015). Differential diagnosis of the swollen red eyelid. *American Family Physician*, *15*(92), 106–112.

Channa, R., Zafar, S., Canner, J., Haring, S., Schneider, E., & Firedman, D. (2016). Epidemiology of eye-related emergency department visits. *JAMA Ophthalmology*, *134*(3), 312–319. doi:10.1001/jamaophthalmol.2015.5778

Strabismus

Jill C. Cash, Nancy Pesta Walsh, and Jenny Mullen

Definition
Strabismus is an eye disorder in which the optic axes cannot be directed toward the same object due to a deficit in muscular coordination. It can be nonparalytic or paralytic.

A. *Esotropia* is a nonparalytic strabismus in which the eyes cross inward.
B. *Exotropia* is a nonparalytic strabismus in which the eyes drift outward. Exotropia may be intermittent or constant.
C. Pseudostrabismus gives a false appearance of deviation in the visual axes.

Incidence
A. Strabismus occurs in approximately 3% of the population.
B. Esotropia (nonparalytic strabismus) is the most common ocular misalignment, representing more than half of all ocular deviations in the pediatric population. Accommodative esotropia typically occurs between 1 and 3 years of age, with an average age of 2.5 years, and it may be intermittent or constant.
C. Intermittent exotropia is the most common type of exotropic strabismus and is characterized by an outward drift of one eye, most often occurring when a child is fixating at distance.

Pathogenesis
A. *Paralytic strabismus* is related to paralysis or paresis of a specific extraocular muscle. *Nonparalytic strabismus* is related to a congenital imbalance of normal eye muscle tone, causing focusing difficulties, unilateral refractive error, nonfusion, or anatomical difference in the eyes.

Predisposing Factors
A. Familial tendencies
B. Congenital defects

Common Complaints
A. Crossing of the eyes
B. Turning in of the eyes
C. Photophobia
D. Diplopia

Other Signs and Symptoms
A. The client's head or chin tilts or the client closes one eye to focus on objects.

Subjective Data
A. Describe the onset, duration, and progression of symptoms.
B. Review any history of eye problems. Ask how were they corrected?
C. Determine whether the client, if a child, has reached the age-appropriate milestones in development.
D. Does the client make faces or move his or her head to see better (tilting the head or chin to improve acuity or to correct diplopia)?
E. Rule out any eye damage, surgery, and so forth.

Physical Examination
A. Inspect:
1. Observe alignment of lids, sclera, conjunctiva, and cornea.
2. Check pupillary response to light, size, shape, and equality.
3. Check the red reflex.

Diagnostic Tests

A. Test visual acuity.

B. Perform the cover–uncover test: In this test, the "lazy eye" drifts out of position and snaps back quickly when uncovered.

C. Corneal light reflex (Hirschberg's) test: Perform the Hirschberg's test for symmetry of the pupillary light reflexes to help detect strabismus. Normally, the light reflexes are in the same position on each pupil, but not with strabismus (positive Hirschberg's test).

D. Test EOMs: If a nerve supplying an extraocular muscle has been interrupted or the muscle itself has become weakened, the eye fails to move in the direction of the damaged muscle. If the right sixth nerve is damaged, the right eye does not move temporally. This is paralytic strabismus.

Differential Diagnoses

A. Pseudostrabismus

B. Ocular trauma

C. Congenital defect

Plan

A. General interventions:

1. When poor fixation is present, patch the stronger, dominant eye to promote vision and muscle strengthening in the weaker eye.

2. Corrective eyeglasses/contacts that promote less focusing efforts and help eyes look straight

3. Prism lenses that bend light entering the eye, which assists with decreasing the amount of eye movement in order to see an object

B. Client teaching:

1. Reinforce the need to consistently wear an eye patch, especially with children.

C. Pharmaceutical therapy:

1. In some cases, injections of botulinum toxin type A (Botox) can weaken eye muscle and be administered by an ophthalmologist in place of surgery.

Follow-Up

A. Monitor progress with eye patch.

B. Surgical intervention depends on the degree of deviation.

Consultation/Referral

A. Additional testing should be done by an ophthalmologist.

B. Pseudostrabismus (a false appearance of strabismus when visual axes are really in alignment) is one of the most common reasons a pediatric ophthalmologist is asked to evaluate an infant.

Individual Considerations

A. Pediatrics:

1. Use the tumbling or illiterate E to test children; for preschoolers, use the Allen picture cards.

2. In very young children, test visual acuity by assessing developmental milestones: Looking at mother's face, responsive smile, reaching for objects. By 3 to 5 years of age, most children can cooperate for performance of accurate visual acuity screening tests.

3. The eyes of the newborn are *rarely aligned* during the first few weeks of life. By the age of 3 months, normal oculomotor behavior is usually established, and an experienced examiner may be able to document the existence of abnormal alignment by that time.

4. Studies have indicated that adolescents and young adults with strabismus often have a predisposition to anxiety and depression disorders. It is recommended that clinicians consider psychiatric evaluation and management.

Bibliography

American Academy of Ophthalmology. (2017c November). *Pediatric ophthalmology strabismus summary benchmarks 2018*. Retrieved from https://www.aao.org/summary-benchmark-detail/pediatric-ophthalmology-strabismus-summary-benchma

Gunton, W. B., Wasserman, B. N., & DeBenedictis, C. (2015). Strabismus. *Primary Care: Clinics in Office Practice, 2*(3), 393–407.

Ozates, S., Ozates, M., Can, C., Polat, S., Yasar, H., Taskale, B., & Gogus, A. (2018). Improvement in psychiatric symptoms after strabismus surgery in adolescent patients in long-term follow-up [Abstract]. *British Journal of Ophthalmology, 102*(8), 1e–5e. doi:10.1136/bjophthalmol-2018-312510

Shaaban, S., MacKinnon, S., Andrews, C., Staffieri, S. E., Maconachie, G., Chan, W., … Whitman, M. (2018). Genome-wide association study identifies a susceptibility locus for comitant esotropia and suggests a parent-of-origin effect. *Investigative Opthalmology & Visual Science, 59*(10), 4054–4064. doi:10.1167/iovs.18-24082. Retrieved from doi:10.1136/bjophthalmol-2018-312510

Subconjunctival Hemorrhage

Jill C. Cash, Nancy Pesta Walsh, and Jenny Mullen

Definition

A. Subconjunctival hemorrhage presents as blood patches in the bulbar conjunctiva. See Figure 5.7.

Incidence

A. Frequently seen in newborns, subconjunctival hemorrhage may also be seen in adults after forceful exertion (coughing, sneezing, childbirth, strenuous lifting).

B. Subconjunctival hemorrhages account for approximately 3% emergent visits in the United States, and males have a higher prevalence than women.

Pathogenesis

A. This disorder is believed to be secondary to increased intrathoracic pressure that may occur during labor and delivery or with physical exertion.

Predisposing Factors

A. Local trauma

B. Systemic hypertension

C. Acute conjunctivitis

D. Vaginal delivery (pushing during delivery)

E. Severe coughing

F. Severe vomiting

G. Long-term hemodialysis

Common Complaint

A. Red-eyed appearance without pain

FIGURE 5.7 Subconjunctival hemorrhage.

Source: Image courtesy of Daniel Flather.

Other Signs and Symptoms
A. Bright red blood in plane between the conjunctiva and the sclera
B. Usually unilateral
C. Normal vision

Subjective Data
A. Identify onset and duration of symptoms.
B. Elicit information about trauma to the eye; is it due to severe coughing or vomiting?
C. Identify history of conjunctivitis or hypertension.

Physical Examination
A. Check temperature, pulse, respirations, and blood pressure (rule out hypertension).
B. Inspect:
 1. Observe eyes.
 2. Inspect ears, nose, and mouth.
 3. Inspect skin for bruises or other trauma.
 4. Assess for signs of trauma or abuse. Blood in the anterior chamber (hyphema) can result from injury or abuse.
C. Other physical examination components are dependent on etiology.

Diagnostic Tests
A. Perform visual screening.
B. Test EOMs and peripheral vision.

Differential Diagnoses
A. Systemic hypertension
B. Blood dyscrasia
C. Trauma to eye
D. Conjunctivitis
E. Hyphema
F. Abuse

Plan
A. General interventions:
 1. Reassure the client. The hemorrhage is not damaging to the eye or vision, and the blood reabsorbs on its own over several weeks.
 2. Teach safety to prevent trauma to the eye.
B. Pharmaceutical therapy: none

Follow-Up
A. If subconjunctival hemorrhage recurs, evaluate the client further for systemic hypertension or blood dyscrasia.

Consultation/Referral
A. Consult or refer the client to a physician if hyphema is noted, if glaucoma is suspected, or if the client has additional eye injuries.

Individual Considerations
A. Pediatrics:
 1. Hemorrhage is common in newborns after vaginal delivery.
B. Adults:
 1. Always measure blood pressure to rule out systemic hypertension.
C. Geriatrics:
 1. Always measure blood pressure to rule out systemic hypertension.
 2. Consider evaluation for blood dyscrasia.
 3. Check clotting times if client is taking warfarin (Coumadin).

Bibliography
Channa, R., Zafar, S., Canner, J., Haring, S., Schneider, E., & Firedman, D. (2016). Epidemiology of eye-related emergency department visits. *JAMA Ophthalmology, 134*(3), 312–319. doi:10.1001/jamaophthalmol.2015.5778
Makino, S. (2018). Massive subjunctive hemorrhage. *Scholars Journal of Medical Case Reports, 11*, 917–918. Retrieved from http://saspjournals.com/wp-content/uploads/2018/12/SJMCR-611-917-918-c.pdf

Uveitis

Jill C. Cash, Nancy Pesta Walsh, and Jenny Mullen

Definition
A. Uveitis, also known as *iritis,* is inflammation of the uveal tract (iris, ciliary body, and choroid) and is usually accompanied by a dull ache and photophobia resulting from the irritative spasm of the pupillary sphincter. See Figure 5.8.

Incidence
A. The true incidence is unknown. Approximately 15% of clients with sarcoidosis present with uveitis.
B. Oder adults, females, smokers, and GI inflammatory diseases have a higher prevalence for uveitis.

Pathogenesis
A. The cause is unknown. Underlying causes include infections, viruses, and arthritis.

Predisposing Factors
A. Collagen disorders
B. Autoimmune disorders
C. Ankylosing spondylitis
D. Sarcoidosis
E. Juvenile rheumatoid arthritis
F. Lupus
G. Reiter's syndrome
H. Behcet's syndrome

FIGURE 5.8 Uveitis.

Source: Image courtesy of Jonathan Trobe, MD.

I. Syphilis
J. Tuberculosis
K. AIDS
L. Crohn's disease
M. Tobacco use
N. Undiagnosed or poorly controlled diabetes

Common Complaints

A. Eye pain: Painless to deep-seated ache
B. Photophobia
C. Blurred vision with decreased visual acuity
D. Black spots
E. Eye redness

Other Signs and Symptoms

A. Unilateral or bilateral symptoms
   1. Unilateral: The pupil is smaller than that of the other eye because of spasm.
B. Ciliary flush
C. Pupillary contraction
D. Nausea and vomiting with vagal stimulation
E. Halos around lights
F. Hypopyon (pus in anterior chamber)
G. Limbal flush with small pupil

Subjective Data

A. Elicit the onset, course, duration, and frequency of symptoms. Are symptoms bilateral or unilateral?
B. Identify the possible causal activity or agent (chemical, traumatic, or infectious etiologies).
C. Review the client's history of previous uveitis and other ophthalmologic disorders.
D. Review any associated fever, rash, weight loss, joint pain, back pain, oral ulcers, or genital ulcers.
E. Review full medical history for comorbid conditions.

Physical Examination

A. Check temperature, pulse, respirations, and blood pressure.
B. Inspect:
   1. Assess both eyes for visual acuity and peripheral fields of vision.
   2. Check sclera and conjunctiva.

C. Other physical components need to be completed related to comorbid conditions.

Diagnostic Tests

A. Slit-lamp test: examination reveals cells in the anterior chamber and "flare," representing increased aqueous humor protein. Inflammatory cells, called *keratic precipitates,* can collect in clusters on the posterior cornea.
B. Penlight examination: shows a slightly cloudy anterior chamber in the uveitic eye

Differential Diagnoses

A. Acute-angle-closure glaucoma
B. Retinal detachment
C. Central retinal artery occlusion
D. Endophthalmitis

Plan

A. General interventions:
   1. Treat underlying cause as indicated.
   2. Provide immediate referral to an ophthalmologist due to possible complications of cataracts and blindness.
B. Client teaching:
   1. Inform the client that recurrent attacks are common and also require immediate attention.
C. Pharmaceutical therapy:
   1. Medications are given per ophthalmologist.
   2. Uveitis and colitis often flare simultaneously; oral steroids are effective for both.

Follow-Up

A. The client with uveitis needs a follow-up with an ophthalmologist.

Consultation/Referral

A. The client should be referred *immediately* to an ophthalmologist for evaluation and intervention.

Individual Considerations

A. Adults:
   1. Recurrent uveitis may be a sign of another systemic condition.
   2. Other conditions to consider:
      a. Infections (bacterial, spirochetal, viral, fungal, and parasitic infections)
      b. Inflammatory diseases, including spondyloarthropathies (ankylosing spondylitis, psoriatic arthritis, reactive arthritis) and inflammatory bowel disease
      c. Multiple sclerosis
      d. Use of new medications

Resources

American Academy of Ophthalmology
P.O. Box 7424
San Francisco, CA 94120–7424
www.aao.org
Phone: 415-561-8500
Fax: +1 415-561-8533
Email: member_services@aao.org

American Council of the Blind
1703 N. Beauregard St.
Suite 420
Arlington, VA 22201
www.acb.org
Phone: 202-467-5081, 1 800-424-8666
Fax: 703-465-5085
Email: info@acb.org

American Foundation of the Blind
2 Penn Plaza, Suite 1102
New York, NY 10121
www.afb.org
Phone: 212-502-7600
Fax: 888-545-8331
Email: afbinfo@afb.net

American Printing House for the Blind
1839 Frankfort Avenue
P.O. Box 6085
www.aph.org
Louisville, KY 40206–6085
Phone: 800-223-1839; 502-895-2405
Fax: 502-899-2284
Email: info@aph.org

Books on Tape
www.booksontape.com
Email: csbot@penguinrandomhouse.com
Phone: 800-733-3000

Glaucoma Research Foundation
251 Post Street, Suite 600
San Francisco, CA 94198
www.glaucoma.org
Phone: 415-986-3162
800-826-6693
Email: questions@glaucoma.org

Guide Dog Foundation for the Blind
371 E Jerico Turnpike
Smithtown, NY 11787
www.guidedog.org
Phone: 631-930-9000; 800-548-4337
Fax: 631-930-9009
9 a.m. to 5 p.m. (Eastern Standard Time),
Monday through Friday, Email: info@guidedog.org

National Service for the Blind and Physically Handicapped
National Library of Congress
1291 Taylor Street NW
Washington, DC 20542
www.loc.gov/nls/
Phone: 800-424-8567; 202-707-5100; TDD 202-707-0744; Fax: 202-707-07128 a.m. to 4:30 p.m. (Eastern Standard Time),
Monday through Friday
Email: nls@loc.gov

National Society to Prevent Blindness
Prevent Blindness America
211 West Wacker Drive
Suite 1700
Chicago, IL 60606
www.preventblindness.org/contact-us
800-331-2020

Bibliography

Dohm, K. D. (2015, January). Practice pearls for managing anterior uveitis. *Review of Optometry, 2015*(1), 58–63.

González, M., Solano, M., Porco, T., Oldenburg, C., Acharya, N., Lin, S., & Chin, M. (2018). Epidemiology of uveitis in a US population-based study. *Journal of Ophthalmic Inflammation and Infection, 8*(6), e1–e15. doi:10.1186/s12348-018-0148-5

Watanabe T., Keino H., Nakayama K., Wakako, T., Echizen, N., & Okada, A. (2019). Clinical features of patients with diabetic anterior uveitis. *British Journal of Ophthalmology. 103*(12), 78–82. doi:10.1136/bjophthalmol-2018-313600

6 Ear Guidelines

Otitis Media (OM)

Jill C. Cash and Ken Watford

Definition
A. Otitis media (OM) is defined as inflammation of the space between the eardrum and the inner ear due to any cause. The two most common variants of OM are acute otitis media (AOM) and otitis media with effusion (OME). It is important for the clinician to understand the differences in these two common middle ear conditions. A characteristic of AOM is rapid onset of symptoms and inflammation of the middle ear. Middle ear effusion (MEE) may or may not be present. OME is characterized by the presence of MEE without the acute symptoms of AOM (see Figures 6.1 and 6.2).

Incidence
A. AOM may occur at any age, but is most commonly seen in children age 12 months or less. OME is seen in clients of all ages. After the onset of AOM, approximately 70% of children have MEE present at 2 weeks, 40% have MEE present at 1 month, 20% have MEE at 2 months, and 10% have MEE at 3 months.

FIGURE 6.2 Otitis media with effusion.

Source: Image courtesy of Michael Hawke, MD.

B. Over two thirds of children have had at least one episode of OM by 3 years of age.
C. One third of children have had three or more episodes by 3 years of age.
D. One third of all pediatric visits are for OM.
E. Approximately 2.2 million new cases of OME are diagnosed in the United States each year.
F. Annual direct costs of OM in the United States are $3 billion to $5 billion.

Pathogenesis
A. Obstruction of the eustachian tube can lead to an MEE and infection. Contamination of this middle ear fluid may result from a backup of nasopharyngeal secretions. The most common bacterial pathogens are *Streptococcus pneumoniae*, *Haemophilus influenzae*, and *Moraxella catarrhalis*.

Predisposing Factors
A. Age less than 12 months, although may occur at any age
B. Recurrent OM (three or more episodes in the last 6 months)
C. Previous episode of OM within the last month

FIGURE 6.1 Otitis media.

Source: Image courtesy of B. Welleschik.

D. Medical condition that predisposes to OM (i.e., Down syndrome, AIDS, cystic fibrosis, cleft palate, and craniofacial abnormalities)

E. Exposure to tobacco smoke and air pollution

F. Day-care attendance

G. Bottle propping

H. Nasal allergies

I. Pacifier use

Common Complaints

A. AOM:
1. Otalgia
2. Pulling ears in children
3. Fever may or may not be present
4. Ear fullness
5. Upper respiratory infection (URI) symptoms
6. Perforated tympanic membrane (TM): sudden severe pain followed by immediate relief of pain with otorrhea

B. OME:
1. New onset hearing loss
2. Tinnitus
3. Unsteadiness
4. Ear pressure
5. Intermittent sharp otalgia
6. URI symptoms

Subjective Data

A. Elicit onset and duration of symptoms.

B. Inquire whether the client recently had (or concurrently has) a URI.

C. Has client/family noticed hearing loss in the affected ear?

D. Elicit for otorrhea (ear drainage), with or without foul odor.

E. Review and inquire regarding risk factors.

F. Identify the client's history of OM.

G. Inquire if the client has flown recently.

Physical Examination

A. Check temperature, pulse, respirations, and blood pressure.

B. Inspect:
1. Observe the canal and auricle for redness, deformity, otorrhea, or foreign body.
2. Inspect the TM position to determine whether landmarks are visible and whether the TM is retracted, bulging, erythematous, or noted with MEE.
3. Observe ears for decreased or absent TM mobility.
4. Inspect nose, mouth, and throat.

C. Auscultate heart and lungs.

Diagnostic Tests

A. Tympanometry is a test that measures how easily the TM vibrates. Type A tympanograms are normal, type B tympanograms indicate MEE, and type C tympanograms indicate TM retraction with or without MEE.

B. A diagnostic audiogram should be done in clients with persistent OM (greater or equal to 3 months' duration), subjective hearing loss, speech delay, or possible cholesteatoma.

C. Consider a complete blood count if the client appears toxic with a high fever.

Differential Diagnoses

A. Red TM secondary to crying (differentiated from AOM by mobility with pneumatic otoscopy)

B. URI

C. Acute mastoiditis and meningitis (rare but serious)

D. Foreign body in the ear

E. Acute otitis externa (AOE)

F. Eustachian tube dysfunction (ETD)

G. Cholesteatoma (saclike structure in the middle ear usually accompanied by chronic foul-smelling otorrhea and progressive hearing loss)

H. Spontaneous TM rupture

Plan

A. General intervention: pain relief with acetaminophen or ibuprofen

B. Client teaching:
1. *See Section III: Client Teaching Guide for this chapter, "Acute Otitis Media."* ◄
2. Educate parents and care providers that children should avoid smoke exposure. Smoke-filled rooms increase the risk of frequent ear infections in children.
3. For young children who use a bottle for feeding, stress the importance of NOT propping bottles at any time for feeding. Propping bottles increases the risk of OM.

C. Pharmaceutical therapy:
1. Intranasal glucocorticoids and intranasal antihistamines (Astelin) used concomitantly are often helpful with improving the underlying ETD, thus resolving the MEE.
2. Oral antihistamines and decongestants are not recommended for routine use for treating OME in children.
3. Oral antibiotics may shorten the duration of symptoms in clients with AOM.
4. The drug of choice is amoxicillin 90 mg/kg/d divided into two daily doses for 10 days, up to a maximum of 3 g/d.
5. For concerns of amoxicillin resistance, treatment failure, recent use of antibiotic in the previous 30 days, and/or concurrent other infections, use an antibiotic with beta-lactamase activity, such as amoxicillin-clavulanate (Augmentin). Other alternatives include cefdinir, cefpodoxime, cefuroxime, and ceftriaxone.
6. For penicillin allergy, alternatives are cefdinir 14 mg/kg/d in one to two doses, maximum dose 600 mg/d; cefpodoxime 10 mg/kg/d, once daily, maximum dose 800 mg/d; *or* cefuroxime suspension, 30 mg/kg/d in two divided doses, maximum dose 1 g/d or capsules, 250 mg every 12 hours.
7. Alternatively, one dose of ceftriaxone 50 mg/kg intramuscularly (IM) may be given. If clinically improved in 48 hours, no further treatment is recommended. If signs/symptoms continue, administer the second dose of ceftriaxone in 48 hours.

8. Other alternatives: macrolides:
   a. Erythromycin plus sulfisoxazole (Pediazole): 50 to 150 mg/kg/d of erythromycin divided into four doses/d for 10 days; maximum dose 2 g erythromycin or 6 g sulfisoxazole/d (**Do not use in children younger than 2 months**)
   b. Azithromycin 10 mg/kg/d, maximum dose 500 mg/d as single dose on day 1, then 5 mg/kg/d, maximum dose of 250 mg/d on days 2 to 5 for 10 days
   c. Clarithromycin 15 mg/kg/d divided into two doses, maximum dose 1 g/d
   d. Trimethoprim with sulfamethoxazole 8 mg/kg/d of trimethoprim (40 mg/kg/d of sulfamethoxazole) divided into two daily doses for 10 days

9. Children younger than 2 years should be treated with antibiotic therapy for 10 days; children older than 2 years without a previous history of OM may be treated for 5 to 7 days: erythromycin with sulfisoxazole 40 mg/kg/d (150 mg/kg/d of sulfisoxazole [Pediazole]) divided into four daily doses for 10 days. **Do not use in children younger than 2 months.**

10. If the client is asymptomatic and AOM is found on examination, consider observation without antibiotics only if child is older than 2 years. Recommend a follow-up examination in 48 hours.

11. Other antibiotics (if first-line antibiotic fails): amoxicillin and clavulanic acid (Augmentin), cefixime (Suprax), azithromycin (Zithromax), and cefprozil (Cefzil)

Follow-Up

A. Check the client with AOM in 2 to 4 weeks or if fever and complaints persist for more than 48 hours if an antibiotic is begun. Documentation of the resolution of the ear infection is valuable information if recurrent infections occur.

B. Recheck the client with OME after 4 to 6 weeks.

Consultation/Referral

A. Refer the client to an otolaryngologist if he or she is less than 6 weeks of age, appears septic, or has mastoiditis.

B. For persistent OM (3 months or longer) and/or documented hearing loss due to MEE, refer to an otolaryngologist for consideration of tympanostomy tube insertion. Also, refer to otolaryngology for suspected speech or learning delay in children with chronic MEE.

C. For complications (abscess, mastoiditis, meningitis, etc.), refer to the EDs for emergent treatment.

Individual Considerations

A. Pregnancy: Do not use sulfa medications (sulfonamides) in pregnant clients.

B. Pediatrics:
   1. Antibiotic therapy should NOT be used to treat OME due to small benefits that are offset by adverse reactions, bacterial resistance, and lack of impact in future ear surgery. Most cases of OME will spontaneously resolve within 3 months. Simply monitor closely. However, OME may become chronic, requiring an otolaryngology consult.
   2. Children of 6 weeks old or younger: Consider a blood culture and lumbar puncture if septicemia is suspected. The client may need intravenous (IV) antibiotics depending on culture results.
   3. Do not use sulfa medications (sulfonamides) in children younger than 2 months.
   4. **The American Academy of Pediatrics does not recommend the use of over-the-counter (OTC) cough and cold medications for children younger than 6 years.** In older children, consider decongestants and/or intranasal steroids for nasal congestion.
   5. Antihistamines are not recommended.

C. Adults:
   1. OME may be present in adults, usually unilaterally, and usually associated with a URI or allergies due to a blocked eustachian tube.
   2. If there is no accompanying URI, a nasopharyngeal mass or adenoid hypertrophy must be ruled out. Otolaryngology consult should be considered for nasopharyngeal endoscopic examination.

Bibliography

American Academy of Otolaryngology Head and Neck Surgery Foundation. (2011). *Primary care otolaryngology* (3rd ed.). Alexandria, VA: Author. Retrieved from https://www.entnet.org/sites/default/files/Oto-Primary-Care-WEB.pdf

Klein, J. O., & Pelton, S. (2015). Acute otitis media in children: Treatment. In M. Edwards & G. Isaacson (Eds.), *UptoDate*. Waltham, MA: Wolters Kluwer. Retrieved from http://www.uptodate.com/contents/acute-otitis-media-in-children-treatment

Klein, J. O., & Pelton, S. (2016). Management of otitis media with effusion (serous otitis media) in children. In S. Kaplan & G. Isaacson (Eds.), *UpToDate*. Waltham, MA: Wolters Kluwer. Retrieved from http://www.uptodate.com/contents/management-of-otitis-media-with-effusion-serous-otitis-media-in-children?source=search_result&search=otitis+meda+with+effusion&selectedTitle=1-48

Lustig, L. R., Limb, C. J., Baden, R., & LaSalvia, M. T. (2015). Chronic otitis media, cholesteatoma, and mastoiditis in adults. In D. Deschler (Ed.), *UpToDate*. Waltham, MA: Wolters Kluwer. Retrieved from http://www.uptodate.com/contents/chronic-otitis-media-choleste-oma-and-mastoiditis-in-adults?source=search_result&search=otitis+media+adult&selectedTitle=2%7E150

Poe, D., & Bassem, M. (2016). Eustachian tube dysfunction. In D. Deschler (Ed.), *UpToDate*. Waltham, MA: Wolters Kluwer. Retrieved from http://www.uptodate.com/contents/eustachian-tube-dysfunction?source=search_result&search=eustachian+tube+dysfunction&selectedTitle=1%7E39

Rosenfeld, R. M., Schwartz, S. R., Cannon, C. R., Roland, P. S., Simon, G. R., Kumar, K. A., . . . Robertson, P. J. (2014). Clinical practice guideline: Acute otitis externa. *Otolaryngology–Head and Neck Surgery, 150*(Suppl. 1), S1–S24. doi:10.1177/0194599813517083

Schilder, A. G. M., Marom, T., Bhutta, M. F., Casselbrant, M. L., Coates, H., Gisselsson-Solén, M., . . . Mandel, E. M. (2017). Panel 7: Otitis media: Treatment and complications. *Otolaryngology–Head and Neck Surgery, 156*(Suppl. 4), S88–S105. doi:10.1177/0194599816633697

Cerumen Impaction (Earwax)

Jill C. Cash and Ken Watford

Definition

A. Cerumen is defined as a mixture of ear secretions and dead epithelial cells which migrates laterally and often mixes with hair. Cerumen occurs naturally in the external auditory canal (EAC) and cleans, lubricates, and protects the EAC. Excessive accumulation of cerumen can cause a partial or complete obstruction of the EAC.

Incidence

A. Cerumen impaction is one of the most common reasons for seeking medical care. Impacted cerumen occurs in one in 10 children, one in 20 adults, and at least one third of geriatric clients. It is also common in developmentally delayed populations.

B. Approximately 12 million office visits per year occur for cerumen extraction in the United States.

Pathogenesis

A. Accumulation of cerumen can be caused by the failure of the self-cleaning mechanism of the EAC. Cilia which have become stiff cannot remove cerumen and dirt from the ear canal. The pushing of cotton swabs, paper clips, bobby pins, and other objects into the EAC may also impact cerumen.

Predisposing Factors

A. Aging
B. Use of hearing aids or earbuds
C. Use of cotton swabs or other objects to clean the EAC

Common Complaints

A. Dryness and itching of EAC
B. Unsteadiness
C. Otalgia
D. Hearing loss
E. Tinnitus

Subjective Data

A. Elicit onset and duration of symptoms.
B. Elicit previous history of cerumen impaction.
C. Question the client regarding the method of cleaning ears.

Physical Examination

A. Check temperature, pulse, respirations, and blood pressure.
B. Inspect:
  1. Observe EACs for occluding cerumen.
  2. Observe the TM if possible. A perforated TM can be associated with OM or use of objects by a client to clean his or her own ears.
  3. Inspect the nose and throat.
C. Auscultate heart and lungs.

Diagnostic Tests

A. None required

Differential Diagnoses

A. Foreign body in the ear canal
B. Otitis externa

Plan

A. General interventions:
  1. If experienced in removal of cerumen impaction and chooses to proceed with cerumenectomy,

the clinician may elect to obtain written informed consent prior to performing this procedure. Remove impaction by means of lavage or curettage. Be sure to inspect the canal and TM after removal of the cerumen. Document the client's hearing before and after removal of cerumen.

  2. If initial management is unsuccessful or for severe cerumen impaction, consider otolaryngology consult for microscopic cerumenectomy.

B. Client teaching:
  1. *See Section III: Client Teaching Guide for this chapter, "Cerumen Impaction (Earwax)."* ◀
  2. Instruct the client to avoid cleaning his or her own ears. Advise not to clean ears with cotton swabs, bobby pins, and so forth. Using these devices pushes the wax further into the ear canal and can worsen symptoms.
  3. Instruct clients to avoid ear candling.

C. Pharmaceutical therapy:
  1. None indicated

Follow-Up

A. No follow-up is needed unless indicated. Recurrence is common.

Consultation/Referral

A. Refer the client to an otolaryngologist when cerumen cannot be safely removed.

Individual Considerations

A. Geriatrics:
  1. Cerumen impaction is very common in the elderly due to atrophic cilia and dry epithelium in the ear canal.
  2. The use of hearing aids and earbuds also can contribute to wax buildup and cause wax to be pushed further into the canal. Persons using hearing aids or earbuds should be evaluated for wax buildup as indicated.

Bibliography

Dinces, E. (2015). Cerumen. In D. Deschler (Ed.), *UpToDate*. Waltham, MA: Wolters Kluwer. Retrieved from https://www.uptodate.com/contents/cerumen?source=machine Learning&search=ear+lavage&selectedTitle=1%7E150&sectionRank=1&anchor=H9#H9

Krouse, H. J., Magit, A. E., O'Connor, S., Schwarz, S. R., & Walsh, S. A. (2017). Plain language summary: Earwax (Cerumen impaction). *Otolaryngology–Head and Neck Surgery, 156*(1), 30–37. doi:10.1177/0194599816680327

Schwartz, S. R., Magit, A. E., Rosenfeld, R. M., Ballachanda, B. B., Hackell, J. M., Krouse, H. J., . . . Cunningham, E. R. (2017). Clinical practice guideline (Update): Earwax (Cerumen impaction). *Otolaryngology–Head and Neck Surgery, 156*(Suppl. 1), S1–S29. doi:10.1177/0194599816671491

Hearing Loss

Jill C. Cash and Ken Watford

Definition

Impaired hearing (complete or partial hearing loss) results from interference with the conduction of sound, its conversion to electrical impulses, or its transmission through the nervous system. It is important to distinguish the type of hearing loss because the treatment options are significantly different based on the type. There are three types of hearing loss:

A. Conductive hearing loss (CHL; defect in the conductive pathway of the ear)
B. Sensorineural hearing loss (SNHL; defect in the inner ear or 8th cranial nerve)
C. Mixed hearing loss (MHL; combined conductive and sensorineural loss)

Incidence

A. Hearing loss is the most prevalent sensory deficit in the United States. Approximately 30 million (12.7%) individuals in the United States have bilateral hearing loss and 48 million (20.3%) have hearing loss in at least one ear.
B. Globally, approximately 360 million individuals experience hearing loss that is considered to be disabling.

Pathogenesis

A. CHL presents with a decrease in hearing volume and/or clarity due to failure of one or more of the conductive components of the external or middle ear. It may be caused by one of the following:
  1. Cerumen impaction
  2. OME
  3. ETD
  4. TM perforation
  5. Cholesteatoma
  6. Otosclerosis: hereditary middle ear disease that involves fixation of the ossicular chain with resulting progressive CHL
  7. Tympanosclerosis: scarring and thickening on the TM after TM injury or surgery
  8. Exostoses of the EAC: bony excrescences of the EAC
  9. Glomus tumors: benign, highly vascular tumors derived from normally occurring glomera of the middle ear and jugular bulb
B. SNHL results from injury to the hair cells in the cochlea and/or the nerves innervating the hair cells. It is usually bilateral and symmetrical. The most common causes are:
  1. Noise-induced hearing loss: due to chronic exposure to loud noises
  2. Presbycusis: age-related damage to the 8th cranial nerve. It is usually bilateral, gradually progressive, and symmetrical.
  3. Genetic factors
  4. Infectious or postinflammatory processes
  5. Drug-induced hearing loss: may be caused by aminoglycoside antibiotics, furosemide, ethacrynic acid, quinidine, and aspirin
  6. Ménière's disease: an inner ear syndrome consisting of fluctuating, unilateral, low-frequency SNHL associated with tinnitus, a sensation of fullness in the ear, and recurring often severe episodes of vertigo lasting at least 20 minutes and up to 12 hours
  7. Acoustic neuroma: benign tumor of the 8th cranial nerve (rare)
  8. Sudden SNHL can derive from head trauma, viral or microvascular events, skull fractures, meningitis, OM, scarlet fever, mumps, congenital syphilis, multiple sclerosis, and perilymph leaks or fistulas. Sudden SNHL can be bilateral or unilateral.

Predisposing Factors

A. Acoustic or physical trauma
B. Ototoxic medications (such as aminoglycosides, aspirin, radiation therapy, and chemotherapy)
C. Recent URI
D. Barotrauma
E. Otosclerosis
F. Nasopharyngeal cancer
G. Cerumen impaction
H. ETD with MEE
I. Foreign body in the EAC
J. Developmental delays

Common Complaints

A. Difficulty understanding words (poor word recognition), especially with background noise present
B. Associated tinnitus
C. Ear pressure and/or otalgia

Subjective Data

A. Elicit the onset, duration, progression, and severity of symptoms. Note whether symptoms are bilateral or unilateral.
B. Obtain the client's history of past or recent trauma
C. Review the client's occupational and recreational exposure to loud noise.
D. Review the client's medical history and medications, including OTC drugs and prescriptions.
E. Review the client's history for recent URI or ear infections, especially for chronic ear infections.
F. Elicit data about any previous hearing loss, how it was treated, and how it affected daily activities. There may be a history of previous ear disease with CHL.
G. Review the client's other symptoms such as dizziness, fullness or pressure in the ears, and noises.
H. Review what causes difficulty with hearing, high tones versus low frequencies. Can the client hear people talking, the television at normal volume, doorbells ringing, telephone ringing, and watch ticking?

Physical Examination

A. Temperature
B. Inspect:
  1. Examine both ears for comparison.
  2. Externally inspect ears for discharge; note color and odor. Check for obstruction of the auditory canal by impacted cerumen, a foreign body, exostoses, AOE, OME, or scarring or perforation of the TM.
  3. Conduct otoscopic examination to observe the EAC for cerumen impaction or foreign body.
  4. Examine TM for color, landmarks, contour, perforation, and AOM. A reddish mass visible through

the intact TM may indicate a high-riding jugular bulb, an aberrant internal carotid artery, or a glomus tumor.
C. Palpate:
1. Palpate auricle and mastoid area for tenderness, swelling, or nodules.
2. Check lymph nodes if infection is suspected.
D. Neurologic testing:
1. Weber test:
a. The Weber test reveals CHL when sound travels toward the poor ear. SNHL is present when sound travels toward the good ear. This screening test is performed by striking a tuning fork and then placing it on the middle of the head. The client is then asked where sound is being heard from—the left ear, the right ear, or equal in both ears. Normal results are reflected by sound being heard equally in both ears.
2. Rinne screen:
a. The Rinne tuning fork test reveals bone conduction greater than air conduction in the affected ear (abnormal). The Rinne test is performed by placing the struck tuning fork against the mastoid bone. Begin counting or timing the interval from the start to when the client can no longer hear. Continue counting or timing the interval to determine the length of time sound is heard by air conduction. Air-conducted sound should be heard twice as long as bone-conducted sound after bone conduction stops.

Diagnostic Tests

A. Audiologic screening in primary setting
B. Air insufflation for TM mobility
C. Diagnostic pure-tone audiometry (hearing test) with tympanometry (used to evaluate the TM and the middle ear status) performed by an audiologist
D. CT of the temporal bones or MRI of the internal auditory canals (IACs) after consultation with an otolaryngologist

Differential Diagnoses

A. Congenital hearing loss
B. Traumatic hearing loss
C. Ototoxicity
D. Presbycusis
E. Ménière's syndrome
F. Acoustic neuroma
G. Cholesteatoma
H. Infection
I. Cerumen impaction
J. Otitis externa
K. Foreign body in the ear
L. Tumors
M. Otosclerosis
N. Perforation of TM
O. Serous OM
P. Hypothyroidism
Q. Paget's disease

Plan

A. General interventions:
1. Treat any primary cause (i.e., remove impacted cerumen, treat ETD, etc.).
2. Inform the client regarding results of screening and indications for further testing.
B. Client teaching:
1. Discuss avoiding loud noises, use of hearing protection, and so forth.
2. Instruct the client not to insert small objects into the ear or to attempt to clean his or her ears.
C. Pharmaceutical therapy: treat primary condition if applicable.

Follow-Up

A. If the primary cause of hearing loss is not identified, refer the client to an otolaryngologist.

Consultation/Referral

A. The client should be referred to an otolaryngologist for an extensive workup when the primary cause cannot be identified. Most types of CHL can be medically or surgically corrected. Both unilateral and bilateral deafness can usually be surgically improved by cochlear implantation.
B. Referral should be made to a hearing aid specialist for hearing evaluation and treatment as indicated (i.e., hearing aids). Both CHL and SNHL can often be improved with hearing aids.

Individual Considerations

A. Pediatrics:
1. Most children are able to respond to a test of gross hearing using a small bell. To determine the client's hearing ability, note if the child stops moving when the bell is rung and if the child turns his or her head toward the sound.
2. When examining children, pull the pinna back and slightly upward to straighten the canal.
B. Adults:
1. The EAC in the adult can best be exposed by pulling the earlobe upward and backward.
C. Geriatrics:
1. Impaired hearing among the elderly is common and can lower the quality of life.
2. Individuals with significantly impaired hearing may become withdrawn or appear confused.
3. Hearing loss can be a contributing cause of depression in the older population.
4. Impacted cerumen is common in the elderly.

Bibliography

American Academy of Otolaryngology – Head and Neck Surgery Foundation. (2011). *Primary care otolaryngology* (3rd ed.). Retrieved from https://www.entnet.org/sites/default/files/Oto-Primary-Care-WEB.pdf

Bhattacharyya, N., & Meyers, A. D. (2015). Auditory brainstem response auditometry. *Medscape*. Retrieved from https://emedicine.medscape.com/article/836277-overview

Centers for Disease Control and Prevention, National Institute for Occupational Safety and Health. (2013). *Noise and hearing loss prevention*. DHHS (NIOSH) Pub. No. 2001-103. Retrieved from www.cdc.gov

Curhan, G., & Curhan, S. (2016). Epidemiology of hearing impairment. In G. Popelka, B. Moore, R. Fay, & A. Popper (Eds.), *Hearing Aids. Springer Handbook of Auditory Research* (vol. 56). Cham, Switzerland: Springer.

Mener, D. J., Betz, J., Genther, D. J., Chen, D., & Lin, F. R. (2013). Hearing loss and depression in older adults. *Journal of the American Geriatrics Society*, 61(9), 1627–1629. doi:10.1111/jgs.12429

National Institutes of Health, National Institute on Deafness and Other Communication Disorders. (2016, March). *NIDCD fact sheet: Hearing and balance: Hearing loss and older adults* (NIH Pub. No. 01-4913). Washington, DC: U.S. Department of Health and Human Services. Retrieved from https://www.nidcd.nih.gov/sites/default/files/Documents/health/hearing/HearingLossOlderAdults.pdf

National Institutes of Health, National Institute on Deafness and Other Communication Disorders. (2015a). *NIDCD fact sheet: Hearing and balance: Pendred syndrome* (NIH Publication No. 06-5875). Washington, DC: U.S. Department of Health and Human Services. Retrieved from https://www.nidcd.nih.gov/health/pendred-syndrome

National Institutes of Health, National Institute on Deafness and Other Communication Disorders. (2015b). Quick statistics about hearing. Retrieved from https://www.nidcd.nih.gov/health/statistics/quick-statistics-hearing

Roland, P. S. (2015). Presbycusis. *Medscape*. Retrieved from https://reference.medscape.com/article/855989-overview

Schubert, C. R., Paulsen, A. J., Nondahl, D. M., Dalton, D. S., Fischer, M. E., Klein, B. E. K., . . . Cruickshanks, K. J. (2018). Association between Cystatin C and 20-year cumulative incidence of hearing impairment in the epidemiology of hearing loss study. *JAMA Otolaryngol Head Neck Surgery*, 144(6), 469–474. doi:10.1001/jamaoto.2018.0041

Otitis Externa

Jill C. Cash and Ken Watford

Definition
A. Otitis externa is the generalized inflammation of the EAC with or without involvement of the TM and/or pinna.

Incidence
A. Otitis externa is seen in clients of all ages. Incidence is higher during summer months. All varieties (with exception of necrotizing otitis externa) are common. It is one of the most common infections treated by the clinician.

Pathogenesis
A. AOE or swimmer's ear: AOE is characterized by rapid onset (1–2 days) of symptoms including otalgia (often severe), EAC swelling, possible otorrhea, and/or cellulitis of the pinna and adjacent skin. It is uncommon before age 2 years. *Pseudomonas* is the most common bacterial infection (67%), followed by *Staphylococcus* and *Streptococcus*. Infection can also be fungal (*Aspergillus*, 90%). Bacterial or fungal invasion is usually preceded by trauma to the ear canal, aggressive cleaning of the natural bactericidal cerumen, or frequent submersion in water (swimming).
B. Chronic otitis externa: generally results from a persistent, low-grade infection and inflammation with *Pseudomonas*
C. Eczematous otitis externa: otitis externa associated with primary coexistent skin disorder such as atopic dermatitis, seborrheic dermatitis, and psoriasis
D. Necrotizing or malignant otitis externa: Invasive *Pseudomonas* infection results in skull base osteomyelitis. It is most commonly seen in the immunocompromised or diabetic geriatric client.

Predisposing Factors
A. Ear trauma from scratching with a foreign object or fingernail, overly vigorous cleaning of cerumen from canal
B. Cerumen impaction
C. Frequent swimming
D. Use of a hearing aid
E. Eczema (eczematous otitis externa)
F. Debilitating disease (necrotizing otitis externa)
G. Humid climates

Common Complaints
A. Otalgia
B. Itching
C. Erythematous and swollen external canal
D. Purulent discharge
E. Hearing loss from edema and obstruction of canal with drainage

Other Signs and Symptoms
A. Plugged ear sensation (aural fullness)
B. Tenderness to palpation (tragus)

Subjective Data
A. Elicit the onset, duration, and intensity of ear discomfort.
B. Inquire into the client's history of previous ear infections.
C. Determine whether the client notes any degree of hearing loss.
D. Question the client about recent exposure to immersion in water (swimming).
E. Question the client as to ear canal cleaning practices and any recent trauma to the canal.

Physical Examination
A. Temperature
B. Inspect:
   1. Carefully examine the ear with an otoscope for extreme tenderness.
   2. Observe the ear for erythematous and edematous EAC; look for otorrhea and debris.
   3. Attempt to visualize the TM, which may appear normal.
   4. Inspect nose and throat.
C. Auscultate heart and lungs.
D. Palpate:
   1. Apply gentle pressure to tragus and manipulate pinna to assess for tenderness.
   2. Palpate cervical lymph nodes.

Diagnostic Tests
A. For persistent or chronic AOE, consider obtaining an otorrhea specimen for culture and sensitivity (C&S) testing and potassium hydroxide (KOH) prep testing.

Differential Diagnoses
A. OM
B. Foreign body
C. Mastoiditis
D. Hearing loss

E. Wisdom tooth eruption

F. Herpes zoster oticus (vesicular eruptions in the ear canal are associated with herpetic otitis externa)

G. Necrotizing or malignant otitis externa (life-threatening condition that occurs in diabetic or immunocompromised clients). Cranial nerve palsies (of the 7th, 9th, and 12th cranial nerves) and periostitis of the skull base have been associated with necrotizing otitis externa.

Plan

A. General interventions:

1. When the client's ear canal is sufficiently blocked by edema or drainage, preventing passage of ear drops, gently insert a cotton ear wick (approximately 1 inch long for adults) to allow passage of drops.

2. Insert the wick by gently rotating it while inserting it into the ear. The client then places ear drops on the wick. The drops are absorbed through the wick, which allows medicine to reach the entire EAC.

B. Client teaching:

1. *See Section III: Client Teaching Guide for this chapter, "Otitis Externa."*

2. The client should be instructed on dry ear precautions until the infection has resolved (usually 7–10 days). The client should not swim until symptoms are completely resolved and the wick is removed.

3. Bathing or showering is permitted with a cotton ball coated with petroleum jelly inserted into the ear to block water passage into the ear canal.

C. Pharmaceutical therapy:

1. For early, mild cases associated with swimming in which the primary symptom is pruritus, acetic acid/aluminum acetate (Domeboro) can be used to create an unsatisfactory environment for *Pseudomonas* growth.

2. Moderate to severe infection: Use of ototopical antibiotics and ototopical glucocorticoid therapy (Cipro Dex) is suggested. Other alternatives include ciprofloxacin (Cipro HC) and ofloxacin (Floxin). Potentially ototoxic ototopical aminoglycosides (Neomycin and Polymyxin) should be avoided if the integrity of the TM is in question.

   a. If fungal infection is suspected, clotrimazole and betamethasone dipropionate lotion (Lotrisone) can also be used for fungal infection if the TM is intact. Apply two drops in the affected ear twice daily for 10 days.

   b. Nystatin 100,000 units/mL or clotrimazole topical solutions may be used for candidal or yeast infections.

3. In general, oral antibiotics are not effective in treating AOE and should not be prescribed. However, for the poorly controlled diabetic client, the immunocompromised client, or for severe infections, additional management with oral antibiotics or oral antifungals may be indicated.

   a. Ciprofloxacin for pseudomonal infections; dicloxacillin or cephalexin for staphylococcal infections

   b. Itraconazole (Sporanox) for treatment of otomycosis (fungal otitis externa)

4. For analgesia, use acetaminophen or ibuprofen. Short-term use of opiates may be necessary when acetaminophen and ibuprofen fail to control pain.

Follow-Up

A. Usual follow-up is within 3 to 5 days to assess improvement. Recheck in 1 to 2 weeks.

B. If an ear wick is inserted, the wick should be removed within 3 to 5 days, once the swelling is reduced. It is common for the wick to spontaneously fall out as the swelling improves. Upon reduction of swelling, ototopical drops can then be directly instilled into the canal, without the need to insert a new wick.

Consultation/Referral

A. Parenteral antibiotics are required for necrotizing otitis externa. Clients with this condition should be immediately referred to an otolaryngologist or ED.

B. Consult or refer the client to an otolaryngologist or ED if osteomyelitis is suspected.

C. For complications (abscess, mastoiditis, meningitis, etc.), refer to the ED for emergent treatment.

Individual Considerations

A. Geriatrics:

1. Persistent otitis externa in the geriatric client (especially those who are immunocompromised or diabetic) may evolve into osteomyelitis of the skull base.

2. The external ear is painful and edematous, and a foul, green discharge is usually present.

3. Treatment may require parenteral gentamicin with a beta-lactam agent. Surgery may be necessary.

4. Oral fluoroquinolones may be useful if infection has not progressed to osteomyelitis.

Bibliography

Rosenfeld, R. M., Schwartz, S. R., Cannon, C. R., Roland, P. S., Simon, G. R., Kumar, K. A., … Robertson, P. J. (2014). Clinical practice guideline: Acute otitis externa. *Otolaryngology–Head and Neck Surgery, 150*(1, Suppl.), S1–S24. doi:10.1177/0194599813517083

Tinnitus

Jill C. Cash and Ken Watford

Definition

A. Tinnitus is the perception of sound heard in the ear and/or head with no external source. It may be described by the client as unilateral, bilateral, or centralized.

Incidence

A. Tinnitus is a very common medical problem that affects an estimated 8% to 25.3% of the population in the United States.

Pathogenesis

A. Tinnitus is poorly understood and there is wide disagreement on the pathophysiology. It is best described as a nonspecific manifestation of pathology of the inner ear, 8th cranial nerve, and/or the central auditory mechanism. There is a strong association between tinnitus, stress, anxiety, and depression.

Predisposing Factors
A. Cerumen impaction
B. Anxiety, depression, or "high stress" (common)
C. TM perforation
D. MEE
E. ETD
F. Acoustic trauma
G. Ototoxic drugs
H. Vascular aneurysm
I. Jugular bulb anomaly. Compression of the ipsilateral jugular vein abolishes the objective tinnitus of a jugular megabulb anomaly.
J. Anemia
K. Temporomandibular joint syndrome
L. Hypertension

Common Complaints
A. Ringing
B. Roaring
C. Buzzing
D. Clicking
E. Hissing
F. Hearing loss
G. Pulsing

Other Signs and Symptoms
A. "Muffled" hearing or ear pressure
B. Change in own voice quality

Subjective Data
A. Review the onset, duration, course, and type of symptoms; note whether the tinnitus is unilateral bilateral, or centralized.
B. Determine the frequency and quality of sound; is the ringing constant, intermittent, or pulsing?
C. Review all medications, including OTC drugs and prescriptions.
D. Determine whether the client has experienced trauma (domestic violence, motor vehicle accident, and so forth).
E. Rule out a recent sinus, oral, or ear infection.
F. Review any previous occurrences.
G. Review work, hobbies, and music habits for noise levels (potential noise-induced SNHL).
H. Assess the date of last hearing examination and determine whether there was any known hearing loss.
I. Review whether the client uses cotton-tipped swabs or other small objects for ear cleaning.
J. Inquire about current stressors the client is experiencing. Is there an active history of depression, anxiety, fatigue, chronic pain, high stress (emotional and physical), worrying, and so on?

Physical Examination
A. Take temperature if infectious cause is suspected.
B. Inspect:
   1. Observe the external ear for discharge; note color and odor.
   2. Conduct otoscopic examination of the auditory canal for cerumen impaction or foreign body.
   3. Inspect TM for color, landmarks, contour, perforation, and AOM.
C. Auscultate:
   1. The skull should be auscultated for a bruit if the origin of the problem remains obscure.
D. Palpate:
   1. Palpate auricle and mastoid area for tenderness, swelling, or nodules.
   2. Check lymph nodes if infection is suspected.
E. Neurologic examination:
   1. The 8th cranial nerve is tested by evaluating hearing.
   2. First evaluate how the client responds to your questions.
   3. Clients who speak in a monotone or with erratic volume may have hearing loss.
   4. Check the client's response to a soft whisper (should respond at least 50% of the time).
   5. Perform the Rinne test.
   6. Perform the Weber test.

Diagnostic Tests
A. Hearing screening is performed in the primary care setting; other more precise audiological testing is performed by an audiologist and/or otolaryngologist.
B. CT scan or MRI after consultation with an otolaryngologist

Differential Diagnoses
A. Cerumen impaction
B. Foreign body in the ear
C. AOM
D. AOE
E. Acoustic traumas
F. Vascular aneurysm
G. Temporomandibular joint syndrome
H. Otosclerosis
I. Ototoxicity
J. Ménière's disease
K. Presbycusis
L. Central nervous system lesion
M. Depression and anxiety

Plan
A. General interventions:
   1. Stress the importance of not placing small objects in the ear and using cotton-tipped applicators to clean external ear only.
   2. Suggest to the client that keeping a radio or sound machine on for background noise often facilitates sleep or work.
   3. Address underlying conditions if present (depression, anxiety insomnia, hearing loss, drug toxicity, etc.).
   4. Consider behavioral therapy, such as biofeedback, mindfulness meditation, or cognitive behavioral therapy, to teach client coping strategies and to treat underlying emotional issues.
   5. Encourage reduction in dietary caffeine, sodium, alcohol, and nicotine, as these substances may exacerbate tinnitus.

B. Client teaching:
1. Educate the client regarding techniques/therapies to improve symptoms of tinnitus.
2. Encourage the client to attend therapy sessions and/or support groups as indicated.
C. Pharmaceutical therapy:
1. No medication "cures" tinnitus.
2. Low-dosage benzodiazepines and insomnia medications may be beneficial for short-term relief of debilitating tinnitus. These medications are generally not advised for long-term management of tinnitus. The client's risk of drug dependency should be carefully evaluated prior to prescribing these medications.

Follow-Up

A. No specific follow-up is required for tinnitus unless a treatable problem is identified.

Consultation/Referral

A. Consult with an otolaryngologist in most cases of tinnitus.

B. Referral of an anxious client to the otolaryngologist may be necessary to satisfy the client that everything has been explored and that there is no serious or correctable underlying condition.
C. Any client with a history of head trauma should be referred to an otolaryngologist because in rare cases tinnitus may be associated with an acoustic neuroma, arteriovenous fistula, or an aneurysm of the intrapetrous portion of the internal carotid artery.

Bibliography

Bhatt, J. M., Bhattacharyya, N., & Harrison, W. L. (2017). Relationship between tinnitus and the prevalence of anxiety and depression. *Laryngoscope, 127*(2), 466–469. doi:10.1002/lary.26107

Kallogjeri, D., Piccirillo, J. F., Spitznagel, E., Hale, S., Nicklaus, J. E., Hardin, F. M., . . . Schlaggar, B. L. (2017). Cognitive training for adults with bothersome tinnitus: A randomized clinical trial. *JAMA Otolaryngology–Head and Neck Surgery, 143*(5), 443–451. doi:10.1001/jamaoto.2016.3779

Tunkel, D. E., Bauer, C. A., Sun, G. H., Rosenfeld R. M., Chandrasekhar, S. S., Cunningham, E. R., . . . Whamond, E. J. (2014). Clinical guidelines: Tinnitus. *Otolaryngology Head Neck Surgery, 151*(Suppl. 2), S1–40. doi:10.1177/0194599814545325

7 Nasal Guidelines

Allergic Rhinitis

Jill C. Cash, Moya Cook, and Sarah Hendershott Taylor

Definition
A. Allergic rhinitis is a chronic or recurring condition characterized by nasal congestion; rhinorrhea; sneezing; pruritus of the nose, palate, and eyes; and watering and redness of the eyes. It can occur seasonally after exposure to allergens, such as tree pollen, grass pollen, and weed pollen. It can also occur perennially related to inhalants, such as dust mites, molds, and pet dander. These classifications can occur distinctly, or clients can have combined seasonal and perennial allergic rhinitis.

Incidence
A. Prevalence varies according to geographic region, affecting 10% to 30% of adults and 40% of children in the United States. Allergic rhinitis accounts for six million missed work days and two million missed school days per year.

Pathogenesis
A. Allergic rhinitis is an immunoglobulin E (IgE)–mediated inflammation of the naso-ocular mucosa. Repeated exposure to aeroallergens leads to allergic sensitization. In subsequent exposure to the aeroallergen, IgE antibodies bind to mast cells in the respiratory epithelium and histamine is released. This results in immediate naso-ocular inflammation leading to congestion, rhinorrhea, sneezing, and pruritus.

Predisposing Factors
A. Genetic predisposition to allergy
B. Exposure to allergic stimuli: pollen, mold, pet dander, dust mites, and indoor inhalants
C. Maternal smoking exposure

Common Complaints
A. Nasal congestion
B. Sneezing
C. Clear rhinorrhea
D. Cough from postnasal drip
E. Pruritis of the nose, eyes, oral mucosa, or face
F. Watering and redness of eyes

Other Signs and Symptoms
A. Dry mouth from mouth breathing
B. Snoring
C. Eczema
D. Hyposmia
E. Shortness of breath, difficulty breathing, and wheezing
F. Headache
G. Halitosis
H. Fatigue

Subjective Data
A. Onset, pattern, and duration of symptoms
B. Characteristics of nasal discharge
C. Exposure to people with similar symptoms or family history of similar symptoms
D. Seasonal impact on symptoms
E. Inquire about other diseases caused by allergens, such as asthma, eczema, and urticaria.
F. Rule out pregnancy.
G. Ask about systemic medications that can induce nasal symptoms (e.g., contraceptives, antihypertensives, erectile dysfunction drugs, and psychiatric drugs).
H. Exposure to irritants
I. Prior nasal trauma

Physical Examination
A. Vitals: make sure to include temperature, as fever would indicate alternate etiology for client symptoms.
B. Inspect:
  1. Examine face:
    a. Note Dennie–Morgan lines (skin folds below lower eyelids), allergic crease (transverse crease on nose from chronic rubbing of nose), and allergic shiners (infraorbital edema and darkening from subcutaneous vasodilation).
  2. Examine eyes:
    a. Conjunctival injection, excess lacrimation, and discharge
  3. Examine ears, nose, and throat:
    a. Ears—red, dull, bulging, perforated tympanic membrane is seen with otitis media.
    b. Nose—look for enlarged and pale (boggy) inferior turbinates, rhinorrhea, septal deviation,

septal perforation, and polyps. Mucosa will appear as pale (blue) and boggy with clear discharge in chronic allergy. Nasal redness, inflammation, enlarged turbinates, and thick/discolored drainage is seen with upper respiratory infection (URI).

  c. Throat—cobblestone appearance ("cobblestoning") in posterior pharynx is seen in chronic allergies. Look for tonsillar hypertrophy and post-nasal drip.

C. Palpate:
  1. Frontal and maxillary sinuses for tenderness
  2. Head and neck for enlarged lymph nodes
D. Percuss:
  1. Frontal and maxillary sinuses for tenderness
  2. Chest for consolidation
E. Auscultate:
  1. Heart and lungs

Diagnostic Tests

A. **Diagnosis may be made from history and physical**
B. Best test: skin prick-puncture method to detect allergen sensitization
C. Serum tests for allergen-specific IgE antibodies (i.e., IgE immunoassay)

Differential Diagnoses

A. Rhinitis caused by systemic medications
B. Rhinitis caused by nasal decongestant or cocaine abuse ("rhinitis medicamentosa")
C. Rhinitis of pregnancy
D. Rhinosinusitis
E. Work related (irritant, corrosive)
F. URI

Treatment

A. General interventions:
  1. Most effective: allergy avoidance
  2. Implement changes in work and home environment to reduce contact with allergens, such as removing upholstery and carpets to reduce reservoirs of dust mites.
▶ B. Client teaching: *See Section III: Client Teaching Guide for this chapter, "Allergic Rhinitis."*
C. Pharmaceutical therapy:
  1. Topical therapy:
    a. Topical corticosteroids offer 70% improvement in 75% of clients with allergic rhinitis; they are single most-effective maintenance therapy for allergy rhinitis.
      i. Fluticasone propionate (Flonase), 50 mcg/spray:
        ▪ not recommended for children under 4 years
        ▪ children 4 to 11 years, one spray each nare daily
        ▪ 12 years to adult, two sprays each nare daily
      ii. Mometasone (Nasonex), 50 mcg/spray:
        ▪ not recommended for children under 2 years

      ▪ children 2 to 11 years, one spray each nare daily
      ▪ 12 years to adult, two sprays each nare daily
    iii. Beclomethasone (Beconase) 42 mcg/spray or (Qnasl) 80 mcg/spray:
      ▪ not recommended for children under 6 years
      ▪ children 6 to 11 years, one to two spray BID with 42 mcg product
      ▪ 12 years to adult, two sprays each nare daily with 80 mcg product
    iv. Budesonide (Rhinocort), 32 mcg/spray:
      ▪ not recommended for children under 6 years
      ▪ children 6 to 11 years, one spray each nare BID
      ▪ 12 years to adult, two sprays each nare daily
    v. Triamcinolone (Nasacort), 55 mcg/spray:
      ▪ not recommended for children under 2 years
      ▪ children 2 to 5 years, one spray each nare daily
      ▪ 6 years to adult, two sprays each nare daily
    vi. Flonase furoate (Veramyst), 50 mcg/spray:
      ▪ not recommended for children under 4 years
      ▪ children 4 to 11 years, one spray each nare daily
      ▪ 12 years to adult, two sprays each nare daily
  b. Topical antihistamine:
    i. Azelastine hydrochloride (Astelin), 137 mcg/spray:
      ▪ not recommended for children under 5 years
      ▪ 6 years to adult, can be administered as needed, one to two sprays each nare, one to two times daily
    ii. Olopatadine, 665 mcg/spray:
      ▪ not recommended for children under 12 years
      ▪ 12 years to adult, may be administered PRN, two sprays each nare, one to two times daily
  c. Other agents:
    i. Nasal saline:
      ▪ nasal spray or irrigations to lavage irritants from the mucosa
      ▪ saline gel can help lubricate nasal mucosa to help prevent dryness
    ii. Ipratropium bromide (Atrovent nasal), 21 mcg/spray:
      ▪ useful for decreasing rhinorrhea
      ▪ 6 years to adult, two sprays each nare, two to three times daily

iii. Oxymetazoline (Afrin), 0.05% spray:
- decongestant NOT recommended as monotherapy in chronic treatment, but can help with severe nasal congestion
- 6 years to adult, one to two sprays each nare, one to two times daily
- MUST NOT USE LONGER THAN 3 DAYS DUE TO REBOUND CONGESTION

iv. Phenylephrine (Neo-Synephrine), 1% spray or drops:
- decongestant NOT recommended as monotherapy in chronic treatment, but can help with severe nasal congestion
- 12 years to adult, one to two spray/drop each nare q4h up to 3 days
- MUST NOT USE LONGER THAN 3 DAYS DUE TO REBOUND CONGESTION

2. Oral therapy:
a. Antihistamines (H_1 receptor antagonists) are drugs of choice. Several may need to be tried before an effective one is found. Drugs may also need to be switched occasionally to prevent tolerance.
  i. Cetirizine (Zyrtec):
  - 6 months to 2 years, 2.5 mg daily
  - children 2 to 5 years, 5 mg daily
  - 6 years to adult, 10 mg daily
  ii. Levocetirizine (Xyzal):
  - children 6 to 11 years, 2.5 mg daily
  - 12 years to adult, 5 mg daily
  iii. Loratadine (Claritin):
  - children 2 to 5 years, 5 mg daily
  - 6 years to adult, 10 mg daily
  iv. Fexofenadine (Allegra):
  - 6 months to 2 years, 15 mg BID
  - children 2 to 11 years, 30 mg BID
  - 12 years to adult, 180 mg daily

Follow-Up

A. Client should return for follow-up visit in 4 to 6 weeks, earlier if symptoms worsen after 3 days of treatment.

Consultation/Referral

A. Refer the client to an allergist if symptoms continue and interfere with daily activities.
B. Allergist may prescribe immunotherapy following identification of offending allergens.

Individual Considerations

A. Pregnancy:
1. Skin testing should be deferred until after delivery.
2. Implement nonpharmacologic therapy first.
3. Cromolyn sodium nasal spray is first line for mild allergic rhinitis during pregnancy/breastfeeding.

4. Budesonide (Rhinocort) is the only pregnancy category B nasal corticosteroid.
5. Immunotherapy should not be initiated during pregnancy, but can be continued at regular dose during pregnancy.

Bibliography

Bunyavanich, S. (2015). Allergic rhinitis. In H. Sampson (Ed.), *Mount Sinai expert guides. Allergy and clinical immunology* (pp. 36–43). Chichester, England: Wiley.

Corren, J. (2017). Allergic rhinitis and conjunctivitis. In R. O'Hehir, S. Holgate, & A. Sheikh (Eds.), *Middleton's allergy essentials* (pp. 205–224). Edinburgh, Scotland: Elsevier.

deShazo, R., & Kemp, S. (2016). Pharmacotherapy of allergic rhinitis. In J. Corren (Ed.), *UpToDate*. Waltham, MA: Wolters Kluwer. Retrieved from http://www.uptodate.com/contents/pharmacotherapy-of-allergic-rhinitis?source=search_result&search=Pharmacotherapy+of+allergic+rhinitis&selectedTitle=1%7E150

deShazo, R. D., & Kemp, S. F. (2018). Allergic rhinitis: Clinical manifestations, epidemiology, and diagnosis. In J. Corren (Ed.) *UpToDate*. Waltham, MA: Wolters Kluwer. Retrieved from https://www-uptodate-com.ckmproxy.vumc.org/contents/allergic-rhinitis-clinical-manifestations-epidemiology-and-diagnosis?search=allergic%20rhinitis&source=search_result&selectedTitle=2-150&usage_type=default&display_rank=2

Lambert, E. M., & Friedman, E. M. (2016). Epistaxis. In J. Teruya (Ed.), *Management of bleeding patients* (pp. 185–190). Cham, Switzerland: Springer.

Pepper, A. N., & Ledford, D. K. (2016). Allergic rhinitis: Diagnosis and treatment. In M. Mahmoudi, T. Craig, & D. K. Ledford (Eds.), *Allergy and asthma* (pp. 63–85). Cham, Switzerland: Springer.

Epistaxis

Jill C. Cash, Moya Cook, and Sarah Hendershott Taylor

Definition

A. Epistaxis is a nosebleed or hemorrhage from the nose. It may be classified as anterior or posterior, depending on the source of bleeding. Up to 90% of nosebleeds are anterior and can often be managed definitely in the primary care setting.

Incidence

A. Epistaxis occurs in up to 60% of the general population; only 10% seek medical attention.

Pathogenesis

A. Epistaxis is caused by disruption of the nasal mucosa. Up to 90% of nosebleeds occur within the vascular area of the anterior nasal septum at the site of anastomosis of three primary vessels (known as Kisselbach's plexus). Anterior epistaxis is mostly self-limited or definitely managed in the primary care setting. Posterior bleeds arise most commonly from the sphenopalatine artery and result in significant hemorrhage. Posterior nosebleeds prompt referral to ED for care by otolaryngologist and possible nasal packing, cautery, and/or hospital admission.

Predisposing Factors

A. Local trauma, usually from nose picking (digital trauma) or vigorous nose blowing
B. Acute inflammation, often from URI, acute sinusitis, allergic rhinitis, or common cold

C. Low moisture causing nasal dryness and irritation
D. Chronic use of nasal corticosteroid spray
E. Inhalation of chemical irritants
F. Presence of foreign body
G. Trauma
H. Cocaine use
I. Pregnancy
J. Neoplasm
K. Systemic causes:
   1. Bleeding disorders (most common)
   2. Hypertension
   3. Anticoagulation

Common Complaints

A. Common complaint is unusually severe or recurrent nosebleeds.

Other Signs and Symptoms

A. Anterior epistaxis:
   1. Unilateral
   2. Continuous, mild/moderate bleeding from nasal septum
B. Posterior epistaxis:
   1. Brisk (arterial) hemorrhage
   2. Blood flowing into pharynx (indicates a more serious problem)

Subjective Data

A. Onset (trigger versus spontaneous), frequency, and duration of bleeding
B. Use of oral anticoagulants, aspirin, or aspirin-containing products (e.g., Pepto-Bismol, aspirin, Excedrin)
C. Recent or current URI, acute sinusitis, and so on
D. Family history of abnormal bleeding, bleeding disorders (such as hemophilia or von Willebrand disease)
E. Recent surgery or trauma
F. Rule out pregnancy.
G. Ask about possible foreign body in the nose.
H. Ask about cocaine use or occupational exposure to irritants or chemicals.
I. If the client has a history of nosebleeds, how did the client treat previous nosebleeds? Has prior cautery or nasal packing been performed?
J. Has the client ever been evaluated for a blood clotting abnormality, such as thrombocytopenia or platelet dysfunction?
K. Does the client complain of bruising easily, melena, or heavy menstrual periods?

Physical Examination

A. Vitals: temperature, blood pressure (check for orthostatic hypertension), pulse, and respirations. Look for signs of airway compromise or hypovolemic shock. If nasal packing is required, take precaution and monitor client closely for vasovagal episode during insertion of nasal packing.
B. Inspect:
   1. Check airway patency with client sitting and leaning forward.
   2. Encourage client to expectorate clots and posterior pharyngeal blood into emesis basin; this will help reduce risk of emesis and aspiration.

   3. Observe skin, mucous membranes, and conjunctiva for rash, pallor, purpura, petechiae, telangiectasias, or ecchymosis.
   4. The nasal cavity should be anesthetized prior to nasal exam with topical lidocaine.
   5. Using nasal speculum, examine nose closely for septal perforation, ulcerations, or erosion. This may indicate cocaine use or can occasionally be associated with certain autoimmune diseases (such as lupus).
   6. Examine nasal discharge. Unilateral bleeding accompanied by purulent discharge indicates a foreign body in the nose. If the discharge is bilateral, sinusitis is also in the differential diagnosis.
   7. After bleeding has stopped:
      a. Inspect nasal mucosa, look closely at nasal vestibule, septum, and turbinates for bleeding source.
      b. Inspect nasal septum for deviation, perforation, and/or crusting.
C. Palpate:
   1. Check for enlarged lymph nodes or masses in the neck to rule out sarcoidosis, tuberculosis, or malignancy.
D. Auscultate heart and lungs

Diagnostic Tests

A. **None are required unless the client has recurrent epistaxis or severe blood loss.**
B. Perform drug screen or pregnancy test, if indicated.
C. Hematocrit and hemoglobin if bleeding is severe
D. Complete blood count (CBC) with differential
E. Platelets, prothrombin time (PT), and partial thromboplastin time (PTT) if bleeding disorder is suspected or if the client is anticoagulated
F. Sinus films if recurrent sinus pain, tenderness, bleeding, or if nasal mass is suspected

Differential Diagnoses

A. Foreign body
B. Septal deviation or perforation
C. Nasal tumors or mass
D. Coagulation disorder (von Willebrand disease)
E. Drug-induced coagulopathy
F. Hypertension
G. Pregnancy

Plan

A. General interventions: Main goal is control of bleeding or reduction of recurrence.
B. Client teaching: *See Section III: Client Teaching Guide for this chapter, "Nosebleeds."* ◄
C. Treatment:
   1. Anterior epistaxis:
      a. Have client sit and lean forward to prevent swallowing of blood.
      b. Initial tamponade:
         i. Soak a cotton pledget in phenylephrine (Neo-Synephrine) or oxymetazoline (Afrin); place this plug into bleeding nostril and hold pressure over nasal alae for 10 to 15 minutes without releasing pressure.

ii. Remove and check for bleeding.

iii. If this fails, chemical cautery may be needed.

c. Cautery:

i. Only do cautery if site of bleeding is visualized.

ii. Warn client that this may be a little painful. Anesthetize mucous membrane by applying cotton soaked with 2% lidocaine, lidocaine with epinephrine, or 4% cocaine.

iii. Apply silver nitrate by applying applicator tip to the site of bleeding for no longer than 10 seconds until a white precipitate forms.

iv. Avoid overzealous cautery, which can lead to ulceration and perforation.

v. Avoid cautery of both sides of the septum, which can lead to tissue necrosis.

vi. If bleeding continues, repeat initial tamponade and cautery, then place a small amount of oxidized regenerated cellulose (Surgicel) against the bleeding artery. **If client continues to have high-flow epistaxis, nasal packing may need to be performed in emergency setting.**

vii. If bleeding stops, give client antibiotic ointment to apply gently with fingertip or cotton swab TID for 3 days.

2. Posterior epistaxis:

a. Have client sit and lean forward to prevent swallowing of blood.

b. As it can be difficult to determine the source of epistaxis, first try to control bleeding with above steps of topical vasoconstrictor and anesthetic then apply pressure.

c. **Consult a physician. The client needs ED care immediately because of rapid blood loss.**

d. Monitor vital signs (blood pressure and pulse); order hematocrit; blood type and crossmatch may be needed.

Follow-Up

A. Anterior epistaxis: as needed

B. Posterior epistaxis: admission to hospital and referral to otolaryngologist is needed.

Consultation/Referral

A. Anterior epistaxis: referral to otolaryngologist is recommended for unsuccessful cessation of hemorrhage or persistent, recurrent epistaxis despite interventions.

B. Posterior epistaxis: refer to a physician and/or otolaryngologist immediately.

Individual Considerations

A. Pregnancy:

1. Nosebleeds are common.

2. Suggest use of saline spray to keep mucous membranes moist throughout the day.

3. Use Vaseline or saline gel applied gently with fingertip or cotton tipped applicator before bed; use humidifier in bedroom.

B. Pediatrics:

1. Commonly occur due to trauma from nose picking or rubbing

2. Advise parents to keep fingernails short.

3. Apply saline gel or spray (avoid Vaseline in children) to rims of nostrils to maintain mucosal moisture.

4. If child is using topical corticosteroid, it should be discontinued.

C. Geriatrics:

1. Monitor elderly clients very closely for airway compromise or hypovolemic shock.

2. Anticoagulated clients are at high risk for nosebleeds.

3. Suggest use of saline spray to keep mucous membranes moist throughout the day.

4. Use Vaseline or saline gel applied gently with fingertip or cotton tipped applicator before bed; use humidifier in bedroom.

Bibliography

Alter, H. (2018). Approach to the adult with epistaxis. In A. B. Wolfson & D. G. Deschler (Eds.), *UpToDate*. Waltham, MA: Wolters Kluwer. Retrieved from https://www-uptodate-com.ckmproxy.vumc .org/contents/approach-to-the-adult-with-epistaxis?search=e pistaxis&source=search_result&selectedTitle=1-150&usage_ type=default&display_rank=1

Messner, A. H. (2018). Management of epistaxis in children. In A. M. Stack & G. C. Isaacson (Eds.), *UpToDate*. Waltham, MA: Wolters Kluwer. Retrieved from https://www-uptodate-com.ckmproxy.vumc.org/ contents/management-of-epistaxis-in-children?search=epistaxis&source =search_result&selectedTitle=2-150&usage_type=default&display_ rank=2

Nonallergic Rhinitis

Jill C. Cash, Moya Cook, and Sarah Hendershott Taylor

Definition

A. Nonallergic rhinitis is rhinitis without an identifiable etiology and without IgE-dependent component. It is characterized by nasal congestion, postnasal drainage, rhinorrhea, and sneezing. It is associated with some degree of autonomic dysregulation. It is classified in various ways: idiopathic, vasomotor, atrophic, geriatric, drug-induced, gustatory, occupational, or rhinitis of pregnancy.

Incidence

A. Nonallergic rhinitis may be responsible for 17% to 52% of all rhinitis cases in adults.

Pathogenesis

A. No single theory of pathogenesis for chronic nonallergic rhinitis has been determined, but it can be divided into noninflammatory and inflammatory. It is a diagnosis of exclusion.

B. Clients exhibit clinical hypersensitivity of nasal mucosa to certain odors and irritants.

C. Atrophic and geriatric rhinitis results from progressive atrophy of nasal mucosa.

D. Overuse of topical nasal decongestants or cocaine and some systemic medications can result in nasal dysfunction.

E. Rhinitis of pregnancy results from hormonal changes; symptoms abate with delivery.

Predisposing Factors

A. Age

B. Abrupt changes in temperature, odors, and emotional stress

C. Other predisposing factors depend on type (e.g., overuse of medications, side effects of systemic medications, and occupational environment).

Common Complaints

A. Nasal congestion

B. Postnasal drainage

C. Rhinorrhea

D. Sneezing

E. Perennial symptoms, often exacerbated by weather conditions

Subjective Data

A. Clinical history is the **most important** tool used to make distinction between allergic and nonallergic rhinitis.

B. Onset, duration, and pattern of symptoms.

C. Inquire about characteristics of nasal discharge, and is it bilateral or unilateral?

D. Ask about potential triggers, including cigarette smoke, strong scents, or fragrances.

E. Ask about exposure to other people with similar symptoms.

F. Inquire about seasonal or weather impact on symptoms, previous treatments, and results.

G. Rule out pregnancy.

H. Ask about use of prescription drugs, over-the-counter (OTC) drugs (Afrin), and illicit drugs (cocaine).

I. Review medical history for other respiratory problems, most importantly asthma.

J. Pediatric consideration: Determine possibility of a foreign object in nostrils.

Physical Examination

A. Vitals: check temperature and blood pressure.

B. Inspect:

  1. Examine general appearance.

  2. Examine eyes:

    a. Inspect conjunctivae for "allergic shiners" (dark circles under eyes), tearing, and eyelid swelling. This would indicate possible allergic rhinitis; nonallergic rhinitis is **not** associated with ocular symptoms.

  3. Examine ears, nose, and throat:

    a. Inspect ears for signs of otitis media (red, bulging, perforated tympanic membrane, and purulent drainage).

    b. Inspect nose for redness, swelling, polyps (soft, pedunculated, nontender, pale, smooth structures), enlarged turbinates, foreign objects,

septal deviation, septal perforation, ischemia, mucosal injury, atrophy, and "cobblestoned" pharyngeal mucosa. Nasal turbinates can appear boggy and edematous in both allergic and nonallergic rhinitis. In nonallergic rhinitis, the mucosa is often more erythematous compared to pale blue in allergic rhinitis. **However, none of these findings are diagnostic, and the mucosa may appear relatively normal in nonallergic rhinitis.**

C. Palpate:

  1. Head and neck

D. Percuss:

  1. Sinuses

E. Auscultate:

  1. Heart and lungs

Diagnostic Test

A. Nonallergic rhinitis is diagnosis of exclusion. Diagnosis is based on characteristic history and physical exam, as well as absence of clinical allergy to aeroallergens.

B. Skin testing for allergies may be done to exclude allergic rhinitis.

Differential Diagnoses

A. Allergic rhinitis

B. URI

C. Foreign body

D. Sinusitis

E. Tumor

F. Deviated septum

G. Nasal polyps

H. Endocrine conditions, such as hypothyroidism and pregnancy

I. Drug use: oral contraceptives, aspirin, alpha-adrenergic blockers, cocaine, and nasal decongestant overuse (rhinitis medicamentosa)

J. Ciliary dysfunction syndrome

K. Cerebral spinal fluid leak

L. Laryngopharyngeal reflux

Plan

A. General interventions:

  1. Identify triggers and address alleviating triggers with avoidance/minimization.

B. Client teaching:

  1. Teach the client the significance of individual triggers for nonallergic rhinitis. Encourage use of a journal to learn personal triggers.

  2. Avoid triggers, such as smoking, smoke-filled rooms, wood-burning stoves/fireplaces, sprays, and perfumes.

  3. Other triggers may include weather changes, hormonal changes, and medications.

  4. Teach methods of treatment and identify treatments that work best for the client.

  5. Encourage use of saline irrigation daily to cleanse nasal and sinus mucosa. Cleansing the mucosa daily will help to remove foreign materials inhaled and will also help with tissue edema. Clean device after each use and allow to air dry.

C. Pharmaceutical therapy:
1. Monotherapy versus combination therapy:
   a. Clients with mild disease may be adequately treated with intranasal corticosteroid or intranasal antihistamine spray. For clients who are more symptomatic, clinical evidence has shown combination therapy to be more effective, with both daily intranasal corticosteroid and antihistamine spray.
   b. Topical corticosteroids:
      i. Fluticasone propionate (Flonase), 50 mcg/spray:
         ▪ not recommended for children under 4 years
         ▪ children 4 to 11 years, one spray each nare daily
         ▪ 12 years to adult, two sprays each nare daily
      ii. Mometasone (Nasonex), 50 mcg/spray:
         ▪ not recommended for children under 2 years
         ▪ children 2 to 11 years, one spray each nare daily
         ▪ 12 years to adult, two sprays each nare daily
      iii. Beclomethasone (Beconase) 42 mcg/spray or (Qnasl) 80 mcg/spray:
         ▪ not recommended for children under 6 years
         ▪ children 6 to 11 years, one to two spray BID with 42 mcg product
         ▪ 12 years to adult, two sprays each nare daily with 80 mcg product
      iv. Budesonide (Rhinocort), 32 mcg/spray:
         ▪ not recommended for children under 6 years
         ▪ children 6 to 11 years, one spray each nare BID
         ▪ 12 years to adult, two sprays each nare daily
      v. Triamcinolone (Nasacort), 55 mcg/spray:
         ▪ not recommended for children under 2 years
         ▪ children 2 to 5 years, one spray each nare daily
         ▪ 6 years to adult, two sprays each nare daily
      vi. Flonase furoate (Veramyst), 50 mcg/spray:
         ▪ not recommended for children under 4 years
         ▪ children 4 to 11 years, one spray each nare daily
         ▪ 12 years to adult, two sprays each nare daily
   c. Topical antihistamine:
      i. Azelastine hydrochloride (Astelin), 137 mcg/spray:
         ▪ not recommended for children under 5 years
         ▪ 6 years to adult, can be administered PRN, one to two sprays each nare, 1 to 2 times daily
      ii. Olopatadine, 665 mcg/spray:
         ▪ not recommended for children under 12 years
         ▪ 12 years to adult, may be administered PRN, two sprays each nare, 1 to 2 times daily
2. If rhinorrhea is the dominant or only symptom (such as in gustatory rhinitis or rhinitis of older adults), recommend anticholinergic nasal spray.
   a. Ipratropium (Atrovent) 0.03% or 0.06%:
      i. Not recommended for children under 6 years
      ii. 6 years to adult, two sprays each nare two to three times daily
3. Oral decongestants:
   a. Oral decongestants can be added to treatment regimen, with dosing of pseudoephedrine 30 or 60 mg PO up to TID on symptomatic days. Do not use in clients with prostatic hyperplasia or hypertension.

Follow-Up
A. Clients receiving chronic therapy for rhinitis should be seen every 3 to 12 months, depending on severity of symptoms.

Consultation/Referral
A. Consult with a physician if symptoms continue despite treatment.
B. If treatment fails, refer the client to the allergist for testing.

Individual Consideration
A. Pregnancy: Reassure pregnant clients that rhinitis is a common hormonal response. Nonallergic rhinitis is not contagious and cannot cross the placenta.

Bibliography
Corn, B. E. (2015). Non-allergic rhinitis. In H. Sampson (Ed.), *Mount Sinai expert guides: Allergy and clinical immunology* (pp. 44–51). Chichester, England: Wiley.

Lieberman, P. L. (2018). Chronic nonallergic rhinitis. In J. Corren (Ed.), *UpToDate.* Waltham, MA: Wolters Kluwer. Retrieved from https://www.uptodate-com.ckmproxy.vumc.org/contents/chronic-nonallergic-rhinitis?search=non%20allergic%20rhinitis&source=search_result&selectedTitle=1-67&usage_type=default&display_rank=1#H8

Sinusitis

Jill C. Cash, Moya Cook, and Sarah Hendershott Taylor

Definition
Sinusitis (often referred to as rhinosinusitis) is the symptomatic inflammation of the mucous membrane lining of one or more paranasal sinuses. It may be acute, subacute, or chronic. Diagnosis is based on subjective and objective findings and depends on duration of symptoms.

A. Acute sinusitis: symptoms lasting up to 4 weeks
B. Subacute sinusitis: symptoms lasting 4 to 12 weeks
C. Chronic sinusitis: symptoms lasting longer than 12 weeks

Incidence

A. Sinusitis is very prevalent, affecting millions of people in the United States each year. It is estimated that 15.2% of the population is affected by sinusitis each year. However, true incidence is unknown because people with sinusitis symptoms often self-medicate with OTC medication.

Pathogenesis

A. Etiology of acute rhinosinusitis involves factors such as environmental, anatomic, and systemic. These factors can occur at the same time and predispose clients not only to acute sinusitis but also to the development of chronic sinusitis.
B. The most common cause of acute sinusitis is viral infection, with 90% to 98% of sinusitis secondary to viral infection. After 10 days, approximately 0.5% of clients will develop acute bacterial rhinosinusitis. The most common bacterial organisms are *Streptococcus pneumoniae*, *Haemophilus influenzae*, and *Moraxella catarrhalis*. If acute sinusitis infections are not resolved or become recurrent, *Staphylococcus aureus* or *Pseudomonas aeruginosa* can become dominant.
C. The transition from viral to bacterial has been studied extensively and it is thought to be secondary to decreased mucociliary clearance and consequent colonization of bacteria on retained mucus secretion from the obstruction of outflow. The sinonasal mucosa inflammation from the triggering agent stuns the cilia and mucus remains trapped in the sinuses, and bacteria proliferate. Anatomical abnormalities can also interfere with normal mucociliary clearance and can prolong illness.
D. Other causes of acute sinusitis are fungi, dental abscess (in 10% of cases), and autoimmune reactions. Fungal sinusitis tends to occur in immunosuppressed clients.

Predisposing Factors

A. Recent URI
B. Allergic rhinitis
C. Cigarette smoke (first or second hand)
D. Air pollutant exposure
E. Sinonasal anatomy (septal deviation, septal spurs, turbinate hypertrophy, Haller cells, adenoidal hypertrophy, or obstructive mass)
F. Ciliary dysfunction (as in Kartagener syndrome and cystic fibrosis)
G. Dental anatomy/abscess
H. Asthma
I. Neoplasms
J. Immunodeficiency (often associated with recurrent acute or chronic sinusitis)
K. Trauma
L. Diving and swimming
M. Flying or rapid changes in altitude

Common Complaints

A. Mucopurulent rhinorrhea
B. Headache and/or facial pain
C. Dental or ear pain
D. Loss of smell (anosmia)
E. Nasal congestion

Other Signs and Symptoms

A. Fever (mostly associated with acute sinusitis)
B. Malaise or fatigue
C. Cough
D. Periorbital edema
E. Halitosis
F. Snoring, mouth breathing
G. Hyponasal speech

Potential Complications to Consider: Immediate Ear, Nose, and Throat Referral

A. Meningitis (symptoms are increased fever, stiff neck)
B. Preseptal or orbital cellulitis
C. Subperiosteal or intracranial abscess
D. Epidural abscess
E. Cavernous sinus thrombosis (acute thrombophlebitis due to infection in the area where veins drain into cavernous sinus)

Subjective Data

A. Onset, duration, and course of symptoms (Have symptoms lasted longer than 10 days, or longer than 12 weeks?)
B. Inquire whether seasons affect symptoms.
C. Ask the client about recent URI and how it was treated:
   1. Did the client receive antibiotics or steroids?
   2. Did the client finish the full course? Any relief from symptoms?
D. Ask about allergies.
E. Inquire about recent dental problems, especially dental abscesses.
F. Find out what home therapies and OTC medications the client tried before the office visit.
G. Ask if the client took a trip recently, especially by airplane.
H. If the client is a child, look for a foreign object up the nose.
I. Inquire whether the client was swimming or diving recently.
J. Review the client's medical history for cystic fibrosis, nasal anatomic abnormalities, asthma, and other respiratory problems.

Physical Examination

A. Vitals: Check temperature, blood pressure, pulse, and respirations.
B. Inspect:
   1. Examine general appearance:
      a. Look for erythema, swelling, or tenderness. Facial cellulitis may be an indication that acute sinusitis has spread outside of the sinuses.
   2. Examine eyes:
      a. Look for periorbital swelling, erythema, epiphora, "allergic shiners," and signs of orbital cellulitis (conjunctival edema, drooping lid, decreased extraocular motion, and vision loss).

b. Thorough ophthalmologic examination with extraocular movements and visual acuity should be performed to rule out subperiosteal or intraorbital abscess.

   3. Examine ears, nose, and throat:

     a. Inspect nose with nasal speculum for erythema, edema, discharge, patency, anatomic abnormalities, polyps, or foreign body.

     b. Inspect oral cavity for evidence of oroantral fistula or dental causes for sinusitis or facial pain.

C. Palpate:

   1. All sinuses for pain and tenderness:

     a. Frontal sinusitis: pain on palpation of forehead

     b. Maxillary sinusitis: the cheeks are tender, or the client may present with jaw and tooth pain

     c. Ethmoid sinusitis: swelling and tenderness in the eyelids and surrounding tissue

   2. Neck for lymphadenopathy

D. Auscultate heart and lungs.

E. Neurologic examination

   1. Evaluate for signs of meningeal irrigation, assessing Brudzinski's sign, Kernig's sign, and nuchal rigidity.

Diagnostic Tests

A. **Diagnosis is usually made through history and physical.**

B. If the disease is refractory to initial treatment or becomes recurrent or chronic, further investigation may be necessary.

   1. Rule out immunodeficiencies (cystic fibrosis, Wegener's granulomatosis, sarcoidosis, Churg–Strauss syndrome).

   2. Skin testing for allergies

   3. Nasal endoscopy to detect abnormalities of the nasal passage (polyps, pus). Culture can be obtained for culture-directed antimicrobial treatment.

   4. Sinus CT is the best imaging method for viewing paranasal sinuses and reveals extent of inflammation and disease. CT is not recommended for routine investigation for acute rhinosinusitis. It is recommended for chronic and recurrent sinusitis, for clients in immunocompromised state, or there is concern for complications (fungal sinusitis, disease extent outside of the sinus cavities, etc.).

Differential Diagnoses

A. Headache (cluster, migraine)

B. Rhinitis (allergic or nonallergic)

C. Nasal polyps

D. Temporomandibular joint disease

E. Trigeminal neuralgia

F. Cerebral spinal fluid rhinorrhea

G. Tumor/neoplasm

H. Autoimmune disease

I. Odontogenic disease

Plan

A. General interventions:

   1. Preventive techniques suggested to avoid getting acute viral sinusitis (hand hygiene, saline irrigations, etc.).

   2. Clients with recurrent sinusitis should be encouraged to keep a log of potential triggers. Avoiding these triggers helps to prevent the onset of acute sinusitis (e.g., avoid smoke, use nasal saline irrigations).

   3. Clients with frequent recurrent sinusitis should have further work up for other causes, such as autoimmune diseases.

B. Client teaching:

   1. Teach client to avoid allergens and irritants, including smoking and secondhand smoke.

   2. Regular use of nasal saline irrigations, especially after exposure to allergens or irritants or with onset of sinusitis symptoms.

   3. Encourage the client to use medications as prescribed. OTC medications, such as pain relievers and decongestants, can be helpful but should be used with caution.

   4. Application of warm, moist compresses to the face several times a day will help with discomfort.

   5. Humidifiers can be helpful, especially in the winter months.

   6. *See Section III: Client Teaching Guide for this chapter, "Sinusitis."* ◄

C. Pharmaceutical therapy:

   1. Acute viral sinusitis

     a. Supportive care, OTC medications (analgesics and decongestants), and saline irrigations.

   2. Acute bacterial sinusitis

     a. Pediatric drugs of choice for acute sinusitis:

       i. First-line treatment: Augmentin 45 mg/kg/d PO in twice-daily dosing for 10 to 14 days.

       ii. Second-line treatment: Augmentin 90 mg/kg/d PO in twice-daily dosing for 10 to 14 days

       iii. Beta-lactam allergy:

         ■ Type I hypersensitivity: Levofloxacin 10 to 20 mg/kg/d PO every 12 or 24 hours for 10 days

         ■ Non–type I hypersensitivity: Cefpodoxime 10 mg/kg/d PO in divided doses every 12 hours *or* Cefdinir 14 mg/kg/d PO in every 12 to 24 hours *or* Levofloxacin 10 to 20 mg/kg in divided doses every 12 to 24 hours

       iv. Risk for antibiotic resistance or failed initial therapy:

         ■ Augmentin 90 mg/kg/d PO twice daily for 10 to 14 days

         ■ Cefpodoxime 10 mg/kg/d PO in divided doses every 12 hours

         ■ Cefdinir 14 mg/kg/d PO divided doses every 12 or 24 hours

         ■ Levofloxacin 10 to 20 mg/kg/d PO divided doses every 12 or 24 hours

         ■ Ceftriaxone 50 mg/kg IM for 1 to 3 days followed by appropriate oral regimen

b. Adult drugs of choice for acute sinusitis. Initial treatment should be 5 to 7 days; if not improving on initial therapy can extend to 10 to 14 days.

    i. First-line treatment: Augmentin 875 mg BID or 500 mg TID

    ii. At risk for pneumococcal resistance or failed initial therapy: Augmentin 2,000 mg BID

    iii. Beta-lactam allergy: Doxycycline 100 mg BID or 200 mg daily

    iv. Respiratory fluoroquinolone can be considered as alternative for penicillin-allergic clients but should be reserved for those who have no alternative treatment options: Levofloxacin 750 mg or 500 mg daily or Moxifloxacin 400 mg daily.

3. The same antibiotics can be used for chronic sinusitis, but treatment should last 3 to 6 weeks.

D. Oral and topical decongestants to correct the underlying edematous mucosa (use cautiously with hypertension)

1. Oxymetazoline (Afrin), 0.05% spray:

a. Decongestant NOT recommended as monotherapy in chronic treatment, but can help with severe nasal congestion

b. 6 years to adult, one to two sprays each nare, one to two times daily

c. MUST NOT USE LONGER THAN 3 DAYS DUE TO REBOUND CONGESTION

2. Phenylephrine (Neo-Synephrine), 1% spray or drops:

a. Decongestant NOT recommended as monotherapy in chronic treatment, but can help with severe nasal congestion

b. 12 years to adult, one to two spray/drop each nare q4h up to 3 days

c. MUST NOT USE LONGER THAN 3 DAYS DUE TO REBOUND CONGESTION

3. Pseudoephedrine 30 or 60 mg PO up to TID for adults

E. Nasal saline:

1. Nasal saline irrigations or spray to nares one to three times daily as needed for hydrating nasal mucosa

F. Nasal corticosteroid sprays may be used to decrease nasal inflammation. Only recommended for children if they have underlying allergic rhinitis.

1. Fluticasone propionate (Flonase), 50 mcg/spray:

a. Not recommended for children under 4 years

b. Children 4 to 11 years, one spray each nare daily

c. 12 years to adult, two sprays each nare daily

2. Mometasone (Nasonex), 50 mcg/spray:

a. Not recommended for children under 2 years

b. Children 2 to 11 years, one spray each nare daily

c. 12 years to adult, two sprays each nare daily

3. Beclomethasone (Beconase) 42 mcg/spray or (Qnasl) 80 mcg/spray:

a. Not recommended for children under 6 years

b. Children 6 to 11 years, one to two spray BID with 42 mcg product

c. 12 years to adult, two sprays each nare daily with 80 mcg product

4. Budesonide (Rhinocort), 32 mcg/spray:

a. Not recommended for children under 6 years

b. Children 6 to 11 years, one spray each nare BID

c. 12 years to adult, two sprays each nare daily

5. Triamcinolone (Nasacort), 55 mcg/spray:

a. Not recommended for children under 2 years

b. Children 2 to 5 years, one spray each nare daily

c. 6 years to adult, two sprays each nare daily

6. Flonase furoate (Veramyst), 50 mcg/spray:

a. Not recommended for children under 4 years

b. Children 4 to 11 years, one spray each nare daily

c. 12 years to adult, two sprays each nare daily

G. Antihistamines are recommended to block histamine production in response to the allergy triggers and prevent allergy symptoms.

1. Cetirizine (Zyrtec):

a. 6 months to 2 years, 2.5 mg daily

b. Children 2 to 5 years, 5 mg daily

c. 6 years to adult, 10 mg daily

2. Levocetirizine (Xyzal):

a. Children 6 to 11 years, 2.5 mg daily

b. 12 years to adult, 5 mg daily

3. Loratadine (Claritin):

a. Children 2 to 5 years, 5 mg daily

b. 6 years to adult, 10 mg daily

4. Fexofenadine (Allegra):

a. 6 months to 2 years, 15 mg BID

b. Children 2 to 11 years, 30 mg BID

c. 12 years to adult, 180 mg daily

Follow-Up

A. Recheck the client in 5 to 7 days after initial therapy; if no improvement consider extending therapy or alternative therapy.

B. Clients not improving may be resistant to antibiotics and may be switched to a different antibiotic for 14 days.

Consultation/Referral

A. Admit clients to the hospital if they have signs and symptoms that the disease has spread intracranially or intraorbitally.

B. Refer clients to an otolaryngologist if they do not improve in 4 weeks or after failed medical therapy.

C. Refer clients to an otolaryngologist for suspected neoplasm, abscess, osteomyelitis, meningitis, or sinus thrombosis.

Individual Considerations

A. Pediatrics:

1. Children with clinical course consistent with acute bacterial rhinosinusitis (purulent drainage, fever, etc., for greater than 7–10 days) should be treated with antimicrobial therapy at time of presentation.

B. Pregnancy:

1. 10% to 30% of pregnant women have worsening rhinitis or sinusitis symptoms due to increase in blood volume and shifts to extravascular space.

2. Antibiotic therapy: Weigh risk and benefit to treat sinusitis during pregnancy. Antimicrobials with category B rating include penicillins, cephalosporins, clindamycin, erythromycin, and azithromycin. Category C antimicrobials include clarithromycin, fluoroquinolones, aminoglycosides, sulfonamides, tetracycline, and vancomycin.

3. Antihistamines: Loratadine and cetirizine are category B.

4. Intranasal steroid: Budesonide is category B.

C. Geriatrics:

1. Chronic sinusitis can affect cognitive functioning in the elderly population.

2. It is important to treat sinusitis in the geriatric population, but considerations need to be made when prescribing antibiotics in the setting of other comorbidities (e.g., renal and hepatic insufficiency).

Bibliography

Cervoni, E., & Leech, K. (Eds.). (2017). Rhinology. In *ENT in primary care* (pp. 39–54). Cham, Switzerland: Springer.

Ho, Y. W., & Govindaraj, S. (2015). Sinusitis. In H. Sampson (Ed.), *Mount Sinai expert guides: Allergy and clinical immunology* (pp. 52–65). Chichester, England: Wiley.

Khasnavis, S. (2018). Sinusitis. In E. Sydney, E. Weinstein, & L. Rucker (Eds.), *Handbook of outpatient medicine* (pp. 215–224). Cham, Switzerland: Springer.

Patel, Z. M., & Hwang, P. H. (2018). Uncomplicated acute sinusitis and rhinosinusitis in adults: Treatment. In T. M. File & D. G. Deschler (Eds.), *UpToDate*. Waltham, MA: Wolters Kluwer. Retrieved from https://www-uptodate-com.ckmproxy.vumc.org/contents/uncomplicated-acute-sinusitis-and-rhinosinusitis-in-adults-treatment?search=sinusitis&sectionRank=1&usage_type=default&anchor=H17857080&source=machineLearning&selectedTitle=1-150&display_rank=1#H17857080

Wald, E. R. (2018). Acute bacterial rhinosinusitis in children: Microbiology and treatment. In S. L. Kaplan, G. C. Isaacson, & R. A. Wood (Eds.), *UpToDate*. Waltham, MA: Wolters Kluwer. Retrieved from https://www-uptodate-com.ckmproxy.vumc.org/contents/acute-bacterial-rhinosinusitis-in-children-microbiology-and-treatment?search=sinusitis&source=search_result&selectedTitle=4-150&usage_type=default&display_rank=4#H3

8 Throat and Mouth Guidelines

Avulsed Tooth

Jill C. Cash, Moya Cook, and Jamie Wiggleton

Definition
A. A tooth that has been completely displaced from its alveolar socket

Incidence
A. Avulsion accounts for 0.5% to 3% of all dental injuries to the permanent teeth. It occurs predominantly in children between ages 7 and 10 years. Multiple studies have shown that this is one of the most serious dental injuries. The upper central incisor is the most frequent tooth that is avulsed.

Pathogenesis
A. Trauma causes a tooth to be completely displaced from its alveolar socket.

Predisposing Factor
A. Erupting teeth are most susceptible to avulsion due to immature periodontal ligaments.

Common Complaints
A. Tooth displaced
B. Pain
C. Bleeding

Subjective Data
A. Ascertain the client's age and note if the avulsed tooth is primary or permanent. Only permanent teeth are considered for reimplantation.
B. Determine the time span for which the tooth has been avulsed (minutes or hours)
C. Ask the client about the underlying cause or trauma. Are there any other injuries that need assessment, such as lacerations or concussion?
D. Did the tooth fall out of the mouth or remain in the mouth?

Physical Examination
A. Check temperature, pulse, respirations, and blood pressure.
B. Inspect:
  1. Observe general appearance:
    a. Check for signs that are secondary to traumatic etiology, such as lacerations, concussion, facial injury, and eye injury.
    b. Keep the client calm. Check to be sure that the client is not in respiratory distress or has not aspirated the tooth.
  2. Inspect gums and avulsed tooth, noting poor dental hygiene. **Do not touch the root surface.**
  3. **If the tooth is not in the mouth, rinse off briefly under cold running water** (<10 seconds)

Diagnostic Tests
A. Dental x-ray should be considered to assess for fracture. Immediate referral to dental specialist for emergency dental evaluation.

Differential Diagnoses
A. Avulsed tooth
B. Luxation injuries: Concussion and subluxation

Plan
A. General interventions:
  1. Refer immediately for emergency dental evaluation and treatment as prognosis is highly dependent on actions taken promptly after the avultion occurs.
  2. Clinician should attempt to reposition the tooth into the socket if there is no concern of the child swallowing the tooth or dropping it. If this is not possible, place the tooth in a glass of milk or another suitable storage medium, such as saline or Hanks balanced storage medium. Avoid storage in water.
B. Client teaching:
  1. If the client or parent is not in a healthcare setting, phone triage should include informing the client not to let the tooth air dry; it may cause permanent destruction of periodontal cells.
  2. Instruct the client to avoid touching the root base, and attempt to insert the tooth in the tooth socket and bite on gauze or a small handkerchief to help hold the tooth in position.

3. If unable to transport inside the tooth socket, as above, advise client to use another medium to transport the tooth, such as milk.

C. Pharmaceutical therapy:

1. Consider administering oral antibiotics prophylactically. Consider tetracycline or doxycycline for adults. Amoxicillin may be used for children.

2. If the tooth had contact with soil, determine tetanus status and administer tetanus booster if necessary.

Follow-Up

A. Follow-up is done with the dentist until stabilization is complete.

Consultation/Referral

A. Immediately refer the client to a dentist or an ED. Teeth replanted within 30 minutes have the best prognosis. Teeth avulsed longer than 2 hours have a poor prognosis.

Individual Consideration

A. Pediatrics: Primary teeth do not need to be replaced.

Bibliography

American Academy of Pediatric Dentistry. (n.d.). Guidelines for the management of traumatic dental injuries: 2. Avulsion of permanent teeth. Retrieved from https://www.aapd.org/globalassets/media/policies_guidelines/e_avulsion.pdf

Doshi, D. (2009). Bet 3. Avulsed tooth brought in milk for replantation. *Emergency Medicine Journal, 26*(10), 736–737.

Dental Abscess

Jill C. Cash, Moya Cook, and Jamie Wiggleton

Definition

A. A dental abscess is a space infection of the gingival or periodontal tissues.

Incidence

A. Incidence is unknown.

Pathogenesis

A. An abscess occurs when bacteria gain access into the gingiva or periodontal tissues. The most common bacteria are *Streptococci viridians*, *Peptostreptococcus*, *Prevotella*, and staphylococci.

Predisposing Factors

A. Poor dental hygiene

B. Dental caries

C. Certain underlying diseases, such as diabetes mellitus, rheumatoid arthritis, and various genetic disorders that impair neutrophil function

Common Complaints

A. Constant, severe jaw pain

B. Swelling

C. Difficulty in chewing with tooth due to pain

Other Signs and Symptoms

A. Fever

B. Warmth, redness

C. Loss of appetite

D. Heat and cold sensitivity

E. Halitosis

Potential Complications

Risk of complications increases with valvular disease.

The following are complications:

A. Extension to potential orofacial space infections (buccal, submental, masticator, and infratemporal fossa) or deep in the head and neck (parapharyngeal space infections)

B. Facial cellulitis

C. Osteomyelitis of the jaw

D. Orocutaneous fistula

E. Sepsis

F. Hematogenous dissemination to native or prosthetic heart valves, joints, or other devices

Subjective Data

A. Elicit information from the client regarding the onset, duration, location, and quality of pain.

B. Note the radiation of pain as well as alleviating or aggravating factors.

C. Note if pain is brought on by contact with hot, cold, or sweet substances; this may indicate periapical abscess or dental caries.

D. Ask if the client has a fever. If so, how high and for how long?

E. Inquire about the history of mitral valve prolapse or rheumatic fever.

Physical Examination

A. Check temperature, pulse, respirations, and blood pressure.

B. Inspect:

1. Inspect teeth for caries, mobility of teeth, or protrusion from sockets, and gum disease.

2. Examine the teeth for erosion, enamel decalcification, diminished tooth size, discoloration, and sensitivity to temperature changes.

C. Palpate neck and submental area for enlarged, tender lymph nodes.

D. Percuss all teeth. Tenderness is diagnostic of an abscess.

E. Auscultate heart, if indicated.

Diagnostic Tests

A. None usually required; however, check white blood cell count (WBC), if cellulitis is suspected.

Differential Diagnoses

A. Periodontal disease

B. Cellulitis

C. Oral cancer

Plan

A. General interventions:

1. Initiate antimicrobial therapy.

2. Refer to the dentist for immediate evaluation and treatment.

B. Client teaching:

1. Advise the client to apply a heating pad to the painful facial area for comfort.

2. Advise a soft diet until pain resolves.

3. Review daily dental care and hygiene with the client.

C. Pharmaceutical therapy:

1. Given increasing resistance due to beta-lactamase production, amoxicillin-clavulanate 875 mg BID for 7 to 14 days (pediatric dosage 25–45 mg/kg/24 hr divided BID, max dosage 1,750 mg/d, using amoxicillin 400 mg/clavulanate 57 mg formulation) is preferred regimen.

2. For penicillin-allergic clients, use clindamycin 450 mg every 8 hours for 7 to 14 days (pediatric dosage 10–30 mg/kg/24 hr divided q6–8 hr).

3. For discomfort and fever, use Ibuprofen (Advil) 400 to 600 mg orally every 6 to 8 hours, not to exceed 1,200 mg/d (pediatric dosage: 10 mg/kg/dose every 6 to 8 hours).

Follow-Up

A. Follow up 2 to 3 days after dental examination to evaluate results.

Consultation/Referral

A. Advise the client to see a dentist promptly, even if pain resolves.

Individual Considerations

A. Pregnancy:

1. It is safe for clients to have dental procedures during pregnancy.

2. X-ray films may be taken with a lead shield over the client's abdomen.

3. Epinephrine and nitrous oxide should not be used during dental procedures.

4. Tetracycline should not be used; it causes staining of fetal bones and teeth.

Bibliography

Ali, A., & Patel, A. (2015). Oral maxillofacial: dangerous dental abscess. *Dental Update, 42*(3), 293. doi:10.12968/denu.2015.42.3.293a

Razzak, A., O'Leary, F., & Ahmed, N. (2017). Facial palsy masquerading as an acute dental abscess. *Dental Update, 44*(3), 241. doi:10.12968/denu.2017.44.3.241

Stephens, M. B., Wiedemer, J. P., & Kushner, G. M. (2018). Dental problems in primary care. *American Family Physician, 98*(11), 654–660.

Epiglottitis

Jill C. Cash, Moya Cook, and Jamie Wiggleton

Definition

A. Epiglottitis is acute, rapidly progressive inflammation and swelling of the epiglottis. Due to dangers of potentially fatal airway obstsruction, it is considered a medical emergency.

Incidence

A. The incidence of epiglottis has decreased dramatically since the *Haemophilus influenzae* type B (Hib) vaccine was introduced.

B. In immunized populations, estimates of epiglottis range from 0.6 to 0.8 cases per 100,000.

C. Epiglottis affects children and adults. It presents more acutely in young children than in adolescents and adults.

D. The median age of children with epiglottitis has increased from 3 years of age to 6 to 12 years of age since the introduction of vaccines against Hib.

Pathogenesis

A. Epiglottitis is most commonly caused by *H. influenzae*. Other pathogens include *Streptococci* (including Group A streptococcus), *Staphylococcus*, and *H. parainfluenzae*.

B. Viruses have not been established as causes of acute epiglottitis.

Predisposing Factor

A. Upper respiratory infection

B. Lack of immunization against Hib

C. Immune deficiency

D. In adults, epiglottitis has been associated with comorbid conditions including hypertension, diabetes mellitus, and substance abuse.

Common Complaints

A. Sudden onset of dysphagia, drooling, and distress ("the three Ds") are hallmarks of epiglottitis in children. Children present in distress and anxious; they may have the classic "tripod" or "sniffing" posture, that is, sitting position with trunk leaning forward, neck hyperextended, and chin thrust forward. Sudden onset of high fever, severe sore throat, stridor, and odynophagia are also common.

B. Adults present with sore throat or odynophagia, fever, muffled voice, drooling, stridor, and hoarseness. Sore throat is the most common presenting complaint in adults.

C. Airway compromise is less common in adults than children.

Subjective Data

A. Determine the onset, duration, and course of illness.

B. Is the client's breathing labored or does the client have stridor?

C. Has the client had a fever?

D. Has the client had trouble swallowing or talking?

Physical Examination

A. Check temperature, pulse, respirations, and blood pressure.

B. Inspect:

1. Observe overall appearance.

2. Check nail beds and lips for cyanosis.

3. Note drooling or difficulty in swallowing.

4. Note breathing pattern and rhythm.

5. Do not examine the throat—airway occlusion may result.

C. Auscultate heart and lungs.

Diagnostic Test

A. Lateral neck radiograph confirms diagnosis, typically revealing enlarged edematous epiglottis (the "thumbprint sign"). However, this test may delay the establishment of an airway.

Differential Diagnoses

A. Epiglottitis

B. Bacterial tracheitis (a pediatric emergency)

C. Laryngotracheitis

D. Angioedema (anaphylaxis)

E. Foreign body aspiration

F. Retropharyngeal or peritonsillar abscess

Plan

A. General interventions:

1. Prompt recognition and appropriate treatment usually result in rapid resolution of swelling and inflammation.

2. Obtain emergency medical transport to ED.

3. Management of the airway is the most critical aspect of initial care when epiglottitis is suspected. While awaiting transport, start oxygen, assemble airway equipment, and move the client as little as possible.

4. If the client is unable to maintain an airway, bag-valve-mask (BVM) ventilation with 100% oxygen should be initiated.

B. Client teaching:

1. Educate the client and the family that epiglottitis is a medical emergency.

C. Pharmaceutical therapy:

1. Defer pharmaceutical therapy with steroids and antibiotics to hospital team.

Follow-Up

A. Follow-up care per hospital discharge instructions

Consultation/Referral

A. Per hospital care team

Individual Considerations

A. Pediatrics:

1. Never place a child in supine position because respiratory arrest has been reported.

2. Airway obstruction can worsen with increased anxiety

3. All close contacts (including children and adults) exposed to a child diagnosed with epiglottitis should be treated with prophylactic antibiotics, such as rifampin, 20 mg/kg, not to exceed 600 mg/d for 4 days.

Bibliography

Lustig, L. R., & Schindler, J. S. (2019). Ear, nose, & throat disorders. In M. A. Papadakis, S. J. McPhee, & M. W. Rabow (Eds.), *Current medical diagnosis & treatment*. New York, NY: McGraw-Hill. Retrieved from https://accessmedicine-mhmedical-com.proxy.library.vanderbilt.edu/content.aspx?bookid=2449&sectionid=194433886

Rubin, M. A., Ford, L. C., & Gonzales, R. (2018). Sore throat, earache, and upper respiratory symptoms. In J. Jameson, A. S. Fauci, D. L. Kasper, S. L. Hauser, D. L. Longo, & J. Loscalzo (Eds.), *Harrison's principles of internal medicine* (20th ed.). New York, NY: McGraw-Hill. Retrieved from http://access-medicine.mhmedical.com.proxy.library.vanderbilt.edu/content.aspx?bookid=2129&sectionid=192012234

Udeani, J. (2016). Pediatric epiglottitis treatment & management. *Medscape*. Retrieved from https://emedicine.medscape.com/article/963773-treatment#d13

Woods, C. (2018a). Epiglottitis (supraglottitis): Clinical features and diagnosis. In M. Edward, G. Isaacson, & G. Fleischner (Eds.), *UpToDate*. Waltham, MA: Wolters Kluwer. Retrieved from http://www.uptodate.com/contents/epiglottitis-supra-glottitis-clinical-features-and-diagnosis?source=search_result&search=epiglottitis&selectedTitle=1%7E44

Woods, C. (2018b). Epiglottitis (supraglottitis): Management. In M. Edward, G. Isaacson, & G. Fleischner (Eds.), *UpToDate*. Waltham, MA: Wolters Kluwer. Retrieved from http://www.uptodate.com/contents/epiglottitis-supraglottitis-clinical-features-and-diagnosis?source=search_result&search=epiglottitis&selectedTitle=1%7E44

Oral Cancer

Jill C. Cash, Moya Cook, and Jamie Wiggleton

Definition

A. Oral cancer is a malignancy of the oral cavity. Subsites include the buccal mucosa, tongue, gingiva, floor of mouth, hard palate, soft palate, and lips. These frequently begin as *leukoplakia* (white, raised patches that do not easily scrape away) or *erythroplakia* (red, velvety patches that are friable with manipulation) and can occur on any of the above listed subsites. Oral cancers are most often squamous cell carcinoma, or cancer of the lining of the mouth. Less common types of malignancy, such as mucoepidermoid carcinoma, adenoid cystic carcinoma, and epithelial/myoepithelial carcinoma, affect the major and minor salivary glands. Mucosal melanoma is rare and account for approximately 1% of all melanomas. They may arise from the mucosal epithelium lining, oral cavity, and oropharynx. See Figure 8.1.

Incidence

A. The average age of most people diagnosed with these cancers is 62. Oral cancer is rare in children, but a little more than one-quarter occur in clients younger than 55 years. Male-to-female predominance is 2 to 1; oral cancer is equal in African Americans and Caucasian adults. The death rate is fairly high for oral cancer secondary to the cancer being diagnosed in the late stages of development.

B. Approximately 51,000 Americans are diagnosed with new cases of oral cancer, and nearly 10,000 deaths occur each year.

C. Oral cancer represents 3% of all newly diagnosed cancers and 1.6% of all cancer-related deaths.

D. Frequency of oral cancer of cheek and gum rises 50-fold among long-term users of smokeless tobacco.

Pathogenesis

A. Pathogenesis is unknown; however, increased risk factors exist which include the following:

1. Tobacco use: Use of tobacco in all its forms is highly correlated with the risk of oral cancer (cigarette

FIGURE 8.1 Tongue cancer.

smoking, smokeless tobacco in western cultures; betel nut quid is a significant factor associated with oral cancer throughout Asia and India).

2. Alcohol consumption: Alcohol by itself or in combination with smoking increases the risk of oral cancer. According to some studies, the risk of these cancers in heavy drinkers and smokers may be as much as 100 times higher than the risk in people who do not smoke or drink.

3. Poor nutrition: Studies have shown that a diet low in fruits and vegetables contributes to oral cancer.

4. Graft versus host disease (GVHD): A condition that sometimes occurs after a stem cell transplant. GVHD occurs when the donor stem cells recognize the client's cells as foreign and launch an attack against them. GVHD can affect many tissues of the body, including those in the mouth. This increases the risk of oral cancer, which can occur as early as 2 years after GVHD.

5. Genetic syndromes: Head and neck cancers are more common in clients diagnosed with genetic syndromes such as Fanconi anemia and Dyskeratosis congenita.

6. Lichen planus: Autoimmune disorder linked to oral squamous cell carcinoma

Predisposing Factors
A. Male gender
B. Age >40 years for men and >50 years for women
C. African American ancestry

Common Complaints
A. Oral sores that do not heal (most common presenting factor)
B. Change in how dentures fit
C. Bleeding mucosa or gingiva without apparent cause
D. Difficulty swallowing, usually indicating more advanced disease
E. Altered sensations: Burning or numbness, usually indicating more advanced disease
F. Leukoplakia or erythroplakia
G. Loosening of teeth

Other Signs and Symptoms
A. Sometimes asymptomatic
B. Decreased appetite related to altered taste
C. Increased salivation
D. Sore throat
E. Foul breath odor
F. Neck mass

Subjective Data
A. Review the onset, course, and duration of symptoms. Question the client regarding altered taste, sensations, difficulty swallowing, and foul breath.
B. Evaluate for risk factors. Review the client's use of tobacco products, including age of onset, amount of daily use, and quit dates. Also review pathogenesis and predisposing factors.

C. Ask the client about any previous history of cancer and treatments.
D. Evaluate the amount of alcohol intake, including age of onset, amount of daily use, and quit dates.
E. Review the client's general health history for other chronic conditions.
F. Review the client's medication history, including prescription and over-the-counter drug use, especially aspirin.
G. Take a dental history, specifically any loose or recently lost teeth, or acute change in denture fitting.
H. Assess for weight loss.

Physical Examination
A. Check temperature, pulse, respirations, blood pressure, and weight.
B. Inspect:
    1. Observe general appearance.
    2. Note quality of voice patterns and articulation.
    3. Note halitosis.
    4. Dentures should be removed. Observe the lips, gums, tongue, and buccal mucosa for swelling, discoloration, bleeding, asymmetry, texture, tongue motion, abnormal ulcerations, leukoplakia, and erythroplakia.
C. Palpate:
    1. Palpate the tongue and any lesions noted on exam. Lesions that are palpable and have submucosal firmness are especially worrisome. Common findings of a malignant oral lesion are central ulceration and firm, rolled borders. Assess flat patches of leukoplakia and/or erythroplakia by scraping them with a tongue blade to assess for removability or friability.
    2. Palpate lymph nodes: Cervical (anterior/posterior chain), submandibular, sublingual, and submental, pre-/postauricular; check nodes for size, texture, mobility, and tenderness.
D. Auscultate lungs and heart. The lungs are the most frequently involved extranodal metastatic site.

Diagnostic Tests
A. Biopsy for persistent lesions (more than 2 weeks)
B. Perform neck soft tissue CT and chest radiography to assess for regional and distant metastasis.

Differential Diagnoses
A. Oral leukoplakia
B. Pulpitis
C. Periapical abscess
D. Gingivitis
E. Periodontitis
F. Lichen planus
G. Oral candidiasis
H. Discoid lupus
I. Pemphigus vulgaris

Plan
A. General interventions:
    1. If oral cancer is suspected, refer to an oral/maxillofacial surgeon or otolaryngologist/head and neck surgeon for biopsy.

B. Client teaching:

1. Advise the client to stop smoking and stop using oral tobacco products.

2. Advise the client to decrease/eliminate alcohol consumption.

3. Encourage routine dental care and examinations.

4. Review dietary intake and educate the client regarding benefits of increasing dietary intake of vitamins A, C, and E. Encourage the client to decrease dietary intake of foods that are high in salt, smoked meats, fats, and oils.

5. Recommend wearing sunscreen/lip balm with sun protection factor (SPF) of 15 or greater.

C. Pharmaceutical therapy:

1. This should focus on symptom management such as topical formulas that have a topical anesthetic or Magic mouthwash (common compounded solution includes Maalox/diphenhydramine/lidocaine combined at a 1:1:1 ratio).

Follow-Up

A. If immediate biopsy is not indicated, ask the client to return for reevaluation in 2 weeks, after eliminating irritants and noxious agents.

Consultation/Referral

A. Refer the client to an otolaryngologist and/or a dentist for immediate biopsy for ulcerative or fungating lesions.

Individual Considerations

A. Adults: The U.S. preventative services task force (USPSTF) has concluded that current evidence is insufficient to assess the balance of benefits and harms of screening for oral cancer in asymptomatic adults. The Oral Cancer Foundation recommends visual and tactile screenings annually starting at age 18 for all adults. If an individual uses tobacco products, screening for them should begin at the age they commence tobacco use.

B. Pediatrics:

1. Currently, the highest rate is in smokeless tobacco use.

2. Oral screening should be considered annually in adolescents who use tobacco and/or alcohol.

Bibliography

American Cancer Society. (2019). About oral cavity and oropharyngeal cancer. Retrieved from https://www.cancer.org/cancer/oral-cavity-and -oropharyngeal-cancer/causes-risks-prevention/risk-factors.html

Carvajal, R., Hamid, O., & Ariyan, C. (2018). Mucosal melanoma. In M. Atkins & R. Berman (Eds.), *UpToDate*. Waltham, MA: Wolters Kluwer. Retrieved from https://www-uptodate-com.ckm proxy.vumc.org/contents/mucosal-melanoma?search=mucosal%20 melanoma&source=search_result&selectedTitle=1~21&usage_ type=default&display_rank=1

Goldstein, B., & Goldstein, A. (2019). Oral lesions. In R. Dellavalle & D. Deschler (Eds.), *UpToDate*. Waltham, MA: Wolters Kluwer. Retrieved from https://www-uptodate-com.ckmproxy.vumc.org/contents/oral -lesions?search=oral%20lesions&source=search_result&selectedTitle=1 ~150&usage_type=default&display_rank=1

Haddad, R. (2018). Human papillomavirus associated head and neck cancer. In B. Brockstein, D. Brizel, & M. Fried (Eds.), *UpToDate*. Retrieved from http://www.uptodate.com/contents/human-papillomavirus-associated -head-and-neck-cancer?source=search_result&search=oral+cancer+and+ hpv&selectedTitle=1%7E150

Oral Cancer Foundation. (2019). Oral cancer screening. Retrieved from https://oralcancerfoundation.org/screening/

Pharyngitis

Jill C. Cash, Moya Cook, and Jamie Wiggleton

Definition

A. Pharyngitis is the inflammation of the throat (oropharynx and hypopharynx) and the surrounding lymph tissue (palatine and lingual tonsils).

Incidence

A. Pharyngitis and tonsillitis account for >10% of all office visits to primary care clinicians and 50% of outpatient antibiotic use.

Pathogenesis

Pharyngitis may be due to viral, bacterial, and fungal agents. Other causes are noninfectious and lead to mucosal irritation.

A. Respiratory viruses, the most common cause of acute pharyngitis, account for approximately 25% to 45% of cases. Most common causative agents are adenovirus, rhinovirus, and coronavirus. Less common are enteroviruses, influenza A and B, parainfluenza viruses, and respiratory syncytial virus.

B. Common bacterial agents include Group A beta-hemolytic Streptococcus, Group C and G Streptococcus, *Neisseria gonorrhoeae*, and *Corynebacterium diphtheriae*.

C. The most common fungal agent is *Candida albicans*.

D. Atypical agents include *Mycoplasma pneumoniae* and *Chlamydia trachomatis* (rare).

E. Noninfectious causes include allergic rhinitis, gastroesophageal reflux, postnasal drip, mouth breathing (especially during dry air months), and trauma.

Predisposing Factors

A. Cigarette smoking

B. Allergies

C. Upper respiratory infections

D. Oral sex

E. Drugs (antibiotics and immunosuppressants)

F. Debilitating illnesses (such as cancer) that can cause candida to proliferate

Common Complaints

A. Sore and/or scratchy throat

B. Fever (>38°C or 100.5°F)

C. Headache

D. Malaise

Other Signs and Symptoms

A. Oral vesicles and/or strawberry tongue

B. Exudate on throat or "beefy" red throat without exudate

C. Painful lymphadenopathy

D. Fatigue

E. Dysphasia
F. Abdominal pain
G. Vomiting

Potential Complications

Without proper antimicrobial treatment, streptococcal pharyngitis can lead to serious complications such as the following:
A. Suppurative adenitis with tender, enlarged lymph nodes
B. Scarlet fever
C. Peritonsillar abscess
D. Glomerulonephritis
E. Rheumatic fever

Subjective Data

A. Assess onset, course, and duration of symptoms.
B. Inquire about mouth lesions, rhinorrhea, cough, drooling, and fever.
C. Ask about malaise, headache, fatigue, and fever; these are symptoms of mononucleosis.
D. Take a sexual history, if indicated. Ask if family members or sexual partners have the same signs and symptoms. Pharyngeal gonorrhea has no symptoms, so high-risk clients should be tested.
E. Ask whether symptoms have caused decreased intake of food and fluid.
F. Determine history of heart disease, previous strep pharyngitis, rheumatic fever, and other respiratory diseases, such as asthma, emphysema, and chronic allergies.
G. If rash is present, find out when it first occurred and if it has spread.
H. Ask about signs and symptoms of urinary tract infection and pyelonephritis.
I. Ask about a history of herpes, immunosuppressive disorders, and steroid use.
J. Review immunization history.

Physical Examination

A. Temperature and blood pressure, if indicated
B. Inspect:
    1. Observe general appearance.
    2. Examine the mouth, pharynx, tonsils, and hard and soft palate for vesicles and ulcers, candidal patches, erythema, hypertrophy, exudate, and stomatitis. Check gum and palate for petechiae and tongue for color and inflammation.
        a. Herpangina are small oral vesicles on the fauces and soft palate and are caused by the coxsackievirus.
        b. Herpes causes vesicles and small ulcers (stomatitis) of the buccal mucosa, tongue, and pharynx.
        c. Trench mouth (gingivitis) and necrotic tonsillar ulcers (Vincent's angina) cause foul breath, pain, pharyngeal exudate, and a gray membranous inflammation that bleeds easily.
        d. *C. albicans* (thrush) may be painful and causes cheesy, white exudate.

        e. Peritonsillar cellulitis causes inflamed, edematous tonsils; grayish-white exudate; high fever; rigors; and leukocytosis. Peritonsillar abscess (palpable mass) may also develop.
        f. Mononucleosis causes tonsillar exudate in 50% of clients; 33% develop petechiae at the junction of the hard and soft palate.
        g. *C. diphtheriae* causes a whitish-blue pharyngeal exudate "pseudomembrane" that covers the pharynx and bleeds if removal is attempted.
    3. Examine the ears, nose, and throat. Assess patency of airway if tonsils are enlarged.
    4. Inspect skin for rashes:
        a. Pastia's lines are petechiae present in a linear pattern along major skin folds in axillae and antecubital fossa that are seen with Group A *Streptococcus*
        b. Erythema marginatum, caused by Group A *Streptococcus*, is an evanescent, nonpruritic, pink rash mainly on the trunk and extremities. It may be brought out by heat application.
C. Auscultate heart and lungs.
D. Percuss:
    1. Abdomen, especially spleen area
    2. Chest
E. Palpate:
    1. Palpate lymph nodes, especially of the anterior and posterior cervical chains, axilla, and groin.
    2. Palpate abdomen for organomegaly and suprapubic tenderness.
    3. Palpate back for costovertebral angle (CVA) tenderness.
F. Neurologic examination: Check for nuchal rigidity and meningeal irritation.

Diagnostic Tests

A. Centor criteria include four clinical indicators of group A beta-hemolytic streptococcal (GABHS) pharyngitis:
    1. Tonsillar exudates
    2. Tender anterior cervical adenopathy
    3. Absence of cough
    4. History of fever (>38°C or 100.5°F)
A. The Centers for Disease Control and Prevention and Infectious Diseases Society of America (IDSA) recommend using two or more Centor criteria as a threshold for selecting clients for rapid antigen detection testing (RADT) and treating only those with positive tests.
B. For children and adolescents, throat culture is recommended by IDSA with a negative RADT. However, a throat culture is not considered necessary for adults with a negative RADT, because of the low likelihood that it will change management.
C. Consider monospot test for infectious mononucleosis (IM) if client has palatal petechiae, splenomegaly, and posterior cervical adenopathy as these are highly suggestive of IM. The absence of cervical lymphadenopathy and fatigue make the diagnosis less likely.
D. Complete blood count with differential.

E. Clients with risk factors for sexually transmitted infections, particularly receptive oral intercourse, should be tested for gonococcal pharyngitis.

F. Take blood cultures if sepsis is suspected.

G. Radiograph neck if there is possible trauma.

Differential Diagnoses

A. Pharyngitis

B. Stomatitis

C. Rhinitis

D. Sinusitis with postnasal drip

E. Epiglottis

F. Peritonsillar abscess

G. Mononucleosis

H. Herpes simplex

I. Coxsackievirus A16

J. *C. diphtheriae*

K. Trench mouth

L. Vincent's angina

M. *C. albicans*

N. HIV

Plan

A. General interventions:

1. Clients with a history of rheumatic fever and those who have a household member with a documented Group A streptococcal infection need immediate treatment without prior testing.

2. Do not put instruments in the airway if you suspect epiglottitis.

▶ B. Client teaching: *See Section III: Client Teaching Guide for this chapter, "Pharyngitis."*

C. Pharmaceutical therapy

1. Treatment of Group A strep pharyngitis—first-line drugs of choice:

a. Penicillin V potassium (Pen-Vee-K):

i. Children under 27 kg: 250 mg orally two to three times daily for 10 days. Children >27 kg, adolescents, and adults: 500 mg, two to three times daily for 10 days.

b. Penicillin G benzathine: Less than 27 kg: 600,000 U × 1 dose intramuscular (IM); ≥27 kg: 1,200,000 U × 1 dose IM

c. Amoxicillin:

i. Children: Amoxcilin 50 mg/kg once daily for 10 days (maximum 1,000 mg); alternative, 25 mg/kg/dose (max = 500 mg) twice daily for 10 days

ii. Adolescents and adults: Amoxicillin 500 mg twice daily for 10 days or 1,000 mg once daily for 10 days

2. Treatment of Group A strep in penicillin-allergic clients:

a. Cephalexin 20 mg/kg/dose twice daily (maximum 500 mg/dose) for 10 days

b. Cefuroxime 10 mg/kg/dose orally twice daily for 10 days (maximum 250 mg/dose)

c. Cefdinir 7 mg/kg/dose orally every 12 hours for 10 days or 14 mg/kg/dose every 24 hours for 10 days (maximum 600 mg/d)

d. Azithromycin: 12 mg/kg once daily (max 500 mg) daily for 5 days

e. Clarithromycin: 7.5 mg/kg/dose twice daily (max 250 mg/dose) for 10 days

f. Clindamycin: 7 mg/kg/dose three times daily (max 300 mg/dose) for 10 days

3. Treatment of recurrent group A strep pharyngitis:

a. If due to noncompliance with oral antibiotics in a client without penicillin allergy, use Penicillin G benzathine; less than 27 kg, use 600,000 U × 1 dose IM; ≥27 kg: 1,200,000 U × 1 dose IM.

b. For clients with persistent infection or an initial recurrence, Amoxicillin-clavulanic acid: 40 mg amoxicillin/kg/d divided every 8 hours (max 2,000 mg amoxicillin/d) for 10 days.

c. For clients with multiple recurrences or penicillin allergy, Clindamycin: 20 to 30 mg/kg/d in three divided doses (max 300 mg/dose) for 10 days.

4. Treatment of pharyngeal gonorrhea:

a. Adults: Ceftriaxone (Rocephin) 500 mg to 1 g by IM injection

b. Children: Ceftriaxone (Rocephin) 50 to 75 mg/kg in one dose by IM injection

5. For *M. pneumoniae* and *C. trachomatis*: Erythromycin (E-Mycin) 250 mg orally three to four times daily for 10 days

6. For pharyngeal candidiasis in the immunocompromised client:

a. Oral nystatin suspension (100,000 U/mL) 15 mL by swish-and-swallow method four times a day

b. Clotrimazole troche 10 mg held in mouth 15 to 30 minutes three times daily

Follow-Up

A. Client should return to clinic if symptoms do not improve in 3 to 4 days.

B. Treat sexual partners of clients with pharyngeal gonorrhea.

Consultation/Referral

A. Consult physician if client has severe dysphagia or dyspnea, signaling possible airway obstruction.

B. Refer the client to an otolaryngologist or ED if peritonsillar abscess is noted.

Individual Considerations

A. Pediatrics:

1. Rheumatic fever follows between 0.5% and 3% of ineffectively treated cases of Group A streptococcal upper respiratory infections.

2. Approximately 20% of children aged 5 to 15 years who are diagnosed with rheumatic fever had pharyngitis in the preceding 3 months.

B. Adults

1. Oral candidiasis may be the first symptom of HIV.

Bibliography

Aronson, M., & Auwaerter, P. (2018). Infectious mononucleosis in adults and adolescents. In M. Hirsch & S. Kaplan (Eds.), *UpToDate*. Retrieved from http://www.uptodate.com/contents/infectious-mononucleosisin-adults-and-adolescents?source=search_result&search=infectious+mononucleosis&selectedTitle=1%7E150

Chow, A., & Doron, S. (2018). Evaluation of acute pharyngitis in adults. In M. Aaronson (Ed.), *UpToDate*. Retrieved from https://www-uptodate-com.ckmproxy.vumc.org/contents/evaluation-of-acute-pharyngitis-in-adults?search=Evaluation%20of%20acute%20pharyngitis%20in%20adults&source=search_result&selectedTitle=1~150&usage_type=default&display_rank=1

Pichichero, M. (2016). Treatment and prevention of streptococcal tonsillopharyngitis. In D. Sexton & M. Edwards (Eds.), *UpToDate*. Retrieved from https://www.uptodate.com/contents/treatment-and-prevention-of-streptococcal-tonsillopharyngitis?source=see_link&sectionName=TREATMENT&anchor=H9#H9

Rubin, M. A., Ford, L. C., & Gonzales, R. (2018). Sore throat, earache, and upper respiratory symptoms. In J. Jameson, A. S. Fauci, D. L. Kasper, S. L. Hauser, D. L. Longo, & J. Loscalzo (Eds.), *Harrison's principles of internal medicine* (20th ed.). New York, NY: McGraw-Hill. Retrieved from http://accessmedicine.mhmedical.com.proxy.library.vanderbilt.edu/content.aspx?bookid=2129&sectionid=192012234

Wald, E. (2016). Approach to diagnosis of acute infectious pharyngitis in children and adolescents. In M. Edwards (Ed.), *UpToDate*. Retrieved from http://www.uptodate.com/contents/approach-to-diagnosis-ofacute-infectious-pharyngitis-in-children-and-adolescents?source=search_result&search=bacterial+pharyngitis+children&selectedTitle=1%7E150

Williams, B. D., Usatine, R.P., & Smith, M. A. (2019). Pharyngitis. In R. P. Usatine, M. A. Smith, E. J. Mayeaux, Jr., & H. S. Chumley (Eds.), *The color atlas and synopsis of family medicine* (3rd ed.). New York, NY: McGraw-Hill. Retrieved from https://accessmedicine-mhmedical-com.proxy.library.vanderbilt.edu/content.aspx?sectionid=206778481&bookid=2547&Resultclick=2

Stomatitis, Minor Recurrent Aphthous Stomatitis

Jill C. Cash, Moya Cook, and Jamie Wiggleton

Definition

A. Stomatitis is a general term indicating inflammation of the oral cavity. It includes the synonyms canker sores, recurrent aphthous ulcer (RAU), aphthous stomatitis, and recurrent aphthous stomatitis (RAS). Typical presentation is that of a discrete round or oval, tender superficial ulcer involving the mucosa of the oral cavity. The ulcers are usually gray, white, or yellow in color and surrounded by erythematous halos.

B. Minor aphthous ulcers are characterized by lesions <1 cm in diameter, mildly painful, and usually lasting 7 to 14 days.

C. Major aphthous ulcers are characterized by lesions >1 cm in diameter, extremely painful, and lasting up to 4 to 6 weeks.

Incidence

A. RAS is estimated to affect approximately 20% of the general population.

Pathogenesis

A. Etiology and pathogenesis are unclear. Host, environmental, and nutritional causes are implicated.

Predisposing Factors

A. Oral trauma
B. History of RAS
C. Possible nutritional deficiency of iron, folic acid, or zinc
D. Hormonal changes
E. Stress and anxiety
F. Food and chemical sensitivities

Common Complaint

A. Painful sore in mouth

Other Signs and Symptoms

A. Prodromal burning sensation in mouth for 24 to 48 hours before lesions appear

Subjective Data

A. Inquire about personal and family history of aphthous stomatitis.
B. Ask the client about prodrome of burning or stinging in the mouth.
C. Elicit information regarding previous illness and trauma.

Physical Examination

A. Check temperature, pulse, respirations, and blood pressure.
B. Inspect:
   1. Mouth for ulcers
   2. Ears, nose, and throat
   3. Skin, especially palms and soles, for lesions; indicates hand, foot, and mouth disease
C. Auscultate heart and lungs.

Diagnostic Tests

A. There is no specific diagnostic testing for stomatitis.
B. Consider herpes simplex virus (HSV) culture if HSV is considered for diagnosis.
C. If syphillis is of concern, order serum rapid plasma reagin (RPR).

Differential Diagnoses

A. Aphthous stomatitis
B. Oral HSV
C. Behçet's disease
D. Crohn's disease
E. HIV
F. Kawasaki syndrome
G. Hand, foot, and mouth disease (Coxsackievirus A16)
H. Consider less common etiologies for large, persistent areas of ulcerative stomatitis such as erythema multiforme or drug allergies, pemphigus, pemphigoid, epidermolysis bullosa acquisita, bullous lichen planus, Behçet disease, or inflammatory bowel disease.

Plan

A. General interventions:
   1. Avoid spicy, salty, or hot foods
   2. Encourage cold foods, such as fluids, ice pops, and so on, to help with pain.
   3. Avoid hard, sharp food that is difficult to chew.
   4. Recommend using a soft bristle toothbrush when brushing teeth.
   5. Avoid toothpaste containing sodium lauryl sulfate (SLS).
B. Client teaching: *See Section III: Client Teaching Guide for this chapter, "Aphthous Stomatitis."* ◀

C. Pharmaceutical therapy:
   1. Magic mouthwash (common compounded solution includes Maalox/diphenhydramine/lidocaine combined at a 1:1:1 ratio).
   2. Sucralfate (Carafate) suspension (1 teaspoon four times a day) may be used to swish in mouth and spit out for oral comfort.
   3. Glucocorticoid gel, such as fluocinonide gel (Lidex), 0.05% may be taken two to four times a day, one of which is always at bedtime.
   4. Orabase with or without triamcinolone acetonide (Kenalog)
   5. Amlexanox 5% paste (Aphthasol) is an over-the-counter product applied directly to ulcers four times a day until ulcers heal.

Follow-Up
A. Follow up as needed for treatment of recurrences.

Consultation/Referral
A. Refer client to an oral/maxillofacial provider or otolaryngologist if ulcers are deeper than 1 to 5 mm, or if lesion(s) last longer than 3 weeks.
B. Cardiology referral is needed if Kawasaki disease is suspected.

Individual Considerations
A. Pregnancy: Avoid use of fluocinonide and triamcinolone acetonide (Kenalog) in pregnant or nursing women.
B. Pediatrics:
   1. Avoid use of fluocinonide and triamcinolone acetonide (Kenalog).
   2. Do not use viscous lidocaine.

Bibliography
Brice, S. (2017). Recurrent aphthous stomatitis. In R. Dellavalle (Ed.), *UpToDate*. Retrieved from https://www.uptodate-com.ckmproxy.vumc.org/contents/recurrent-aphthous-stomatitis?search=stomatitis&source=search_result&selectedTitle=3-150&usage_type=default&display_rank=3

Usatine, R. P., Gonsalves, W. C., & Diaz, D. (2019). Aphthous ulcer. In R. P. Usatine, M. A. Smith, E. J. Mayeaux, Jr., & H. S. Chumley (Eds.), *The color atlas and synopsis of family medicine* (3rd ed.). New York, NY: McGraw-Hill. Retrieved from https://accessmedicine-mhmedical-com.proxy.library.vanderbilt.edu/content.aspx?bookid=2449&sectionid=194433886

Thrush

Jill C. Cash, Moya Cook, and Jamie Wiggleton

Definition
A. Thrush is a fungal infection of the oral cavity and/or the pharynx caused by *Candida* species.

Incidence
A. It is estimated that 5% to 7% of babies younger than 1 month, both bottle-fed and breastfed infants, will develop oral candidiasis. Approximately 9% to 31% of AIDS clients and 20% of clients diagnosed with cancer will have thrush. It is also common in older adults who wear dentures, clients with cellular immune deficiency states, such as AIDS. Clients with pulmonary disorders treated with inhaled corticosteroids are also at risk.

Pathogenesis
A. Thrush is an overgrowth of yeast cells, *C. albicans*, on the oral mucosa, which leads to desquamation of the epithelial cells.
B. Pseudomembranous thrush is the most common form; it appears as white plaques on the oral mucosa and/or oropharynx.
C. Atrophic thrush, also called denture stomatitis as it occurs most frequently in denture wearers, is typically found on the maxillary gingiva and is characterized by erythema without the usual white plaques of the pseudomembranous type.

Predisposing Factors
A. Use of broad-spectrum antibiotics
B. Adults:
   1. HIV
   2. Prolonged steroid use (systemic or inhaled corticosteroids)
   3. Cancer treatments (radiation/chemotherapy)
   4. Dentures
   5. Malnutrition
   6. Diabetes mellitus
C. Children:
   1. Endocrine disorders (thyroid disease, diabetes mellitus, and Addison's disease)
   2. HIV
   3. Cancer

Common Complaint
A. Soreness, pain of the mouth

Other Signs and Symptoms
A. Irritability in infants
B. Refusal to eat in infants
C. White plaques coating buccal mucosa

Subjective Data
A. Determine the onset, duration, and course of illness.
B. Inquire about oral intake or refusal to eat.
C. Has the client used antibiotics or other medications in the previous weeks?
D. Does the client use inhaled or systemic steroids on a daily basis?
E. Is the client currently receiving chemotherapy and/or radiation treatment for cancer?

Physical Examination
A. Check temperature, pulse, respirations, and blood pressure.
B. Inspect:
   1. Oral cavity for white, curd-like plaques that cannot be removed
   2. Erythematous changes of the gingiva in denture wearers
   3. Ears, nose, and throat

Diagnostic Tests
A. If diagnosis is certain, no testing recommended.
B. If uncertain of diagnosis, swab lesion for KOH testing.
C. If treatment prescribed is not working, fungal culture should be sent for diagnosis.

Differential Diagnoses
A. Leukoplakia
B. Lichen planus
C. Stomatitis
D. Aphthous ulcer
E. Hairy leukoplakia

Plan
A. General interventions:
   1. If the infant is breastfeeding, instruct the mother to clean breasts and nipples well with warm water between feedings to prevent contamination. Consider prescribing antifungal cream to be applied to breasts; this should be washed off before feedings.
   2. If bottle feeding, boil all bottles, nipples, and pacifiers to kill the organism.
   3. Instruct caregiver to attempt removal of large plaques with a moistened cotton-tipped applicator and/or small, moist gauze pad before inserting medication in mouth.
   4. If thrush is recurrent or resistant, consider checking the mother for candidal vaginitis.
   5. For adults, instruct the client/family on proper use and cleaning/rinsing of inhalers/dentures to prevent reoccurrence of thrush.
▶ B. Client teaching: *See Section III: Client Teaching Guide for this chapter, "Oral Thrush in Children"*

C. Pharmaceutical therapy:
   1. Oral candidiasis: Nystatin (Mycostatin) oral suspension 1 mL four times a day for 1 week. Place medication in front of mouth on each side. Rub directly on plaques with a cotton swab. Adults: Pastilles: 200,000-unit lozenge four times a day for 14 days, or swish-and-swallow 500,000 units four times a day for 14 days or two 500,000-unit tablets three times daily for 14 days.
   2. Clotrimazole troche (Mycelex): 10 mg five times daily for 14 days; monitor for side effects.
   3. Fluconazole: Adults: 200 mg × 1, then 100 mg daily for 5 to 7 days. Children: 5 mg/kg by mouth every day for 5 days or 6 to 12 mg/kg on first day, then 3 to 6 mg/kg for 10 days.

Follow-Up
A. Instruct caregiver to telephone the office if the child refuses to eat, if there is no improvement, if thrush lasts more than 10 days, or if there is unexplained fever.

Consultation/Referral
A. Consult an oral surgeon or otolaryngologist if thrush does not resolve with adequate antifungal treatment.

Bibliography
Kauffman, C. (2018). Treatment of oropharygneal and esophageal candidiasis. In K. Marr (Ed.), *UpToDate*. Retrieved from http://www.uptodate.com/contents/treatment-of-oropharyngeal-and-esophageal-candidiasis?source=search_result&search=oral+candidiasis&selectedTitle=1%7E150
Papadakis, M. A., McPhee, S. J., & Bernstein, J. (Eds.). (2019). Candidiasis, mucocutaneous. In *Quick medical diagnosis & treatment*. New York, NY: McGraw-Hill. Retrieved from https://accessmedicine-mhmedical-com.proxy.library.vanderbilt.edu/content.aspx?bookid=2566&sectionid=206879921

9 Respiratory Guidelines

Asthma

Mellisa A. Hall and Cheryl A. Glass

Definition

Pathophysiologically, asthma is defined by airway inflammation, intermittent airflow obstruction secondary to increased smooth muscle tone, and bronchial hyperresponsiveness. Episodes are associated with widespread, variable, often reversible airflow obstruction and bronchial hyperresponsiveness when airways are exposed to various stimuli or triggers. Asthma is responsible for lost school days, lost productivity, and presentism.

Asthma is classified into four categories:

A. *Step 1—Mild intermittent*: Symptoms less than or equal to twice per week; asymptomatic with normal peak expiratory flow rate (PEFR) between attacks; nighttime symptoms less than or equal to twice per month; PEFR greater than 80% is predicted with a variability of less than 20%

B. *Step 2—Mild persistent*: Symptoms greater than twice per week but less than once per day; exacerbations may affect activity; nighttime symptoms greater than twice per month; PEFR greater than or equal to 80% is predicted with variability of 20% to 30%

C. *Step 3—Moderate persistent*: Daily symptoms require beta-2 agonist use; attacks affect activity; exacerbations greater than or equal to twice per week; nighttime symptoms greater than once per week; PEFRs between 60% and 80% with a variability greater than 30%

D. *Step 4—Severe persistent*: Continuous symptoms with limited physical activity, frequent exacerbations, frequent nighttime symptoms, PEFR less than or equal to 60% is predicted with greater than 30% variability

Incidence

A. Asthma affects 25 million people in the United States, or 300 million worldwide.

B. Asthma is the most common chronic disease of childhood, affecting 15% of children.

C. Up to 95% of clients with asthma also suffer from persistent rhinitis.

D. Asthma is often associated with other comorbid conditions, including gastroesophageal reflux disease (GERD) and obesity.

E. Although asthma can present at any age, the peak age of diagnosis is before age 5 years.

Pathogenesis

A. Asthma arises from a complex cycle of processes initiated by airway inflammation resulting from physical, chemical, and pharmacological agents (such as environmental irritants, allergens, furry animals, cockroaches, dust mites, pollen and mold, cold air, viral respiratory infections, and exercise). It progresses to airway hyperresponsiveness, bronchoconstriction, airway wall edema, chronic mucus plug formation, and chronic airway remodeling.

Predisposing Factors

A. In children:
  1. Allergy or family history of allergy
  2. Atopy
  3. Ethnicity (Puerto Rican descent, non-Hispanic Black)
  4. Gender: Male during childhood

B. In adults:
  1. Family history
  2. Coexisting sinusitis, nasal polyps, and sensitivity to aspirin or other nonsteroidal anti-inflammatory drugs (NSAIDs)
  3. Exposure in workplace to wood dust, metals, and animal products
  4. Premenstrual asthma (PMA)
  5. Gender: Female in adulthood
  6. Ethnicity: Non-Hispanic Black for persistent asthma
  7. Occupational exposures
  8. Comorbidities in older adults

C. In all ages:
  1. Inhalation of irritants such as tobacco smoke
  2. Viral respiratory infections
  3. Gastroesophageal reflux
  4. Obesity
  5. Lower socioeconomic level

D. Triggers:
1. Allergen exposure
2. Viral infections of the upper airways
3. Medication (potential risk with beta-blockers, angiotensin-converting enzyme [ACE] inhibitors, cyclo-oxygenase [COX] inhibitors, aspirin [ASA], NSAIDs)
4. Exercise
5. Situational factors: Cold air, laughter, strong odors, air pollution, smoke exposure, pregnancy
6. Foods
7. Hormones
8. Gastrointestinal (GI) reflux
9. Stress
10. Alternative/herbal remedies
11. Dander/saliva from animals with fur or feathers
12. Mold
13. Dust mites, rodents, cockroaches

Common Complaints

A. Recurrent cough (worse at night and early morning)
B. Recurrent wheezing
C. Recurrent shortness of breath (SOB)
D. Dyspnea (less likely to be reported in the elderly)
E. Recurrent chest tightness (may worsen with moderate activity)

Other Signs and Symptoms

A. Nocturnal awakening from symptoms
B. Variation of symptoms with seasons or environment
C. Chest discomfort, tightness with moderate activity

Subjective Data

A. Ask about the onset, duration, and course of symptoms.
B. Inquire about sudden severe episodes of coughing, wheezing, and SOB and whether precipitating factors can be identified.
C. Ask whether the client has chest colds that take more than 10 days to resolve.
D. Ask if the client is a smoker, how much, and for how long he or she has smoked.
E. Ask whether symptoms seem to occur during certain seasons or during exposure to the following environmental irritants:
1. Tobacco smoke, including e-cigarettes/vaping
2. Perfume
3. Household pets
4. Fireplaces
5. Woodburning stoves
6. Mold
7. Dust mites
8. Cockroaches
F. Find out how often coughing, wheezing, or SOB awaken the client.
G. Ask if symptoms are caused or exacerbated by moderate exercise or physical activity.
H. Determine the family history of asthma, allergies, and eczema.
I. Determine whether the client is pregnant or has medical problems. If so, do not prescribe long-term beta-2 adrenergics or NSAIDs. The safest medications are short-acting beta-2 agonists (SABA), cromolyn sodium, and anti-cholinergic drugs.
J. Administer the asthma control test for adults or the childhood asthma control test for children aged 4 to 11 years. This test is for self-report (or parent-report) to determine whether asthma symptoms are under control. Both tests are available online from www.asthmacontrol.com. A score greater than 20 points indicates the client's asthma is well controlled. Scores of 5 to 19 points indicate the client's asthma is not well controlled.
K. Evaluate whether the client has ever been tested for allergies.
L. Ask whether the client has ever needed to go to the emergency department or had to be hospitalized for an asthma attack.
M. Review all medications, including over-the-counter (OTC) and herbal supplements.

Physical Examination

A. Check temperature (if indicated), blood pressure (BP), pulse, respirations, and pulse oximetry. Measure the client's height and weight to calculate body mass index (BMI) because obesity is associated with asthma, and evaluate failure to thrive if suspected.
B. Inspect:
1. Especially in children, observe for hyperexpansion of thorax and signs that accessory muscles are being used (retractions, nasal flaring) or stridor.
2. Note appearance of hunched shoulders and/or chest deformity.
3. In children, inspect the nose for a foreign body
4. In all clients, inspect ears, nose, and throat. Evaluate the presence of enlarged tonsils and adenoids, and nasal polyps.
5. Inspect skin for eczema, dermatitis, or other irritation that might signal allergy.
6. Observe for allergic shiners and pebbled conjunctiva.
7. Observe for digital clubbing.
C. Auscultate:
1. Auscultate lung sounds. Note wheezing during normal expiration and prolonged expiration, which is seen with asthma.
2. Listen to all lung fields for an asymmetric wheeze.
3. Auscultate heart.
D. Percuss:
1. Lung fields

Diagnostic Tests

A. Spirometry is the gold standard. Peak flow meter measurements are not a substitute for spirometry. Evaluate the forced vital capacity (FVC) and forced expiratory volume in 1 second (FEV_1) before and after the client inhales a short-acting bronchodilator.
B. Evaluate chest radiograph (CXR) and complete blood count (CBC) to exclude other diagnoses and infection.
C. Allergy testing is recommended for children with persistent asthma.

D. Check PEFR after inhalation of SABA. Diagnosis is confirmed if:

1. There is a 15% increase in PEFR after 15 to 20 minutes.

2. PEFR varies more than 20% between arising and 12 hours later in clients taking bronchodilators (or 10% without bronchodilators).

3. There is a greater than 15% decrease in PEFR after 6 minutes of running or exercise.

E. Consider a bronchial provocation test with histamine or methacholine for nondiagnostic spirometry.

Differential Diagnoses

A. In infants and children:
1. Asthma
2. Pulmonary infections:
   a. Pneumonia
   b. Respiratory syncytial virus (RSV)
   c. Viral bronchiolitis
   d. Tuberculosis (TB)
3. Allergic rhinitis and sinusitis
4. Foreign body in the nose, trachea, or bronchus
5. GERD
6. Cystic fibrosis (CF)
7. Bronchopulmonary dysplasia
8. Vocal cord dysfunction
9. Enlarged lymph nodes or tumors

B. In adults:
1. Asthma
2. Chronic obstructive pulmonary disease (COPD)
3. GERD
4. Congestive heart failure (CHF)
5. Cough secondary to medications such as ACE inhibitors or beta-blockers
6. Pneumonia, including aspiration pneumonia in elderly or post-cerebrovascular accident (CVA)
7. Pulmonary embolism
8. Laryngeal dysfunction
9. Benign and malignant tumors
10. Vocal cord dysfunction

Plan

A. General interventions:

1. Review proper medication dosages. Short- and long-term agents come in several formulations, such as nebulizer, metered-dose inhaler (MDI), and a dry powder inhaler (DPI). Young children should have medication via a nebulizer using an appropriate-size face mask. The "blow-by" technique is not an appropriate means of administering medication.

2. Demonstrate correct use of inhalers, spacers, and nebulizers. If the client does not use correct technique when using these devices, medication does not get delivered to the bronchioles, and therefore the client may believe that the medication does not work. Most often, the medication works well when delivered to the bronchioles correctly.

3. Stress the importance of using a peak flow monitor at home to monitor progress of the disease.

4. For rescue from acute symptoms, use SABAs.

5. The use of a SABA more than twice a week for symptom relief would indicate the client has inadequate asthma control and needs an inhaled corticosteroid (ICS) as controller therapy.

6. Stress the need for an asthma action plan.

B. Client teaching:
1. *See Section III: Client Teaching Guide for this chapter, "Asthma."*
2. *See Section III: Client Teaching Guide for this chapter, "Asthma: Action Plan and Peak Flow Monitoring."*
3. *See Section III: Client Teaching Guide for this chapter, "Asthma: How to Use a Metered-Dose Inhaler."*

C. Pharmaceutical therapy:

1. Drugs are prescribed in a stepwise fashion for the type of asthma. The amount of medication used depends on the severity of the asthma (Steps 1–6 in the following list). Before any medication/dosage changes, monitor the client's compliance (see Table 9.1).

2. The following treatments are recommended for children aged 5 years and older and for adults:
   a. Step 1: Mild:
      i. No long-term preventive medications are needed.
      ii. Use SABAs as rescue medication. May be used up to four times a day to treat exacerbations
      iii. Alternative medications include cromolyn, nedocromil, leukotriene modifier, or theophylline.
   b. Step 2: Mild to moderate:
      i. Low-dose ICSs are used daily as a long-term preventive medication.
      ii. Only budesonide inhalation suspension is approved by the Food and Drug Administration (FDA) for use in infants and children younger than 4 years.
      iii. Alternative medications include an ICS plus either a leukotriene modifier or theophylline.
   c. Step 3: Moderate:
      i. Consider referral to asthma specialist at Step 3.
      ii. Use low-dose ICS plus a long-acting beta-2 agonist (LABA) *or* a medium-dose ICS.
      iii. Use ICS plus either a leukotriene modifier or theophylline or zileuton.
   d. Step 4: Moderate to severe:
      i. Medium- to high-dose ICS plus either a LABA or montelukast
      ii. Medium-dose ICS plus either a leukotriene modifier or theophylline
      iii. Second alternative: Medium-dose ICS plus either leukotriene modifier, theophylline, or zileuton
   e. Step 5: Severe:
      i. High-dose ICS plus LABA and consider omalizumab for clients with allergies

TABLE 9.1   MEDICATIONS FOR ASTHMA AND COPD (BY CLASS/ALPHABETICAL ORDER)

Brand	Generic	Drug Classification	Availability
SABA, for Rescue/Fast-Acting Rescue			
Accuneb	Albuterol	Beta-2 agonist	Nebulizer
Albuterol	Albuterol sulfate	Beta-2 agonist	Inhaler, solution
			Nebulizer
			Syrup
Combivent	Ipratropium + albuterol	Combination anticholinergic + beta-2 agonist	MDI
Fenoterol	Ipratropium + fenoterol	Beta-2 agonist	Inhaler, MDI, and oral syrup
Maxair Autohaler	Pirbuterol acetate	Beta-2 agonist	MDI
ProAir HFA inhaler	Albuterol	Beta-2 agonist	MDI
Proventil HFA inhaler	Albuterol	Beta-2 agonist	MDI
Terbutaline sulfate	Brethine	Beta-2 agonist	Tablet
Ventolin HFA	Albuterol sustained release	Beta-2 agonist	MDI
Vospire ER	Albuterol	Beta-2 agonist	Extended-release tablet
Xopenex	Levalbuterol tartrate	Beta-2 agonist	HFA inhaler
			Concentrate solution for nebulizer
Long-Acting Beta-2 Agonist (LABA), for Maintenance/Long-Acting Control			
Advair Diskus	Fluticasone + salmeterol	Combination-steroid + LABA	Dry powder diskus
			MD–HFA inhaler
Arcapta	Indacaterol	LABA	Nebulizer
Brovana	Arformoterol	Beta-2 agonist	Nebulizer
Foradil Aerolizer	Formoterol fumarate	LABA	Nebulizer
			Dry powder diskus
Perforomist	Formoterol solution	Beta-2 agonist	Nebulizer
Serevent Diskus	Salmeterol	LABA	Dry powder diskus
Striverdi Respimat	Olodaterol	LABA	MDI
Inhaled CS Anti-Inflammatory (ICS), for Maintenance or Long-Term Control			
Aerobid and Aerobid M	Flunisolide	ICS	MDI
			MDI with menthol
Aerospan	Flunisolide	ICS	MDI
AirDuo RespiClick	Fluticasone propionate/ salmeterol	ICS + LABA	DPI
Alvesco	Ciclesonide	ICS	MDI
Arnuity Ellipta	Fluticasone furoate	ICS	DPI
ArmonAir RespiClick	Fluticasone propionate	ICS	DPI
Asmanex	Mometasone	ICS	Twisthaler dry powder
Beclovent	Beclomethasone dipropionate	ICS	Dipro powder inhaler
Breo Ellipta	Fluticasone furoate/ vilanterol	ICS + LABA	DPI
Dulera	Mometasone furoate + formoterol	Combination CS + LABA	MDI
Flovent HFA	Fluticasone	ICS	MDI (also available as a DPI as Flovent diskus)
Pulmicort	Budesonide	ICS	Flexhaler and respules
QVAR	Beclomethasone	ICS	MDI
Symbicort	Budesonide + formoterol	Combination CS + LABA	MDI

(*continued*)

TABLE 9.1   MEDICATIONS FOR ASTHMA AND COPD (BY CLASS/ALPHABETICAL ORDER) *(continued)*

Brand	Generic	Drug Classification	Availability
Leukotriene Modifiers—Nonsteroidal Anti-Inflammatory			
Accolate	Zafirluklast	Leukotriene modifier	Tablet
Singulair	Montelukast	Leukotriene modifier	Chew tablet
			Tablet granules
Zyflo	Zileuton	Leukotriene modifier	Filmtab
Interleukin-5 agonist			
Cinqair	Reslizumab	Interleukin-5 agonist	Intravenous infusion
Dupixent	Dupilumab	Interleukin-5 agonist	Subcutaneous injection
Fesenra	Benralizumab	Interleukin-5 agonist	Subcutaneous injection
Nucala	mepolizumab	Interleukin-5 agonist	Subcutaneous injection
Anticholinergics			
Atrovent HFA	Ipratropium	Antimuscarinic/antispasmodic	MDI and nebulized
DuoNeb	Ipratropium + albuterol	Combination antimuscarinic/ antispasmodic + beta-2 agonist	Nebulizer
Spiriva with HandiHaler	Tiotropium	Antimuscarinic/antispasmodic	Dry powder diskus
Mast Cell Stabilizer			
Intal	Cromolyn sodium	Mast cell stabilizer	MDI
Tilade	Nedocromil	Mast cell stabilizer	MDI
Methylxanthine			
Aminophylline	Theophylline	Methylxanthines respiratory smooth muscle relaxant	Tablet
Theo-24	Theophylline sustained-release	Methylxanthines respiratory smooth muscle relaxant	Tablet
Anti-IgE (Immunoglobulin E Blocker) Monoclonal Antibody			
Xolair	Omalizumab	IgE blocker-immunomodulator	Subcutaneous injection
Systemic CSs—Used as a Short-Term "Burst" for Control			
Deltasone	Prednisone	Systemic CS	Tablet
Medrol	Methylprednisolone	Systemic CS	Tablet
Prelone	Prednisolone	Systemic CS	Tablet
Phosphodiesterase-4 Inhibitors (PDE4)			
Ariflo	Cilomilast	Selective PDE4	Tablet
Daliresp	Roflumilast	Selective PDE4	Tablet

CS, corticosteroid; DPI, dry powder inhaler; HFA, hydrofluoroalkanes; ICS, inhaled corticosteroid; LABA, long-acting beta-2 agonist; MDI, metered-dose inhaler; SABA, short-acting beta-2 agonist.

f. Step 6: Severe:
   i. High-dose ICS plus LABA plus oral corticosteroid (CS) and consider omalizumab for clients who have allergies
g. Exercise-induced bronchospasm:
   i. Short-acting inhaled beta-2 agonist: Two inhalations shortly before exercise are effective for 2 to 3 hours
   ii. LABA, two inhalations are effective for 10 to 12 hours. No immediate effect
h. Hypertension and asthma: Drug of choice is a calcium channel blocker. Asthmatics also tolerate diuretics well.
i. Theophylline can cause cardiac arrhythmias; therefore, use it with caution and always follow up with theophylline levels.

j. Vaccinations:
   i. Inhaled flu vaccine is not used in clients with asthma. Inactivated influenza vaccine is safe, including for children with severe asthma.
   ii. Pneumococcal vaccines are recommended for children and adults with asthma.
D. Goal of asthma therapy:
   1. Minimal to no chronic symptoms, including night-time symptoms
   2. Minimal exacerbations
   3. No emergency department visits
   4. Minimal use of SABA
   5. No limitations of activities
   6. Peak expiratory flow maintained in normal range
   7. Minimal adverse effects of medications

Follow-Up

A. After acute episodes, follow up within 1 to 2 hours or next day to monitor improvement until client is stable.

B. For clients with mild intermittent or mild persistent asthma under control for at least 3 months, assess and follow up at least every 6 months to provide education and reinforce positive behaviors. Gradually reduce medication dosage. If control is not achieved, consider increasing the dosage after reviewing medication technique, compliance, and environmental control.

Consultation/Referral

A. Consider hospitalization for clients with acute episodes who do not completely respond to treatment within 1 to 2 hours.

B. If all therapies fail—including a short burst of prednisone—refer the client to an asthma specialist.

C. Consult with a physician when the client is pregnant or has other medical problems, or when standard treatment is ineffective.

D. Refer if the client presents with atypical symptoms.

Individual Considerations

A. Pregnancy:
1. Risks of uncontrolled asthma far outweigh risks to the mother or fetus from drugs used to control the disease.
2. Most drugs used to treat asthma and rhinitis, with the exception of brompheniramine and epinephrine, pose little increased risk to the fetus.
3. Classes of drugs that do cause risk include decongestants, antibiotics (tetracycline, sulfonamides, and ciprofloxacin), live virus vaccines, immunotherapy (if doses are increased), and iodides. Always weigh benefits against risks, because adequate fetal oxygen supply is essential.
4. If CSs are necessary, recommend aerosolized forms due to their lower systemic effects. Prednisone or methylprednisolone is preferred and should be prescribed at minimum effective doses.
5. Do not prescribe inhaled triamcinolone because it is teratogenic.
6. Inhaled budesonide is the preferred ICS for treatment of asthma in pregnancy. Ipratropium is generally considered less effective than ICS and is therefore a second-line agent in pregnancy (https://acaai.org/asthma/who-has-asthma-and-why/pregnancy-and-asthma).
7. Drugs recommended during pregnancy:
   a. A SABA, such as albuterol, is preferred; two inhalations every 4 hours as needed. Regular daily use suggests a need for additional medications. If a daily LABA is needed, budesonide is preferred.
   b. Ipratropium: Two inhalations four times daily may be used in step therapy.
   c. Regular inhaled budesonide is considered a first-line agent if an inhaled glucocorticoid is needed.
   d. The leukotriene modifiers montelukast or zafirlukast may be considered as add-ons to inhaled glucocorticoids.
   e. Oral prednisone if all other therapies fail; 1 week of 40 mg/d, followed by 1 to 2 weeks of tapering. Recommend obstetric consult before prescribing.

B. Geriatrics:
1. Asthma in the elderly is often associated with other comorbidities such as COPD, cardiac conditions, or dementia.
2. Half of elderly clients with asthma have the first onset after age 65. Respiratory viruses are a common trigger.
3. Recurrent episodes of SOB may be primary symptom.
4. Treatment is the same as with younger clients, with inhaled SABA as needed and step therapy with daily inhaled steroids. Oral steroids are reserved for severe episodes. The elderly have more adverse effects from inhaled ICS.
5. If steroids are prescribed, carefully monitor the client for complications, including cataracts, increased intraocular pressure, hyperglycemia, and accelerated loss of bone mass.
6. Inhaled anticholinergics and LABAs are second-line treatments.
7. The elderly may have difficulty with inhaling medications or activating inhaler devices and may require a nebulizer.
8. Theophylline is rarely effective in the elderly. Asthma medications may have increased adverse effects in the elderly or may aggravate coexisting medical conditions, requiring medication adjustments. Also consider drug interactions and drug-and-disease interactions.

C. Pediatrics
1. Spacing chambers are recommended to assist in proper delivery of medication.

Resources

Adult and Children Asthma Control tests: www.asthmacontrol.com

American Lung Association: www.lungusa.org

Asthma & Allergy Foundation of America: www.aafa.org

Global Initiative for Asthma (GINA) Instructions for Inhaler and Spacer Use: www.ginasthma.com

National Heart Lung and Blood Institute (NHLBI): www.nhlbi.nih.gov

Bibliography

Barnes, P. J. (2015). Asthma. In D. L. Kasper, A. S. Fauci, S. L. Hauser, D. L. Longo, & J. L. Jameson (Eds.), *Harrison's principles of internal medicine* (19th ed., pp. 1669–1680). New York, NY: McGraw-Hill. Retrieved from http://accessmedicine.mhmedical.com/book.aspx?bookid=1130

Centers for Disease Control and Prevention. (2017, March 31). *FastStats: Asthma.* Retrieved from www.cdc.gov/nchs/fastats/asthma.htm

Fanta, C. H. (2017a, October). An overview of asthma management. *UpToDate.* Waltham, MA: Wolters Kluwer. Retrieved from http://www.uptodate.com/contents/an-overview-of-asthma-management

Fanta, C. H. (2017b, March). Diagnosis of asthma in adolescents and adults. *UpToDate*. Waltham, MA: Wolters Kluwer. Retrieved from http://www.uptodate.com/contents/diagnosis-of-asthma-in-adolescents-and-adults

Harding, S. M. (2017, November). Gastroesophageal reflux and asthma. *UpToDate*. Retrieved from http://www.uptodate.com/online/contents/gastroesophageal-reflux-and-asthma

Medscape Drug Reference. (n.d.). Theophylline oral. *Medscape*. Retrieved from http://www.medscape.com/druginfo/dosage?drugid=3591&drugname=Theophylline+Oral&monotype=default

Monthly Prescribing Reference. (2018, July). Asthma treatment: Inhalations. Retrieved from https://www.empr.com/home/clinical-charts/asthma-treatments-inhalations/

Prescriber's letter. (2019, March). Inhaled corticosteroid dose comparison in asthma. Retrieved from prescribersletter.therapeuticresearch.com

Rains, S. G. (2020). Fifteen-to-eighteen-month visit. In B. Richardson (Ed.), *Pediatric primary care: Practice guidelines for nurses* (4th ed., pp. 117–127, 113–124). Burlington, MA: Jones & Bartlett Learning.

Resnick, B. (Ed.). (2017). *GNRS geriatric nursing review syllabus: A core curriculum in advanced practice geriatric nursing* (5th ed.). New York, NY: American Geriatrics Society.

Sawicki, G., & Haver, K. (2019, March). Acute asthma exacerbations in children younger than 12 years: Home/office management and severity assessment. *UpToDate*. Retrieved from http://www.uptodate.com/contents/acute-asthma-exacerbations-in-children-home-office-management-and-severity-assessment?source=search_result&search=acute+asthma+exacerbations+in+children&selectedTitle=3%7E150

Schatz, M., & Weinberger, S. E. (2018, May). Management of asthma during pregnancy. *UpToDate*. Retrieved from http://www.uptodate.com/contents/management-of-asthma-during-pregnancy

Terry, E. G. (2020). Seven-to-ten-year visit (school age). In B. Richardson (Ed.), *Pediatric primary care: Practice guidelines for nurses* (4th ed., pp. 147–162). Burlington, MA: Jones & Bartlett Learning.

Vaz Fragoso, C. (2018, May). Diagnosis and management of asthma in older adults. *UpToDate*. Retrieved from http://www.uptodate.com/contents/diagnosis-and-management-of-asthma-in-older-adults?source=search_result&search=diagnosis+and+management+in+older+adults&selectedTitle=1%7E150

Zachary, K. C. (2019, February). Treatment of seasonal influenza in adults. *UpToDate*. Retrieved from http://www.uptodate.com/contents/treatment-of-seasonal-influenza-in-adults

Bronchiolitis: Child

Mellisa A. Hall and Cheryl A. Glass

Definition

A. Bronchiolitis is a narrowing and inflammation of the bronchioles, causing wheezing and mild to severe respiratory distress. Infants are affected most often because of their small airways and insufficient collateral ventilation. It is one of the most common causes of acute hospitalizations in infants, especially in the fall and the winter. A small decrease in a bronchiole's already small airway will lead to a fourfold increase in airway resistance and accounts for this pathologic manifestation in this age group.
B. The average length of illness with bronchiolitis is 12 days.

Incidence

A. Respiratory infection is seen in one third of children younger than 12 months, with one in 10 requiring hospitalization.
B. Bronchiolitis occurs most often in infants and children aged 1 to 2 years. Approximately 2% to 4% of adults with respiratory illnesses, comorbidity of immunosuppression, and the elderly will also be diagnosed with bronchiolitis.

Pathogenesis

A. The pathology results in obstruction of bronchioles from inflammation, edema, and debris, leading to hyperinflation of the lungs, increased airway resistance, atelectasis, and ventilation–perfusion mismatching.
B. RSV is the most common cause (50%–80%) of bronchiolitis.
C. Human metapneumovirus (HMPV) is the second most common cause (3%–19%).
D. Other causes include parainfluenza virus, adenovirus, influenza *Chlamydia pneumoniae*, *Mycoplasma pneumoniae*, and human bocavirus (HBoV).

Predisposing Factors

A. Low birth weight, particularly in premature infants
B. Chronic lung disease (CLD; formerly bronchopulmonary dysplasia)
C. Parental smoking
D. Congenital heart disease
E. Immunodeficiency
F. Lower socioeconomic group
G. Crowded living conditions and day care
H. Gender: Bronchiolitis occurs in males 1.25 times more frequently than in females.

Common Complaints

Clinical manifestations are initially subtle.
A. Infants who become increasingly fussy
B. Difficulty feeding during the 2- to 5-day incubation period. This is because infants prefer to breathe through their nose (obligate nasal breathing) as opposed to their mouths; significant nasal edema and/or rhinorrhea may force mouth breathing and disturb feedings.
C. Low-grade fever (usually less than 101.5°F)
D. Cough
E. Tachypnea
F. Wheezing
G. Retractions
H. Nasal flaring and grunting

Other Signs and Symptoms

A. Coryza
B. Irritability
C. Lethargy
D. Respiratory distress
E. Nasal flaring and grunting
F. Hypothermia (infants younger than 1 month)

Subjective Data

A. Determine the onset, course, and duration of illness
B. Are breathing problems affecting the ability to eat and drink? Is the baby able to be breastfed?
C. Evaluate a history of fever, nausea, vomiting, or diarrhea
D. Does the client or any family members have asthma?
E. Are there any other family members who are ill?
F. Are there smokers in the family environment or exposures to other types of inhaled toxins?

Physical Examination

A. Check temperature, BP, and respirations:
1. Count respirations for 1 full minute.
2. Respirations greater than 70 breaths per minute in an infant may be associated with risk for severe disease and warrant further evaluation for pneumonia.
3. Tachypnea at any age is a concern for severe lower respiratory illness.

B. Inspect:
1. Observe overall appearance.
2. Note respiratory pattern and nasal flaring.
3. Note the use of accessory muscles for breathing.
4. Check for tachypnea, which differentiates bronchiolitis from upper respiratory infections. (URI) and bronchitis.
5. Examine the eyes, ears, and throat, noting other potential infections.
6. Inspect the nose for nasal flaring.

C. Auscultate:
1. Heart
2. Lungs. On examination there are fine inspiratory crackles and/or high-pitched expiratory wheezes. A prolonged expiration phase is seen with bronchiolitis.

D. Palpate:
1. Liver and spleen

E. Percuss:
1. Chest/lungs for hyperresonance

F. Neurologic examination:
1. Assess for irritability and lethargy

Diagnostic Tests

A. Diagnosis is made based on age and seasonal occurrence, tachypnea, and the presence of profuse coryza and fine rales, wheezes, or both on auscultation.

B. Viral isolation from nasopharyngeal secretions or rapid antigen detection (enzyme-linked immunosorbent assay [ELISA], immunofluorescence) for RSV can confirm the diagnosis.

C. Consider pulse oximetry.

D. Routine use of CXR is not recommended by the American Academy of Pediatrics (AAP).

Differential Diagnoses

A. Viral bronchiolitis
B. Asthma
C. Viral or bacterial pneumonia
D. Aspiration syndromes
E. Pertussis
F. CF
G. Cardiac disease
H. Reflux
I. Aspiration
J. Tracheoesophageal fistula
K. Foreign body

Plan

A. General interventions:
1. Use a humidifier in the client's bedroom.
2. Clear stuffy nose with saline solution drops and suction out nares with bulb syringe.
3. Infants should not be exposed to secondhand smoking.
4. Monitor respiratory pattern.
5. Use good hygiene practices—handwashing.

B. Client teaching: *See Section III: Client Teaching Guide for this chapter, "Bronchiolitis: Child."* ◀

C. Pharmaceutical therapy:
1. Bronchodilators should not be routinely used. They do not shorten the duration of illness or lessen the risk of hospitalization.
2. CSs should not be routinely used. They do not shorten the duration of illness or lessen the risk of hospitalization.
3. Antibacterials should be used only with proven coexistence of a bacterial infection.
4. There is no vaccine against bronchiolitis. A vaccine against HMPV is currently in the early stages of development. HMPV, which is most closely related to avian metapneumovirus, has been in existence in humans for more than 60 years, but is only newly categorized. The virus most frequently infects young children and the elderly, and it is most common in late winter and early spring, a timing associated with up to 25% of respiratory infections. Palivizumab (Synagis) prophylaxis should be administered to selected children following the AAP guidelines. HMPV has a worldwide distribution and is responsible for the majority of viral URIs in children and adults.
5. Use of the montelukast (Singulair) has not proven beneficial in resolution of symptoms.

D. Dietary management:
1. Encourage fluids, such as juice and water. Dilute juice for younger infants.
2. Offer small, frequent feedings.
3. Breastfeeding should continue.

E. Medical/surgical management:
1. Clients may require only supportive care. Clients with respiratory distress require hospitalization.
2. Hypoxemic clients need oxygen therapy and possibly mechanical ventilation.
3. Chest physiotherapy is not recommended.

Follow-Up

A. Contact the client within 12 to 24 hours for evaluation.

Consultation/Referral

A. Notify a doctor if the client's breathing becomes labored, his or her wheezing becomes worse, and/or respiratory distress is suspected.

B. Refer clients with RSV to the emergency department if moderate respiratory distress, dehydration, or hypoxemia occurs.

C. Hospitalization recommended for:
1. Younger clients in moderate to severe respiratory distress
2. Infants less than 3 months of age
3. Clients with pulmonary hypertension, CLD (formerly bronchopulmonary dysplasia), or CF if their

respiratory rate is greater than 60 breaths/min, their pulse oximetry is less than 92%, or they eat poorly

Individual Considerations

A. High-risk chronic conditions:
1. Clients with pulmonary hypertension, bronchopulmonary dysplasia, or CF may have prolonged courses with high morbidity and mortality. Some may have reactive airway diseases in the future.
B. Pediatrics:
1. Young children are most susceptible to HMPV infection. The majority of children are seropositive for HMPV infection by age 5. History of prematurity and asthma increase risk for hospitalization in children.
C. Adults:
1. Human pneumovirus was identified in 8% of adults requiring hospitalization for lower respiratory infections.
D. Geriatrics:
1. Geriatric clients are most susceptible to HMPV infection.

Bibliography

Barr, F., & Graham, B. (2020). Immunoprophylactic agents: Palivizumab. *UpToDate*. Retrieved from https://www.uptodate.com/contents/respiratory-syncytial-virus-infection-prevention

Crow, J. E. (2018, July). Human metapneumovirus infections. *UpToDate*. Retrieved from http://www.uptodate.com/contents/human-metapneumo-virus-infections

Munoz, F. M., & Flomenberg, P. (2018, June). Diagnosis, treatment, and prevention of adenovirus infection. *UpToDate*. Retrieved from http://www.uptodate.com

Piedra, P. A. (2019, January). Bronchiolitis in infants and children: Clinical features and diagnosis. *UpToDate*. Retrieved from http://www.uptodate.com/contents/bronchiolitis-in-infants-and-children-clinical-features-and-diagnosis

Weiner, D. L. (2018, August). Causes of acute respiratory distress in children. *UpToDate*. Retrieved from http://www.uptodate.com/contents/causes-of-acute-respiratory-distress-in-children

Bronchitis, Acute

Mellisa A. Hall and Cheryl A. Glass

Definition

Acute bronchitis is inflammation of the tracheobronchial tree. Bronchitis is nearly always self-limited in the otherwise healthy individual. Generally, the clinical course of acute bronchitis lasts 10 to 14 days. The cause is usually infectious, but allergens and irritants may also produce a similar clinical profile. Asthma can be mistaken as acute bronchitis if the client has no prior history of asthma.

Incidence

Bronchitis is more common in fall and winter in relation to the common cold or other respiratory illness. It occurs in both children (younger than 5 years of age) and adults and is diagnosed in men more frequently than in women. Fewer than 5% of clients with bronchitis develop pneumonia.

Pathogenesis

A. Most attacks are caused by viral agents, such as adenovirus, influenza, parainfluenza viruses, and RSV.
B. Bacterial causes include *Bordetella pertussis, Mycobacterium tuberculosis, Corynebacterium diphtheriae,* and *M. pneumoniae. B. pertussis* should be considered in children who are incompletely vaccinated.

Predisposing Factors

A. Viral infection
B. URI
C. Smoking
D. Exposure to cigarette smoke
E. Exposure to other irritants
F. Allergens
G. Chronic aspiration/GERD

Common Complaint

The most common symptom initially is a dry, hacking, or raspy-sounding cough. The cough then loosens and becomes productive.

Other Signs and Symptoms

A. Sore throat
B. Rhinorrhea or nasal congestion
C. Rhonchi during respiration
D. Low-grade fever
E. Malaise
F. Retrosternal pain during deep breathing and coughing
G. Decreased/lack of appetite

Subjective Data

A. Ask about the onset, duration, and course of symptoms.
B. Is the cough productive?
C. Is there substernal discomfort?
D. Is there malaise or fatigue?
E. Has the client had a fever?
F. Does the client smoke, including e-cigarettes? (Smoking aggravates bronchitis.)
G. A review of occupational history may be important in determining whether irritants play a role in symptoms.
H. Assess for symptoms of gastroesophageal reflux.

Physical Examination

Examinations of children may best be completed with the child sitting on the parent's lap.
A. Check temperature, pulse, and BP. Always check a pulse oximeter.
B. Inspect:
1. Observe overall appearance.
2. Inspect the eyes, ears, nose, and throat (the pharynx may be injected).
3. Transilluminate the sinuses.
C. Palpate:
1. Lymph nodes
2. Maxillary and frontal sinuses
D. Auscultate:
1. Lung fields for crackles, wheezing, and rhonchi

Diagnostic Test

A. Consider chest x-ray to exclude pneumonia.

Differential Diagnoses

A. Pneumonia
B. URI
C. Asthma
D. Sinusitis
E. CF
F. Aspiration
G. Respiratory tract anomalies
H. Foreign-body aspiration
I. Pneumonia
J. COPD and emphysema
K. Pediatrics and adults with persistent cough: Pertussis

Plan

A. General interventions are primarily supportive and should ensure the client is adequately oxygenated:
   1. Tell the client to increase fluid intake.
   2. Suggest cool mist humidity and mist therapy.
   3. Avoid irritants, such as smoke.
▶ B. Client teaching: *See Section III: Client Teaching Guide for this chapter, "Bronchitis, Acute."*
C. Pharmaceutical therapy:
   1. Acetaminophen (Tylenol) for fever and malaise:
      a. Adults: 500 to 1,000 mg orally every 6 hours; not to exceed 4 g/d
      b. Pediatrics: For those younger than 12 years: 10 to 15 mg/kg/dose by mouth every 4 to 6 hours max: 75 mg/kg/d and up to 4 g/d; for children older than 12 years: 325 to 650 mg by mouth every 4 to 6 hours; not to exceed 4 g/d
   2. Expectorants, such as guaifenesin with dextromethorphan (Robitussin DM, Humibid DM, Mytussin), can be used to treat minor cough from bronchial/throat irritation:
      a. Adults and children older than 12 years: 10 mL by mouth every 4 hours
      b. Children younger than 4 to 6 years: Not recommended
      c. Children 6 to 12 years: 5 mL by mouth every 4 hours as needed

> In response to child safety concerns, the American Academy of Pediatrics states that cough and cold medications should not be used for children younger than 6 years.

   3. Among otherwise healthy individuals, antibiotics have not demonstrated benefit for acute bronchitis, as the etiology is usually viral. However, oral antibiotics should be considered if symptoms persist for 2 weeks with treatment (indicates bacterial infection).
      a. Erythromycin (EES, E-Mycin, Ery-Tab):
         i. Adults: 250 to 500 mg by mouth four times a day or 333 mg by mouth three times a day
         ii. Pediatrics: 30 to 50 mg/kg/d by mouth divided four times a day
      b. Clarithromycin (Biaxin):
         i. Adults: 250 to 500 mg by mouth twice a day
         ii. Pediatrics: 7.5 mg/kg by mouth twice a day
      c. Azithromycin (Zithromax):
         i. Adults: Day 1: 500 mg by mouth, then 250 mg by mouth on days 2 to 5
         ii. Pediatrics: 12 mg/kg by mouth every day; do not exceed 500 mg/dose
   4. Albuterol (Ventolin) for clients with wheezes or rhonchi, or for clients with a history of bronchoconstriction:
      a. Adults: 2 puffs every 4 to 6 hours *or* 2 to 4 mg by mouth for three to four times a day
      b. Pediatrics: 0.1 to 2 mg/kg by mouth three times daily

Follow-Up

A. Follow up if client does not improve in 48 hours.
B. Recommend yearly influenza vaccinations.

Consultation/Referral

A. In uncomplicated cases, mucus production decreases and cough disappears in 7 to 10 days. If symptoms persist, refer the client to a physician.
B. Refer the client if you note respiratory distress or if the client appears ill and you suspect pneumonia

Individual Considerations

A. Pediatrics:
   1. Children who have repeated episodes of bronchitis should be evaluated for congenital defects of the respiratory system.
   2. Instruct clients regarding the need for immunization against pertussis, diphtheria, and influenza, which reduces the risk of bronchitis.
   3. Children may attend school or day care without restrictions except during acute bronchitis with fever.
B. Geriatrics:
   1. Monitor elderly clients for complications such as pneumonia. The elderly have a greater morbidity and mortality rate.

Bibliography

American Academy of Pediatrics. (2018, June). *Cough and cold medicine: Not for children.* Retrieved from http://www.choosingwisely.org/clinician-lists/american-academy-pediatrics-cough-and-cold-medicines-for-children-under-four/

Centers for Disease Control and Prevention. (n.d.). *Bronchitis (chest cold).* Retrieved from https://www.cdc.gov/getsmart/antibiotic-use/url/bronchitis.html

Centers for Disease Control and Prevention. (2010). Infant deaths associated with cough and cold medications: Two states, 2005. *Morbidity and Mortality Weekly Report, 56*(1), 1–4. Retrieved from https://www.cdc.gov/mmwr/preview/mmwrhtml/mm5601a1.htm

Centers for Disease Control and Prevention. (2017a). Adverse drug events in children. *Medication Safety Program,* Retrieved from https://www.cdc.gov/medicationsafety/parents_childrenadversedrugevents.html

Centers for Disease Control and Prevention. (2017b, August 7). *Pertussis (whooping cough) surveillance & reporting.* Retrieved from https://www.cdc.gov/pertussis/surv-reporting.html

Chang, A., Oppenheimer, J., Weinberger, M., Rubin, B. K., Grant, C. C., Weir, K., … CHEST Expert Cough Panel. (2017). Management of children with chronic wet cough and protracted bacterial bronchitis. *Chest, 151*(4), 884–890. doi:10.1016/j.chest.2017.01.025

CNBC News. (2016, March 17). *Cold remedies and kids: Study finds some parents ignoring warnings against use.* Retrieved from http://www.cbc.ca/news/health/cold-medicines-children-1.3496164

File, T. M. (2018, November). Acute bronchitis in adults. *UpToDate.* Retrieved from http://www.uptodate.com/contents/acute-bronchitis-in-adults

Bronchitis, Chronic

Mellisa A. Hall and Cheryl A. Glass

Definition
A. Chronic bronchitis is excessive mucus secretion with chronic or recurrent productive cough occurring three successive months a year for two consecutive years.
B. Others limit the definition to a productive cough that lasts more than 2 weeks despite therapy.
C. Clients with chronic bronchitis have more mucus than normal because of either increased production or decreased clearance. Coughing is the mechanism for clearing excess secretion.

Incidence
The incidence of chronic bronchitis is uncertain secondary to underreporting of symptoms; many clients remain undiagnosed. There is a lack of definitive diagnostic criteria, as well as considerable overlap with asthma. Visits for bronchitis are second only to visits for otitis media and are slightly more common than visits for asthma.

Pathogenesis
A. Mucociliary clearance is delayed because of excess mucus production and loss of ciliated cells, leading to a productive cough. This is usually secondary to the number of years of cigarette smoke–induced damage. In children, chronic bronchitis follows either an endogenous response to an acute airway injury or continuous exposure to noxious environmental agents such as allergens or irritants.
B. Bacteria most often implicated are *Streptococcus pneumoniae, Haemophilus influenzae, M. pneumoniae,* and *Moraxella catarrhalis.* The most common causes of chronic bronchitis in the pediatric population include viral infections such as adenovirus, RSV, rhinovirus, and HBoV.
C. Specific occupational exposures are associated with symptoms of chronic bronchitis, including coal, cement, welding fumes, organic dusts, engine exhausts, fire smoke, and secondhand smoke.

Predisposing Factors
A. Cigarette smoking
B. Cold weather
C. Acute viral infection
D. COPD/emphysema
E. Occupational exposure to other airborne irritants
F. Chronic, recurrent aspiration or gastroesophageal reflux
G. Allergies

Common Complaints
A. Worsening cough: Hacking, harsh, or raspy sounding
B. Changes in color (yellow, white, or greenish), amount, and viscosity of sputum
C. Children younger than 5 years rarely expectorate, and sputum is usually seen in vomitus
D. "Rattling" sound in chest
E. Dyspnea/breathlessness
F. Wheezing

Other Signs and Symptoms
A. Difficulty breathing, retrosternal pain during a deep breath or cough
B. Rapid respirations
C. Fatigue
D. Headache
E. Loss of appetite
F. Fever
G. Myalgias
H. Arthralgias

Subjective Data
A. Determine the onset, course, and duration of illness
B. Is the client having trouble breathing?
C. Has there been a fever?
D. How is the client's appetite? Is the client drinking enough fluids?
E. Does the client smoke, use vapor cigarettes (vaping), or is the client exposed to secondhand smoke?
F. Review occupational history to evaluate exposure to irritants
G. Does the client have a history of asthma?
H. How often is the client currently using his or her SABA inhaler?

> Chronic bronchitis has a long history of a productive cough and late-onset wheezing. Patients with asthma with a chronic obstruction have a long history of wheezing with a late-onset of productive cough.

Physical Examination
Examinations of children may best be started with the child sitting on the parent's lap.
A. Check temperature, pulse, BP, and pulse oximetry.
B. Inspect:
   1. Observe overall appearance/mentation/ease of respirations.
   2. Inspect the eyes, ears, nose, and throat:
      a. The pharynx may be injected.
      b. Conjunctivitis suggests adenovirus.
   3. Transilluminate the sinuses.
C. Auscultate:
   1. Lungs in all fields; lung sounds may sound normal to scattered, rhonchi, or large airway wheezing
   2. Heart
D. Percuss:
   1. Chest

E. Palpate:
  1. Lymph nodes
  2. Maxillary and frontal sinuses

Diagnostic Tests
A. Clients with uncomplicated respiratory illness need little, if any, laboratory evaluation.
B. Pulse oximetry can help diagnose the issue.
C. Sputum culture is used to identify bacteria.
D. CXR may help exclude other diseases or complications.
E. Pulmonary function studies may be indicated.
F. EKG and pulmonary function tests (PFTs) may be required for clients with COPD.
G. Sweat test may be necessary to rule out CF.

Differential Diagnoses
A. Acute bronchitis
B. Pneumonia
C. Asthma
D. Sinusitis
E. CF
F. Bronchiectasis
G. Central airway obstruction
H. Lung cancer
I. Aspiration syndrome
J. Gastroesophageal reflux
K. TB
L. Foreign body

Plan
A. General interventions:
  1. Rest during early phase of illness.
  2. Encourage smoking cessation and staying away from secondhand smoke.
  3. Suggest exercise for clients with COPD.
  4. The client's goal is to improve symptoms and to decrease cough and production of sputum.
  5. Inform clients that increased sputum production may occur after smoking cessation and the client may have airway reactivity (wheezing), which is especially seen in clients with asthma.
▶ B. Client teaching: *See Section III: Client Teaching Guide for this chapter, "Bronchitis, Chronic."*
C. Pharmaceutical therapy:
  1. Bronchodilators should be considered for bronchospasm:
    a. Albuterol sulfate (Proventil, Ventolin, ProAir):
      i. Adults: MDI-2 actuations (90 mcg/actuation) inhaled every 4 to 6 hours
      ii. Pediatrics: MDI or nebulizer:
        1) Younger than 1 year: 0.05 to 0.15 mg/kg dose every 4 to 6 hours
        2) 1 to 5 years old: 1.25 to 2.5 mg/kg dose every 4 to 6 hours
        3) 5 to 12 years old: 2.5 mg/kg dose every 4 to 6 hours
        4) Older than 12 years: 2.5 to 5 mg/kg dose every 6 hours

2. Analgesics and antipyretics are used to control fever, myalgias, and arthralgias.
3. Consider oral steroids to decrease inflammation:
  a. Adults: 5 to 60 mg/d by mouth
  b. Pediatrics: 1 to 2 mg/kg by mouth daily or in twice a day divided dosing; do not exceed 80 mg/d
  c. Tapering steroids is not necessary with steroid courses of 10 days' duration or less
4. ICS may be effective:
  a. Budesonide (Pulmicort) is available as an MDI that delivers 90 or 180 mcg/actuation:
    i. Adult MDI: 90 to 180 mcg inhaled by mouth twice a day, not to exceed 1440 mcg/d. Use lowest effective dosage.
    ii. Pediatric MDI: 90 mcg inhaled by mouth twice a day, not to exceed 720 mcg/d
  b. Fluticasone (Flovent HFA, Flovent Diskus): Available as MDI (44 mcg, 110 mcg, or 220 mcg per actuation) and diskus powder for inhalation (50 mcg, 100 mcg, or 250 mcg per actuation)
    i. Adults:
      1) MDI: 88 mcg inhaled by mouth twice a day; dosage not to exceed 440 mcg twice a day
      2) Diskus: 100 mcg inhaled by mouth twice a day; dosage not to exceed 500 mcg twice a day
    ii. Pediatrics:
      1) MDI: Ages 4 to 11 years: 88 mcg inhaled by mouth twice a day; older than 11 years, administer as adults
      2) Diskus: Ages 4 to 11 years: 50 mcg inhaled by mouth twice a day; older than 11 years, administer as adults
5. Antibiotics for bacterial infection:
  a. Erythromycin (EES, E-Mycin, Ery-Tab):
    i. Adults: 250 to 500 mg by mouth four times a day or 333 mg by mouth three times daily
    ii. Pediatrics: 30 to 50 mg/kg/d by mouth divided four times a day; do not exceed 2 g/d
  b. Clarithromycin (Biaxin):
    i. Adults: 250 to 500 mg by mouth twice a day
    ii. Pediatrics: 7.5 mg/kg by mouth twice a day
  c. Azithromycin (Zithromax):
    i. Adults: 500 mg by mouth on day 1, then 250 mg by mouth on days 2 to 5
    ii. Pediatrics: 10 mg/kg/d by mouth on day 1, then 5 mg/kg on days 2 to 5; do not exceed adult dose
  d. Amoxicillin–clavulanic acid (Augmentin):
    i. Adult: 250 to 500 mg by mouth every 8 hours
    ii. Pediatrics
      1) Younger than 3 months: 30 mg/kg/d by mouth divided to every 12 hours

2) 3 months or older: 40 to 80 mg/kg/d by mouth divided to every 12 hours

6. OTC cold and cough products: The AAP does not recommend use of cold and cough products in children 6 years of age or younger. These products have been associated with serious adverse effects.

D. Dietary management:
1. Increase fluids.
2. Eat nutritious food.

Follow-Up
A. Follow up if there is no improvement in 3 to 4 days after starting therapy.
B. Recommend yearly influenza vaccinations.

Consultation/Referral
A. Refer clients with respiratory distress to a physician. If respiratory failure occurs (rare), hospitalization may be needed.
B. Refer clients with COPD to a physician or pulmonary specialist.
C. Referral to a pediatric pulmonologist should be considered when symptoms persist and do not respond to initial therapy.

Individual Considerations
A. Pediatrics:
1. Recurrent acute or chronic bronchitis should alert the clinician to the diagnosis of asthma.
2. Recurrent episodes of acute or chronic bronchitis may also be associated with immunodeficiencies.
3. Discuss the need for immunization against pertussis, diphtheria, and influenza, which reduces the risk of bronchitis.
4. Children may attend school or day care without restrictions except during fever.
5. In children, a foreign body needs to be ruled out either radiographically or by bronchoscopy.
B. Geriatrics:
1. Age-specific changes in elderly include changes in airway size due to connective tissue changes, including shallow alveolar sacs.
2. Chest wall compliance is reduced, with diaphragmatic strength reduction of 25%.
3. Older adults may adjust their lifestyle to compensate due to declining lung function.
4. Dyspnea should be addressed and not associated only with deconditioning with age.

Bibliography
Centers for Disease Control and Prevention. (n.d.). *Bronchitis (chest cold)*. Retrieved from https://www.cdc.gov/getsmart/antibiotic-use/url/bronchitis.html
Centers for Disease Control and Prevention. (2017a, May 3). *FastStats chronic obstructive pulmonary disease (COPD) includes: Chronic bronchitis and emphysema*. Retrieved from www.cdc.gov/nchs/fastats/copd.htm
Centers for Disease Control and Prevention. (2017b, August 7). *Pertussis (whooping cough) surveillance & reporting*. Retrieved from https://www.cdc.gov/pertussis/surv-reporting.html
Epocrates Online. (2019). *Pulmicort Flexhaler*. Retrieved from https://online.epocrates.com/drugs/464802/Pulmicort-Flexhaler/Peds-Dosing
Resnick, B. (Ed.). (2017). *GNRS geriatric nursing review syllabus: A core curriculum in advanced practice geriatric nursing* (5th ed.). New York, NY: American Geriatrics Society.
Weiner, D. L. (2018, August). Causes of acute respiratory distress in children. *UpToDate*. Retrieved from http://www.uptodate.com/contents/causes-of-acute-respiratory-distress-in-children
Zachary, K. C. (2019, February). Treatment of seasonal influenza in adults. *UpToDate*. Retrieved from http://www.uptodate.com/contents/treatment-of-seasonal-influenza-in-adults

Chronic Obstructive Pulmonary Disease

Mellisa A. Hall and Cheryl A. Glass

Definition
COPD is progressive, chronic, expiratory airway obstruction due to chronic bronchitis or emphysema. The relief of bronchoconstriction due to inflammation has some reversibility. Chronic bronchitis is a chronic productive cough lasting 3 months during two consecutive years, after all causes of chronic cough have been excluded. Emphysema is an abnormal, permanent enlargement (hyperinflation) and destruction of the alveoli air sacs, as well as the destruction of the elastic recoil. Many clients have both types of air-restriction symptoms of chronic bronchitis and emphysematous destruction leading to COPD. Clients with asthma whose airflow obstruction is completely reversible are not considered to have COPD. When asthmatic clients do not have complete reversible airflow obstruction, they are considered to have COPD.

Irreversible airflow obstruction is a key factor in the client's disability. The goal of COPD management is to improve daily quality of life (QOL) and the recurrence of exacerbations. Smoking cessation continues to be the most important therapeutic intervention.

The Global Initiative for Chronic Obstructive Lung Disease (GOLD) staging criteria are:
A. Stage I—Mild obstruction: FEV_1 greater than 80% of predicted value, some sputum, and chronic cough
B. Stage II—Moderate obstruction: FEV_1 between 50% and 80% of predicted value, SOB on exertion, and chronic symptoms
C. Stage III—Severe obstruction: FEV_1 between 30% and 50% of predicted value, dyspnea, reduced exercise tolerance, and exacerbations affecting QOL
D. Stage IV—Very severe obstruction chronic respiratory failure: FEV_1 less than 30% of predicted value or moderate obstruction FEV_1 less than 50% of the predicted value, dyspnea at rest, and chronic respiratory failure. Fourteen percent of clients admitted for COPD exacerbation die within 3 months of admission.
E. Comorbidities commonly seen with COPD include hypertension; cardiac disorders, including atrial fibrillation and heart failure; diabetes/metabolic syndrome; GI disorders; lung cancer; depression; and osteoporosis

Incidence
The National Heart, Lung and Blood Institute reported that 16 million Americans are affected with COPD, and millions more do not know they have it. COPD is still an

underrecognized diagnosis although it is the third leading cause of death in the United States. COPD is more commonly seen in males than females, but gender differences are lessening as more females are smoking. The Global Burden of Disease Study reported a prevalence of 251 million cases of COPD globally, and that number is predicted to increase annually secondary to higher smoking prevalence (tobacco, vaping, and marijuana) in many countries.

Pathogenesis

A. Chronic bronchitis leads to the narrowing of the airway caliber and increase in airway resistance. Mucous gland enlargement is the histologic hallmark of chronic bronchitis.

B. In emphysema, loss of the air sac's elastic recoil and alveoli destruction causes air limitation. Emphysema caused by smoking is the most severe in the upper lobes. Most clients with COPD have smoked one pack of cigarettes a day for 20 or more years before the symptomatic dyspnea, cough, and sputum appear.

Predisposing Factors

A. Cigarette smoking

B. Occupational, environmental, or atmospheric pollutants:
   1. Dust
   2. Chemical fumes
   3. Secondhand smoke
   4. Air pollution

C. Genetic factor: Alpha-1 antitrypsin (AAT) deficiency

D. Recurrent or chronic lower respiratory infections or disease

E. Age (most common in fifth decade of life)

Common Complaints

A. Chronic cough and colorless sputum, usually worse in morning

B. Dyspnea with exertion, progressing to dyspnea at rest

C. Wheezing

D. Difficulty speaking or performing tasks

E. Weight loss (decrease in fat-free mass)

Other Signs and Symptoms

A. Pursed-lip breathing: induces auto-peeping and hence helps keep alveoli open

B. Use of accessory muscles

C. Tripod position

D. Barrel chest

E. Cyanosis (fingertips, tip of nose, around lips)

F. Tachypnea

G. Tachycardia

H. Difficulty speaking or performing tasks

I. Distended neck veins

J. Abnormal, diminished, or absent lung sounds

K. Mental status changes

L. Anxiety and depression

M. Pulmonary hypertension

N. Cor pulmonale

O. Left-sided heart failure

Subjective Data

A. Ask the client about past respiratory problems and infections. Does he or she currently have fever, chills, or other signs of infection?

B. Ask about the onset of cough and characteristics of sputum (amount, color, and presence of blood).

C. Determine cigar use and cigarette pack-year history (pack/day × number of years smoked).

D. Inquire about exposure to occupational or environmental irritants.

E. How far can the client walk before becoming breathless? Is there more breathlessness when the client walks on a slight incline?

F. Does the client become breathless or tired when performing activities of daily living (ADLs)?

G. Ask about insomnia, anxiety, restlessness, edema, and weight change.

H. How many pillows does the client sleep on? Does he or she have to sleep in a recliner or sitting up?

I. Assess the client's ability to perform ADLs and instrumental activities of daily living (IADLs), including grooming and personal hygiene, performing chores around the house, shopping, cooking, and driving.

J. Ask about alcohol use.

K. Review all medications, including OTC and herbal products.

L. Review further assessment questions based on existing comorbidities.

Physical Examination

A. Record temperature (if indicated), BP, pulse, respirations, and pulse oximetry:
   1. The respiratory rate increases proportionally to disease severity
   2. Take height and weight to calculate the BMI
   3. The client may have a fairly normal examination early in the disease course.

B. Inspect:
   1. Observe general appearance: Skin color, affect, posture, gait, amount of respiratory effort when walking; note increased anterior–posterior chest diameter.
   2. Examine sputum: Frothy pink signals pulmonary edema. Hemoptysis as seen in TB
   3. Examine the lips, fingertips, and nose for cyanosis (finger clubbing is not characteristic of COPD).
   4. Observe the neck for distended veins and peripheral edema (advanced disease).
   5. Check for pursed-lip breathing and use of accessory muscles.

C. Auscultate:
   1. Auscultate the heart.
   2. Auscultate the lungs for wheezes, crackles, decreased breath sounds, and prolonged forced expiratory rate.
   3. Assess for vocal fremitus (vibration) and egophony (increased resonance and high-pitched bleating quality). Air trapping causes air pockets that do not

transmit sound well. Absent ventricular lung sounds are a distinctive characteristic of COPD.

  4. Auscultate the carotid arteries and the abdomen for bruits.

D. Percuss:

  1. Chest for the presence of hyperresonance and for signs of consolidation

E. Palpate:

  1. Palpate the neck for lymphadenopathy.

  2. Palpate the chest.

  3. Evaluate the abdomen for organomegaly.

  4. Evaluate pedal edema.

F. Mental status: Assess for decreased level of consciousness.

G. Six-minute walking distance (6MWD) test to evaluate desaturation. A medical 6MWD may be found at https://www.mdcalc.com/6-minute-walk-distance.

H. Further physical examinations are dependent on comorbidities.

Diagnostic Tests

A. Spirometry is the gold standard for diagnosing COPD. PFTs are used to diagnose, determine severity, and follow the disease progression of COPD. Perform spirometry before and after the client uses a bronchodilator.

  1. FEV_1 is used as an index to airflow obstruction and evaluates the prognosis in emphysema.

  2. FVC

  3. FEV_1/FVC ratio less than 0.70

B. Chest radiograph: CXR is not required to diagnose COPD but rules out other diagnoses

C. CBC: Evaluate polycythemia due to chronic hypoxia

D. Sputum specimen for culture

E. If the client is younger than age 40 years or has a family history of early onset of emphysema, measure AAT levels. Clients with a family history of AAT deficiencies are at risk of lung damage early in life, as AAT serves to protect lower lung tissue from damage by proteolytic enzymes.

F. Arterial blood gas (ABG)

G. EKG: Note sinus tachycardia, atrial arrhythmias

H. Two-dimensional echocardiogram is used to evaluate secondary pulmonary hypertension.

I. Chest CT is an alternative imaging study for emphysema; however, it is not required as a diagnostic tool

J. Perform a purified protein derivative (PPD) skin test or Quantiferon TB Gold blood test if TB is suspected.

K. Brain natriuretic peptide (BNP)

L. Theophylline level (if applicable)

Differential Diagnoses

A. Asthma

B. Heart failure

C. Bronchiectasis

D. Pulmonary edema

E. TB

F. AAT deficiency

G. Pneumonia

H. Pulmonary embolism

I. CF

J. Cancer

Plan

A. General interventions:

  1. A smoking-cessation plan is an essential part of a comprehensive treatment plan. Develop a smoking-cessation plan; assess readiness to quit. Set a quit date; encourage a group smoking-cessation program. Discuss smoking at every subsequent visit. (*See Section III: Client Teaching Guide for this chapter, "Nicotine Dependence."*) ◀

  2. Advise client to stay away from secondhand smoke and limit exposure to other pulmonary irritants, including extreme temperature changes.

  3. Advise exercise including lung exercises/pulmonary rehabilitation.

  4. Consider pulmonary rehabilitation for all stages of COPD.

  5. The selection of inhalers is dependent on the client's age and ability to use the inhaler. Clients should be evaluated as to their coordination and inspiration abilities necessary to use inhalers; otherwise, aerosol medication via nebulizer is the best delivery method.

  6. Have clients bring in their medication/spacers to demonstrate correct use

B. Client teaching:

  1. *See Section III: Client Teaching Guide for this chapter, "Chronic Obstructive Pulmonary Disease."* ◀

  2. Educate and encourage active participation in the plan of care, including medication adherence

  3. Educate and counsel clients regarding advance directives.

  4. Consider group visits for teaching sessions.

C. Dietary management:

  1. About 25% of clients with COPD are malnourished because of coexisting medical conditions, depression, and inability to shop for or prepare food.

  2. Suggest a low-carbohydrate diet. High-carbohydrate intake may increase respiratory work by increasing CO_2 production.

D. Pharmaceutical therapy: Treatment guidelines are based on spirometry.

> Peak flow meters should not be used to diagnose or monitor COPD.

  1. Stage I (mild FEV_1 80% or greater): The client may be unaware that he or she has COPD. Give influenza vaccine and use SABA bronchodilators as needed.

  2. Stage II (moderate FEV_1 between 50% and 79%): Give influenza vaccine, plus SABA bronchodilators, as needed, plus long-acting bronchodilator(s) plus cardiopulmonary rehabilitation.

  3. Stage III (severe FEV_1 between 30% and 49%): Give influenza vaccine, plus SABA bronchodilators as needed, plus long-acting bronchodilator(s)—for example, a long-acting antimuscarinic antagonist (LAMA), plus cardiopulmonary rehabilitation, plus inhaled glucocorticoid steroids if client has repeated exacerbations.

4. Stage IV (very severe FEV_1 less than 30%): Give influenza vaccine, plus SABA bronchodilator, as needed, plus long-acting bronchodilator(s) (e.g., LAMA), plus cardiopulmonary rehabilitation, plus inhaled glucocorticoid steroids if repeated exacerbations plus long-term oxygen therapy (if the client meets the criteria for O_2). Medicare guidelines require a client's PaO_2 (partial pressure of oxygen) to be less than 55 mmHg or the resting oxygen saturation to be less than 88% on room air.

5. Encourage utilization of a spacer/holding chamber for inhalers.

6. Administer pneumonia vaccines for clients 65 years and older. Prevnar 13 or Pneumovax 23 should be administered according to Centers for Disease Control and Prevention (CDC) recommendations and based on the individual client's vaccine history. See the CDC website for current recommendations.

> Administer yearly flu vaccine. Quadrivalent influenza vaccine is essential for all COPD clients. Give the vaccine each year as soon as it is available.
>
> Prescribe pharmacological agents/nicotine replacement therapy for smoking cessation.

    a. Nicotine chewing gum produces better quit rates than counseling alone.

    b. Transdermal nicotine patches have a long-term success rate of 22% to 42%.

    c. Use of an antidepressant such as Zyban (150 mg twice a day) has been shown to be effective for smoking cessation and may be used in combination with nicotine replacement therapy.

    d. Chantix is a partial agonist selective for alpha-4, beta-2 nicotinic acetylcholine receptors.

7. Antibiotics are not recommended in clients with COPD except with acute exacerbation; with symptoms of increased dyspnea, increased sputum volume, and increased sputum purulence; or with changes in cough, fever, or other evidence of an infection such as an infiltrate on CXR. Antibiotics are prescribed for clients with COPD on mechanical ventilation.

8. Consider phosphodiesterase-4 (PDE-4) inhibitors (Roflumilast or Cilomilast) as needed when necessary.

9. Mucolytic agents have small benefits and are not usually recommended.

10. Antitussives are not recommended.

11. Long-term oxygen has been shown to increase survival in clients with severe resting hypoxemia. Target oxygen saturation is 88% to 92% (Long-Term Oxygen Treatment Trial Research Group, 2016).

12. Cardioselective beta-blockers are not contraindicated in COPD. Cardioselective beta-blockers at low dosages do not cause bronchospasm. A noncardioselective beta-blocker or a cardioselective beta-blocker (B_1-blocker) at higher dosages may contribute to bronchospasm.

13. Methylxanthines (e.g., theophylline) have a risk for toxicity in all clients; this risk is higher in elderly populations. Although methylxanthines have many drug-to-drug interactions, adding theophylline to salmeterol has suggested improvements in FEV_1. Adverse effects could include cardiac arrhythmias and seizure activity.

Follow-Up

A. For acute exacerbations, follow up on the same day or the following day.

B. Reassess stable, chronic COPD every 1 to 2 months, depending on the client's needs.

C. Serial PFTs may help guide therapy and offer prognostic information.

D. Monitor serum theophylline levels. Theophylline has a narrow therapeutic window and the potential for toxicity. Nausea and nervousness are the most common adverse effects. Other adverse effects include abdominal pain with cramps, anorexia, tremors, insomnia, cardiac arrhythmias, and seizures.

E. Reevaluate clients on oxygen therapy 1 to 3 months after starting oxygen.

F. Evaluate for osteoporosis; bone mineral density is lower in clients with COPD, and they are at risk for vertebral fractures.

G. Monitor the client's body weight.

Consultation/Referral

A. Consult with a physician if the client has acute respiratory decompensation, or severe cor pulmonale (distended neck veins, hepatomegaly, dependent peripheral edema, ascites, and pleural effusion).

B. Refer the client to a pulmonary specialist for rehabilitation, if available:

    1. Outpatient education for the client and the family

    2. Exercise training

    3. Breathing retraining—that is, pursed-lip breathing, huff coughing

    4. Correct administration of medications

C. Refer to a registered dietitian (RD) to provide medical nutrition therapy (MNT). RDs focus on the prevention and treatment of weight loss associated with COPD and other comorbidities.

D. Send to a pulmonologist for evaluation for continuous positive airway pressure (CPAP) or bilevel positive airway pressure (BiPAP).

E. Send to a pulmonologist to evaluate for surgical intervention such as bullectomy, lung volume reduction surgery, or lung transplantation.

Individual Considerations

A. Pregnancy:

    1. In pregnancy, COPD is rare except in AAT deficiency.

    2. Monitor drug treatment for potential teratogenic effects.

B. Adults:
  1. Sexual dysfunction is common in clients with COPD; encourage other ways to display affection.
C. Geriatrics:
  1. Presentation may be atypical.
  2. Clients should have annual flu vaccinations and pneumococcal vaccination every 5 years.
  3. Clients may not have the ability to use inhaler devices because of tremors, muscle weakness, poor hand–eye coordination, and/or poor memory.
  4. Theophylline is on the Beers list of drugs to use with caution in the geriatric population related to cardiovascular, renal, and hepatic concerns; insomnia; and peptic ulcers.
  5. Discuss the course of disease, living wills, advance directives, and resuscitation status early, before a crisis occurs.

Resource

Global Initiative for Chronic Obstructive Lung Disease (GOLD) guidelines: www.goldcopd.org

Bibliography

Ball, J. W., Dains, J. E., Flynn, J. A., Solomon, B. S., & Stewart, R. W. (2018). *Seidel's guide to physical examination: An interprofessional approach* (9th ed.). St. Louis, MO: Mosby-Elsevier.

Bartlett, J. G., & Sethi, S. (2018, November). Management of infection in exacerbations of chronic obstructive pulmonary disease. *UpToDate*. Retrieved from http://www.uptodate.com/contents/management-of-infection-in-exacerbations-of-chronic-obstructive-pulmonary-disease?source=search_result&search=Management+of+infection+in+exacerbations+of+chronic+obstructive+pulmonary+disease&selectedTitle=1~150

Centers for Disease Control and Prevention. (2017, May 3). *FastStats chronic obstructive pulmonary disease (COPD) includes: Chronic bronchitis and emphysema.* Retrieved from www.cdc.gov/nchs/fastats/copd.htm

COPD Foundation. (2019). *COPD across America: How does your state compare?* Retrieved from https://www.copdfoundation.org/What-is-COPD/Understanding-COPD/Statistics.aspx

Emanuel, E. J. (2015). Palliative and end-of-life care. In D. L. Kasper, A. S. Fauci, S. L. Hauser, D. L. Longo, & J. L. Jameson (Eds.), *Harrison's principles of internal medicine* (19th ed.). New York, NY: McGraw-Hill. Retrieved from http://accessmedicine.mhmedical.com/book.aspx?bookid=1130

Ferguson, E., & Make, B. (2019, January 21). Management of stable chronic obstructive pulmonary disease. *UpToDate*. Retrieved from http://www.uptodate.com/contents/management-of-stable-chronic-obstructive-pulmonary-disease

Global Initiative for Chronic Obstructive Lung Disease. (2019). *Global strategy for the diagnosis, management, and prevention of COPD.* Retrieved from https://goldcopd.org/

Han, M. K., Dransfield, M. T., & Martinez, F. J. (2018, May). Chronic obstructive pulmonary disease: Definition, clinical manifestations, diagnosis, and staging. *UpToDate*. Retrieved from http://www.uptodate.com/contents/chronic-obstructive-pulmonary-disease-definition-clinical-manifestations-diagnosis-and-staging

Long-Term Oxygen Treatment Trial Research Group; Albert, R. K., Au, D. H., Blackford, A. L., Casaburi, R., & Cooper, J. A. Jr. (2016, October). A randomized trial of long-term oxygen for COPD with moderate desaturation. *New England Journal of Medicine, 375*(17), 1617–1627. doi:10.1056/NEJMoa1604344

Medscape Drug Reference. (n.d.). Theophylline oral. *Medscape.* Retrieved from http://www.medscape.com/druginfo/dosage?drugid=3591&drugname=Theophylline+Oral&monotype=default

National Heart, Lung and Blood Institute, Department of Health and Human Services. (2017). *COPD national action plan.* Retrieved from https://www.nhlbi.nih.gov/sites/default/files/media/docs/COPD%20National%20Action%20Plan%20508_0.pdf

Prescriber's letter. (2018, November). Talk to kids about the harms of e-cigs and vaping. Retrieved from https://prescriber.therapeuticresearch.com/Content/Articles/PRL/2018/Nov/Talk-to-Kids-About-the-Harms-of-E-Cigs-and-Vaping

Rains, S. G. (2020). Fifteen-to-eighteen-month visit. In B. Richardson (Ed.), *Pediatric primary care: Practice guidelines for nurses* (2nd ed., pp. 117–127). Burlington, MA: Jones & Bartlett Learning.

Reilly, J. J., Silverman, E. K., & Shapiro, S. D. (2015). Chronic obstructive pulmonary disease. In D. L. Kasper, A. S. Fauci, S. L. Hauser, D. L. Longo, & J. L. Jameson (Eds.), *Harrison's principles of internal medicine* (19th ed., pp. 1700–1707). New York, NY: McGraw-Hill. Retrieved from http://accessmedicine.mhmedical.com/book.aspx?bookid=1130

Resnick, B. (Ed.). (2017). *GNRS geriatric nursing review syllabus: A core curriculum in advanced practice geriatric nursing* (5th ed.). New York, NY: American Geriatrics Society.

Terry, E. G. (2020). Seven-to-ten-year visit (school age). In B. Richardson (Ed.), *Pediatric primary care: Practice guidelines for nurses* (3rd ed., pp. 147–162). Burlington, MA: Jones & Bartlett Learning.

Weiss, S. T. (2018, August). Chronic obstructive pulmonary disease: Risk factors and risk reduction. *UpToDate.* Retrieved from http://www.uptodate.com/contents/chronic-obstructive-pulmonary-disease-risk-factors-and-risk-reduction

Zachary, K. C. (2019, February). Treatment of seasonal influenza in adults. *UpToDate.* Retrieved from http://www.uptodate.com/contents/treatment-of-seasonal-influenza-in-adults

Common Cold/Upper Respiratory Infection

Mellisa A. Hall and Cheryl A. Glass

Definition

The common cold is a self-limiting acute respiratory tract infection (ARTI) resulting from viral infection of the upper respiratory tract. It is also called *acute nasopharyngitis*. Symptoms of ARTI include mild coryzal symptoms, rhinorrhea, nasal obstruction, and sneezing.

Incidence

ARTIs are among the most frequent reasons for office visits. However, the true incidence is not known because clients treat themselves with OTC and home remedies, as well as seasonal and locational variability. Most children have six to eight colds a year; most adults have two to four.

Pathogenesis

A. More than 25% to 80% of ARTIs are caused by a rhinovirus (greater than 100 antigenic serotypes). Other viral agents include coronavirus (10%–20%), RSV, adenoviruses (5%), influenza viruses (10%–15%), and parainfluenza viruses. The incubation period is 1 to 5 days, with viral shedding lasting up to 2 weeks.
B. Rhinoviral infections are chiefly limited to the upper respiratory tract but may cause otitis media and sinusitis

Predisposing Factors

A. Exposure to airborne droplets
B. Direct contact with virus by touching hands or skin of infected people, or by touching surfaces they touched, and then touching eyes or nose.
C. Very young or old ages
D. Smoking, which increases risk by 50%
E. Crowded conditions such as day-care centers and schools

Common Complaints

A. Low-grade fever
B. Generalized malaise
C. Nasal congestion and discharge (initially clear, then yellow and thick)
D. Sneezing
E. Sore throat or hoarseness
F. Watery and/or inflamed eyes

Other Signs and Symptoms

A. Headache
B. Cough

Subjective Data

A. Elicit the onset, course, and duration of symptoms.
B. Inquire about color and other characteristics of nasal discharge and sputum. Purulent nasal discharge after 14 days signals bacterial sinusitis.
C. Inquire about other discomforts and exposure to people with similar symptoms.
D. Review allergens, seasonal problems, and exposure to irritants and smoke.
E. Review history for other respiratory problems, such as asthma, chronic bronchitis, and emphysema.

Physical Examination

A. Check temperature, pulse, respirations, and BP. Carry out pulse oximetry if difficult respiratory symptoms are noted.
B. Inspect:
   1. Observe general appearance.
   2. Inspect eyes. Note "allergic shiners," tearing, and eyelid swelling.
   3. Observe ears, throat, and mouth. Otitis media is indicated by redness and bulging of tympanic membrane, or by membrane perforation with drainage.
   4. Inspect nose for nasal redness, swelling, polyps, enlarged turbinates, septal deviation, and foreign bodies.
   5. Transilluminate the sinuses:
      a. Group A *Streptococcus*: Tonsilar enlargement, exudate, petechiae
      b. Allergies: "Cobblestoned" pharyngeal mucosa
      c. Mononucleosis: About half of clients with mononucleosis develop tonsillar exudates, and about one third develop petechiae at the junction of the hard and soft palates, which is highly suggestive of the disease.
C. Auscultate:
   1. All lung fields
   2. Heart
D. Percuss:
   1. Sinus cavities and mastoid process of temporal bone to rule out otitis media
   2. Chest for consolidation
E. Palpate:
   1. Palpate face for sinus tenderness.
   2. Examine head and neck for enlarged, tender lymph nodes.

Diagnostic Tests

A. Diagnosis may be made from history and physical examination. Because common cold manifestations are so prevalent, an aggressive workup is rarely necessary.
B. Consider rapid strep test if the client has symptoms or was exposed to group A *Streptococcus*.
C. Consider throat culture if negative rapid strep test and client is symptomatic.

Differential Diagnoses

A. URI
B. Allergic rhinitis
C. Foreign body
D. Sinusitis
E. Influenza
F. Group A strep pharyngitis
G. Otitis media
H. Pneumonia

Plan

A. General interventions:
   1. Controlled trials reveal minimal therapeutic benefits of vitamin C for the treatment and prevention of colds.
   2. Zinc has no proven benefit. Echinacea has not shown any differences in rates of infection or severity of symptoms when compared with placebo.
   3. Validation and standardization of herbal products have not been completed.
B. Client teaching: *See Section III: Client Teaching Guide for this chapter, "Common Cold."* ◀
C. Pharmaceutical therapy:
   1. In a report by Irwin et al. (2018), the American College of Chest Physicians updated 2006 clinical practice guidelines with management algorithms for the management of cough in adults. Healthcare providers should refrain from recommending cough suppressants and OTC cough medicines for young children because of associated morbidity and mortality. The AAP reminds consumers to avoid the use of OTC cough and cold products in children younger than 4 years.
   2. Antibiotics are ineffective in treating viral infection.
   3. CSs may actually increase viral replication and have no impact on cold symptoms.
   4. Topical decongestants for rhinorrhea and nasal congestion
      a. Adults and children older than 6 years: Pseudoephedrine (Afrin) nasal spray 0.05% two to three sprays per nostril twice daily, or phenylephrine (Neo-Synephrine) nasal spray 0.25% to 1% two to three sprays per nostril every 4 hours as needed. Using decongestant-type nasal sprays longer than 2 to 3 days can result in rebound congestion and abuse of the drug.
      b. Children younger than 6 years: Saline nasal drops 2 to 3 drops per nostril two to three times daily.

c. As an alternative to pseudoephedrine and other nasal decongestants, consider clearing nasal congestion in infants with a rubber suction bulb; secretions can be softened with saline nose drops or a cool-mist humidifier.

5. Oral decongestants are available such as pseudo-ephedrine (Sudafed). Side effects include tachycardia, palpitations, and elevated BP.

   a. Adults: Pseudoephedrine (Sudafed) 60 mg every 4 to 6 hours or 120 mg every 12 hours

   b. Children older than 12 years: Pseudoephedrine (Sudafed) liquid 5 mL every 4 to 6 hours, or pseu-doephedrine (Sudafed) 30 mg every 4 to 6 hours

6. Analgesics, such as acetaminophen (Tylenol) and ibuprofen (Advil), may be used for headache relief.

   a. Ibuprofen: Adults: 200 to 400 mg by mouth while symptoms persist; not to exceed 3.2 g/d

   b. Ibuprofen: Pediatrics:

      i. Younger than 6 months: Not established

      ii. 6 months to 12 years: 4 to 10 mg/kg/dose by mouth three to four times a day

      iii. Children older than 12 years: Administered as adults

7. Cough suppressants, if necessary: Dextromethor-phan (Benylin DM, Robitussin, Vicks Formula 44 pediatric formula):

   a. Adults and children older than 12 years: 10 to 20 mg orally every 4 hours, or 30 mg every 6 to 8 hours, or 60 mg extended-release liquid twice daily, to a maximum of 120 mg/d

   b. Elderly: Anticholinergic effects from antihis-tamines may be associated with side effects includ-ing confusion, cognitive impairment, delirium, dry mouth, constipation, urinary retention, and sedation. Diphenhydramine may be appropriate in acute treatment of severe allergic reactions.

8. Colds have no allergic mechanism, so antihista-mines are ineffective. The atropine-like drying effect from antihistamines may exacerbate congestion and obstruct the upper airway by impairing mucus flow.

Follow-Up

A. None is recommended unless symptoms persist lon-ger than 7 days from onset.

B. Parents should return to the doctor's office if their child's fever exceeds 102°F, if respiratory symptoms increase, or if symptoms do not resolve in 10 to 14 days.

Consultation/Referral

A. Consult a physician if the client has been reevaluated and given a new treatment plan but still has symptoms.

B. Refer the client to an otolaryngologist if tonsillary abscess is suspected.

Individual Considerations

A. Pediatrics:

   1. Oral decongestants are not recommended for children younger than 6 years of age.

2. The most common calls to poison control centers that involve OTC medications concern the ingestion of acetaminophen and cough and cold preparations

   a. Accidental pediatric toxic ingestion is reported in children younger than 6 years; intentional toxic ingestion is more common in adolescents aged 13 to 19 years.

   b. Adolescents have used dextromethorphan as a recreational drug.

B. Geriatrics:

   1. Use of antihistamines with anticholinergic prop-erties may cause side effects of confusion and delir-ium as listed earlier, along with increased rates of hospitalization.

Bibliography

American Academy of Pediatrics. (2018, June). *Cough and cold medicine: Not for children.* Retrieved from http://www.choosingwisely.org/clinician -lists/american-academy-pediatrics-cough-and-cold-medicines-for -children-under-four/

Centers for Disease Control and Prevention. (2017). Adverse drug events in children. *Medication Safety Program.* Retrieved from https://www.cdc .gov/medicationsafety/parents_childrenadversedrugevents.html

Dolin, R. (2015). Common viral respiratory infections. In D. L. Kasper, S. L. Hauser, J. L. Jameson, A. S. Fauci, D. L. Longo, & J. Loscalzo (Eds.), *Harrison's principles of internal medicine* (19th ed., pp. 225–227). New York, NY: McGraw-Hill. Retrieved from http://accessmedicine .mhmedical.com/book.aspx?bookid=1130

Irwin, R., French, C., Chang, A., & Altman, K. (2018). Classification of cough as a symptom in adults and management algorithms. *CHEST Journal, 153*(1), 196–209. doi:10.1016/j.chest.2017.10.016

Larson, L., & File. T. M. (2018, July). *Treatment of respiratory infec-tions in pregnant women.* Retrieved from https://www.uptodate.com/ treatment-of-respiratory-infections-in-pregnant-women

Munoz, F. M., & Flomenberg, P. (2018, June). Diagnosis, treatment, and prevention of adenovirus infection. *UpToDate.* Waltham, MA: Wolters Kluwer. Retrieved from http://www.uptodate.com/contents/ diagnosis-treatment-and-prevention-of-adenovirus-infection

Pappas, D. E. (2019, February). *Client information: The common cold in children (Beyond the Basics).* Retrieved from http://www.uptodate.com/ contents/the-common-cold-in-children-beyond-the-basics

Cough

Mellisa A. Hall and Cheryl A. Glass

Definition

A. Coughing is a mechanism that clears the airway of secretions and inhaled particles. The act of coughing has the potential to traumatize the upper airway (e.g., vocal cords). A chronic cough is one that lasts longer than 8 weeks.

B. Coughing can be an affective behavior; psychological issues must be considered as a cause or effect of coughing.

Incidence

A. Data on the incidence of coughing are not available. However, most healthy people do not cough, and the main reason for coughing is airway clearance. A chronic cough is the most common presenting symptom in adults who seek medical treatment in an ambulatory setting.

B. Pertussis affects infants and young children; however, the incidence is increasing in adults secondary to the lack of booster vaccination.

Pathogenesis

A. Stimulation of mucosal neural receptors in the naso-pharynx, ears, larynx, trachea, and bronchi can produce a cough, as can acute inflammation and/or irritation of the respiratory tract. Cough is a reflex response that is mediated by the medulla but is subject to voluntary control. There is clear evidence that vagal afferent nerves regulate involuntary coughing.

B. Pertussis (whooping cough) is caused by the bacterium *B. pertussis*.

C. The pathogenic triad of chronic cough responsible for 92% to 100% of chronic cough is as follows:

    1. Upper airway cough syndrome (UACS), previously referred to as postnasal drip syndrome

    2. Asthma

    3. GERD

Predisposing Factors

A. Pharyngeal irritants

B. Foreign-body aspiration

C. TB (prominent in prisons and nursing homes). Evaluate immigrants from areas where TB is endemic.

D. Psychogenic factors (more common in children and those with emotional stress)

E. Mediastinal or pulmonary masses

F. CHF

G. CF

H. Congenital malformations

I. Viral bronchitis

J. Asthma (sole symptom in 28%)

K. *Mycoplasma* infection

L. UACS, previously referred to as postnasal drip

M. Chronic sinusitis

N. Allergic rhinitis

O. Environmental irritants

P. GERD

Q. Chronic bronchitis

R. Pulmonary edema

S. Medications, including ACE inhibitors

T. Impacted cerumen and external otitis

U. Nonasthmatic eosinophilic bronchitis (NAEB; 13%–33%)

Common Complaints

A. Common complaint is a cough that interferes with ADLs and sleeping, leading to a decrease in a client's QOL.

B. The pertussis cough is uncontrollable and violent. Following coughing, a "whooping" sound follows with a deep breath.

Other Signs and Symptoms

A. Fatigue

B. Rhinitis

C. Epistaxis

D. Tickle in throat

E. Pharyngitis

F. Night sweats

G. Dyspnea

H. Fever

I. Sputum production

J. Hoarseness

K. Postnasal drip

Subjective Data

A. Elicit information about the onset, duration, and course of the cough.

B. Was the onset recent or gradual? Does the cough occur at night? Nocturnal cough may be caused by chronic interstitial pulmonary edema and may signal left-sided heart failure. Cough caused by asthma is also worse at night. Morning cough with sputum suggests bronchitis.

C. Inquire about the cough's characteristics. For example, is it productive, dry, bronchospastic, brassy, wheezy, strong, or weak? If it is productive, is it bloody or mucoid? Note the color, consistency, odor, and amount of sputum or mucus. Dry, irritative cough suggests viral respiratory infection. Severe or changing cough should be evaluated for bronchogenic carcinoma. Rusty-colored sputum suggests bacterial pneumonia. Green or very purulent sputum is due to degeneration of white cells. HIV cough produces purulent sputum.

D. Inquire whether the cough is associated with eating and choking episodes. Wheezing or stridor with coughing may indicate a foreign body or aspiration.

E. Ask whether the cough is associated with postnasal drip, which produces a chronic cough, clear sputum, edematous nasal mucosa, and a "cobblestoned" pharyngeal mucosa.

F. Find out whether the cough is associated with heartburn or a sour taste in the mouth, indicating GERD

G. Ask about precipitating factors, such as exercise, cold air, or laughing.

H. Ask about alleviating factors. Cough from asthma can be triggered or exacerbated by exposure to environmental irritants, allergens, cold, or exercise.

I. Ask about current and previous work. Is the client exposed to occupational and environmental irritants, such as dust, fumes, or gases? If so, what are the type, level, and duration of exposures?

J. Ask about family history of respiratory illness, such as CF or asthma.

K. Is the client a smoker? If so, how much does he or she smoke, and how long has he or she smoked? Is he or she exposed to secondhand smoke? How much of the day? Smoking is the main cause of chronic cough.

L. Find out the date of the client's last tuberculin skin test. Note recent exposure to TB.

M. Inquire about any exposure to the flu.

N. Does the client have a history of heart problems?

O. Does the client have a history of respiratory problems or other medical problems? Chronic bronchitis is a major cause of chronic cough and sputum production. Cough may also be an early sign of lung cancer; in late stages, cough occurs along with weight loss, anorexia, and dyspnea.

P. Review medications such as ACE inhibitors. Cough related to ACE inhibitors usually subsides within 2 weeks, but the median time is up to 26 days.

Q. Common causes of chronic cough in the elderly include postnasal drip, asthma, and gastroesophageal reflux.

Physical Examination

A. Record temperature and BP if indicated.
B. Inspect:
   1. Observe general appearance for cyanosis, difficulty breathing, use of axillary muscles, and finger clubbing.
   2. Examine ears, nose, and throat.
C. Auscultate:
   1. Heart and lungs
D. Percuss:
   1. Sinus cavities and mastoid process
   2. Chest and lungs for consolidation
E. Palpate:
   1. Palpate face for sinus tenderness.
   2. Examine head and neck for lymph nodes, masses, and jugular vein distention (JVD).

Diagnostic Tests

Testing can be held to a minimum by careful review of history and physical examination. Children with chronic cough should undergo, at a minimum, a chest x-ray and spirometry (if age appropriate).

A. White blood cell (WBC) if infection suspected
B. HIV test if suspected
C. Sputum for eosinophils, Gram stain, and/or culture
D. Mantoux test if indicated or Quantiferon TB Gold
E. CXR
F. Sweat chloride test to rule out CF
G. Pulmonary function testing/spirometry
H. Methacholine challenge to rule out asthma
I. Esophageal pH monitoring to rule out GERD
J. CT scan if necessary

Differential Diagnoses

A. Environmental irritants:
   1. Cigarette, cigar, or pipe smoking
   2. Pollutants (e.g., wood smoke, smog, burning leaves)
   3. Dust
   4. Lack of humidity
B. Lower respiratory tract problems:
   1. Lung cancer
   2. Asthma
   3. Chronic obstructive lung disease (includes bronchitis)
   4. Interstitial lung disease
   5. CHF
   6. Pneumonitis
   7. Bronchiectasis
C. Upper respiratory tract problems:
   1. Chronic rhinitis
   2. Chronic sinusitis
   3. Disease of external auditory canal
   4. Pharyngitis
D. Medication-induced cough from ACE inhibitors

E. Extrinsic compression lesions:
   1. Adenopathy
   2. Malignancy
   3. Aortic aneurysm
F. Psychogenic factors, more common in children and those with emotional stress
G. GI problems such as reflux esophagitis
H. Genetic problems such as CF

Plan

A. General intervention:
   1. If sputum is purulent, obtain a sample for examination.
   2. Clients with COPD and CF should be taught huffing as an adjunct to other methods of sputum clearance.
B. Client teaching: *See Section III: Client Teaching Guide for this chapter, "Cough."* ◄
C. Pharmaceutical therapy:
   1. In 2018, the American College of Chest Physicians updated 2006 clinical practice guidelines with management algorithms for the management of cough in adults. Healthcare providers should refrain from recommending cough suppressants and OTC cough medicines for young children because of associated morbidity and mortality. The AAP reminds consumers to avoid the use of OTC cough and cold products in children younger than 4 years.
   2. Antibiotics should not be prescribed for cough unless a bacterial infection is suspected.
   3. Therapy depends on various acute inflammatory and chronic irritating processes and on the cause of the cough. Refer to applicable sections of this chapter, such as "Asthma" and "Tuberculosis," and see Chapter 11, "Gastrointestinal Guidelines."

Follow-Up

A. The client with a normal CXR and no risk factors for lung cancer (e.g., smoking or occupational exposure) can be followed expectantly without further testing.
B. In clients whose cough resolves after the cessation of ACE inhibitors, and for whom there is a compelling reason to treat with these agents, a repeat trial of ACE inhibitors may be attempted.
C. See applicable sections for specific diagnoses.
D. Pertussis vaccination is available for infants, children, preteens, adults, and the elderly. Pertussis cases should be reported to the local health department.

Consultation/Referral

A. Consult a physician if symptoms persist after treatment. Reevaluate the client in 2 weeks if he or she is no better.
B. When a cough lasts more than 2 weeks without another apparent cause and it is accompanied by paroxysms of coughing, post-tussive vomiting, and/or an inspiratory whooping sound, the diagnosis of a *B. pertussis* infection should be made unless another diagnosis is proven.
C. Clients whose condition remains undiagnosed after a workup and therapy may need referral to a cough specialist.

Individual Considerations

A. Pregnancy:
  1. Cough may be an early symptom of pulmonary edema. Watch intrapartum clients for signs of edema.
B. Pediatrics:
  1. The most common calls to poison control centers involve the ingestion of acetaminophen and cough and cold preparations. Accidental pediatric toxic ingestion is reported in children younger than 6 years; intentional toxic ingestion is more common in adolescents aged 13 to 19 years. Adolescents have used dextromethorphan as a recreational drug.
  2. Children with chronic productive purulent cough should always be investigated to document the presence or absence of bronchiectasis and to identify underlying and treatable causes such as CF and immune deficiency.
C. Geriatrics:
  1. Aspiration should be considered in the elderly with chronic cough, as well as heart failure, laryngeal dysfunction, bronchiectasis, or tumors of the central airway.

Bibliography

American Academy of Pediatrics. (2018, June). *Cough and cold medicine: Not for children*. Retrieved from http://www.choosingwisely.org/clinician-lists/american-academy-pediatrics-cough-and-cold-medicines-for-children-under-four/

Centers for Disease Control and Prevention. (2017). Adverse drug events in children. *Medication Safety Program*. Retrieved from https://www.cdc.gov/medicationsafety/parents_childrenadversedrugevents.html

Gibson, P., Wang, G., McGarvey, L., Vertigan, A. E., Altman, K. W., Birring, S. S., & Chest Expert Cough Panel. (2016). Treatment of unexplained chronic cough: CHEST guideline and Expert Panel report. *Chest, 149*, 27–44. doi:10.1378/chest.15-1496. Retrieved from https://www.ncbi.nlm.nih.gov/pmc/articles/PMC5831652/

Kritek, P. A., & Fanta, C. H. (2015). Cough and hemoptysis. In D. L. Kasper, A. S. Fauci, S. L. Hauser, D. L. Longo, J. L. Jameson, & J. Loscalzo (Eds.), *Harrison's principles of internal medicine* (19th ed., pp. 243–247). New York, NY: McGraw-Hill. Retrieved from http://accessmedicine.mhmedical.com/book.aspx?bookid=1130

Rains, S. G. (2020). Fifteen-to-eighteen-month visit. In B. Richardson (Ed.), *Pediatric primary care: Practice guidelines for nurses* (2nd ed., pp. 117–127). Burlington, MA: Jones & Bartlett Learning.

Resnick, B. (Ed.). (2017). *GNRS geriatric nursing review syllabus: A core curriculum in advanced practice geriatric nursing* (5th ed.). New York, NY: American Geriatrics Society.

Terry, E. G. (2020). Seven-to-ten-year visit (school age). In B. Richardson (Ed.), *Pediatric primary care: Practice guidelines for nurses* (3rd ed., pp. 147–162). Burlington, MA: Jones & Bartlett Learning.

Zachary, K. C. (2019, February). Treatment of seasonal influenza in adults. *UpToDate*. Retrieved from http://www.uptodate.com/contents/treatment-of-seasonal-influenza-in-adults

Croup, Viral

Mellisa A. Hall and Cheryl A. Glass

Definition

A. Viral croup is an acute inflammatory disease of the larynx, also called *laryngotracheobronchitis*. Croup is the most common cause of stridor in febrile children. The uncomplicated disease usually wanes in 3 to 5 days but may persist up to 10 days. Croup is most often self-limited, but occasionally is severe and rarely fatal. Lethargy, cyanosis, and decreasing retractions are indications of impending respiratory failure.
B. Inspiratory stridor suggests a laryngeal obstruction.
C. Poiseuille's equation states that flow (air, fluid) is directly proportional to the radius of the chamber to the fourth power and inversely proportional to the length. Realizing that pediatric airways are relatively small compared to adult counterparts, a twofold decrease in airway radius decreases the airflow by 16-fold. Therefore, airway resistance is exquisitely sensitive to changes in radius in the pediatric population.
D. Expiratory stridor suggests tracheobronchial obstruction.
E. Spasmodic croup may be a noninfectious variant with symptoms always occurring at night and has the hallmark of reoccurring in children. Although viral illness may trigger this variant, the reaction may be allergic.

Incidence

The most common form of acute upper airway obstruction, croup, generally affects children aged 6 months to 3 years. Croup has a peak incidence during the second year of life and is more common in boys than girls (1.5:5 ratio). In the United States, it accounts for 7% of pediatric hospitalizations in children younger than 4 years, and it is most prevalent in younger children in fall and early winter.

Pathogenesis

Parainfluenza viruses types 1, 2, and 3 cause about 80% of croup. The initial port of entry is the nose and nasopharynx. Other viral causes include enterovirus and rhinovirus. Influenza A and B, RSV, adenovirus, coronavirus, herpes simplex virus (HSV), and measles are less common causes. In a small number of cases, croup may be caused by *M. pneumoniae*. Inflammation usually occurs in the entire airway, and edema formation in the subglottic space accounts for the predominant signs of upper airway obstruction.

Predisposing Factors

A. URI
B. Male-to-female ratio of 1.4:1
C. Ages 6 months to 3 years (mean onset: 18 months)
D. Hyperactive airway
E. Anatomic narrowing of the airway
F. Acquired airway narrowing (from intubation, GERD scarring, or human papillomavirus [HPV] papillomas)

Common Complaints

A. Hoarseness
B. Cough progressing to a seal-like barking cough
C. Stridor, especially during sleep
D. Fever, usually absent or low grade, but may be high
E. Runny nose

Subjective Data

A. Determine the onset, duration, and course of illness
B. Has the child been exposed to respiratory illness?
C. Is the child coughing? Having trouble breathing?

D. Has the child had fever, nausea, vomiting, or diarrhea?

E. Are immunizations up to date?

Physical Examination

Have the child sit upright in a parent's lap to perform the physical examination. Persistent crying increases oxygen demand and respiratory muscle fatigue.

A. Record temperature, pulse, respirations, and BP.

B. Inspect:

1. Observe overall appearance, noting respiratory pattern, retractions, nasal flaring, and air hunger. Children often sound terrible but do not look very ill.

2. Check nail beds and lips for cyanosis (ominous sign).

3. Assess skin and mucous membranes for signs of dehydration.

4. Observe for drooling or difficulty swallowing.

5. Inspect throat for foreign body.

6. Inspect eyes, ears, nose, and throat for infection.

C. Auscultate:

1. Auscultate heart. Tachycardia is out of proportion to fever.

2. Auscultate lungs for unequal breath sounds (signals foreign-body aspiration). Stridor is an audible harsh, high-pitched musical sound that may be noted on inspiration or heard during both inspiration and expiration. Stridor is audible without a stethoscope.

3. The Westley score is a way to quantify the severity of respiratory compromise. The severity of croup is evaluated by assessing inspiratory stridor, air entry, retractions, cyanosis, and level of consciousness (see Table 9.2).

D. Percuss chest.

E. Palpate neck to evaluate lymph nodes.

F. Neurologic examination: Assess level of alertness.

Diagnostic Tests

The diagnosis of croup is largely clinical, based on the presenting history and physical examination findings.

A. Pulse oximetry assesses respiratory status.

B. Laboratory testing is usually not needed for croup in a well-hydrated client. However, a CBC may be indicated.

C. Imaging is not required in mild cases with a typical history that responds appropriately to treatment.

D. CXR may show the "steeple or pencil sign."

E. Anterior–posterior (AP) soft-tissue neck radiography may show subglottic narrowing.

F. Bronchoscopy or laryngoscopy may be required in unusual circumstances.

G. ABGs are unnecessary as they do not indicate hypoxia or hypercarbia unless respiratory fatigue is present.

Differential Diagnoses

A. Bacterial croup

B. Epiglottitis

C. Spasmodic croup

D. Membranous croup

E. Bacterial tracheitis

F. Retropharyngeal abscess

TABLE 9.2   WESTLEY SCORING FOR CROUP

Symptom	Scoring
Inspiratory stridor	No inspiratory stridor = 0 points
	Stridor upon agitation = 1 point
	Stridor at rest = 2 points
Retractions	Mild = 1 point
	Moderate = 2 points
	Severe = 3 points
Air entry	Normal = 1 point
	Mild decrease = 1 point
	Marked decrease = 2 points
Cyanosis	None = 0 points
	Cyanosis upon agitation = 4 points
	Cyanosis at rest = 5 points
Level of consciousness	Normal = 0 points
	Disoriented = 5 points

Mild disease = A score of less than 2 points. Occasional barking coughs, no stridor at rest, and mild to no suprasternal or subcostal retraction.

Moderate disease = A score of 3 to 7 points. Frequent cough, audible stridor at rest, visible retractions, but little distress or agitation.

Severe disease = A score of 8 or greater. Frequent cough, prominent inspiratory (occasional expiratory) stridor, obvious retraction, decreased air entry on auscultation, and significant distress and agitation.

Source: Adapted from Woods, C. R. (2019, January). Croup: Approach to management. *UpToDate*. Waltham, MA: Wolters Kluwer. Retrieved from http://www.uptodate.com/contents/croup-approach-to-management.

G. Diphtheria

H. Foreign bodies (GI or trachea)

I. RSV

J. Measles

K. Varicella

L. Influenza A or B

M. Mechanical trauma or lesions

Plan

A. General interventions:

1. Treatment is supportive for clients without stridor at rest.

2. Stress rest and minimal activity.

3. Cool-mist therapy has not been shown to be clinically effective.

4. Hot steam should be avoided due to the potential of scalding.

B. Client teaching: *See Section III: Client Teaching Guide for this chapter, "Croup, Viral."*

C. Pharmaceutical therapy:

1. Antibiotics are not indicated for the treatment of croup

2. Acetaminophen (Tylenol) 5 to 15 mg/kg/dose for fever

3. In moderate to severe cases requiring hospitalization: Nebulized racemic epinephrine (asthmanefrin solution) 0.5 mL of 2.25% solution in 2.5 mL sterile water may relieve airway obstruction up to 2 hours. Treatment may be repeated three times.

4. Steroid use is controversial but may be considered if the preceding therapy is ineffective. Steroids are used to decrease subglottic edema by suppressing the local inflammatory process. CSs should not be given to children with untreated TB.

    a. Decadron (dexamethasone) is the drug of choice. Pediatric dosing is 0.6 mg/kg in a single dose orally or intramuscularly. Maximum 16 mg

    b. Budesonide (Pulmicort Respules inhalation suspension) has been shown to be equivalent to oral dexamethasone. Pediatric dosing is 2 mg (2 mL of suspension) nebulized.

    c. Prednisone (Deltasone) pediatric dosing is 1 to 2 mg/kg/d orally daily or in a divided dose twice a day for 5 days

    d. Observation for 3 to 4 hours is recommended following the initial treatment.

D. Dietary management: Give plenty of fluids.

E. Medical/surgical management: If pulse oximetry shows desaturation, administer oxygen and monitor carefully.

Follow-Up

Call the parent in 12 to 24 hours to evaluate client status.

Consultation/Referral

A. Consultation with an otolaryngologist and anesthetist before rapid-sequence induction may be necessary if the client is exhibiting rapid deterioration.

B. Refer the client to a physician if he or she is a child who is severely ill with respiratory distress or dehydration.

C. Refer the client to a physician if there is no improvement in 12 to 24 hours.

D. Clients with stridor at rest should be admitted to the hospital.

Individual Considerations

A. Pediatrics:

    1. Most children improve within a few days.

    2. Virus is most contagious during the first few days of fever.

    3. Children may return to day care or school when temperature is normal and they feel better, even if cough lingers.

    4. Children older than 5 years of age with recurrent croup should be referred to an otolaryngologist for evaluation.

Bibliography

Dolin, R. (2015). Common viral respiratory infections: Croup. In D. L. Kasper, S. L. Hauser, J. L. Jameson, A. S. Fauci, D. L. Longo, & J. Loscalzo (Eds.), *Harrison's principles of internal medicine* (19th ed., p. 1208). New York, NY: McGraw-Hill. Retrieved from http://accessmedicine.mhmedical.com/book.aspx?bookid=1130

Epocrates Online. (2019). Pulmicort Flexhaler. Retrieved from https://online.epocrates.com/drugs/464802/Pulmicort-Flexhaler/Peds-Dosing

Munoz, F. M., & Flomenberg, P. (2018, June). Diagnosis, treatment, and prevention of adenovirus infection. *UpToDate*. Retrieved from http://www.uptodate.com

Sizar, O., & Carr, B. (2019, April 1). Croup. *StatPearls*. Retrieved from https://www.ncbi.nlm.nih.gov/books/NBK431070/

Weiner, D. L. (2018, August). Causes of acute respiratory distress in children. *UpToDate*. Retrieved from http://www.uptodate.com/contents/causes-of-acute-respiratory-distress-in-children

Woods, C. R. (2018, June). Croup: Clinical features, evaluation, and diagnosis. *UpToDate*. Retrieved from http://www.uptodate.com/contents/croup-clinical-features-evaluation-and-diagnosis

Woods, C. R. (2019, January). Croup: Approach to management. *UpToDate*. Retrieved from http://www.uptodate.com/contents/croup-approach-to-management

Emphysema

Mellisa A. Hall and Cheryl A. Glass

Definition

A. Emphysema is an abnormal dilation and destruction of alveolar ducts and air spaces distal to the terminal bronchioles. Lung function slowly deteriorates over many years before the illness develops. COPD—a term that refers to conditions characterized by continued increased resistance to expiratory airflow—encompasses chronic bronchitis, emphysema, and asthma. Chronic bronchitis and emphysema with airflow obstruction commonly occur together, and as such are usually discussed together in terms of treatment.

B. There are three morphological types of emphysema:

    1. Centriacinar emphysema is associated with long-term smoking and primarily involves the upper half of the lungs.

    2. Panacinar emphysema is predominant in the lower half of the lungs. Panacinar emphysema is observed in clients with AAT deficiency.

    3. Paraseptal emphysema involves the distal airway.

Incidence

A. Emphysema typically occurs in people older than 50 years, with peak occurrence between ages 65 and 75 years.

B. Approximately 14 million people in the United States have emphysema.

Pathogenesis

Decreased gas exchange occurs due to focal destruction limited to the air spaces distal to the respiratory bronchioles, causing airway obstruction, hyperinflation, loss of lung recoil, and destruction of the alveolar–capillary interface.

Predisposing Factors

A. Long-term cigarette smoking

B. Occupational and environmental exposure to toxic agents:

    1. Dust

    2. Chemical fumes

    3. Secondhand smoke

    4. Air pollution

    5. Gases

    6. Respiratory infection

C. Alpha-1 protease inhibitor deficiency

D. Intravenous (IV) drug use secondary to pulmonary vascular damage from the insoluble fillers (e.g., cornstarch, cotton fibers, cellulose, talc)

E. Connective tissue disorders (e.g., Marfan syndrome, Ehlers-Danlos syndrome)

F. HIV

Common Complaints
A. Gradually progressing exertional dyspnea
B. Chronic cough
C. Wheezing
D. Fatigue
E. Weight loss

Other Signs and Symptoms
A. Cough with mild to moderate sputum production and clear to mucoid sputum
B. Early-morning cough
C. SOB
D. Tachypnea
E. Use of accessory muscles for breathing; pursed-lip breathing; *prolonged* expiration
F. Barrel chest (increased anterior-to-posterior chest diameter)
G. Flushed skin
H. Clubbed fingers
I. Decreased libido
J. Thin, wasted appearance
K. Wheezing, particularly during exertion and exacerbations of emphysema

Subjective Data
A. Elicit information about the onset, duration, and course of symptoms.
B. Determine whether the client is a smoker. If so, how much and for how long? Evaluate exposure to second-hand smoke. How much of the day?
C. Ask about current and previous work. Is the client exposed to occupational and environmental irritants, such as dust, fumes, or gases? If so, what are the type, level, and duration of exposures?
D. Inquire about the cough's characteristics. Is it productive, dry, bronchospastic, brassy, wheezy, strong, or weak?
E. Question the client about episodes of tachypnea, frequency of respiratory infections, and incidence of angina during exertion.
F. Does the client have a hereditary disease (e.g., CF or AAT deficiency), asthma, nasal abnormalities (e.g., deviated septum), or other respiratory problems?
G. When was the client's last tuberculin skin test done?
H. Find out the client's usual weight and assess how much weight loss has occurred and over what time period.
I. Evaluate current vaccination status for pneumonia and influenza.
J. Review all medications, including OTC and herbal products.
K. Assess the client's ability to perform ADLs and IADLs, including grooming and personal hygiene, performing chores around the home, shopping, cooking, and driving.
L. Ask about alcohol use.

Physical Examination
A. Temperature (if indicated), pulse, respirations, BP, and weight. Consider pulse oximetry.
B. Inspect:
　1. Observe general appearance; note flushed skin color, use of accessory muscles, pallor around lips, pursed-lip breathing, barrel chest (lung hyperinflation), and thinness.
　2. Assess for peripheral edema.
　3. Dermal examination: Note finger clubbing and cyanosis.
C. Auscultate:
　1. Auscultate heart.
　2. Auscultate lungs for wheezes, crackles, decreased breath sounds (generally diffuse decreased breath sound).
　3. Assess for vocal fremitus (vibration) and egophony (increased resonance and high-pitch bleating quality). Air trapping causes air pockets that do not transmit sound well.
　4. Auscultate carotid arteries and abdomen for bruits.
D. Percuss:
　1. Chest for presence of hyperresonance and signs of consolidation
E. Palpate:
　1. Palpate abdomen.
　2. Evaluate pedal edema.
　3. Evaluate the abdomen for organomegaly.
F. Further physical examinations are dependent on comorbidities.

Diagnostic Tests
A. Pulse oximetry: Blood gases if indicated
B. AAT deficiency to rule out hereditary deficiency
C. Tuberculin skin test or Quantiferon TB Gold blood test
D. PFTs reveal increased total lung capacity with poor respiratory expulsion and increased respiratory volume.
E. EKG reveals sinus or supraventricular tachycardia.
F. CXR reveals hyperinflation, flat diaphragm, and enlarged heart.
G. Sputum evaluation and/or culture

Differential Diagnoses
A. Emphysema
B. Chronic bronchitis
C. Chronic asthma
D. Bronchiectasis
E. CF
F. Chronic asthmatic bronchitis
G. TB
H. AAT deficiency
I. CHF

Plan
A. General interventions:
　1. Medical management: Supplemental oxygen therapy is indicated if the client has a resting PaO_2 less than 55 mmHg or a PaO_2 less than 60 mmHg, along with right-heart failure or secondary polycythemia. Goals are to achieve a PaO_2 of greater than 55 mmHg (usually 1–3 L/min).
　2. Develop a smoking-cessation plan: Assess readiness to quit. Set a quit date and encourage a group

smoking-cessation program. A smoking-cessation plan is an essential part of a comprehensive treatment plan.

   a. Nicotine chewing gum produces better quit rates than counseling alone.

   b. Transdermal nicotine patches have a long-term success rate of 22% to 42%.

   c. The use of an antidepressant, such as Zyban (150 mg twice a day), has been shown to be effective for smoking cessation and may be used in combination with nicotine replacement therapy.

   d. Chantix is a partial agonist selective for alpha-4, beta-2 nicotinic acetylcholine receptors

▶ B. Client teaching: *See Section III: Client Teaching Guide for this chapter, "Emphysema."*

C. Pharmaceutical therapy:

1. Drugs of choice are inhaled beta-2 agonists. Beta-2 agonists are used primarily for relief of symptoms and, in stable clients, have an additive effect when used with an anticholinergic agent (e.g., ipratropium bromide). A spacer/chamber device should be used to improve delivery and reduce adverse effects. The following inhaled preparations have rapid action and fewer cardiac side effects:

   a. Ipratropium bromide (Atrovent) has bronchodilatory activity with minimum side effects.

      i. MDI: Two to four puffs every 4 to 6 hours

      ii. Nebulizer: 250 mcg diluted with 2.5 mL normal saline every 4 to 6 hours

   b. Tiotropium (Spiriva) is a bronchodilator similar to ipratropium. Available in a capsule form containing a dry powder or oral inhalation via a HandiHaler inhalation device. Adults: 1 capsule (18 mcg) inhaled every day via the inhaler device.

   c. Metaproterenol sulfate (Alupent) is available as a liquid for nebulizer and MDI.

      i. MDI: Two puffs every 3 to 4 hours

      ii. Nebulizer: 0.2 to 0.3 mL of 5% solution diluted to 2.5 mL with normal saline three to four times a day

   d. Albuterol (Proventil, Ventolin) is available as a liquid for nebulizer, MDI, and DPI.

      i. MDI: One to four puffs every 3 to 4 hours

      ii. Nebulizer: 0.2 to 0.3 mL of 5% solution diluted to 2.5 mL with normal saline three to four times a day

2. If improvement is not satisfactory or tachyphylaxis occurs, consider theophylline. Theophylline improves respiratory muscle function, stimulates the respiratory center, and bronchodilates. It has a narrow therapeutic index and many drug-to-drug interactions. Side effects may include tachycardia, arrhythmias, and seizure activity. Toxicity is more common in elderly.

   a. Initial dose: 10 mg/kg daily divided in oral doses every 8 to 12 hours

   b. Maintenance: 10 mg/kg daily divided in oral doses every day or twice a day; adjust doses in 25% increments to maintain serum theophylline level of 5 to 15 mcg/mL—not to exceed 800 mg/d

3. Oral steroids should be used to treat outpatients with acute exacerbations. CSs reduce mucosal edema, inhibit prostaglandins that cause bronchoconstriction, and increase responsiveness to bronchodilators. Taper the dose as soon as bronchospasm is controlled. A minority of clients who respond to oral steroids can be maintained on long-term inhaled steroids.

4. In clients with COPD, chronic infection or colonization of the lower airways is common. The goal of antibiotic therapy is not to eliminate organisms, but rather to treat acute exacerbations. If infection is present, give one of the following:

   a. Doxycycline 100 mg twice daily

   b. Trimethoprim–sulfamethoxazole 160/800 mg twice daily

   c. Clarithromycin 250 to 500 mg orally twice daily

   d. Cefaclor (Ceclor) 250 to 500 mg orally every 8 hours; this drug is active against *Pneumococcus* and *H. influenzae*

5. Mucolytic agents in clinical practice are not recommended because of a lack of evidence for their benefit.

6. Quadrivalent influenza vaccine is essential for all clients with COPD. Give the client the vaccine each October, at least 6 weeks before the onset of flu season.

7. Pneumococcal vaccines are essential for clients with COPD. Administer according to the CDC adult immunization recommendations.

8. Clients with AAT deficiency (antitrypsin deficiency lab value is less than 80 mg/dL) must receive weekly or monthly infusions. Consult with a physician before therapy. A history of smoking rules out candidacy.

Follow-Up

A. If the client is acutely ill, contact him or her by phone in 24 to 48 hours and consider immediate referral.

B. Monitor the client's body weight.

C. Serial PFTs may help guide therapy and offer prognostic information.

D. Monitor theophylline levels because of the drug's potential for toxicity. Nausea and nervousness are the most common adverse effects. Other adverse effects include abdominal pain with cramps, anorexia, tremors, insomnia, cardiac arrhythmia, and seizures. Theophylline doses: 100 to 200 mg every 6 to 8 hours.

Consultation/Referral

A. If the client's condition remains acute after 48 hours of treatment, consider immediate referral to a physician.

B. Refer the client to a social worker for help in getting "Meals on Wheels," handicapped parking, and finding other community resources.

C. A consultation with a pulmonary specialist is recommended.

Individual Considerations
A. Adults:
   1. Sexual dysfunction is common in clients with COPD; encourage other ways to display affection.
   2. Depression is a common comorbidity with COPD. Clients should be screened and treated appropriately.
B. Geriatrics:
   1. Discuss course of disease, living wills, advance directives, and resuscitation status early, before a crisis occurs.
   2. Theophylline is on the Beers list of drugs to use with caution in the geriatric population related to cardiovascular, renal, and hepatic effects; insomnia; and peptic ulcers.

Resources
A Patient's Guide to Aerosol Drug Delivery: www.aarc.org/resources/clinical-resources/aerosol-resources
A Guide to Aerosol Delivery Devices for Respiratory Therapists: www.aarc.org/app/uploads/2015/04/aerosol_guide_rt.pdf
National Emphysema Foundation: www.emphysema-foundation.org
Global Initiative for Chronic Obstructive Lung Disease (GOLD) Guidelines: www.goldcopd.org

Bibliography
Centers for Disease Control and Prevention. (2017, May 3). *FastStats chronic obstructive pulmonary disease (COPD) includes: Chronic bronchitis and emphysema*. Retrieved from www.cdc.gov/nchs/fastats/copd.htm
Parul, P., & Sharma, S. (2019, February 23). Emphysema. *StatPearls*. Retrieved from https://www.ncbi.nlm.nih.gov/books/NBK482217/

Obstructive Sleep Apnea

Mellisa A. Hall and Cheryl A. Glass

Definition
Obstructive sleep apnea (OSA) is the periodic reduction (hypopnea) or cessation (apnea) of breathing due to a narrowing or occlusion of the upper airway during sleep. OSA has been linked to traffic accidents, cardiac diseases, stroke, diabetes, and visceral obesity. It is also associated with nocturnal cardiac arrhythmias and chronic and acute cardiac events, and is a risk factor for strokes. When in the supine sleeping position, symptoms of OSA may worsen. The following are diagnostic criteria for OSA if either of these two conditions exists:
A. The presence of 15 or more apneas, hypopneas, or respiratory effort-related arousals per hour of sleep in an asymptomatic client. More than 75% of the apneas and hypopneas must be obstructive.
B. Five or more obstructive apneas, obstructive hypopneas, or respiratory effort-related arousals per hour of sleep in a client with symptoms or signs of disturbed sleep. More than 75% of the apneas or hypopneas must be obstructive.

Incidence
A. The incidence of OSA attributed to obesity has increased steadily over the past 30 years and is estimated at 58% in the morbidly obese population. Generally, in the middle-aged population, the incidence of moderate to severe OSA in males is 50% and in females is 25%.
B. In nonobese and otherwise healthy children younger than 8 years, incidence is between 1% and 3%. Obesity adds a fourfold added risk for disordered breathing.
C. Most children with OSA are aged 2 to 10 years, coinciding with adenotonsillar lymphatic tissue growth. (Surgical removal of enlarged tonsils and adenoids usually results in a complete cure.)
D. Most cases in adults are undiagnosed.

Pathogenesis
Increased tissue thickness of the structures of the tongue and soft tissues in the pharyngeal cavity, which decreases the passageway for air to the trachea, is thought to be the mechanism of OSA. During the night, the muscles of the oropharynx relax, which results in the relative obstruction of the airway. Obesity and hypertrophy of tonsils and/or adenoids account for most cases of OSA in children. Poor neurocognitive performance and increased risk for mortality, including cardiovascular disease, is associated with OSA.

Predisposing Factors
A. Obesity
B. Increased neck circumference
C. Age: Increases in older persons (older than 65 years)
D. Gender: Males
E. Postmenopause
F. Hypothyroidism
G. Tonsillar hypertrophy
H. Alcohol
I. Craniofacial abnormalities
J. Medications:
   1. Benzodiazepines
   2. Antipsychotics
   3. Opioid analgesics
   4. Beta-blockers
   5. Barbiturates
   6. Antihistamines
   7. Sedative antidepressants
K. Allergic rhinitis
L. Genetic conditions (e.g., Down syndrome, Pierre Robin anomalies, Marfan syndrome)
M. Ethnicity (e.g., Black, Asian, Hispanic)
N. Acromegaly
O. Family history
P. Diabetes
Q. Hypertension

Common Complaints
A. Daytime sleepiness
B. Loud snoring, gasping, or snorting during sleep
C. Fatigue

Other Signs and Symptoms
A. Adults:
   1. Asymptomatic: Clients may not recognize they have OSA because they are able to go to sleep anytime.
   2. Restless sleep

3. Dry mouth or sore throat
4. Lack of physical or mental energy
5. Falling asleep when watching TV, reading, driving/riding in a car
6. Morning headaches
7. Decreased libido and impotence
8. Cognitive deficits
B. Children:
1. Short attention span
2. Emotional lability
3. Behavioral problems
4. Enuresis

Subjective Data

A. Does the client feel sleepy during the day? Is daytime sleepiness a problem?
B. Does the client struggle to stay awake during the day?
C. Does the client take naps? How often and how long does the client sleep?
D. Does the client feel physically and mentally exhausted?
E. Does the client's bed partner complain about snoring, gasping, or snorting?
F. Ask the Epworth Sleepiness Scale questions related to how often the client dozes off or falls asleep (in contrast to just feeling tired). Each situation is scored from 0 = would never doze, to 1 = a slight change of dozing, 2 = moderate chance of dozing, and 3 = a high chance of dozing. There are eight situations to which the client should respond:
1. Sitting and reading
2. Watching TV
3. Sitting inactive in a public place (e.g., a theater or meeting)
4. As a passenger in a car for an hour without a break
5. Lying down to rest during the day when circumstances permit
6. Sitting and talking to someone
7. Sitting quietly after lunch without alcohol
8. In a car, while stopped for a few minutes in traffic
G. Ask the client to list all medications currently being taken, particularly substances not prescribed, including OTC and herbal products.
H. Review alcohol use.
I. Men who present with sleep disorders should also be questioned about the presence of erectile dysfunction.

Physical Examination

A. BP, pulse, respirations, height and weight to calculate BMI, and waist measurement
B. Inspect:
1. Oropharynx examination for:
   a. Peritonsillar narrowing or hypertrophy
   b. Tongue (evaluate for macroglossia)
   c. Elongated or enlarged uvula
   d. Palate (high arch or narrow palate)
2. Nasal examination; look for septal deviation and nasal polyps
3. Inspect for signs of pulmonary hypertension or cor pulmonale
   a. Jugular venous distention
   b. Peripheral edema
C. Palpate:
1. Thyroid gland
D. Auscultate:
1. Heart and lungs
E. Mental status:
1. Assess for confusion.

Diagnostic Tests

A. Polysomnography (PSG) is the standard method of diagnosis. The apnea hypopnea index (AHI) or the respiratory disturbance index (RDI) is used to quantify hypopneas and classify the degree of sleep disturbance.
1. Full-night PSG
2. Split-night PSG
3. Home testing with portable monitors
B. Routine laboratory work is not helpful in the confirmation or exclusion of OSA.

Differential Diagnoses

A. OSA
B. Primary snoring
C. Narcolepsy
D. Restless leg syndrome
E. Swallowing disorder
F. Nocturnal seizures
G. GERD
H. Obesity hypoventilation syndrome
I. Sleep deprivation
J. Neurodegenerative disease (e.g., Parkinson's disease, dementia, Alzheimer's disease)
K. Substance abuse
L. Tonsillar hypertrophy

Plan

A. General interventions:
1. CPAP or BiPAP is the mainstay of treatment for moderate to severe OSA
B. Client teaching: *See Section III: Client Teaching Guide for this chapter, "Sleep Apnea."* ◀
1. Educate the client about modifying controllable risk factors such as keeping diabetes and hypertension under control, healthy diet, exercise, and stopping smoking.
2. Treatment with CPAP and BiPAP is required at all times during the night and during naps.
3. Behavioral strategies include sleeping in a non-supine position using a positioning device (e.g., alarm, pillow, backpack, tennis ball are used for positional therapy).
4. Give the client a teaching sheet on sleep apnea.
C. Dietary management:
1. Even a modest weight loss of 10% to 20% has been associated with an improvement.
D. Nonsurgical treatment:
1. Oral appliances (OAs): Require a thorough dental examination.

a. Custom-made OAs may improve airway patency during sleep by enlarging the upper airway and/or by decreasing the upper airway collapse.

b. Mandibular repositioning appliances (MRAs) cover the upper and lower teeth and hold the mandible in an advance position.

c. Tongue retaining devices (TRDs) hold the tongue in a forward position without mandibular repositioning.

E. Surgical treatment:

1. Tracheostomy can eliminate OSA but not central hypoventilation syndromes. This procedure should be considered only when other options have failed or when it is considered necessary by clinical urgency.

2. Maxillomandibular advancement (MMA) is indicated when the client cannot tolerate/refuses CPAP and an OA is not appropriate/effective

3. Surgical treatment should be considered after using an OA or positive airway pressure for 3 months. Surgical treatment has been shown to benefit clients with tonsillar or adenoid hypertrophy, or craniofacial deformities (www.uptodate.com/contents/management -of-obstructive-sleep-apnea-in-adults#H15).

4. Weight loss resulting from bariatric surgery has been effective in improving sleep efficiency and increasing amounts of REM sleep. The severity of pre-surgical OSA determines the degree to which OSA improves post bariatric surgery.

5. Radiofrequency ablation (RFA) is for treatment of mild to moderate OSA when the client cannot tolerate/refuses CPAP and an OA is not appropriate/effective.

6. Laser-assisted uvulopalatoplasty is not recommended for OSA.

Follow-Up

There is no standard for recommending repeat PSG testing or a CPAP titration study after significant weight loss.

Consultation/Referral

A. Refer to a dentist for an OA.

B. Refer to a pulmonologist for management of therapy and/or surgical treatment.

C. Refer the client to a cardiologist as needed.

Bibliography

Center for Medicare & Medicaid Services. (n.d.). *Medicare coverage of durable medical equipment and other coverage*. Retrieved from https://www .medicare.gov/coverage/durable-medical-equipment-dme-coverage

Czeisler, C. A., Scammell, T. E., & Saper, C. B. (2015). Sleep disorders. In D. L. Kasper, S. L. Hauser, J. L. Jameson, A. S. Fauci, D. L. Longo, & J. Loscalzo (Eds.), *Harrison's principles of internal medicine* (19th ed., pp. 184–190). New York, NY: McGraw-Hill.

Kline, L. R. (2018, November). Clinical presentation and diagnosis of obstructive sleep apnea in adults. *UpToDate*. Retrieved from http:// www.uptodate.com/contents/clinical-presentation-and-diagnosis-of -obstructive-sleep-apnea-in-adults

Kondamudi, N., & Khetarpal, S. (2019, March 6). Apnea in children. *StatPearls*. Retrieved from https://www.ncbi.nlm.nih.gov/books/ NBK441894/

McNellis, R. J., & Thomas, S. (2017). Screening for obstructive sleep apnea in adults. *American Family Physician*, 96(2), 123–124.

Memon, J., & Manganaro, S. (2019, February 21). Obstructive sleep-disordered breathing. *StatPearls*. Retrieved from https://www.ncbi .nlm.nih.gov/books/NBK441909/

Schwartzstein, R. M. (2017, November). Physiology of dyspnea. *UpToDate*. Retrieved from http://www.uptodate.com/contents/ physiology-of-dyspnea

Schwartzstein, R. M. (2018, June). Approach to the patient with dyspnea. *UpToDate*. Retrieved from http://www.uptodate.com/contents/approach -to-the-patient-with-dyspnea

Schwartzstein, R. M., & Adams, L. (2016). Dyspnea. In V. C. Broaddus, R. J. Mason, J. D. Ernst, T. E. King, S. C. Lazarus, J. F. Murray, . . . M. B. Gotway (Eds.). *Murray & Nadel's textbook of respiratory medicine* (6th ed., pp. 485–496). Philadelphia, PA: Elsevier–Saunders.

Strohl, K. P. (2018, April). An overview of sleep apnea in adults. *UpToDate*. Retrieved from http://www.uptodate.com/contents/overview -of-obstructive-sleep-apnea-in-adults?source=search_result&search= sleep+apnea&selectedTitle=1%7E150

U.S. Preventive Services Task Force. (2017). *Obstructive sleep apnea in adults: Screening*. Retrieved from https://www.uspreventiveservicestaskforce.org/ Page/Document/UpdateSummaryFinal/obstructive-sleep-apnea-in-adults -screening

Weinburger, S. E. (2018, January). Maternal adaptations to pregnancy: Physiologic respiratory changes and dyspnea. *UpToDate*. Retrieved from http://www.uptodate.com/contents/dyspnea-during -pregnancy

Pneumonia (Bacterial)

Mellisa A. Hall and Cheryl A. Glass

Definition

A. Pneumonia is inflammation and consolidation of lung tissue caused by a bacterial pathogen. The causative agent and the anatomic location classify pneumonia. It is not uncommon to have acute viral and bacterial pneumonia concurrently.

B. Other types of pneumonia and pulmonary inflammation occur secondary to smoking, exposure to chemicals, fungi, near-drowning, and from recurrent aspiration with gastroesophageal reflux.

C. The CURB acronym represents the assessments for confusion, urea, respiratory rate, and BP. The CURB-65 severity score for community-acquired pneumonia (CAP) is a tool to estimate pneumonia mortality and assist in determining whether the client should best be treated in the inpatient or outpatient setting. Each parameter is given a score = 1 if present. There are five parameters: confusion, blood urea nitrogen (BUN) greater than 19 mg/ dL, respiratory rate greater than 30/min, systolic BP less than 91 mmHg or diastolic BP less than 60 mmHg, and age greater than 65 years (https://www.mdcalc.com/ curb-65-score-pneumonia-severity).

Incidence

Pneumonia is the leading cause of death of children worldwide. Approximately 4 million children younger than 5 years worldwide die per year secondary to pneumonia. Pneumonia is also a leading cause of death for clients older than 65 years.

A. Bacterial pneumonia is more prevalent in the very old and the very young.

B. A higher mortality rate occurs in young infants, persons with immunodeficiency, and adults with abnormal vital signs and certain pathogens.

C. The incidence rate varies by pathogen.

Pathogenesis

Pneumonia results from inflammation of the alveolar space and anatomically can be thought of as an alveolitis. Lobar pneumonia has four stages:

A. Vascular congestion and alveolar edema within the first 24 hours of infection.

B. Red hepatization (2–3 days), characterized by erythrocytes, neutrophils, and fibrin within the alveoli.

C. Gray hepatization (2–3 days), characterized by a gray-brown to yellow color secondary to exudate.

D. Resorption and restoration of the pulmonary architecture; a rub may still be auscultated due to the fibrinous inflammation.

Bacterial causes include *S. pneumoniae* (the most common pathogen), *H. influenzae* type b (Hib; the second most common pathogen), *Staphylococcus aureus*, *Legionella*, *Chlamydia trachomatis*, *Chlamydia pneumoniae*, *M. pneumoniae* (most common pathogen in school-age children and adolescents), and *Pneumocystis jirovecii* pneumonia previously known as *Pneumocystis carinii* pneumonia (PCP) in clients with HIV.

Predisposing Factors

A. Age extremes
B. COPD
C. Alcoholism
D. Cigarette smoking
E. Aspiration
F. Heart failure
G. Diabetes
H. Heart failure/heart disease
I. Crowded conditions (day care, dormitories)
J. Immunodeficiency
K. Congenital anomalies
L. Abnormal mucus clearance
M. Lack of immunization
N. Measles
O. Indoor air pollutants from cooking or heating with wood
P. Prematurity

Common Complaints

Acute onset of these symptoms:
A. Fever
B. Shaking chills
C. Dyspnea; rapid, labored breathing
D. Cough
E. Rust-colored sputum

Other Signs and Symptoms

A. Increased respiratory rate (tachypnea)
B. Chest pain
C. URI symptoms such as pharyngitis
D. Headache
E. Nausea
F. Vomiting
G. Vague abdominal pain
H. Diarrhea
I. Myalgia
J. Arthralgias
K. Poor feeding
L. Lethargy in infants

Subjective Data

A. Determine the onset, duration, and course of illness.

B. Has the client had fever or shaking chills?

C. Has there been breathing trouble? Are the breathing problems interfering with eating and drinking?

D. If a child, review the presence of acute onset of fever, cough, tachypnea, dyspnea, and grunting.

E. Is there a cough? Is the cough productive? What color is the sputum?

F. Are any other family members ill?

G. If a child, has he or she been hospitalized for pneumonia or respiratory distress before?

H. Review the history for any chronic diseases.

I. Has the client been immunized for pneumonia?

J. Review all medications, including OTC and herbal products. Specifically review whether the client has been on any antibiotics in the past 3 months. Recent exposure to an antibiotic is a risk factor for antibiotic resistance, as is recent hospitalization. Continued or repeated use of that class of antibiotics is not recommended.

Physical Examination

A. Temperature, BP, pulse, and weight. Count respirations for a full minute.

   1. Tachypnea is the single best predictor of pneumonia in children and the elderly.

   2. In the elderly the BP is usually low.

B. Inspect:

   1. Observe overall appearance. Does the client appear ill? Consider the clinical presentation, age of the person, and history.

   2. Observe breathing pattern and the use of accessory muscles, grunting, retractions, and tachypnea.

   3. Obtain pulse oximetry to assess oxygen saturation. Oxygen saturation less than 92% is an indicator of severity and the need for oxygen therapy.

   4. Check nail beds and lips for cyanosis.

   5. Examine the eyes, nose, ears, and throat.

C. Auscultate:

   1. Heart

   2. Lungs for the following (auscultate bases first in geriatric clients):

      a. Crackles represent fluid in the alveolar sacs (present in 80% of clients), wheezes, and decreased breath sounds.

      b. Whispered pectoriloquy (increased loudness of whisper during auscultation)

      c. Egophony (client's "e" sounds like "a" during auscultation)

      d. Bronchophony (voice sounds louder than usual)

   3. Abdomen (usually hypoactive bowel sounds)

D. Percuss:
  1. Chest to identify areas of consolidation
E. Palpate:
  1. Chest for tactile fremitus (increased conduction when client says "99")
  2. Lymph nodes for adenopathy
  3. Sinuses for tenderness; sinusitis is a sign of *Mycoplasma* infection

Diagnostic Tests

A. The British Thoracic Society, in its 2011 guideline update for CAP in children, notes that no diagnostic tests are necessary in the community, but emphasizes the importance of education on management, signs of deterioration, and the need for reassessment.
B. The World Health Organization (WHO) defines pneumonia solely on the basis of clinical finding observed by inspection and timing of respirations.
C. CXR:
  1. Infiltrates confirm diagnosis. False negatives result from dehydration, evaluation in first 24 hours, and infection.
  2. Ordering a posterior, anterior, and lateral CXR ensures adequate visualization for diagnosis.
D. CBC with differential
E. BUN is needed to calculate the CURB-65 score.
F. Cultures:
  1. Blood cultures if critically ill, immunocompromised, or for persistent symptoms.
  2. Sputum cultures are reserved for very ill clients with unusual presentations.
G. Consider rapid viral testing.
H. Consider skin testing for TB for high-risk exposure.

Differential Diagnoses

A. Pneumonia:
  1. Viral pneumonia
  2. Aspiration pneumonia
  3. Chemically induced pneumonia
B. Asthma
C. Bronchitis/bronchiolitis
D. Pertussis
E. Heart failure
F. Pulmonary embolus
G. Empyema and abscess
H. Aspiration of foreign body

Plan

A. General interventions:
  1. Encourage rest during acute phase.
  2. Encourage clients to avoid smoking/secondhand smoke.
  3. A vaporizer may be used to increase humidity.
  4. Encourage good handwashing or use of hand sanitizer.
  5. Chest physiotherapy is not prescribed for pneumonia.
▶ B. Client teaching: *See Section III: Client Teaching Guides for this chapter, "Bacterial Pneumonia: Adult" and "Bacterial Pneumonia: Child."*
C. Pharmaceutical therapy:

  1. Treatment with antibiotics is empirical. Oral therapy should continue for 7 to 10 days (see Table 9.3).
    a. Amoxicillin is considered a first-line therapy in pediatrics.
    b. Macrolide antibiotics should not be the first-line therapy, but can be added if there is no response to first-line empirical therapy.
    c. Macrolides are the first choice in otherwise healthy adults.
  2. Administer acetaminophen (Tylenol) for fever.
  3. Avoid cough suppressants. Suppression of a cough may interfere with airway clearance.
  4. Vaccines:
    a. Children: Heptavalent pneumococcal vaccine is recommended for all children in the United States.
    b. Geriatrics: Pneumococcal 13 and 23 vaccines are recommended for the elderly, ages 65 years or older and/or adults older than 19 years of age with risk factors and with a compromised immune system.
D. Dietary management: Encourage a nutritious diet with increased fluid intake.

Follow-Up

A. Clients/parents should know the signs of increasing respiratory distress and seek immediate medical attention.
B. Follow up with a telephone call in 24 hours.
C. If there is no improvement after 48 hours on antibiotics, the client is advised to return to the office.
D. Schedule a return visit in 2 weeks for evaluation.
E. Follow up with a CXR in 4 to 6 weeks for clients older than 60 years and for those who smoke. However, if the client is younger than 60 years, a nonsmoker, and feels well at 6-week follow-up, there is no need to follow up with a CXR.

Consultation/Referral

A. Clients who are immunocompromised or have signs of toxicity or hypoxia may need hospitalization. Refer them to a physician.
B. If the child is in moderate respiratory distress, dehydrated, or hypoxemic, consult with or refer the client to a physician/hospital.
C. Poor prognostic signs that require referral are age greater than 65 years, respiration rate greater than or equal to 30 breaths per minute, systolic BP less than 90 mmHg or diastolic BP less than 60 mmHg, temperature greater than 101°F, altered mental status, extrapulmonary infection, and WBCs less than 4,000 or greater than 30,000.
D. Physician consultation is needed for suspected PCP.

Individual Considerations

A. Pregnancy:
  1. The annual U.S. rate of antepartum CAP is 0.5 to 1.5 per 1,000 pregnancies.
  2. Perinatal mortality may increase slightly due to an associated increase in prematurity. Pneumonia puts older mothers at high risk of maternal death.

TABLE 9.3 ANTIBIOTIC THERAPIES FOR PNEUMONIA

Antibiotic	Adult Dosages	Pediatric Dosages
Amoxicillin: Oral	250–500 mg TID	90 mg/kg/d divided TID (5 years and older) not to exceed 4,000 mg/d
Amoxil, Trimox	Not to exceed 1,500 mg/d	
Clarithromycin: Oral (Biaxin)	250–500 mg BID	15 mg/kg/d divided every 12 hours
		Not recommended for children <6 months
Cefotaxime: Intramuscular (Claforan)	>50 kg: 1–2 g IM every 6–8 hours; not to exceed 12 g/d	<50 kg: 100 mg–200 mg/kg/d IM divided doses every 6–8 hours
Doxycycline: Oral (Doryx)	200-mg loading dose, then 100 mg BID	>8 years and <100 lb
		2 mg/lb divided in 2 doses for 2 days, then 1–2 mg/lb daily in two divided doses
		>100 lb: 100 mg orally every 12 hours
		Not recommended for children < 9 years
Azithromycin: Oral (Zithromax)	500 mg loading dose, then 250 mg daily on days 2–5	10 mg/kg initial dose (not to exceed 500 mg/d), then 5 mg/kg daily on days 2–5 (not to exceed 250 mg/d)
Moxifloxacin: Oral (Avelox)	400 mg once a day	Not recommended for children < 18 years
Levofloxacin (Levaquin) Adults > 18 years of age	500 mg once a day for 7–14 days OR 750 mg once a day for 5 days Other regimens depend on the pathogen	Not recommended for children < 18 years. Limit use to areas that have resistance to previously mentioned antibiotics. Quinolones are associated with aortic aneurysm rupture, hypo/hyperglycemia, QT prolongation, tendonopathies, psychiatric reactions.

Note: Renal dosing should be considered in elders.

3. The symptoms of bacterial pneumonia are the same in pregnancy.

4. CXRs are acceptable in pregnancy to diagnose pneumonia.

B. Pediatrics:

1. Hospitalization is recommended in infants aged 6 months and younger and also in very severe cases of pneumonia.

2. Immunization against *H. influenzae* type B (Hib), pneumococcus, measles, and whooping cough (pertussis) is the most effective way to prevent pneumonia.

C. Geriatrics:

1. Depending on the frailty status of the client, hospitalization may be required. A calculation to objectively determine client risk has been developed (CURB-65 Severity Score) and is available at www.mdcalc.com/curb-65-severity-score-community-acquired-pneumonia/.

Bibliography

Bradley, J., Byington, C., Shah, S., Alverson, B., Carter, E., Harrison, C., … Moore, M. (2011). The management of community-acquired pneumonia in infants and children older than 3 months of age: Clinical practice guidelines by the Pediatric Infectious Diseases Society and the Infectious Diseases Society of America. *Clinical Infectious Diseases, 53*(7), e25–e76. doi:10.1093/cid/cir625. Retrieved from https://academic.oup.com/cid/article/53/7/e25/424286

Centers for Disease Control and Prevention. (2018, August 17). *Adults with chronic conditions: Get vaccinated.* Retrieved from https://www.cdc.gov/features/vaccineschronicconditions/index.html

Centers for Disease Control and Prevention. (2019). *Recommended adult immunization schedule. U.S.—2019.* Retrieved from http://www.cdc.gov/vaccines/schedules/downloads/adult/adult-schedule.pdf

Mandell, L. A., & Wunerink, R. G. (2015). Pneumonia. In D. L. Kasper, S. L. Hauser, J. L. Jameson, A. S. Fauci, D. L. Longo, & J. Loscalzo (Eds.), *Harrison's principles of internal medicine* (19th ed., pp. 803–812). New York, NY: McGraw-Hill.

MPR: Nurse practitioner's edition. (2019, Spring). New York, NY: Haymarket Media.

Prescriber's letter. (2018, May). Analgesics for acute pain. Retrieved from https://prescriber.therapeuticresearch.com/Content/Segments/PRL/2014/Nov/Analgesics-for-Acute-Pain-7707

Rains, S. G. (2020). Fifteen-to-eighteen-month visit. In B. Richardson (Ed.), *Pediatric primary care: Practice guidelines for nurses* (2nd ed., pp. 117–127). Burlington, MA: Jones & Bartlett Learning.

Resnick, B. (Ed.). (2017). *GNRS geriatric nursing review syllabus: A core curriculum in advanced practice geriatric nursing* (5th ed.). New York, NY: American Geriatrics Society.

Terry, E. G. (2020). Seven-to-ten-year visit (school age). In B. Richardson (Ed.), *Pediatric primary care: Practice guidelines for nurses* (3rd ed., pp. 147–162). Burlington, MA: Jones & Bartlett Learning.

Weiner, D. L. (2018, August). Causes of acute respiratory distress in children. *UpToDate.* Retrieved from http://www.uptodate.com/contents/causes-of-acute-respiratory-distress-in-children

World Health Organization. (2016, November). *Pneumonia fact sheet N331.* Retrieved from http://www.who.int/mediacentre/factsheets/fs331/en

Pneumonia (Viral)

Mellisa A. Hall and Cheryl A. Glass

Definition

Viral pneumonia is inflammation and consolidation of lung tissue due to a viral pathogen.

Incidence

A. Viral pneumonia is most common in the pediatric and elderly populations. There has been a sharp decline its incidence in the adolescent through middle-aged populations, except when related to immunosuppression. It is not uncommon to have concurrent viral and bacterial infections.

B. Children younger than 5 years and elderly persons have the highest rate of influenza-associated hospitalizations.

C. Pneumonia is the leading cause of death in children worldwide.

Pathogenesis

A. Pneumonia results from inflammation of the alveolar space and may compromise air at the alveoli–pulmonary capillary interface. Viral pneumonia is caused by influenza viruses, parainfluenza virus, and adenovirus and RSV.

B. RSV is the most common viral cause of pneumonia.

C. Viruses and bacteria are spread from a cough or sneeze.

D. Pneumonia can also be spread via blood, especially during and shortly after birth.

Predisposing Factors

A. Age extremes
B. Prematurity
C. Exposure to viral illness
D. Lack of immunization
E. Frailty
F. Immunocompromise

Common Complaints

A. Fever
B. Cough
C. Dyspnea
D. Tachypnea
E. Wheezing (more common in viral pneumonia)

Other Signs and Symptoms

A. Upper respiratory prodrome
B. Poor appetite
C. Malaise/lethargy in pediatrics
D. Myalgia
E. Muscle aches
F. Headache
G. Fatigue
H. Chest pain/tightness

Subjective Data

A. Determine the onset, duration, and course of illness.
B. Has the client had fever, cough, and URI?
C. Have there been any flulike symptoms?
D. Has there been any labored breathing?
E. Has there been a cough? Is it a productive cough? What color is the sputum?
F. Are the breathing problems affecting the ability to eat or drink?
G. Has the child had nausea, vomiting, or diarrhea?
H. Review if the client is up to date on immunizations.
I. Review all medications, including OTC and herbal products.

Physical Examination

A. Temperature, BP, pulse, and respirations. Count respirations for a full minute. **Tachypnea is the single best predictor of pneumonia in children.**

B. Inspect:
    1. Observe overall appearance. Does the client appear ill? Consider the clinical presentation, age of person, and history.
    2. Observe respiratory pattern, grunting, nasal flaring, retractions, and use of accessory muscles.
    3. Check pulse oximetry. **Oxygen saturation less than 92% is an indicator of severity and the need for oxygen therapy.**
    4. Check nail beds and lips for cyanosis.
    5. Examine eyes, ears, nose, and throat.

C. Auscultate:
    1. Heart
    2. Lungs for the following (auscultate bases first in geriatric clients):
        a. Crackles, decreased breath sounds
        b. Whispered pectoriloquy (client's whispered sounds are louder than normal)
        c. Egophony (client's "e" sounds like "a")
        d. Bronchophony (voice sounds louder than usual)

D. Percuss chest for dull sound (consolidation).

E. Palpate:
    1. Lymph nodes for swelling
    2. Chest for tactile fremitus (increased conduction when client says "99")
    3. Sinuses

Diagnostic Tests

A. CXR, which reveals interstitial, perihilar, or diffuse infiltrates
B. CBC with differential
C. Rapid viral tests per nasal swab
D. Sputum Gram stain if indicated

Differential Diagnoses

A. Bacterial pneumonia
B. Varicella pneumonia
C. Herpes pneumonia
D. Cytomegalovirus pneumonia
E. Pertussis
F. Asthma
G. Bronchitis/bronchiolitis
H. Sinusitis
I. Foreign-body obstruction (usually in small children and mentally handicapped persons)
J. Aspiration

Plan

A. General interventions:
    1. Recommend to the client to rest during acute phase.
    2. Avoid smoking or secondhand smoke.
    3. Respiratory isolation; may use facial masks

4. Encourage good handwashing or use of hand sanitizer.

5. Chest physiotherapy is not recommended for pneumonia.

▶ B. Client teaching: *See Section III: Client Teaching Guides for this chapter, "Pneumonia, Viral: Adult" and "Pneumonia, Viral: Child."*

C. Pharmaceutical therapy:

1. Antiviral agents should be considered in immunocompromised clients, those at high risk for complications, or those requiring hospitalization. High risk includes age greater than 65 years; pregnancy or up to 2 weeks postpartum; long-term care residents; pulmonary disease, including asthma; diabetes; cardiovascular disease, excluding hypertension; chronic kidney disease; hepatic dysfunction; and active malignancy.

 a. Oseltamivir, Peramivir, Baloxavir, and Zanamivir are the recommended initial choices. Antivirals should be started within the first 12 to 24 hours when possible.

2. Post-exposure prophylaxis should be considered for children at high risk for complications of influenza. Post-exposure prophylaxis should be initiated for these high-risk children within 48 hours of exposure.

3. Avoid cough suppressants. The suppression of a cough may interfere with airway clearance.

4. Acetaminophen (Tylenol) can be used to treat myalgias and to prevent fever.

5. Immunizations:

 a. Recommend the influenza vaccine for prevention.

 b. Consider RSV vaccine prophylaxis for pediatric clients following the current AAP recommendations.

 c. The measles vaccine is recommended except during pregnancy and in immunocompromised clients.

D. Dietary management: Encourage fluids and a nutritious diet.

E. Clients with viral pneumonia who are superinfected with bacterial organisms require antibiotic therapy

Follow-Up

Signs and symptoms may vary greatly according to the viral pathogen, severity of disease, and client's age.

A. Recommend the client to return to the clinic if no improvement is seen after 48 hours on antiviral agents.

B. Follow up with a phone call in 24 hours.

C. Consider follow-up at 2 weeks if bronchoconstriction is noted on examination.

Consultation/Referral

A. Consult a physician if viral pneumonia is suspected.

B. Consult a physician if the client is pregnant.

C. Consult a physician or transfer to the hospital if the client is in respiratory distress, dehydrated, or hypoxemic.

D. Consider consultation with a pulmonologist.

Individual Considerations

A. Pregnancy:

1. Ribavirin is contraindicated in pregnancy; it is a class X drug.

2. Varicella-zoster pneumonia is associated with 40% mortality.

3. Varicella-zoster immune globulin (VZIG) may be considered in pregnancy. Consultation with a physician is recommended.

4. If herpes pneumonia is suspected, a physician consult should be obtained immediately.

5. The measles vaccine contains a live-attenuated virus and should not be given during pregnancy.

B. Pediatrics:

1. Hospitalization is recommended in infants aged 2 months and younger and also in very severe cases of pneumonia.

Bibliography

Centers for Disease Control and Prevention. (2019). *Recommended adult immunization schedule. U.S.—2019*. Retrieved from http://www.cdc.gov/vaccines/schedules/downloads/adult/adult-schedule.pdf

Freeman, A., & Leigh, T. (2018, November 11). Pneumonia, viral. *StatPearls*. Retrieved from https://www.ncbi.nlm.nih.gov/books/NBK513286/

Mandell, L. A., & Wunerink, R. G. (2015). Pneumonia. In D. L. Kasper, S. L. Hauser, J. L. Jameson, A. S. Fauci, D. L. Longo, & J. Loscalzo (Eds.), *Harrison's principles of internal medicine* (19th ed., pp. 803–812). New York, NY: McGraw-Hill.

Rains, S. G. (2020). Fifteen-to-eighteen-month visit. In B. Richardson (Ed.), *Pediatric primary care: Practice guidelines for nurses* (2nd ed., pp. 117–127). Burlington, MA: Jones & Bartlett Learning.

Terry, E. G. (2020). Seven-to-ten-year visit school age. In B. Richardson (Ed.), *Pediatric primary care: Practice guidelines for nurses* (3rd ed., pp. 147–162). Burlington, MA: Jones & Bartlett Learning.

Weiner, D. L. (2018, August). Causes of acute respiratory distress in children. *UpToDate*. Retrieved from http://www.uptodate.com/contents/causes-of-acute-respiratory-distress-in-children

World Health Organization. (2016, November). *Pneumonia fact sheet N331*. Retrieved from http://www.who.int/mediacentre/factsheets/fs331/en

Respiratory Syncytial Virus Bronchiolitis

Mellisa A. Hall and Cheryl A. Glass

Definition

RSV is the most frequent cause of viral respiratory tract infection in infants. Most infants develop upper respiratory tract symptoms; 20% to 30% develop lower respiratory tract disease with their first infection. Infection with RSV may produce minimal respiratory symptoms. Most previously healthy infants who develop RSV bronchiolitis do not require hospitalization. Preterm infants with respiratory symptoms with lethargy, irritability, and poor feeding may require admission for treatment. There is no specific treatment for RSV infection.

Incidence

A. RSV is prevalent worldwide and affects all age groups. Infants, the elderly, and adults with chronic heart or lung disease or weakened immune systems are at high risk. Annual epidemics occur in winter and early spring, usually in temperate climates. The peak season in North America is between November and March. Most infants are infected during the first year of life. Peak incidence of occurrence of severe RSV disease is observed at ages of 2 to 8 months. Virtually all children have been infected at least once by their third birthday. Reinfection with RSV throughout life is common.

B. The period of viral shedding usually is 3 to 8 days, but shedding may continue up to 4 weeks. The incubation period ranges from 2 to 8 days.

C. Full recovery from RSV illness occurs in about 1 to 2 weeks.

Pathogenesis

A. RSV is an enveloped, nonsegmented, negative-strand RNA virus of the *Paramyxoviridae* family. Two major strains (Groups A and B) have been identified, and strains of both often circulate concurrently.

B. Humans are the only source of infection. Transmission is by direct or close contact with contaminated secretions of RSV. It can persist on environmental surfaces for several hours and for a half hour or more on hands.

Predisposing Factors

A. Prematurity
B. Congenital heart disease
C. CLD
D. Immunodeficiency
E. Child-care centers
F. Two or more siblings younger than 5 years
G. Hospitalization

Common Complaints

A. Pediatrics:
  1. Fever (less than 101°F); 20% of clients have higher temperatures
  2. Decreased appetite
  3. Irritability
  4. Lethargy
  5. Rapid respirations
  6. Cough
  7. Coryza
  8. Decreased activity
  9. Wheezing
B. Adults:
  1. Rhinorrhea
  2. Pharyngitis
  3. Cough
  4. Headache
  5. Fatigue
  6. Fever

Other Signs and Symptoms

A. Tachypnea or apnea
B. Nasal flaring
C. Retractions
D. Crackles
E. Wheezes

Subjective Data

A. Ask about the onset, duration, and course of illness.
B. Inquire whether the child is having trouble eating or drinking because of breathing problems.

C. Review other symptoms, including fever, nausea, vomiting, or diarrhea.
D. Are there any labored breathing patterns?
E. Calculate the child's age—how old the baby is and birth date—if palivizumab (Synagis) is prescribed.
F. Was the baby born preterm and at what gestational age?
G. Has the client ever been diagnosed with any cardiac or lung problems, including CF?
H. Do the client's siblings attend day care?

Physical Examination

A. Record temperature, pulse, respirations, BP, and pulse oximetry.
B. Inspect:
  1. Observe general appearance.
  2. Note respiratory pattern, retractions, nasal flaring, grunting, and circumoral cyanosis.
  3. Inspect eyes, ears, nose, and throat. As many as 40% of clients have an associated viral and/or bacterial otitis media.
  4. Assess hydration status: Skin turgor, capillary refill, mucous membranes
C. Auscultate:
  1. Heart
  2. Lungs for crackles and mild to moderate respiratory distress with scattered wheezes
D. Percuss:
  1. Chest
E. Palpate:
  1. Lymph nodes for adenopathy
  2. Head and fontanelles (if applicable)

Diagnostic Tests

A. Rapid diagnostic assay of nasopharyngeal secretions is reliable in infants and young children.
B. Laboratory studies are frequently not indicated in the infant who is comfortable in room air, is well hydrated, and is feeding adequately. Nonspecific laboratory tests may include CBC, serum electrolytes, and urinalysis.
C. CXR may show hyperexpansion, atelectasis, and/or infiltrates in a specific nonlobar (bacterial) viral pattern.
D. ABGs or pulse oximetry may show hypoxemia.

Differential Diagnoses

A. Viral or bacterial pneumonia
B. Asthma
C. Croup
D. Influenza
E. Neonatal sepsis
F. Foreign-body aspiration

Plan

A. General interventions:
  1. Most infants require only supportive care, such as nasal suctioning.
  2. Infants should never be exposed to cigarette smoke.
  3. Hydration is important.

4. Contact precautions are recommended for the duration of RSV-associated illness among infants and young children. Adhere to appropriate hand-hygiene practices.

5. Prevention includes limiting exposure to contagious settings (e.g., child-care centers).

▶ B. Client teaching: *See Section III: Client Teaching Guide for this chapter, "Respiratory Syncytial Virus."*

C. Pharmacological therapy:

1. The use of CSs is controversial, but might reduce bronchial reactivity in children with asthma.

2. Bronchodilators are not recommended.

3. Antibiotics are not indicated for RSV bronchiolitis or pneumonia unless there is a secondary bacterial infection.

4. Palivizumab (Synagis) immunoprophylaxis is extremely costly and should be limited to infants at risk for RSV infection. The decision to recommend palivizumab should be made in association with a collaborating physician. Dosing: Palivizumab 15 mg/kg intramuscularly every 30 days. Immunizations are given from 3 to 5 months depending on the gestational age, risk factors, and month that prophylaxis is started. The 2014 AAP eligibility criteria for palivizumab prophylaxis criteria includes:

a. Infants born at ≤28 weeks 6 days gestational age and infants < 12 months at the start of the RSV season

b. Infants < 12 months of age with CLD of prematurity

c. Infants ≤ 12 months of age with hemodynamically significant CHD

d. Infants and children < 24 months of age with CLD of prematurity necessitating medical therapy (e.g., supplemental oxygen, bronchodilator, diuretic, or chronic steroid therapy) within 6 months prior to the beginning of RSV season

5. AAP also suggests that palivizumab prophylaxis may be considered in the following circumstances:

a. Infants < 12 months of age with congenital airway abnormality or neuromuscular disorder that decreases the ability to manage airway secretions

b. Infants < 12 months of age with CF with clinical evidence of CLD and/or nutritional compromise

c. Children < 24 months with CF with severe lung disease: Previous hospitalization for pulmonary exacerbation in the first year of life or abnormalities on chest radiography or chest CT that persist when stable) or weight for length less than the 10th percentile

d. Infants and children < 24 months who are profoundly immunocompromised

e. Infants and children < 24 months undergoing cardiac transplantation during RSV season

Follow-Up

Call the client's caregiver in 12 to 24 hours to assess feeding and respiratory status.

Consultation/Referral

A. Refer the client to a physician or emergency department if the infant is in moderate respiratory distress, is dehydrated, is hypoxemic, or is younger than 6 months of age.

B. Admit hypoxemic infants to the hospital for hydration, oxygen therapy, and, possibly, mechanical ventilation.

Individual Considerations

A. Adults: Palivizumab (Synagis) is not approved for adults.

B. Pediatrics:

1. Age is a significant factor in the severity of infection: The younger the client is, the more severe the infection/hypoxemia tends to be. Infants younger than 6 months are most severely affected secondary to their smaller, more easily obstructed airways and their decreased ability to clear secretions.

2. All high-risk infants 6 months of age and older and their contacts should be administered the influenza vaccine as well as other recommended age-appropriate immunizations.

3. Palivizumab does not interfere with response to vaccines.

C. Pregnancy:

1. Ribavirin is contraindicated during pregnancy. A negative pregnancy test and assurance of contraception should be obtained before prescribing.

Bibliography

American Academy of Pediatrics. (2018–2021). Respiratory syncytial virus. In D. Kimberlin, M. T. Brady, M. A. Jackson, & S. S. Long (Eds.), *Red book: 2018–2021 report of the Committee on Infectious Diseases* (31st ed., pp. 682–692). Elk Grove Village, IL: Author. Retrieved from https://redbook.solutions.aap.org/book.aspx?bookid=2205

Barr, R. G., & Graham, B. S. (2018a, December). Respiratory syncytial virus: Prevention. *UpToDate*. Retrieved from http://www.uptodate.com/contents/respiratory-syncytial-virus-infection-prevention

Barr, R. G., & Graham, B. S. (2018b, June). Respiratory syncytial virus: Treatment. *UpToDate*. Retrieved from https://www.uptodate.com./respiratory-syncytial-virus-infection-treatment

Barr, R. G., & Graham, B. S. (2019, January). Respiratory syncytial virus: Clinical features and diagnosis. *UpToDate*. Retrieved from https://www-uptodate-com.respiratory-syncytial-virus-infection-clinical-features-and-diagnosis

Centers for Disease Control and Prevention. (2018a, June). *For parents: Young children and adverse drug events*. Retrieved from https://www.cdc.gov/MedicationSafety/parents_childrenAdverseDrugEvents.html

Centers for Disease Control and Prevention. (2018b, August). *Prevention and control of influenza with vaccines: Recommendations of the Advisory Committee on Immunization Practices, United States, 2018–2019 influenza season*. Retrieved from https://www.cdc.gov/flu/professionals/acip/index.htm

Centers for Disease Control and Prevention. (2018c, June). *Respiratory syncytial virus infection (RSV)*. Retrieved from www.cdc.gov/rsv

Lexicomp Inc. (2019). Palivizumab: Drug information. *UpToDate*. Retrieved from https://www-uptodate-com./palivizumab-drug-information

Munoz, F. M. (2019). *Seasonal influenza in children: Prevention and treatment with antiviral drugs*. Retrieved from https://www-uptodate-com./seasonal-influenza-in-children-prevention-and-treatment-with-antiviral-drugs

Rains, S. G. (2020). Fifteen-to-eighteen-month visit. In B. Richardson (Ed.), *Pediatric primary care: Practice guidelines for nurses* (2nd ed., pp. 117–127). Burlington, MA: Jones & Bartlett Learning.

Terry, E. G. (2020). Seven-to-ten-year visit school age. In B. Richardson (Ed.), *Pediatric primary care: Practice guidelines for nurses* (3rd ed., pp. 147–162). Burlington, MA: Jones & Bartlett Learning.

Weiner, D. L. (2018, August). Causes of acute respiratory distress in children. *UpToDate*. Retrieved from http://www.uptodate.com/contents/causes-of-acute-respiratory-distress-in-children

Zachary, K. C. (2019, February). Treatment of seasonal influenza in adults. *UpToDate*. Retrieved from http://www.uptodate.com/contents/treatment-of-seasonal-influenza-in-adults

Shortness of Breath

Mellisa A. Hall

Definition

SOB (dyspnea) is derived from the Greek terms for *difficult* and *breath*. Dyspnea may be experienced by clients with or without respiratory disorders. SOB/dyspnea is clinically significant when it interferes with normal functioning. Dyspnea is considered chronic when it persists longer than 4 to 8 weeks. SOB is a subjective symptom, reported by the client. As self-reported, SOB may cause greater distress than pain.

Incidence

Dyspnea affects millions of people and is commonly associated with pulmonary disease, cardiovascular disease, anemia, obesity, and deconditioning. Dyspnea is reported in more than one fourth of the elderly. An estimated 25 million people with asthma or COPD experience SOB during the course of their illness. SOB is reported in more than 95% of clients in terminal stages of lung cancer, COPD, and heart failure.

Pathogenesis

A. The sensation of SOB can involve psychological, physical, social, and environmental factors. A sensation of SOB is stimulated by chemoreceptors that respond to changes in pH and carbon dioxide. Mechanoreceptors are located in upper airways, lungs, and the chest wall.
B. A sensation of SOB occurs with ventilation–perfusion mismatch, metabolic acidosis, increase in respiratory dead space, or stimulation of chest wall or pulmonary respiratory receptors.
C. SOB is perceived more by clients with existing lung disease.
D. Anemia and cardiovascular disease compromise the amount of oxygen delivered to tissues, worsening the sensation of dyspnea.
E. Interstitial lung disease associated with autoimmunity increases dyspnea/SOB, and with disease progression tissue oxygenation is reduced

Predisposing Factors

A. Exertion
B. Asthma
C. COPD
D. CHF
E. Cardiac valve disorders
F. Cardiac anomalies
G. Pulmonary embolism
H. High altitudes
I. Environmental air pollution
J. Respiratory muscle weakness or paralysis, including neuromuscular disorders
K. Metabolic acidosis (renal failure)
L. Hemoglobinopathies
M. Hyperventilation syndrome, anxiety disorder, panic episodes
N. Reduced vital capacity and thoracic expansion with aging
O. Severe kyphoscoliosis
P. Obesity
Q. Pregnancy
R. Pleural effusions
S. Pulmonary hypertension
T. Foreign-body aspiration
U. OSA
V. End-stage terminal illness (lung cancer, COPD, CHF)

Common Complaint

Discomfort with breathing or air hunger, worsening with positioning or activity

Subjective Data

A. How long have the symptoms been present?
B. How do they interfere with functioning?
C. What worsens and what improves the SOB?
D. Associated with syncope?
E. Associated with palpitations?
F. Increased anxiety before episodes?
G. History of similar symptoms?
H. Associated with odors (including household cleaners)?
I. Associated with certain social environments?
J. Weight changes since symptoms began?
K. History of lung or cardiac disease?
L. Treatments used to relieve the SOB?
M. Family history of similar issues?
N. If using a SABA, how often, and has it helped?
O. Is cough associated more with some activities than others?
P. Is it hemoptysis?
Q. Is the client smoking now or ever? Pack-years? E-cigarettes?
R. Did the client use illicit substances? What type? In what amount? When was the most recent use?
S. Has the client taken any new medications, eaten new foods, or been stung by an insect?
T. Has the client been injured in the chest or neck?
U. Does the client's chest hurt anywhere?
V. What is the client's history of sickle cell disease?
W. What does the client feel is causing the SOB?

Physical Examination

A. Record temperature, pulse, respirations, BP, and pulse oximetry. Compare weight to last visit.
B. Inspect:
    1. Observe general appearance—including morbid obesity, gravid uterus, skin tones, and use of accessory muscles of breathing—and facial appearance for fear or reduced level of consciousness, as well as tobacco or other chemical odors.

2. Use of the tripod position to be able to speak in complete sentences.

3. Assess hydration status: Skin turgor, capillary refill, and mucous membranes. Note distal fingers for clubbing.

4. Pharynx and tonsils for erythema or hypertrophy

5. Trachea for deviation

6. Chest for barrel appearance or obvious trauma

7. Spine for scoliosis or kyphosis

8. Abdomen for distention

9. Infants: Note respiratory pattern, retractions, nasal flaring, grunting, and circumoral cyanosis

C. Auscultate:

1. Heart for murmur, rate, irregular rhythm, S_3 or S_4

2. Lungs for crackles and mild to moderate respiratory distress with wheezing

D. Percuss:

1. Chest

E. Palpate:

1. Palpate lymph nodes for adenopathy.

2. Perform strength testing against resistance of upper and lower extremities to assess for lethargy/atonia

F. Neurological examination:

1. Assess mentation

Diagnostic Tests

A. Labs: CBC, BUN, creatinine, electrolytes, cardiac troponin, BNP, D-dimer, carbon monoxide levels

B. EKG

C. CXR

D. PFTs

E. Echocardiogram if heart failure is suspected

F. Anxiety and depression scales as indicated

Differential Diagnoses

A. Cardiovascular anomalies, dysfunction, or acute ischemia

B. Pulmonary disease, including autoimmune disorders affecting lung tissue

C. Anxiety

D. Foreign-body or other aspiration syndromes

E. Anaphylaxis

F. Airway trauma

G. Infection of upper or lower airways

H. Pulmonary hypertension

I. IV Fluid overload

Plan

A. General interventions:

1. The underlying etiology of the SOB should be considered and treated.

2. Severe airway compromise should be considered in clients with stridor or change in level of consciousness. Emergency medical services (EMS) should be activated immediately with airway support, including supplemental oxygen.

▶ B. Client teaching: *See Section III: Client Teaching Guide for this chapter, "Shortness of Breath."*

1. Discuss the underlying etiology of SOB with the client and family and establish strategies to prevent further episodes of SOB.

C. Pharmaceutical therapy:

1. Medications should be prescribed according to the underlying etiology. Products specific for dyspnea relief in terminal illness in clients under hospice care are outlined here. Medication adjustments should follow dyspnea assessment scales.

2. Weak opioids: Codeine (30 mg q 4 hours)

3. Strong opioids: Morphine 5–10 mg q 3 hours

4. Anxiolytics: Lorazepam 0.5–2 mg PO/SL/IV q hour

5. Anxiolytics: Clonazepam 0.25–2 mg q 12 hours

D. Dietary management:

1. Foods associated with worsening SOB should be avoided.

2. Swallowing studies should be considered for clients at risk for aspiration.

Follow-Up

Follow-up should occur frequently until symptoms of SOB have been controlled and the underlying etiology treated.

Consultation/Referral

A. Activate EMS for clients in acute respiratory distress.

B. Provide supplemental oxygen for clients of all ages until EMS has transported the client.

C. Refer to appropriate specialty care depending on underlying cause of SOB.

D. Consultation with palliative care or hospice services should be considered to relieve dyspnea based on clients' advance care planning.

Individual Considerations

A. Pediatrics:

1. Acute respiratory distress should be immediately ruled out in infants and children in an emergency department setting.

B. Pregnancy:

1. Dyspnea occurs in up to two thirds of clients beginning in the first or second trimester of pregnancy. Underlying pathology during pregnancy should be considered, just as with clients of all ages.

C. Geriatrics:

1. Avoid sedating medications that would increase the risk for hypoventilation or aspiration.

2. Physical changes associated with aging increase the risk for hypoxia.

3. Elderly clients may report SOB less frequently and assume it is an expectation of aging.

Bibliography

Schwartzstein, R. M. (2018, June). Approach to the patient with dyspnea. *UpToDate.* Retrieved from http://www.uptodate.com/contents/approach-to-the-patient-with-dyspnea

Valentine, N. (2020). Respiratory disorders. In B. Richardson (Ed.), *Pediatric primary care: Practice guidelines for nurses* (4th ed., pp. 325–370). Burlington, MA: Jones & Bartlett Learning.

Tuberculosis

Mellisa A. Hall and Cheryl A. Glass

Definition

A. Tuberculosis (TB) is an infectious, granulomatous disease caused by *M. tuberculosis*, *Mycobacterium bovis*, and other mycobacteria. Humans are the only reservoirs for *M. tuberculosis*. In many cases, TB involves multiple organs, including the lungs, liver, spleen, lymph nodes, kidney, brain, eyes, and bone. WHO has estimated that one third of all people in the world are infected with *M. tuberculosis.*

B. In most immunocompetent individuals, macrophages are successful in containing the bacilli, and the infection is self-limited and often subclinical. As many as 60% of children and 5% of adults with primary TB are asymptomatic. When the pulmonary macrophages are unable to contain the bacilli, this leads to clinically apparent infection—progressive primary TB.

C. Post-primary (reactivation) TB occurs when the initial infection was successfully contained by the pulmonary macrophages, with bacilli remaining viable within the macrophages. Infection results when the host's immune status (T cells) is compromised.

D. Clients with fever of unknown origin, failure to thrive, significant weight loss, or unexplained lymphadenopathy should be evaluated for TB.

E. The lungs are the most common site for the development of TB; 85% of clients present with pulmonary complaints.

Incidence

A. Tuberculosis is a worldwide infection and is considered a global public health emergency by WHO.

 1. WHO reports more than 9 million new cases of TB every year.

 2. Generally, TB affects any age group: More than 60% of cases are in those 25 to 40 years old; TB is uncommon in children between ages 5 and 15 years.

 3. Child-to-child transmission is not common because children rarely develop a cough and the sputum is scant.

 4. The incidence of TB in the United States is 2.8 cases per 100,000 population.

 5. Due to the high risk among immigrants, California, New York, Texas, and Florida account for half of the TB cases reported in the United States.

B. Post-primary TB (reactivation of tuberculosis or secondary tuberculosis) is a significant cause of worldwide morbidity and mortality. Pulmonary morbidity results from a chronic cough, hemoptysis, fibrosis, superinfection, bronchial stenosis, repeated pulmonary infections, or empyema. Morbidity also arises from chronic TB osteomyelitis, chronic renal insufficiency, and central nervous system (CNS) TB.

Pathogenesis

Mycobacteria are non-spore-forming, slow-growing bacilli. TB infection occurs by means of inhalation of airborne bacillus droplets from an infected host. The development of an infection depends on prolonged exposure (weeks) to an individual with active pulmonary TB. Bacilli travel through the pulmonary lymphatics or enter the vascular system and are disseminated to the brain, meninges, eyes, bones, joints, lymph nodes, kidneys, intestines, larynx, pericardium, genitourinary system, and skin. The incubation period from infection to positive skin test reaction is 2 to 10 weeks, although disease may not occur for many years or may never occur. The risk of disease is greatest within 2 years following infection.

Predisposing Factors

A. Exposure to someone with active disease

B. High-risk groups: Minorities, young children (before age 5 years) and the elderly, foreign-born people, prisoners, nursing home residents, teachers, indigents, migrant workers, and healthcare providers

C. HIV infection is one of the most significant risk factors for TB.

D. Steroid therapy, cancer chemotherapy, and hematologic malignancies increase the risk of TB

E. Tumor necrosis factor-alpha (TNF-alpha) antagonist is used for rheumatoid arthritis, psoriasis, and other autoimmune disease associated with a significant risk for TB. Before beginning any TNF-alpha treatment, a TB skin test should be given.

F. Non-TB infections, such as measles, varicella, and pertussis, may activate quiescent TB.

G. Smoking

H. Malnutrition

I. Alcoholism

J. IV drug abuse

K. Congenital TB (rare)

Common Complaints

A. Fever (usually low grade at onset but becoming marked with progression of disease)

B. Malaise

C. Weight loss/difficulty gaining weight

D. Cough

E. Night sweats

F. Chills

G. Occasional hemoptysis

H. Fatigue

I. Pediatric symptoms:

 1. Nonproductive cough

 2. Failure to thrive

 3. Difficulty gaining weight

 4. Fever

 5. Night sweats

 6. Anorexia

Other Signs and Symptoms

A. Pulmonary TB: Fatigue, irritability, undernutrition, with or without fever and cough
B. Glandular TB: Chronic cervical adenitis
C. Meningeal TB: Fever and meningeal signs, positive cerebrospinal fluid
D. Failure to thrive
E. Anorexia

Subjective Data

A. Determine the onset, duration, and course of illness.
B. Review symptom history: Fever, night sweats, chills, or cough.
C. Review history of weight loss.
D. Review exposure history to someone who has TB.
E. What is the client's living situation (including past history of homelessness)?
F. Review travel history to endemic areas with TB, including China, Pakistan, the Philippines, Thailand, Indonesia, Bangladesh, and the Democratic Republic of Congo.
G. Review HIV status or need for testing.

Physical Examination

A complete physical examination is mandatory. Physical findings of pulmonary TB are not specific and usually are absent in mild or moderate disease.

A. Record temperature, respirations, pulse, BP, and weight.
B. Inspect:
    1. Observe overall appearance.
    2. Check skin for pallor.
    3. Inspect eyes, ears, nose, and throat.
C. Auscultate:
    1. Heart
    2. Lungs and chest for the following:
        a. Rales in upper posterior chest
        b. Bronchophony: Voice sounds louder than usual
        c. Whispered pectoriloquy: Client's whispered sounds are louder than normal
D. Percuss:
    1. Chest
E. Palpate:
    1. With lymphadenopathy, usually anterior or posterior cervical and supraclavicular nodes are involved.

Less commonly involved lymph nodes include submandibular, axillary, and inguinal lymph nodes.
    2. Abdomen to evaluate hepatosplenomegaly.
F. Neurologic examination:
    1. Evaluate the presence of nuchal rigidity.
    2. Assess deep tendon reflexes.

Diagnostic Tests

Diagnosis is based on a combination of tuberculin skin testing, PPD or serum Quantiferon TB Gold testing, and sputum cultures. Bronchoscopy may be required to obtain specimens. Clients with primary TB may not undergo imaging. However, conventional CXR may be performed; 15% of clients with primary TB have normal CXR findings.

Clients with progressive primary or post-primary TB may need a CT to evaluate parenchymal involvement, satellite lesions, bronchogenic spread, and miliary disease. Magnetic resonance imaging (MRI) may be ordered to evaluate complications, such as the extent of thoracic wall involvement with empyema.

A. Tuberculin skin test using the Mantoux test is the recommended method. The dosage of 0.1 mL or 5 tuberculin units (TU) of PPD should be injected intradermally into the volar aspect of the forearm using a 27-gauge needle. A wheal should be raised and should measure approximately 6 to 10 mm in diameter. Skilled personnel should read the test in 48 to 72 hours after administration. Measure the amount of induration and note the erythema. Measure transverse to the long axis of the forearm (see Table 9.4).
B. Quantiferon TB Gold is an alternative TB test for detecting both TB and latent TB infection.
C. Annual Mantoux tests are given for those at high risk. There is no need to repeat PPD once the client has reacted and had a positive PPD.
D. AP and lateral CXR films: "Snowstorm" appearance indicates miliary TB; segmental consolidation and hilar adenopathy are common; pleural effusion may be present.
E. CBC with differential may be performed.
F. Sputum culture with acid-fast smear:
    1. Nasopharyngeal secretions and saliva are not acceptable.

TABLE 9.4	INTERPRETATION OF MANTOUX TUBERCULIN SKIN TEST
Positive Reaction— Induration Size	**Risk Factors**
5 mm or more	Close contact with a known or suspected TB; immunosuppressive conditions (e.g., HIV); on immunosuppressive medications; or an abnormal CXR—consistent with active TB, previously active TB, or clinical evidence of the disease, children, organ transplant recipients, other immunosuppressive illnesses or high-risk medical conditions (silicosis and end-stage renal disease on dialysis).
10 mm or more	High-risk categories (i.e., homeless, HIV infected, users of illicit drugs, residents in nursing homes, incarcerated, or institutionalized); travel histories or recent immigration to high-prevalence areas of world; mycobacteriology lab personnel, employees of high-risk settings).
15 mm or more	Low-risk persons

TB, tuberculosis.

Source: Adapted from Centers for Disease Control and Prevention. (2016). Tuberculosis: Fact sheets tuberculin skin testing. Retrieved from https://www.cdc.gov/tb/publications/factsheets/testing/skintesting.htm

2. Gastric aspirate specimens for children younger than 6 years old. (Young children do not have a cough deep enough for a sputum specimen.)

G. Interferon-gamma release assay (IGRA) test

H. HIV testing as indicated by risk factors to guide management

I. Pregnancy test (if indicated) to guide management

Differential Diagnoses

A. TB

B. Bronchiectasis

C. Asthma

D. Histoplasmosis

E. Coccidioidomycosis

F. Blastomycosis

G. Malignancies

H. Other pulmonary infections

I. Aspiration pneumonia

Plan

A. General interventions:

1. Report all suspected and confirmed cases of TB to the local health department.

2. Directly observed therapy (DOT) is mandatory for the treatment of clients with coexistent HIV disease, those with multidrug-resistant (MDR) TB, and those who may be noncompliant.

B. Client teaching:

1. Educate clients regarding compliance to therapy, adverse effect of medications, and follow-up care.

C. Pharmaceutical therapy: The American Thoracic Society (ATS) and the CDC provide the standard guidelines for therapy.

1. Contact public health authorities for up-to-date recommendations on medications. Medication protocols vary and include the following first-line agents: isoniazid (INH), rifampin (Rifadin), pyrazinamide (Tebrazid), and ethambutol (Etibi) (see Table 9.5).

a. Isoniazid (Laniazid, Nydrazid) dosing:

i. Adults: 5 mg/kg by mouth (not to exceed 300 mg/d)

ii. Pediatrics: 10 to 20 mg/kg by mouth every day; not to exceed 300 mg/d

b. Rifampin (Rifadin) dosing:

i. Adults: 10 mg/kg, maximum of 600 mg/d

ii. Pediatrics: 10 to 20 mg/kg by mouth every day; not to exceed 600 mg/d

c. Pyrazinamide (Tebrazid) dosing:

i. Adults: 25 mg/kg by mouth every day; not to exceed 2 g/d

ii. Pediatrics: Not routinely recommended in children receiving INH. Public health authorities should be contacted for current guidelines.

d. Ethambutol (Myambutol) dosing:

i. Adults with no previous anti-TB therapy: 15 mg/kg by mouth every day

ii. Pediatrics: For those older than 13 years administer as in adults; not recommended for those younger than 13 years.

2. Compliance with drug regimen is most important.

3. Drug resistance averages 5% to 10% nationally and is increasing.

4. The bacilli Calmette–Guérin (BCG) vaccine is available for the prevention of disseminated TB. BCG is a live vaccine. BCG does not prevent infection with *M. tuberculosis*.

Follow-Up

A. Regular follow-up every 4 to 8 weeks to ensure compliance and to monitor the adverse effects and response of the medications.

B. Repeat CXR may be performed after 2 to 3 months of therapy to observe the response to treatment for clients with pulmonary TB.

C. Consider monitoring liver enzymes monthly in the following clients:

1. Severe or disseminated TB

2. Concurrent or recent hepatic disease or hepatobiliary tract disease from other causes

3. Those receiving high doses of INH (10 mg/kg/d) in combination with rifampin, pyrazinamide, or both drugs

4. Women who are pregnant or within the first 6 weeks postpartum

5. Clinical evidence of hepatotoxic effects

TABLE 9.5   TREATMENT OF TUBERCULOSIS

Tuberculosis	Regimen	Duration
Pulmonary and cervical lymphadenopathy	Isoniazid (INH) + rifampin	6 months
	Supplement with pyrazinamide	First 2 months only
Hilar adenopathy	Isoniazid + rifampin daily or INH + rifampin daily then INH + rifampin twice a week	9 months 1 month 8 months
Bone and joint disease and miliary disease	INH + rifampin + pyrazinamide and streptomycin once a day then INH + rifampin once a day	2 months 7–10 months
TB in clients with HIV	Consult with a specialist	

Note: Current guidelines should be in accordance with the Centers for Disease Control and Prevention (CDC).

TB, tuberculosis.

Consultation/Referral

An infectious diseases consultation for the management of affected clients.

Individual Considerations

A. Pregnancy:

1. Manage TB on a case-by-case basis with a physician.

2. Chemotherapy must be started immediately after the first trimester to protect both mother and fetus.

    a. First-line agents recommended by the AAP include INH, rifampin, and ethambutol.

    b. Streptomycin is contraindicated in pregnancy.

3. All pregnant women on INH therapy should receive pyridoxine.

4. The mother who has current disease but is non-contagious at delivery does not require separation of the infant and the mother. The mothers can also breastfeed.

    a. Evaluation of the infant includes CXR and Mantoux test at age 4 to 6 weeks.

    b. If the Mantoux test is negative, a repeat test is warranted at age 3 to 4 months and at age 6 months.

    c. INH should be administered even if the Mantoux results and CXR do not suggest TB because sufficient cell-mediated immunity to prevent progressive disease may not develop until age 6 months.

5. The mother who has current disease and is contagious at delivery requires separation of the mother and the infant until the mother is noncontagious. The management is the same as noted earlier.

B. Pediatrics:

1. Most children and adolescents with positive skin tests are asymptomatic.

2. Mantoux tests are given at ages 1 year, between 4 and 6 years, between 11 and 16 years, and annually to children at risk.

3. Neonatal symptoms of TB typically develop in the second or third week of life and include poor feeding, poor weight gain, cough, lethargy, and irritability.

4. The AAP recommends administration of 9 months of therapy for latent TB. The drug of choice is INH.

5. INH tablets can be crushed and added to food. Isoniazid liquid without sorbitol should be used to avoid osmotic diarrhea.

6. Rifampin capsules can be opened and the powder added to food.

7. Young children are at high risk of disseminated TB and permanent sequela. Timely treatment is essential.

8. TB is commonly diagnosed clinically and should be considered in children presenting with superficial lymph adenopathy and CNS dysfunction.

C. Geriatrics:

1. The majority of cases of TB in older adults are due to reactivation of previous TB exposure.

2. Most cases of TB in older adults have pulmonary involvement (75%).

3. For long-term care, use a two-step TB PPD test for initial screening of newly admitted residents.

4. Treatment of active TB is the same as in younger adults. Renal and hepatic labs should be monitored according to the manufacturer's recommendations.

5. Adult clients who have recently converted to positive TB status should receive prophylaxis with INH for 9 months.

Bibliography

Adams, L. V., & Starke, J. R. (2018, October). Tuberculosis disease in children. *UpToDate*. Retrieved from http://www.uptodate.com/contents/tuberculosis-disease-in-children

American Lung Association. (n.d.). *Tuberculosis*. Retrieved from http://www.lung.org/lung-health-and-diseases/lung-disease-lookup/tuberculosis

Clinical Infectious Diseases, Infectious Diseases Society of America. (2017). *Official American Thoracic Society/Infectious Diseases Society of America/Centers for Disease Control and Prevention clinical practice guidelines: Diagnosis of tuberculosis in adults and children*. Retrieved from https://www.cdc.gov/tb/publications/guidelines/pdf/ciw778.pdf

Hopewell, P. C., Kato-Maeda, M., & Ernst, J. D. (2016). Tuberculosis. In V. C. Broaddus, R. J. Mason, J. D. Ernst, T. E. King, S. C. Lazarus, J. F. Murray, … M. B. Gotway (Eds.), *Murray & Nadel's textbook of respiratory medicine* (6th ed., Vol. 1, pp. 593–628). Philadelphia, PA: Elsevier Saunders.

Horsburgh, C. R. Jr. (2019, January). Treatment of latent tuberculosis infection in HIV-uninfected nonpregnant adults. *UpToDate*. Retrieved from https://www-uptodate-com/treatment-of-latent-tuberculosis-infection-in-hiv-uninfected-nonpregnant-adults

Pozniak, A. (2019, March). Clinical manifestations and complications of pulmonary tuberculosis. *UpToDate*. Retrieved from http://www.uptodate.com/contents/clinical-manifestations-and-complications-of-pulmonary-tuberculosis

Raviblione, M. C. (2015). Tuberculosis. In D. L. Kasper, A. S. Fauci, S. L. Hauser, D. L. Longo, & J. L. Jameson (Eds.), *Harrison's principles of internal medicine* (19th ed., pp. 1102–1121). New York, NY: McGraw-Hill. Retrieved from http://accessmedicine.mhmedical.com/book.aspx?bookid=1130

Resnick, B. (Ed.). (2017). *GNRS geriatric nursing review syllabus: A core curriculum in advanced practice geriatric nursing* (5th ed.). New York, NY: American Geriatrics Society.

Sterling, T. R. (2018, October). Treatment of pulmonary tuberculosis in HIV-uninfected adults. *UpToDate*. Retrieved from http://www.uptodate.com/contents/treatment-of-pulmonary-tuberculosis-in-hiv-uninfected-adults

10 Cardiovascular Guidelines

Acute Myocardial Infarction

Jill C. Cash and Debbie Gunter

Definition
A. Acute myocardial infarction (MI) is a prolonged lack of myocardial oxygenation leading to necrosis of a portion of the heart muscle. It is caused by atherosclerotic coronary artery disease (CAD), which alone or in association with other factors causes complete blockage of one of the coronary arteries.

Incidence
A. According to the Centers for Disease Control and Prevention (CDC) in 2017, approximately 790,000 Americans experience an acute MI annually in the United States (Benjamin & Blaha, 2017). Of these, 580,000 MIs are a first-time event, and 210,000 are a subsequent MI. Despite a marked decrease in incidence and mortality during the past three decades, MI continues to be the leading cause of death in the United States, accounting for one-fourth of all fatalities. More women die from heart disease than do men.

Pathogenesis
A. Abrupt coronary artery occlusion is the primary cause of most MIs. Occlusions can result from atherosclerotic plaque, intracoronary thrombus formation, or arterial spasm.

Predisposing Factors
A. Hypercholesterolemia: Increased low-density lipoprotein (LDL) and decreased high-density lipoprotein (HDL)
B. Hypertriglyceridemia
C. Premature familial onset of coronary heart disease (CHD), formerly called CAD, before age 55 years
D. Smoking
E. Hypertension (HTN)
F. Obesity
G. Sedentary lifestyle
H. Diabetes mellitus
I. Aging
J. Stress

Common Complaints
A. Primary complaint: Pain somewhere in chest, described as worst pain ever experienced
B. Nausea
C. Vomiting
D. Diaphoresis
E. Indigestion

Other Signs and Symptoms
A. Pain in abdomen, arm, back, jaw, and neck
B. Chest heaviness or tightness
C. Anxiety
D. Cough
E. Dyspnea
F. HTN or hypotension
G. Weakness, light-headedness, syncope
H. Pallor
I. Orthopnea
J. Fatigue
K. Malaise

Potential Complications
A. Arrhythmias
B. Heart failure (HF)
C. Cardiogenic shock
D. Rupture of left ventricular (LV) papillary muscle
E. Ventricular septal rupture
F. Pericarditis or Dressler's syndrome
G. Ventricular aneurysm
H. Thromboembolism
I. Death

Subjective Data
A. Ask the client what activity brought about or preceded the episode of chest pain.
B. Ask the client to describe the duration of pain and what time of day symptoms began.
C. Ask the client to describe the pain—for example, crushing, stabbing, or burning.
D. Ask the client where sensation began and in what direction it radiates.
E. Identify the degree of pain by using a pain scale of 1 to 10, with 1 being the least painful.

F. Ask the client to list all medications currently being taken, particularly substances not prescribed and illicit drugs such as cocaine.

Physical Examination

Clients presenting with acute chest pain should be quickly assessed for the need to call emergency services/911 for immediate transport to the hospital.

A. Check pulse, respirations, blood pressure (BP), and pulse oxygenation.

B. Inspect:
1. General appearance, noting dyspnea and weakness
2. Skin for pallor and diaphoresis
3. Legs for edema
4. Chest wall for visible pulsations
5. Neck for jugular vein distention
6. Nail beds for signs of cyanosis and note capillary filling time

C. Palpate:
1. Abdomen for organomegaly
2. Peripheral pulses in legs
3. Femoral pulses

D. Auscultate:
1. Auscultate carotid arteries.
2. Auscultate abdomen.
3. Conduct a complete heart examination, checking for dysrhythmias.
4. Conduct a complete lung examination.

E. Mental status: Assess for confusion and anxiety.

Diagnostic Tests

A. EKG shows inverted T waves and ST-segment elevation; depending on the timing, Q waves may also be present. One normal EKG initially does not always rule out MI; perform serial EKGs if MI is suspected.

B. Laboratory testing:
1. Cardiac biomarkers/enzymes
2. Troponins: Troponins increase within 3 to 4 hours of injury and may remain elevated for 1 to 2 weeks
3. Creatine kinase (CK): Creatine kinase—muscle and brain (CK-MB) levels increase 3 to 12 hours after the chest pain begins, peak at 24 hours, and return to normal in 48 to 72 hours
4. Myoglobin: Urine myoglobin levels rise 1 to 4 hours after the chest pain begins
5. Complete blood count (CBC)
6. Chemistry profile
7. Lipid profile
8. C-reactive protein (CRP) and inflammatory markers

C. Cardiac imaging: Coronary angiogram

Differential Diagnoses

A. Acute MI
B. Unstable angina pectoris
C. Aortic dissection
D. Pulmonary embolism (PE)
E. Pericarditis
F. Esophageal spasm
G. Pancreatitis
H. Biliary tract disease

Plan

A. General interventions:
1. Educate the client and family regarding the signs and symptoms of an acute MI.
2. Long-term care and treatment should be reinforced at each client visit.

B. Client teaching:
1. Educate the client about modifying controllable risk factors, such as keeping diabetes and HTN under control, diet, exercise, and smoking cessation.
2. If known CHD is present:
   a. Instruct the client on signs and symptoms of an acute MI.
   b. Advise the client to have a plan for seeking medical attention or dialing 911 if signs and symptoms occur.
   c. Advise the client to carry nitroglycerin at all times and to take the nitroglycerin at the first sign of chest pain. If there is no relief after 5 minutes, 911 should be called. Nitroglycerin may be repeated every 5 minutes, up to a total of three doses.
   d. Encourage CPR training for family members and close friends.
   e. Exercise regimen: Encourage routine exercise for the client most days of the week, such as walking, treadmill use, and so on, once released by the cardiologist.
   f. Advise smoking cessation as indicated. Encourage support groups, classes, and smoking-cessation aids as indicated (*see Section III: Client Teaching Guide for Chapter 9, Nicotine Dependence*). ◄

C. Dietary management: Counsel the client on nutrition and a low-fat, low-cholesterol, low-sodium diet. Recommend the Dietary Approaches to Stop Hypertension (DASH) diet and lifestyle changes. Provide dietary handouts on the DASH diet, a low-fat, low-cholesterol, low-sodium diet. See Appendix B for the DASH diet.

D. Pharmaceutical therapy:
1. When MI is suspected: Aspirin 160 to 325 mg (four 81-mg baby aspirin) chewed or swallowed as soon as possible. Enteric-coated aspirin delays absorption and therefore is not recommended.
2. Instruct the client on how to take sublingual nitroglycerin tablets and other medications
3. Nitrates: Nitroglycerin sublingual 0.2 to 0.6 mg every 5 minutes for ischemic chest pain in the absence of hypotension up to three doses. Monitor side effects: headache and hypotension.
4. If pain persists after three doses of nitroglycerin:
   a. Morphine sulfate IV: 2 to 4 mg IV, repeating every 5 minutes until pain resolves. Dose may be increased at 2 to 8 mg per dose as tolerated. Monitor side effects: nausea/vomiting, dizziness, hypotension.
5. Oxygen therapy: 2 to 4 L per nasal cannula
6. If there are no contraindications (bradycardia, HF, second- or third-degree heart block, asthma, shock), beta-blockers may be started IV during the acute phase and changed to oral therapy during the course of the treatment.

7. Fibrinolytic therapy may be used for clients with suspected MI with ST-elevation myocardial infarction (STEMI) or non-ST-elevation myocardial infarction (NSTEMI) with left bundle branch block.

8. After an MI, if the client is not currently on a statin, a statin should be started.

Follow-Up

A. Follow-up is determined by the client's needs, severity of acute MI, and whether complications are present.

Consultation/Referral

A. If MI is suspected, call 911 and refer the client for immediate hospitalization.

B. According to the 2015 American College of Cardiology/American Heart Association (ACC/AHA) guidelines, a client who is a candidate for reperfusion and who is seen at a percutaneous coronary intervention (PCI)–capable hospital should be sent to the catheterization lab for primary PCI in 90 minutes or less. If the client is at a facility that is non-PCI capable, then a transfer should be made to a PCI-capable facility as soon as possible in 120 minutes or in less than or equal to 120 minutes. If the time lapse will be more than 120 minutes, then it is recommended to administer fibrinolytic therapy within 30 minutes of arrival.

C. Follow up with cardiologist as scheduled when discharged from the hospital.

Individual Considerations

A. Adults:

1. Women do not always complain of typical chest pain. Suspect MI in clients who complain of shortness of breath (SOB), back pain, jaw pain, nausea, just not feeling right, or profound fatigue. Men may also exhibit these symptoms.

B. Geriatrics:

1. Consider MI in clients complaining of atypical chest pain. Symptoms may include dyspnea, fatigue, dizziness, confusion, altered mental state, indigestion, jaw pain, and nausea.

2. Older adults may not perceive chest pain as being severe and may not consider that symptoms may be related to a heart attack because of an altered pain perception. Educate older adults that pain perception may be diminished as one ages.

Bibliography

American Diabetes Association. (2019). Cardiovascular disease and risk management: Standards of medical care in diabetes—2019. *Diabetes Care, 42*(suppl 1), S103–S123. doi:10.2337/dc19-S010

Amsterdam, E. A., Wenger, N. K., Brindis, R. G., Casey, D. E., Ganiats, T. G., Holmes, D. R., & Zieman, S. J. (2014). AHA/ACC guideline for the management of patients with non-ST-elevation acute coronary syndromes: A report of the American College of Cardiology/American Heart Association Task Force on Practice Guidelines and the Heart Rhythm Society. *Circulation, 130*(25), e344–e426. doi:10.1161/CIR.0000000000000133

Drug information. (2019). *Prescribers' digital reference.* Retrieved from www.pdr.net

Eckel, R. H., Jakicic, J. M., Ard, J. D., deJesus, J. M., Houston-Miller, N., Hubbard, V. S., & Yanovski, S. Z. (2014). 2013 AHA/ACC guideline on lifestyle management to reduce cardiovascular risk: A report of the American College of Cardiology/American Heart Association

Task Force on practice guidelines. *Circulation, 129*(25), S76–S99. doi:10.1161/01.cir.0000437740.48606.d1. Retrieved from http://circ.ahajournals.org/content/129/25_suppl_2/S76

Food and Drug Administration. (2018, June 12). *Use the nutrition facts label to reduce your intake of sodium in your diet.* Retrieved from https://www.fda.gov/food/nutrition-education-resources-materials/use-nutrition-facts-label-reduce-your-intake-sodium-your-diet

Goff, D. C., Lloyd-Jones, D. M., Bennett, G., Coady, S., & D'Agostino, B. R. Sr. (2014). 2013 ACC/AHA guideline on the assessment of cardiovascular risk: A report of the American College of Cardiology/American Heart Association Task Force on practice guidelines. *Circulation, 129*(25, Suppl. 2), S49–S73. doi:10.1161/01.cir.0000437741.48606.98

O'Gara, P. T., Kushner, F. G., Ascheim, D. D., Casey, D. E., Chung, M. K., de Lemos, J. A., & Zhao, D. X. (2013, January). 2013 ACCF/AHA guideline for the management of ST-elevation myocardial infarction: A report of the American College of Cardiology Foundation/American Heart Association Task Force on Practice Guidelines. *Journal of the American College of Cardiology, 61*(4), e78–e140. Retrieved from http://content.onlinejacc.org/article.aspx?articleid=1486115

O'Gara, P. T., Kushner, F. G., Ascheim, D. D., Casey, D. E., Chung, M. K., de Lemos, J. A., . . . Zhao, D. X. (2016, March). 2015 ACC/AHA/SCAI focused update on primary percutaneous coronary intervention for patients with ST-elevation myocardial infarction. *Journal of the American College of Cardiology, 67*(10), 1235–1250. Retrieved from http://www.onlinejacc.org/content/67/10/1235?_ga=2.97161503.1451040440.1555197207-1269255221.1523817965

Arrhythmias

Jill C. Cash and Debbie Gunter

Definition

Arrhythmias are abnormal heart rhythms. Common types are the following:

A. Bradycardia: Heart rate less than 60 beats per minute (bpm); impulse originates in sinoatrial (SA) node

B. Tachycardia: Heart rate greater than 100 to 160 bpm; impulse originates in SA node

C. Supraventricular tachydysrhythmias (SVTs): Heart rate greater than 100 bpm; the origin of impulse is listed as follows:

1. Atrioventricular (AV) nodal reentrant tachycardia (NRT): Intranodal reentry by means of fast and slow conduction pathways within the AV junction

2. Orthodromic atrioventricular reentrant tachycardia (AVRT): Tachycardia across accessory pathways associated with preexcitation

D. Atrial fibrillation (AF): Chaotic electrical activity caused by rapid discharges from numerous ectopic foci in atria. Atrial rate is difficult to count. There are three types of AF:

1. Paroxysmal AF occurs in clients who usually have normal sinus rhythm (NSR), but then have an episode of faulty electrical signals and rapid heart rate. It usually starts suddenly and stops on its own. Symptoms can be mild or severe and usually stop in less than 24 hours, but may last for several days.

2. Persistent AF is a condition in which the abnormal heart rhythm continues for more than a week. It may stop on its own, or it can be stopped with treatment.

3. Permanent AF is a condition in which a normal heart rhythm cannot be restored with treatment. Both paroxysmal and persistent AF may become more frequent and, over time, result in permanent AF.

E. Premature ventricular contractions (PVCs) are impulses that form within the Purkinje network.

Incidence

A. SVTs are the most common cardiac arrhythmias presenting to healthcare providers.

B. AVNRT accounts for 60% to 70% of all SVTs.

C. AVRTs account for 30% to 40% of all SVTs. More than 90% of younger children who present with SVTs are likely to have an AVRT, but once they reach adolescence, AVNRT is the primary cause of SVT in about one-third of these clients.

D. AF is the most common cardiac tachydysrhythmia, affecting approximately 2% of the general population. Prevalence increases with age to 5% of those older than 69 years. The presence of AF is associated with a fivefold increase in the risk of morbidity, a twofold increase in mortality, and an increased incidence of embolic stroke. It is estimated that AF will affect more than 7.5 million people by 2050.

E. PVCs are common, and their frequency increases with age.

Pathogenesis

A. Bradycardia: Dominance of the parasympathetic nervous system, with excessive vagal stimulation to the heart, causes a decreased heart rate of sinus node discharge.

B. Tachycardia: Dominant sympathetic nervous system stimulation of the heart or vagal inhibition results in positive chronotropic, dromotropic, and inotropic effects.

C. AVRT: The most classic form of this SVT is Wolff–Parkinson–White (WPW) syndrome. Reentry occurs in a loop using the atrial myocardium, AV node–His–Purkinje system, ventricular myocardium, and an accessory AV connection. During sinus rhythm, antegrade conduction through the accessory connection depolarizes the myocardium earlier than would occur by conduction through the AV node–His–Purkinje system, preexcitation is present, and a delta wave (slurring of initial deflection of the QRS complex) is usually seen on the surface 12-lead EKG.

D. AVNRT: The most common form is antegrade conduction, which occurs through a pathway with a short effective refractory period (ERP) and a longer conduction time. This pathway is often referred to as the *slow pathway*.

E. AF: Multiple, rapid impulses from many foci depolarize the atria in a totally disorganized manner. In the chaos, no P waves, no atrial contraction, no atrial kick, and a totally irregular ventricular response occur. The atria quiver, which leads to formation of mural thrombi and potential embolic events.

F. PVCs: These originate in the ventricles as a result of increased irritability in those cells.

Predisposing Factors

A. Bradycardia:
1. Increased vagal tone
2. Decreased sympathetic drive
3. Ischemia to SA node

4. Drugs: Digitalis, propranolol, sedatives, propylthiouracil (PTU) or Tapazole, aminophylline, caffeine, alcohol, nicotine, and sympathomimetics
5. Normal variant in athletes
6. Normal body response to insult
7. Atrial enlargement
8. Acute MI
9. Congestive heart failure (CHF)
10. Rheumatic heart disease
11. Hypertensive heart disease
12. Hypothyroidism
13. Hypothermia
14. Electrolyte abnormality
15. Acidosis
16. Infection

B. Tachycardia:
1. Decreased vagal tone
2. Increased sympathetic tone
3. MI
4. Hyperthyroidism

C. SVT:
1. Digitalis toxicity
2. Catecholamine surge

D. AF:
1. Myocardial ischemia
2. Thyrotoxicosis

E. PVC: Stress

Common Complaints

A. Symptoms may not be present; however, client may note irregular heartbeat
B. Palpitations
C. Chest discomfort
D. SOB
E. Dizziness
F. Diaphoresis
G. Weakness
H. Syncope
I. Nausea

Subjective Data

A. Obtain an accurate health and medical history.
B. Explore precipitating factors such as emotional stress, alcohol or drug use, or hot tub or bath use.
C. Inquire about the onset and duration of symptoms, also noting the client's age when symptoms began.
D. Explore whether the client has had concomitant weight loss, mood changes, and tremor, which are often associated with hyperthyroidism.
E. Carefully determine the number of previous episodes of palpitations or symptoms and what treatment, if any, was initiated.
F. Review all medications, including prescription, over-the-counter (OTC), and herbal products.

Physical Examination

A. Check pulse, respirations, BP, and weight:
1. Sinus bradycardia: Pulse rate decreased below 60 bpm
2. EKG: Normal

3. Sinus tachycardia: Pulse rate increased above 100 bpm:
   a. Pulse regular
   b. Systolic BP (SBP) constant
4. AF:
   a. Pulse irregular
   b. SBP changing
5. AVNRT:
   a. Pulse regular; AV block usual
   b. SBP constant; electrical alternans rare
6. AVRT:
   a. Pulse regular; AV block not present
   b. SBP constant; electrical alternans common, especially at high heart rates
7. PVC: Pulse diminished or absent during the PVC

B. Inspect:
1. General appearance:
   a. Is the client in respiratory distress? Note SOB, chest pain, dyspnea.
   b. Does the client look apathetic? This is a sign of a thyroid problem.
2. Inspect the skin for flushing or pallor.
3. Examine the eyes, noting lid lag.
4. Assess the neck for jugular vein distention or thyromegaly.
   a. With sinus tachycardia, neck vein pulsation is normal.
   b. With AF, neck vein pulsation is irregular; assess for thyromegaly.
   c. AVNRT: Assess the neck veins for "frog sign," in which the atria contract against closed AV valves, producing rapid, regular, expansive venous pulsation in the neck, resembling the rhythmic puffing motion of a frog.
   d. AVRT: Assess for frog sign.

C. Auscultate the neck for carotid artery bruits and the heart for abnormal heart sounds. Heart rhythm may be regular or irregular, depending on type of dysrhythmia. Have the client perform a vagal maneuver (Valsalva maneuver). If the rapid heart rate responds to the vagal maneuver and the cycle is broken, it is likely the client has AVRT. If it does not respond, it is possible the client has AVNRT.
1. Sinus bradycardia:
   a. Rate less than 60 bpm
   b. Rhythm regular
2. Sinus tachycardia:
   a. Rate greater than 100 bpm
   b. Rhythm regular; gradual onset and cessation
   c. Constant loudness of first heart sound
3. AF:
   a. Rate: Atrial rate is nonmeasurable; ventricular rate is variable, usually rapid at onset.
   b. Rhythm: Atrial and ventricular rhythms are irregular.
   c. Loudness of first heart sound changes.
4. AVNRT:
   a. AV block is usually present.
   b. Loudness of first heart sound is constant.

5. AVRT:
   a. AV block is not present.
   b. Constant loudness of first heart sound
6. PVC:
   a. Rate depends on underlying rhythm.
   b. Rhythm: Prematurity interrupts regularity of rhythm.

Diagnostic Tests
A. EKG
B. Drug screen:
   1. Digitalis
   2. Aminophylline
   3. Illicit drugs
C. Electrolytes
D. Arterial blood gases (ABGs) if indicated

Differential Diagnoses
A. Multifocal atrial tachycardia
B. Sinus tachycardia with multiple premature atrial contractions
C. Atrial flutter
D. Ventricular tachycardia
E. AV blocks

Plan
A. General interventions:
   1. Remove as many predisposing factors as possible.
   2. Stop smoking.
   3. Decrease or stop caffeine use.
B. Client teaching:
   1. Teach relaxation techniques.
   2. Teach the client and his or her family signs of hemodynamic compromise, including rapid heart rate, unexplained weight gain or loss, worsening dyspnea on exertion, and decreased exercise tolerance.
   3. Teach and reassure the client about long-term medication therapy and its side effects.
   4. Educate the client and family regarding safety, dietary restrictions, and complications that may occur (bleeding) with the use of anticoagulant therapy.
   5. Discuss the need for a pacemaker/defibrillator or surgical ablation.
C. Pharmaceutical therapy:
   1. Initial treatment usually is prescribed by a physician/cardiologist.
   2. Selection of treatment modality should be based on underlying pathophysiology
   3. For reentrant cases (AVNRT, AVRT), agents that block the reentrant circuit are more effective:
      a. Calcium channel blockers (CCBs)
      b. Beta-blockers—long acting
      c. Digitalis
   4. Episodes caused by increased automaticity are treated with antiarrhythmic therapy.
   5. Chronic AF is treated with anticoagulants such as warfarin sodium (Coumadin) or direct thrombin inhibitors.

a. Start therapy as soon as possible if a history of underlying heart disease is present.

b. Evaluate prothrombin time/international normalized ratio (PT/INR) on a regular basis to monitor for therapeutic response to warfarin sodium treatment.

Follow-Up

A. Clients who have their first episode of AF should return to the clinic within 24 to 48 hours for reevaluation.
B. Clients on antiarrhythmic agents should have liver enzymes measured during the first 4 to 8 weeks of therapy.
C. Clients with risk factors for developing cardiac complications to therapy, such as QT prolongation, should have an EKG during the first weeks of therapy and every 3 to 6 months thereafter.
D. Clients on digitalis should be carefully monitored for signs of toxicity. Caution the client regarding interactions of medication with digitalis.

Consultation/Referral

A. Clients with hemodynamic instability should be referred to a hospital or 911 immediately.
B. Clients unable to tolerate their dysrhythmia should be hospitalized immediately.
C. Consult a physician if the client has an abnormal EKG pattern, refractory AF, suspicion of WPW syndrome, or sick sinus syndrome.
D. Consult a physician when questions arise about the difference between a narrow and wide QRS complex.

Individual Considerations

A. Pregnancy: Digitalis is safe during pregnancy.
B. Pediatrics:
  1. Paroxysmal supraventricular tachycardia (PSVT) is probably the most common pediatric arrhythmia.
  2. Instruct young adult clients without underlying heart disease to quit/avoid smoking, avoid sleep deprivation, and limit use of alcohol and stimulants.
C. Geriatrics:
  The incidence of AF increases with age to 5% of those older than 69 years of age and should be suspected with any complaint of SOB, breathlessness, or fluttering sensation.

Bibliography

Benjamin, E. J., Blaha, M. J., Chiuve, S., Cushman, M., Das, S., Deo, R., . . . American Heart Association Statistics Committee and Stroke Statistics Subcommittee. (2017). Heart disease and stroke statistics—2017 update: A report from the American Heart Association. *Circulation, 135*(1), e1–e603. doi:10.1161/CIR.0000000000000485

Drug information. (2019). *Prescribers' digital reference.* Retrieved from www.pdr.net

Kusumoto, F., Shoenfeld, M., & Barrett, C. (2018). 2018 ACC/AHA/HRS guideline on the evaluation and management of patients with bradycardia and cardiac conduction delay. *Journal of the American College of Cardiology, 74*(7), e51–e156. doi:10.1016/j.jacc.2018.10.044

Mozaffarian, D., Benjamin, E. J., & Go, A. S. (2016). Heart disease and stroke statistics—2016 update: A report from the American Heart Association. *Circulation, 133*(4), 447–454. doi:10.1161/CIR.0000000000000350

Prutkin, J. (2019, January). Overview of the acute management of tachyarrhythmias. *UpToDate.* Retrieved from https://www.uptodate.com/contents/overview-of-the-acute-management-of-tachyarrhythmias

Atherosclerosis and Hyperlipidemia

Jill C. Cash and Debbie Gunter

Definition

A. Atherosclerosis is a systemic disease characterized by lipid deposition and smooth muscle cell migration and proliferation in the intima of the larger arteries. Atheromatous changes lead to thrombotic stroke, peripheral vascular disease (PVD), atherosclerotic cardiovascular disease (ASCVD), and MI (see Figure 10.1).

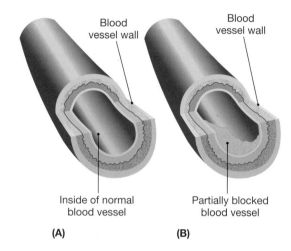

FIGURE 10.1 Atherosclerosis. (A) Normal blood vessel. (B) Partially blocked blood vessel.

B. Hyperlipidemia is an elevation in serum lipoproteins and a major risk factor in the development of cardiovascular disease (CVD). The two main lipids in blood are cholesterol and triglyceride. Cholesterol is a relatively insoluble lipid that is necessary for cell membrane formation, steroid and bile salt production, and the development of nerve sheaths. Cholesterol is composed of three clinically significant components: high-density lipoprotein cholesterol (HDL-C), low-density lipoprotein cholesterol (LDL-C), and very-low-density lipoprotein (VLDL). Triglyceride is found in VLDL particles, but its role in atherosclerosis is not clear.
C. The atherosclerotic buildup of lipids, cholesterol, calcium, and cellular debris within the intima of the blood vessels causes plaque formation, vascular remodeling, and acute and chronic obstruction of the lumen of the blood vessels. This decreases blood flow, causing myocardial ischemia and decreased oxygen to other vital organs.
D. In 2018, the ACC/AHA published an updated guideline on the assessment of cardiovascular risk, lifestyle management, and treatment of cholesterol to reduce ASCVD risks. A web-based calculator is available to help estimate 10-year and lifetime risks for ASCVD in individuals without a history of ASCVD (tools.acc.org/ASCVD-Risk-Estimator-Plus/#!/calculate/estimate/). These tools can be used to drive conversations about client risk factors for ASCVD, potential benefits, negative aspects of risk, and client preferences regarding initiation of relevant therapies. The assessment of ASCVD risk factors is recommended every 4 to 6 years in adults 20 to 79 years of

age who are free from ASCVD; the 10-year ASCVD risk should be estimated every 4 to 6 years in adults aged 40 to 79 years who are free from ASCVD. Long-term and lifetime risk information may be used to motivate therapeutic lifestyle changes (TLCs) and encourage adherence to these changes and pharmacological therapies.

Incidence

A. Atherosclerosis begins in childhood with the development of fatty streaks. The incidence of atherosclerotic diseases increases with age. CVD causes one in three deaths reported each year in the United States. CVD claims more lives each year than all forms of cancer and chronic lower respiratory disease combined. Direct and indirect costs of CVD and stroke are estimated to total more than $316 billion.

B. The leading risk factors for CVD are HTN, high cholesterol, and smoking.

1. HTN can increase arterial wall tension, potentially leading to disturbed repair processes and aneurysm formation.

2. Cigarette smoking is associated with an increase in multiple inflammatory markers, including CRP, interleukin-6, and tumor necrosis factor.

Pathogenesis

A. Atherosclerosis is in part attributed to the deposition of cholesterol and lipoproteins in arterial smooth muscle cells. Dietary factors, obesity, drugs, and genetic defects in lipoprotein particle metabolism influence lipid and lipoprotein concentrations in blood.

B. Primary hyperlipoproteinemias are caused by either single-gene disorders transmitted by simple dominant or recessive mechanisms or multifactorial disorders with complicated inheritance patterns

C. Secondary hyperlipoproteinemias (such as in thyroid disease and diabetes mellitus) occur as part of a constellation of abnormalities in certain metabolic pathways. The associations among atherosclerosis, CVD, and hypercholesterolemia are well documented. HDL-C accounts for about one-fourth of the total serum cholesterol and acts as a scavenger, removing cholesterol from peripheral tissues and returning it to the liver, which produces a favorable cardioprotective effect. Elevated HDL-C levels are desirable. HDL-C levels greater than 60 mg/dL are a negative risk factor for CVD; those below 35 mg/dL are a major risk factor for CVD.

D. LDL-C constitutes 70% of the total serum cholesterol. It is the most atherogenic cholesterol subgroup. LDL-C particles interact with platelets, damaged arterial endothelium, and smooth muscle cells in the process of plaque formation. LDL-C levels of 160 mg/dL or greater are associated with an increased number of cardiac events.

E. VLDL accounts for a small amount of total serum cholesterol and is responsible for carrying triglycerides from the liver. Its role in atherogenesis is uncertain, but an inverse relationship has been observed between VLDL and HDL-C.

Predisposing Factors

A. High-risk factors for CVD events (CVD risk equivalent):
1. Clinical CVD
2. Symptomatic carotid artery disease
3. Peripheral arterial disease (PAD)
4. Abdominal aortic aneurysm

B. Presence of major risk factors (other than LDL-C):
1. **Age is the strongest risk factor for the development of CVD:**
   a. Age greater than 45 years for men and greater than 55 years for women
   b. Elderly persons experience a higher morbidity and mortality.
2. Cigarette smoking
3. Low HDL-C level, less than 40 mg/dL
4. Family history of early CVD: MI or sudden cardiac death at younger than 55 years in father or other male first-degree relative, or before age 65 years in mother or other female first-degree relative
5. HTN (BP > 140/90 mmHg or on antihypertensive medication)
6. Sedentary lifestyle
7. Obesity
8. Metabolic syndrome
9. Diabetes
10. Chronic inflammation

> HDL-C greater than 60 mg/dL is equal to a "negative" risk factor and removes one risk factor from the total count.

Common Complaints

There are no complaints or symptoms associated with atherosclerosis and hyperlipidemia. Most lipid abnormalities are detected by routine laboratory testing or as part of a cardiovascular evaluation.

Subjective Data

A. Ask the client if there is a history of CVD.
B. Discuss his or her past medical history, including predisposing factors for CVD.
C. Have the client list current medications, including OTC and herbal products.
D. Have the client discuss his or her current diet and exercise routine.
E. Explore the client's social habits, including use of alcohol and tobacco.

Physical Examination

A. Check pulse, respirations, BP, height, and weight. Calculate body mass index (BMI) at each subsequent visit. An adult BMI calculator and a child and teenage BMI calculator are located at www.cdc.gov/healthyweight/assessing/bmi.
B. Inspect:
1. Funduscopic examination: Examine eyes for premature arcus cornealis, which is a gray opaque line

around the cornea caused by lipoid degeneration, and for lipemia retinalis, which is a pale retina with white blood vessels caused by excess serum lipids because of VLDL of more than 2,000 mg/dL or alcoholism.

2. Inspect skin for xanthomas, which appear as red-brown or yellow papules, nodules, or plaque, caused by lipid deposits from high VLDL. Tendinous xanthomas are found on Achilles tendons, patellae, and hands.

3. Inspect joints for Achilles tendonitis and arthritis.

C. Palpate:
   1. Palpate abdomen for hepatomegaly or splenomegaly.
   2. Palpate neck and thyroid.

D. Auscultate:
   1. Perform a complete heart examination.
   2. Perform a complete vascular examination.

Diagnostic Tests

A. Laboratory testing:
   1. Lipid profile and lipoprotein analysis (see Table 10.1).
   2. CBC
   3. Complete metabolic panel (CMP)
   4. Thyroid function studies to exclude disorders of the thyroid

   5. CRP
   6. Hemoglobin (Hgb) A1C (if appropriate)

B. Tests/imaging:
   1. Treadmill stress test
   2. Nuclear stress test
   3. Echocardiogram
   4. Ultrasound
   5. CT
   6. Coronary angioplasty

Differential Diagnoses

Assess the client for the following secondary causes of ASCVD and hyperlipidemia:

A. Atherosclerosis
B. Hyperlipidemia
C. Diabetes mellitus
D. Hypothyroidism
E. Nephrotic syndrome
F. Porphyria
G. Obesity
H. Obstructive liver disease
I. Diuretic use

TABLE 10.1   ATP III CLASSIFICATION OF LDL-C, TOTAL CHOLESTEROL, AND HDL-C (MG/DL)

Determine lipoprotein levels. In adults who are 20 years of age or older and not on lipid-lowering therapy, measurement of either a fasting or a nonfasting plasma lipid profile is effective in estimating ASCVD risk and documenting baseline. In adults who are 20 years of age or older and without a personal history of ASCVD but with a family history of premature ASCVD or genetic hyperlipidemia, measurement of a fasting plasma lipid profile is reasonable as part of an initial evaluation to aid in the understanding and identification of familial lipid disorders.

LDL-C—primary target of therapy	
<100	Optimal
<70	If coronary heart disease is present
130–159	Borderline high
160–189	High
≥190	Very high
Total cholesterol	
<200	Desirable
200–239	Borderline high
≥240	High
HDL-C	
<40	Low
≥60	High or ideal
Triglycerides	
<149	Good
150–199	Borderline
>200	High
500>	Very high

ATP, Adult Treatment Panel; HDL-C, high-density lipoprotein cholesterol; LDL-C, low-density lipoprotein cholesterol.

Plan

A. General interventions:

1. TLCs, including exercise, diet, and weight management, are recommended for all clients.

2. Increased physical activity. The 2018 ACC/AHA cholesterol and lifestyle management guidelines outline the physical activity recommendations; they advise adults to engage in 40 minutes of aerobic physical activity three to four times a week. The aerobic exercise should involve moderate to vigorous intensity to reduce BP, LDL-C, and non-HDL-C.

B. Dietary management:

1. Advise the client that diet modification is the first line of therapy for hyperlipidemia.

2. Explain the cholesterol-lowering diet. Give dietary recommendation sheets. See Appendix B for low-fat/low-cholesterol and DASH dietary approaches to stop HTN.

C. Client teaching:

1. Weight reduction: Explain that weight reduction in clients greater than 20% over ideal body weight can lower LDL-C and triglyceride levels.

2. Other key dietary recommendations:

   a. Reduce intake of saturated fats and trans fats. Aim for 5% to 6% of calories from saturated fat.

   b. Increase intake of polyunsaturated and monounsaturated fats.

   c. Increase intake of soluble fiber (psyllium supplement).

   d. Limit intake of alcohol: One drink per day for women and two drinks per day for men.

   e. Increase intake of plant stanols and sterols (1 oz of Promise Activ or Benecol spread per day).

   f. Increase intake of omega-3 fatty acids from marine sources (salmon or tuna twice a week or supplements).

   g. Follow the DASH, Mediterranean, or AHA diet.

   h. Lower sodium intake. Consume no more than 2,400 mg/d of sodium. Further reductions to 1,500 mg/d of sodium are associated with greater reduction in BP and may be recommended with concomitant HF and/or CKD.

3. Discuss smoking cessation (*see Section III: Client Teaching Guide for Chapter 9, Nicotine Dependence*).

D. Pharmaceutical therapy: Use clinical judgment when deciding potential benefits, possible side effects, and costs of drug treatment.

1. Drug of choice: HMG-CoA reductase inhibitors (statins):

   a. Statins suppress the activity of the key enzyme in cholesterol synthesis in the liver; they are highly effective in lowering LDL-C but can cause liver toxicity, myositis, rhabdomyolysis, and low HDL-C.

   b. There are four major statin benefit groups:

      i. Individuals with the presence of clinical ASCVD, including acute coronary syndromes, a history of MI, stable or unstable angina, coronary or other arterial revascularization, stroke, transient ischemic attack (TIA), or PAD

      ii. Individuals with primary elevations of LDL-C ≥ 190 mg/dL

      iii. Individuals 40 to 75 years of age with diabetes and LDL-C 70–189 mg/dL and without clinical ASCVD (refer to Chapter 20, "Endocrine Guidelines")

      iv. Individuals without clinical ASCVD or diabetes who are 40 to 75 years of age with an LDL-C 70–189 mg/dL and an estimated 10-year ASCVD risk of 7.5% or higher

   c. ASCVD events are reduced by using the maximum tolerated statin intensity in those groups shown to benefit. The expert panel defines intensity of statin therapy on the basis of the average expected LDL-C response to a specific statin and dose. The intensity levels are "high-intensity," "moderate-intensity," and "low-intensity" statin therapy. Full statin treatment recommendations for primary and secondary prevention as well as the high-, moderate-, and low-intensity statin therapy levels from the 2018 ACC/AHA guidelines on the treatment of cholesterol are available at www.onlinejacc.org/content/early/2018/11/02/j.jacc.2018.11.003?_ga=2.70988304.1451040440.1555197207-1269255221.1523817965.

   d. Monitor liver function tests (LFTs) before therapy begins, then 4 to 6 weeks after starting drug therapy. Check at 6- to 12-month intervals or more frequently, if necessary.

   e. Discontinue medications if abnormal laboratory values or adverse symptoms appear.

   f. Use caution with the use of statins and other medications. Avoid concomitant drugs such as erythromycin, nicotine, azole antifungals, clofibrate, and gemfibrozil.

2. Category X drugs: Statins are category X drugs and are contraindicated in pregnancy.

3. Nonstatin drug therapy (see Table 10.2 for the nonstatin drugs that affect cholesterol):

   a. Bile acid sequestrants bind bile acids in the gastrointestinal (GI) tract; lower moderately elevated LDL-C by 20%; and may cause constipation, bloating, and poor absorption of other drugs. Bile acid sequestrant therapy is not recommended if triglycerides are greater than 300 mg/dL.

   b. Nicotinic acid or niacin: Broad-spectrum lipid-regulating agent. Niacin has been documented to exhibit anti-inflammatory properties (reduction of lipoprotein-associated phospholipase A_2 and CRP).

      i. Discuss possibilities of flushing. Contraindicated with chronic liver disease and severe gout. The niacin-treated subjects in the Atherothrombosis Intervention in Metabolic Syndrome with Low HDL/High Triglycerides: Impact on Global Health (AIM-HIGH)

TABLE 10.2 NONSTATIN DRUGS AFFECTING LIPOPROTEIN METABOLISM

Drug Class	Agents and Daily Doses	Lipid/Lipoprotein Effects	Side Effects	Contraindications
Bile acid sequestrants	Cholestyramine (4–16 g), Colestipol (5–30 g), Colesevelam (1,875–3,750 mg)	LDL-C ↓ 15%–30% HDL-C ↑ 3%–5% TG No change or increase	GI distress Constipation Decreased absorption of other drugs	Absolute: • Dysbeta-lipoproteinemia • TG > 400 mg/dL Relative: • TG > 200 mg/dL
Nicotinic acid	Immediate-release (crystalline) nicotinic acid (1.5–3 g), extended-release nicotinic acid (Niaspan; 500–2,000 mg), sustained-release nicotinic acid (1–2 g)	LDL-C ↓ 5%–25% HDL-C ↑ 15%–35% TG ↓ 20%–50%	Flushing Hyperglycemia Hyperuricemia (or gout) Upper GI distress Hepatotoxicity	Absolute: • Chronic liver disease • Severe gout Relative: • Diabetes • Hyperuricemia • Peptic ulcer disease
Fibric acids	Gemfibrozil (600 mg BID); Fenofibrate (145–200 mg) Clofibrate (500–2,000 mg)	LDL-C ↓ 5%–20% (may be increased in clients with high TG) HDL-C ↑ 10%–20% TG ↓ 20%–50%	Dyspepsia Gallstones Myopathy	Absolute: • Severe renal disease • Severe hepatic disease
PCSK9 inhibitors	Alirocumab (75–150 mg q 2 weeks or 300 mg q 4 weeks) Evolocumab (140 mg q 2 weeks or 420 mg q 4 weeks)	LDL-C ↓ 43%–64%	Arthralgias Headache Limb pain Fatigue	Absolute: Prior hypersensitivity reaction to either medication
Cholesterol absorption inhibitor	Ezetimibe (Zetia) 10 mg q day	LDL-C ↓ 13%–20%	Diarrhea Back pain Abdominal pain	Absolute: None Serious: Cyclosporin

GI, gastrointestinal; HDL-C, high-density lipoprotein cholesterol; LDL-C, low-density lipoprotein cholesterol; TG, triglyceride.

clinical trial had a trend toward increased stroke incidence.

ii. The combination of niacin with other lipid-lowering drugs has been shown to reduce progression and promote regression of coronary and carotid atherosclerosis and improve clinical outcomes.

c. Fibric acid derivatives: Highly effective in lowering triglycerides; lower VLDL-C, cause modest reduction in LDL-C, and raise HDL-C.

i. Fibrates may cause GI distress, rash, pain, blurred vision, anemia, and gallstones.

ii. Fibrates may inhibit insulin and oral hypoglycemic absorption, and potentiate oral anticoagulants.

d. PCSK9 inhibitors: Fully human monoclonal antibodies that bind to PCSK9 and decrease degradation of the LDL receptor:

i. Indicated as adjunct to diet and maximally tolerated statin therapy for the treatment of adults with heterozygous familial hypercholesterolemia (HeFH) or clinical ASCVD, who require additional lowering of LDL-C

ii. Long-term safety remains to be determined.

e. Cholesterol absorption inhibitors: Mild decreases in LDL-C, may be used in conjunction with statins and fibrates

Follow-Up

A. Measure client's total cholesterol 4 weeks after initiation of diet and then at 3- to 4-month intervals.

B. If initiating medication therapy, obtain baseline blood work, including fasting or nonfasting lipid profile with LFTs and a CBC. In adults who are 20 years of age or older and not on lipid-lowering therapy, measurement of either a fasting or a nonfasting plasma lipid profile is effective in estimating ASCVD risk and documenting baseline. In adults who are 20 years of age or older and without a personal history of ASCVD but with a family history of premature ASCVD or genetic hyperlipidemia, measurement of a fasting plasma lipid profile is reasonable as part of an initial evaluation to aid in the understanding and identification of familial lipid disorders. Recheck tests 4 to 6 weeks after starting drug therapy. Then check at 6- to 12-month intervals or more frequently, if necessary.

Consultation/Referral

A. Refer to dietitian for nutritional counseling for dietary modifications.

Individual Considerations

A. Adults:

1. Clients with high cholesterol who are otherwise at low risk for ASCVD (particularly men older than age 35 years and premenopausal women) are candidates for primary prevention emphasizing diet modification and increased physical activity. It is recommended that drug therapy be used sparingly in these clients.

2. Lowering serum cholesterol reduces morbidity and mortality in clients with ASCVD, and reduces the number of new cardiac events in clients without known ASCVD

3. Elevated triglycerides increase the risk of pancreatitis and diabetes.

B. Children:

1. It is uncommon for children to have events secondary to atherosclerosis during childhood; however, the build-up of plaque begins during childhood and progressive changes can lead to heart events during early adulthood. Risk factors for children for this to occur include obesity, high BP, family history of heart disease, depression/bipolar disorder, exposure to cigarette smoking, and underlying chronic conditions.

2. Education and lifestyle changes during childhood are imperative to prevent these events in children and early adulthood. Education should include healthy diet, exercise, and avoiding exposures (cigarette smoke) that increase risk factors.

3. Guidelines for screening children have been developed according to risk factors. In 2016, the U.S. Preventive Services Task Force (USPSTF) concluded that the current evidence is insufficient to assess the balance of benefits and harms of screening for lipid disorders in children and adolescents 20 years or younger.

C. Geriatrics:

1. The decision to implement statin therapy for the high-risk very elderly client (>80 years) with ASCVD should include a shared decision-making approach with an honest discussion of benefits and risks, and consideration of client perceptions, comorbidities, concurrent medications, frailty, and cost concerns.

2. The majority of studies show overall a very favorable cardiovascular benefit with low associated risk that may help preserve quality of life.

3. The decision to prescribe high-intensity statin therapy needs to take into account many factors that may predispose the elderly client to increased risk.

Bibliography

American Diabetes Association. (2019). Cardiovascular disease and risk management: Standards of medical care in diabetes—2019. *Diabetes Care, 42*(suppl 1), S103–S123. doi:10.2337/dc19-S010

Boudi, F. B. (2016, April 25). Coronary artery atherosclerosis. *Medscape.* Retrieved from http://emedicine.medscape.com/article/153647-overview

Collins, J., (2018). Statin therapy for the very elderly >80 with ASCVD: Balancing the benefits and risks. *National Lipid Association.* Retrieved from https://www.lipid.org/node/1901

Drug information. (2019). *Prescribers' digital reference.* Retrieved from www.pdr.net

Eckel, R. H., Jakicic, J. M., Ard, J. D., deJesus, J. M., Houston-Miller, N., Hubbard, V. S., & Yanovsk, S. Z. (2014). 2013 AHA/ACC guideline on lifestyle management to reduce cardiovascular risk: A report of the American College of Cardiology/American Heart Association Task Force on practice guidelines. *Circulation, 129*(25), S76–S99. doi:10.1161/01.cir.0000437740.48606.d1. Retrieved from http://circ.ahajournals.org/content/129/25_suppl_2/S76

Food and Drug Administration. (2018, June 12). *Use the nutrition facts label to reduce your intake of sodium in your diet.* Retrieved from https://www.fda.gov/food/nutrition-education-resources-materials/use-nutrition-facts-label-reduce-your-intake-sodium-your-diet

Goff, D. C., Lloyd-Jones, D. M., Bennett, G., Coady, S., & D'Agostino, B. R. Sr. (2014). 2013 ACC/AHA guideline on the assessment of cardiovascular risk: A report of the American College of Cardiology/American Heart Association Task Force on practice guidelines. *Circulation, 129,* S49–S73. doi:10.1161/01.cir.0000437741.48606.98

Grundy, S., Stone, N., & Bailey, A. (2018, November). AHA/ACC/AACVPR/AAPA/ABC/ACPM/ADA/AGS/APhA/ASPC/NLA/PCNA guideline on the management of blood cholesterol. *Journal of the American College of Cardiology, 73*(24), e235–e350. doi:10.1016/j.jacc.2018.11.003. Retrieved from https://www.sciencedirect.com/science/article/pii/S073510971839034X?via%3Dihub

Kastelein, J. (2017). PCSK9 inhibitors: Pharmacology, adverse effects, and use. *UpToDate.* Retrieved from https://www.uptodate.com/contents/pcsk9-inhibitors-pharmacology-adverse-effects-and-use

Lavigne, P. M., & Karas, R. H. (2013). The current state of niacin in cardiovascular disease prevention: A systematic review and meta-regression. *Journal of the American College of Cardiology, 61*(4), 440–446. doi:10.1016/j.jacc.2012.10.030

Stone, N. J., Robinson, J., Lichtenstein, A. H., Bairey-Merz, C. N., Lloyd-Jones, D. M., Blum, C. B., & Wilson, P. W. (2013, November 7). 2013 ACC/AHA guidelines on the treatment of blood cholesterol to reduce atherosclerotic cardiovascular risk in adults: A report of the American College of Cardiology/American Heart Association Task Force on practice guidelines. *Journal of the American College of Cardiology, 53*(25), 2889–2934. Retrieved from https://www.ahajournals.org/doi/full/10.1161/01.cir.0000437738.63853.7a

Summary of the second report of the National Cholesterol Education Program Expert Panel on Detection, Evaluation, and Treatment of High Blood Cholesterol in Adults (Adult Treatment Panel II). (1993). *Journal of the American Medical Association, 269,* 3015–3023. doi:10.1001/jama.269.23.3015

Third report of the National Cholesterol Education Program (NCEP) Expert Panel on Detection, Evaluation, and Treatment of High Blood Cholesterol in Adults (Adult Treatment Panel III): Final report 2018. (2002). *Circulation, 106*(25), 3157–3160. Retrieved from https://www.ncbi.nlm.nih.gov/pubmed/12485966

Yang, E. (2018, November 30). Lipid management guidelines. *Medscape.* Retrieved from https://emedicine.medscape.com/article/2500032-overview

Atrial Fibrillation

Laura A. Petty

Definition

A. AF is the irregular and rapid heart rhythm caused by abnormal electrical impulse formation and/or propagation. These impulses make the heart's upper chambers (the atria) beat chaotically and out of sync with the heart's lower chambers (the ventricles), resulting in poor circulation of blood throughout the body.

B. Classification of AF:

1. Paroxysmal AF:

   a. Also called *intermittent AF*

b. Two or more episodes of AF that end spontaneously within 7 days or less and usually last less than 24 hours

2. Persistent AF:

a. AF that does not end spontaneously within 7 days

b. Usually requires pharmacological interventions and/or cardioversion to restore sinus rhythm

3. Permanent AF:

Persistent AF in which rhythm control strategies are no longer effective (such strategies are not utilized to restore sinus rhythm)

4. "Lone" AF:

The term used to reference clients with paroxysmal, persistent, or permanent AF who do not have structural heart disease

Incidence

A. The CDC notes that as of 2005, AF is the most frequently managed cardiac arrhythmia in the United States, with an estimated 2.7 to 6.1 million clients affected

B. AF is more common in women than in men. Men of any age are more likely than women to develop AF. However, because AF occurs much more often in older adults, and because there are more women than men older than age 75, the total numbers of women and men with AF in this age group are essentially the same.

C. By comparison, AF is more common in Caucasians.

Pathogenesis

A. Multiple impulses travel throughout the atria, yielding continuous electrical activity and an atrial rate in excess of 300 bpm. The impulses enter the AV node in a completely random manner. A small percentage of the impulses are conducted to the ventricle, which results in a lower ventricular rate, usually 100 to 180 bpm, and an irregularly irregular rhythm. This leads to ineffective atrial contractions, a decreased cardiac output, and an increased risk of thrombus formation.

Predisposing Factors

A. Age, increased occurrence after age 65 years

B. CAD

C. HTN, accounts for 14% to 22% of AF cases

D. Diabetes

E. Rheumatic heart disease

F. Valvular heart disease:

1. Mitral valve stenosis

2. Mitral regurgitation

3. Tricuspid regurgitation

G. Fibrosis or calcification in the vicinity of the AV node

H. Left ventricular hypertrophy (LVH)

I. HF

J. MI

K. Sick sinus syndrome

L. Hyperthyroidism

M. Infection

N. Pericarditis

O. Obstructive sleep apnea (OSA)

P. Obesity

Q. Recent cardiac surgery, including heart transplantation

R. Pulmonary diseases (related to hypoxia):

1. Chronic obstructive pulmonary disease (COPD)

2. Bronchitis, acute or chronic

3. Asthma

4. Emphysema

S. Electrolyte imbalances:

1. Hyperkalemia and hypokalemia

2. Hypercalcemia and hypocalcemia

3. Hypermagnesemia and hypomagnesemia

T. Factors that can trigger episodes of AF:

1. Physical or emotional stress

2. Nicotine

3. Caffeine

4. Alcohol

5. Exercise

Common Complaints

A. Palpitations

B. Angina

C. Fatigue

D. Dyspnea at rest or on exertion

E. Vertigo or dizziness

F. Disorientation

G. Confusion

H. Syncope

I. Headache

J. Urinary frequency or urgency

K. Anxiety

L. Asymptomatic presentation, most often seen in the elderly and in clients with permanent AF

Potential Complications

A. Stroke: The risk for stroke increases five times during an episode of AF.

B. PE

C. Peripheral emboli: May present as an ischemic extremity or ischemic bowel

Subjective Data

A. Ask the client what activity brought about or preceded the episode.

B. Have the client describe the duration of pain, if any, and what time of day the symptoms began.

C. Ask the client to describe his or her symptoms.

D. Ask the client whether any previous episodes have occurred.

E. Ask the client to list all medications, OTC products, and herbal products currently being taken or recently stopped.

1. Medications with links to AF:

a. Common complications with AF:

i. Theophylline (theophylline anhydrous, Theo-24, Elixophyllin)

ii. Digoxin (Lanoxin)

iii. Quinidine (quinidine gluconate, Nuedexta)

iv. Tricyclic antidepressants (TCAs)

b. Rare complications with AF:

i. Aricept (donepezil hydrochloride)

   c. Questionable complications with AF:
     i. Bisphosphonates (alendronate, risedronate, etidronate)

F. Ask the client to quantify his or her smoking history, alcohol history, and caffeine intake.

Physical Examination

A. **Clients presenting with an acute cardiovascular episode should be quickly assessed for the need to call emergency services/911 for immediate transport to the hospital.**

B. Vital signs: Check BP, pulse, and respirations. Count heart rate for 1 full minute.
   1. Check orthostatic BP: Sitting, standing, and lying down

C. Inspect:
   1. Inspect overall physical appearance, noting any distress.
   2. Inspect the neck: Check jugular vein distention and pulsations.
     a. Provoking maneuvers (i.e., carotid massage) should be performed only by a cardiologist.
   3. Inspect extremities: Note edema, pallor, and cyanosis.
   4. Perform a funduscopic examination: Note hemorrhage, exudates, and papilledema to determine the presence of malignant HTN.

D. Palpate:
   1. Palpate extremities for peripheral pulses in arm and groin; determine rate and regularity.
   2. Assess capillary refill.
   3. Palpate carotid arteries for thrills and heaves.

E. Auscultate:
   1. Heart: While the client is in sitting, standing, and left lateral recumbent positions, note normal and extra heart sounds (S_3 and S_4).
     a. S_4 is not present during AF.
   2. Neck for carotid bruits.
   3. Lungs: Note the presence of wheezing and crackles.

F. Additional areas for physical examination:
   1. Assess for focal neurological deficits (orientation, unilateral weakness, dysarthria).

Diagnostic Tests

A. CBC, basic metabolic panel (BMP; including electrolytes, blood glucose, blood urea nitrogen [BUN], creatinine), magnesium, and LFTs

B. Thyroid profile and lipid profile

C. Brain natriuretic peptide (BNP) and N-terminal pro b-type natriuretic peptide (NT-proBNP)

D. Cardiac profile (including troponin, creatine phosphokinase test [CPK], CK-MB)

E. Serum drug levels, digoxin, amiodarone, quinidine (if applicable)

F. INR, if applicable

G. Creatinine clearance (CrCl)

H. EKG

I. 2-D echocardiogram

J. Chest x-ray

K. Exercise stress test or thallium stress test if exercise-induced arrhythmia or CAD is suspected

L. Holter monitoring

M. Evaluation of sleep apnea

Differential Diagnoses

A. AF
B. MI
C. CAD
D. HF
E. Mitral stenosis
F. HTN
G. Hyperthyroidism
H. Digitalis intoxication
I. Acute infections

Plan

A. General interventions:
   1. The goal of therapy is to improve the client's quality of life by reducing morbidity and prolonging survival.

B. Client teaching:
   1. Encourage weight loss, smoking cessation, and stress management. *See Section III: Client Teaching Guide for this chapter, "Atrial Fibrillation."*
   2. Educate clients about the adverse effects of their anticoagulant and antiarrhythmic medications.
   3. Instruct clients taking Coumadin (warfarin) to take steps to lessen their risk of falls.
   4. Educate clients with implanted defibrillators and pacemakers about their susceptibility for external electrical fields and avoidance of exposure.
   5. Advised clients regarding the importance of controlling other chronic medical conditions, such as hypertension, diabetes, HF, pulmonary diseases, and hyperlipidemia.

C. Dietary management:
   1. Counsel clients on proper nutrition, specifically a low-fat, low-cholesterol, low-sodium diet. Give diet handouts.
   2. Clients taking Coumadin should be educated regarding foods that are high in vitamin K. Some foods will interfere with clotting factors. See Appendix B, "Foods to Avoid While Taking Warfarin (Coumadin, Jantoven)," for common foods that interfere with clotting factors.

D. Pharmaceutical therapy:
   1. Anticoagulant therapy:
     a. Goal of therapy: Prevention of thromboembolism
       i. Coumadin (warfarin sodium, Jantoven):
        1) Doses: 1 mg, 2 mg, 2.5 mg, 3 mg, 4 mg, 5 mg, 6 mg, 7.5 mg, and 10 mg tablets
        2) Warfarin Dose Calculator: www.globalrph.com/warf-maint.htm
        3) Review all medications that may affect the anticoagulant effects of warfarin. GlobalRPH is a resource with a list

of medications that both increase and decrease the INR (www.globalrph.com/warfarin_calc.htm).

  ii. Non-vitamin K oral anticoagulants (NOACs):

    1) Pradaxa (dabigatran etexilate mesylate):

      a) 75 mg and 150 mg tablets

      b) Dosage indications based on CrCl:

        i) CrCl > 30 mL/min: 150 mg, taken twice a day

        ii) CrCl of 15 to 30 mL/min: 75 mg, taken twice a day

    2) Xarelto (rivaroxaban):

      a) 10 mg, 15 mg, and 20 mg tablets

      b) Dosage indications based on CrCl:

        i) CrCl > 50 mL/min: 20 mg with evening meal

        ii) CrCl of 15 to 50 mL/min: 15 mg with evening meal

    3) Eliquis (apixaban):

      a) 2.5 mg and 5 mg tablets

      b) Dosage indications:

        i) Recommended dose is 2.5 mg, taken twice a day in clients who fit any of the following criteria:

          (1) 80 years of age or older

          (2) Weight ≥ 60 kg (132 lb)

          (3) Serum creatinine ≥ 1.5 mg/dL

    4) Savaysa (edoxaban):

      a) 15 mg, 30 mg, and 60 mg tablets

      b) Dosage indications:

        i) CrCl between 15 and 50 mL/min: 30 mg, once daily

        ii) CrCl > 95 mL/min: Do not prescribe.

2. Antiplatelet therapy:

  a. Goal of therapy: Prevention of thromboembolism; modest preventive effect:

    i. Aspirin: 81 mg and 325 mg tablets

    ii. Plavix (clopidogrel bisulfate): 75 mg and 300 mg

3. Combined anticoagulant and antiplatelet therapies:

  a. Prescription of both antiplatelet medications (Plavix and aspirin) in addition to an anticoagulant is referred to as *triple therapy*. Triple therapy is commonly used to prevent complications when two or more of the following conditions are present:

    i. AF

    ii. Mechanical valve prosthesis

    iii. Drug-eluting coronary stent

  b. Triple therapy is linked with an increase in bleeding complications ranging from mild to life-threatening.

4. Heart rate control therapy:

  a. Goal of therapy: Varies based on client age, but typically involves achieving a ventricular rate between 60 and 80 bpm at rest and between 90 and 115 bpm during moderate exercise.

  b. Beta-blockers:

    i. Acebutolol (Sectral, acebutolol hydrochloride):

      1) 200 mg and 400 mg capsules

    ii. Atenolol (Tenormin):

      1) 25 mg, 50 mg (scored), and 100 mg tablets

    iii. Betaxolol (Betoptic, Betoptic S, betaxolol hydrochloride):

      1) 10 mg and 20 mg tablets, all scored

    iv. Bisoprolol (Zebeta, bisoprolol fumarate):

      1) 5 mg (scored) and 10 mg tablets

    v. Metoprolol (Lopressor, Toprol-XL, metoprolol tartrate):

      1) 50 mg and 100 mg tablets, all scored

    vi. Nadolol (Corgard):

      1) 20 mg, 40 mg, and 80 mg tablets, all scored

    vii. Nebivolol (Bystolic):

      1) 2.5 mg, 5 mg, 10 mg, and 20 mg tablets

    viii. Propranolol (propranolol hydrochloride):

      1) 10 mg, 20 mg, 40 mg, 60 mg, and 80 mg tablets, all scored

    ix. Sotalol (Betapace, sotalol hydrochloride):

      1) 80 mg, 120 mg, and 160 mg tablets, all scored

    x. Timolol (timolol maleate):

      1) 5 mg, 10 mg (scored), and 20 mg (scored) tablets

  c. CCBs:

    i. Diltiazem (Cardizem, diltiazem hydrochloride)

      1) 30 mg, 60 mg (scored), 90 mg (scored), 120 mg (scored) tablets

    ii. Verapamil (Calan, verapamil hydrochloride, Tarka)

      1) 40 mg, 80 mg (scored), and 120 mg (scored) tablets

  d. Fourth-generation CCBs:

    i. Cilnidipine (Cilacar):

      1) 5 mg, 10 mg, and 20 mg tablets

    ii. Digoxin (Lanoxin):

      1) 0.125 mg and 0.25 mg tablets, all scored

5. Heart rhythm control therapy:

  a. Goal of therapy: The maintenance of a normal rhythm and suppression of AF:

    i. Sodium channel blockers:

      1) Disopyramide (Norpace): 100 mg and 150 mg capsules

      2) Quinidine (quinidine gluconate): 200 mg and 300 mg tablets, all scored

        ii. Potassium channel blockers:
            1) Amiodarone (Cordarone, Pacerone, Nexterone, amiodarone hydrochloride): 200 mg tablet, scored
            2) Dofetilide (Tikosyn): 125 mcg, 250 mcg, and 500 mcg capsules
            3) Dronedarone (Multaq): 400 mg tablet
            4) Sotalol (Betapace, sotalol hydrochloride): 80 mg, 120 mg, and 160 mg tablets, all scored
E. Surgical therapies:
    1. Ablation therapy:
        a. Goal of therapy: Prevention of recurrent AF
        b. Preferred clinical characteristics include the following:
            i. Symptomatic paroxysmal AF
            ii. Failure of one or more antiarrhythmic medications
            iii. Normal to mildly dilated atria
            iv. Normal to mildly reduced ventricular function
            v. Absence of severe pulmonary disease
        c. The long-term efficacy of ablation therapy requires further study, especially with regard to clients with HF and structural heart disease.

Follow-Up

A. Clients with AF should be comanaged with a physician.
B. AF that is resistant to routine therapy should always be followed by a cardiologist.
C. Laboratory monitoring as indicated by the client's anticoagulant and antiarrhythmic medications:
    1. CrCl for clients taking Pradaxa and Xarelto
    2. INR for clients taking Coumadin. Multiple medications affect the anticoagulant property of Coumadin.
        a. The INR labs are located on GlobalRPH: www.globalrph.com/warfarin_drug_interactions.htm
D. Follow-up is determined by the client's needs, frequency of AF reoccurrence, and the presence of other medical conditions.
E. After defibrillator or pacemaker placement, monitor the client using regular follow-up appointments and EKGs to identify failure of the implanted device, thromboembolism, lead dislodgement, infection, and complicating arrhythmias.

Consultation/Referral

A. If you suspect an acute cardiovascular episode, refer the client for immediate hospitalization to initiate thrombolytic therapy, cardioversion, hypertensive management, and additional diagnostic testing
B. Refer to cardiology as indicated by the client's clinical situation, specifically the frequency of AF reoccurrence and the presence of other complex medical conditions.
C. AF that is resistant to routine therapy should always be followed by a cardiologist.

Individual Considerations

Pediatrics: AF is uncommon in the pediatric population; however, when present, AF occurs secondary to structural heart disease.

Bibliography

Andrade, J. G., Verma, A., Mitchell, L, Parkash, R., Leblanc, K., Atzema, C., . . . Macle, L. (2018). 2018 focused update of the Canadian Cardiovascular Society guidelines for the management of atrial fibrillation. *Canadian Journal of Cardiology, 34*(11), 1371–1392. doi:10.1016/j.cjca.2018.08.026

Batra, G., Svennblad, B., Held, C., Jernberg, T., Johanson, P., Wallentin, L., & Oldgren, J. (2016). All types of atrial fibrillation in the setting of myocardial infarction are associated with impaired outcome. *Heart (British Cardiac Society), 102*(12), 926–933. doi:10.1136/heartjnl-2015-308678

Centers for Disease Control and Prevention. (2017, August 22). *Atrial fibrillation fact sheet.* Retrieved from http://www.cdc.gov/dhdsp/data_statistics/fact_sheets/fs_atrial_fibrillation.htm

Chao, T.-F., Liu, C.-J., Tuan, T.-C., Chen, S.-J., Wang, K.-L., Lin, Y.-J., & Chen, S.-A. (2015). Rate-control treatment and mortality in atrial fibrillation. *Circulation, 132,* 1604–1612. doi:10.1161/CIRCULATIONAHA.114.013709. Retrieved from http://circ.ahajournals.org/content/early/2015/09/17/CIRCULATIONAHA.114.013709.abstract

Cheng, A., & Kumar, K. (2019, February 5). Overview of atrial fibrillation. *UpToDate.* Retrieved from www.uptodate.com/contents/overview-of-atrial-fibrillation

Dima, C. (2018, February 2). Mitral stenosis. *Medscape.* Retrieved from https://emedicine.medscape.com/article/155724-overview

Drug information. (2019). *Prescribers' digital reference.* Retrieved from www.pdr.net

Dubin, A. (2018, July). Management of supraventricular tachycardia in children. *UpToDate.* Retrieved from https://www.uptodate.com/contents/management-of-supraventricular-tachycardia-in-children

Fawzy, A. M., Yang, W.-Y. & Lip, G. Y. H. (2019, January 31). Safety of direct oral anticoagulants in real-world clinical practice: Translating the trials to everyday clinical management. *Expert Opinion of Drug Safety, 18*(3), 187–209. doi:10.1080/14740338.2019.1578344

Food and Drug Administration. (2018, June 12). *Use the nutrition facts label to reduce your intake of sodium in your diet.* Retrieved from https://www.fda.gov/food/nutrition-education-resources-materials/use-nutrition-facts-label-reduce-your-intake-sodium-your-diet

Ganz, L. (2019, March). Epidemiology of and risk factors for atrial fibrillation. *UpToDate.* Retrieved from http://www.uptodate.com/contents/epidemiology-of-and-risk-factors-for-atrial-fibrillation

Gugneja, M. (2017, April). Paroxysmal supraventricular tachycardia. *Medscape.* Retrieved from https://emedicine.medscape.com/article/156670-overview

Hanson, I. (2018, November 28). Mitral regurgitation. *Medscape.* Retrieved from https://emedicine.medscape.com/article/155618-overview

January, C. T., Wann, L. S., Alpert, J. S., Calkins, H., Cigarroa, J. E., Cleveland, J. C., . . . Yancy, C. W. (2019). 2019 AHA/ACC/HRS focused update of the 2014 AHA/ACC/HRS guideline for the management of patients with atrial fibrillation: A report of the American College of Cardiology/American Heart Association Task Force on Practice Guidelines and the Heart Rhythm Society. *Circulation, 139,* 1–49. doi:10.1161/CIR.0000000000000665. Retrieved from http://www.ahajournals.org/doi/pdf/10.1161/CIR.0000000000000665

Milling, T. J. Jr., & Frontera, J. (2017). Exploring indications for the use of direct oral anticoagulants and the associated risks of major bleeding. *American Journal of Managed Care, 23*(4 suppl), S67–S80. Retrieved from https://www.ncbi.nlm.nih.gov/pubmed/28581331

Moss, J. D., Cifu, A. S., & ACC/AHA Task Force on Practice Guidelines. (2015). Management of anticoagulation in patients with atrial fibrillation. *Journal of the American Medical Association, 314*(3), 291–292. doi:10.1001/jama.2015.3088

Nishimura, R., Otto, C., & Bonow, R. (2017). 2017 AHA/ACC focused update of the 2014 AHA/ACC guideline for the management of patients with valvular heart disease. *Journal of the American College of Cardiology, 70*(2), 252–289. doi:10.1161/CIR.0000000000000503

Palmer, S. (2015). Atrial fibrillation. *British Journal of Cardiac Nursing, 10*(11), 567. doi:10.12968/bjca.2015.10.11.567

Chest Pain

Cheryl A. Glass and Debbie Gunter

Definition

A. Chest pain is a localized sensation of distress or discomfort that may or may not be associated with actual tissue damage.

Incidence

A. Chest pain is one of the most common complaints of adult clients. Causes can range from minor disorders to life-threatening diseases; every client must be assessed carefully.

Pathogenesis

A. Cardiac etiology: Ischemia, atherosclerosis, inflammation, or valvular problems caused by angina, MI, pericarditis, endocarditis, dissecting aortic aneurysm, or mitral valve prolapse (MVP; see Table 10.3)

B. Musculoskeletal etiology: Muscle strain and inflammation caused by costochondritis, chest wall syndrome, cervicodorsal arthritis, or intercostal myositis

C. Neurological etiology: Nerve inflammation and/or compression caused by herpes zoster and nerve root compression

D. GI etiology: Structural defects, inflammation, or infection caused by gastroesophageal reflux disease (GERD), hiatal hernia, esophageal spasm, pancreatitis, cholecystitis, or peptic ulcer disease (PUD)

E. Pleural etiology: Inflammation, distention, or compression of pleural membranes caused by pneumonia, pulmonary embolus, pulmonary HTN, spontaneous pneumothorax, and lung and mediastinal tumors

F. Psychogenic etiology: Stress caused by anxiety, depression, or panic disorders

Predisposing Factors

A. These vary depending on the etiology of pain.

Common Complaints

A. Primary complaint: Pain somewhere in the chest

B. "Levine's sign": Placing the fist on the center of the chest to demonstrate pain

C. Fatigue

D. Cough

E. Indigestion

F. Dyspnea

G. Syncope

H. Palpitations

I. Profound fatigue

Other Signs and Symptoms

A. Pain may be typical of angina and MI.

B. Musculoskeletal pain may be relieved by position change, aggravated by body movement, reproducible, or caused by injury or trauma.

C. Neurological pain is associated with skin lesion if herpes zoster is the causative agent.

D. GI pain may be associated with meals, certain positions, belching, or an acid "brash" taste in mouth, or it may be referred to other sites.

E. Pleural pain is accompanied by cough, upper respiratory infection (URI) symptoms, or SOB.

F. Psychogenic pain or pressure along with SOB and dizziness may be associated with a specific event or time.

Subjective Data

A. How long has the client had chest pain?

B. Has the client ever been treated for chest pain? What treatment, tests, and medications (such as nitroglycerin) were used?

C. What precipitates and relieves the client's chest pain?

   1. Precipitates pain: Exertion, taking a deep breath, eating, cold, stress, and sexual intercourse

   2. Relieves pain: Resting, eating, taking an antacid, taking nitroglycerin, and positional change

D. Inquire about character of pain:

   1. Location: Neck, throat, chest, epigastric area, and shoulder

   2. Radiation: Neck, throat, shoulder, lower jaw, and upper extremity:

      a. **Radiation to both arms is a predictor of acute MI.**

      b. **Chest pain that radiates between the scapulae may indicate thoracic aortic dissection.**

   3. Quality: Squeezing, pressure, strangling, fullness, heavy weight, tightening, constriction, and ripping/tearing (acute aortic dissection)

   4. Intensity: Abrupt onset, gradually getting worse, dull, or insidious

   5. How long has the pain been occurring? Seconds, minutes, hours, or years?

   6. Frequency: Intermittent, occurs every morning/evening

E. Are other associated symptoms present?

F. Discuss any risk factors the client may have for cardiac disease: Smoking, hyperlipidemia, HTN, sedentary lifestyle, diabetes, and family history.

G. Review medical history as noted earlier.

H. Review all medications including prescription (such as sildenafil), OTC, and herbal products.

I. Review recreational/illicit drug use.

J. Inquire about any new physical labor if musculoskeletal etiology is suspected.

K. Has the client had any trauma (including domestic violence)?

L. Has the client had a recent infection?

Physical Examination

A. Check temperature (if infection is suspected), pulse, respirations, BP, and pulse oximetry.

B. Inspect:

   1. Inspect general appearance:

      a. Appearance of discomfort/distress

      b. Any appearance of respiratory distress

      c. Evaluate jugular venous distention (JVD).

      d. Note client position: Sitting, lying, squatting. Relief of chest pain with recumbency suggests MVP; relief with squatting suggests hypertrophic cardiomyopathy. Noncardiac chest pain may be present along with cardiac chest pain.

TABLE 10.3 COMPARISON OF COMMON CHEST PAIN ETIOLOGIES

Condition	Pain Findings	Associated Symptoms	Precipitating Factors	Relieving Factors	Physical Findings	Diagnostic Tests	Treatment Modalities
Cardiac–stable angina	Substernal, tight, dull pressure, usually lasts longer than 15 minutes		Exertion, cold, emotional stress	Rest, nitroglycerin, Valsalva maneuver	Sinus tachycardia, bradycardia, xanthomas, signs of HF	Resting EKG, stress EKG, cardiac enzymes, echocardiogram, angiogram	ASA, BB, nitrate, CCB
Prinzmetal's angina (variant)	Substernal, achy, tight, dull pressure		Often occurs at rest; may awaken from sleep	Nitroglycerin	Same as stable angina	Resting EKG, angiogram	ASA, nitrate, CCB
MI	Precordial, substernal, severe, crushing, squeezing, lasts >15 minutes	Dyspnea, sweating, dizzy, pain radiates to neck/arm/jaw, N&V, cough, fever, unstable V/S	Oxygen	Not relieved by nitroglycerin	S_3 or S_4 murmur, tachycardia, bradycardia, pericardia, friction rub, hyper/hypotension	EKG, serial CK enzymes, echo, radio nuclide studies	Analgesia, reperfusion, prevention, and treatment complications limit infarcts Thrombolytic therapy for acute MI
MVP	Usually not substernal, often knife-like, may last 1 to 3 hours	Palpitations, fatigue, light-headed, arrhythmia, syncope		Recumbent position, BB, nitroglycerin	Midsystolic click and/or murmur, thin body status, SOB	Echo, EKG	Usually none, BB if palpitations or ventricular ectopy becomes disabling
Hypertrophic cardiomegaly	Similar to angina	Dyspnea with exertion, arrhythmias, light-headed syncope	May be increased by nitroglycerin, exertion	BB, squatting	Systolic murmur, increased upright position, Valsalva maneuver, more forceful PMI	EKG, CXR, echo, Doppler, cardiac catheterization	BB, CCB, possible pacing and myomectomy, exercise restriction
Pericarditis	Retrosternal, sharp or dull; sudden onset; long duration; radiates to one side of the trapezius	Fever, myalgia, anorexia, anxiety, recent viral infection		Sitting up, leaning forward	Friction rub, SVT1, tachypnea, crackles, signs of cardiac tamponade	EKG, echo, CBC, ESR	Hospitalize: rule out purulent process Analgesics
Endocarditis	Usually dull, retrosternal, may radiate to back	Fever, night sweats, joint pain, back pain, weight loss, headache, murmur			Systolic–diastolic murmur, petechiae, Osler's modes, Roth spots, neck vein distention, pleural or pericardia rub, pain in extremities, splenomegaly, hematuria	CBC, ESR blood cultures, echo	Hospitalize, for antibiotic therapy
GI esophageal spasm	May be identical to angina		Alcohol or cold liquids	May be relieved by nitroglycerin		Esophageal manometry	Nitroglycerin anticholinergics, esophageal dilation
Esophagitis	Burning, tightness	Heartburn, water brash	Overeating, alcohol, recumbent position	Antacids	May have slight to moderate epigastric tenderness	Esophago-scopy	Lifestyle modification, antacid, H_2 blocker, PPI, promotility agent
Musculoskeletal costochondritis	Sharp, sometimes pleuritic, parasternal costochondral pain		Sneezing, cough on deep inspiration, or twisting motions, reaching overhead		Erythema at sites of tenderness; positive pinpoint tenderness at costochondral junctions	CXR to rule out other causes	NSAIDs, ASA, ibuprofen, naproxen, heat application

ASA, acetylsalicylic acid; BB, beta-blocker; CBC, complete blood count; CCB, calcium channel blocker; CK, creatine kinase; CXR, chest x-ray; ESR, eosinophilic sedimentation rate; GI, gastrointestinal; HF, heart failure; MI, myocardial infarction; MVP, mitral valve prolapse; NSAIDs, nonsteroidal anti-inflammatory drugs; N&V, nausea and vomiting; PMI, point of maximal impulse; PPI, proton pump inhibitor; SOB, shortness of breath; SVT, supraventricular tachydysrhythmias; VS, vital signs.

Chest Pain

2. Inspect skin for diaphoresis, jaundice, pallor, herpes zoster lesions, rash, or cyanosis.

3. Inspect chest wall for herpes zoster lesions or signs of trauma.

4. Inspect eyes by performing funduscopic examination.

5. Inspect legs for signs of phlebitis: Unilateral swelling, cyanosis, venous stasis, and diminished pulses.

6. Inspect neck for enlarged thyroid and lymph nodes, midline trachea, and JVD.

C. Palpate:

1. Palpate chest wall for tenderness and swelling. Chest pain present in only one body position is usually not cardiac in origin.

2. Palpate abdomen for masses, tenderness, bounding pulses, organomegaly, and ascites.

3. Palpate femoral and distal pulses.

D. Auscultate:

1. Auscultate carotid arteries for bruits.

2. Auscultate lungs for crackles, wheezes, equal breath sounds, and pleural rub.

3. Auscultate abdomen for bruits and bowel sounds.

4. Auscultate heart for murmurs, rubs, clicks, irregularities, or extra sounds.

E. Neurological examination: Perform this examination if neurological etiology is suspected.

Diagnostic Tests

A. Testing depends on information collected in the examination. A normal physical examination, EKG, and/or laboratory test results in a client with chest pain do not rule out CHD. Typical tests include the following:

1. EKG

2. Chest radiography, whenever diagnosis of chest pain is not clear

3. Echocardiogram

4. Stress test

5. Cardiac catheterization

6. Barium tests

7. Endoscopy to rule out GI etiology

8. Esophageal pH, low

9. Laboratory tests:

   a. Troponin I or T

   b. Myoglobin

   c. CK

   d. CK-MB

   e. CRP

   f. BNP for clinical findings/risk of HF

   g. D-dimer for suspected venous thrombotic event (deep vein thrombosis [DVT] or PE)

Differential Diagnoses

A. Cardiac causes:

1. CHD:

   a. Acute MI: Chest pain lasting more than 15 minutes

   b. Unstable angina pectoris

   c. Stable angina pectoris

   d. Prinzmetal's or variant angina

2. Valvular heart disease:

   a. MVP

   b. Aortic stenosis

3. Hypertrophic cardiomyopathy

4. Pericarditis

5. Endocarditis

6. Aortic dissection

B. Noncardiac causes:

1. Pulmonary causes:

   a. Pneumonia

   b. Pleurisy

   c. PE

   d. Pulmonary HTN

   e. Pneumothorax

   f. Tracheobronchitis

   g. Lung cancer

2. GI causes:

   a. GERD

   b. Esophageal spasm

   c. PUD

   d. Pancreatitis

   e. Cholecystitis

   f. Flatulence

3. Rheumatology causes:

   a. Fibromyalgia

   b. Costochondritis

   c. Arthritis

4. Chest wall causes:

   a. Rib fracture

   b. Muscle strain

   c. Cervical or thoracic spine disease

   d. Metastatic bone disease

   e. Breast conditions

5. Neurological causes:

   a. Herpes zoster

   b. Postherpetic pain syndrome

   c. Nerve root compression

6. Psychogenic causes:

   a. Panic disorder

   b. Generalized anxiety

   c. Depression

   d. Somatoform disorders

Plan

A. General interventions: Direct management toward primary disorder causing the symptom

B. Client teaching:

1. Teach the client about medications.

2. Encourage CPR training for the client's family and/or close friends if chest pain is cardiac in origin.

3. Explain to the client and family when and how to call 911 and the importance of going to the ER immediately so that thrombolytic therapy can be considered. A positive response to nitroglycerin does not confirm the presence of CAD.

C. Pharmaceutical therapy:

1. Cardiac pain: Nitroglycerin

2. GI pain: H_2 blocker, proton pump inhibitor (PPI)

3. Musculoskeletal pain: Nonsteroidal anti-inflammatory drugs (NSAIDs)
4. Psychogenic pain:
   a. Selective serotonin reuptake inhibitors (SSRIs)
   b. TCAs
   c. Benzodiazepines

Follow-Up
A. Follow-up of clients with CAD to be carried out for an indefinite period of time to detect the recurrence or progression of disease.
B. Other follow-ups depend on the etiology of chest pain.

Consultation/Referral
A. Consult a physician when chest pain is cardiac in origin. If a cardiac origin is found in a pregnant client, schedule a cardiology consultation as soon as possible for comanagement.

Individual Considerations
A. Pregnancy:
   1. Evaluate chest pain in the same manner as in non-pregnant clients.
   2. Rule out pregnancy-induced hypertension (PIH) and hemolysis, elevated liver enzymes, low platelets (HELLP) syndrome when a third-trimester client presents with upper epigastric/chest pain
B. Pediatrics:
   1. Chest pain usually does not represent serious CVD.
   2. Pericarditis is one of the most frequent causes of chest pain associated with a febrile illness.
   3. Exercise-induced chest pain may be indicative of asthma.
   4. A chest wall syndrome, such as costochondritis, is another frequent etiology.

C. Geriatrics:
   1. Frail elderly clients usually do not present with the "typical" symptom complex of chest pain. Often, the only symptoms of acute MI are lethargy, decreased level of consciousness (LOC), crackles, CHF, persistent cough, or hypotension.
   2. Prescribe medications for frail elderly clients in half the usual dosage and then slowly taper upward to the desired effect.

Bibliography
Abid, S., & Shuaib, W. (2015). Chest pain assessment and imaging practices for nurse practitioners in the emergency department. *Advanced Emergency Nursing Journal, 37*, 12–22. doi:10.1097/TME.0000000000000048
Alaeddini, J. (2018, July). Angina pectoris. *Medscape*. Retrieved from https://emedicine.medscape.com/article/150215-overview
Drug information. (2019). *Prescribers' digital reference*. Retrieved from www.pdr.net
Nishimura, R., Otto, C., & Bonow, R. (2017). 2017 AHA/ACC focused update of the 2014 AHA/ACC guideline for the management of patients with valvular heart disease. *Journal of the American College of Cardiology, 70*(2), 252–289. doi:10.1161/CIR.0000000000000503
Ren, X. (2017, March 23). Aortic stenosis. *Medscape*. Retrieved from https://emedicine.medscape.com/article/150638-overview

Chronic Venous Insufficiency and Varicose Veins

Laura A. Petty

Definition
Peripheral vascular disease (PVD) is a general term that encompasses all occlusive or inflammatory diseases that occur within the peripheral arteries, veins, and lymphatics. These conditions include PAD, DVT, superficial thrombophlebitis, lymphedema, and chronic venous diseases. Chronic venous diseases include chronic venous insufficiency (CVI) and varicose veins (see Figure 10.2).

FIGURE 10.2 Varicosities. (A) Vein with normal blood flow. (B) Varicose vein.
Source: Adapted from the National Heart, Lung, and Blood Institute.

Incidence

A. CVI:
  1. An estimated 20% of adults in the United States have CVI; it is twice as common in females as in males.
  2. Peak incidence is seen in women older than 50 years.
  3. CVI is the most common cause of the 2.5 million leg ulcerations in the United States.
B. Varicose veins: This is the most common circulatory condition of the lower extremities, affecting more than 20 million Americans. Varicose veins are usually thought to be more common in females; however, in certain populations the rate is higher in males.

Pathogenesis

A. CVI: Venous insufficiency is caused by incompetent valves that allow valvular reflux and subsequently venous HTN. In CVI, venous HTN leads to obstruction of venous flow, which produces local tissue anoxia, inflammation, and at times even tissue necrosis. This process eventually causes subcutaneous fibrosing panniculitis and additional venous and lymphatic outlet obstruction.
B. Varicose veins: Varicose veins are a form of CVI. The same incompetent valves that cause valvular reflux and subsequently venous HTN in CVI also cause varicose veins. This influx of volume and pressure causes the vessels to dilate, twist, and bulge.

Predisposing Factors

A. CVI:
  1. Age > 30 years
  2. Female gender
  3. Prolonged standing or sitting
  4. Prior history of DVT
  5. Stature—more common in tall persons
  6. Obesity
  7. Sedentary lifestyle
  8. Family history
  9. History of multiple pregnancies, if female
  10. HTN
B. Varicose veins:
  1. Genetics
     a. Risk increases to 90% if both parents have varicose veins.
     b. If one parent is affected, the risk increases by 25% for men and by 62% for women.
  2. Age
  3. History of multiple pregnancies
  4. Prolonged standing
  5. Restrictive clothing
  6. Obesity
  7. Ligamentous laxity:
     A history of hernia(s) or flat feet
  8. Smoking
  9. History of superficial or deep vein clots

Common Complaints

A. CVI:
  1. Extremity edema
  2. Pain worse when standing, usually dull, aching, or cramping
  3. Pain improved with elevation
  4. Itching sensation
  5. Feeling of heaviness in extremity
  6. Hyperpigmentation
  7. Thickening and hardening of the skin
  8. Ulcerations (see Figure 10.3)

FIGURE 10.3   Venous ulcerations.

B. Varicose veins:
  1. Pain, usually burning, aching, or itching
  2. Blue veins that protrude above the surface of the skin
  3. Leg fatigue
  4. Edema
  5. Symptoms worsened toward the end of the day
  6. Leg heaviness

Potential Complications

A. CVI:
  1. Cellulitis
  2. Peripheral neuropathy
  3. Varicose veins
  4. Abscess
  5. Ulceration
  6. Stasis dermatitis
  7. DVT
B. Varicose veins:
  1. Stasis dermatitis
  2. Stasis ulceration
  3. Petechial hemorrhage
  4. Chronic edema
  5. Superficial thrombophlebitis
  6. Hyperpigmentation
  7. Eczema
  8. DVT

Subjective Data

A. Ask the client when the symptom(s) were first noticed.
B. Have the client describe the duration of symptoms.

C. Ask the client to describe the pain—for example, crushing, stabbing, or burning.

D. Ask the client what makes the symptoms better and what makes them worse.

E. Have the client rate the pain on a scale of 1 to 10, with 1 being the least painful.

F. Ask the client to list all medications currently being taken, particularly substances not prescribed and illicit drugs such as cocaine.

G. Review recent history of invasive procedures or surgery.

Physical Examination

A. CVI:
1. Vital signs: BP, resting heart rate, respirations, temperature, height, and weight.
2. Inspect:
  a. Inspect extremity for edema, hyperpigmentation, erythema, and difference in temperature.
  b. Inspect and document any varicosities.
3. Palpate:
  a. Palpate distended veins, noting tenderness.
  b. Perform the cough impulse test to determine turbulent retrograde flow.
  c. Perform the tap test to determine if the great saphenous vein is distended with blood.
4. Auscultate:
  a. Heart: Rate rhythm, heart sounds, murmur, and gallops
  b. Lungs: Assess lung sounds in all fields.

B. Varicose veins:
1. **Clients presenting with any of the following should be quickly assessed for the need to call emergency services/911 for immediate transport to the hospital:**
  a. **A bleeding varicosity with eroded surrounding skin**
  b. **A varicosity that has bled and is at risk of bleeding again**
  c. **An ulceration that is worsening and/or painful despite treatment**
2. Vital signs: BP, resting heart rate, respirations, temperature, height, and weight
3. Inspect:
  a. Inspect skin for superficial veins that are raised above the skin's surface; client should be standing.
  b. Inspect extremity for edema, hyperpigmentation, and eczema.
4. Palpate:
  Palpate distended veins, noting tenderness.
5. Auscultate:
  a. Heart: Rate rhythm, heart sounds, murmur, and gallops.
  b. Lungs: Assess lung sounds.

Diagnostic Tests

A. CVI:
1. Trendelenburg test
2. Perthes test
3. Doppler ankle/brachial index (ABI)
4. Duplex ultrasound
5. Venography—not utilized often because of expense and risk of phlebitis

B. Varicose veins:
1. Trendelenburg test
2. Perthes test
3. Duplex ultrasound

Differential Diagnoses

A. CVI:
1. DVT
2. Ulceration
3. Infection
4. PAD
5. Varicose veins with risk of hemorrhage

B. Varicose veins:
1. Arthritis
2. Peripheral neuritis
3. Nerve root compression
4. Telangiectasia
5. DVT
6. Inflammatory liposclerosis

Plan

A. Prevention: General:
1. Avoid prolonged standing or sitting.
2. Exercise on a regular basis.
3. Encourage smoking cessation, weight loss, and exercise, if applicable.
4. Encourage strategies to better manage other chronic medical conditions that directly affect the progression of PAD—for example, diabetes, dyslipidemia, obesity, and HTN.

B. CVI:
1. Nonpharmaceutical therapy
  a. Extremity elevation
  b. Compression stockings
  c. Exercise
  d. Venous ulcerations treated with wound care and compression therapy
    i. Compression therapy is the primary mode of management and has demonstrated venous ulcer healing rates as high as 97%.
2. Pharmaceutical therapy:
  Diuretics: Management of edema, short-term administration
    i. Hydrochlorothiazide
    ii. Antiplatelet: May increase the speed of healing to ulcerations
      1) Aspirin: 325 mg tablet
      2) Systemic antibiotics: Management of infection in persons demonstrating an increase in pain, erythema, or size of ulceration
3. Surgery:
  a. Venous ablation for clients who continue to be symptomatic after 6 months of nonpharmacological therapies
  b. Types of ablation: Chemical, thermal, and mechanical

C. Varicose veins:
1. Client teaching: *See Section III: Client Teaching Guides for this chapter, "Chronic Venous Insufficiency" and "Varicose Veins."*
   a. If prolonged standing is required, shift weight from one leg to the other.
   b. Do not sit with legs dependent.
2. Nonpharmaceutical therapy:
   a. Extremity elevation
   b. Compression stockings
   c. Exercise
3. Surgery:
   a. Superficial vein
      i. Vein stripping, ligation, varicectomy
      ii. Sclerotherapy
      iii. Endovascular heat ablation (EVHA)
      iv. Radiofrequency ablation
   b. Deep vein:
      i. Valvuloplasty
      ii. Valvuloconstruction
      iii. Valve transplantation
      iv. Valve transposition
   c. Perforating vein:
      i. Subfascial endoscopic perforator surgery (SEPS)
      ii. Linton's operation
      iii. Percutaneous ablation of perforators (PAPs)

Follow-Up

A. Follow-up is determined by the client's needs, frequency and intensity of symptoms, and the presence of other medical conditions.
B. PVD manifesting persistent symptoms should always be followed by a cardiologist.

Consultation/Referral

A. If you suspect acute limb ischemia (ALI), refer the client for immediate hospitalization to obtain diagnostic testing to determine the presence of a thrombus and restore circulation to the affected extremity.
B. If chronic limb ischemia (CLI) has led to ulceration and/or superimposed infection, hospitalization is indicated to initiate a wound care consultation and diagnostic testing to determine the degree of arterial occlusion.
C. Referral to a cardiologist is indicated in the presence of persistent PVD symptoms.
D. Referral to a podiatrist becomes necessary to trim toenails and assess the client for proper-fitting shoes.
E. Referral to pain management is indicated if pain is resistant to treatment.

Individual Considerations

A. Nonambulatory clients:
1. Using rocking chairs is a possible substitute for persons unable to participate in a walking program.
B. Geriatrics:
1. Be alert to signs and symptoms of depression related to immobility and pain.

Bibliography

Alguire, P. C., & Mathes, B. M. (2017, December 4). Diagnostic evaluation of chronic venous insufficiency. *UpToDate*. Retrieved from http://www.uptodate.com/contents/diagnostic-evaluation-of-chronic-venous-insufficiency

Alguire, P. C., & Scovell, S. (2018, May 29). Overview and management of lower extremity chronic venous disease. *UpToDate*. Retrieved from www.uptodate.com/contents/overview-and-management-of-lower-extremity-chronic-venous-disease

Al-Shammeri, O., Al-Hamdan, N., Al-Hothaly, B., Midhet, F., Hussain, M., & Al-Mohaimeed, A. (2014). Chronic venous insufficiency: Prevalence and effect of compression stockings. *International Journal of Health Sciences, 8*(3), 231–236. doi:10.12816/0023975

Armstrong, D. G. & Meyr, A. J. (2018, January 29). Compression therapy for the treatment of chronic venous insufficiency. *UpToDate*. Retrieved from http://www.uptodate.com/contents/compression-therapy-for-the-treatment-of-chronic-venous-insufficiency

Barstow, C., & Kassop, D. (2019, April). Cardiovascular disease: Chronic venous insufficiency and varicose veins. *Family Practice Essentials, 479*, 16–20. Retrieved from https://www.ncbi.nlm.nih.gov/pubmed/30995000

Drug information. (2019). *Prescribers' digital reference*. Retrieved from www.pdr.net

Haruta, N. (2018, March 25). Recent progress of varicose vein treatment especially about endovascular heat ablation, SEPS, and foam sclerotherapy. *Annals of Vascular Diseases, 11*(1), 66–71. doi:10.3400/avd.ra.18-00005

Rooke, T. W., & Felty, C. L. (2014). A different way to look at varicose veins. *Journal of Vascular Surgery. Venous and Lymphatic Disorders, 2*(2), 207–211. doi:10.1016/j.jvsv.2013.08.006

Trayes, K. P., Studdiford, J. S., Pickle, S., & Tully, A. S. (2013). Edema: Diagnosis and management. *American Family Physician, 88*(2), 102–110. doi:10.1097/ACM.0b013e318277d5b2

Vascular Cures. (2016). *Chronic venous insufficiency*. Retrieved from http://www.vascularcures.org/about-vascular-disease/2011-05-05-02-02-59/chronic-venous-insufficiency

Vascular Cures. (2017a). Chronic venous insufficiency. Retrieved from http://vascularcures.org/chronic-venous-insufficiency/

Vascular Cures. (2017b). Varicose veins. Retrieved from http://vascularcures.org/varicose-veins/

Wittens, C., Davies, A. H., Bækgaard, N., Broholm, R., Cavezzi, A., & Chastanet, S. (2015). Editor's choice: Management of chronic venous disease: Clinical practice guidelines of the European Society for Vascular Surgery (ESVS). *European Journal of Vascular and Endovascular Surgery, 49*(6), 678–737. doi:10.1016/j.ejvs.2015.02.007

Zhang, S., & Melander, S. (2014). Varicose veins: Diagnosis, management, and treatment. *Journal for Nurse Practitioners, 10*(6), 417–424. doi:10.1016/j.nurpra.2014.03.004

Deep Vein Thrombosis

Laura A. Petty

Definition

Peripheral vascular disease (PVD) is a general term that encompasses all occlusive or inflammatory diseases that occur within the peripheral arteries, veins, and lymphatics. DVT is included with PVD, and is a condition in which a thrombus forms in one or more veins. It greatly increases the risk of PE (see Figure 10.4).

Incidence

The CDC estimates that between 350,000 and 900,000 Americans are affected by DVT or PE for the first time annually. Between 60,000 and 180,000 deaths are directly or indirectly attributed to DVT or PE.

Pathogenesis

Changes within the venous system precipitate the formation of a DVT. These changes, formally called Virchow's triad, include hypercoagulability, stasis, and endothelial

FIGURE 10.4 Deep vein thrombosis.

Source: Image courtesy of Dr. Sellers/Emory University/Centers for Disease Control and Prevention. Retrieved from https://phil.cdc.gov/Details.aspx?pid=1345

cell injury. At least two of the three must be present for a DVT to form. Essentially, an injury to the vessel wall causes inflammation that attracts platelets, especially in a state of altered coagulation. The thrombus that forms spreads in the direction of blood flow, and additional layers of platelets are added to the thrombus as time progresses. As it grows, the vessel becomes more occluded and symptoms worsen.

Predisposing Factors
A. Age: 60 years and older
B. Hip or femur fracture
C. Recent surgery, especially cardiac or extremity surgery
D. Prolonged inactivity/immobility
E. Pregnancy
F. Medication:
  1. Hormone replacement therapy (HRT)
  2. Oral contraceptives
  3. Tamoxifen
G. Current or recent hospitalization
H. Smoking
I. Obesity
J. Cancer
K. Inherited hypercoagulable conditions

Common Complaints
Symptoms are usually unilateral and have a sudden onset.
A. Extremity edema
B. Extremity pain
C. Increased temperature of extremity
D. Change in color or extremity
E. Asymptomatic, depending on the size and location of the thrombus

Potential Complications
A. PE
B. Arterial embolism with AV shunting
C. MI
D. CVI
E. Postphlebitic syndrome
F. Phlegmasia cerulea dolens

Subjective Data
A. Ask the client when the symptom(s) were first noticed.
B. Have the client describe the duration of the symptoms.
C. Ask the client to describe the pain—for example, crushing, stabbing, or burning.
D. Ask the client what makes the symptoms better and what makes them worse.
E. Have the client rate the pain on a scale of 1 to 10, with 1 being the least painful.
F. Ask the client to list all medications currently being taken, particularly substances not prescribed and illicit drugs such as cocaine.
G. Review recent history of invasive procedures or surgery.

Physical Examination
Clients presenting with acute SOB and/or chest pain should be quickly assessed for the need to call emergency services/911 for immediate transport to the hospital. Clients presenting with symptoms of DVT that include cyanosis of the distal extremity should be quickly assessed for the need to call emergency services/911 for immediate transport to the hospital.
A. Vital signs:
  1. Check BP and document resting heart rate, respirations, height, and weight.
B. Inspect:
  1. Assess for signs of erythema, increased temperature, and edema.
  2. Assess for Homans' sign—calf pain with forced plantar flexion.
  3. Assess for Moses' or Bancroft's sign—pain when calf muscle is compressed forward against the tibia.
  4. Assess for Lisker's sign—pain upon tibial percussion.
C. Palpate:
  1. Pulses distal to affected area, noting symmetry
  2. Capillary refill
  3. Extremity for tenderness. Do not perform deep palpation.
D. Auscultate:
  1. Heart: Rate, rhythm, heart sounds, murmur, and gallops
  2. Lungs: Assess lung sounds in all fields

Diagnostic Tests
A. DVT:
  1. Serum laboratory testing:
    a. D-dimer
    b. CBC with differential
    c. Coagulation panel (PT, partial thromboplastin time [PTT], INR)
    d. Testing for idiopathic DVT: Add factor V Leiden, homocysteine, G20210A prothrombin, factor VIII, lupus anticoagulant antibody, protein C and protein S levels, anticardiolipin antibodies, and antithrombin
  2. Compression ultrasound

3. MRI, if thrombus is suspected in the pelvic veins or vena cava

4. Venography—not utilized often because of expense and risk of phlebitis

Differential Diagnoses

A. DVT

B. Cellulitis

C. Fracture

D. Lymphedema

E. CHF

F. Vein compression (caused by enlarged lymph nodes or mass)

G. Filariasis (parasitic disease)

H. Allergic reaction, localized

I. Compartment syndrome

Plan

A. General interventions:

1. Encourage strategies to better manage other chronic medical conditions that directly affect the progression of PAD. Examples of these conditions include diabetes, dyslipidemia, obesity, and HTN.

B. Client teaching:

1. Client teaching: *See Section III: Client Teaching Guide for this chapter, "Deep Vein Thrombosis."*

2. Clients taking Coumadin should be educated regarding foods that are high in vitamin K. Some foods will interfere with clotting factors. See Appendix B, "Diet Recommendations" for common foods that interfere with clotting factors.

3. Teach the client to perform activities that can help prevent DVT.

   a. Avoid prolonged standing or sitting.

   b. Avoid crossing the legs.

   c. Gradually resume normal activity after a period of inactivity.

   d. Avoid immobility.

   e. Exercise on a regular basis.

   f. Stop smoking.

   g. Wear compression stockings frequently.

C. Pharmaceutical therapy:

1. Thrombolytics: Administered in the inpatient setting

2. Anticoagulants:

   a. Heparin, intravenous (IV), administered in the inpatient setting

   b. Coumadin (warfarin sodium, Jantoven)

      i. Doses: 1 mg, 2 mg, 2.5 mg, 3 mg, 4 mg, 5 mg, 6 mg, 7.5 mg, and 10 mg tablets

      ii. See "Atrial Fibrillation" section in this chapter for specifics on Coumadin therapy

3. Low-molecular-weight heparin (LMWH):

   a. Lovenox (enoxaparin sodium):

      i. Doses: 300 mg/3 mL multidose vial

      ii. Doses: 30 mg/0.3 mL, 40 mg/0.4 mL, 60 mg/0.6 mL, 80 mg/0.8 mL, 100 mg/mL, 120 mg/0.8 mL, and 150 mg/mL prefilled syringes

   b. Fragmin (dalteparin sodium):

      i. Doses: 95,000 IU/9.5 mL multidose vial

      ii. Doses: 2,500 IU/0.2 mL, 5,000 IU/0.2 mL, 7,500 IU/0.3 mL, 10,000 IU/0.4 mL, 10,000 IU/mL, 12,500 IU/0.5 mL, 15,000 IU/0.6 mL, 18,000 IU/0.72 mL by injection

4. NOACs:

   a. Xarelto (rivaroxaban):

      i. 10 mg, 15 mg, and 20 mg tablets

      ii. Dosage indications based on CrCl

         1) CrCl > 50 mL/min: 20 mg with evening meal

         2) CrCl of 15 to 50 mL/min: 15 mg with evening meal

   b. Eliquis (apixaban):

      i. 2.5 mg and 5 mg tablets

      ii. Dosage indications:

         1) Recommended dose is 2.5 mg, taken twice a day in clients who fit any of the following criteria:

            a) 80 years of age or older

            b) Weight ≥ 60 kg (132 lb)

            c) Serum creatinine ≥ 1.5 mg/dL

   c. Savaysa (edoxaban):

      i. 15 mg, 30 mg, and 60 mg tablets

      ii. Dosage indications:

         1) CrCl between 15 and 50 mL/min: 30 mg, once daily

         2) CrCl > 95 mL/min: Do not prescribe

   d. Bevyxxa (betrixaban):

      i. 40 mg and 80 mg

      ii. Initial dose of 160 mg, then maintenance dose of 80 mg daily with duration of therapy being 35 to 42 days

5. Thrombin inhibitors:

   a. Angiomax (bivalirudin): 250 mg per vial, add 5 mL of sterile water for injection

   b. Acova (argatroban): 2 mcg/kg/min in constant infusion until PTT is 1.5 to 3 times the initial baseline PTT value

   c. Pradaxa (dabigatran etexilate mesylate):

      i. 75 mg and 150 mg tablets

      ii. Dosage indications based on CrCl:

         1) CrCl > 30 mL/min: 150 mg, taken twice a day

         2) CrCl of 15 to 30 mL/min: 75 mg, taken twice a day

   d. Thrombate III (antithrombin III)

D. Surgery:

1. Insertion of vena cava filter to prevent PE

2. Venous thrombectomy

Follow-Up

A. Follow-up is determined by the client's needs, frequency and intensity of symptoms, and the presence of other medical conditions.

B. Persistent symptoms of a DVT should be managed by a cardiologist.

C. Clients taking anticoagulants are best followed by an anticoagulant clinic and/or cardiologist.

Consultation/Referral

A. If you suspect ALI, refer the client for immediate hospitalization to obtain diagnostic testing to determine the presence of a thrombus and restore circulation to the affected extremity.

B. If CLI has led to ulceration and/or superimposed infection, hospitalization is indicated to initiate a wound care consultation and diagnostic testing to determine the degree of arterial occlusion.

C. Referral to a cardiologist is indicated in the presence of persistent PVD symptoms.

D. Refer to pain management if pain is resistant to treatment.

E. Refer to a registered dietitian as indicated by the client's understanding of the dietary modification necessary to improve his or her status in terms of risk factors.

Individual Considerations

A. Nonambulatory clients:
1. Using rocking chairs is a possible substitute for persons unable to participate in a walking program.

B. Geriatrics:
1. Be alert to signs and symptoms of depression related to immobility and pain.

Bibliography

Brenner, B., Hull, R., Arya, R., Beyer-Westendorf, J., Douketis, J., Elalamy, I., . . . Zhai, Z. (2019, April 15). Evaluation of unmet clinical needs in prophylaxis and treatment of venous thromboembolism in high-risk patient groups: Cancer and critically ill. *Thrombosis Journal*, 17(6), 1–12. doi:10.1186/s12959-019-0196-6

Centers for Disease Control and Prevention. (2018, February 8). *Data and statistics on venous thromboembolism*. Retrieved from http://www.cdc.gov/ncbddd/dvt/data.html

Chang, S., Huang, Y., Lee, M., Hu, S., Hsiao, Y., Chang, C., & Chen, P. (2019, February 27). Association of varicose veins with incident venous thromboembolism and peripheral artery disease. *Journal of the American Medical Association*, 319(8), 807–817. doi:10.1001/jama.2018.0246

Faiz, A. S., Khan, I., Beckman, M. G., Bockenstedt, P., Heit, J. A., Kulkarni, R., & Philipp, C. S. (2015). Characteristics and risk factors of cancer associated venous thromboembolism. *Thrombosis Research*, 136(3), 535–541. doi:10.1016/j.thromres.2015.06.036

Fawzy, A. M., Yang, W.-Y., & Lip, G. Y. H. (2019, January 31). Safety of direct oral anticoagulants in real-world clinical practice: Translating the trials to everyday clinical management. *Expert Opinion of Drug Safety*, 18(3), 187–209. doi:10.1080/14740338.2019.1578344

Fernandez, L., & Scovell, S. (2016, April). Superficial thrombophlebitis of the lower extremity. *UpToDate*. Retrieved from http://www.uptodate.com/contents/superficial-thrombophlebitis-of-the-lower-extremity

Gordon, R. J., & Lombard, F. W. (2017, August). Perioperative venous thromboembolism: A review. *Anesthesia & Analgesia*, 125(2), 403–412. doi:10.1213/ANE.0000000000002183

Kaufman, C., Kinney, T., & Quencer, K. (2018, March 29). Practice trends of fibrinogen monitoring in thrombolysis. *Journal of Clinical Medicine*, 7(5), 111. doi:10.3390/jcm7050111

Kearon, C., Akl, E. A., Ornelas, J., Blaivas, A., Jimenez, D., Bounameaux, H., & Moores, L. (2016). Antithrombotic therapy for VTE disease: *Chest* guideline and expert panel report. *Chest*, 149(2), 315–352. doi:10.1016/j.chest.2015.11.026

Lip, G., & Hull, R. (2016, May). Overview of the treatment of lower extremity deep vein thrombosis (DVT). *UpToDate*. Retrieved from http://www.uptodate.com/contents/overview-of-the-treatment-of-lower-extremity-deep-vein-thrombosis-dvt

Piran, S., & Schulman, S. (2016, October 4). Management of venous thromboembolism: An update. *Thrombosis Journal*, 14(suppl 1), 23. doi:10.1186/s12959-016-0107-z. Retrieved from http://thrombosis-journal.biomedcentral.com/articles/10.1186/s12959-016-0107-z

Trayes, K. P., Studdiford, J. S., Pickle, S., & Tully, A. S. (2013). Edema: Diagnosis and management. *American Family Physician*, 88(2), 102–110. doi:10.1097/ACM.0b013e318277d5b2

Vascular Cures. (2017c). *Deep vein thrombosis*. Retrieved from http://vascularcures.org/deep-vein-thrombosis-dvt/

Heart Failure

Cheryl A. Glass and Debbie Gunter

Definition

HF is failure of the heart to pump sufficient blood to meet the metabolic demands of the tissues. However, the 2017 guidelines from the ACC/AHA address management of HF with reduced ejection fraction (HFrEF) and preserved ejection fraction (HFpEF).

The 2017 ACC/AHA guidelines for HF are available at www.onlinejacc.org/content/70/6/776?_ga=2.71537939.1451040440.1555197207-1269255221.1523817965.

A. HFrEF:
1. Ejection fraction (EF) less than 40% because of weak, inefficient systolic contractions. The left ventricular ejection fraction (LVEF) is a measurement of systolic failure.
2. An S_3 ventricular gallop rhythm commonly occurs.
3. Systolic failure is often the result of CHD and/or MI.
4. It can result from right- or left-sided failure, or both.

B. HFpEF:
1. EF is greater than 50%, but with poor compliance of the ventricle, which impedes ventricular diastolic filling (the ventricle is unable to relax).
2. There are two subgroups:
   a. HFpEF borderline (or intermediate): Clients with an EF of 41% to 49%
   b. HFpEF with an EF greater than 40% who previously had HFrEF (EF < 40%) but improvement or recovery was noted in EF
3. The client may be asymptomatic for years. HFpEF presents with the same symptoms of systolic failure, pulmonary congestion, and peripheral edema.
4. An S_4 atrial gallop rhythm commonly occurs.

Incidence

A. HFrEF incidence is higher in older women, chronic HTN, obesity, LVH, cardiomyopathy, excessive alcohol use, end-stage COPD, valvular disorders, anemia, renal failure, AF, CAD, or diabetes.

B. Approximately 6.5 million people in the United States have HF. By the year 2030, the AHA estimates that more than 8 million people will be affected by HF.

C. The costs of direct client care (e.g., healthcare services, hospitalization, medications) for these clients with chronic disease are projected to increase to approximately $69.7 billion by the year 2030.

Pathogenesis

Injuries to the myocardium may cause loss of functioning muscle. Compensatory mechanisms, including cardiac hypertrophy and neurohumoral processes, lead to adverse long-term effects. An inotropic insult results in incomplete emptying (systolic failure), and a compliance abnormality results in incomplete filling (diastolic failure). Most clients with HF have some degree of both abnormalities.

Predisposing Factors

A. Atherosclerotic heart disease
B. MI
C. Rheumatic heart disease involving mitral and aortic valves
D. Cardiomyopathies
E. Hypertensive heart disease
F. Aortic stenosis or regurgitation
G. Thyrotoxicosis
H. Pregnancy-related disorders such as multiple births with preexisting heart disease
I. Volume overload
J. Beta-blockers or other cardiac depressants
K. PE
L. Systemic infection
M. Arrhythmias
N. Renal disease

Common Complaints

Clients are assigned the New York Heart Association classifications based on their tolerance of physical activity and SOB. This classification may change according to the progression or regression of their CVD (Table 10.4).
A. Dyspnea on exertion
B. Hemoptysis
C. Fatigue
D. Cough
E. Orthopnea
F. Edema/weight gain
G. Paroxysmal nocturnal dyspnea
H. Nausea
I. Right upper abdominal pain or fullness

J. Chest pain
K. Palpitations

Other Signs and Symptoms

A. Hemoptysis
B. Bibasilar crackles
C. S_3 gallop
D. Murmurs
E. Exercise intolerance
F. Weakness
G. Cough
H. Orthopnea
I. Nocturnal dyspnea
J. Tachycardia
K. Pallor
L. Cyanosis
M. Anorexia
N. Constipation
O. JVD
P. Hepatomegaly
Q. Hepatojugular reflux (HJR)
R. Murmurs
S. Exercise intolerance

Subjective Data

A. Ask the client if he or she has difficulty breathing.
B. Ask how many pillows he or she sleeps on. Does the client need to sit up in a recliner to sleep?
C. Inquire about how often the client wakes up at night with SOB.
D. Inquire about how far the client can walk without getting SOB. Have the client describe his or her routine activities of daily living (ADLs) and how well the client tolerates each activity.
E. Discuss the client's history of heart disease, heart attack, HTN, or hyperlipidemia.
F. Ask the client about all current medications—prescription, OTC, and herbal products.
G. Question the client regarding all symptoms found in the "Common Complaints" section.
H. Discuss drug and alcohol history.

TABLE 10.4   NEW YORK HEART ASSOCIATION FUNCTIONAL CLASSIFICATION FOR HEART FAILURE

Functional Class	Activities	Objective Assessment
AHA Class I ACCF Stage A	No limitation. Ordinary activity does not cause undue fatigue, palpitation, dyspnea, or angina.	No objective evidence of CVD
AHA Class II ACCF Stage B	Slight limitations. Fatigue, palpitation, SOB, angina with ordinary physical activity.	Objective evidence—minimal CVD
AHA Class III ACCF Stage C	Marked limitations. No discomfort at rest. Fatigue, palpitation, SOB, and angina with less than usual activities.	Objective evidence—moderately severe CVD
AHA Class IV ACCF Stage D	Inability to do physical activity without discomfort. Symptoms of heart failure are present at rest and become worse with activity.	Objective evidence—severe CVD

ACCF, American College of Cardiology Foundation; AHA, American Heart Association; CVD, cardiovascular disease; SOB, shortness of breath.

Source: Data from the American Heart Association and includes staging by the American College of Cardiology Foundation.

I. Has the client ever been treated for cancer/chemotherapy, and how long ago?

J. What is the client's usual weight? Has he or she experienced more symptoms if he or she has pedal edema?

K. Does the client have a cough (consider angiotensin-converting enzyme inhibitors [ACEI] as the cause)?

Physical Examination

A. Check pulse, respirations, BP, height, and weight:
  1. Check BP while client is sitting, standing, and lying down.
  2. Be alert for abnormal vital signs: Hypotension, narrow or wide pulse pressure, tachycardia, bradycardia, and tachypnea.
  3. Calculate BMI.
  4. On all subsequent visits, note weight gain of more than 1 lb per day over 3 consecutive days or 3 lb in 1 day.

B. Inspect:
  1. Overall physical appearance. Is the client in distress?
  2. Skin: Note pallor, cyanosis, and temperature.
  3. Neck: Check jugular veins for distention.
  4. Extremities: Note edema, cyanosis, pallor, and ulcers.

C. Auscultate:
  1. Heart for murmurs; tachycardia; S_3 or S_4 gallops; and other abnormalities
  2. Lungs: Note moderate to severe crackles/rales and other abnormal sounds
  3. Neck and carotid arteries

D. Palpate:
  1. Abdomen for hepatomegaly and HJR
  2. Extremities for peripheral pulses
  3. Chest wall for displaced point of maximal impulse (PMI), lifts, heaves, and thrills

E. Mental status: Check mental status because confusion may occur, especially in the elderly.

Diagnostic Tests

A. Two-dimensional echocardiography with Doppler to evaluate LVEF

B. Radionuclide ventriculography may be used to measure LVEF and LV volumes.

C. Coronary angiography

D. Anterior/posterior chest x-ray

E. EKG for clients with suspected arrhythmia, ischemia, or cardiac disease. Identify acute and old EKG changes to rule out pathologic Q wave, ST-segment elevation, and LV hypertrophy.

F. Natriuretic peptides (BNP or NT-proBNP)

Differential Diagnoses

A. HF
  1. HFrEF less than or equal to 40%
  2. HFpEF:
    a. HFpEF borderline clients with an EF of 41% to 49%
    b. HFpEF clients with an EF greater than 40% who previously had HFrEF (EF, 40%) with improvement noted in EF

B. Renal disease or nephrotic syndrome
C. Liver disease
D. Asthma
E. COPD

> To distinguish between progressing HF and a COPD exacerbation when both conditions are present, note that the presence of weight gain and an S_3 gallop indicates HF, not COPD.

Plan

A. General interventions:
  1. Determine the etiology of the failure state and treat appropriately.
  2. Treat HF stages:
    a. Stage A: Treat/manage the client's underlying conditions (HTN, AF, hyperlipidemia, diabetes, tobacco cessation, obesity, substance abuse [e.g., alcohol, cocaine]).
    b. Stage B: Begin ACEI with beta-blockers for clients with HFrEF. Add statin therapy if the client has a history of MI.
    c. Stage C: HFrEF: Implantable cardioverter defibrillators and consider cardiac resynchronization therapy
      i. Digoxin may be used to manage symptoms. Hydralazine and isosorbide dinitrate are indicated for African American clients with HFrEF, clients with kidney dysfunction, or clients who cannot take ACEI or angiotensin receptor blocker (ARB) therapy. A diuretic agent is also recommended.
    d. Stage D: Provide advanced treatment such as cardiac transplant, mechanical support, and/or palliative care.
  3. The goals of therapy are to improve the client's quality of life by reducing symptoms, decreasing morbidity, and prolonging survival.

B. Client teaching:
  1. Teach the client to weigh self daily at the same time, on the same scale, and in the same clothing. Instruct the client to call if there is a weight gain of more than 3 lb in 1 day or more than 1 lb a day over a 3-day period.
    a. Develop a plan of care for the increase of diuretic dosing in case of edema/weight gain to decrease dyspnea and prevent hospitalization.
  2. Encourage weight loss.
  3. Recommend regular, moderate exercise as long as dyspnea is not induced. Encourage exercise to increase endurance and strengthen muscles even though the client may tolerate only a few minutes of walking.
  4. Encourage smoking cessation.
  5. Encourage medication adherence. Instruct the client about all medications and possible side effects. Do not use OTC medicines without consulting the provider. NSAIDs are contraindicated in HF.
  6. Use continuous positive airway pressure (CPAP) or bilevel positive airway pressure (BiPAP) for nighttime sleep and naps for the treatment of OSA.

7. Educate the client and family about biventricular pacing or an implantable defibrillator that may be necessary for advanced HF.

8. Discuss the need for palliative/hospice care when HF does not respond despite maximal therapy.

9. Discuss the client's desire for advanced therapies, which might include an evaluation for heart transplant or ventricular assist device.

C. Dietary management:

1. Read food labels for sodium content.

2. Teach dietary modifications, especially salt restriction of 2,000 to 3,000 mg/d for HFrEF and HFpEF. Less than 2,000 mg sodium per day is recommended in clients with moderate to severe HF symptoms.

3. Fluid restriction is not recommended unless the client is classified as Stage D or is diagnosed with hyponatremia with sodium levels less than 130 mEq/L. Restrict fluid intake to 2,000 mL/d or less for clients with chronic fluid retention despite use of diuretics and sodium restrictions.

4. Alcohol consumption should be limited to one glass of beer or wine per day. This amount should be counted in the daily fluid restriction.

5. See Appendix B for the DASH diet (Tables B.3 and B.4).

6. Other diet changes include low-fat/low-cholesterol foods and the use of the following:

a. Monounsaturated fats, which decrease cholesterol:
   i. Canola oil
   ii. Olive oil

b. Polyunsaturated fats, which decrease cholesterol but not as well as monounsaturated fats:
   i. Vegetable and fish oils
   ii. Corn, safflower, peanut, and soybean oils

c. Avoid saturated fats.
   i. Animal fats and some plant fats
   ii. Butter and lard
   iii. Coconut oil and palm oil

D. Pharmaceutical therapy:

1. Therapy is based on the extent of cardiac impairment and severity of symptoms. Medication regimens include a combination of the following classes: diuretics, ACEI (ARB if unable to tolerate ACEI), cardioselective beta-blockers, inotropic agents such as digoxin, vasodilators, nitrates, and anticoagulants if there is an increased risk of thrombus formation. In general, CCBs are not used in HF management.

2. Drug classifications for antihypertensive and cardiac medication are noted in Table 10.5.

TABLE 10.5   ANTIHYPERTENSIVE AND CARDIAC MEDICATIONS (SORTED ALPHABETICALLY)

Brand Name	Generic Name	Drug Class
Accupril	Quinapril	ACEI
Accuretic	Quinapril	ACEI/diuretic
Aceon	Perindopril erbumine	ACEI
Adalat CC	DHP/nifedipine	CCB
Aldactazide	Spironolactone + HCTZ	Combination: K$^+$ sparing + thiazide
Aldactone	Spironolactone	Diuretic—K$^+$ sparing
Altace	Ramipril	ACEI
Amiloride/HCTZ	Amiloride/HCTZ	Combination + diuretic
Amturnide	Aliskiren/amlodipine/HCTZ	CCB/renin inhibitor/HCTZ
Atacand	Candesartan cilexetil	Angiotensin II receptor blocker
Atacand HCT	Candesartan + HCTZ	Combination: ARB + diuretic
Avalide	Irbesartan + HCTZ	Combination: ARB + diuretic
Avalide Avapro	Irbesartan + HCTZ irbesartan	Combination: ARB + diuretic angiotensin II receptor blocker
Azor	Amlodipine + olmesartan	CCB + ARB
Benicar	Olmesartan medoxomil	Angiotensin II receptor blocker
Benicar HCT	Olmesartan + HCTZ	Combination: ARB + diuretic
Betapace	Sotalol	Beta-blocker/class II and III antiarrhythmic
Betapace AF	Sotalol	Class II and III antiarrhythmics
Betaxolol Bidil	Betaxolol HCl isosorbide dinitrate + hydralazine	Beta-blocker (cardioselective) nitrate + diuretic
Bumex	Bumetanide	Loop diuretic
Bystolic	Nebivolol	Beta-blocker (cardioselective)

(continued)

TABLE 10.5 ANTIHYPERTENSIVE AND CARDIAC MEDICATIONS (SORTED ALPHABETICALLY) (continued)

Brand Name	Generic Name	Drug Class
Byvalson	Nebivolol and valsartan	Beta-blocker + ARB
Caduet	Amlodipine + atorvastatin	CCB/amlodipine/atorvastatin
Calan	Verapamil	CCB/antianginal
Calan SR	Verapamil	CCB
Capoten	Captopril	ACEI/CHF
Capozide	Captopril + HCTZ	Combination: ACE + diuretic
Cardizem LA	Diltiazem	CCB
Cardura	Doxazosin	Alpha-2 blocker AAB
Catapres	Clonidine	Central alpha agonist
Chlorothiazide	Various	Thiazide diuretic
Chlorthalidone	Various	Monosulfamyl diuretic
Cleviprex	Clevidipine	CCB
Clorpres	Clonidine/chlorthalidone	Central alpha agonist + thiazide diuretic
Cordarone	Amiodarone	Class II and III antiarrhythmics
Coreg CR	Carvedilol	Beta-blocker (noncardioselective)/CHF
Corgard	Nadolol	Beta-blocker (noncardioselective)/antianginal
Corlanor	Ivabradine	Hyperpolarization-activated cyclic nucleotide-gated channel blocker
Corzide	Nadolol + HCTZ	Combination: beta-blocker (noncardioselective) + diuretic
Covera-HS	Verapamil	CCB/antianginal
Cozaar	Losartan	Angiotensin II receptor blocker (ARB)
Demadex	Torsemide	Loop diuretic
Dilacor XR	Diltiazem	CCB/antianginal
Dilatrate SR	Isosorbide dinitrate	Nitrate
Diovan	Valsartan	Angiotensin II receptor blocker/CHF class II–IV
Diovan HCT	Valsartan + HCTZ	Combination: ARB + diuretic
Diuril	Chlorothiazide	Thiazide diuretic
Dutoprol Dyazide	Metoprolol ext. release + HCTZ triamterene + HCTZ	Beta-blocker (cardioselective) + thiazide combination—K+ sparing + thiazide
Dynacirc CR	Isradipine controlled release	CCB
Edarbi	Azilsartan	Angiotensin II receptor blocker
Edarbyclor	Azilsartan + chlorthalidone	Angiotensin II receptor blocker + diuretic
Edecrin	Ethacrynic acid	Loop diuretic
Entresto	Sacubitril/valsartan	Angiotensin Receptor-Neprilysin Inhibitors (ARNi)
Epaned	Enalopril	ACEI
Exforge	Amlodipine + valsartan	CCB + ARB
Exforge HCT	Valsartan/amlodipine/HCTZ	CCB + ARB + diuretic
Fosinopril HCTZ	Various HCTZ	ACEI thiazide diuretic
Hytrin	Terazosin	Alpha-1 blocker
Hyzaar	Losartan potassium + HCTZ	Combination ARB + diuretic
Imdur	Isosorbide dinitrate	Nitrate
Inderal	Propranolol	Beta-blocker (noncardioselective)/antianginal/antiarrhythmic
Inderide	Propranolol + HCTZ	Combination: beta-blocker (noncardioselective) + diuretic
Innopran XL	Propranolol HCL ext. release	Beta-blocker (noncardioselective)

(continued)

TABLE 10.5   ANTIHYPERTENSIVE AND CARDIAC MEDICATIONS (SORTED ALPHABETICALLY) *(continued)*

Brand Name	Generic Name	Drug Class
Inspra	Eplerenone	Aldosterone receptor blocker—mineralocorticoid selective/CHF
ISMO	Isosorbide mononitrate	Nitrate
Isoptin SR	Verapamil	CCB
Isordil	Various	Nitrate
Kerlone	Betaxolol	Beta-blocker (cardioselective)
Lanoxin	Digoxin	Cardiac glycoside/antiarrhythmic
Lasix	Furosemide	Loop diuretic
Levatol	Penbutolol sulfate	Beta-blocker (noncardioselective)
Lopressor	Metoprolol tartrate	Beta-blocker (cardioselective)/antianginal
Lopressor HCT	Metoprolol + HCTZ	Combination: beta-blocker (cardioselective) + diuretic
Lotensin	Benazepril	ACEI
Lotensin HCT	Benazepril + HCTZ	Combination: ACE + diuretic
Lotrel	Amlodipine + benazepril	Combination: CCB + ACEI
Mavik	Trandolapril	ACE inhibitor/CHF
Maxide	Triamterene + HCTZ	Combination—K^+ sparing + thiazide
Micardis	Telmisartan	Angiotensin II receptor blocker
Micardis HCT	Telmisartan + HCTZ	Combination: ARB + diuretic
Microzide	HCTZ	Diuretic
Minitran	Nitroglycerin	Nitrate
Monoket	Isosorbide dinitrate	Nitrate
Monopril	Fosinopril	ACEI/CHF
Multaq	Dronedarone	Antiarrhythmic
Nicardipine	Various	CCB
Nitro-BID	Nitroglycerin	Nitrate
Nitro-Dur	Nitroglycerin	Nitrate
Nitrolingual	Nitroglycerin	Nitrate
Nitrostat	Nitroglycerin	Nitrate
Normodyne	Labetalol	Beta-blocker
Norpace	Disopyramide	Antiarrhythmics—class 1 ventricular
Norvasc	Amlodipine	CCB/antianginal
Pindolol	Pindolol	Beta-blocker (noncardioselective)
Plendil	Felodipine	CCB
Prestalia	Perindopril arginine/amlodipine	ACEI/CCB
Prinivil	Lisinopril	ACEI/CHF
Prinzide	Lisinopril + HCTZ	Combination: ACE inhibitor + thiazide diuretic
Procanbid	Procainamide	Antiarrhythmics—class 1a ventricular
Procardia XL	Nifedipine	CCB/antianginal
Quinidine gluconate	Various	Antiarrhythmics—class 1 atrial and ventricular ACEI
Quinidine sulfate	Various	Antiarrhythmics—class 1 atrial and ventricular
Ranexa	Ranolazine	Antianginal
Rythmol	Propafenone	Antiarrhythmics—class 1c ventricular
Sectral	Acebutolol	Beta-blocker (cardioselective)
Sular	Nisoldipine	CCB

(continued)

TABLE 10.5   ANTIHYPERTENSIVE AND CARDIAC MEDICATIONS (SORTED ALPHABETICALLY) (*continued*)

Brand Name	Generic Name	Drug Class
Tambocor	Flecainide	Antiarrhymics—class 1c-ventricular
Tarka	Trandolapril + verapamil	Combination: ACE + CCB
Tekamlo	Aliskiren + amlodipine	Direct renin inhibitor + DHP CCB
Tekturna	Aliskiren	Direct renin inhibitor
Tekturna HCT	Aliskiren + HCTZ	Direct renin inhibitor + thiazide diuretic
Tenex	Guanfacine	Central alpha agonist
Tenoretic	Atenolol + chlorthalidone	Combination: beta-blocker (cardioselective) + diuretic
Tenormin	Atenolol	Beta-blocker (cardioselective)/antianginal
Teveten	Eprosartan	Angiotensin II receptor blocker
Teveten HCT	Eprosartan + HCTZ	Combination: ARB + diuretic
Thalitone	Chlorthalidone	Antihypertensive/diuretic
Tiazac	Diltiazem	CCB/antianginal
Timolide	Timolol maleate + HCTZ	Combination: beta-blocker (noncardioselective) + diuretic
Toprol-XL	Metoprolol	Beta-blocker (cardioselective)/antianginal/CHF class II or III
Trandate	Labetalol	Beta-blocker (noncardioselective)
Tribenzor	Olmesartan + amlodipine + HCTZ	ARB + CCB + thiazide diuretic
Twynsta	Telmisartan + amlodipine	ARB + CCB
Uniretic	Moexipril + HCTZ	Combination: ACE + diuretic
Univasc	Moexipril	ACEI
Valturna	Aliskiren + valsartan	Direct renin inhibitor + ARB
Vaseretic	Enalapril + HCTZ	Combination: ACE + diuretic
Vasotec	Enalapril	ACEI/CHF with digitalis and diuretics
Verelan PM	Verapamil	CCB
Zaroxolyn	Metolazone	Diuretic: Quinazoline
Zebeta	Bisoprolol	Beta-blocker (cardioselective)
Zestoretic	Lisinopril + HCTZ	Combination: ACE + diuretic
Zestril	Lisinopril	ACEI/CHF with digitalis and diuretics
Ziac	Bisoprolol + HCTZ	Combination: beta-blocker (cardioselective) + diuretic

AAB, alpha-adrenergic blocker; ACEI, angiotensin-converting enzyme inhibitor; ARB, angiotensin receptor blocker; CCB, calcium channel blocker; CHF, congestive heart failure; DHP, dihydropyridine; HCTZ, hydrochlorothiazide.

3. Drugs that should be avoided and/or used with caution in HF because they cause exacerbations or are at high risk of adverse reactions include:

a. NSAIDs: Increased renal dysfunction, edema, impaired response to ACEI

b. Cyclooxygenase (COX-2) inhibitors: Increased rate of HF and increased mortality

c. Aspirin: Interaction between ASA and ACEI; interference with benefits of beta-blockers on LVEF

d. Metformin: Increased risk of lethal lactic acidosis

e. Thiazolidinediones: Cause fluid retention that may precipitate HF

f. CCBs: Some data exist on possible effects on systolic dysfunction.

g. Antidepressants (TCAs) and SSRIs: Major adverse cardiovascular events, including HF, MI, stroke, and cardiovascular death

h. Phosphodiesterase inhibitors (PDE-3, PDE-4, and PDE-5): Increased mortality

i. Antiarrhythmic: Negative inotropic activity and further reduction in LV function can impair the elimination and result in toxicity of the antiarrhythmic agent.

j. Chemotherapy: Many are cardiotoxic.

k. Androgen–testosterone patch: Edema may increase the rate of HF.

l. Theophylline-serum levels may increase and cause toxicity because of acute decompensation of HF.

m. Sodium bicarbonate and Fleet Phospho-Soda contain significant quantities of sodium.

n. Herbal/supplements may also affect HF.

4. Pneumonia vaccination and annual influenza immunization should be encouraged.

Follow-Up

A. HF clients should be comanaged with a cardiologist.

B. Close follow-up is essential if the client is to be maintained as an outpatient.

C. Appointments every 1 to 2 weeks may be necessary, with additional appointments depending on the client's symptoms such as increasing SOB, inability to lie flat to sleep, nocturnal moist cough, and increase in daily weight.

D. Laboratory monitoring is required for electrolytes, BUN, creatinine, proteinuria, and digoxin level.

Consultation/Referral

A. Consult a physician when the client requires the next level up in pharmacological management.

B. Consult a cardiologist for staging and hospital management.

Individual Considerations

A. Pregnancy:

1. HF is uncommon in healthy women without coexisting heart disease.

2. Pregnancy in a client with heart disease is considered high risk.

3. Refer to a high-risk obstetrician/perinatologist for care during pregnancy.

B. Pediatrics: HF is usually associated with congenital heart defects.

C. Adults:

1. The 5-year survival rate is 25% for men and 38% for women.

2. Predictors of poor outcome include an EF less than 25%, ischemic etiology, ventricular arrhythmias, serum sodium less than 130 mEq/L, poor functional class, low cardiac index, and high filling pressures.

D. Geriatrics:

1. In very frail elderly clients or those in long-term care settings, the only sign may be increased agitation or acute change in LOC.

Bibliography

American Diabetes Association. (2019). Cardiovascular disease and risk management: Standards of medical care in diabetes—2019. *Diabetes Care, 42*(suppl 1), S103–S123. doi:10.2337/dc19-S010

American Heart Association. (2017). *Top ten things to know: 2017 ACC/AHA/HFSA focused update of the 2013 ACCF/AHA guideline for the management of heart failure.* Retrieved from https://www.heart.org/-/media/data-import/downloadables/hfsa-focused-update-for-the-management-of-heart-failure-ucm_493382.pdf

Benjamin, E. J., Blaha, M. J., Chiuve, S., Cushman, M., Das, S., Deo, R., . . . American Heart Association Statistics Committee and Stroke Statistics Subcommittee. (2017). Heart disease and stroke statistics—2017 update: A report from the American Heart Association. *Circulation, 135*(1), e1–e603. doi:10.1161/CIR.0000000000000485

Centers for Disease Control and Prevention. (2019, January 8). *Heart failure fact sheet.* Retrieved from https://www.cdc.gov/dhdsp/data_statistics/fact_sheets/fs_heart_failure.htm

Dumitru, I. (2018, May 7). Heart failure. *Medscape.* Retrieved from https://emedicine.medscape.com/article/163062-overview

Eckel, R. H., Jakicic, J. M., Ard, J. D., deJesus, J. M., Houston-Miller, N., Hubbard, V. S., & Yanovsk, S. Z. (2014). 2013 AHA/ACC guideline on lifestyle management to reduce cardiovascular risk: A report of the American College of Cardiology/American Heart Association Task Force on Practice Guidelines. *Circulation, 129*(25), S76–S99. doi:10.1161/01.cir.0000437740.48606.d1. Retrieved from http://circ.ahajournals.org/content/129/25_suppl_2/S76

Goff, D. C., Lloyd-Jones, D. M., Bennett, G., Coady, S., & D'Agostino, B. R. Sr. (2014). 2013 ACC/AHA guideline on the assessment of cardiovascular risk: A report of the American College of Cardiology/American Heart Association Task Force on Practice Guidelines. *Circulation*, S49–S73. doi:10.1161/01.cir.0000437741.48606.98

Jackson, S. M. (2013). Diastolic heart failure. *Advance for NPs & PAs, 4*(2), 23–25, 34. Retrieved from http://citeseerx.ist.psu.edu/viewdoc/download;jsessionid=0CE1906640AD9C67C63BA30A5A32A475?doi=10.1.1.370.1815&rep=rep1&type=pdf

Kusumoto, F., Shoenfeld, M., & Barrett, C. (2018). 2018 ACC/AHA/HRS guideline on the evaluation and management of patients with bradycardia and cardiac conduction delay. *Journal of the American College of Cardiology, 74*, e51–e156. doi:10.1016/j.jacc.2018.10.044

Mozaffarian, D., Benjamin, E. J., & Go, A. S. (2016). Heart disease and stroke statistics—2016 update: A report from the American Heart Association. *Circulation, 133*(4), 447–454. doi:10.1161/CIR.0000000000000350

Murphy, N., Shanks, M., & Alderman, P. (2019, January). Management of heart failure with outpatient technology. *Journal for Nurse Practitioners, 15*(1), 12–18. doi:10.1016/j.nurpra.2018.07.004

Ren, X. (2017, March 23). Aortic stenosis. *Medscape.* Retrieved from https://emedicine.medscape.com/article/150638-overview

Trayes, K. P., Studdiford, J. S., Pickle, S., & Tully, A. S. (2013). Edema: Diagnosis and management. *American Family Physician, 88*(2), 102–110. doi:10.1097/ACM.0b013e318277d5b2

Yancy, C. W., Jessup, M., Bozkurt, B., Butler, J., Casey, D. E., Drazner, M. H., . . . Wilkoff, B. L. (2017). 2017 ACC/AHA/HFSA focused update of the 2013 ACCF/AHA guideline for the management of heart failure: A report of the American College of Cardiology Foundation/American Heart Association Task Force on Practice Guidelines. *Journal of the American College of Cardiology, 70*(6), 776–803. doi:10.1161/CIR.0000000000000509

Hypertension

Jill C. Cash, Cheryl A. Glass, and Debbie Gunter

Definition

A. Discord exists between the ACC/AHA (2017) and the JNC 8 guideline (2014) as to the definition and stages of HTN. The JNC 8 guideline provided more permissive (higher) BP goals, especially for those 60 and older. The newer AHA/ACC guideline defines HTN as an SBP of 130 mmHg or more, a diastolic blood pressure (DBP) of 80 mmHg or more, or describes a condition in which a person is taking antihypertensive medications. (Table 10.6; For more information go to https://www.ahajournals.org/doi/10.1161/HYP.0000000000000065.)

B. Resistant HTN is defined as:

1. BP that is not at target despite a three-drug regimen, with one of the agents being a diuretic appropriate for the client's glomerular filtration rate (GFR)

2. BP that is controlled while taking four or more medications is also considered resistant HTN

C. Standing and supine BPs should be measured before the initiation of combination antihypertensive therapy. Orthostatic (postural) hypotension is diagnosed when, within 2 to 5 minutes of quiet standing, one or more of the following is present:

1. At least a 20 mmHg fall in systolic pressure

2. At least a 10 mmHg fall in diastolic pressure

3. Symptoms of cerebral hypoperfusion, such as dizziness

D. The average nocturnal BP is approximately 15% lower than daytime values. Failure of the BP to fall by at least 10% during sleep is called "nondipping" and is

TABLE 10.6   WHELTON 2017 HIGH BP CLINICAL PRACTICE GUIDELINE

Ethnicity/ Population	Age (Years)	Begin Initiation of Pharmacological Treatment to Lower BP	BP Goals for Treatment	Other Comments
General population	≥60	Initiate therapy for SBP ≥ 130 mmHg *or* DBP ≥80 mmHg	Treat to goal of SBP < 130 mmHg *and* DBP < 80 mmHg	If pharmacological treatment results in a lower achieved SBP and treatment is well tolerated, treatment does not need to be adjusted.
	<60	Initiate therapy to lower BP at SBP ≥ 130 mmHg	Treat to goal of SBP < 130 mmHg	
		Initiate therapy to lower BP at DBP ≥ 80 mmHg	Treat to goal of DBP < 80 mmHg	
Clients with chronic kidney disease	≥18	Initiate therapy to lower BP at SBP ≥ 130 mmHg *or* DBP ≥ 80 mmHg	Treat to goal of SBP < 130 mmHg *and* DBP < 80 mmHg	
Clients with chronic kidney disease (regardless of race or diabetes status)	≥18			Initial or add-on antihypertensive therapy should include an ACEI or ARB to improve kidney outcomes.
Clients with diabetes	≥18	Initiate therapy to lower BP at SBP ≥ 130 mmHg *or* DBP ≥ 80 mmHg	Treat to goal of SBP < 130 mmHg *and* DBP < 80 mmHg	The American Diabetes Association criteria differ from all others, in that these guidelines advocate treating toward a SBP goal of <140 mmHg and to a DBP of <80 mmHg.
General non-Black population, including those with diabetes				Initial antihypertensive therapy should include a thiazide-type diuretic, CCB, ACEI, or ARB.
General Black population, including those with diabetes				Initial antihypertensive therapy should include a thiazide-type diuretic *and* CCB.

ACEI, angiotensin-converting enzyme inhibitor; ARB, angiotensin receptor blocker; BP, blood pressure; CCB, calcium channel blocker; DBP, diastolic blood pressure; SBP, systolic blood pressure.

Source: Data from Whelton, P. K., et al. (2017). ACC/AHA/AAPA/ABC/ACPM/AGS/APhA/ASH/ASPC/MNA/PCN guideline for the prevention, detection, evaluation, and management of high blood pressure in adults. *Hypertension*. doi:HYP.0000000000000065

a stronger predictor of adverse cardiovascular outcomes than daytime BP.

E. *Isolated systolic HTN (ISH)* is when the SBP is greater than or equal to 130 mmHg with DBP normal or below normal (<80 mmHg). ISH usually affects the elderly, increasing their risk of stroke or MI.

F. *Isolated diastolic HTN (IDH)* is defined as a diastolic pressure greater than or equal to 80 mmHg with a systolic pressure less than 130 mmHg. IDH is more common in younger men who are overweight/obese and in individuals younger than 40 years.

G. Malignant HTN is marked HTN with retinal hemorrhages, exudates, or papilledema. It is usually associated with pressures above 180/120 mmHg with evidence of end-organ damage.

Incidence

A. Worldwide, HTN affects about 975 million people.

B. Approximately 75 million people, equivalent to one in three adults, in the United States have HTN.

C. The incidence of resistant HTN is being studied more closely; the current rate is about 12% of all clients with HTN.

D. High BP was a primary or contributing cause of death for more than 410,000 Americans in 2014—that is more than 1,100 deaths each day.

Pathogenesis

More than 90% of cases have no identifiable cause, thus constituting the category of primary or essential HTN. The remaining 10% of cases have the following secondary causes:

A. Renal causes:
   1. Glomerulonephritis
   2. Pyelonephritis
   3. Polycystic kidney disease

B. Endocrine causes:
   1. Primary hyperaldosteronism
   2. Pheochromocytoma
   3. Hyperthyroidism
   4. Cushing's syndrome

C. Vascular causes:
1. Coarctation of aorta
2. Renal artery stenosis
D. Chemical/medication induced:
1. Oral contraceptives
2. NSAIDs
3. Decongestants
4. Antidepressants
5. Sympathomimetics
6. Corticosteroids
7. Lithium
8. Ergotamine alkaloids
9. Cyclosporine
10. Monoamine oxidase inhibitors (MAOIs), in combination with certain drugs or foods
11. Appetite suppressants, in combination with certain drugs or foods
12. Cocaine
13. Amphetamines
E. OSA

Predisposing Factors

When making a diagnosis, consider not only the absolute BP reading, but also the presence or absence of other cardiovascular risk factors (Table 10.7). Factors include the following:
A. Family history of HTN
B. Obesity
C. Alcohol consumption
D. Stress
E. Sedentary lifestyle
F. African American ancestry
G. Male gender
H. Age greater than 30 years
I. Excessive salt intake
J. Medications
K. Drug use

Common Complaint

A. HTN is asymptomatic in the majority of clients.

Other Signs and Symptoms

A. Headaches
B. Advanced disease: Organ-specific complaints with end-organ damage
C. Retinopathy

TABLE 10.7 MODIFIABLE AND NONMODIFIABLE RISK FOR CONTROL OF HTN

Modifiable	Nonmodifiable
Sedentary lifestyle	Age
Smoking	Gender
Diet	Ethnicity
Lipid control	Diabetes
Sodium intake	Postmenopausal
Alcohol intake	Family history
Obesity	

Potential Complications

A. Cerebral vascular accident (CVA)
B. MI
C. Renal failure
D. HF
E. PAD

Subjective Data

A. Ask the client about any family history of HTN or cardiac or renal disease.
B. Ask if the client has ever been diagnosed with HTN or cardiac or renal disease.
C. Ask if the client ever had any high-BP readings.
D. Ask if the client has ever been treated for any of the aforementioned problems.
E. Ask the client about other risk factors such as smoking, drinking, high-fat intake, obesity, and/or diabetes.
F. Inquire about the client's lifestyle, exercise regimen, work environment, and stress level.
G. Ask the client about symptoms that suggest secondary etiology:
1. Palpitations, headache, diaphoresis (pheochromocytoma)
2. Anxiety, weight gain or loss (thyroid abnormality)
3. Muscle weakness, polyuria (primary hyperaldosteronism)
H. Find out if the client is taking drugs that elevate BP (noted under "Pathogenesis").
I. Ask whether the client feels nervous when having his or her BP taken in the office ("white coat HTN").
J. Review current medications, including prescription, OTC, and herbal products.
K. Review current recreational/illicit drug use.

Physical Examination

A. Check pulse, BP, height, weight, waist circumference, and distribution of body fat. Calculate BMI.
1. The diagnosis of HTN is made after averaging two or more properly measured readings at each of two or more visits after an initial screen. Compare both upper extremes during the first visit; if they are unequal, use the higher value.
2. When the client's SBP and DBP fall into two different categories, use the higher category to classify his or her BP.
3. For accurate measurement, use the correct size cuff for the client (adult, large adult, or thigh cuff). Compare the home cuff's reading with the office cuff's reading to verify the accuracy of the home cuff's measurements.
4. Perform manual vital signs with irregular rhythms.
5. If there are still problems diagnosing true HTN, consider a 24-hour ambulatory BP monitor.
B. Inspect:
1. Observe overall appearance.
2. Conduct funduscopic examination; look for papilledema, exudates, AV nicking, anterior nicking.
3. Inspect the neck for jugular vein distention.

4. Observe for lower-extremity edema.

C. Auscultate:
  1. Heart: Note the PMI.
  2. Lungs: Check for bronchospasm and rales.
  3. Neck: Assess carotid arteries for bruits.

D. Palpate:
  1. Palpate the neck; check thyroid for enlargement.
  2. Palpate the abdomen for masses or organomegaly.
  3. Palpate the extremities; assess peripheral pulses and note edema.
  4. Assess deep tendon reflexes (DTRs).

Diagnostic Tests

A. Hematocrit

B. LFTs, lactate dehydrogenase (LDH) test, and uric acid test

C. Chemistry profile

D. Lipid profile (total and HDL cholesterol and triglycerides)

E. Urinalysis for proteinuria

F. Estimated GFR

G. EKG

H. If history, physical examination, or laboratory tests indicate the need, obtain the following:
  1. Intravenous pyelography (IVP)
  2. Renal arteriogram
  3. Plasma renin
  4. Catecholamines
  5. Chest radiography
  6. Aortogram
  7. Ultrasonography
  8. Sleep study

I. Monitor potassium levels if client is on an ACEI/ARB or spironolactone.

Differential Diagnoses

A. Primary HTN

B. Secondary HTN

C. Drug-induced HTN

D. White coat syndrome

Plan

A. General interventions (see Table 10.7):
  1. Advise overweight clients to lose weight. Loss of as little as 10 pounds reduces BP in many clients.
  2. Advise the client to limit or discontinue alcohol intake.
  3. Encourage the client to stop smoking.
  4. Encourage increased physical activity. The 2017 ACC/AHA guidelines on lifestyle management outline the optimal physical activity recommendation, which advises adults to engage in 40 minutes of aerobic physical activity three to four times a week (Table 10.7). The aerobic exercise should involve moderate to vigorous intensity.
  5. Encourage some form of relaxation technique.

B. Client teaching:
  1. Stress the asymptomatic nature of the disease.
  2. Stress the importance of ongoing monitoring and treatment under the direction of a healthcare provider.

3. Review risk factors for cardiac, renal, and cerebrovascular disease and possible preventive measures.

4. The ACC maintains the CardioSmart Patient Education Portal as an online BP management tool to educate and motivate clients. ACC's CardioSmart is a free resource located at www.cardiosmart.org. CardioSmartTXT PREVENT is a 6-month program of health tips and reminders sent via two text messages a week. CardioSmartTXT QUIT is a 2-month program to assist clients in smoking cessation. Four text messages are sent a day with information and assistance with smoking cessation. Clients can sign up at author.cardiosmart.org/Tools/CardioSmartTXT-Prevent.

C. Dietary management: Review specific dietary measures. Give dietary recommendation sheets. See Appendix B for low-fat/low-cholesterol and DASH dietary approaches to stop HTN.
  1. Diet alone will make only the lowest incremental change in BP; therefore, it should be combined with lifestyle modification. Lower sodium intake, smoking cessation, weight loss, and exercise are all essential.
  2. It is essential for the client/family to read labels for sodium, fat content, and serving sizes.
  3. Other dietary changes include low-fat/low-cholesterol diets and limiting fat consumption.
    a. Use monounsaturated fats to decrease cholesterol:
      i. Canola oil
      ii. Olive oil
    b. Use polyunsaturated fats in limited quantities: Polyunsaturated fats decrease cholesterol, but not as well as monounsaturated fats:
      i. Vegetable and fish oils
      ii. Corn, safflower, peanut, and soybean oils
    c. Limit saturated fats:
      i. Animal fats and some plant fats
      ii. Butter and lard
      iii. Coconut oil and palm oil

D. Pharmaceutical therapy:
  1. If lifestyle changes alone are not adequate to control HTN, consider drug therapy. Medication doses are dependent on age, ethnicity, and comorbid conditions. Most clients will require two or more medications to control their BP. Consider starting antihypertensives and/or diuretics (see Table 10.5 for drugs and classifications) as outlined by the current guidelines. An extensive guideline is available at www.thecardiologyadvisor.com/home/clinical-charts/hypertension-treatment-algorithm.
  2. The 2017 Science Advisory recommendations from the AHA, ACC, and CDC provide medication classifications for the treatment of HTN in the presence of medical conditions (see Table 10.8).
  3. ACEIs, ARBs, CCBs, and thiazide diuretics should be used as first-line options, either as single agents or in combination

TABLE 10.8   AHA, ACC, AND CDC 2013 SUGGESTED HYPERTENSIVE MEDICATIONS BY MEDICAL CONDITION

Medical Condition	BB	ACEI or ARB	Aldo Antag	Thiazide	CCB
Coronary artery disease/post-MI	X	X			
Systolic heart failure	X	X	X	X	
Diastolic heart failure	X	X		X	
Diabetes	X	X		X	X
Kidney disease		X			
Stroke or TIA		ACEI		X	

ACC, American College of Cardiology; ACEI, angiotensin-converting-enzyme inhibitor; AHA, American Heart Association; Aldo Antag, aldosterone antagonist; ARB, angiotensin II blocker; BB, beta-blocker; CCB, calcium channel blocker; CDC, Centers for Disease Control and Prevention; MI, myocardial infarction; TIA, transient ischemic attack.

4. Antihypertensives/diuretics should be started at low doses and then the doses increased if there is inadequate response to initial therapy and nonadherence is ruled out. Consider the following:

   a. Increasing drug dose

   b. Substituting another drug

   c. Adding a second drug from another class; a diuretic is recommended if one is not already being used.

   d. Beta-blockers are no longer first-line antihypertensive agents. A beta-blocker can be used in clients who have any of the following: CAD, post-MI, dysrhythmia, and HF. Those older than 60 years, however, should not use a beta-blocker as the initial agent. Atenolol should not be used for HTN treatment, as it has been shown to be less effective in the prevention of events compared with all other agents.

   e. ACEIs and ARBs are critical medications to prescribe and titrate to maximum dose as a first-line medication in people with renal disease, diabetes, and proteinuria.

5. If response is still inadequate, add a second or third drug or a diuretic if one has not already been tried.

6. Evaluate the client for secondary causes if severe HTN is resistant to therapy.

7. Resistant HTN: Rule out all inadequate responses to the three-drug therapy (ACEI or ARB or CCB + diuretic):

   a. "White coat HTN": Have the client begin to take and record his or her BP at home and report the values.

   b. Use size-appropriate BP cuffs on obese clients.

   c. Nonadherence to therapy, including side effects, medication regimen too complex, and/or cost/affordability

   d. Volume overload because of excessive salt intake, progressive renal damage, fluid retention

from BP reduction, and inadequate diuretic therapy

   e. Drug problems: Dose too low, wrong type of diuretic, inappropriate combinations, rapid inactivation, drug actions, and interactions

   f. Associated conditions: Smoking, obesity, sleep apnea, insulin resistance, ethanol intake more than 30 mL (1 oz) per day, panic attacks, chronic pain, and organic brain syndrome

   g. Adding spironolactones can decrease SBP by 25 mmHg on average and DBP by 12 mmHg on average in clients with resistant hypertension

8. Treat with decongestants very cautiously. Pseudoephedrine HCl (Sudafed) has the least cardiovascular effect.

9. Diuretics may worsen gout and diabetes.

10. Beta-blockers are contraindicated in clients with asthma, HF, and heart block.

11. Use diltiazem HCl (Cardizem) and verapamil HCl (Calan) cautiously in clients with HF or block

12. ACEIs may cause coughing.

13. Abrupt cessation of therapy with a short-acting beta-blocker, such as propranolol, or the short-acting alpha-2 agonist clonidine, can lead to a potentially fatal withdrawal syndrome. Gradual discontinuation of these agents over a period of weeks should prevent this syndrome.

14. A suggested treatment protocol for moderate HTN of >20 mm Hg above goal is:

   a. An ACE inhibitor or an ARB with a diuretic or a dihydropyridine (DHP) calcium channel blocker (such as amlodipine, felodipine, or nifedipine) combination

   b. Start with a low dose and titrate upward.

15. If HTN is not controlled, the following may be added in stepwise order:

   a. A DHP CCB or a thiazide diuretic (chlorthalidone is more potent than hydrochlorothiazide [HCTZ]; add whichever has not yet been used);

can use combination low-dose amiloride/HCTZ in appropriate clients

    b. A vasodilating beta-blocker (such as carvedilol or nebivolol) and/or an aldosterone blocker

    c. Alpha-blockers and direct vasodilators

    d. Consider referral to HTN specialist.

16. Differences in ARBs and diuretics:

    a. Losartan (Cozaar) is weakest ARB; may require twice a day dosing

    b. More potent ARBs include olmesartan and azilsartan (most potent).

    c. Chlorthalidone is more potent than HCTZ.

17. For HTN that is difficult to treat:

    a. Make sure client is on a sodium-restricted diet of 1,500 mg to 2,000 mg of sodium per day and not taking OTC NSAIDs or drinking excessively.

    b. If a client is already on an ACEI or ARB with a thiazide diuretic and SBP remains elevated, first try changing ACEI to ARB; if on losartan, try changing to a more potent once-daily ARB.

    c. If client is already on a beta-blocker for another reason, may change to a vasodilating beta-blocker

    d. If client is on HCTZ, change to chlorthalidone, which is a more potent diuretic.

    e. May add an aldosterone blocker if BP remains uncontrolled

    f. May add a DHP CCB

Follow-Up

A. If drug therapy is initiated, see the client again in 2 to 4 weeks for follow-up.

B. Once the client is stable, see him or her every 3 to 6 months.

C. Evaluate the client yearly, including uric acid, creatinine, and potassium.

D. Review and discuss drug therapy compliance, effectiveness, and adverse reactions (including effect on sexual activity) at each visit.

E. Home and ambulatory blood pressure monitoring (ABPM) is an adjunctive tool for the management of HTN.

    1. BP tracking apps are available at online app stores for smartphones, MP3 players, and tablets.

    2. The AHA/American Stroke Association has BP tracker instructions located at www.heart.org/idc/groups/heart-public/@wcm/@hcm/documents/downloadable/ucm_305157.pdf

    3. A printable BP tracker log is located at www.organizedhome.com/sites/default/files/image/pdf/health_blood_pressure_tracker.pdf

F. Consider a sleep study for the diagnosis of OSA (see "Obstructive Sleep Apnea" section in Chapter 9).

G. Clients with pre-HTN without diabetes, chronic kidney disease (CKD), or CVD should be treated with nonpharmacological therapy (i.e., diet, sodium reduction, weight loss, exercise, smoking cessation) and should be evaluated annually.

Consultation/Referral

A. If the client is pregnant, consult a physician before prescribing medications. Many antihypertensive drugs are harmful to the fetus.

B. Consult a physician if the client is having an acute hypertensive emergency: DBP greater than 130 mmHg.

C. Consult/comanage with a physician if the client needs more than three drugs for therapy.

Individual Considerations

A. Pregnancy: Refer to Chapter 13, "Obstetrics Guidelines."

    1. HTN may be either chronic or pregnancy-induced.

    2. HTN is considered chronic if it is present before pregnancy or diagnosed before the 20th week of gestation.

    3. PIH is diagnosed if SBP increases 30 mmHg or more or if DBP increases 15 mmHg or more over baseline when compared with BP readings before the 20th week of gestation. When BP readings are not known, a reading of 140/90 mmHg or higher is considered abnormal.

    4. Maternal as well as fetal mortality and morbidity improve with treatment.

B. Pediatrics:

    1. Evaluate BP at every visit starting at the age of 3 years.

    2. HTN can occur in many acute illnesses, or it may be a chronic problem.

    3. Determine high BP by correlating height indexes with BP readings.

C. Geriatrics:

    1. The optimal BP treatment goal in the elderly has not been determined, as there is no consensus among various national and international organizations. In the most recent JNC 8 guideline, treatment goals for individuals older than 60 years were changed to a goal of less than 150/90 mmHg. HTN in the elderly places the client at risk of coronary events, stroke, HF, and PAD.

    2. Elderly persons with HTN are more likely to develop orthostatic and postprandial hypotension, which may result in falls or syncope.

        a. Evaluate side effects, including dizziness and sedation.

        b. Beta-blockers may cause depression or confusion in the elderly.

    3. The general approach to drug therapy in the geriatric population is to start low and go slow.

    4. Check the Beers list for harmful drugs in the geriatric population. The 2019 American Geriatrics Society's Updated Beers Criteria for Potentially Inappropriate Medication Use in Older Adults is available at geriatricscareonline.org/ProductAbstract/american-geriatrics-society-updated-beers-criteria-for-potentially-inappropriate-medication-use-in-older-adults/CL001. A printable pocket card is available for download at www.americangeriatrics.org/publications-tools.

5. To avoid hyperkalemia in the elderly, potassium-sparing diuretics should not be given with ACEI or ARBs.

Resource

The National Kidney Foundation provides online calculators: www.kidney.org/professionals/KDOQI/gfr_calculator

Bibliography

Alexander, M. (2019, February 22). Hypertension. *Medscape.* Retrieved from https://emedicine.medscape.com/article/241381-overview

American Geriatrics Society. (2019, April). Updated AGS Beers criteria for potentially inappropriate medication use in older adults. *Journal of the American Geriatrics Society, 67*(4), 674–694. doi:10.1111/jgs.15767

American Heart Association. (2017). *Monitoring your blood pressure at home.* Retrieved from heart.org/en/health-topics/high-blood-pressure/understanding-blood-pressure-readings/monitoring-your-blood-pressure-at-home

Benjamin, E. J., Blaha, M. J., Chiuve, S., Cushman, M., Das, S., Deo, R., . . . American Heart Association Statistics Committee and Stroke Statistics Subcommittee. (2017). Heart disease and stroke statistics—2017 update: A report from the American Heart Association. *Circulation, 135*(1), e1–e603. doi:10.1161/CIR.0000000000000485

Crawford, C. (2017, November 15). *AAFP to review AHA/ACC redefinition of high blood pressure; Academy continues to endorse JNC8 hypertension guideline.* American Academy of Family Physicians. Retrieved from https://www.aafp.org/news/health-of-the-public/20171115ahaacchbpguideline.html

Davis, L. L. (2013, November). Using the latest evidence to manage hypertension. *Journal for Nurse Practitioners, 9,* 621–628. doi:10.1016/j.nurpra.2013.08.013

Davis, L. L. (2019, January). Hypertension: How low to go when treating older adults. *Journal for Nurse Practitioners, 15*(1), 1–6. doi:10.1016/j.nurpra.2018.10.010

Fihn, S., Blankenship, J. C., Alexander, K. P., Bittl, J. A., Byrne, J. G., Fletcher, B. J., . . . Smith, P. K. (2014). 2014 ACC/AHA/AATS/PCNA/SCAI/STS focused update of the guideline for the diagnosis and management of patients with stable ischemic heart disease. *Journal of the American College of Cardiology, 130*(19), 1749–1767. doi:10.1161/CIR.0000000000000095

Food and Drug Administration. (2018, June 12). *Use the nutrition facts label to reduce your intake of sodium in your diet.* Retrieved from https://www.fda.gov/food/nutrition-education-resources-materials/use-nutrition-facts-label-reduce-your-intake-sodium-your-diet

Go, A. S., Bauman, M. C., King, S. M., Fonarow, G. C., Lawrence, W., Williams, K. A., & Sanchez, E. (2013, November 15). An effective approach to high blood pressure control: A science advisory from the American Heart Association, the American College of Cardiology, and the Centers for Disease Control and Prevention. *Journal of the American College of Cardiology, 63*(12), 1230–1238. doi:10.1016/j.jacc.2013.11.007

James, P. A., Oparil, S., Carter, B. L., Cushman, W. C., Dennison-Himmelfarb, C., Handler, J., & Ortiz, E. (2014). 2014 evidence-based guideline for the management of high blood pressure in adults: Report from the panel members appointed to the Eighth Joint National Committee (JNC 8). *Journal of the American Medical Association, 311*(5), 507–520. doi:10.1001/jama.2013.284427

Jeffery, S. (2017, November 13). New ACC/AHA hypertension guidelines make 130 the new 140. *Medscape.* Retrieved from https://www.medscape.com/viewarticle/888560#vp_2

Judd, E., & Calhoun, D. A. (2014). Apparent and true resistant hypertension: Definition, prevalence and outcomes. *Journal of Human Hypertension, 28*(8), 463–468. doi:10.1038/jhh.2013.140

Madhur, M. S. (2013, December 3). Hypertension. *Medscape.* Retrieved from http://emedicine.medscape.com/article/241381-overview

Mann, J. F. E. (2018, September 19). Choice of therapy in primary (essential) hypertension: Recommendations. *UpToDate.* Retrieved from www.uptodate.com

Mann, J. F. E., & Hilgers, K. F. (2015, January 20). Hypertension: Who should be treated? *UpToDate.* Retrieved from http://www.uptodate.com/contents/hypertension-who-should-betreated?topicKey-NEPH

Mozaffarian, D., Benjamin, E. J., & Go, A. S. (2016). Heart disease and stroke statistics—2016 update: A report from the American Heart Association. *Circulation, 133*(4), 447–454. doi:10.1161/CIR.0000000000000350

On, R., & Arakelians, S. (2018). Hypertension treatment guidelines update. *Pharmacy Times.* Retrieved from https://www.pharmacytimes.com/publications/issue/2018/december2018/hypertension-treatment-guidelines-update

Papadopolou, E., Angeloudi, E., Karras, S., & Sarafidis, P. (2018, June 22). The optimal blood pressure target in diabetes mellitus: A quest coming to an end? *Journal of Human Hypertension, 32*(10), 641–650. doi:10.1038/s41371-018-0079-5

Robert, L. (2013, May 15). *Hypertension meeting has primary care track.* Retrieved from https://www.patientcareonline.com/ash2013/hypertension-meeting-has-primary-care-track

Rutecki, G. W. (2013a, May 16). *Some do's and don'ts for tough-to-treat hypertensives.* Retrieved from https://www.patientcareonline.com/hypertension/some-dos-and-donts-tough-treat-hypertensives

Rutecki, G. W. (2013b, May 22). *Lessons in quality improvement: Reflections on ASH 2013.* Retrieved from https://www.patientcareonline.com/sleep-disorders/reflections-ash-2013-lessons-quality-improvement

Sheppard, J. P., Martin, U., & McManus, R. J. (2017). Diagnosis and management of resistant hypertension. *Heart, 103*(16), 1295–1302. doi:10.1136/heartjnl-2015-308297

Spencer, A., Jablonski, R., & Loeb, S. J. (2012). Hypertensive African American women and the DASH diet. *Nurse Practitioner, 37*(2), 41–46. doi:10.1097/01.NPR.0000410278.75362.a2

U.S. Department of Health and Human Services. (2017). *The seventh report of the Joint National Committee on Prevention, Detection, Evaluation, and Treatment of High Blood Pressure* (pp. 1–63). National Institutes of Health: National Heart, Lung, and Blood Institute. Bethesda, MD: Author. Retrieved from https://www.nhlbi.nih.gov/files/docs/guidelines/jnc7full.pdf

U.S. Department of Health and Human Services, National Institutes of Health, & National Heart, Lung, and Blood Institute. (2006). *Your guide to lowering your blood pressure with DASH* (NIH Publication No. 06-4082). Washington, DC: U.S. Government Printing Office. Retrieved from https://www.nhlbi.nih.gov/files/docs/guidelines/jnc7full.pdf

Varon, J. (2019, February 13). Management of severe asymptomatic hypertension (hypertensive urgencies) in adults. *UpToDate.* Retrieved from https://www.uptodate.com/contents/management-of-severe-asymptomatic-hypertension-hypertensive-urgencies-in-adults

Vongpatanasin, W. (2014). Resistant hypertension: A review of diagnosis and management. *Journal of the American Medical Association, 311*(21), 2216–2224. doi:10.1001/jama.2014.5180

Wright, B. M., Rutecki, G. W., & Bellone, J. (2013, January). Resistant hypertension: An approach to diagnosis and treatment. *Consultant, 53*(1), 9–16. Retrieved from www.Consultant360.com

Lymphedema

Laura A. Petty

Definition

A. PVD is a general term that encompasses all occlusive or inflammatory diseases that occur within the peripheral arteries, veins, and lymphatic system. Lymphedema is a chronic condition caused by the accumulation of lymphatic fluid in the interstitial tissue.

Incidence

The Vascular Disease Foundation reports that almost 1 million Americans have lymphedema. The incidence worldwide is projected to approach 100 million.

Pathogenesis

Lymphedema occurs when lymph fluid is unable to flow in a normal manner and accumulates in an extremity. The propensity for lymphedema can be inherited or caused by another condition such as lymphangitis, malignancy, filariasis, or removal of lymph nodes.

Predisposing Factors

A. Cancer
B. Radiation therapy
C. Surgical removal of lymph nodes
D. Parasitic infection (filariasis)
E. Congenital disorders involving the structure of the lymph system:
    1. Milroy's disease
    2. Meige's disease
F. Obesity
G. Surgical implantation of pacemaker or arteriovenous shunt
H. Systemic diseases (hyperthyroidism, HTN, renal or cardiac disease)
I. Vascular disease (CVI or postthrombotic syndrome)

Common Complaints

A. Severe edema that is consistent to the distal aspect of the extremity
B. Hard skin over edematous area
C. Loss of range of motion

Potential Complications

A. Infection, including lymphangitis and cellulitis
B. Lymphangiosarcoma

Subjective Data

A. Ask the client when the symptom(s) were first noticed
B. Have the client describe the duration of symptoms
C. Review any history of cancer, radiation, and chemotherapy
D. Review recent history of invasive procedures or surgery
E. Ask the client to list all medications currently being taken, particularly substances not prescribed and illicit drugs
F. Ask the client to describe any pain
G. Ask the client what makes the symptoms better and what makes them worse
H. Have the client rate discomfort on a scale of 1 to 10, with 1 being the least uncomfortable

Physical Examination

A. Vital signs: Check BP and document resting heart rate, respirations, temperature, height, and weight
B. Inspect: Assess for signs of erythema, increased temperature, and edema.
C. Auscultate:
    1. Heart: Rate, rhythm, heart sounds, murmur, and gallops
    2. Lungs: Assess lung sounds in all fields
D. Palpate:
    1. Lymph nodes distal and proximal to the site
    2. Pulses distal and proximal in all extremities
    3. Extremity for tenderness

Diagnostic Tests

A. Serum laboratory tests (CBC with differential and BNP)
B. CT scan of the affected extremity
C. Doppler ultrasound of the affected extremity

D. Testing to assess the extent of the lymphedema or to rule in/out an etiology: CT scan, MRI, and/or Doppler
E. Lymphoscintigraphy
F. Additional tests to monitor coexisting systemic and/or vascular disease

Differential Diagnoses

A. Unilateral limb edema:
    1. Lymphedema
    2. Venous insufficiency
    3. DVT or postthrombotic syndrome
    4. Arthritis
    5. Baker's cyst
    6. Presence or reoccurrence of cancer
B. Symmetrical limb edema:
    1. CHF
    2. CVI
    3. Renal dysfunction
    4. Hepatic dysfunction
    5. Hypothyroidism (myxedema)
    6. Medication-induced edema
    7. Lipedema

Plan

A. General interventions:
    1. Protect the arm or leg while recovering from cancer treatment.
    2. Suggest strategies to protect the extremity from developing a blood clot.
B. Client teaching:
    1. *See Section III: Client Teaching Guide for this chapter, "Lymphedema."* ◄
    2. Avoid heavy lifting, if an arm is affected.
    3. Avoid strenuous exercise.
    4. Avoid heat on the arm or leg.
    5. Avoid tight clothing.
    6. Inspect the affected limb daily. Note any cracks or cuts that increase the risk of infection, and treat as directed.
    7. Apply lotion daily to protect and prevent dry skin.
    8. Avoid burns to the skin.
    9. Take extra care when shaving and use a clean razor on clean skin.
    10. Use insect repellent to prevent insect bites, which could become infected.
C. Nonpharmaceutical therapy:
    1. Extremity elevation
    2. Compression stockings or wrapping of affected limb
    3. Pneumatic compression boot
    4. Therapeutic massage, specifically manual lymph drainage
D. Surgery:
    1. Lymphaticovenular bypass
    2. Lymphovenous bypass

Follow-Up

A. Follow-up is determined by the client's needs, frequency and intensity of symptoms, and presence of other medical conditions.

B. When PVD manifests with persistent symptoms, it must be followed by a cardiologist.

Consultation/Referral

A. When ALI is suspected, refer the client for immediate hospitalization to obtain diagnostic testing to determine the presence of a thrombus and restore circulation to the affected extremity.

B. If CLI has led to ulceration and/or superimposed infection, then hospitalization is indicated to initiate a wound care consultation, along with diagnostic testing to determine the degree of arterial occlusion.

C. Referral to a cardiologist is indicated in the presence of persistent PVD symptoms.

D. Referral to a lymphedema therapist to manage chronic lymphedema.

E. Referral to physical therapy is indicated to teach a home exercise program.

Bibliography

Executive Committee. (2016, December). The diagnosis and treatment of peripheral lymphedema: 2016 consensus document of the International Society of Lymphology. *Lymphology, 49*(4), 170–184. Retrieved from https://journals.uair.arizona.edu/index.php/lymph/article/download/20106/19734

Nudelmann, J. (2016, September 1). Do no harm: Lymphedema risk reduction behaviors. *Journal of Clinical Oncology, 34*(25), 3109–3110. doi:10.1200/JCO.2016.67.9928. Retrieved from http://communities.ons.org/HigherLogic/System/DownloadDocumentFile.ashx?DocumentFileKey=03d70adb-4663-4142-8132-76d26b4e642c

Scheer, R. (2017, April 27). Clinical innovation: Compression garments for managing lymphoedema. *Wounds International, 8*(2), 34–38. Retrieved from https://lymphoedemaeducation.com.au/resources/clinical-innovation-compression-garments-managing-lymphoedema/

Trayes, K. P., Studdiford, J. S., Pickle, S., & Tully, A. S. (2013). Edema: Diagnosis and management. *American Family Physician, 88*(2), 102–110. doi:10.1097/ACM.0b013e318277d5b2

Vascular Cures. (2016b). *Lymphedema.* Retrieved from http://vasculardisease.org/images/VDF-Diseases-Flyers/lymphedemaflyer%20Vascular%20Cures.pdf

Murmurs

Jill C. Cash and Debbie Gunter

Definition

A murmur is turbulent blood flow through the heart as a result of one or more of the following etiologies:

A. Narrow valve opening, stenosis

B. Incomplete valve closure, regurgitant or insufficient blood flow

C. Abnormal opening through chambers, atrial or ventricular septal defect (VSD)

D. Rapid blood flow through normal valve structures; occurs during pregnancy, with increased physiological demand states, and in children

E. No abnormality; occurs in clients with thin chest walls and in children

Incidence

A. Approximately 80% of children have a physiological murmur at one time or another. Four percent of women studied in the Framingham Heart Study had a murmur related to MVP.

Pathogenesis

A. Pathogenesis depends on specific etiology, but rheumatic disease, calcific changes, ischemic insults, congenital abnormalities, and degenerative diseases all contribute to the development of a murmur

Common Complaints

A. Often no symptoms are present, and murmur is found on routine examination.

B. Complaints with advanced valvular disease:
1. Chest pain
2. Dyspnea
3. Palpitations
4. SOB
5. Exercise intolerance
6. Postural light-headedness

Subjective Data

A. Has the client ever been diagnosed with a murmur?

B. Did the client have frequent strep infections as a child?

C. Ask the client about any recent viral infections.

D. Question the client about chest pain; SOB; palpitations; diaphoresis; light-headedness; or syncope, especially with exertion.

E. Ask the client whether any family members had sudden cardiac death before the age of 55 years.

Physical Examination

A. Check temperature, if indicated, pulse, respirations, and BP.

B. Inspect: Chest for lifts and heaves

C. Palpate: Chest for lifts, heaves, and thrills.

D. Auscultate:

1. Heart for splitting of heart sounds, clicks, rubs, and murmurs; use the bell and diaphragm of the stethoscope to auscultate the client in the left lateral, supine, standing, sitting (and leaning forward), and squatting positions and after having client run in place or do jumping jacks for 2 to 3 minutes.

   a. A new, systolic, regurgitant murmur in the setting of an acute MI may indicate a ruptured papillary muscle and possible cardiogenic shock.

   b. When a new murmur is audible, differentiate location, timing, quality, intensity, and duration. Note if radiation to the neck, axilla, or back is present.

   c. Note location of murmur:

      i. Aortic: Second right intercostal space (ICS) next to sternum

      ii. Pulmonic: Second left ICS next to sternum

      iii. Tricuspid: Fifth left ICS next to sternum

      iv. Mitral: Fifth left ICS at midclavicular line

   d. If murmur is heard, have the client squat, stand, and/or perform the Valsalva maneuver. Squatting will increase the blood to the heart and increase the LV blood volume and stroke volume, which will increase the sound of the murmur. Standing and the Valsalva maneuver will provide the opposite, in which the venous return will drop and decrease the ventricle size and stroke volume and soften the sound of the murmur.

e. If the sound of the murmur occurs during the opposite action, becoming softer when squatting and louder when standing or during the Valsalva maneuver, consider hypertrophic cardiomyopathy or MVP as the diagnosis.

2. Assess the neck and axilla for radiation.

Diagnostic Tests

A. EKG
B. Echocardiogram
C. Chest radiography

Differential Diagnoses

Major differentiation should be in the description of murmur, as this aids in the identification of the murmur.

A. Timing:
1. Identify when the murmur occurs in the cardiac cycle.
2. Systolic murmurs may or may not be normal. Occurs between the S_1 "lub" and the S_2 "dub"
3. Diastolic murmurs are always abnormal and need further evaluation:
   Occurs between the S_2 "dub" and the S_1 "lub"

B. Quality: Is the sound harsh, blowing, musical, rumbling, vibratory, or soft?

C. Intensity: Murmurs are usually graded on a six-point scale:

- Grade I: Barely audible
- Grade II: Audible but soft
- Grade III: Easily audible without thrill
- Grade IV: Easily audible, thrill usually palpable
- Grade V: Audible with only the rim of the stethoscope on the chest wall; thrill present
- Grade VI: Audible with the stethoscope barely off the chest wall; thrill present

D. Duration: Identify location and timing in the specific phase of the cardiac cycle:
1. Holosystolic: Throughout systole
2. Holodiastolic: Throughout diastole
3. Midsystolic: Midway between S_1 and S_3
4. Mid-diastolic: Midway between S_2 and S_1
5. Decrescendo: Starts loud at the beginning, then tapers off
6. Crescendo: Starts soft at the beginning, then gets louder

E. Radiation: Murmur can be heard in another place, such as the neck, back, left axilla, or across precordium. Sound usually radiates in the direction of blood flow.

F. Location: Identify location on chest wall where murmur is heard the best. Identify site: apex, pulmonary area, tricuspid, and aortic areas. Radiation murmur may also include axilla, left fourth ICS, or base of heart.

G. Configuration: Assess the intensity of the murmur over time. Does it plateau, crescendo, decrescendo, or crescendo–decrescendo?

H. Systolic murmurs: Systolic murmurs are benign or pathologic.
1. Early systolic murmurs:
   a. Mitral regurgitation: Holosystolic, blowing may be loud. Located at fifth ICS and radiates to left axilla/back. Heard best in left lateral position and with sudden squatting; intensity decreases with the Valsalva maneuver and standing.
   b. Tricuspid regurgitation: Holosystolic, heard in left lower sternal border or apex when right ventricle is enlarged. Intensity increases with inspiration and decreases with expiration. Straight-leg raises may increase intensity. May also see HJR.
   c. Physiological: Early to midsystolic, low-pitch normal S_1–S_2, located at left lower sternal edge at third to fourth ICS. Heard best with bell and supine; disappears when sitting up or holding breath. Commonly seen in children, pregnancy, and infection.
2. Midsystolic to late systolic murmurs:
   a. Aortic stenosis: Loud, hard crescendo–decrescendo at second-right ICS that radiates to the neck. Heard best when client is leaning forward; increases with leg raise and lying flat. Decreases with Valsalva and handgrip standing.
   b. Pulmonic stenosis: Prolonged, loud S_2 or crescendo–decrescendo, usually greater than 3/6 at second ICS and radiates to neck; increases with inspiration
   c. Hypertrophic cardiomyopathy (aortic outflow obstruction): Peaks at midsystole; loud, harsh tone at left, lower sternal border that may radiate to neck. Increases with Valsalva maneuver and standing, decreases with sudden squatting. Note brisk carotid upstroke.
3. Late systolic murmurs:
   a. MVP: Midsystolic click heard before late systolic murmur, heard best at fifth left ICS. Heard best with diaphragm; sitting or squatting may increase intensity.
   b. Tricuspid valve prolapse: Heard over the left lower sternal border, delayed onset of murmur with inspiration secondary to an increase in the right ventricular volume

I. Diastolic murmurs: Murmurs are always pathologic.
1. Early diastolic murmur:
   a. Aortic regurgitation: High-pitch faint, decrescendo may start with S_2, at third left ICS and radiate down sternal edge. Heard best when client is leaning forward, holding breath. Increases with sudden squatting or handgrip. May hear displaced PMI, S_3, bounding pulse.
   b. Pulmonary regurgitation: Valvular, dilation of valve annulus, congenital defect (tetralogy of Fallot VSD), pulmonic stenosis. Best heard over second/third left ICS. May be a high-pitched, "blowing" sound in clients with HTN. May be pansystolic, having decrescendo configuration.

2. Mid-diastolic murmur:

a. Mitral stenosis: Rumbling extends beyond mid-diastole at fifth ICS; heard best using the bell of the stethoscope. Increases with left lateral position. May hear snap after S_2.

b. Tricuspid stenosis: Increased flow across the tricuspid valve, heard best at the left sternal border. Identified by its increase in intensity of the murmur with inspiration (Carvallo's sign). Commonly seen with mitral stenosis.

Plan

A. General interventions:

1. Major therapeutic goals are to preserve quality of life, increase life expectancy and exercise capacity, and reduce risk of complications.

2. Activity restriction is not necessary in clients with asymptomatic valvular disease.

B. Client teaching:

1. Reassure the client regarding specific diagnosis.

2. Counsel the client regarding his or her specific condition. Teach the client signs and symptoms to report to the health provider, including chest pain, SOB, difficulty breathing, and so forth.

C. Medical and surgical management: Clients who need progressive increases in medications to control symptoms may be candidates for valve replacement surgery.

D. Pharmaceutical therapy:

1. The 2017 focused update of the AHA guideline does not recommend routine endocarditis antimicrobial prophylaxis treatment for common valvular lesions, which include bicuspid aortic valve, acquired aortic or mitral valve disease (including MVP with regurgitation), and hypertrophic cardiomyopathy with latent or resting obstruction.

2. The European Society of Cardiology (ESC) published a guideline in 2015, which continued to support the recommendations from the AHA 2007 guideline.

E. Endocarditis prophylaxis treatment: Cardiac conditions:

1. It is recommended that clients with high-risk cardiac condition abnormalities receive prophylactic treatment. Specific cardiac conditions are as follows:

a. Prosthetic cardiac valves including transcatheter-implanted prostheses and homografts or prosthetic material used for cardiac valve repair, such as annuloplasty rings and cords

b. Previous infective endocarditis

c. Certain congenital heart diseases such as cyanotic congenital heart disease that has not been repaired; a congenital heart disease that has been repaired with an artificial material or device for 6 months after repair; and repaired congenital heart defects with continued problems, such as leaks or insufficient flow at the prosthetic device or adjacent to the repair endocarditis prophylaxis treatment

d. Postcardiac transplant valvulopathy

2. Procedures for the high-risk clients mentioned earlier that require prophylaxis treatment:

a. All dental procedures that involve manipulation of gingival tissue or the periapical region of the teeth or perforation of oral mucosa

b. Incision or biopsy of respiratory mucosa or any invasive procedure of the respiratory tract system

c. Procedures that include infected skin or musculoskeletal tissue

d. Preventive treatment with antibiotics is not recommended for procedures that include the reproductive tract, urinary tract, or GI tract.

3. Antibiotic prophylactic regimens include a single dose 30 to 60 minutes before procedure:

a. Amoxicillin single dose: 2 g by mouth, intramuscular (IM), or IV for adults or 50 mg/kg for children

b. Ampicillin 2 g IM or IV or 50 mg/kg IM or IV

c. Allergy to penicillin (PCN): Cephalexin 2 g by mouth for adults or 50 mg/kg for children

d. Azithromycin or clarithromycin 500 g for adults or 15 mg/kg for children

e. Allergic to azithromycin or clarithromycin: Consider cefazolin or ceftriaxone 1 g IM or IV for adults or 50 mg/kg IM or IV for children, or clindamycin 600 mg IM or IV for adults or 20 mg/kg IM or IV children

4. Other pharmaceutical treatments depend on the specific valvular abnormality:

a. Mitral stenosis: The mitral valve has a narrowing that does not allow adequate blood to enter the LV during diastole, usually because of rheumatic heart disease. Mitral heart disease is the most commonly seen valve effect with rheumatic heart disease.

b. Diuretics, such as furosemide (Lasix) or HCTZ (HydroDiuril), are used to control edema

c. Digoxin (Lanoxin) or beta-blockers are used to control AF and irregular heart rate.

d. Warfarin (Coumadin) and the antiplatelet agent aspirin (Bayer) are used to prevent clotting

e. MVP: The echocardiogram is the recommended test for the diagnosis of MVP. Usually no medications are recommended except when clients are symptomatic or meet EKG requirements within current cardiology guidelines.

i. Beta-blockers (such as Atenolol) may be used for palpitations.

ii. Diuretics should be avoided in clients who are volume reserved.

iii. Oral contraceptives should be avoided in women who exhibit neurological symptoms.

f. Mitral regurgitation: Diuretics, digitalis, and afterload-reducing agents for CHF:

i. Used in clients with aortic stenosis

ii. Diuretics are used for CHF.

iii. Avoid vasodilators; they may result in profound, irreversible hypotension.

iv. Echocardiograms should be performed every 6 to 12 months to follow the progression of narrowing of the LV across the aortic valve

g. Aortic regurgitation: Afterload-reducing agents, digitalis, and diuretics are recommended.

Follow-Up

A. Most clients with valvular disease should be evaluated at least once a year.

B. Clients on oral anticoagulation drugs need monthly follow-up or as-needed PT/INRs if on warfarin.

Consultation/Referral

A. Consult a physician if the client is diagnosed with a new murmur or exercise-induced symptoms during a sports physical examination.

B. Refer clients with newly diagnosed murmurs to a cardiologist after obtaining echocardiogram results. Drug therapy should be initiated according to diagnosis and symptoms.

C. Onset of AF with rapid ventricular response is an indication for immediate hospitalization.

D. Refer clients with systemic embolization to a physician for emergent anticoagulation therapy and chronic oral anticoagulant therapy. Discuss the possibility of valve replacement with a cardiologist.

E. If a new murmur is diagnosed in a pregnant client with a history of cardiac disease, refer her to a physician immediately.

F. All diastolic murmurs in pediatric clients indicate pathology and need to be evaluated by a physician.

Individual Considerations

A. Pregnancy:
  1. The development of a new, "high-flow" murmur in a healthy woman is not uncommon because of physiological changes occurring during pregnancy

B. Pediatrics:
  1. Perform a thorough cardiac examination on clients from the time they are newborns through adolescence, so that if a murmur is detected, it can be compared.

C. Geriatrics:
  1. A systolic murmur heard best in the aortic area may indicate aortic sclerosis because of aging of the aortic valve rather than true aortic stenosis.

Bibliography

Ajam, T. (2018, June 28). Pulmonary regurgitation. *Medscape*. Retrieved from https://emedicine.medscape.com/article/157639-overview

Alguire, P. C., & Mathes, B. M. (2017, December 4). Diagnostic evaluation of chronic venous insufficiency. *UpToDate*. Retrieved from http://www.uptodate.com/contents/diagnostic-evaluation-of-lower-extremity-chronic-venous-insufficiency

American Heart Association. (2019). *Infective endocarditis*. Retrieved from https://www.heart.org/en/health-topics/infective-endocarditis

Baddour, L., Wilson, W., & Bayer, A. (2015). Infective endocarditis in adults: Diagnosis, antimicrobial therapy, and management of complications. A scientific statement for healthcare professionals from the American Heart Association. *Circulation, 132*(15), 1435–1486. doi:10.1161/CIR.0000000000000296

Brusch, J. (2019, January 3). Infective endocarditis. *Medscape*. Retrieved from https://emedicine.medscape.com/article/216650-overview

Dima, C. (2018, February 2). Mitral stenosis. *Medscape*. Retrieved from https://emedicine.medscape.com/article/155724-overview

Drug information. (2019). *Prescribers' digital reference*. Retrieved from www.pdr.net

Hanson, I. (2018, November 28). Mitral regurgitation. *Medscape*. Retrieved from https://emedicine.medscape.com/article/155618-overview

National Institute for Health and Care Excellence. (2016, July). *Prophylaxis against infective endocarditis: Clinical guideline 64.1: Methods, evidence and recommendations*. Retrieved from https://www.nice.org.uk/guidance/cg64

Ren, X. (2017, March 23). Aortic stenosis. *Medscape*. Retrieved from https://emedicine.medscape.com/article/150638-overview

Wang, S. (2018). Aortic regurgitation. *Medscape*. Retrieved from https://emedicine.medscape.com/article/150490-overview

Palpitations

Jill C. Cash and Debbie Gunter

Definition

A. Palpitations are a feeling or an unpleasant awareness of the heartbeat in the chest. They may be described as feeling a sensation of the heart "flip-flopping" or feeling a "rapid flutter" of the heart.

Incidence

A. The incidence of palpitations may range from 1% to 8% of clients in a general practice setting.

Pathogenesis

Palpitations may be caused by the following:

A. Increase in stroke volume or contractility

B. Sudden change in heart rate or rhythm

C. Unusual cardiac movement within the thorax

D. Hyperkinetic states, which cause constant pounding; hyperthyroidism; late-stage pregnancy

E. Valvular heart disease that produces large stroke volumes

F. Catecholamine release during anxiety or panic attacks

Predisposing Factors

A. Cardiac defects

B. Severe anemia

C. Hyperthyroidism

D. Pregnancy

E. Fever

F. Anxiety

G. Stimulants such as caffeine and certain drugs

H. Emotions such as fear

I. Exertion

J. Diabetes mellitus and insulin reaction

Common Complaints

A. Palpitations are often described as a turning over or flopping sensation in the chest, but symptoms vary enormously.

B. Most clients are free of palpitations at the time of the examination.

Other Signs and Symptoms

A. Fluttering in the chest

B. SOB

C. Pounding in the chest and neck

D. Diaphoresis
E. Light-headedness
F. Anxiety or fear

Subjective Data

A. Ask the client when symptoms first presented, including age, and how they have changed.
B. Have the client describe the characteristics of the palpitations, such as rapid, regular, irregular, or slow.
C. Ask the client what precipitates the palpitations. Does anything terminate them, or do they go away on their own?
D. Inquire whether symptoms occur or change with position (standing, bending over, lying down, left lateral decubitus position) and/or exercise.
E. Ask the client about other symptoms associated with the palpitations such as dizziness or syncope.
F. Ask how often the episodes occur and how long each lasts.
G. Discuss any previous treatments for this condition and the results.
H. Ask the client about risk factors for CHD and prior cardiac history.
I. Question the client's use of OTC decongestants and diet pills. Are there any new medications or change in routine medications? Obtain a complete list of medications the client is currently taking.

Physical Examination

A. Check pulse (count the pulse for 1 full minute), respirations, and BP.
B. Inspect:
    1. Overall appearance
    2. The skin for diaphoresis and pallor
    3. The neck for thyromegaly or jugular vein distention
    4. The legs for edema
C. Palpate:
    1. The skin for temperature and dryness
    2. The lower extremities for edema and calf tenderness
    3. The neck for thyroid enlargement
D. Auscultate:
    1. The heart for abnormal rhythms. Auscultate the heart with the client in the sitting, standing, and left lateral decubitus positions. Ask the client to walk quickly down the hallway and back, and then auscultate the heart in all positions again.
    2. The lungs
    3. The neck and carotid arteries for bruits
E. Mental status: Does the client appear light-headed, anxious, or fearful?

Diagnostic Tests

Diagnostic testing is highly recommended for clients who have an arrhythmia or who are at risk of an arrhythmia, and clients who are anxious and want to explore causes for their symptoms.
Testing recommended:
A. Hgb to rule out anemia if suggestive on examination
B. Thyroid-stimulating hormone (TSH) to rule out hyperthyroidism if suggestive on examination

C. EKG during episode if possible
D. Ambulatory monitoring if symptoms continue, either 24-hour Holter monitoring or client-activated transtelephonic monitoring
E. Treadmill test if palpitations are provoked by exercise

Differential Diagnoses

A. Palpitations are secondary to the underlying problem such as anxiety, medications, or cardiac or pulmonary origin.

Plan

A. General interventions:
    1. Provide reassurance if the palpitations result from a neurotic concern.
B. Client teaching:
    1. Caution the client to avoid any factors that trigger episodes. Factors may include stress, exercise, foods, and medications.
    2. Teach the client a vagal maneuver, which is effective in halting palpitations.
C. Medical and surgical management: Correct any underlying problem (e.g., cardiac or pulmonary). Treat medical conditions accordingly. Management of arrhythmias should be monitored by a cardiologist.
D. Pharmaceutical therapy: Discontinue all nonessential medications that could cause palpitations.

Follow-Up

A. Depending on the etiology of palpitations and the existence of comorbid conditions, the prognosis in clients with no underlying cardiac disease is generally favorable.

Consultation/Referral

A. Consult a physician if the client has a history of palpitations leading to syncope or near syncope, angina-like chest pain, or dyspnea. These clients are candidates for referral to a cardiologist and/or inpatient evaluation. Refer any client with an arrhythmia to a cardiologist.
B. Hemodynamically compromised clients need prompt hospital admission.

Bibliography

Benjamin, E. J., Blaha, M. J., Chiuve, S., Cushman, M., Das, S., Deo, R., . . . American Heart Association Statistics Committee and Stroke Statistics Subcommittee. (2017). Heart disease and stroke statistics—2017 update: A report from the American Heart Association. *Circulation*, *135*(1), e1–e603. doi:10.1161/CIR.0000000000000485

Mozaffarian, D., Benjamin, E. J., & Go, A. S. (2016). Heart disease and stroke statistics—2016 update: A report from the American Heart Association. *Circulation*, *133*(4), 447–454. doi:10.1161/CIR.0000000000000350

Nishimura, R., Otto, C., & Bonow, R. (2017). 2017 AHA/ACC focused update of the 2014 AHA/ACC guideline for the management of patients with valvular heart disease. *Journal of the American College of Cardiology*, *70*(2), 252–289. doi:10.1161/CIR.0000000000000503

Trayes, K. P., Studdiford, J. S., Pickle, S., & Tully, A. S. (2013). Edema: Diagnosis and management. *American Family Physician*, *88*(2), 102–110. doi:10.1097/ACM.0b013e318277d5b2

Wexler, R., & Pleister, A. (2017). Palpitations: Evaluation in the primary care setting. *American Family Physician*, *96*(12), 784–789. Retrieved from https://www.aafp.org/afp/2017/1215/p784.html

Peripheral Arterial Disease

Laura A. Petty

Definition

A. PAD is a circulatory disorder generally characterized by the build-up of plaques on the interior surface of arteries. These plaques harden and narrow the diameter of the arteries, which reduces the volume of blood circulating to the internal organs and extremities. The arteries affected by PAD include all arteries in the body with the exception of the cerebral and coronary arteries. The decreased circulation seen in PAD can also be caused by nonatherosclerotic conditions. Some of these conditions are arteritis, trauma, radiation damage, and fibromuscular dysplasia. Symptoms of PAD can occur in the upper or lower extremities (see Figure 10.5).

FIGURE 10.5 Peripheral artery disease.

B. Classification of PAD:
  1. Asymptomatic PAD:
     No symptoms but the presence of risk factors or a new diagnosis of a common coexisting disease (CAD or cerebrovascular disease) should prompt further evaluation
  2. Intermittent claudication (IC):
     Discomfort including cramping or pain with physical exertion that remits within 10 minutes of rest
  3. CLI:
     a. Pain at rest with a nonhealing wound, skin ulceration, or gangrene
     b. Onset is defined as chronic (i.e., ≥ 2 weeks)
  4. ALI:
     a. Pain at rest in a pale, pulseless extremity that is usually cold (poikilothermia) and has paresthesias and/or paralysis
     b. Onset is defined as acute (i.e., <2 weeks)
C. Other conditions contained within PAD:
  1. Buerger's disease (thromboangiitis obliterans): A disease manifested by inflammation, peripheral edema, and microthrombi leading to gangrene of the hands and feet. Usually caused by tobacco abuse; clients are thought to have a genetic predisposition to develop this condition.

  2. Raynaud's disease/phenomenon: A vasospastic disorder manifested by a response in the extremities to cold temperatures or stress during which pallor, cyanosis, numbness, and/or pain are experienced
  3. Leriche syndrome: Involves the triad of claudication, absent or diminished femoral pulses, and erectile dysfunction

Incidence

A. Approximately 8 million adults in the United States have PAD. This correlates to between 12% and 20% of Americans older than 60 years of age.
B. PAD is more common in men than in women.
C. People of Hispanic origin have a higher rate of PAD compared to nonwhite populations.

Pathogenesis

PAD is most commonly precipitated by atherosclerosis. An atherosclerotic plaque develops in response to turbulent blood flow on the endothelial cells of the vessel wall. The plaque contains inflammatory cells and a thrombogenic lipid core that is covered by a fibrous cap. When the fibrous cap is disturbed, the lipid core can precipitate to development of a thrombus and lead to occlusion of the vessel.

Predisposing Factors

A. Smoking
B. Diabetes
C. Dyslipidemia
D. HTN
E. Obesity
F. Atherosclerotic disease in another vascular bed (i.e., coronary, carotid, subclavian, renal, mesenteric artery stenosis, or abdominal aortic aneurysm)
G. Age:
  1. Age ≥ 65 years—increased occurrence
  2. Age 50 to 64 years—with family history of PAD or risk factors for atherosclerosis (i.e., diabetes, smoking history, hyperlipidemia, and/or HTN)
  3. Age <50 years—with diabetes and one additional risk factor for atherosclerosis

Common Complaints

A. Pain with activity is commonly characterized as cramping and/or aching:
  1. Upper-extremity pain in the forearm, hand, and digits
  2. Lower-extremity pain in the foot, calf, hip, thigh, and/or buttocks:
     a. Foot pain is most common in tibial or peroneal artery stenosis.
     b. Calf pain is most common with superficial femoral or popliteal artery stenosis.
     c. Thigh pain is most common in aortoiliac and common femoral artery stenosis.
     d. Hip and buttock pain are most common with aortoiliac arterial stenosis.
B. Pain at rest
C. Calf weakness or fatigue
D. Numbness or tingling

E. Dizziness with upper-extremity exertion

F. Syncope with upper-extremity exertion

G. Extremity ulceration

Other Signs and Symptoms

A. Decreased peripheral pulses

B. Blanching of the affected limb with elevation

C. Ulcerations or infection on distal aspects of extremities

D. Erectile dysfunction

Potential Complications

A. Nonhealing lower-extremity ulcerations

B. Infection

C. Amputation

D. Common coexisting diseases:
1. CAD; also known as CHD
2. Cerebrovascular disease
3. Subclavian artery stenosis

Subjective Data

A. Ask the client what activity brought about or preceded the episode or whether it occurs at rest. If ambulation was the precipitating factor, how far was the client able to walk?

B. Have the client describe the duration of pain and what time of day symptoms began.

C. Ask the client what alleviates his or her pain.

D. Ask the client whether any previous episodes have occurred.

E. Ask the client to list all medications, including OTC and herbal products, currently being taken or recently stopped.

F. Ask the client to quantify his or her smoking history.

G. Ask the client if he or she has a past medical history of an MI or cerebrovascular accident.

H. If the client is male, ask if he has any history of impotence or erectile dysfunction.

Physical Examination

A. Clients presenting with ALI should be quickly assessed for the need to call emergency services/911 for immediate transport to the hospital.
1. Symptoms of ALI as evidenced by the six Ps—pain, pallor, paresthesia, paralysis, pulselessness, and poikilothermia (the inability to maintain a constant core temperature).

B. Vital signs:
1. Check BP in both upper extremities.
    a. A difference in SBP of 10 mmHg or greater in the upper extremities is associated with upper-extremity PAD and cerebrovascular disease.
    b. A difference in SBP of 15 mmHg or greater in the upper extremities is associated with lower-extremity PAD.
    c. A difference in SBP of 15 to 20 mmHg is suggestive of subclavian artery stenosis.
2. Check BP in both lower extremities.
3. Document resting heart rate, respirations, height, and weight.

C. Inspect:
1. Perform a funduscopic examination: Check for retinal vascular changes that indicate a retinal vascular occlusion such as macular edema and neovascularization.
    a. Macular edema is the swelling of the central part of the retina.
    b. Neovascularization is the growth of abnormal vessels secondary to decreased perfusion of the retina.
2. Inspect the abdomen for a pulsating abdominal mass.
3. Inspect the extremities. Note edema, pallor, and cyanosis. Note the color of the extremities in dependent and elevated positions (i.e., elevation pallor and dependent rubor).
4. Inspect the distal skin, hair, and nails. Note any temperature discrepancies or trophic changes that are indicative of ischemia.
5. Assess the lower extremities for any ulcerations or diffuse erythema.
6. Assess for Homans' sign (i.e., calf pain with forced dorsiflexion).
7. Assess whether pain occurs when affected limb is elevated.

D. Auscultate:
1. Heart: Assess the rate, rhythm, heart sounds, murmur, and gallops
2. Carotids, abdomen, and bilateral groin for bruits
3. Lungs: Assess lung sounds, noting any sign of HF.

E. Palpate:
1. Palpate pulses, noting symmetry.
    a. Bilateral upper extremities (brachial and radial)
    b. Abdominal (aorta)
    c. Bilateral groin (femoral)
    d. Bilateral lower-extremity pulses (popliteal, dorsalis pedis, and posterior tibialis)
2. Palpate capillary refill.
3. Perform an Allen test: Occlude the radial and ulnar arteries with the fist closed. Open the hand and then release one of the occluded arteries. Repeat but release the other artery. Each time, prompt capillary refill should occur.
4. Palpate neck for carotid bruits.
5. Palpate the abdominal aorta noting any lateral pulsation, indicative of an aortic aneurysm.

Diagnostic Tests

A. Doppler ABI:
1. Interpretation of ABI ratios:
    a. 1.00 to 1.40: Normal
    b. 0.91 to 0.99: Borderline PAD
    c. 0.41 to 0.90: Mild to moderate PAD
    d. 0.00 to 0.40: Severe PAD

B. BMP (including BUN, creatinine, sodium, and potassium)

C. Lipid profile

D. CRP, homocysteine, D-dimer

E. EKG 12 lead
F. Duplex ultrasound
G. Abdominal ultrasound
H. Treadmill testing
I. CT angiography (CTA)
J. Magnetic resonance angiography (MRA)
K. Angiography, ordered and performed by a surgeon

Differential Diagnoses
A. PAD
B. Venous stasis
C. Venous obstruction/claudication
D. Spinal stenosis
E. Nerve root compression
F. Arthritis of the hip
G. Peripheral neuropathy
H. Arteritis

Plan
A. General interventions:
  1. The goal of therapy is to improve the client's quality of life by reducing morbidity and prolonging survival.
  2. Encourage preventive measures such as controlling other chronic medical conditions, such as diabetes, dyslipidemia, HTN, and obesity.

▶ B. Client teaching: *See Section III: Client Teaching Guide for this chapter, "Peripheral Arterial Disease."*
  1. Encourage smoking cessation, weight loss, and exercise if applicable.
  2. Encourage strategies to better manage other chronic medical conditions that directly affect the progression of PAD—that is, diabetes, dyslipidemia, obesity, and HTN.
  3. Proper foot care:
    a. Instruct the client to wear proper-fitting shoes that protect the feet.
    b. Inspect the inside of the shoes before donning them.
    c. Encourage the client to inspect the feet daily for signs of trauma or infection.
    d. Instruct the client to dry the feet well, including between the toes, after bathing.

C. Pharmaceutical therapy:
  1. Goal of therapy: Prevention of thromboembolism:
    a. Trental (pentoxifylline):
      i. 400 mg tablet
      ii. Dosage indications based on CrCl:
        1) CrCl < 10 mL/min: 400 mg, taken once a day
        2) CrCl = 10 to 50 mL/min: 400 mg, taken twice daily
        3) CrCl > 50 mg/min: 400 mg, taken three times a day
    b. Pletal (cilostazol):
      i. 50 mg and 100 mg tablets:
        1) Warning: Metabolites of Pletal are inhibitors of phosphodiesterase III and

are contraindicated in clients with CHF of any severity.
        2) Dosage indications:
          a) 50 mg, taken twice daily when coadministered with ketoconazole, itraconazole, erythromycin, and diltiazem
          b) 100 mg, taken twice daily at least half an hour before or 2 hours after breakfast and dinner
    c. Aspirin (acetylsalicylic acid, Ecotrin): 81 mg, 325 mg tablets, taken once daily
    d. Plavix (clopidogrel bisulfate) 75 mg, taken once daily
  2. Risk factor reduction:
    a. Manage dyslipidemia:
      i. LDL-C goal: Less than 100 mg/dL
      ii. LDL-C goal in clients at high risk of CAD: Less than 70 mg/dL
    b. Manage HTN:
      i. BP goal in clients without diabetes: Less than 140/90 mmHg
      ii. BP goal in clients with diabetes or CKD: Less than 130/80 mmHg
    c. Manage diabetes:
      i. Hgb A1C goal: Less than 7.0%

D. Dietary management:
  1. To manage dyslipidemia and HTN: Counsel client on nutrition and low-fat, low-cholesterol, low-sodium diet.
  2. To manage diabetes: Counsel client on diabetic diet and carbohydrate counting.
  3. To manage infection related to PAD: Counsel client on high-calorie, high-protein diet. Consider the addition of vitamins and minerals to promote wound healing—specifically, zinc, vitamin A, and vitamin C.
  4. Give diet handouts and/or refer to a registered dietitian.

E. Surgical therapies: These are considered in clients with pain at rest, tissue loss, or significant physical limitations that prevent exercise.
  1. Bypass
  2. Stenting
  3. Angioplasty/percutaneous transluminal angioplasty

F. Nonsurgical therapies:
  1. Smoking-cessation program
  2. Daily walking program
    a. Instruct client to walk to the point of pain, then stop and resume walking when pain remits.
    b. May need to obtain medical clearance for the client to exercise

Follow-Up
A. When PAD manifests with persistent symptoms, the client should be followed by a cardiologist.
B. Follow-up is determined by the client's needs, the frequency and intensity of symptoms, and the presence of other medical conditions.

Consultation/Referral

A. When ALI is suspected, refer the client for immediate hospitalization to obtain diagnostic testing to determine the presence of a thrombus and restore circulation to the affected extremity.

B. If CLI has led to ulceration and/or superimposed infection, then hospitalization is indicated to initiate a wound care consultation and diagnostic testing to determine the degree of arterial occlusion.

C. Refer to a cardiologist in the presence of persistent PAD symptoms.

D. Refer to a vascular surgeon for further evaluation of angioplasty, stenting, or bypass surgery.

E. Refer to a podiatrist to trim toenails and assess the client for proper-fitting shoes.

F. Refer to pain management if pain is resistant to treatment.

G. Refer to a registered dietitian as indicated by the client's understanding of the dietary modifications necessary to improve status of risk factors.

Individual Considerations

A. Nonambulatory clients:

    1. Using rocking chairs is a possible substitute for persons unable to participate in a walking program.

B. Geriatrics:

    1. Be alert to signs and symptoms of depression related to immobility and pain.

Bibliography

American Diabetes Association. (2019). Cardiovascular disease and risk management: Standards of medical care in diabetes—2019. *Diabetes Care, 42*(suppl 1), S103–S123. doi:10.2337/dc19-S010

Anderson, J. L., Halperin, J. L., Albert, N. M., Bozkurt, B., Brindis, R. G., Curtis, L. H., & Shen, W. K. (2013). Management of patients with peripheral artery disease (compilation of 2005 and 2011 ACCF/AHA guideline recommendations): A report of the American College of Cardiology Foundation/American Heart Association Task Force on Practice Guidelines. *Circulation, 127*(13), 1425–1443. doi:10.1161/CIR.0b013e31828b82aa

Barshes, N. R. (2017, November 11). Overview of upper extremity peripheral artery disease. *UpToDate.* Retrieved from http://www.uptodate.com/contents/overview-of-upper-extremity-peripheral-artery-disease

Centers for Disease Control and Prevention. (2016, June 16). *Peripheral arterial disease (PAD) fact sheet.* Retrieved from http://www.cdc.gov/DHDSP/data_statistics/fact_sheets/fs_PAD.htm

Chang, S., Huang, Y., Lee, M., Hu, S., Hsiao, Y., Chang, C., & Chen, P. (2019, February 27). Association of varicose veins with incident venous thromboembolism and peripheral artery disease. *Journal of the American Medical Association, 319*(8), 807–817. doi:10.1001/jama.2018.0246

Drug information. (2019). *Prescribers' digital reference.* Retrieved from www.pdr.net

Food and Drug Administration. (2018, June 12). *Use the nutrition facts label to reduce your intake of sodium in your diet.* Retrieved from https://www.fda.gov/food/nutrition-education-resources-materials/use-nutrition-facts-label-reduce-your-intake-sodium-your-diet

Gerhard-Herman, M. D., Gornik, H. L., Barrett, C., Barshes, N. R., Corriere, M. A., Drachman, D. E., . . . Walsh, M. E. (2017, March 21). 2016 AHA/ACC guideline on the management of patients with lower extremity peripheral artery disease: Executive summary: A report of the American College of Cardiology/American Heart Association Task Force on Clinical Practice Guidelines. *Circulation, 135*(12), e686–e725. Retrieved from http://www.ahajournals.org/doi/10.1161/CIR.0000000000000470

Goff, D. C., Lloyd-Jones, D. M., Bennett, G., Coady, S., & D'Agostino, B. R. Sr. (2014). 2013 ACC/AHA guideline on the assessment of cardiovascular risk: A report of the American College of Cardiology/American Heart Association Task Force on Practice Guidelines. *Circulation, 129,* S49–S73. doi:10.1161/01.cir.0000437741.48606.98

Harris, L., & Dryjski, M. (2018, October). Epidemiology, risk factors, and natural history of peripheral artery disease. *UpToDate.* Retrieved from http://www.uptodate.com/contents/epidemiology-risk-factors-and-natural-history-of-peripheral-artery-disease

Kastelein, J. (2017). PCSK9 inhibitors: Pharmacology, adverse effects, and use. *UpToDate.* Retrieved from https://www.uptodate.com/contents/pcsk9-inhibitors-pharmacology-adverse-effects-and-use

Kohlman-Trigoboff, D. (2019, January). Update: Diagnosis and management of peripheral arterial disease. *Journal for Nurse Practitioners, 15*(1), 87–95. doi:10.1016/j.nurpra.2018.09.008

Mohler, E. III. (2015, October). Overview of upper extremity peripheral artery disease. *UpToDate.* Retrieved from http://www.uptodate.com/contents/overview-of-upper-extremity-peripheral-artery-disease

Morcos, R., Louka, B., Tseng, A., Misra, S., McBane, R., Esser, H., & Shamoun, F. (2018, January 9). The evolving treatment of peripheral arterial disease through guideline-directed recommendations. *Journal of Clinical Medicine, 7*(1), 9. doi:10.3390/jcm7010009

Neschis, D. G., & Golden, M. A. (2018, June 11). Clinical features and diagnosis of lower extremity peripheral artery disease. *UpToDate.* Retrieved from http://www.uptodate.com/contents/clinical-features-and-diagnosis-of-lower-extremity-peripheral-artery-disease

Patel, M. R., Conte, M. S., Cutlip, D. E., Dib, N., Geraghty, P., Gray, W., & Krucoff, M. W. (2015). Evaluation and treatment of patients with lower extremity peripheral artery disease: Consensus definitions from Peripheral Academic Research Consortium (PARC). *Journal of the American College of Cardiology, 65*(9), 931–941. doi:10.1016/j.jacc.2014.12.036. Retrieved from http://content.onlinejacc.org/article.aspx?articleid=2174621#tab1

Trayes, K. P., Studdiford, J. S., Pickle, S., & Tully, A. S. (2013). Edema: Diagnosis and management. *American Family Physician, 88*(2), 102–110. doi:10.1097/ACM.0b013e318277d5b2

Vascular Cures. (2017). *Critical limb ischemia.* Retrieved from http://vascularcures.org/critical-limb-ischemia-cli/

Superficial Thrombophlebitis

Cheryl A. Glass and Laura A. Petty

Definition

A. Superficial thrombophlebitis is inflammation of a vessel wall accompanied by blood stasis in varicose veins, which may also have clot formation in a vein close to the surface.

    1. Most superficial thrombophlebitis occurs in the lower extremity, but may also occur in the breast and in the penis (Mondor disease).

    2. Superficial thrombophlebitis may also occur in the upper extremities and in the neck after invasive IV catheters are used in medical procedures.

    3. Generally superficial thrombophlebitis is self-limiting but may persist for a period of time (3–4 weeks or longer) before resolution.

B. Superficial phlebitis with an infection is referred to as *septic thrombophlebitis.*

Incidence

A. Pregnancy carries an increased risk of phlebitis. Eighty percent of thromboembolic events in pregnancy are venous. The incidence of PE in pregnancy accounts for 1.1 deaths per 100,000 deliveries.

B. The prevalence of superficial thrombophlebitis ranges from 4% to 8% of clients with an indwelling IV catheter.

C. Superficial phlebitis after a vein radiofrequency or laser ablation is common.

Pathogenesis

A. Superficial thrombosis is caused by infection, abuse of IV drugs, chemical irritation from overuse of an IV route for diagnostic tests and drugs, and/or trauma. Several episodes can signal an underlying problem such as carcinoma of the pancreas.

B. A common cause of varicose veins is blood-flow stasis, basically caused by valvular incompetence and/or dilation of the vessel lumen.

C. Thrombi in the upper extremities commonly have iatrogenic causes such as IV catheters.

D. Thrombophlebitis during pregnancy through the first 6 weeks postpartum is linked to a reduced fibrinolytic state.

Predisposing Factors

A. Previous thrombophlebitis is the highest risk factor for recurrence.

B. Hypercoagulability states such as pregnancy (50% of events) through 6 weeks postpartum (50% of events)

C. Hemoglobinopathies:
1. Factor V Leiden mutation
2. Protein C deficiency
3. Protein S deficiency
4. Prothrombin gene mutation
5. Antithrombin III deficiency
6. Factor XII deficiency

D. Estrogen therapy:
1. Oral contraceptives
2. High-dose HRT

E. Malignancy (especially in the tail of the pancreas)

F. Lupus, positive anticardiolipin antibody

G. Sepsis

H. Surgery

I. Long bone trauma

J. Recent IV catheter access

K. Prolonged immobilization

L. Obesity

M. Varicose veins

N. Age older than 60 years

O. Stroke

P. MI

Q. Family history of DVT

R. Smoking

S. HTN

T. Infection

Common Complaints

A. Warm, tender, inflamed vessel with palpable cord

B. Redness along the course of the superficial vein

C. Tenderness or pain localized to the affected vein

Other Signs and Symptoms

A. Fever/no fever

B. Localized edema

Potential Complications

A. Superficial thrombophlebitis extending into the deep venous system

B. DVT

C. Conversion to suppurative thrombophlebitis:
1. Metastatic abscess formation
2. Septicemia
3. Septic emboli

Subjective Data

A. Query the client regarding the onset, duration, and intensity of symptoms.

B. Ask the client about fever or other related symptoms.

C. Obtain a thorough medical history and account of recent physical activity.

D. Ask the client about any recent experience of any type of injury.

E. Inquire whether the client has ever had similar symptoms or history of previous thrombophlebitis. If so, discuss previous treatment and therapy used and the results.

F. Review current medications: Prescription, OTC, and herbal products.
1. Ask specifically about oral contraceptives and hormone therapy.

G. Review the client's occupation for sedentary lifestyle.

H. Review any recent plane travel.

I. Review history for recent invasive procedures.

Physical Examination

A. Check temperature (if indicated with inflammation), pulse, respirations, and BP.

B. Inspect:
1. Assess overall appearance. Evaluate for the presence of respiratory distress.
2. Inspect extremities, noting erythema and edema.
3. Assess for increased warmth over the affected vein.

C. Auscultate:
1. Heart, noting rate, rhythm, heart sounds, murmurs, and gallops
2. Lungs for lung sounds in all fields

D. Palpate:
1. Palpate extremities; check all pulses, including femoral, post-tibial, pedal, and radial.
2. Palpate extremities for tenderness and palpable cord.
3. Palpate lymph nodes distal and proximal to the site.
4. Test for Homans' sign in lower extremities bilaterally if DVT is suspected.

Diagnostic Tests

A. Duplex ultrasound identifies the presence, location, and extent of venous thrombosis.

B. Doppler ultrasound

C. Laboratory tests are ordered dependent on the clinical situation:
1. CBC with differential
2. Screening for hypercoagulability should not be considered for one episode of superficial thrombophlebitis.
3. Screening for hypercoagulability should be considered for recurrent superficial thrombophlebitis.
4. Blood cultures

Differential Diagnoses

A. Thrombophlebitis
B. Varicose veins
C. Cellulitis
D. Strained muscle
E. Insect bites
F. Erythema nodosum
G. Cutaneous polyarteritis nodosa
H. Kaposi's sarcoma
I. Hyperalgesic pseudothrombophlebitis

Plan

A. General interventions:
   1. Prescribe supportive hose/compression stockings.
   2. Prescribe bed rest for superficial thrombophlebitis.
   3. DVT: Hospitalization is required.
B. Client teaching:
   1. Tell the client to avoid prolonged sitting or standing and not to cross or massage legs. *See Section III: Client Teaching Guides for this chapter, "Superficial Thrombophlebitis" and "Varicose Veins."*
   2. Advise the client to avoid constrictive clothing such as knee-high hosiery.
   3. Have the client apply heat and elevate the extremity for varicose veins or superficial thrombophlebitis.
   4. Advise clients with thrombophlebitis to discontinue oral contraceptives and hormone replacement. Alternative forms of birth control recommended by the American College of Obstetricians and Gynecologists (ACOG) include:
      a. Intrauterine devices (IUDs), including IUDs that contain progestin
      b. Progestin-only oral contraceptives
      c. Progestin-only implants
      d. Barrier methods
      e. Surgical procedures: Vasectomy and tubal ligation
C. Pharmaceutical therapy for superficial thrombophlebitis:
   1. NSAIDs are used for the treatment of pain. No NSAID has been identified as superior for treatment.
   2. The use of anticoagulation therapy for the treatment of lower-extremity superficial thrombophlebitis is controversial. Unfractionated heparin and LMWH are both used for the treatment to reduce risk of DVT and/or recurrent phlebitis.
   3. Anticoagulation is an option for clients with lower-extremity superficial thrombophlebitis at increased risk of thromboembolism. This is defined as having an affected venous segment greater than or equal to 5 cm in proximity (less than or equal to 5 cm) to the deep venous system and positive medical risk factors. The American College of Chest Physicians' full evidence-based clinical practice guidelines on antithrombotic therapy are available at journal.chestnet.org/issue/S0012-3692(12)X6003-3.
   4. Antibiotics, if infection is suspected
D. Surgery:
   1. Biopsy
   2. Vein ablation, but only if symptoms are significant and persistent
   3. Vein ligation, but only if symptoms are significant and persistent

Follow-Up

A. Schedule an appointment for clients with superficial thrombophlebitis to return in 7 to 10 days or earlier as needed. Repeat physical examination as needed to evaluate resolution or progression of the thrombophlebitis.
B. Periodic follow-up is needed to monitor clients on anticoagulation therapy.
C. After an acute problem is resolved, consider laboratory evaluation for hypercoagulation syndrome (protein C, protein S, and antithrombin III).
D. Monitor bone loss with a dual-energy x-ray absorptiometry (DEXA) scan with prolonged use of heparin.
E. ACOG does not recommend screening all women for thrombophilias before starting oral contraceptives.
F. Women with a history of thrombosis who have not had a complete evaluation should be tested for both antiphospholipid antibodies and inherited thrombophilias.

Consultation/Referral

A. If septic thrombophlebitis or DVT is diagnosed, refer the client to a physician.
B. Hospitalization is required to initiate heparin therapy.
C. Comanage pregnancy with an obstetrician.

Individual Considerations

A. Pregnancy:
   1. Routine anticoagulation therapy for all pregnant women is not recommended. Therapeutic anticoagulation is recommended for women with acute thromboembolism during the current pregnancy or those at high risk of thrombosis such as women with mechanical heart valves.
   2. Warfarin and NSAIDs are contraindicated.
   3. Heparin is the preferred anticoagulant in pregnancy. Neither unfractionated heparin nor LMWH crosses the placenta.
   4. Warfarin, LMWH, and unfractionated heparin do not accumulate in breast milk and do not induce an anticoagulant effect in the infant; therefore they are considered compatible with breastfeeding.
B. Geriatrics:
   1. Prognosis is poor for clients with septic thrombophlebitis.
   2. Using a rocking chair is a possible substitute for persons unable to participate in a walking program.
   3. Be alert to signs and symptoms of depression related to immobility and pain.

Bibliography

Di Nisio, M., Wickers, I., & Middeldorp, S. (2018, December 11). Treatment of lower extremity superficial thrombophlebitis. *Journal of the American Medical Association, 320*(22), 2367–2368. doi:10.1001/jama.2018.16623

Fernandez, L., & Scovell, S. (2016, April). Superficial thrombophlebitis of the lower extremity. *UpToDate.* Retrieved from http://www.uptodate.com/contents/superficial-thrombophlebitis-of-the-lower-extremity

Klever, R. G. (2015, June). Superficial thrombophlebitis. *Medscape.* Retrieved from http://emedicine.medscape.com/article/463256-overview

Nasr, H., & Scriven, J. M. (2015). Superficial thrombophlebitis (superficial venous thrombosis). *BMJ, 350,* h2039. doi:10.1136/bmj.h2039. Retrieved from http://www.bmj.com/content/350/bmj.h2039

Scovell, S. (2019, March). Phlebitis and thrombosis of the superficial lower extremity veins. *UpToDate*. Retrieved from http://www.uptodate.com/contents/phlebitis-and-thrombosis-of-the-superficial-lower-extremity-veins

Trayes, K. P., Studdiford, J. S., Pickle, S., & Tully, A. S. (2013). Edema: Diagnosis and management. *American Family Physician*, 88(2), 102–110. doi:10.1097/ACM.0b013e318277d5b2

Syncope

Jill C. Cash and Debbie Gunter

Definition
A. Syncope is a brief, sudden loss of consciousness and muscle tone secondary to cerebral ischemia, or inadequate oxygen or glucose delivery to brain tissue. Recovery is spontaneous.

Incidence
A. Syncope is a common problem in all age groups. An estimated 15% of children experience an episode by adulthood. Between 12% and 48% of healthy young adults have lost consciousness (one third following trauma), but most do not seek medical attention. Adults older than age 75 years in long-term care facilities have a 6% annual incidence of syncope, and 23% have had previous episodes. Syncopal episodes account for approximately 1% to 6% of hospital admissions and 3% of ED visits.

Pathogenesis
The most common cause of syncope is inadequate cerebral perfusion caused by one of the following:
A. Vasomotor instability associated with a decrease in systemic vascular resistance and/or venous return. The following may cause syncope:
  1. Vasovagal episodes
  2. Situational syncope, from coughing, micturition, and defecation
  3. Medications:
    a. Vasodilators
    b. Antiarrhythmics
    c. Diuretics
    d. Neurological agents
    e. Glucose-regulating drugs
    f. Impotence therapy
B. Decrease in cardiac output caused by blood-flow obstruction within the heart or pulmonary circulation or by arrhythmias. This may be caused by the following:
  1. Aortic, pulmonic, and mitral stenosis
  2. Idiopathic hypertrophic subaortic stenosis (IHSS)
  3. Pump failure
  4. Subclavian steal syndrome
  5. Seizures
C. Focal or generalized decrease in cerebral perfusion leading to transient ischemia because of cerebrovascular disease.
D. Metabolic abnormalities:
  1. Hypoglycemia
  2. Hypocarbia and hypoxia usually do not result in syncope unless they are profound, although consciousness may be altered

E. Psychiatric illnesses associated with syncope include:
  1. Generalized anxiety
  2. Panic attacks
  3. Major depressive disorders
F. Unexplained cause

Predisposing Factors
A. Advanced age, caused by altered regulation of cerebral blood flow and/or systemic arterial pressure because of aging process and increased medication use
B. Other factors, depending on etiology
C. Medication use (noted earlier)

Common Complaints
A. Dizziness
B. Light-headedness
C. Fainting with no memory of events

Other Signs and Symptoms
A. Neuroautonomic regulations:
  1. Event triggered by changing position, turning head, wearing tight collars
  2. Nausea, warmth, diaphoresis, weakness 1 hour after eating
B. Cardiac causes: Exercise-induced palpitations, chest pain, SOB with no warning before episode
C. Neurological causes:
  1. Vertigo
  2. Diplopia
  3. Facial paresthesias
  4. Ataxia
  5. Auditory, visual, or vestibular disturbances
D. Metabolic or endocrine causes:
  1. Restlessness
  2. Anxiety
  3. Confusion
  4. No recent food intake, low glucose level
E. Psychiatric: Graceful fainting in presence of an audience

Subjective Data
A. Inquire if the client ever experienced similar symptoms or episodes before. If so, when and at what age did it begin?
B. Ask the client or witness of the episode to give a detailed description of the loss of consciousness. Was loss of consciousness complete, and, if so, for how long? What was the posture of the client before, during, and after the event? Did it occur abruptly, or were there symptoms leading up to the event?
C. Question the client regarding events leading up to the episode, noting prodromal symptoms such as headache, aura, nausea/vomiting, light-headedness, diaphoresis, feeling of warmth
D. Obtain a detailed account of symptoms during and after the episode, noting mental status. Did the client recover on his or her own, or did the client require assistance? Were there any associated symptoms that occurred during the event—SOB, chest pain, loss of bowel, or bladder control?

E. If syncope has occurred in the past, are there any events that precipitate an episode? Exertion, exercise, coughing, standing quickly?

F. Obtain a detailed medication history, addressing prescribed and OTC drugs, alcohol, and illicit preparations.

G. Review the client's past medical history.

Physical Examination

A. Check temperature, if indicated, pulse, respirations, and BP.
   1. Measure BP and pulse in both arms and legs. Note BP differences between the arms.
   2. Measure BP several times during a 2-minute period with the client standing.
   3. Check for orthostatic hypotension, which is defined as a drop of 20 mmHg or more in SBP on standing:
      a. First, measure BP after the client lies supine for 5 to 10 minutes.
      b. Then have the client stand and measure BP several times during a 2-minute period.
B. Inspect:
   1. Assess overall appearance of the client, skin color
   2. Note the range of motion in the neck.
C. Auscultate:
   1. The heart with position changes. Note murmurs or extra heart sounds to rule out structural disease.
   2. The carotid arteries
   3. The abdomen for bruits
D. Palpate:
   1. The abdomen, noting pulsatile expansion
E. Neurological examination:
   1. Perform a complete examination, if indicated, including assessing 2nd to 12th cranial nerves, Babinski's reflex, and gait.
F. Mental status:
   1. Assess mental health if indicated.

Diagnostic Tests

The following tests are performed depending on history and physical examination results.

The ESC published new guidelines and the ESC guidelines of 2018 recommend the following work-up:

A. Carotid sinus massage in client older than 40 years of age. Avoid if the client has a history of TIA or stroke in the past 3 months and in clients with carotid bruits. Recommend physician or cardiology specialist assistance when performing carotid massage. Use caution when performing carotid sinus massage. Consider contraindications, complications, and protocol for performing this procedure.

B. Echocardiogram for clients with a history of heart disease, structural heart disease, or syncope secondary to cardiovascular cause (known heart disease, family history of unexplained sudden death, syncope with exertion or supine, abnormal EKG, sudden onset of palpitation before syncope, or arrhythmia on EKG)

C. EKG for clients with suspected arrhythmia or cardiac disease. Identify acute and old EKG changes to rule out pathologic Q waves, ST-segment elevation, and LVH.

D. Orthostatic challenge test if syncope is related to position change or a suspected reflex mechanism

E. Neurological/serum laboratory testing for other concerns of nonsyncopal loss of consciousness. Laboratory testing includes chemistry profile, TSH, and free T_4. Consider a glucose tolerance test if diabetes is suspected. BNP may be useful to evaluate cardiac versus noncardiac cause for syncope.

F. Chest radiography, for essential baseline data. Wide mediastinum signals aortic dissection.

G. In-hospital monitoring recommended for unstable, life-threatened clients

H. Holter monitoring for 24 to 48 hours

I. External event monitoring

J. Exercise testing is recommended for clients with syncope that occurs during, or quickly after, cessation of exercise. Echocardiogram is recommended before this testing.

K. Cardiac catheterization

L. Lung scan

M. Treadmill test

N. Electrophysiological studies are recommended for clients with unexplained syncope

Differential Diagnoses

A. Irregular neuroautonomic regulations:
   1. Neurocardiogenic causes
   2. Situational causes, such as coughing, defecation, diving, micturition, sneezing, swallowing, trumpet playing, vagal stimulation, weight lifting, postprandial state
   3. Orthostatic causes:
      a. Hyperadrenergic state
      b. Hypoadrenergic state, primary or secondary autonomic insufficiency
      c. Carotid sinus syncope
      d. Cardioinhibitory state
      e. Vasodepressor stimulation
      f. Mixed
B. Cardiac causes:
   1. Mechanical causes such as aortic dissection, aortic stenosis, atrial myxoma, cardiac tamponade, global myocardial ischemia, hypertrophic cardiomyopathy, mitral stenosis, MI, prosthetic valve dysfunction, PE, pulmonary HTN, pulmonary stenosis, and Takayasu's arteritis
   2. Electrical causes, such as AV block, long QT syndrome, pacemaker, sick sinus syndrome, supraventricular tachyarrhythmias, and ventricular tachyarrhythmias
C. Neurological causes:
   1. Neuralgias: Glossopharyngeal, trigeminal
   2. Normal-pressure hydrocephalus
   3. Subclavian steal
   4. Vertebrobasilar artery disease: Compression, migraine, TIA
D. Metabolic or endocrine causes: Hypoadrenalism, hypoglycemia, hyponatremia, hypothyroidism, and hypoxia
E. Psychiatric causes: Anxiety, hysteria, major depression, panic disorder, somatization, and hyperventilation syndrome

Plan

A. General interventions:
  1. Management is directed at the primary cause of the episode.
B. Client teaching:
  1. If the client has orthostatic hypotension, suggest that he or she wear elastic stockings, change positions slowly, sleep with the head of the bed elevated, and exercise legs before standing.
  2. If syncope is induced by situations, warn the client to avoid or alter his or her approach to such precipitating events.
  3. If the client has prodromal symptoms, such as nausea, light-headedness, pallor, sweating, or palpitations, advise him or her to lie down when they occur.
  4. If the client has hypersensitive carotid sinus reflex, recommend that he or she loosen his or her collar.
  5. Tell clients to avoid prolonged standing. If they cannot avoid it, they should contract their calf muscles to increase venous blood flow.
  6. Some driving restrictions exist for clients at risk of recurrent syncope. Driving restrictions are enforced by state law. Review these restrictions with the client and family as indicated by diagnosis.
C. Dietary management:
  1. If not contraindicated, instruct clients with orthostatic hypotension to use salt liberally.
D. Pharmaceutical therapy for neurocardiogenic syncope:
  1. Nonpharmacological methods suggested: Avoid volume depletion. Maintain adequate sodium levels by increasing salt intake in the diet. Wear thigh-high elastic support hose with 30- to 40-mmHg pressure. Orthostatic training is also recommended two times a day.
  2. Drugs of choice: Beta-blockers (propranolol 80–160 mg/d, metoprolol 50–100 mg/d)
  3. Fludrocortisone acetate (Florinef Acetate), a corticosteroid, may be used alone or with beta-blockers. Initial dosage is 0.1 to 0.4 mg/d; this may be increased gradually to 1.0 to 2.0 mg/d.
  4. Other drugs include anticholinergic agents (disopyramide 100 to 200 mg twice daily sustained release) and SSRIs (sertraline 50 mg/d, fluoxetine 20 mg/d, paroxetine 20 mg/d).

Follow-Up

Scheduling of return visits depends on the etiology and severity of syncope and whether the client has been placed on medications.

Consultation/Referral

A. Consult with or refer the client to a physician when cardiac or neurological involvement is suspected.
B. Consult with or refer the client to a physician if medication therapy is required.

Individual Considerations

A. Adults:
  1. In young adult athletes, be aware of symptoms of Marfan syndrome.
  2. In older adults, coronary atherosclerosis may present along with syncope.
B. Geriatrics:
  1. Elderly clients may have multiple comorbid conditions such as decreased cerebral blood flow and acute viral illness.

Bibliography

Benditt, D. (2018, September 28). Syncope in adults: Clinical manifestations and diagnostic evaluation. *UpToDate*. Retrieved from https://www.uptodate.com/contents/syncope-in-adults-clinical-manifestations-and-diagnostic-evaluation

Brignole, M., Moya, A., de Lange, F., Deharo, J., Elliot, P., Fanciulli, A., . . . van Dijk, J. (2018). 2018 ESC guidelines for the diagnosis and management of syncope. *European Heart Journal*, *39*(21), 1883–1948. doi:10.1093/eurheartj/ehy037

Dima, C. (2018, February 2). Mitral stenosis. *Medscape*. Retrieved from https://emedicine.medscape.com/article/155724-overview

Drug Information. (2019). *Prescribers' digital reference*. Retrieved from www.pdr.net

Morag, R. (2017, January 13). Syncope. *Medscape*. Retrieved from https://emedicine.medscape.com/article/811669-overview

Saklani, P., Krahn, A., & Klein, G. (2013). Syncope. *Circulation*, *127*(12), 1330–1339. doi:10.1161/CIRCULATIONAHA.112.138396

Shen, W., Sheldon, R., & Benditt, D. (2017). 2017 ACC/AHA/HRS guideline for the evaluation and management of patients with syncope: A report of the American College of Cardiology/American Heart Association Task Force on Clinical Practice Guidelines and the Heart Rhythm Society. *Circulation*, *136*(5), e60–e122. doi:10.1161/CIR.0000000000000537. Retrieved from https://www.ahajournals.org/doi/10.1161/CIR.0000000000000499

Walsh, K., Hoffmayer, K., & Hamdan, M. H. (2015). Syncope: Diagnosis and management. *Current Problems in Cardiology*, *40*(2), 51–86. doi:10.1016/j.cpcardiol.2014.11.001

11 Gastrointestinal Guidelines

Abdominal Pain

Cheryl A. Glass, Audra Malone, and Doncy Eapen

Definition

A. Abdominal pain is a common nonspecific complaint. The clinician's responsibility is to determine whether clients can be safely observed and treated symptomatically or whether they require further investigation or a specialist referral. Pain in the abdomen is most commonly secondary to problems relating to abdominal organs, and it is categorized as follows:

    1. Acute pain: Pain of less than a few days that has worsened progressively until presentation

    2. Chronic pain: Interval of 12 weeks can be used to separate acute from chronic pain (i.e., pain has remained unchanged for months or years)

    3. Emergent: Pain that lasts 3 hours or longer, accompanied by fever or vomiting

B. Pain may be categorized by description:

    1. Visceral pain is usually dull and aching in character and poorly localized.

    2. Parietal pain is sharp and well localized.

    3. Referred pain is aching and perceived as originating from distant from its source.

Incidence

Abdominal pain is very common. On questioning, abdominal pain is present in 75% of adolescents and in about 50% of all adults. Gastroenteritis and irritable bowel syndrome (IBS) are the most common causes of acute pain, and chronic stool retention is the most common cause of chronic pain. Other causes of abdominal pain include the following:

A. Acute appendicitis: Incidence is 10 per 100,000 population.

B. Acute cholecystitis: Varies according to age and ethnic origin

C. Intestinal obstruction, usually small intestines: Accounts for 20% of acute abdominal conditions

D. Pancreatitis: Incidence of acute pancreatitis ranges from 4.9 to 35 per 100,000 population

E. Inflammatory bowel disease (IBD): Incidence is approximately 1.3% in the United States, which has increased from 0.9% in 1999

F. Abdominal pain associated with pregnancy: Ectopic pregnancy (1 per 200 pregnancies), miscarriage, and abruptio placenta

Pathogenesis

A. Pathogenesis depends on the origin of pain. Pain may result from inflammation, ischemia, distention, altered motility, obstruction, or ulceration.

Predisposing Factors

A. Abdominal trauma

B. Motor vehicle accidents

C. Lactose intolerance

D. Pregnancy

E. Testicular/ovarian torsion

F. Psychogenic pain

G. Sickle cell disease

H. Infection

I. Neoplasms

Common Complaints

The clinical presentation of abdominal pain is determined in part by the site of the involvement.

A. Acute or chronic onset of pain

B. Vomiting

C. Diarrhea

Other Signs and Symptoms

A. Blood in stool/emesis

B. Referred shoulder pain

C. Fever

D. Nausea and/or projectile vomiting

E. Rigid abdomen

F. Changes in vital signs

G. Abdominal distention

H. Constipation

I. Guarding

J. Rebound tenderness

K. Biliary pain and right subcostal tenderness

L. Anorexia

M. Periumbilical discomfort; consider appendicitis if within 2 to 12 hours, pain localizes in right lower quadrant (RLQ) at McBurney's point.

N. Dysuria

O. Abdominal mass: Do not overlook the possibility of pregnancy as the cause of a mass.

P. Melena (most common in peptic ulcer disease [PUD])

Subjective Data

> Evaluate for a "surgical abdomen," defined as a rapidly worsening prognosis in the absence of surgical intervention. Clients should not eat or drink while a diagnosis of a surgical abdomen remains under consideration. Once a surgical abdomen has been excluded, the remainder of the evaluation will be guided by the chronicity of symptoms along with the location of pain.

A. Review the onset, duration, course, and quality of pain:
1. When did the pain start?
2. What were you doing when the pain started?
3. What does the pain feel like?
4. Has this ever occurred before?
5. What was the primary diagnosis?
6. What was the previous treatment, and was it effective?
7. Is there anyone else in your home having the same symptoms?
8. Review the progression of pain.

B. Determine the pain rating on a 10-point scale, with 0 being no pain and 10 being equivalent to the worst pain the client has ever felt.

C. Qualify the duration of pain in minutes, hours, days, weeks, or months. Does the pain interfere with sleep?

D. Review the pattern of pain:
1. Review aggravating factors.
2. Review alleviating factors.
3. Does the pain radiate?
4. Does the pain have any relationship to food intake?
5. What other symptoms occur with pain?

E. Questions specific to females:
1. Determine the client's last menstrual period (LMP).
2. Has she had a hysterectomy or tubal ligation?
3. Does she have a recent history of dyspareunia or dysmenorrhea that suggests pelvic pathology?
4. Is there any history of physical abuse?
5. **What type of contraception is used? Specifically evaluate for an intrauterine device (IUD).**

F. Review the client's current medications and drug history, especially antibiotic, laxative, acetaminophen, aspirin, and nonsteroidal anti-inflammatory drug (NSAID) use. Pain may be significantly masked in clients taking corticosteroids.

G. Rule out abdominal trauma from domestic violence, motor vehicle accidents, falls, or assaults.

H. Review bowel habits and note changes: Constipation, diarrhea, change in bowel pattern, urgency, color of stools

I. Review the client's history for sickle cell disease. Any individual of African American or Mediterranean descent presenting with leg or abdominal pain should be questioned regarding sickle cell disease or trait.

J. Review urinary function. Is there any urinary frequency, urgency, dysuria, flank pain, or back pain? If the client is male, does he have any hesitancy, difficulty starting the urine stream, nocturia, low urinary volume, or any lower abdominal distention indicating urinary retention?

K. Review alcohol intake/history.

L. Has the client had any unexplained weight loss?

M. Evaluate sexual activity to rule out potential sexually transmitted infection (STI):
1. Evaluate whether the client has new partners.
2. Are the partners experiencing any symptoms?

Physical Examination

A. Check temperature, pulse, respirations, and blood pressure (BP); include orthostatic BP.

> Tachycardia or hypotension may be signs of a ruptured aortic aneurysm, septic shock, gastrointestinal (GI) hemorrhage, or volume depletion. Absence of a fever in the elderly or immunosuppressed client does not exclude a serious illness.

B. Inspect:
1. Observe general appearance: Facial expressions, gait, skin turgor, refusal to move/writhing; note grimace or guarding during the examination.
2. Perform eye and mouth examination to rule out iritis and aphthous ulcers of the mouth (extraintestinal manifestations of IBD). Examine eyes for jaundice.
3. Examine the abdomen for the presence of hernia at the umbilicus, groin, or near the site of prior surgical incisions.
4. Examine the abdomen for overt masses or pulsations.
5. Examine the skin for jaundice. Observe for any bruising or other signs of domestic violence in the "bathing suit" areas—breasts, abdomen, and back—that would be easily covered with clothes.

C. Auscultate:
1. Auscultate for bowel sounds in all four quadrants of the abdomen.
2. Evaluate the heart and lungs.
3. Check for aortic, iliac, and renal bruits.

D. Percuss:
1. Abdomen for tympany and dullness

E. Palpate:
1. Abdomen for masses, rebound tenderness, hepatomegaly or splenomegaly, and peritoneal signs:
   a. Before palpating the abdomen, ask the client to bend the knees to help with relaxation of the wall musculature.
   b. Elderly clients may lack classical peritoneal signs of rebound and guarding.
   c. Begin palpation gently, starting from the area of the least pain, and advancing to the area of the greatest pain.

2. Check the abdomen for a tender pulsatile mass at midline; it may indicate abdominal aortic aneurysm (AAA).

3. Examine the back, assessing for costovertebral angle tenderness (CVAT).

4. Perform a bimanual examination in women regardless of whether the client has had a hysterectomy or is postmenopausal:

a. Evaluate the size and symmetry of the uterus.

b. Evaluate the adnexal areas for the presence of appropriately sized mobile ovaries. A fixed, painful adnexal mass is suggestive of an endometrioma or tubo-ovarian abscess.

c. Endometriosis is suggested by localized tenderness in the cul-de-sac or uterosacral ligaments, palpable tender nodules, pain with uterine movement, and tenderness fixation of adnexal mass or uterus in a retroverted position.

5. Check for the obturator sign, which is abdominal pain in response to passive internal rotation of the right hip from a 90° angle knee–hip flexion position; perform this when an inflamed appendix is suspected.

6. Check for the psoas sign, which is a pain response to the iliopsoas group of hip flexor muscles when an inflamed appendix is suspected. A positive psoas sign is the presence of lower quadrant pain noted as the supine client raises his or her right leg from the hip while the examiner pushes downward against the client's lower thigh.

F. Perform a rectal examination, including testing of stool for occult blood. **Failure to perform a rectal examination in clients with abdominal pain may be associated with an increased rate of misdiagnosis and should be considered a medicolegal pitfall.**

Diagnostic Tests

Diagnostic testing is ordered based on the following differential diagnoses:

A. **In all women of childbearing age, assume the woman is pregnant until proven otherwise. Vaginal bleeding with or without abdominal pain should prompt a transvaginal ultrasound and a serum human chorionic gonadotropin (HCG) test. HCG should be tested before performing the transvaginal ultrasound.**

B. Complete blood count (CBC) with differential

C. Electrolytes

D. Complete metabolic panel

E. Blood urea nitrogen (BUN)

F. Amylase and lipase

G. Aminotransferases, alkaline phosphatase (ALP), and bilirubin

H. Urinalysis; save the sample for culture

I. Free erythrocyte protoporphyrin (FEP) or zinc protoporphyrin (ZPP) if lead poisoning is suspected in adults

J. Plain x-ray films of the abdomen to rule out obstruction

K. CT of the abdomen with or without contrast

L. Abdominal ultrasonography

M. GI series radiography

N. Upper endoscopy; consider *Helicobacter pylori* testing

O. Sigmoidoscopy

P. Barium enema (BE): Avoid with suspected obstruction

Q. Stool guaiac test for occult blood

R. Consider endoscopic retrograde cholangiopancreatography (ERCP) to visualize the distal common bile duct.

S. EKG to rule out cardiac pain

T. Consider blood cultures for elderly clients who present with abdominal pain associated with either fever or hypothermia or when sepsis is suspected.

U. Chest radiography

Differential Diagnoses

The location and duration of abdominal pain can often significantly help in narrowing the differential diagnosis.

A. Right upper quadrant (RUQ) pain:

1. Acute cholecystitis and biliary colic:

a. Biliary tract disorders: Biliary duct stones, gallstones, tumor, and sphincter of Oddi dysfunction. A slightly increased serum amylase of 140 IU/L may suggest bile duct obstruction associated with acute cholecystitis; however, a level ≥ 500 IU/L might indicate pancreatitis.

b. Ascending cholangitis presents with fever and jaundice in a client with RUQ pain

c. In acute cholecystitis, the typical pain is maximal in the RUQ or epigastrium, radiating to the scapular region, and is accompanied by nausea, vomiting, and fever without jaundice. Murphy's sign, or inspiratory arrest in response to upper quadrant palpation, may be seen with acute cholecystitis. RUQ tenderness to percussion or pressure of the gallbladder is also a suggestive finding.

2. Acute hepatitis

3. Hepatic abscess

4. Hepatomegaly due to congestive heart failure (CHF)

5. Perforated duodenal ulcer (DU)—epigastric and generalized abdominal pain

> A perforated ulcer is accompanied by an increased serum amylase.

6. Acute pancreatitis: Bilateral pain—RUQ and left upper quadrant (LUQ) pain

> Pancreatitis is accompanied by an increased serum amylase and lipase.

7. Herpes zoster

8. Myocardial ischemia

9. Pleural or pulmonary pathology (e.g., pneumonia, pulmonary embolism, or empyema)

B. RLQ pain:

1. Appendicitis often begins with symptoms of dull, steady, periumbilical pain, and anorexia before localizing to the RLQ at McBurney's point.

2. Regional enteritis

3. Leaking aneurysm
4. Ruptured ectopic pregnancy
5. Ovarian cyst
6. Ovarian torsion
7. Pelvic inflammatory disease (PID)
8. Ureteral calculi
9. Incarcerated, strangulated inguinal hernia
10. Endometriosis
11. Meckel's diverticulitis
12. Abdominal wall hematoma
13. Pyelonephritis
14. Infectious colitis

C. LUQ pain:
1. Gastritis
2. Acute pancreatitis: Epigastric pain that is relatively sudden, bores in to the back, and is associated with nausea, vomiting, and anorexia
3. Splenic enlargement, rupture, abscess, infarction, aneurysm
4. Myocardial ischemia
5. Left lower lobe pneumonia
6. Renal colic: Radiates to the groin

D. Left lower quadrant (LLQ) pain:
1. Sigmoid and/or descending diverticulitis
2. Regional enteritis
3. Leaking aneurysm

> AAA may present with a tender pulsatile mass at the abdominal midline. Vascular disorders such as acute arterial insufficiency due to atherosclerosis or embolus may present with severe abdominal pain; however, mild, constant pain may be the only symptom for several days. Dissection or rupture of an AAA produces severe acute abdominal pain and often radiates to the back or genitalia.

4. Ruptured ectopic pregnancy

> Rupture of the fallopian tube generally causes sudden, acute, and localized abdominal pain. Internal hemorrhage causes syncope and referred shoulder pain, caused by phrenic nerve irritation. Diagnosis before tubal rupture may be difficult because symptoms and physical findings mimic other conditions such as appendicitis.

5. Ovarian cyst
6. Ovarian torsion
7. PID
8. Ureteral calculi
9. Incarcerated, strangulated inguinal hernia
10. Pyelonephritis
11. Infectious colitis

E. Generalized abdominal pain:
1. Trauma:
   a. **Any person with a possible blow to the abdomen should have orthostatic BP taken, careful palpation of the abdomen, and measurement of serial abdominal circumferences, and should be considered for abdominal imaging.**

Serial hemoglobin (Hgb) and hematocrit (Hct) measurements should be obtained if necessary.
   b. In abdominal trauma, the spleen is the most commonly injured organ, especially in blunt abdominal trauma; the onset can be immediate or delayed.
   c. Nontraumatic splenic rupture is often associated with acute infectious mononucleosis
2. Intestinal obstruction: Obstruction that develops slowly over weeks to months may be relatively subtle in presentation.

> Acute obstruction presents with severe "colicky" pain or pain that is wavelike in nature; it makes the pain relentless.

3. Peritoneal irritation: Severe pain due to the rich innervation of the parietal peritoneum. Focal injury results in well-localized discomfort that is described as a sharp aching or burning sensation.
4. Metabolic disturbances may mimic intra-abdominal etiologies.

> Porphyria and lead poisoning sometimes simulate bowel obstruction because they can cause cramping, abdominal pain, and hyperperistalsis.

5. Nonspecific dysfunctional abdominal pain and psychogenic abdominal pain are diagnoses of exclusion.
6. Mesenteric ischemia: Clients may present with acute onset of severe diffuse abdominal pain, often described as pain out of proportion to examination.
7. IBD—Ulcerative colitis (UC) and Crohn's disease (CD)
8. Ketoacidosis—Clients may have diffuse abdominal pain in diabetic/alcoholic ketoacidosis.
9. Viral gastroenteritis

Plan
A. General interventions:
1. If necessary, prepare the client for emergency transport and hospitalization.
2. Management and follow-up of other causes of abdominal pain are variable and depend on diagnosis.
B. Client teaching:
1. *See Section III: Client Teaching Guides for this chapter, "Abdominal Pain: Adults" and "Abdominal Pain: Children."* ◀
2. Counsel the client to keep a pain diary, including information on activity, foods, and other pain triggers (duration of pain and what provides relief of symptoms).
C. Pharmaceutical therapy:
1. Treatment depends on the findings from the history, physical examination, and testing, as well as the clinical diagnosis.

Follow-Up

A. Variable: Depends on diagnosis
B. Review the pain diary.

Consultation/Referral

A. Consult the physician for the client with acute abdominal pain and pain related to abdominal trauma.
B. For the obstetrical client, consult a physician for any bleeding or abdominal pain.
C. Surgical consultation when a surgical abdomen is suspected.

Individual Considerations

A. Pregnancy: There is no evidence that acute intra-abdominal surgical emergencies are more common during pregnancy if ectopic pregnancy is excluded.
　1. The presence of peritoneal signs, rebound tenderness, and abdominal guarding is never normal in pregnancy.
　2. Bleeding complications include the following:
　　a. First trimester: Miscarriage and ectopic pregnancy
　　b. Second and third trimesters: Abruptio placenta
　3. Physiological changes of pregnancy may affect the presentation and evaluation of abdominal pain. The enlargement of the uterus can impede physical examination, affect the normal location of pelvic and abdominal organs, and mask or delay peritoneal signs.
　4. Severe preeclampsia: The clinical manifestations of liver involvement include RUQ or midepigastric pain, elevated transaminases, and, in severe cases, subcapsular hemorrhage or hepatic rupture.

B. Pediatrics:
　1. The caregiver's lap makes the best examining surface. It is much better than having the child lie fixed and supine on a table.
　2. Observe the child's interaction and gait prior to examination. If able to stand, ask the child to hop as an assessment of peritoneal irritation. If the child is unwilling to stand, then shaking the examination table or pelvis can also evaluate for peritoneal signs.
　3. An infant's abdomen should be examined during a time of relaxation and quiet. It is often best to do this at the start of the overall examination, especially before initiating any procedure that may cause distress.
　4. Allowing an infant to suck on a pacifier may help relax him or her.
　5. Tenderness or pain on palpation may be difficult to detect in an infant. However, pain and tenderness are assessed by such behaviors as change in the pitch of crying, facial grimacing, rejection of opportunity to suck, and drawing the knees to the abdomen with palpation.
　6. Urinary tract infections (UTIs) can cause abdominal pain; often the child with a UTI does not complain of dysuria and frequency as adults typically do.
　7. Young children have inaccurate body perceptions and are inaccurate historians. The practitioner must rely on the caregiver and the examination for data.

Consider psychosocial aspects of child care and possible abuse.
　8. Appendicitis is the most common pediatric surgical emergency. The diagnosis can be difficult, because the classic symptoms are often not present.
　9. Intestinal malrotation must be considered when a healthy infant suddenly refuses to eat, vomits, becomes inconsolable, and develops abdominal distention.
　10. Intussusception presents as paroxysmal, colicky pain, and the infant often has currant-jelly stools; a palpable RUQ abdominal mass; and, ultimately, distention.
　11. Young male clients may hesitate to report testicular pain.
　12. Use of toys, and distracting objects and pictures help in gaining cooperation of young children, infants, and toddlers.

C. Adults:
　1. Obesity distorts the abdominal examination, making organ palpation or pelvic examination difficult
　2. With men older than age 40 and women older than age 50, suspect cardiac origin when presenting with epigastric pain. Consider obtaining an EKG for clients in this age group.

Although myocardial infarction (MI) "classically" presents with anterior chest pressure or pain, the client may also have a gastritis or heartburn sensation, coupled with nausea and diaphoresis.

D. Geriatrics:
　1. Elderly clients may have a vague or atypical presentation of pain, varying in location, severity, and presence of a fever or nonspecific findings on examination:
　　a. Classic findings of acute peritonitis, rebound tenderness, and local rigidity occur less often in the elderly.
　　b. After abdominal palpation, look for responses in facial expressions: confusion, surprise, or worry. Often geriatrics may not physically feel discomfort, yet they sense something is not normal for them.
　2. Elderly clients have a diminished sensorium, which may allow pathology to advance to a dangerous point prior to symptom development:
　　a. The level of pain is much less severe at presentation and continues to be at a lower level of pain.
　　b. Elderly clients may present with altered mental status.
　3. In an older client, a presentation similar to IBD with abdominal pain and a change in bowel habits can be the first sign of colon cancer.
　4. AAA is observed almost exclusively in elderly clients. Maintain a high index of suspicion in clients who present with a clinical picture suggestive of renal colic or musculoskeletal back pain:
　　a. Approximately 5% of men 65 years and older have AAA.

b. Maintain a high index of suspicion in clients who present with a clinical picture suggestive of renal colic or musculoskeletal back pain.

5. Elderly clients with UTI are less likely to have dysuria, frequency, or urgency.

6. Clients older than 65 years have a 30% to 50% risk of gallstones and may not present with significant pain; fewer than half have fever, vomiting, or leukocytosis.

7. Fever and an elevated white blood cell (WBC) count occur in fewer than half of all elderly clients with diverticulitis. Only about 25% of the elderly with diverticulitis present with a guaiac-positive stool.

8. The incidence of PUD is more common in the elderly due to the availability and use of NSAIDs. The most common presenting symptom with PUD in the elderly is melena.

Resource

Rome Foundation: https://theromefoundation.org

Bibliography

American College of Obstetricians and Gynecologists. (2018). Tubal ectopic pregnancy. *Clinical Management Guidelines for Obstetrician–Gynecologists, 193*(2018), 1e–10e. Retrieved from https://www.acog.org/Clinical-Guidance-and-Publications/Practice-Bulletins/Committee-on-Practice-Bulletins-Gynecology/Tubal-Ectopic-Pregnancy?IsMobileSet=false

American College of Physicians. (2019). Laboratory values. *ACP: Leading Internal Medicine, Improving Lives.* Retrieved from https://annualmeeting.acponline.org/sites/default/files/shared/documents/for-meeting-attendees/normal-lab-values.pdf

Ansari, P. (2018). Acute abdominal pain. In *Merck manual professional version.* Retrieved from https://www.merckmanuals.com/professional/gastrointestinal-disorders/acute-abdomen-and-surgical-gastroenterology/acute-abdominal-pain

Cartwright, S. L., & Knudson, M. P. (2015). Diagnostic imaging of acute abdominal pain in adults. *American Family Physician, 91,* 452–460. Retrieved from https://www.aafp.org/afp/2015/0401/p452.html

Crocket, J. R., Bastian, L. A., & Chireau, M. V. (2013). Does this woman have an ectopic pregnancy? The rational clinical examination systematic review. *Journal of the American Medical Association, 309,* 1722–1729. doi:10.1001/jama.2013.3914

Goldman, R. H., & Howard, H. (2016). Adult occupational lead poisoning. *UpToDate.* Retrieved from https://www.uptodate.com/contents/adult-occupational-lead-poisoning

Kendall, J. K., & Moreira, M. E. (2018, October 12). Evaluation of the adult with abdominal pain in the emergency department. *UpToDate.* Retrieved from https://www.uptodate.com/contents/evaluation-of-the-adult-with-abdominal-pain-in-the-emergency-department#H14

Lautenbacher, S., Walz, A., & Kunz, M. (2018). Using observational facial descriptors to infer pain in persons with and without dementia. *BMC Geriatrics, 18*(88), e1–e10. https://doi.org/10.1186/s12877-018-0773-8

Lowry, J. A. (2019, February 12). Childhood lead poisoning: Clinical manifestations and diagnosis. *UpToDate.* Retrieved from https://www.uptodate.com/contents/childhood-lead-poisoning-clinical-manifestations-and-diagnosis?search=coproporphyrin%20in%20lead%20poisoning&source=search_result&selectedTitle=1~150&usage_type=default&display_rank=1#H10

Nettina, S. (2010). *The Lippincott manual of nursing practice* (9th ed.). Philadelphia, PA: Wolters Kluwer Lippincott Williams & Wilkins.

Neuman, M. I. (2018, April 2). Causes of acute abdominal pain in children and adolescents. *UpToDate.* Retrieved from https://www.uptodate.com/contents/causes-of-acute-abdominal-pain-in-children-and-adolescents

Penner, R. M., & Fishman, M. B. (2017, November 2). Evaluation of the adult with abdominal pain. *UpToDate.* Retrieved from https://www.uptodate.com/contents/evaluation-of-the-adult-with-abdominal-pain#H23

Penner, R. M., & Fishman, M. B. (2019, April 3). Causes of abdominal pain in adults. *UpToDate.* Retrieved from https://www.uptodate.com/contents/causes-of-abdominal-pain-in-adults#H629462043

Reust, C., & Williams, A. (2016). Acute abdominal pain in children. *American Family Physician, 93,* 830–837.

Solomkin, J. S., Mazuski, J. E., Bradley, J. S., Rodvold, K. A., Goldstein, E. J., Baron, E. J., . . . Bartlett, J. G. (2010). Diagnosis and management of complicated intra-abdominal infection in adults and children: Guidelines by the Surgical Infection Society and the Infectious Diseases Society of America. *Clinical Infectious Disease, 50*(2), 133–164. doi:10.1086/649554

Vege, S. S. (2019, January 9). Etiology of acute pancreatitis. *UpToDate.* Retrieved from https://www.uptodate.com/contents/etiology-of-acute-pancreatitis

Zakko, S. F. (2018, February 21). Patient education: Gallstones (beyond the basics). *UpToDate.* Retrieved from https://www.uptodate.com/contents/gallstones-beyond-the-basics

Appendicitis

Cheryl A. Glass, Audra Malone, and Doncy Eapen

Definition

A. Appendicitis is acute inflammation of the appendix caused by the obstruction of the appendiceal lumen. Perforation is rare in the first 12 hours, but the rate of possible perforation increases after 72 hours. Prompt, early diagnosis and intervention are the goal of treatment. The differential diagnoses for appendicitis include all abdominal sources of pain.

Incidence

A. Acute appendicitis occurs at a rate of 10 per 100,000 population; 250,000 cases are reported annually in the United States. It is the most common condition in children (1%–8%) and during pregnancy (0.06%–0.1%) that requires emergency abdominal surgery. One in every 2,000 adults older than age 65 years will develop appendicitis.

Pathogenesis

A. Foreign bodies, fecal material, tissue hypertrophy, strictures, or a bend or twist on the organ may cause obstruction of the appendix. The obstruction causes colicky pain. Bacterial invasion causes inflammation and leads to gangrene and perforation. The most common bacteria are *Escherichia coli*, *Pseudomonas*, *Bacteroides fragilis*, and *Peptostreptococcus* species.

Predisposing Factors

A. Pregnancy
B. Torsion
C. Abdominal trauma
D. Male; ages 10 to 30 years

Common Complaints

> The classic history of anorexia and periumbilical pain followed by nausea, RLQ pain, and vomiting occurs in only 50% of cases.

A. Adults:

1. Generalized or localized abdominal pain in the epigastric or periumbilical areas. Within 2 to 12 hours, pain localizes in RLQ at McBurney's point, and intensity increases.

2. The location of the appendix is altered in pregnancy and with anatomical variations.
3. Pain typically develops before vomiting.
4. Nausea and/or vomiting (may be projectile)
5. Anorexia signals an organic cause of abdominal pain.
6. Elderly clients may present with confusion. The duration of symptoms is longer than 48 hours in elderly persons.
B. Pediatrics:
  1. Children younger than 2 years:
    a. Abdominal distention
    b. Irritability
    c. Lethargy
    d. Fever
  2. Children older than 2 years:
    a. Vomiting is often the first symptom.
    b. Abdominal pain in RLQ
    c. Fever

Other Signs and Symptoms
A. Rigid abdomen
B. Changes in pulse (tachycardia), breathing (tachypnea), or skin temperature
C. Involuntary guarding
D. Rebound tenderness

Subjective Data
Evaluate for a "surgical abdomen," defined as a rapidly worsening prognosis in the absence of surgical intervention. Clients should not eat or drink while a diagnosis of a surgical abdomen remains under consideration. Once a surgical abdomen has been excluded, the remainder of the evaluation will be guided by the chronicity of symptoms along with the location of pain.
A. Review the onset, duration, course, and quality of pain. Has pain ever occurred before? If so, what was the primary diagnosis? What was the previous treatment, and was it effective?
B. Qualify the duration of pain in minutes, hours, days, weeks, or months. Does it interfere with sleep? Is there a pattern to the pain?
C. Have the client rate the pain on a 10-point pain scale, with 0 being no pain and 10 being the worst pain the client has ever felt.
D. Review the pattern of pain:
  1. Review aggravating factors.
  2. Review alleviating factors.
  3. Does the pain radiate?
  4. Does the pain have any relationship to food?
E. Questions specific to females:
  1. Determine the client's LMP to rule out pregnancy.
  2. What type of contraception is used? Specifically evaluate for an IUD.
  3. Has she had a hysterectomy or tubal ligation?
  4. Does she have a recent history of dyspareunia or dysmenorrhea that suggests pelvic pathology?
F. Review current medications and drug history, especially antibiotic and laxative use. Clients taking corticosteroids may have a significant masking of pain.

G. Rule out abdominal trauma, motor vehicle accidents, falls, and assault.
H. Discuss bowel habits, including any changes, such as constipation or diarrhea, anorexia, food intolerance, nausea and vomiting, and bloating.
I. Ask the client about urinary frequency, urgency, dysuria, flank pain, and back pain. In males, ask about hesitancy, difficulty starting the urine stream, nocturia, low urinary volume, or lower abdominal distention (urinary retention).

Physical Examination
A. Check temperature, pulse, respirations, and BP, including orthostatic BP.
B. Inspect:
  1. Observe general appearance: Facial expressions (grimace during examination), walk, skin color and turgor, level of consciousness, and acuity level of pain.
  2. Inspect the abdomen for surgical scars.
  3. Observe for any bruising or other signs of domestic violence in the "bathing suit" area—breasts, abdomen, or back—that would be easily covered by clothes.
C. Auscultate:
  1. Abdomen for bowel sounds in all quadrants
  2. Heart and lungs
D. Percuss:
  1. Abdomen for tympany
E. Palpate:
Palpate at the end of the examination because a positive response produces pain and muscle spasm that can interfere with subsequent examination. Note guarding during the exam.
  1. Ask the client to bend his or her knees to help relax abdominal wall musculature.
  2. Assess for McBurney's point tenderness—tenderness at 1.5 to 2 inches on a straight line from the anterior superior iliac spine (ASIS) to the umbilicus.
  3. Check for Murphy's sign, which is inspiratory arrest in response to RUQ palpation, seen in acute cholecystitis.
  4. Check for rebound tenderness.
  5. Check for jar tenderness—pain elicited in the lower area of the abdomen when the standing client drops from standing on toes to the heels with a jarring landing.
  6. Palpate the back; note CVAT.
  7. Check for the obturator sign, or abdominal pain in response to passive internal rotation of the right hip from a 90° angle hip–knee flexion position. A positive sign indicates pain secondary to irritation of the obturator muscle with an inflamed appendix.
  8. Assess for the psoas sign, or increased abdominal pain occurring when the client attempts to raise his or her right thigh against the pressure of the clinician's hand placed over the client's right knee. Pain is caused by inflammation of the psoas muscle in acute appendicitis.
  9. Check for the Apley rule: The farther the pain from the navel, the more likely it is organic in origin.

FIGURE 11.1 The position of the appendix is altered during pregnancy, and likewise for the site of incision to gain access.

10. Check for Rovsing's sign, or pain in the RLQ on palpation of the left side, suggesting appendicitis.
11. Anatomical variations of the appendix may lead to differences in the location of the pain. For example, the location of the appendix changes with pregnancy (Figure 11.1); a retrocecal appendix (inflamed appendix located behind cecum) may lead to right groin pain.
12. Perform rectal or pelvic examination if needed. Clients may have right-side pain with a subcecal or pelvic appendix.

Diagnostic Tests

A. **Serum HCG: Pregnancy should be excluded in all women of childbearing age. Assume that the woman is pregnant until proven otherwise.**
B. CBC with differential
C. C-reactive protein (CRP)
D. Urinalysis, to rule out urinary disorders
E. Abdominal ultrasonography; any person with trauma to the abdomen should have an abdominal ultrasound.
F. CT scan with or without contrast
G. MRI may be used as an alternative diagnostic test in pregnancy to avoid exposure to ionizing radiation.
H. Stool guaiac test for occult blood

Differential Diagnoses

The appendix has no fixed position. The duration of pain can significantly help in narrowing the differential diagnosis. Nonspecific dysfunctional abdominal pain and psychogenic abdominal pain are diagnoses of exclusion.

A. Appendicitis
B. Regional enteritis
C. Leaking aneurysm
D. Ruptured ectopic pregnancy
E. Ovarian cyst
F. Ovarian torsion
G. PID
H. Mittelschmerz (ovulatory bleeding or pain)
I. Endometriosis
J. Ureteral calculi
K. Incarcerated, strangulated groin hernia
L. Meckel's diverticulitis
M. Abdominal wall hematoma
N. Bowel obstruction
O. Intestinal malrotation
P. Intussusception
Q. Testicular torsion
R. IBD/CD
S. Parasites
T. IUD
U. Constipation

Plan

A. General interventions:
   1. **Consult with the physician and prepare the client for admission to the hospital for surgery.**
   2. Surgical management: Open versus laparoscopic appendectomy is the standard treatment for acute appendicitis.
B. Client teaching: *See Section III: Client Teaching Guides for this chapter, "Abdominal Pain: Adults" and "Abdominal Pain: Children."*
C. Pharmaceutical therapy:
   1. Antibiotics are used to treat uncomplicated, nonsurgical appendicitis; however, there is a 5% to 15% rate of complications and a 15% to 30% recurrence rate. More studies are needed to determine the efficacy of antibiotic therapy alone. Prophylactic antibiotic are also used perioperatively and postoperatively to prevent wound infection and intra-abdominal abscess following appendectomy.
   2. Do not give antipyretics to mask fever.
   3. Do not administer cathartics because they may cause rupture.

Follow-Up

A. Postoperative follow-up is with the surgeon.

Consultation/Referral

A. Physician consultation and possible emergency transport and hospitalization are often required.

Individual Considerations

A. Pregnancy:
   1. Any abdominal pain or bleeding in the first 8 weeks after a missed menstrual period must be considered a symptom of possible *ectopic pregnancy.*
   2. The identification of intra-abdominal masses may be compromised by the enlarged uterus, but this problem may be partially obviated by examining the woman in the lateral position.

3. The intestinal tract is progressively displaced upward, outward, and backward during pregnancy; bowel sounds are best heard lateral or superior to the uterus.

B. Pediatrics:

1. The caregiver's lap makes the best examining surface. It is much better than having the child lie fixed and supine on a table.

2. If possible, examine the infant's abdomen during a time of relaxation and quiet. It is often best to do this at the start of the overall examination, especially before initiating any procedure that might cause distress. Allowing the infant to suck on a bottle or pacifier may help relax him or her.

3. Tenderness or pain on palpation may be difficult to detect in the infant. However, pain and tenderness are assessed by such behaviors as change in the pitch of crying, facial grimacing, rejection of the opportunity to suck, and drawing knees to the abdomen with palpation.

4. Intestinal malrotation must be considered when a healthy infant suddenly refuses to eat, vomits, becomes inconsolable, and develops abdominal distention.

5. Young children have inaccurate body perceptions and are inaccurate historians, so rely on caregivers and examination for data, and consider psychosocial aspects such as child care and child abuse.

6. Intussusception presents as paroxysmal, colicky pain, and the infant often has currant-jelly stools, a palpable RUQ, abdominal mass, and ultimately distention.

C. Adults:

1. Obesity distorts the abdominal examination, making organ palpation or pelvic examination difficult.

2. Immunocompromised clients are susceptive to infection. They may not exhibit the typical signs and symptoms of appendicitis, but rather show only mild tenderness on examination.

3. To make a diagnosis in the immunocompromised client, a CT examination is useful.

D. Geriatrics:

1. The elderly tend to have a diminished inflammatory response, resulting in a less remarkable history and physical examination. Be aware of vague symptoms, such as milder pain, less pronounced fever, and leukocytosis with shift to left on differential.

2. Confusion is a common presenting symptom.

3. A redundant sigmoid colon may also cause right-sided pain from sigmoid disease.

4. Prompt CT scan is used for diagnosis and differential.

Bibliography

American College of Obstetricians and Gynecologists. (2018). Tubal ectopic pregnancy. *Clinical Management Guidelines for Obstetrician–Gynecologists*, *193*(2018), 1e–10e. Retrieved from https://www.acog.org/Clinical-Guidance-and-Publications/Practice-Bulletins/Committee-on-Practice-Bulletins-Gynecology/Tubal-Ectopic-Pregnancy?IsMobileSet=false

Craig, S. (2018, July 23). Appendicitis: Epidemiology. *Medscape*. Retrieved from https://emedicine.medscape.com/article/773895-overview#a6

Crocket, J. R., Bastian, L. A., & Chireau, M. V. (2013). Does this woman have an ectopic pregnancy? The rational clinical examination systematic review. *Journal of the American Medical Association*, *309*, 1722–1729. doi:10.1001/jama.2013.3914

Ehlers, A. P., Talan, D. A., Moran, G. J., Flum, D. R., & Davidson, G. H. (2016). Evidence for an antibiotics first strategy for uncomplicated appendicitis in adults: A systematic review and gap analysis. *Journal of the American College of Surgeons*, *222*, 309–314. doi:10.1016/j.jamcollsurg.2015.11.009

Martin, R. F. (2018, April 27). Acute appendicitis in adults: Clinical manifestations and differential diagnosis. *UpToDate*. Retrieved from https://www.uptodate.com/contents/acute-appendicitis-in-adults-clinical-manifestations-and-differential-diagnosis

Nettina, S. (2010). *The Lippincott manual of nursing practice* (9th ed.). Philadelphia, PA: Wolters Kluwer Lippincott Williams & Wilkins.

Smink, D., & Soybel, D. I. (2019, April 1). Management of acute appendicitis in adults. *UpToDate*. Retrieved from https://www.uptodate.com/contents/management-of-acute-appendicitis-in-adults?topicRef=1386&source=see_link

Celiac Disease

Cheryl A. Glass, Audra Malone, and Doncy Eapen

Definition

A. Celiac disease, previously known as *celiac sprue*, is an autoimmune disorder triggered by a well-defined environmental factor, gluten. Celiac disease is a permanent sensitivity to gluten; specifically, affected people are unable to tolerate gliadin, the alcohol-soluble fraction of gluten. Three cereals contain gluten and are considered toxic for clients with celiac disease: wheat, rye, and barley. The disease primarily affects the small intestine and is characterized by mucosal inflammation, villous atrophy, and crypt hyperplasia that occur upon exposure to dietary gluten. Onset of symptoms depends on the amount of gluten in the diet. Dietary nonadherence is the chief cause of persistent or recurrent symptoms (see Appendix B, Table B.5).

B. Celiac disease is one of the most common causes of chronic malabsorption as a result of injury to the small intestine with loss of absorptive surface area, reduction of digestive enzymes, and consequential impaired absorption of micronutrients such as fat-soluble vitamins, iron, and potentially vitamin B_{12} and folic acid.

C. Celiac disease is strongly associated with autoimmune conditions, including type 1 diabetes, Addison disease, and thyroiditis, as well as genetic syndromes, including Down syndrome, Williams syndrome, and Turner syndrome. Complications from celiac disease include osteopenia, osteoporosis, infertility, short stature, delayed puberty, anemia, GI malignancies, and non-Hodgkin's lymphoma (NHL).

D. After GI symptoms, the second most common manifestation of celiac disease in clients with type 1 diabetes is diminished or impaired bone mineralization.

E. Celiac disease is the most common cause of steatorrhea in people older than 50 years and the second most common cause in people older than 65 years.

F. A substantial number of clients are misdiagnosed as having IBS for years before the diagnosis of celiac disease is made.

Incidence

A. Celiac disease can occur at any stage of life. The prevalence of celiac disease in children is unknown. Its prevalence is approximately 1% of the general population in North America. The highest incidence (5%) is noted in the sub-Saharan African population. The true incidence is undetermined due to asymptomatic disease and underdiagnosis. It is estimated that 75% of those affected by celiac disease remain underdiagnosed or misdiagnosed.

B. **Screening of the general population is not recommended.**

C. Newly diagnosed clients with celiac disease should inform their first-degree family members of their increased risk of celiac disease and the American College of Gastroenterology (ACG) recommendation for testing.

Pathogenesis

A. Interactions between gluten and immune and genetic factors result in celiac disease. Gluten is poorly digested. The enzyme tissue transglutaminase (tTG) is the autoantigen against which abnormal immune response is directed. The immune responses promote an inflammatory reaction. Celiac disease primarily affects the mucosal layer of the small intestine. The classic celiac lesion is noted in the proximal small intestine.

B. **A hallmark on histology is the presence of villous atrophy.** The Marsh classification is used to describe the progressive histological stages of celiac disease. Marsh 1 and Marsh 2 may be seen in sow and cow's milk allergies:

Marsh 0: Pre-infiltrative stage (normal)

Marsh 1: Infiltrative lesion (increased intraepithelial lymphocytes)

Marsh 2: Hyperplastic lesion (type 1 plus hyperplastic crypts)

Marsh 3: Destructive lesion (type 2 plus villous atrophy of progressively more severe degrees [termed 3a, 3b, and 3c])

Marsh 4 (atrophic-hypoplastic): Total villous atrophy, crypt hypoplasia

Predisposing Factors

A. Female gender

B. May be precipitated by an infectious diarrheal episode or other intestinal disease (e.g., rotavirus)

C. Genetic disorders:
1. Down syndrome (8%–12%)
2. Type 1 diabetes (10%)
3. Turner syndrome (2%–10%)
4. Williams syndrome (8.2%)

D. Strong hereditary component (10% in first-degree relatives)

E. The introduction of gluten before 4 months of age is associated with increased disease development.

F. Autoimmune thyroiditis

G. Selective immunoglobulin A (IgA) deficiency

Common Complaints

A. Asymptomatic

B. Chronic diarrhea or explosive watery diarrhea

C. Foul-smelling voluminous stools

D. Anorexia

E. Abdominal distention

F. Abdominal pain

G. Poor weight gain or weight loss

H. Vomiting

I. Steatorrhea (malabsorption of ingested fat)

J. Refusal to eat (children)

Other Signs and Symptoms

A. Behavioral changes, including irritability

B. Dehydration

C. Lethargy

D. Constipation

E. Failure to thrive (FTT)

F. Short stature and delayed puberty

G. Dermatitis herpetiformis

H. Arthritis

I. Seizures

J. Weakness and fatigue

K. Dental enamel hypoplasia of permanent teeth

L. Iron-deficiency anemia unresponsive to treatment

M. Bruising/bleeding tendency

N. Osteopenia/osteoporosis

O. Hair loss

P. Lactose intolerance

Q. Aphthous stomatitis

R. Ataxia

S. Neuropathy

T. Migraines/headaches

Subjective Data

A. Review the onset, duration, course, and type of symptoms.

B. Review the client's weight history.

C. Evaluate family history for celiac disease or members with similar histories.

D. Review current medications and drug history, especially antibiotic, laxative, and herbal products.

E. Review bowel habits and note changes: Constipation, diarrhea, anorexia, and/or food intolerance

F. Review the client's tolerance of lactose products.

Physical Examination

A. Check vital signs, including height and weight. Follow serial weights and plot serial height/weight on growth charts.

B. Inspect:
1. Observe general overall appearance.
2. Oral examination to evaluate for glossitis, dry mucosal membranes (dehydration), and the presence of oral aphthae
3. Examine the skin for the presence of dermatitis herpetiformis: A blistering rash involving the scalp, neck, elbows, knees, and buttocks.
4. Evaluate the abdomen for the presence of bloating and protuberant "potbelly."
5. Evaluate the client's weight loss, including muscle wasting.

C. Auscultate:
1. For bowel sounds in all four quadrants of the abdomen

D. Percuss:
1. Abdomen: May present with tympanic sounds, especially in children.

E. Palpate:
1. Palpate the abdomen for masses, rebound tenderness, and peritoneal signs.
   a. Before palpating the abdomen, ask the client to bend his or her knees to help with relaxation of the wall musculature.
2. Perform a rectal examination, including testing stool for occult blood.

Diagnostic Tests

The confirmation of a diagnosis of celiac disease is based on the combination of findings from the medical history, physical examination, serology, and upper endoscopy, with histological analysis of multiple biopsies of the duodenum. **All testing should be performed while clients are following a gluten-rich diet.**

A. **Endoscopy for duodenal biopsies is the standard and a critical component for diagnosing celiac disease.**

B. Screening and monitoring tests for celiac disease (see Table 11.1 for celiac disease tests and possible results):
1. tTG antibody, IgA class:
   a. Primary test ordered to screen for celiac disease
   b. Used for monitoring and evaluating the effectiveness of treatment
   c. Antibody levels should fall when gluten is removed from the diet
2. Anti-tTG antibodies, immunoglobulin G (IgG)
3. Anti-tTG, IgG class
4. Deamidated gliadin peptide antibodies (anti-DGP, IgA)
5. Antigliadin antibodies (AGAs) IgG (gliadin is a component of wheat-storage protein gluten)
6. AGA IgA

7. IgA endomysial antibody (EMA): Less frequently ordered; measures the same thing as the anti-tTG test
8. Antireticulin antibody (ARA): Rarely ordered
9. Anti-F-actin: Ordered if the disease has been diagnosed; evaluates the severity of intestinal damage. May be used for monitoring

C. CBC and electrolytes

D. Aspartate transaminase (AST) and alanine transaminase (ALT): Liver enzymes normalize on a gluten-free diet.

E. Prothrombin time (PT): May be prolonged with malabsorption of vitamin K

F. CRP

G. Erythrocyte sedimentation rate (ESR)

H. Total protein

I. Albumin

J. Calcium

K. Iron, transferrin, and ferritin

L. Vitamin B_{12} and folate levels

M. Thyroid screen: Autoimmune thyroid disorders and hypothyroidism are common in the elderly.

N. Stool tests: Culture, ova, and parasites; 72-hour fecal fat collection to detect steatorrhea

O. Fecal fat

P. Bone density: Bone mineral density improves on a gluten-free diet

Q. HLA haplotypes

R. Colonoscopy if the client has bloody stools or symptoms of colitis

S. Sweat test to exclude cystic fibrosis (CF)

T. Other testing specific to nutritional deficiencies as needed (vitamins D, B_{12}, folate)

U. Radiograph, including barium swallow study with a small-bowel follow-through, is usually nonspecific and is not indicated.

TABLE 11.1   SOME CELIAC DISEASE TESTS AND POSSIBLE RESULTS

tTG, IgA	Total IgA	tTG, IgG	DGP, IgA	DGP, IgG	Diagnosis
Positive	Normal	Not performed	Not performed	Not performed	Presumptive celiac disease
Negative	Normal	Negative	Negative	Negative	Symptoms not likely due to celiac disease
Negative	Low	Positive	Negative	Positive	Possible celiac disease (false negative anti-tTG, IgA, and anti-DGP, IgA are due to total IgA deficiency)
Negative	Normal	Negative	Positive	Positive (or not performed)	Possible celiac disease (may be seen in children younger than 3 years old)

AGA, antigliadin antibodies; DGP, deamidated gliadin peptide; IgA, immunoglobulin A; IgG, immunoglobulin G; tTG, tissue transglutaminase.

Source: American Association for Clinical Chemistry. (2018, October 28). Celiac disease antibody tests. *Lab Tests Online*. Retrieved from https://labtestsonline.org/tests/celiac-disease-antibody-tests. Reprinted with permission from Lab Tests Online.

Differential Diagnoses

A. Celiac disease
B. Child or adult FTT
C. Food allergies
D. IBD:
   1. CD
   2. UC
E. Immunodeficiency disorders
F. Gastroenteritis (viral or bacterial)
G. Parasites
H. Fungal infection
I. IBS
J. Malabsorption
K. Lymphomas of the small intestine

Plan

A. General interventions:
   1. Nutritional therapy is the only accepted treatment for celiac disease.
   2. Gluten-free dietary instructions should be given and clients advised of the need to read all food labels.
   3. Genetic testing does not diagnose celiac disease.
   4. Screen for osteoporosis: As many as 70% of adult and elderly clients with celiac disease have osteopenia.
   5. Gluten rechallenge is not generally recommended unless the diagnosis remains uncertain:
      a. The rechallenge is not mandatory for clients with good improvement of symptoms.
      b. HLA-DQ2/DQ8 genotyping for genetic risk factors should be used to try to exclude celiac disease prior to a formal gluten challenge.
B. Client teaching:
   1. The ACG recommends a referral to a registered dietitian so that the client can receive a thorough nutritional assessment and education on a gluten-free diet. Stress that "wheat-free" is not the same as "gluten-free."
   2. A gluten-free diet should be maintained for life.
   3. Nutriguides "nutrition guides" apps are available from the iTunes Store for iPhone and iPad and from Google Play for Android products.
   4. Monitor for iron and vitamin deficiencies because substitute flours are not fortified with B vitamins. Supplement with iron, folate, and vitamin B_{12} as needed.
   5. Keep a food/symptom diary to help identify and eliminate trigger foods. See Appendix B, Table B.5.
   6. Gluten has been identified in dietary supplements, over-the-counter (OTC) medications, and nonfood items such as lipstick and envelope adhesive, and in food items with gluten additives such as condiments.
C. Pharmaceutical therapy:
   1. Corticosteroids may be prescribed for rapid control of symptoms: Prednisone (Deltasone, Orasone, Sterapred):
      a. Adults: 30 to 40 mg/d; taper off completely in 6 to 8 weeks
      b. Pediatrics: 1 mg/kg/d; not to exceed 30 mg/d. Taper off completely in 6 to 8 weeks. Children with celiac disease are rarely given steroids.
   2. Bisphosphonates for osteoporosis

Follow-Up

A. After the diagnosis of celiac disease is made and a strict diet has been started, follow up in 4 to 8 weeks or earlier if the client has other comorbidities.
B. The Celiac Disease Guideline Committee recommends the measurement of tTG after 6 months of a gluten-free diet.
C. Newly diagnosed clients with celiac disease should undergo testing and treatment for micronutrient deficiencies. Deficiency testing should include, but not be limited to, iron, folic acid, vitamin D, and vitamin B_{12}.
D. Refer the client for dietary consultation with a nutritionist with experience in gluten-free diets.
E. Consider allergy testing.

Consultation/Referral

A. If the gluten-free diet fails or the client experiences new symptoms, a systematic evaluation is required.
B. Endocrine consultation for clients with Hashimoto thyroiditis and celiac disease
C. Consultation with a pediatric gastroenterologist

Individual Considerations

A. Pregnancy:
   1. Women with untreated celiac disease are at risk for preterm birth, low-birth-weight babies, recurrent loss, and reduced fertility.
B. Pediatrics:
   1. Children may appear to have a "potbelly" with muscle wasting from malnutrition.
   2. Monitor growth and development. Utilize a growth chart to plot growth rates. As many as 10% of children with idiopathic short stature may have celiac disease.
   3. Breastfeeding has a protective role even if gluten is introduced while breastfeeding.
   4. Biliary sludge and/or gallstones are likely to form in one in five children with hemolytic anemia before the adolescent years.
C. Geriatrics:
   1. The elderly may present with nonspecific GI symptoms, abdominal discomfort, bloating, constipation, or dyspepsia.
   2. Diarrhea may be mild or intermittent in the elderly.
   3. Iron-deficiency anemia may also be a presenting symptom. Anemia is present in 60% to 80% of elderly clients with celiac disease.
   4. The elderly are at increased risk for falls related to osteopenia, ataxia, and neuropathy.
   5. Autoimmune thyroid disorders are common with elderly clients with celiac disease. The majority present with hypothyroidism.
   6. The risk for NHL is increased in people with celiac disease aged 50 years and older.

Resources

www.celiac.com
www.celiac.com/categories/Gluten-Free--Recipes-c-3400
   .html
www.celiac.org
www.gluten-freedrugs.com

Bibliography

Academy of Nutrition and Dietetics. (n.d.). *Celiac disease evidence-based nutrition practice guideline*. Retrieved from http://www.adaevidencelibrary.com/topic.cfm?cat=3677

American Association for Clinical Chemistry. (2015, February 24). Celiac disease antibody tests. *Lab Tests Online*. Retrieved from http://labtestsonline.org/understanding/analytes/celiac-disease/tab/test

American Association for Clinical Chemistry. (2019). *Lab tests online: Patient test information*. LabCorp. Retrieved from https://www.labcorp.com

Centers for Disease Control and Prevention. (2018, July 25). *Rotavirus vaccination*. Celiac Disease Foundation. Retrieved from https://www.cdc.gov/vaccines/vpd/rotavirus/index.html

Goebel, S. U. (2018, October 10). Celiac disease (sprue). *Medscape*. Retrieved from http://emedicine.medscape.com/article/171805-overview

Hammer, H., & Hogenauer, C. (2020). Lactose intolerance: Clinical manifestations, diagnosis, and management. *UpToDate*. Retrieved from https://www.uptodate.com/contents/lactose-intolerance-clinical-manifestations-diagnosis-and-management

Husby, S., Murray, J. A., & Katzka, D. A. (2019). AGA clinical practice update on diagnosing and monitoring of celiac disease: Changing utility of serology and histologic measures: Expert review. *Gastroenterology*, *156*(4), 885–889. doi:10.1053/j.gastro.2018.12.010

Kelly, C. P. (2018, November 28). Diagnosis of celiac disease in adults. *UpToDate*. Retrieved from https://www.uptodate.com/contents/diagnosis-of-celiac-disease-in-adults

Kelly, C. P., & Dennis, M. (2018, October 8). Patient education: Celiac disease in adults: Beyond the basics. *UpToDate*. Retrieved from https://www.uptodate.com/contents/celiac-disease-in-adults-beyond-the-basics#H21

Nettina, S. (2010). *The Lippincott manual of nursing practice* (9th ed.). Philadelphia, PA: Wolters Kluwer Lippincott Williams & Wilkins.

RotaTeq (rotavirus vaccine, live, oral, pentavalent). (2017). *Highlights of prescribing information*. Retrieved from http://www.fda.gov/downloads/BiologicsBloodVaccines/Vaccines/ApprovedProducts/UCM142288.pdf

Rubio-Tapia, A., Hill, I. D., Kelly, C. P., Calderwood, A. H., & Murray, J. A. (2013, May). ACG clinical guidelines: Diagnosis and management of celiac disease. *American Journal of Gastroenterology*, *108*(1), 656–676. doi:10.1038/ajg.2013.79. Retrieved from http://gi.org/guideline/diagnosis-and-management-of-celiac-disease

Sharma, G. D. (2019, May 2). Cystic fibrosis. *Medscape*. Retrieved from http://emedicine.medscape.com/article/1001602-overview

Trandafir, L., Tesariu, O., Diaconescu, I. M., Miron, I., Sârbu, I., & Ciongradi, I. (2016). Unusual presentation of celiac disease in a toddler from a pediatric surgery unit. *International Journal of Celiac Disease*, *4*(2), 74–76. doi:10.12691/ijcd-4-2-8

University of Chicago Celiac Disease Center. (n.d.). *Gluten free diet*. Retrieved from http://www.celiacdisease.net/glutenfree-diet

Zakko, S. F. (2018, February 21). Patient education: Gallstones (beyond the basics). *UpToDate*. Retrieved from https://www.uptodate.com/contents/gallstones-beyond-the-basics

Cholecystitis

Cheryl A. Glass, Audra Malone, and Doncy Eapen

Definition

A. Cholecystitis is acute or chronic inflammation of the gallbladder. Acute cholecystitis has associated stone formation (cholelithiasis) in 90% of all cases, causing obstruction and inflammation. Biliary sludge is a feature of chronic cholecystitis.

Incidence

A. Gallstones affect approximately 10% to 20% of Americans and one-third of these people develop acute cholecystitis. The exact frequency of cholecystitis in children is not known, but the overall incidence in children has increased in the past three decades due to high fat consumption. Most clients with an acute attack of cholecystitis have complete remission in 1 to 5 days; however, approximately 20% require surgical intervention. Mortality related to acute cholecystitis is 5% to 10%, with the highest risk for clients older than 60 years. The most common complication is the development of gallbladder gangrene in up to 20% of cases, with the potential for subsequent perforation in approximately 10% of cases. Gangrenous cholecystitis is most common in older clients, clients with diabetes, and clients who delay treatment.

B. Cholecystectomy for recurrent biliary colic or acute cholecystitis is the most common major surgical procedure performed by general surgeons.

Pathogenesis

A. Cholecystitis occurs subsequent to bile stasis, bacterial infection, ischemia, or obstruction by a gallstone. Acute cholecystitis is related to the impaction of a calculus in the neck of the gallbladder in approximately 90% of cases. This can lead to gallbladder distention and compromise of blood flow and lymphatic drainage, leading to mucosal ischemia and necrosis. Spontaneous resolution may occur after the reestablishment of cystic duct patency.

B. *E. coli* is the primary microorganism in 80% of cholecystitis infections.

C. Estrogen-induced alteration in bile salts may favor stone formation. Stones occur when cholesterol supersaturates the bile in the gallbladder and precipitates out of the bile. Cholesterol stones are the most common type of gallstones in the United States.

D. Pigment stones occur when free bilirubin combines with calcium. Pigment stones are found in clients with cirrhosis, hemolysis, and infections in the biliary tree.

E. Acalculous cholecystitis is associated with infection and local inflammation. Formation of gallstones is not necessary for the obstruction of the bile duct.

Predisposing Factors

A. Female gender
B. Ethnic groups: Northern European and Hispanic
C. Sudden starvation/prolonged fasting
D. Medications:
 1. Cholesterol-lowering drugs: Stone formation increases in users of cholesterol-lowering drugs, which are known to increase biliary cholesterol saturation.
 2. Estrogen usage (oral contraceptives [OCPs] and hormone replacement therapy [HRT]): Stone formation increases in users of contraceptives and estrogens, which are known to increase biliary cholesterol saturation.
 3. Furosemide
 4. Ceftriaxone
 5. Cyclosporine
 6. Opiate narcotic analgesics
 7. Octreotide
E. Bile acid malabsorption
F. Genetic predisposition: Native Americans and those of Chinese or Japanese descent have a high incidence
G. Total parenteral nutrition (TPN)

H. Obesity
I. Status post bariatric surgery
J. Pregnancy secondary to elevated progesterone
K. Increasing age
L. Hemolytic anemia
M. Diabetes
N. High serum triglyceride and low high-density lipo-protein (HDL) levels
O. High-caloric and refined-carbohydrate diet
P. Cirrhosis, CD, and gallbladder stasis

Common Complaints

A. Abrupt, severe abdominal pain lasting 24 hours
B. Constant aching pain in the RUQ, right subcostal region, with radiation to the back and right shoulder
C. Nausea and vomiting
D. Acalculous cholecystitis may present with fever and sepsis alone

Other Signs and Symptoms

A. Anorexia
B. Heartburn
C. Upper abdominal fullness
D. Biliary colic: Sudden onset of severe pain in the epigastrium or right hypochondrium that subsides relatively slowly. Tenderness may remain for days.
E. Fat intolerance
F. Fever (low grade)
G. Mild jaundice (20%)
H. Complicated disease such as an abscess or perforation; symptoms include more severe localized persistent pain, tenderness, fever, chills, and leukocytosis.

Subjective Data

A. Review the onset, location, duration, course, and quality of pain.
B. Use a pain-rating scale, such as a 10-point pain scale, with 0 being no pain and 10 being equivalent to the worst pain the client has ever felt. Determine the progression of the pain as well.
C. Review any alleviating factors, such as antacids, and any worsening factors, such as deep inspiration.
D. Review any pain radiating to the jaw, neck, shoulder, or arm.
E. Review the onset of pain in relation to the last meal and foods ingested.
F. Ask the client about recurrent history of epigastric pain.
G. Obtain a history and demographic data that may indicate the risk factors for biliary disease.
H. Review the date of the client's LMP, and, if she is pregnant, establish gestational age.

Physical Examination

The absence of physical findings does not rule out the diagnosis of cholecystitis.
A. Check temperature, pulse (tachycardia), respirations, and BP.
B. Inspect:
  1. Observe the client's general appearance, facial expressions, gait, skin color (15% have jaundice)

and turgor, and grimace during examination. Overall appearance is generally unremarkable between attacks; ill appearance occurs during an acute attack.
C. Auscultate:
  1. Heart
  2. Lung fields
  3. Abdomen for bowel sounds in all four quadrants
D. Percuss the abdomen.
E. Palpate:
  1. Palpate the abdomen; check for tenderness in the RUQ, especially with inspiration; assess for guarding and rebound tenderness.
  2. Check Murphy's sign. Ask the client to inspire deeply while the examiner palpates the area of the gallbladder fossa just beneath the liver edge. A positive Murphy's sign is an inspiratory pause secondary to extreme tenderness during palpation.

Diagnostic Tests

A. Laboratory tests:
  1. Amylase: Will be normal in classic cholecystitis
  2. CBC with differential: Leukocytosis
  3. Alkaline phosphate: Normal in classic cholecystitis; elevated in 25% of clients with cholecystitis
  4. Bilirubin: Normal to mildly elevated in classic cholecystitis
  5. AST: Slightly elevated to normal
  6. ALT: Slightly elevated to normal
  7. Urinalysis to rule out pyelonephritis and renal calculi
  8. Pregnancy test if childbearing age
  9. Stool guaiac test for occult blood to rule out bleeding
B. Radiography:
  1. **Ultrasonography: Study of choice; can often establish the diagnosis. Positive findings include the presence of stones, gallbladder wall thickening, or enlargement and fluid. Sonographic Murphy's sign is defined as an inspiratory pause with a deep breath while the gallbladder is being insonated.**
  2. Cholescintigraphy (hepatobiliary [HIDA]) scan is indicated if the diagnosis is uncertain after an ultrasound. However, it is not recommended in critically ill clients, as the test takes hours to perform and a delay in therapy can be potentially fatal.
  3. Magnetic resonance cholangiopancreatography (MRCP): Noninvasive technique to evaluate intrahepatic or extrahepatic bile ducts
  4. CT scan: Can identify extrabiliary disorders and complications of acute cholecystitis
  5. ERCP: Useful in clients with signs of common bile duct obstruction
  6. Chest radiography to rule out pneumonia
C. EKG to rule out MI

Differential Diagnoses

A. Acute cholecystitis
B. Biliary colic
C. Acute pancreatitis
D. Appendicitis
E. PUD/perforation

F. Acute hepatitis, hepatic abscess
G. Pneumonia or pleurisy
H. MI
I. Renal calculi
J. Gastroesophageal reflux disease (GERD)
K. Pregnancy
L. Pyelonephritis

Plan

A. General interventions:
1. Clients with a single episode of biliary colic are reasonable candidates for expectant management, as long as they continue to be free of recurrent pain.
B. Client teaching:
1. No activity restriction is required.
2. Treatment depends on acuteness of the attack. If pain continues to worsen, have the client contact his or her healthcare provider. Hospitalization and/or surgery may be required depending on the severity of the attack.
3. Counsel the client to avoid fatty foods.
4. Encourage the client to avoid fasting and starvation diets, which make the bile even more lithogenic.
C. Pharmaceutical therapy:
1. Acetaminophen (Tylenol) may be used as needed for pain.
2. Anticholinergics are not helpful.
3. Oral bile acid therapy decreases the amount of cholesterol produced by the liver and absorbed by the intestines:
   a. Actigall (Ursodiol):
      i. Dissolution of stones: 8 to 10 mg/kg/d in two or three divided doses. Many months of treatment may be required for dissolution of gallstones.
      ii. Urso (Ursodiol) 250 mg tablets also available as Urso Forte 500 mg tablets
4. Antibiotics:
As per the Infectious Diseases Society of America (IDSA):
   a. Cefazolin, cefuroxime, or ceftriaxone: For clients with community-acquired acute cholecystitis of mild-to-moderate severity
   b. Imipenem–cilastatin, meropenem, doripenem, piperacillin–tazobactam, ciprofloxacin plus metronidazole, levofloxacin plus metronidazole, or cefepime plus metronidazole: For clients with community-acquired acute cholecystitis of severe physiological disturbance, advanced age, or immunocompromised state
   c. Imipenem–cilastatin, meropenem, doripenem, piperacillin–tazobactam, ciprofloxacin plus metronidazole, levofloxacin plus metronidazole, or cefepime plus metronidazole, with vancomycin added to each regimen: For clients with healthcare-associated biliary infection of any severity
5. Antiemetics for nausea and vomiting
6. Drug dissolution therapy with ursodeoxycholic acid and extracorporeal shock-wave lithotripsy have lower cure rates.

D. Surgical management:
1. Cholecystectomy may be recommended for symptomatic clients. **The standard of care is the laparoscopic cholecystectomy** The conversion rate from a laparoscopic procedure to an open surgical procedure is approximately 5%.

Follow-Up
A. See the client at the next pain attack to reevaluate.
B. Surgical follow-up in 2 weeks

Consultation/Referral
A. For an acute attack, consult a physician for possible surgical consultation referral.
B. Refer the client for elective cholecystectomy when he or she has documented gallstones and recurrent biliary colic or a history of complication of gallstone disease such as pancreatitis.
C. Refer the client to a gastroenterologist for consideration of ERCP.

Individual Considerations
A. Pregnancy:
1. The RUQ or epigastric pain in pregnancy differential includes preeclampsia, pancreatitis, hemolysis, elevated liver enzymes, low platelet count (HELLP) syndrome, acute fatty liver, abruptio placentae, uterine rupture, intraamniotic infection, and appendicitis
2. In the absence of pancreatitis, maternal mortality should be rare, and fetal loss is generally estimated to be no more than 5%. However, if secondary pancreatitis is present, maternal mortality is 15%, and fetal loss is reported to be as high as 60%.
B. Pediatrics:
1. Clients with sickle cell disease are at higher risk for developing cholecystitis.
2. Infants with cholecystitis may present with irritability, jaundice, and acholic (pale white) stools.
3. The most common complication of gallstones in children is pancreatitis.
C. Geriatrics:
1. Signs and symptoms may be nonspecific and vague.
2. Localized tenderness may be the only presenting sign.
3. The Murphy's sign response may be diminished in the elderly.
4. Early cholecystectomy is advocated for elderly clients with gallstone disease. The most important risk factor for postoperative morbidity and mortality is advanced age.
5. Biliary sludge and/or gallstones are likely to form in one in five children with hemolytic anemia before their adolescent years.

Bibliography
Afdhal, N. H. (2019, March 11). Acalculous cholecystitis: Clinical manifestations, diagnosis, and management. *UpToDate*. Retrieved from https://www.uptodate.com/contents/acalculous-cholecystitis-clinical-manifestations-diagnosis-and-management#H231456978
Arain, M. A., & Freeman, M. L. (2017, August 10). Choledocholithiasis: Clinical manifestations, diagnosis, and management. *UpToDate*. Retrieved from https://www.uptodate.com/contents/choledocholithiasis-clinical-manifestations-diagnosis-and-management#H972627867

Bloom, A. A. (2016, April 15). Cholecystitis. *Medscape*. Retrieved from http://emedicine.medscape.com/article/171886-overview

Brooks, D. C. (2019, April 15). Gallstones in pregnancy. *UpToDate*. Retrieved from https://www.uptodate.com/contents/gallstones-in-pregnancy?search=ursodiol%20adult&topicRef=673&source=see_link

Nettina, S. (2010). *The Lippincott manual of nursing practice* (9th ed.). Wolters Kluwer Lippincott Williams & Wilkins.

Prescriber's Digital Reference. (2019). Ursodiol-drug summary. Retrieved from https://www.pdr.net/drug-summary/Actigall-ursodiol-1231

Schwarz, S. M. (2017, October 20). Pediatric cholecystitis. *Medscape*. Retrieved from https://emedicine.medscape.com/article/927340-overview#a5

Steel, P. A. D. (2017, January 18). Acute cholecystitis and biliary colic. *Medscape*. Retrieved from https://emedicine.medscape.com/article/1950020-overview#a2

Vege, S. S. (2019, January 9). Etiology of acute pancreatitis. *UpToDate*. Retrieved from https://www.uptodate.com/contents/etiology-of-acute-pancreatitis

Zakko, S. F. (2018, February 21). Patient education: Gallstones (beyond the basics). *UpToDate*. Retrieved from https://www.uptodate.com/contents/gallstones-beyond-the-basics

Zakko, S. F., & Afdhal, N. M. (2018, November 8). Acute calculous cholecystitis: Clinical features and diagnosis. *UpToDate*. Retrieved from https://www.uptodate.com/contents/acute-calculous-cholecystitis-clinical-features-and-diagnosis

Colic

Doncy Eapen and Cheryl A. Glass

Definition

A. Colic is a benign disorder characterized by abdominal spasms and rigidity that result in abdominal pain. Infants with colic exhibit persistent, unexplained, and inconsolable crying, lasting more than 3 hours a day, occurring more than 3 days in a week for 3 weeks in an otherwise healthy infant less than 3 months of age. The infant is in good health, eats well, and gains weight appropriately, despite the daily crying episodes. Colic is self-limited.

Incidence

A. Between 8% and 40% of all infants exhibit colic, regardless of ethnicity, gender, gestational age, breastfed versus bottle-fed, or socioeconomic status.

Pathogenesis

A. Research has never conclusively identified a cause for colic, and many interventions are based on hypothesized causes, such as immature GI function, milk allergy to casein or whey, and maternal anxiety. Exposure to cigarette smoke may be linked to colic. There has been a causal relationship between colic and family stress.

Predisposing Factors

A. Age: 2 weeks to 4 months; usually resolves by 6 months of age
B. Generally colic is equally frequent in males and females.
C. First in birth order
D. Fruit juice intolerance (sorbitol-containing fruit juices)
E. Faulty feeding techniques: Underfeeding, overfeeding, or infrequent burping and swallowing air

Common Complaints

Crying characteristics:
A. Intense crying: Louder, higher, and more variable in pitch
B. The cry may sound like the baby is in pain or is screaming rather than crying.
C. Inconsolable

Other Signs and Symptoms

A. Hands clenched
B. Abdominal distention
C. Legs flexed over abdomen
D. Short sleep cycles
E. Flatus
F. Fussiness
G. No disease process found on examination
H. Red flags include distended abdomen, fever, and lethargy.

Subjective Data

A. Review when the crying occurs and how long it lasts. What techniques help?
B. Review basic infant needs with caregivers, such as determining whether the infant is hungry or wet, has air bubbles, or is in an uncomfortable position.
C. Review feeding methods, technique, and burping. Crying that occurs directly after feeding may be associated with swallowing too much air or gastroesophageal reflux.
D. If the infant is breastfed, review the maternal diet for offending foods, including chocolate, pizza, spicy foods, cabbage, and so forth.
E. If the infant is breastfed, review prescribed maternal drugs and any OTC medications that she is taking, such as laxatives.
F. If the infant is bottle-fed, review preparation of formula and type of formula.
G. Rule out the early introduction of solid foods.
H. Review any history of fever and high-pitched or shrill cry
I. Have the caregiver describe the color, frequency, and softness of stools.
J. Review secondhand smoke exposure: There is an association between maternal smoking and colic.

Physical Examination

A. Check temperature, pulse, respirations, BP, and weight.
  1. Children: Plot growth parameters including length, head circumference, and weight. **Note signs of FTT. Failure to gain approximately 1 oz/d may indicate FTT.**
B. Inspect:
  1. Evaluate the skin for signs of abuse.
  2. Check the fontanelles for bulge.
  3. Conduct ear, eye, nose, and throat examinations.
  4. Evaluate the skin and mucosa for signs of dehydration.
  5. Evaluate the perineum for diaper rash, meatal ulcer, or inguinal hernia.

C. Auscultate:
1. Abdomen
2. Heart and lungs
D. Percuss:
1. Abdomen
E. Palpate:
1. Palpate the abdomen for tenderness, masses, and distention.
2. Feel the anterior and posterior fontanelles.
3. Perform a testicular examination to evaluate torsion.

Diagnostic Tests
A. Colic is a diagnosis of exclusion and must be differentiated from identifiable causes of prolonged crying.
B. Laboratory tests and radiographic examination are not required if the infant is gaining weight and has a normal physical examination.
C. Consider urinalysis.
D. Check the infant's stool for occult blood to rule out cow's milk allergy.

Differential Diagnoses
A. Colic
B. Infection
C. Obstruction
D. Injury
E. Abuse
F. FTT
G. GERD
H. Intussusception
I. Meningitis
J. Otitis media
K. Protein intolerance
L. Testicular torsion
M. Strangulated inguinal hernia

Plan
A. General interventions:
1. Reassure the family that the baby has no evidence of infant developmental problems and the problem is not related to poor parenting skills.
2. Reassure the family that colic does resolve over time.
3. Encourage parents to take time away from the infant to rest and recoup the energy needed to deal with the demands of a crying baby.
4. Empathize with parental frustration and provide coping techniques.

> Physical abuse of the infant with colic may occur when crying is prolonged and parents have inadequate resources to cope.

5. Consider a hypoallergenic diet (e.g., protein hydrolysate formula such as Alimentum, Nutramigen, or Pregestimil). The literature does not support the use of fiber-enriched formulas.
B. Client teaching:
1. Encourage parents and caregivers to keep a diary on crying and fussing spells for review.
2. Review feeding and burping techniques, making sure the baby is not overfed or underfed.
3. *See Section III: Client Teaching Guide for this chapter, "Colic: Ways to Soothe a Fussy Baby."*
4. Teach caregivers to assess the child for signs of emergent abdominal problems such as fever, pallor, sweating, vomiting, diarrhea, and a rigid and tender abdomen.
C. Pharmaceutical therapy:
1. Simethicone has little therapeutic benefit versus a placebo for treating colic according to randomized controlled trials.
2. Antispasmodics have adverse effects, including apnea, seizures, and coma. Dicyclomine is contraindicated in infants younger than 6 months of age and is not considered for the indication of colic by the manufacturer.
3. Lactase is not a therapeutic option for colic.
4. For breastfed infants, consider five drops of *Lactobacillus reuteri* DSM 17938 per day. Evidence does not support other forms of probiotics or prebiotics.
5. Sedatives should not be used for the treatment of colic.
6. Herbal remedies are common in many cultures, but few herbal products have been evaluated for colic.
D. Dietary management:
1. Dietary changes such as eliminating cow's milk proteins are indicated only in cases of suspected intolerance to protein (e.g., positive family history, eczema, onset after the first month, association with other GI symptoms such as vomiting or diarrhea).
2. Use of soy-based formula is not recommended because many infants who are allergic to cow's milk protein also develop an intolerance to soy protein.
3. For breastfeeding mothers, suggest a period of elimination of allergic foods (e.g., dairy, nuts, soy, citrus) to evaluate the baby's response.
4. For formula-fed infants, consider hydrolyzed formula.
5. Educate caregivers to avoid the use of home-grown mint teas for fussy babies. Fatalities have been reported secondary to ingestion of the pennyroyal form of mint, which produces a toxic oil.

Follow-Up
A. Reevaluate the child periodically to provide support and assess for other problems.
B. Review signs of emergent abdominal problems such as fever, pallor, sweating, vomiting, diarrhea, and rigid and tender abdomen.

Consultation/Referral
A. Refer to a behavioral/developmental pediatrician or mental health provider as needed.
B. Consider a home-based nursing consultation.
C. Refer the breastfeeding mother for an observational feeding.

Bibliography

Deshpande, P. G. (2015, September 3). Colic. *Medscape*. Retrieved from http://emedicine.medscape.com/article/927760

Nettina, S. (2010). *The Lippincott manual of nursing practice* (9th ed.). Philadelphia, PA: Wolters Kluwer Lippincott Williams & Wilkins.

Turner, T. L., & Palamountain, S. (2018, November 20). Infantile colic: Clinical features and diagnosis. *UpToDate*. Retrieved from https://www.uptodate.com/contents/infantile-colic-clinical-features-and-diagnosis

Turner, T. L., & Palamountain, S. (2019, January 22). Patient education: Colic (excessive crying) in infants (beyond the basics). *UpToDate*. Retrieved from https://www.uptodate.com/contents/colic-excessive-crying-in-infants-beyond-the-basics

Colorectal Cancer Screening

Doncy Eapen and Cheryl A. Glass

Definition

Screening for colorectal cancer (CRC) has increased early detection and the ability to engage in early intervention of premalignant localized cancer. There are multiple screening guidelines; the U.S. Preventive Services Task Force's (USPSTF) recommendations are presented in this review (see Table 11.3). Screening is done for men and women between the ages of 50 and 75 years. There are two categories of screening:

A. Stool-based testing
B. Endoscopic and radiological testing

Incidence

A. In the United States, CRC is the second leading cause of cancer-related death in both men and women.
B. Americans have a 4.4% lifetime risk of CRC.
C. CRC is infrequent before age 40 years. It is most frequently diagnosed among adults aged 65 to 74 years. Consider screening in older clients if symptoms are present and life expectancy is greater than 10 years.
D. Approximately 90% of all CRC cases occur after age 50 years.
E. Up to 20% of CRC in the United States is associated with smoking.
F. Obesity is associated with colon cancer but not an increase in rectal cancer. Abdominal obesity is a stronger risk factor than truncal obesity or body mass index (BMI).

Pathogenesis

A. The usual pathogenesis is an adenomatous polyp that grows slowly, followed by dysplasia and final cancerous cells.

Predisposing Factors

A. Age: 50 years and older
B. African American: Screening is recommended at age 40 years.
C. Gender: Risk is higher in men (4.49%) than in women (4.15%).
D. IBDs: CD and UC
E. Family history/genetic:
   1. Familial adenomatous polyposis (FAP)
   2. Nonpolyposis CRC (Lynch syndrome)
F. Smoking
G. Obesity
H. Diet high in red meat and fats

Common Complaints

A. Asymptomatic
B. Routine screening after the age of 50 years. See guidelines for routine colonoscopy screening.

Subjective Data

A. Review the client's age and risk factors to discuss screening for CRC.
B. Review family history of CRC.
C. Review smoking history.
D. Review the client's diet, evaluating intake of red meat; processed meats; and lack of grains, fruits, and vegetables.
E. Review all medications currently being taken, including OTC medications and herbal products.

Physical Examination

A. Examinations are not required for discussion of colorectal screening testing.
B. A physical examination should be performed and vital signs taken as indicated for other presenting complaints.

Diagnostic Tests

See Table 11.2 for frequency of tests.
A. Stool-based testing:
   1. Guaiac-based fecal occult blood test (FOBT)
   2. **Fecal immunochemical test (FIT) is replacing the FOBT as the preferred cancer detection test.**
   3. FIT DNA panel
B. Endoscopic and radiological:
   1. Flexible sigmoidoscopy
   2. **Colonoscopy: The ACG recommends colonoscopy as the preferred strategy for screening**
   3. **Double-contrast barium enema (DCBE): The ACG recommends the DCBE as a screening test; however, it has limited effectiveness for polyp detection**
   4. Computed tomography colonography (CTC) every 5 years

Differential Diagnosis

A. None related to screening

Plan

A. Client teaching:
   1. Educate the client about modifying controllable risk factors with diet, exercise, and smoking cessation.
   2. Discuss the procedures and the preparation needed for each test.
B. Pharmaceutical therapy:
   1. Bowel prep depends on the test, the client's age, and other comorbidities.

Follow-Up

A. Follow-up and consultations are determined by the client's needs, severity, and whether complications are present.
B. Clients with classic FAP (> 100 adenomas) should be advised to have genetic counseling.
C. NSAIDs have been associated with a decrease in the risk of developing CRC. There is insufficient evidence to recommend the use of NSAIDs as a prevention strategy.

TABLE 11.2   SCREENING TESTS AT A GLANCE BASED ON U.S. PREVENTIVE SERVICES TASK FORCE (USPSTF) COLORECTAL CANCER SCREENING

Name	Preparation	What Happens?	Frequency
High-sensitivity FOBT or stool test; or FIT Note: There are two types of FOBT: One uses the chemical guaiac to detect blood. The other—an FIT—uses antibodies to detect blood in the stool. Ask your doctor for a *high-sensitivity* FOBT or FIT.	Your doctor may recommend that you follow a special diet before taking the FOBT.	You receive a test kit from your healthcare provider. At home, you use a stick or brush to obtain a small amount of stool. You may be asked to do this for several bowel movements in a row. You return the test kit to the doctor or a lab, where stool samples are checked for blood.	This test should be done every year. (If anything unusual is found, your doctor will recommend a follow-up colonoscopy.)
The one-time FOBT done by the doctor in the doctor's office is *not* appropriate as a screening test for colorectal cancer. FIT-DNA is an emerging screening strategy. It is a multitargeted stool DNA test combined with FIT testing.			The FIT-DNA test should be done every year or once in 3 years (suggested by the manufacturer).
Flexible sigmoidoscopy (flex sig) Note: This is sometimes done in combination with *high-sensitivity* FOBT.	Your doctor will tell you what foods you can and cannot eat before the test. The evening before the test, you use a strong laxative and/or enema to clean out the colon.	During the test, the doctor puts a short, thin, flexible, lighted tube into the rectum. This tube allows the doctor to check for polyps or cancer inside the rectum and lower third of the colon.	This test should be done every 5 years. When it is done in combination with high-sensitivity FIT, the FIT should be done every year and flexible sigmoidoscopy every 10 years. (If anything unusual is found, your doctor will recommend a follow-up colonoscopy.)
Colonoscopy Note: Colonoscopy also is used as a follow-up test if anything unusual is found during one of the other screening tests.	Before this test, your doctor will tell you what foods you can and cannot eat. You use a strong laxative to clean out the colon. Some doctors recommend that you also use an enema. Make sure you arrange for a ride back home, as you will not be allowed to drive.	You will receive medication during this test to make you more comfortable. This test is similar to flex sig, except the doctor uses a longer, thin, flexible, lighted tube to check for polyps or cancer inside the rectum and the entire colon. During the test, the doctor can find and remove most polyps and some cancers.	This test should be done every 10 years. If polyps or cancers are found during the test, you will need more frequent colonoscopies in the future.

FIT, fecal immunochemical test; FOBT, fecal occult blood test.

Source: Adapted from U.S. Preventive Services Task Force. (2016, June). *Final recommendation statement: Colorectal cancer screening*. Retrieved from www.uspreventiveservicestaskforce.org/Page/Document/RecommendationStatementFinal/colorectal-cancer-screening2#tab

D. The USPSTF has made a recommendation on aspirin use for primary prevention of cardiovascular disease and CRC in average-risk adults (www.uspreventiveservices-taskforce.org).

Consultation/Referral

A. Referral to a gastroenterologist and/or surgeon as indicated.

Individual Considerations

A. Geriatrics:

1. The benefit of early detection of and intervention for CRC declines after age 75 years. Screening for adults aged 76 to 85 years should be made on an individual basis (see Table 11.3), taking into account the client's overall health and prior screening history.

2. Medicare Part B covers several colorectal screening tests:

   a. Medicare covers a screening BE when used instead of a flexible sigmoidoscopy or colonoscopy once every 48 months for clients 50 years or older and once every 24 months if at high risk.

   b. Screening colonoscopy is covered every 24 months if at high risk for CRC. If not at high risk, Medicare covers the colonoscopy once every 120 months, or 48 months after a previous flexible sigmoidoscopy.

3. FOBT is covered by Medicare once every 12 months for clients ages 50 years or older.

4. Flexible sigmoidoscopy is covered by Medicare every 48 months for most people older than 50 years. If not at high risk, Medicare covers the flexible sigmoidoscopy every 120 months after a previous screening colonoscopy.

5. Multitarget stool DNA at-home test is covered once every 3 years for people who meet *all* of the following criteria:

    a. Between ages 50 and 85 years

    b. No signs or symptoms of colorectal disease, including, but not limited to, lower GI pain, blood in stool, positive guaiac FOBT, or FIT

    c. Average risk for developing CRC:

       i. No personal history of adenomatous polyps, CRC, or IBD, including CD and UC

       ii. No family history of CRCs or adenomatous polyps, FAP, or hereditary nonpolyposis CRC

Resources

Centers for Disease Control and Prevention—Screening Tests at-a-Glance includes the 2008 recommendations on screening for CRC from the USPTF website: www.cdc.gov/cancer/colorectal/pdf/SFL_inserts_screening.pdf

Medicare.gov, Your Medicare coverage—colorectal cancer screenings: www.medicare.gov/coverage/screening-colono-scopies

---

TABLE 11.3   CRC SCREENING RECOMMENDATIONS FOR ADULTS AT AVERAGE RISK

	U.S. Preventive Task Force—2016	American Cancer Society—2018	U.S. MTSF[a] on CRC—2017
Ages for screening	• Start screening at age 50 • Stop screening at 75 • The decision to be screened after 75 to 85 should be made on an individual basis taking into account the patient's overall health and prior screening history • Screening after age 85 is not recommended	• Start screening at age 45 • For adults with average CRC risk, in good health, and with a life expectancy of more than 10 years, screening should continue through age 75 years • The decision to be screened for patients aged 76 to 85 years should be individualized to patient preference, life expectancy, health status, and prior history of screen • Screening after 85 is not recommended	• Start screening at age 50 • Limited evidence supports screening African Americans at 45 years • Stop screening at age 75 or have <10 years of life expectancy • Persons without prior screening should be con- sidered for screening up to age 85, depending on age and comorbidities • Colonoscopy and FIT are recommended as thecornerstones of screening regardless of how screening is offered
Highly sensitive gFOBT	Annual	Annual	No recommendation
Highly sensitive FIT	Annual	Annual	Annual
FIT fecal DNA	Every 1 or 3 years[b]	No recommendation	Every 3 years
MT-s DNA test		Every 3 years	No recommendation
FSIG	Every 5 years OR the FSIG and FIT DNA recommendation	Every 5 years	Every 5 to 10 years
FSIG and FIT DNA	FSIG every 10 years plus FIT every year	No recommendation	No recommendation
Colonoscopy	Every 10 years	Every 10 years	Every 10 years[c]
CT colonography (virtual colonoscopy)	Every 5 years	Every 5 years	Every 5 years

[a]MSTF represents the American College of Gastroenterology, the American Gastroenterological Association, and the American Society for Gastrointestinal Endoscopy.

[b]FIT DNA testing suggested by manufacturer.

[c]Colonoscopy offered first, FIT should be offered to patients who decline colonoscopy.

CRC, colorectal cancer; FIT, fecal immunochemical test; FSIG, flexible sigmoidoscopy; gFOBT, guaiac-based fecal occult blood test; MT-s DNA, multi-targeted stool DNA; MTSF, Multi-Society Task Force.

Source: Reproduced from Cash, J. C., & Glass, C. A. (2019). *Adult-gerontology practice guidelines* (2nd ed.). New York, NY: Springer Publishing Company.

National Cancer Institutes, National Institutes of Health—Colon and rectal cancer: www.cancer.gov/cancertopics/types/colon-and-rectal

National Cancer Institute, National Institutes of Health—Rectal cancer treatment for professionals (PDQ): www.cancer.gov

National Cancer Institutes, National Institutes of Health—Tests to detect colorectal cancer and polyps: www.cancer.gov/cancertopics/factsheet/detection/colorectal-screening

National Comprehensive Cancer Network: www.nccn.org

Bibliography

American Cancer Society. (2019). *Key statistics for colorectal cancer.* Retrieved from https://www.cancer.org/cancer/colon-rectal-cancer/about/key-statistics.html

Centers for Disease Control and Prevention. (n.d.). *Screening tests at-a-glance.* Retrieved from https://www.cdc.gov/cancer/colorectal/pdf/SFL_inserts_screening.pdf

Doubeni, C. (2018, June 7). Screening for colorectal cancer: Strategies in patients at average risk. *UpToDate.* Retrieved from https://www.uptodate.com/contents/screening-for-colorectal-cancer-strategies-in-patients-at-average-risk#H4220220052

Huguet, J. M., Suárez, P., Ferrer-Barceló, L., Ruiz, L., Monzó, A., Durá, A. B., & Sempere, J. (2017). Endoscopic recommendations for colorectal cancer screening and surveillance in patients with inflammatory bowel disease: Review of general recommendations. *World Journal of Gastrointestinal Endoscopy, 9*(6), 255–262. doi:10.4253/wjge.v9.i6.255

Medicare.gov. (n.d.). *Your Medicare coverage: Colorectal cancer screening.* Retrieved from www.medicare.gov/coverage/colorectal-cancer-screenings.html

Nettina, S. (2010). *The Lippincott manual of nursing practice* (9th ed.). Philadelphia, PA: Wolters Kluwer Lippincott Williams & Wilkins.

Qaseem, A., Denberg, T. D., Hopkins, R. H., Humphrey, L. L., Levine, J., Sweet, D. E., & Shekelle, P. (2012). Screening for colorectal cancer: A guidance statement from the American College of Physicians. *Annals of Internal Medicine, 156,* 378–386. doi:10.7326/0003-4819-156-5-201203060-00010. Retrieved from https://annals.org/aim/fullarticle/1090694/screening-colorectal-cancer-guidance-statement-from-american-college-physicians

U.S. Preventive Services Task Force. (2016, June). *Final recommendation statement: Colorectal cancer screening.* Retrieved from https://www.uspreventiveservicestaskforce.org/Page/Document/RecommendationStatementFinal/colorectal-cancer-screening2#tab

Constipation

Cheryl A. Glass, Audra Malone, and Doncy Eapen

Definition

Constipation is infrequent and difficult defecation of hard stools and a sensation of incomplete evacuation or straining. Constipation may also refer to a decrease in the volume or weight of stool, and the need for enemas, suppositories, or laxatives to maintain bowel regularity. Constipation is a symptom, not a disease. The lower limit of normal stool frequency is three bowel movements (BMs) a week. The Rome consensus criterion defines constipation as two or fewer stools weekly, lumpy/hard stools, straining, sensation of incomplete evacuation/obstruction or blockage, and/or the need for digital removal of stool. Classification of constipation includes:

A. Normal-transit constipation (most common)
B. Functional constipation (slow transit)
C. IBS (constipation dominant)
D. Outlet obstruction (sudden onset)

Incidence

A. The incidence of constipation is unknown due to frequent self-treatment. Constipation is commonly self-reported. Constipation occurs in more than 50% of clients with CRC; it may be an early symptom of rectal cancer or a symptom of advanced disease in colon cancer.

Pathogenesis

A. Constipation can be caused by an alteration of the filling of the rectum by colonic transportation and/or reflex defecation of stool.
B. Lack of exercise decreases propulsion of bowel contents.
C. During pregnancy, progesterone has a relaxing effect on the muscles of the GI tract and causes a decrease in peristalsis. The compression of the intestines by the enlarging uterus causes constipation during pregnancy.
D. Habitual use of laxatives is associated with impaired motor activity and has the potential of producing hypokalemia.
E. Severe hypokalemia can produce a generalized ileus and is most often seen in clients who take diuretics.
F. Psychiatric disease and psychosocial distress have important roles. The exact mechanisms by which emotional difficulties lead to constipation remain unclear, but their contribution is widely recognized.
G. Drugs (see Table 11.4)

Predisposing Factors

A. Insufficient nutrition:
 1. Low-fiber diet
 2. Low fluid intake
B. Neurological causes:
 1. Spinal cord injury
 2. Parkinson's disease
 3. Multiple sclerosis
 4. Aganglionosis (Hirschsprung's disease [HD])
 5. Sacral nerve trauma/tumor
C. Sedentary lifestyle
D. Laxative abuse
E. Travel

TABLE 11.4 DRUGS/DRUG CLASSIFICATIONS THAT CAUSE AND INCREASE CONSTIPATION

Anticholinergics (atropine, antidepressants, neuroleptics, antiparkinsonian drugs)	Opiates
Antipsychotics	Cholestyramine (binds bile salts)
Anticonvulsants	Antacids (aluminum hydroxide and calcium carbonate)
Antihistamines	Iron supplements
Antihypertensives (calcium-channel blockers, clonidine, hydralazine, MAOIs, methyldopa)	NSAIDs
Diuretics	Ganglionic blockers

MAOIs, monoamine oxidase inhibitors; NSAIDs, nonsteroidal anti-inflammatory drugs.

F. Ignoring urge to defecate
G. Drug use: Individual medications and polypharmacy
H. Pregnancy, especially third trimester
I. Psychosocial problems:
 1. Depression
 2. Sexual abuse
 3. Unusual attitudes to food and bowel function
J. Extremes of ages: Infants and geriatrics
K. Hypothyroidism
L. CRC
M. IBS
N. Pelvic floor disorders:
 1. Impaired function of the pelvic floor and/or external sphincter
 2. Pelvic floor obstruction
 3. Rectal prolapse
 4. Enterocele and/or rectocele
 5. Rectal intussusception

Common Complaints
A. Hard, infrequent stools
B. Straining
C. Inability to defecate when desired
D. Need for digital manipulation to facilitate evacuation

Other Signs and Symptoms
A. Hard, pebbly, rocklike stools
B. Painful defecation
C. Abdominal pain
D. Weight loss
E. Blood in stools

Potential Complications
A. A rectal prolapse of the mucosa is pink and looks like a doughnut or rosette. Complete prolapse involving the muscular wall is larger and red, and has circular folds.

Subjective Data
A. Review the onset, duration, and course of symptoms:
 1. Is constipation a chronic or acute problem?
 2. If there has been a change in bowel habits, was it gradual or sudden?
 3. What feature does the client rate as most distressing?
B. Review bowel habits:
 1. Does the client have a regular time for defecation?
 2. Review size, color, consistency, and frequency of stools. Has there been a change in the caliber of stools?
 3. Is there any blood?
 4. Are there any periods of diarrhea?
 5. How often are laxatives being used, and at what doses?
 6. Are suppositories and enemas also required?
 7. Does the client have the urge to defecate?
 8. Does the client have a sensation of incomplete evacuation?
 9. Does the client need to digitally remove stool?
 10. Does the client have fecal incontinence?
C. Review the client's daily diet and fluid intake. Has there been any dietary change?

D. Review the client's medication history: Prescription and OTC drugs (refer to Table 11.4)
E. Review the client's daily physical activity.
F. Review the client's psychosocial history of stress, depression, anxiety, and coping mechanisms.
G. Review the client's other health problems, such as diabetes, depression, hypothyroidism, and hypercalcemia.
H. Review family history of constipation and CRC.
I. Review surgical history.

Physical Examination
A. Check pulse, respirations, BP, and weight. Check temperature if indicated.
B. Inspect:
 1. General overall assessment of nutritional status.
 2. Examine the skin, especially the rectum, for pallor and signs of dehydration and hypothyroidism.
 3. Evaluate for the presence of hernias.
 4. Inspect the anus, including the position, anal wink, prolapse, presence of excoriation, presence of perianal erythema, hemorrhoids, fissures, and skin tags.
 5. Examine the lower back to rule out spinal lesions—hairy or hyperpigmented patches, gluteal fold asymmetry, cutaneous dimples, sinus tracts, and lipomas.
C. Auscultate:
 1. Abdomen: Four abdominal quadrants for bowel sounds. Bowel sounds may be high pitched or absent.
D. Percuss:
 1. Abdomen: Constipation will present changes from tympanic to dull.
E. Palpate:
 1. The abdomen for masses, tenderness, distention, and fecal mass
F. Digital rectal examination:
 1. Examine the rectum for an anorectal mass, stricture, hemorrhoids, fissures, fistula, prolapse, inflammation, and anal warts.
 2. Evaluate for impaction, hard stool in ampulla.
 3. Perform an anal reflex test by a light pinprick or scratch.
 4. Evaluate sphincter tone:
  a. Disordered innervation of the anus is indicated by finding that the anal canal opens wide when the puborectalis muscle is pulled posteriorly.
  b. Evaluate the resting tone of the sphincter and squeezing effort.
  c. Instruct the client to "expel the examination finger" to evaluate the force of expulsion.
  d. Have the client do a Valsalva maneuver to diagnose a rectocele, prolapse, pelvic floor descent, or puborectalis dysfunction.
  e. In women, the vagina should also be evaluated for rectocele and cystocele.
G. Neurological examination: Assess for tone, strength, and reflexes to search for focal deficits and the delayed relaxation phase of the ankle jerks, suggestive of hypothyroidism.
H. Pelvic examination: Evaluate for prolapse or rectocele. Evaluate when the client is at rest and with straining.
I. Psychiatric examination: Assess mental status for signs of depression and somatization.

Diagnostic Tests

A. No tests are required for *common* constipation.
B. Tests to rule out differential diagnoses:
  1. CBC with differential
  2. Thyroid studies
  3. Potassium and calcium: Clients taking diuretics should have serum potassium checked. Hypokalemia may reduce bowel contractility and produce an ileus.
  4. Urinalysis
  5. Serum glucose to rule out diabetes
  6. BE to evaluate for megacolon and redundant sigmoid colon
  7. Flexible sigmoid or colonoscopy is recommended if the client meets the guidelines for general screening or weight loss greater than 10 pounds, anemia, or blood in the stool; or clients with family history of CRC or IBD
  8. Stool for occult blood
  9. Anorectal function tests:
    a. Manometry
    b. Electromyography

Differential Diagnoses

A. Constipation
B. Intestinal obstruction: Acute onset of constipation requires ruling out an ileus, especially when accompanied by abdominal discomfort
C. Hypothyroidism
D. Psychosocial dysfunction
E. Fecal impaction
F. Neurological disorders
G. Multiple sclerosis
H. Spinal cord injury
I. CRC
J. Drug use
K. CD: Constipation is often the presenting complaint.
L. Diabetes (chronic dysmotility)
M. HD

Plan

A. General interventions:
  1. Reassure the client that recommended dietary changes and exercise can help with constipation.
  2. Ask the client to keep a stool diary and bring the diary to the next appointment.
B. Client teaching:
  1. *See Section III*: *Client Teaching Guide for this chapter, "Constipation Relief."*
  2. Encourage the client to exercise. Both exercise and dietary fiber stimulate the natural wavelike contraction of the colon that triggers the urge to defecate.
  3. Warn chronic laxative users that it may take 4 to 6 weeks before spontaneous BMs return.
  4. Teach the client about potential complications of long-term constipation.
C. Pharmaceutical therapy:
  1. Bulk-forming agents decrease abdominal pain and improve stool consistency. They should be used if an increase in dietary fiber does not work. They act by causing retention of fluid and increasing fecal mass. They must be taken with plenty of fluids to prevent formation of an obstructing bolus. Flatulence and abdominal distention may occur, but long-term use is safe.
  2. Stimulant laxatives act by directly stimulating the colonic nerves. Suppositories are faster (20–60 minutes) versus oral laxatives (8–12 hours).
  3. Osmotic laxatives act by retaining fluid in the bowel by osmosis, changing the water distribution in the feces. Good hydration is important (Table 11.5).
  4. Lubiprostone (Amitiza) 24 mcg orally twice a day is approved for treatment of chronic idiopathic constipation (CIC) in adults, opioid-induced constipation in adults with chronic noncancer pain, and IBS–constipation predominant in women 18 years or older in age.
  5. Linaclotide (Linzess) has been approved by the Food and Drug Administration (FDA) for the treatment of CIC at a dose of 145 mcg orally daily.
  6. Methylnaltrexone bromide (Relistor) 450 mg tablet once per day is currently approved by the

TABLE 11.5   LAXATIVES

Bulk laxatives	Psyllium (Konsyl, Metamucil) Polycarbophil Methylcellulose (Citrucel)
Lubricating agents	Mineral oil[a]
Stimulant laxatives	Docusate Bile acids Bisacodyl[b] Castor oil Senna[a] Cascara Aloes Rhubarb
Osmotic agents	Magnesium and phosphate salts Lactulose (Kristalose)[a] Sorbitol[a] Polyethylene glycol (Colyte, Glycolax, Miralax)[b] Glycerin suppositories[a]
Selective 5-HT$_4$ receptor agonists	Prucalopride
Type-2 chloride channel	Tegaserod (Zelnorm, HTF-919)[c]
Activator	Lubiprostone (Amitiza)
Guanylate cyclase C agonist	Linaclotide (Linzess)[d]

[a]Considered safe and effective in children.

[b]After a thorough evaluation, use in low doses for selected children when constipation is hard to manage.

[c]Tegaserod is prescribed under limited restrictive authority.

[d]The safety and efficacy of Linzess have not been established in pediatric clients younger than 18 years. Contraindicated in pediatric clients up to 6 years of age.

FDA for treatment of opioid-induced constipation in adult clients with chronic noncancer pain.

7. When severe depression requires the use of anti-depressants, the least constipating agent should be selected (i.e., one with minimal anticholinergic activity).

8. Treat other identified causes, such as hypo-thyroidism.

D. Dietary management: See Appendix B.

E. Surgical and medical management:

1. Treatment of constipation is symptomatic and should begin with lifestyle and dietary changes.

2. Evaluate and stop medications, if possible, that cause constipation.

3. Glycerin suppositories may be needed for rectal disimpaction in infants. Enemas are to be avoided.

4. Fecal impaction may require enemas or manual removal to relieve the situation. Enemas should not be given routinely to treat constipation because they disrupt normal defecation reflexes and the client becomes dependent. Disimpaction by enema treatments includes three enemas per day.

    a. The first enema of the day includes the use of a phosphate-based enema:

        i. Clients older than 12 years: One adult phosphate-based enema, plus 1 L of saline solution

        ii. Clients aged 4 to 12 years: One pediatric phosphate-based enema, plus 1 L of saline solution

        iii. Clients younger than 4 years: One half of a pediatric phosphate-based enema, plus 500 mL of saline solution

    b. The second and third enemas of the day include only the saline solution and no phosphate-based enema.

    c. Clients should never receive more than one phosphate enema per day because of the risk of phosphate intoxication, hypoglycemia, and hyponatremia.

    d. Soap suds, tap water, and magnesium enemas in children are not recommended because of potential toxicity.

5. Pelvic floor physiotherapy may be offered.

6. Biofeedback has been effective for short-term treatment of intractable constipation.

7. Manual removal of fecal impaction can stimulate the vagus nerve and cause syncope and tachycardia. It is contraindicated in the following conditions:

    a. Pregnancy

    b. After genitourinary, rectal, perineal, abdominal, or gynecological surgery

    c. MI, coronary insufficiency, pulmonary embolus, CHF, or heart block

    d. GI or vaginal bleeding

    e. Blood dyscrasias or bleeding disorders

    f. Hemorrhoids, fissures, and rectal polyps

Follow-Up

A. Repeat assessment in 4 to 6 weeks. Ask the client to keep a stool diary and bring it for subsequent appointments.

B. If there is no evidence of obstruction, anemia, or occult blood loss, follow the client expectantly for a few weeks on a conservative program that includes increased dietary fiber and increased exercise, and follow stool guaiac.

C. Failure to improve may indicate a serious underlying cause and need for referral.

Consultation/Referral

A. Consider consultations with a gastroenterologist (adult or pediatric), pediatrician, gynecologist, surgeon, or psychologist/psychiatrist as indicated.

Individual Considerations

A. Pregnancy:

1. Constipation is very common in pregnancy secondary to progesterone and the enlarging uterus (see the "Pathogenesis" section).

2. Constipation that results from iron supplementation can be avoided by increasing the intake of fluid and high-fiber foods, and increasing physical activity such as walking.

3. Bulking agents and lactulose will not enter breast milk. Senna, in large doses, will enter breast milk and may cause diarrhea and colic in infants.

B. Pediatrics:

1. In infancy and childhood, most constipation is functional. Constipation can be associated with coercive toilet training, sexual abuse, excessive parental interventions, and toilet phobia.

2. An empty contracted anal canal in a constipated child may suggest HD.

    a. Bloody mucoid diarrhea in an infant with a history of constipation could be an indication of enterocolitis complicating HD.

    b. If HD is suspected, the client should be evaluated by a pediatric gastroenterologist and a pediatric surgeon.

3. Reinforce the idea that each infant has individual stool patterns. Formula-fed infants generally pass at least one stool each day, whereas breastfed infants may pass a stool after every feeding or, occasionally, only one every 2 to 3 days.

4. Teach parent(s) and care givers that regular BMs are different for each child (once or twice a day or every other day). Explain the stool consistency and appearance (dry, hard, and marblelike stools) that could suggest the child is constipated.

5. Infants may get red in the face and appear to be straining when having a BM, but it is normal behavior and does not indicate constipation.

6. Rectal prolapse in children has been associated with CF.

7. Use a high-fiber diet and fluids first before other therapies. Prune, pear, and apple juices may decrease constipation.

8. Common times when constipation is likely to occur in the pediatric population:

a. Upon introduction of solid foods or cow's milk:

i. Recommended fiber intake is 20 g/d.

ii. Minimum fluid intake depends on the child's age.

iii. Consumption of cow's whole milk should be limited to 24 oz/d.

b. During toilet training: A potty seat that provides appropriate foot support and leverage for elimination should be used.

c. On school entry: Establish regular and routine toilet times; at least twice daily for 5–10 minutes.

C. Adults:

1. The most common cause of chronic constipation in adults is failure to initiate defecation.

2. Clients with diabetes should avoid stimulant laxatives such as lactulose and sorbitol. Their metabolites may influence blood glucose levels.

D. Geriatrics:

1. Constipation in older people is not a result of aging; it is usually related to an increase in constipating factors such as chronic illnesses, immobility, dietary factors, medications, neurological factors, and psychiatric conditions. **Acute onset of constipation is considered a red flag in the geriatric population.**

2. An important diagnostic concern in the elderly is the possibility of constipation due to a colonic neoplasm. More than 25% of clients with colorectal carcinomas present with constipation.

3. Check for a fecal impaction, especially in elderly clients with a history of chronic constipation. Fecal impaction ranks as one of the major sources of anorectal discomfort among the elderly and bedridden. Chronic, incomplete evacuation leads to the formation of an obstructing bolus of desiccated hard stool in the rectum. Fecal incontinence may be a sign of fecal impaction.

4. Diarrhea, rather than constipation, is sometimes the only complaint because of the collection of liquid stool distending the proximal colon and passing around the obstructing bolus.

5. Dietary fiber supplementation has been shown to allow discontinuation of laxatives in 59% to 80% of elderly clients with CIC.

Resource

Rome Foundation: https://theromefoundation.org

Bibliography

Borowitz, S. M. (2018, December 14). Pediatric constipation treatment and management. *Medscape.* Retrieved from https://emedicine.medscape.com/article/928185-treatment#d10

Levitt, M. A. (2015, August 28). Management of severe pediatric constipation. *Medscape.* Retrieved from http://emedicine.medscape.com/article/937030-overview

Mason, D., Tobias, N., Lutkenhoff, M., Stoops, M., & Ferguson, D. (2004). The APN's guide to pediatric constipation management. *Nurse Practitioner, 29*(7), 13–21. doi:10.1097/00006205-200407000-00003

Nettina, S. (2010). *The Lippincott manual of nursing practice* (9th ed.). Philadelphia, PA: Wolters Kluwer Lippincott Williams & Wilkins.

North American Society for Pediatric Gastroenterology Hepatology and Nutrition. (2006). Clinical practice guideline: Evaluation and treatment of constipation in infants and children: Recommendations of the North American Society for Pediatric Gastroenterology, Hepatology and Nutrition. *Journal of Pediatric Gastroenterology and Nutrition, 43,* e1–e13. doi:10.1097/01.mpg.0000233159.97667.c3

Paquette, I. M., Varma, M., Ternent, C., Melton-Meaux, G., Rafferty, J. F., Feingold, D., & Steele, S. R. (2016). The American Society of Colon and Rectal Surgeons' clinical practice guidelines for the evaluation and management of constipation. *Diseases of the Colon & Rectum, 59,* 479–492. doi:10.1097/DCR.0000000000000599

Sharma, G. D. (2019, May 2). Cystic fibrosis. *Medscape.* Retrieved from http://emedicine.medscape.com/article/1001602-overview

Vargas, H. D. (n.d.). *Constipation expanded version.* Retrieved from https://www.fascrs.org/patients/disease-condition/constipation-expanded-version

Wald, A. (2018, September 6). Etiology and evaluation of chronic constipation in adults. *UpToDate.* Retrieved from https://www.uptodate.com/contents/etiology-and-evaluation-of-chronic-constipation-in-adults#H13

Wald, A. (2019, March 5). Management of chronic constipation in adults. *UpToDate.* Retrieved from https://www.uptodate.com/contents/management-of-chronic-constipation-in-adults#H3625634867

Crohn's Disease

Cheryl A. Glass, Audra Malone, and Doncy Eapen

Definition

A. CD is a chronic IBD of the GI tract that produces ulceration, fibrosis, and malabsorption. CD can involve any segment of the GI tract from the mouth to the anus; the terminal ileum and colon are the most common sites. Pediatric clients are more likely to present with the disease limited to the small intestine.

1. In 2003, CD was subclassified based on age, location (ileal, colonic, ileocolonic, or upper GI), and clinical presentation (nonstricturing/nonpenetrating to penetrating) using the Montreal classification

2. Elderly clients with IBD can be subdivided into two groups:

a. Elderly clients with onset of IBD at a late age (late-onset IBD)

b. Elderly clients with long-standing IBD; first diagnosed as having IBD at a younger age (long-standing IBD)

B. The disease is chronic, relapsing, and incurable. CD is characterized by episodes of remission and exacerbation. The most frequent cause of death in persons with IBD is the primary disease, followed by malignancy and thromboembolic disease. In most cases, symptoms do correspond well with the degree of inflammation present. The diagnosis is usually established with endoscopic findings in a client with a compatible clinical history. Objective evidence for disease activity should be sought before administering medication with significant adverse effects.

C. More than 70% of clients with CD undergo surgery within 20 years of the diagnosis. Indications for surgery include stricture, intractable or fulminant disease, anorectal disease, and intra-abdominal abscess. Approximately 30% of clients who have surgery for CD have a recurrence within 3 years, and up to 60% will have a recurrence within 10 years.

D. The lifetime risk of fistula development is 20% to 40%.

E. The incidence of small bowel and colorectal adenocarcinoma in clients with CD is higher than that in the general population. Lymphoma is also increased, especially for clients with IBD treated with azathioprine (AZA; 6-mercaptopurine [6-MP]).

Incidence

A. The incidence rate ranges from 3.1 cases per 100,000 to 20.2 cases per 100,000. An estimated 1 to 2 million people in the United States have UC or CD. The incidence of IBD has been reported to be highest in Jewish populations. IBD is very prevalent among the American Jewish population—prevalence is four to five times that of the general population.

B. The peak incidence of CD typically occurs in late adolescence to the third decade of life. A second peak in incidence of CD is with children younger than 5 years and elderly persons aged 70 to 80 years. CD may involve the entire GI tract; note the incidence according to the location.

1. About 80% have small-bowel involvement, usually in the distal ileum. In severe cases of ileitis, complications may include fistulas or an abscess in the RLQ of the abdomen.

2. About 50% have ileocolitis, involving both the ileum and the colon. This type is associated with significant weight loss.

3. About 20% have disease limited to the colon, with roughly one half having sparing of the rectum.

4. Approximately 5% to 15% have predominant involvement of the mouth (aphthous ulcers) or gastroduodenal area; fewer have involvement of the esophagus (odynophagia and dysphagia) and proximal small bowel.

5. One-third have perianal disease (perianal pain, drainage from large skin tags, anal fissures, perirectal abscesses, and anorectal fistulae).

6. Approximately 15% to 20% have arthralgias. Arthritis is the most common complication.

Pathogenesis

Pathogenesis is unknown. The common end pathway is inflammation of the mucosal lining of the intestinal tract, causing ulceration, edema, bleeding, and fluid and electrolyte loss. Speculation for the pathogenesis includes:

A. Pathogenic organism (remains unidentified)

B. Immunological response

C. Autoimmune process

D. Potential genes linked to IBD:

1. Chromosome 16 (*IBD1* gene)

2. *CARD15* gene, which is noted to be a susceptibility gene for CD

3. Susceptibility genes on chromosomes 5 (5q31) and 6 (6p21 and 19p)

Predisposing Factors

A. Age between 15 and 40 years

B. Gender: Slight female predominance

C. Genetic predisposition/family history of CD:

1. First-degree relatives: 5- to 20-fold increased risk

2. Children of a parent with IBD: 5% risk

3. About 70% incidence in identical twins versus 5% to 10% in nonidentical twins

D. Race and ethnicity: More common in Jewish populations

E. Smoking: Increased risk for CD, but reduced risk for UC

Common Complaints

The following cardinal symptoms occur in about 80% of clients.

A. Chronic or nocturnal diarrhea

B. Abdominal pain, with the classic location being in the RLQ (appendicitis-like)

C. Fatigue, commonly related to pain, inflammation, and anemia

Other Signs and Symptoms

Symptoms vary depending on the location of the intestinal tract and extent of disease.

A. Constipation: Early sign

B. Weight loss

C. Abdominal mass

D. Cramping with BM

E. Urgent need to move bowels

F. Rectal bleeding or blood in stools

G. Perianal discomfort or soft or semiliquid irritating rectal discharge

H. Vomiting

I. Low-grade fever

J. Folate deficiency

K. Anorexia

L. Fissures and fistulas, abscesses sometimes extending to the skin

M. Weight loss, diarrhea, and growth retardation may be presenting signs in children.

N. Extraintestinal symptoms:

1. Arthritis or arthropathy: Most common extraintestinal symptoms; involve large joints in approximately 20% of clients

2. Inflammation of the eyes; uveitis, iritis, episcleritis

3. Skin disorders: Erythema nodosum and pyoderma gangrenosum

4. Venous or arterial thromboembolism resulting from hypercoagulability

5. Pulmonary involvement: Chronic bronchitis, bronchiectasis, interstitial lung disease, sarcoidosis, and pulmonary embolism

O. Pediatric:

1. Failure to grow

2. Delayed development of secondary sex characteristics

P. Loss of normal menstrual cycle

Subjective Data

A. Ask about the onset, duration, and course of symptoms. Have any of the presenting symptoms occurred at any time in the past? (Flares of CD may have gone undiagnosed in the past.)

B. Review the client's history and extent of diarrhea, including frequency, consistency, color, quantity, and odor of stools. Evaluate if there is blood, mucus, pus, or food particles in the stools.

C. Inquire about recent travel to foreign countries.

D. Ask the client if diarrhea represents a change in bowel habits. Is there nocturnal diarrhea?

E. Ask the client what makes the diarrhea worse or better.

F. Inquire about previous GI surgery.

G. Review the client's usual weight and any history of weight loss. If weight loss has occurred, how many pounds? How is the client's appetite?

H. Review family history of CD, colon cancer, UC, and malabsorption syndrome.

I. How has the duration of the current complaints affected the client's work or usual social activities?

J. Review for duration and extraintestinal symptoms:

   1. Urinary complications: Renal calculi

   2. Sclerosing cholangitis: Fatigue and jaundice

   3. Skin diseases:

     a. Erythema nodosum: Painful, tender, raised, purple lesion on the tibia

     b. Pyoderma gangrenosum: Inflamed patch of skin that has progressed to ulceration

     c. Herpetic lesions related to immune suppression

   4. Arthritic symptoms

   5. Ocular inflammation

   6. Hypercoagulability

K. Review the client's medications, especially antibiotics and NSAIDs.

L. Review the client's current tobacco/cigarette use.

Physical Examination

A. Check temperature, pulse, respirations, BP, and weight. Pediatrics: Plot height/weight on growth curves to follow growth failure.

B. Inspect:

   1. Observe the client's general appearance, noting pallor, wasting, apathetic appearance, ecchymosis, skin ulcerations, jaundice, and signs of Kaposi's sarcoma.

   2. Inspect the head and neck for aphthous ulcers, glossitis, stomatitis, and poor dentition.

   3. Inspect the abdomen for surgical scars.

   4. Order an eye examination for uveitis.

   5. Inspect the joints for warmth and redness.

C. Auscultate:

   1. Abdomen in all quadrants for altered bowel sounds (obstruction)

D. Palpate:

   1. Palpate the neck for goiter and lymphadenopathy.

   2. Palpate the abdomen for distention, ascites, tenderness rebound, guarding, and masses.

   3. Palpate for hepatomegaly in the RLQ.

   4. Palpate the joints for tenderness.

E. Rectal examination:

   1. Check the anal sphincter for tags, control, and discharge.

   2. Palpate for masses, fissures, fistulas, tags, and inflammation.

   3. Perform a digital rectal examination to assess for anal strictures and rectal mass.

F. Neurological examination:

   1. Assess for signs of vitamin B12 deficiency, including tingling sensation and numbness in the hands or feet

Diagnostic Tests

A. Laboratory tests:

   1. CBC with differential

   2. Electrolytes and albumin

   3. ESR

   4. Serum cobalamin (vitamin B_{12})

   5. Serum iron studies

   6. Folate

   7. Liver enzymes and functioning tests, including international normalized ratio (INR) and bilirubin (refer to the "Elevated Liver Enzymes" section in this chapter)

   8. HIV

   9. Celiac antibody testing should be considered

   10. Thiopurine methyltransferase (TPMT) activity should be assessed before AZA or 6-MP therapy is implemented.

   11. Vitamin D level

B. Stool studies:

   1. Guaiac

   2. Stool culture

   3. *Clostridium difficile* toxin assay

   4. Ova and parasites

C. Imaging:

   1. Abdominal flat plate

   2. BE:

     a. Classic "string sign": Narrow band of barium flowing through an inflamed or scarred area in the terminal ileum; differentiates CD from UC

     b. "Rectal sparing": Suggests CD in the presence of inflammatory changes in other parts of the colon

     c. "Thumbprinting": Indicates mucosal inflammation (may be seen on the flat plate of the abdomen)

     d. "Skip lesions": Areas of inflammation with normal-appearing areas

   3. Small-bowel follow-through GI series

   4. Fistulogram: Used to guide the surgical correction

   5. CT scan of the abdomen and pelvis. Standard CT and CT enterography are useful in evaluating the small bowel and complications such as intra-abdominal abscesses.

   6. MRI and magnetic resonance (MR) enterography for visualization of the small bowel and identification of extraluminal findings and complications

D. Procedures with/without biopsy:

   1. Colonoscopy: Mucosa has a characteristic cobblestone appearance

   2. Flexible sigmoidoscopy with biopsy: Reveals "skip areas" in the colon, significant small-bowel involvement, fistulas, and granulomas

   3. Upper endoscopy: Aphthous ulcerations occur in the stomach and duodenum in 5% to 10% of clients.

   4. Capsule enteroscopy: Detects small-bowel CD. The major risk is the potential for the camera to become lodged at the point of stricture, requiring operative intervention.

   5. Biopsy of the colon and/or small intestine

E. Tuberculin purified protein derivative (PPD) skin test

Differential Diagnoses

A. UC
B. Appendicitis
C. Colon cancer
D. IBS
E. Anorexia nervosa
F. Perianal abscess
G. Intestinal protozoan and bacterial infection
H. Food poisoning
I. Cytomegalovirus (CMV)
J. Intestinal tuberculosis (TB)
K. Other forms of colitis (ischemic, medication induced)
L. Gastroenteritis
M. Celiac disease

Plan

A. General interventions:
  1. **A gastroenterologist, colorectal surgeon, and specialists such as a rheumatologist and a nutritionist should jointly manage CD**
▶ B. *Client teaching: See Section III: Client Teaching Guide for this chapter, "Crohn's Disease."*
C. Pharmaceutical therapy:
  1. The medical management of CD can be divided into treatment of an acute exacerbation and maintenance of remission. In acute exacerbation, triggers, such as underlying infection, fistula, perforation, and other pathology, must be ruled out prior to the intravenous (IV) administration of glucocorticoids. The goal of chronic therapy is the remission of bowel inflammation. Therapies include the following:
    a. Vitamin, mineral, and folic acid supplements are necessary for proper healing and avoidance of secondary complications, such as bone disease and anemia:
      i. The client should take a multiple-vitamin supplement containing about five times the normal daily vitamin requirements.
      ii. Folic acid supplementation is required for clients on sulfasalazine because it impairs folic acid absorption.
      iii. Vitamin B12 replacement is required for clients who have ileal surgery.
      iv. Vitamin D, 4,000 international units (IU), is required for clients with steatorrhea.
    b. Opiates provide symptomatic relief of diarrhea during acute phases of illness and chronic active colitis. Diphenoxylate and atropine (Lomotil), codeine, tincture of opium (Paregoric), and loperamide (Imodium A–D) all limit the number of BMs. Tincture of belladonna and other anticholinergics help control cramping.
    c. In CD, inflamed areas can occur intermittently between the mouth and the anus, whereas inflammation of UC is continuous and limited within the colon. The following is a stepwise medication approach for CD (see Table 11.6 for adult dosing for CD and UC medications):
      i. Aminosalicylates (5-ASA) are a mainstay of therapy because of their anti-inflammatory

activities and rapid absorption throughout the small intestines. Several formulations are available for targeting a specific region of the bowel. The 5-ASA drugs are not specifically approved by the FDA for use in CD:
        1) Sulfasalazine and balsalazide are primarily released in the colon:
          a) Pediatrics: 50 to 75 mg/kg/d is given in three or four divided doses of with a maximum dose of 1 g/dose.
          b) **Reduced absorption of folic acid and digoxin has been reported when administered with sulfasalazine.**
        2) Mesalamine (Pentasa) can be released in the duodenum to the distal colon:
          a) Pediatrics: 50 to 75 mg/kg/d is given in three or four divided doses with a maximum dose of 1 g/dose.
        3) Asacol is targeted for release in the distal ileum and colon:
          a) Pediatrics: For clients 5 years or older, dose is weight based (up to a maximum of 2.4 g/d), divided into two daily doses for a duration of 6 weeks
          b) **Two Asacol 400 mg tablets are not interchangeable or substitutable with one mesalamine delayed-release 800 mg tablet.**
        4) Multi-Matrix System (MMX; marketed as Lialda) releases mesalamine in the colon. *Lialda is not recommended for children younger than 18 years.* Dosage is 2.4 to 4.8 mg once a day with meals, taken for 8 weeks.
        5) Mesalamine (Rowasa) is specific for the rectum and distal colon. Mesalamine 800 mg tablets are given three times daily for a total of 2.4 g/d for 6 weeks. Alternatively, 1 g control-release capsule four times daily for a total of 4 g/d for up to 8 weeks; or 40 g/60 mL as a retention enema or suppository once daily, preferably at bedtime. The rectal formulation should be retained overnight, for about 8 hours. The usual course of therapy for the rectal formulation is 3 to 6 weeks.
    d. Corticosteroids are used to provide immediate symptom relief in clients experiencing a flare. Glucocorticoids should not be used on a long-term basis because of the adverse effects and are not used for maintaining remission.
      i. Budesonide (Entocort) is designed to be effective only in the treatment of disease involving the ileum and ascending colon. Budesonide is effective in the maintenance of short-term (3 months) but not long-term (1 year) remission.
        1) Pediatrics: For children 6 years of age and older: The dose is 0.45 mg/kg/d

TABLE 11.6   MEDICATIONS FOR CROHN'S DISEASE AND ULCERATIVE COLITIS—ADULT DOSING

		Induction Therapy	Maintenance Therapy
5-ASA drugs have anti-inflammatory activities and rapid absorption throughout the GI tract. The 5-ASA drugs are not specifically approved by the FDA for CD			
Sulfasalazine (Azulifidine)	Treatment of mild-to-moderate UC, and as adjunctive therapy in severe UC. Converted to mesalamine in the colon.	**UC and CD** Initial 1 to 2 g/d in divided doses. Gradual increase to 3 to 4 g/d in divided doses.	**UC** For the prolongation of the remission period between acute attacks: 2 to 4 g/d in divided doses
Olsalazine (Dipentum)	Release is delayed in the colon. Converted to mesalamine in the colon.	**UC** Maintenance of remission of UC in clients intolerant of sulfasalazine	**UC** Maintenance: 500 mg orally. Take with food in evenly divided doses.
Balsalazide (Colazal)	Mild-to-moderately active CD. Release is delayed until the terminal ileum and cecum. Converted to mesalamine in the colon.	**UC and CD** 6.75 g/d in divided doses Duration 8 to 12 weeks	**UC and CD** Safety and effectiveness have not been established beyond 12 weeks
Mesalamine (Asacol)	Targeted for release in the distal ileum and colon	**UC and CD** 2.4 to 4.8 g/d in divided doses	**UC and CD** Maintenance: 2.4 to 4.8 g/d in divided doses
Mesalamine (Pentasa)	Mild-to-moderate disease. Released in the duodenum to the distal colon.	**UC and CD** 4 g/day in divided doses for up to 8 weeks	**UC and CD** 2 to 4 g/d in divided doses
Mesalamine (Apriso)	Locally acting 5-ASA, 24-hour delayed and extended release. Release occurs at a pH ≥ 6, then is prolonged throughout the colon.	**UC** 1.5 to 3 g/d in divided doses	**Maintenance of remission of UC.** 1.5 g every day
Mesalamine suppository	Specific to the rectum and distal colon	**Ulcerative proctitis** **Rectal suppository** One 500-mg suppository rectally twice a day **OR** one 1,000 mg suppository rectally at night. Suppositories should be retained 1 to 3 hours to achieve maximal benefit.	**Maintaining remission of ulcerative proctitis** **Rectal suppository** One 500 mg suppository rectally twice a day **OR** one 1,000 mg suppository rectally at night. Suppositories should be retained 1 to 3 hours to achieve maximal benefit.
Mesalamine retention enema (Rowasa)	Specific to the rectum and distal colon	**Retention enema**—60 mL (4 g) at bedtime, retained overnight (8 hours)	**Retention enema**—60 mL (4 g) at bedtime, retained overnight (8 hours)
Corticosteroids nonspecifically suppress the immune system. They are the mainstay of treatment for active flares			
Budesonide (Uceris, Entocort EC)	Treatment of mild-to-moderate CD involving the ileum and/or ascending colon Released in the distal small intestine and right colon **Rectal 5-ASA is the first-line therapy in distal UC**	**UC and CD** 9 mg daily for up to 8 weeks Taper to 6 mg daily for 2 weeks prior to complete cessation For recurring episodes of active CD, a repeat 8-week course can be given	**UC and CD** Maintenance of clinical remission of mild-to-moderate CD of ileum and/or ascending colon 6 mg/d up to 3 months Maintenance treatment beyond 3 months has no proven substantial clinical benefit
Prednisone (most common oral steroid used) Methylprednisolone (IV)	Used in acute treatment but is not preventive IV steroids are used in clients in severe disease who require hospitalization	**UC and CD** Dosage and length of treatment vary Steroids should not be stopped abruptly; tapering should begin concomitant with initiating other treatments to maintain remission	**UC and CD** Not for maintenance therapy

(continued)

TABLE 11.6   MEDICATIONS FOR CROHN'S DISEASE AND ULCERATIVE COLITIS—ADULT DOSING (continued)

		Induction Therapy	Maintenance Therapy
Hydrocortisone enemas (Cortenema) Hydrocortisone acetate foam and steroid suppositories (Cortifoam, ProctoFoam-HC)	Colonic disease—proctitis requiring topical/rectal formulations	**UC and CD** **Enema**—One nightly at HS; usual length of treatment 2 to 3 weeks **Suppository**—One twice a day (a.m. and p.m.). Severe proctitis may require using a suppository three times a day or using two suppositories twice a day. **Foam**—One applicator once daily or every 12 hours for 2 to 3 weeks, then one applicator every other day if needed	**UC and CD** Dosage and length of treatment are based on medical treatment and response to treatment

Immunomodulatory agents: Thiopurines—The 2013 AGA recommends against using thiopurine monotherapy to induce remission with clients with moderately severe CD. Because of the delay in the onset of action of 6-thiopurines, concomitant therapy with systemic corticosteroids or an anti-TNF-α drug is required for rapid system relief in clients with moderately severe CD.
The AGA suggests against using MTX to induce remission in clients with moderately severe CD.
The AGA suggests using MTX over no immunomodulator therapy to maintain corticosteroid-induced remission in clients with CD.

6-MP (Purinethol)	Slow onset: The onset of therapy is noted after 3 to 6 months.	**CD** Weight-based dosage and response to therapy: 1.5 mg/kg/d	**CD** Weight-based dosage and response to therapy: 1.5 mg/kg/d
Azathioprine (Imuran) Used off-label for UC and CD	Converts to its active form, 6-MP. Slow acting; can take up to 3 months to work.	**UC and CD** Weight-based dosage and response to therapy: 2.5 mg/kg/day	**UC and CD** Weight-based dosage and response to therapy: 2.5 mg/kg/day
MTX folic acid antagonist	Improvement generally in 3 to 6 weeks; full benefit may not be seen for 12 weeks	**CD** 15 to 25 mg once a week by injection Clients also need to take folic acid: 1 mg/d	**CD** 15 mg per week Clients also need to take folic acid: 1 mg/d

Biologics—TNF-alpha blocker
The AGA recommends using anti-TNF-α monotherapy to induce remission in clients with moderately severe CD.
The AGA recommends using anti-TNF-α with thiopurines over thiopurine monotherapy to induce remission in clients with moderately severe CD.
The AGA recommends using anti-TNF-α over no anti-TNF-α to maintain corticosteroid- or anti-TNF-α-induced remission in clients with CD

Infliximab (Remicade) IV infusion	Moderate-to-severe CD with fistulizing CD or resistance to steroids and conventional therapy	**CD** 5 mg/kg IV over 2 hours at 0, 2, and 6 weeks	**CD** 5 mg/kg every 6 to 8 weeks thereafter. If no response by week 14, consider discontinuing therapy.
Infliximab-dyyb (Inflectra)	Approved for adult and pediatric clients with moderate-to-severe CD.	**CD** IV infusion given at 2 to 4 hours at 0, 2, and 6 weeks	**CD** Every 8 weeks thereafter
Certolizumab Pegol (Cimzia) Subcutaneous (subq) in the abdomen or thigh	Moderate-to-severe CD resistance to steroids and conventional therapy	**CD** 400 mg (two 200 mg) subcutaneous injections on day 1, then at 2 weeks, and at 4 weeks	**CD** 400 mg every 4 weeks
Adalimumab (Humira) Subcutaneous in the abdomen or thigh	Moderate-to-severe CD resistance to steroids and conventional therapy	**CD** Prefilled syringes: On day 1, four injections are self-administered. On day 15, two injections are self-administered.	**CD** One injection every 2 weeks
Golimumab (Simponi)	Moderate-to-severe UC resistance to steroids and conventional therapy	**UC** 200-mg injections are self-administered at initiation, 100-mg subq at week 2	**UC** 100-mg injection every 4 weeks

(continued)

TABLE 11.6   MEDICATIONS FOR CROHN'S DISEASE AND ULCERATIVE COLITIS—ADULT DOSING (*continued*)

		Induction Therapy	Maintenance Therapy
Vedolizumab (Entyvio)	Moderate-to-severe CD and UC resistance to steroids and conventional therapy	**UC and CD** 300 mg IV infused over 30 minutes at initiation, week 2, and week 6	**UC and CD** 300-mg IV every 8 weeks thereafter
Antiadhesion molecule			
Natalizumab (Tysabri)[a] **Distribution is restricted and infusion is available only through a closely monitored infusion center program known as TOUCH**	Moderate-to-severe CD for adults who failed anti-TNF therapy.	**CD** 300 mg every 4 weeks. Given by IV infusion over 1 hour. Discontinue after 12 weeks based on individual response/protocol	**CD** 300-mg IV monthly— **Restricted distribution**
Antibiotics—Used for treatment of bacterial infections that cause abscesses and can be helpful with treatment of fistulas			
Ciprofloxacin (Cipro)		**UC and CD** Dosage and length of treatment vary	**UC and CD** Dosage and length of treatment vary
Metronidazole (Flagyl)		**UC and CD** Dosage and length of treatment vary	**UC and CD** Dosage and length of treatment vary

AGA, American Gastrenterology Association; CD, Crohn's disease; FDA, Food and Drug Administration; 5-ASA, aminosalicylates; GI, gastrointestinal; HS, bedtime; IV, intravenous; 6-MP, 6-mercaptopurine; MTX, methotrexate; TNF, tumor necrosis factor; TOUCH, Tysabri Outreach: Unified Commitment to Health; UC, ulcerative colitis.

[a]Natalizumab use carries an increased risk of a severe brain condition called *progressive multifocal leukoencephalopathy (PML)*, resulting from infection with the John Cunningham (JC) virus. It is important to be tested for JC virus prior to starting natalizumab; clients who are negative for JC virus have a much lower risk of developing PML.

Source: Adapted from the American College of Gastroenterology Guidelines (2013): gastro.org/guidelines

(maximum of 9 mg/d), tapered by 3-mg increments.

ii. Prednisone or prednisolone:

1) Pediatrics: Prednisone or prednisolone 1 to 2 mg/kg/d (maximum 60 mg/d) given orally or IV brings rapid improvement but should serve as a short-term induction therapy due to its long-term side effects, including growth failure, osteopenia, hirsutism, diabetes, psychosis, cataracts, and altered body shape and image. As soon as the acute disease subsides, steroid taper for 2 weeks to minimum is necessary to control symptoms.

2) Adults: Start prednisone with 40–60 mg PO daily and then taper 5 to 10 mg weekly for a total duration of 4 to 8 weeks.

e. Immunomodulatory agents may be initiated for IBD refractory to corticosteroids or frequent flares that require steroids. These agents require monitoring of blood counts due to hematological toxicity. A 3% incidence of pancreatitis, allergic reactions, infections, and marrow toxicity is associated with their use. The main drawback to the use of AZA and 6-MP is their slow onset. The effect of therapy is noted after 3 to 6 months of treatment. The FDA recommends that individuals should have TPMT genotype or phenotype assessment before initiation of therapy with AZA or 6-MP to detect individuals who have low-enzyme activity or who are homozygous deficient in TPMT:

i. 6-MP:

1) Pediatrics: 1.0 to 2.0 mg/kg/d orally (maximum of 150 mg/d)

2) Clients with inherited little or no TPMT activity are at increased risk for severe Purinethol toxicity and generally require substantial dose reduction.

ii. AZA (Imuran):

1) Monitoring includes CBC, including platelet counts weekly during the first month, twice monthly for the second and third months of therapy, then monthly or more frequently if dosage alteration is necessary.

2) TPMT testing: Testing is recommended or considered to either genotype or phenotype clients for TPMT.

3) Pediatrics: 1.5 to 2.5 mg/kg/d orally (maximum 200 mg/d)

4) Doses for adults and pediatrics must be lowered for clients with reduced TPMT activity.

iii. Methotrexate (MTX; folic acid antagonist) has adverse effects, including leukopenia, GI upset, and hypersensitivity pneumonitis:

1) Pediatrics: Doses typically start at 15 mg/m² per week and are advanced as

tolerated to a maximum of 25 mg/m² per week. Subcutaneous dosing for children is recommended to ensure absorption until the client enters remission; then switch to oral MTX.

    2) Folic acid supplement (1 mg/d) may reduce the likelihood of oral ulcers.

  f. Tumor necrosis factor (TNF)-alpha blocker:

   i. Infliximab (Remicade) is a chimeric monoclonal antibody to TNF-alpha. Infliximab is effective for moderate-to-severe CD and for clients with fistulizing CD or who are resistant to steroids and conventional therapy. Infliximab can close perianal fistulas refractory to therapy with antibiotics and 6-MP. Infliximab has a half-life of approximately 10 days.

    1) Pediatrics: Recommended for people ages 6 to 17 years with severe active CD whose disease has not responded to conventional therapy, including corticosteroids, immunomodulators, and conventional therapy; 5 mg/kg in a single IV dose

   ii. Certolizumab (Cimzia) is given subcutaneously in the abdomen or thigh.

    1) *Pediatrics: Not recommended*

   iii. Adalimumab (Humira) is an antibody directed against TNF. It is also administered subcutaneously in the abdomen or thigh.

    1) *Pediatrics: Not recommended for clients younger than 18 years*

  g. Natalizumab (Tysabri), a monoclonal antibody, is an effective induction agent for CD in adults. It is given in a certified TOUCH center. IV infusion is given over 1 hour and requires a 1-hour observation period post infusion.

    1. *Pediatrics: Not recommended for those younger than 18 years.*

  h. Antibiotics are utilized in adults for perianal disease or inflammatory mass. Pediatric doses have not been established in either metronidazole or ciprofloxacin for CD.

  i. Thalidomide, an inhibitor of both TNF and angiogenesis, has been used off-label to treat refractory IBD.

Follow-Up

A. Have the client record his or her weight daily to monitor changes.

B. Assess frequency and consistency of stools to evaluate volume losses and effectiveness of therapy.

C. Instruct clients on self-medication to call the healthcare provider's office if fever develops, diarrhea worsens, bleeding occurs, or abdominal pain becomes marked.

D. Monitoring of clients on 5-ASA should include a CBC at least twice a year and urinalysis at least annually.

E. Clients on 6-MP require frequent monitoring, including CBC and aminotransferase levels (ALT and AST) before treatment, and again at 2, 3, 8, and 12 weeks after initiating therapy. When stable, monitor every 3 months thereafter, and 2 to 3 weeks after a change in dosage.

F. Monitoring of clients on MTX includes a CBC and aminotransferases, just as with 6-MP/thiopurine therapies.

G. Periodic bone mineral density assessment is recommended for clients on long-term corticosteroid therapy (longer than 3 months). Osteopenia should be treated aggressively. The primary intervention includes dietary counseling and supplementation to ensure adequate intake of vitamin D and calcium.

H. Annual ophthalmological examinations are recommended for clients on long-term corticosteroids.

I. Clients who are using corticosteroids should be monitored for glucose intolerance and other metabolic abnormalities.

Consultation/Referral

A. Refer the client to a gastroenterologist initially for evaluation. Treatment requires multidisciplinary management with the gastroenterologist and other subspecialists, including a nutritionist, ophthalmologist, and social workers.

B. Promptly hospitalize for parenteral management those clients who are toxic, bleeding heavily, in severe pain, or too sick to obtain adequate nutrition orally.

C. Consider a referral for genetic testing.

Individual Considerations

A. Pregnancy:

  1. Active disease at the time of conception is associated with increased incidence of miscarriage and postpartum exacerbation. It may also predispose the client to other maternal and prenatal risks, such as premature labor, small-for-gestational-age babies, and stillbirth.

  2. Oral and topical mesalamine, oral balsalazide, sulfasalazine, corticosteroids, and ciprofloxacin (after the first trimester) are safe and effective during nursing or pregnancy.

  3. Women on prednisone should receive supplementary steroids during labor and delivery as well as during other highly stressful times.

  4. Counsel women to attempt pregnancy only when the disease has been quiescent for several months.

  5. Withholding sulfasalazine for 2 to 3 days before delivery may be advisable to minimize neonatal jaundice due to bilirubin displacement.

  6. MTX is an FDA category X drug.

B. Pediatrics:

  1. Approximately 30% of children with CD are refractory to or dependent on steroids despite concomitant use of 6-MP. These clients may require conversion from thiopurine to MTX maintenance therapy, or treatment with a biological agent.

  2. Sulfasalazine and olsalazine can be compounded into a suspension for young children to drink. It is recommended that other 5-ASA agents be swallowed whole; however, Pentasa may be opened and administered by sprinkling the granules on soft food.

  3. Psychological counseling may be required for children secondary to the chronic relapsing nature of the illness, effects on body appearance and image such as short stature, and pubertal delay.

  4. Children with CD should undergo colonoscopy for cancer screening beginning 8 to 10 years after the

diagnosis of CD. The frequency of screening should be determined by the findings on the initial colonoscopy (around every 1–3 years).

5. The National Institute for Health and Clinical Excellence (NICE) clinical guideline recommendations include consideration of monitoring for changes in bone mineral density in children and young people with risk factors, such as low BMI, low-trauma fracture, or continued or repeated glucocorticoid use.

C. Geriatrics:
1. **Unexplained diarrhea, weight loss, and perianal disease in the elderly should arouse suspicions regarding CD. Elderly clients have worse outcomes because of delayed presentation and comorbid conditions.**
2. Elderly clients tend to have CD confined to the distal colon, with only 40% having proctitis.
3. With an increase in cancers in elderly clients with CD, it is imperative to evaluate and exclude cancer before beginning immunosuppressant or biological therapies.
4. Review CD therapies, with comorbid conditions in mind, for side effects, interactions, need for increased laboratory monitoring (e.g., INR, as well as digoxin levels and phenytoin levels), and risk of infection
5. Anti-TNF-α agents are contraindicated in clients with New York Heart Association (NYHA) class III and IV heart failure (HF).

Resource
Crohn's and Colitis Foundation of America: www.ccfa.org

Bibliography
Crohn's and Colitis Foundation of America. (n.d.[a]). *Crohn's disease medication options.* Retrieved from http://www.ccfa.org/what-are-crohns-and-colitis/what-is-crohns-disease/crohns-medication.html
Crohn's and Colitis Foundation of America. (n.d.[b]). *Crohn's treatment options.* Retrieved from http://www.ccfa.org/what-are-crohns-and-colitis/what-is-crohns-disease/crohns-treatment-options.html
Crohn's and Colitis Foundation of America. (n.d.[c]). *Types of Crohn's disease and associated symptoms.* Retrieved from http://www.ccfa.org/what-are-crohns-and-colitis/what-is-crohns-disease/types-of-crohns-disease.html
Global RPH. (2016, March 10). *TNF inhibitors: Biological response modifiers (BRMs).* Retrieved from http://www.globalrph.com/TNFinhibitors.htm
Hashash, J., & Regueiro, M. (2019, January 15). Overview of medical management of high risk adult patients with moderate to severe Crohn's disease. *UpToDate.* Retrieved from https://www.uptodate.com/contents/overview-of-medical-management-of-high-risk-adult-patients-with-moderate-to-severe-crohn-disease
McDonald, L., Gerding, D., Johnson, S., Bakken, J., Carroll, K., Coffin, S., . . . Wilcox, M. (2018, December). Clinical practice guidelines for *Clostridium difficile* infection in adults and children: 2017 update by the Infectious Diseases Society of America and Society for Healthcare Epidemiology of America. *IDSA Clinical Practice Guidelines, 2018,* 1–48. doi:10.1093/cid/ciy149. Retrieved from http://www.uphs.upenn.edu/bugdrug/antibiotic_manual/C%20difficile%20guidelines%20IDSA2017.pdf
Nettina, S. (2010). *The Lippincott manual of nursing practice* (9th ed.). Philadelphia, PA: Wolters Kluwer Lippincott Williams & Wilkins.
Peppercorn, M. A., & Cheifetz, A. S. (2018, November 12). Definition, epidemiology and risk factors in inflammatory bowel disease. *UpToDate.* Retrieved from https://www.uptodate.com/contents/definition-epidemiology-and-risk-factors-in-inflammatory-bowel-disease#H531113302
Peppercorn, M. A., & Kane, S. V. (2018, May 18). Patient education: Crohn disease (beyond the basics). *UpToDate.* Retrieved from https://www.uptodate.com/contents/crohn-disease-beyond-the-basics

Cyclosporiasis

Cheryl A. Glass, Audra Malone, and Doncy Eapen

Definition
A. Cyclosporiasis is an infection caused by a one-cell parasite that affects the upper small intestines. Causes of cyclosporiasis include ingesting infected water or produce (fresh fruits, especially raspberries, and vegetables) or exposure to the organism during travel to countries where it is endemic.
B. Cyclosporiasis manifests as protracted and relapsing gastroenteritis. The clinical syndrome consists of explosive watery diarrhea, nausea, anorexia, weight loss, fatigue, low-grade fever, flatulence, myalgias, bloating and abdominal cramps that may persist for 7 days to several weeks, with a waxing and waning course.
C. In an immunocompromised host, onset is insidious; the condition becomes chronic with symptoms, and the shedding of oocysts continues indefinitely.
D. The oocysts are resistant to most disinfectants used in food and water processing and can remain viable for prolonged periods.

Incidence
A. The incidence of infection is unknown, although it is common around the world.
B. Most outbreaks in the United States and Canada have been associated with consumption of imported fresh produce, including raspberries, basil, snow peas, and mesclun lettuce.

Pathogenesis
A. Infection is caused by an 8- to 10-μm, spore-forming coccidian protozoan called *Cyclospora cayetanensis.* Transmission of oocysts is by the oral–fecal route. The incubation period ranges from 2 days to 2 weeks after excretion, depending on temperature and humidity.

Predisposing Factors
A. Incompetent or compromised immune system (e.g., infection with AIDS)
B. Travel to underdeveloped or tropical countries
C. Ingestion of contaminated food or water
D. Contact with animals that carry the parasite

Common Complaints
A. Abrupt, profuse, malodorous, watery diarrhea
B. Nausea
C. Vomiting
D. Anorexia
E. Substantial weight loss
F. Flu-like symptoms
G. Abdominal cramps and bloating

Other Signs and Symptoms
A. Asymptomatic
B. Low-grade fever
C. Nausea and vomiting
D. Profound fatigue

E. Yellow- to khaki-green stools

F. Flatus

G. Dehydration

Subjective Data

A. Review the onset, duration, and course of symptoms. Is diarrhea acute or chronic?

B. Question the client about travel to areas known for cyclospora, such as Haiti, Puerto Rico, Pakistan, India, Mexico, Nepal, New Guinea, and Peru. The protozoan has also been seen in Chicago, Los Angeles, New York, Florida, and Massachusetts.

C. Review the client's intake of medications and other substances that can cause diarrhea (e.g., antibiotics, laxatives, quinidine, magnesium-containing antacids, digitalis, loop diuretics, antihypertensives, alcohol, caffeine, herbal teas, and sorbitol-containing [sugar-free] gum and mints).

D. Ask about the nature of the client's BMs, including frequency, consistency, and volume; and presence of blood, pus, or mucus.

E. Review associated symptoms that need evaluation: Fever, abdominal pain, and anorexia.

F. Ask the client if other family members or sexual contacts are also ill.

G. Establish the client's normal weight and any recent weight loss. How much weight was lost and over what period of time?

Physical Examination

A. Check temperature, pulse, respirations, BP, and weight (vital signs are normal in most cases).

B. Inspect:
1. General appearance for signs of illness and dehydration:
   a. Inspect mucous membranes.
   b. Inspect infants' fontanelles.
   c. Note decreased skin turgor.

C. Auscultate:
1. Abdomen for bowel sounds in all quadrants

D. Palpate:
1. The abdomen for masses, rebound tenderness, and guarding; may exhibit RUQ pain (biliary disease)
2. Lymph nodes for enlargement

E. Rectal examination:
1. Perform this evaluation if other symptoms indicate a need for it (e.g., rectal bleeding, pelvic lymphadenopathy).

Diagnostic Tests

Identification may be made by microscopic examination of stool under UV light, by modified acid-fast staining, or by review of wet mounts of stool by experienced microscopists. Finding large numbers of white blood cells suggests an inflammatory or invasive diarrhea. The following tests are done:

A. Acid-fast Ziehl–Neelsen stained slide of stool

B. Stool culture for ova and parasites: Parasites are passed intermittently, so three or more stools on alternating days should be examined.

C. Endoscopy with small-bowel biopsy if stool tests are negative and other signs/symptoms indicate a need for this evaluation.

Differential Diagnoses

A. Cyclosporiasis

B. Giardiasis

C. Malabsorption

D. *E. coli* infection: *E. coli* causes diarrhea within hours of ingesting contaminated food. Confirm by checking if others were affected.

E. IBS: Leukocyte-free mucus is the hallmark of IBS

F. Viral diarrhea

G. Lactose intolerance

H. Other bacterial infections—for example, *Shigella*, *Salmonella*, and *Campylobacter*

I. Cholera

J. IBD (CD or UC)

K. Cryptosporidiosis

Plan

A. General interventions:
1. Avoid food and water that is contaminated with feces.
2. Fresh produce should always be washed thoroughly before it is eaten.

B. Client teaching:
1. *See Section III: Client Teaching Guide for this chapter,* ◄ *"Diarrhea."*
2. Teach contact precautions to those caring for diapered and/or incontinent children.

C. Pharmaceutical therapy:
1. Drugs of choice are trimethoprim with sulfamethoxazole (TMP–SMZ). They can reduce shedding, and stop diarrhea within 2 days.
   a. Adults:
      i. Immunocompetent host: TMP 160 mg/SMZ 800 mg tablet orally twice a day for 7 to 10 days
      ii. Immunocompromised host: TMP 160 mg/SMZ 800 mg tablet orally four times a day for 10 days, followed by prophylaxis with TMP 160 mg/SMZ 800 mg orally three times per week
   b. Children:
      i. For those younger than 2 months, do not prescribe TMP/SMZ.
      ii. For those older than 2 months: TMP 8 mg/kg, SMZ 40 mg/kg orally twice a day for 7 days for acute infections
2. Ciprofloxacin (Cipro) is the alternative treatment for clients with allergies to sulfamethoxazole:
   a. Adults: Cipro 500 mg orally twice a day for 5 to 7 days for acute infection
   b. Adults: Prophylaxis in HIV: Cipro 500 mg orally three times a week
   c. Pediatrics: Not recommended for those younger than 18 years

D. Dietary management:

1. Tell the client to increase fluids. Fluid replacement is the basic approach to prevent dehydration from diarrhea.

2. Tell the client to restrict milk products to rule out lactose intolerance.

3. Give the client a copy of a diet plan to control nausea and vomiting (children and adults).

Follow-Up

A. See the client in 1 week to verify continuing clinical improvement.

B. If diarrhea persists 2 weeks or longer, a second evaluation is indicated.

C. Retest stools for blood and leukocytes; do a stool culture for ova and parasites.

D. Report cases of cyclosporiasis to the health department.

Consultation/Referral

A. Consult an infectious disease specialist and/or gastroenterologist if the client has no symptom relief after completing therapies or has a prolonged or severe case.

Individual Considerations

A. Pregnancy:

1. TMP–SMZ is a pregnancy category C drug. Use it during pregnancy only if the potential benefits outweigh the risk to the fetus.

2. TMP–SMZ should be avoided near term because of the potential for hyperbilirubinemia and kernicterus in the newborn.

Bibliography

Centers for Disease Control and Prevention. (2015, February 28). *Parasites: Cyclosporiasis (cyclospora infection)*. Retrieved from www.cdc.gov/parasites/cyclosporiasis

Gupta, S. (2017, August 8). Cyclosporiasis clinical presentation. *Medscape*. Retrieved from https://emedicine.medscape.com/article/996978-clinical

Hammer, H., & Hogenauer, C. (2020). Lactose intolerance: Clinical manifestations, diagnosis, and management. *UpToDate*. Retrieved from https://www.uptodate.com/contents/lactose-intolerance-clinical-manifestations-diagnosis-and-management

Nettina, S. (2010). *The Lippincott manual of nursing practice* (9th ed.). Philadelphia, PA: Wolters Kluwer Lippincott Williams & Wilkins.

Diarrhea

Cheryl A. Glass, Audra Malone, and Doncy Eapen

Definition

A. Diarrhea is an abnormally high fluid content in the stool. Generally, diarrhea also involves an increase in the frequency of BMs, which can range from four to five to more than 20 times a day. Diarrhea may be an acute-onset or chronic/persistent condition.

B. Acute diarrhea is usually self-limited; the most common complication is dehydration.

C. Chronic diarrhea is defined as lasting longer than 14 days.

Incidence

A. The incidence of diarrhea is unknown; however, it is responsible for 20% of pediatric referrals in children younger than 2 years and for 10% in children younger than 3 years. Morbidity has decreased because of the use of oral rehydration solutions; however, the global rate of mortality from acute diarrhea is 18% in children younger than age 5 years.

B. The incidence of *Clostridium difficile* infection is approximately 7%, and 28% of clients who were hospitalized have positive cultures for this organism. *C. difficile–*associated diarrhea has a mortality rate as high as 25% in the frail elderly.

C. 20% to 27% of cases of *C. difficile* are community acquired.

Pathogenesis

A. The increased water content in diarrhea stools is due to an imbalance in the physiology of the small and large intestinal processes. A bacterial infection is usually the cause of acute diarrhea in children (Table 11.7). Other causes of diarrhea in children include malabsorption syndrome.

Predisposing Factors

A. Enteric infections from organisms that cause diarrhea

B. Females have a higher incidence of *Campylobacter* species infections.

C. Young children

D. Institutional: Day care and skilled nursing facilities

E. Food: Raw or contaminated food

F. Contaminated water or inadequate chlorinated water supply

G. Travel

H. Chemotherapy or radiation induced

I. Vitamin deficiencies (niacin and folate)

J. Vitamin toxicity (vitamin C, niacin, and vitamin B_3)

K. Ingestion of heavy metals (copper, tin, or zinc) or toxins

L. Ingestion of plants, mistletoe, or mushrooms

TABLE 11.7   ORGANISMS THAT CAUSE DIARRHEA

Viral organisms	Rotavirus Norovirus Adenovirus Calicivirus Astrovirus
Invasive bacteria	*Escherichia coli* *Klebsiella* *Clostridium difficile* *Clostridium perfringens* *Shigella* *Salmonella* *Campylobacter* *Cholera* *Yersinia* *Plesiomonas* *Aeromonas*
Parasites	*Giardia* *Entamoeba* organisms *Cryptosporidium* *Giardia lamblia*

M. Antibiotics
N. Antacids containing magnesium

Common Complaints
A. Frequent watery stool
B. Foul-smelling stools (fat malabsorption)
C. Flatulence
D. Abdominal cramping

Other Signs and Symptoms
A. Lethargy
B. Fever
C. Nausea and vomiting
D. Currant-jelly stool (blood and mucus)
E. Anorexia
F. Dehydration in adults:
    1. Thirst
    2. Less frequent urination
    3. Dark urine
    4. Dry skin
    5. Fatigue
    6. Dizziness
    7. Lightheadedness
G. Dehydration in infants and young children:
    1. Dry mouth and tongue
    2. No tears when crying
    3. No wet diapers for 3 hours or more
    4. Sunken eyes, cheeks, or fontanelles
    5. High fever
    6. Listlessness or irritability

Subjective Data
A. Review the onset of diarrheal stools. What is the normal stool pattern?
B. Review the consistency, color, volume, and frequency of the stools.
C. Review dietary intake of raw foods, contaminated food, and nonabsorbable sugars, including lactulose or lactose in lactose malabsorbers.
D. Review any contact with others who may have the same symptoms.
E. Have any of the stools contained blood? Bloody stool may be an indication of bacterial infection.
F. Review travel history, including camping vacations.
G. Review any exposure to turtles or young dogs or cats.
H. Review medication history, including antibiotics, vitamins, herbal production, laxatives, antacids that contain magnesium, opiate withdrawal, Olestra, and methyl-xanthines (caffeine, theobromine, and theophylline).
I. Review any food allergies and history of lactose intolerance.
J. Evaluate the client for the presence of other symptoms such as fever, nausea, vomiting and abdominal pain, or tenesmus.
K. Evaluate the client for symptoms of dehydration, including thirst, dizziness, mental status changes, and decreased urine output.

Physical Examination
A. Check temperature, pulse, respirations, BP (standing and sitting), and weight.

B. Inspect:
    1. Observe the client's general overall appearance, the presence of lethargy or depressed consciousness, or grimace during examination.
    2. Evaluate muscle tone, skin turgor, reduced muscle, and fat mass.
    3. Examine the mouth, lips, and mucous membranes for signs, symptoms, and severity of dehydration.
    4. Perform a perianal examination for skin breakdown, erythema, and fissures.
C. Auscultate:
    1. Heart
    2. Lungs
    3. Abdomen in all four quadrants
    4. Assess the presence of borborygmi (significant increase in peristaltic action that may be audible and/or palpable)
D. Percuss:
    1. Abdomen tends to be round and tympanic with diarrhea.
E. Palpate:
    1. Palpate the abdomen for masses, guarding, rebound tenderness, and peritoneal signs. Most often a doughy consistency is palpated when clients have diarrhea.
    2. For a newborn, palpate the fontanelles.
    3. Palpate for lymphadenopathy.
    4. Perform a rectal examination, including testing of stool for occult blood.

Diagnostic Tests
A. Stool specimens for the evaluation of:
    1. *C. difficile*
    2. Fecal leukocytes
    3. Blood
    4. Culture
    5. Ova and parasites
    6. Fecal alpha-1 antitrypsin levels
    7. Viral antigen testing
B. Specific enzyme immunoassay (EIA) and direct fluorescence antibody (DFA) assays are becoming the standard for the diagnosis of giardiasis.
C. CBC: WBC may be elevated.
D. Albumin
E. Electrolytes
F. A colonoscopy for intestinal biopsy for clients with chronic or protracted diarrhea or clients with AIDS should be done. A sigmoidoscopy alone may not reveal any abnormality.
G. Abdominal ultrasound to identify intussusception
H. Abdominal CT

Differential Diagnoses
A. Diarrhea: Infectious etiology
B. IBD:
    1. CD
    2. UC
C. CF
D. Giardiasis
E. Protozoan

F. Malabsorption syndromes

G. Intussusception

H. Stool impaction

I. IBS

J. Meckel's diverticulum

K. Intolerance of lactose, carbohydrates, and protein

L. Medication induced:
1. Antibiotic-associated diarrhea
2. Antacids containing magnesium
3. Cancer drugs

M. Pseudomembranous colitis

N. Toxic megacolon

O. Appendicitis

Plan

A. General interventions:
1. Examination of stools for ova and parasites should be done every other day or every 3 days.
2. Rehydrate with oral fluids for each diarrheal stool. Administer small amounts of fluids at frequent intervals.
3. Hold foods until hydration is completed. No evidence shows that bananas, rice, applesauce, and toast (BRAT) are useful; these foods are not currently recommended.

B. Client teaching:
1. Encourage proper hygiene and food preparation to prevent spread and future infections.
2. Water should be boiled for at least 1 minute if contamination is suspected.
▶ 3. Client teaching: *See Section III: Client Teaching Guide for this chapter, "Diarrhea."*

C. Pharmaceutical therapy:
1. Use antibiotics (or discontinue antibiotics in the case of *C. difficile*) or use antiparasitic agents, depending on the etiology.
2. The use of probiotics, *Lactobacillus GG* (I, A) and *S. boulardii* (II, B), has been found to be effective and may reduce the spread of rotavirus.

Follow-Up

A. Follow-up depends on the severity of diarrhea and the age of the client. Neonates require strict follow-up within a few days of illness.

B. Monitor children who require labor-intensive oral hydration. Hospitalization for IV hydration may be required.

C. Rotavirus vaccine is available for the prevention of rotavirus gastroenteritis. RotaTeq oral solution is administered in a three-dose series for infants aged 6 to 12 weeks and completed before 32 weeks. *Alternatively,* Rotarix prefilled oral applicator vaccine is available as a two-dose regimen for clients aged 6 to 24 weeks.

Consultation/Referral

A. Evaluate the need for a surgical consultation (fulminant colitis, peritonitis, and toxic megacolon) or a consultation with an infectious-disease specialist or a gastroenterologist.

Individual Considerations

A. Pediatrics:
1. Stool patterns vary widely. Breastfed children may have up to five to six stools per day. Breastfed infants with acute diarrhea should continue on breast milk.
2. The younger the child, the higher the risk for severe, life-threatening dehydration and nutrient malabsorption is.

B. Geriatrics
1. Review any hospitalizations within the last 72 hours as a cause of diarrhea.
2. Advanced age is a risk factor for *C. difficile* infection.
3. Diarrhea may be related to fecal impaction.
4. Dehydration is more common in the elderly.
5. Because of polypharmacy risk in the elderly, review all medications for drug-to-drug interactions.

Resources

Drugs.com Drug Interaction Checker: www.drugs.com/drug_interactions.html

Epocrates Medical Reference APP: www.epocrates.com

Medscape Drug Interaction Checker: reference.medscape.com/drug-interactionchecker

RxList Drug Interaction Checker: www.rxlist.com/drug-interaction-checker.htm

Bibliography

Hammer, H., & Hogenauer, C. (2020). Lactose intolerance: Clinical manifestations, diagnosis, and management. *UpToDate.* Retrieved from https://www.uptodate.com/contents/lactose-intolerance-clinical-manifestations-diagnosis-and-management

LaRoque, R., & Harris, J. B. (2018, March 17). Patient education: Acute diarrhea in adults (beyond the basics). *UpToDate.* Retrieved from https://www.uptodate.com/contents/acute-diarrhea-in-adults-beyond-the-basics

McDonald, L., Gerding, D., Johnson, S., Bakken, J., Carroll, K., Coffin, S., . . . Wilcox, M. (2018, December). Clinical practice guidelines for *Clostridium difficile* infection in adults and children: 2017 update by the Infectious Diseases Society of America and Society for Healthcare Epidemiology of America. *IDSA Clinical Practice Guidelines, 2018*, 1–48. doi:10.1093/cid/ciy149. Retrieved from http://www.uphs.upenn.edu/bugdrug/antibiotic_manual/C%20difficile%20guidelines%20IDSA2017.pdf

Nettina, S. (2010). *The Lippincott manual of nursing practice* (9th ed.). Philadelphia, PA: Wolters Kluwer Lippincott Williams & Wilkins.

RotaTeq (rotavirus vaccine, live, oral, pentavalent). (2017). *Highlights of prescribing information.* Retrieved from http://www.fda.gov/downloads/BiologicsBloodVaccines/Vaccines/ApprovedProducts/UCM142288.pdf

Sharma, G. D. (2019, May 2). Cystic fibrosis. *Medscape.* Retrieved from http://emedicine.medscape.com/article/1001602-overview

Diverticulosis and Diverticulitis

Cheryl A. Glass, Audra Malone, and Doncy Eapen

Definition

A. Diverticula are saclike protrusions of mucosa through the muscular colonic wall. Protrusions can occur in weakened areas of the bowel wall and blood vessels. Diverticulosis is the presence of diverticula, but it does not imply a pathological condition. Diverticulitis occurs when the diverticula become plugged and inflamed. Surgery is indicated when diverticulitis is refractory to medical treatment. Diverticular disease is one of the most common causes of lower GI hemorrhage and a leading consideration in clients who present with brisk rectal bleeding.

B. There is no evidence of a relationship between the development of diverticula and smoking, caffeine, and alcohol consumption. However, an increased risk of developing diverticular disease is associated with a diet that is high in red meat and total fat content. This risk can be reduced by consuming a diet high in fiber content, especially with fruits and vegetables (cellulose) (see Appendix B, Table B.6).

C. Diverticulosis is often diagnosed as an incidental finding on a BE or sigmoidoscopy/colonoscopy

D. Recurrent attacks of diverticulitis can result in the formation of scar tissue, leading to narrowing and obstruction of the colonic lumen.

E. Complicated diverticulitis includes those episodes associated with free perforation, abscess, fistula, obstruction, or stricture.

Incidence

Diverticulosis is very common and increases with age.

A. Prevalence by age:
   1. Age 40 years: 5%
   2. Age 60 years: 30%
   3. Age 80 years: 65% to 80%

B. No significant difference in prevalence by gender. Diverticulosis is symptomatic in 70% of cases. It leads to diverticulitis in 5% to 25% of cases, and is associated with bleeding in 5% to 15%. The sigmoid colon is commonly affected. There are two types of diverticular disease and diverticulitis:
   1. Simple, with no complications; responds to treatment such as dietary changes without the need for surgery
   2. Complicated, with abscesses, fistula, obstruction, perforation, and peritonitis leading to sepsis; usually requires surgery

Pathogenesis

A. The exact etiology of diverticular disease is not known.

B. The present theory is that fiber is a protective agent against the development of diverticula and subsequent diverticulitis; insoluble fiber causes the formation of more bulky stool, which leads to decreased effectiveness in colonic segmentation. The overall result is that intracolonic pressure remains close to the normal range during colonic peristalsis. Diverticular sacs can become inflamed when undigested food residues and bacteria get trapped in the thin-walled sacs. If this occurs, blood supply is mechanically compromised and bacterial invasion ensues.

Predisposing Factors

A. Advanced age

B. Obesity (84%–96%)

C. Low-residue diet

D. Complicated diverticular disease is exacerbated by:
   1. Smoking
   2. NSAIDs
   3. Opioids
   4. Steroids

E. Genetics may be a predisposing factor:
   1. Left-sided diverticula is predominant in the United States.
   2. Right-sided (cecal) diverticula is predominant in Asia.

Common Complaints

A. Diverticulosis is usually asymptomatic.

B. Painless rectal bleeding is the hallmark of diverticular bleeding, with intermittent passage of maroon or bright red blood.

C. Common diverticulitis symptoms:
   1. LLQ pain
   2. Constipation

Other Signs and Symptoms

A. Back pain

B. Flatulence

C. Periodic abdominal distention

D. Borborygmi, or loud, prolonged gurgles caused by hyperactive intestinal peristalsis

E. Diarrhea

F. Nausea or vomiting

G. Dysuria

H. Tenderness on palpation, possible guarding

I. Fever, low grade

Subjective Data

A. Review the onset, duration, and course of symptoms, including size, color, consistency, and frequency of stools.

B. Ask the client if constipation is a chronic or acute problem, and if it alternates with diarrhea. Has the client ever had a bowel obstruction?

C. Review the client's daily diet and fluid intake.

D. Ask the client about medication use, including iron supplements, NSAIDs, acetaminophen in high doses, and steroids.

E. Inquire about the color, amount, and frequency of rectal bleeding. Does the client strain when having a BM?

F. Review the client's history of pain with defecation.

G. Review the client's history of kidney stones, as this condition can mimic diverticulitis.

Physical Examination

The constellation of LLQ tenderness with or without peritoneal findings, fever, and leukocytosis is suggestive of sigmoid diverticulitis.

A. Check temperature, pulse, respirations, BP, and weight.

B. Inspection:
   1. Observe the client's general overall appearance for signs of pain.
   2. Inspect the abdomen in detail, assessing for distention and guarding.

C. Auscultate:
   1. All four quadrants of the abdomen; bowel sounds may be decreased or normal in early diverticulitis.

D. Percuss:
1. Abdomen
E. Palpate:
1. The physical examination may be relatively unremarkable but most commonly reveals abdominal tenderness or a mass:
a. Palpate the abdomen for rebound tenderness or masses signaling possible abscess and tenderness.
b. Palpate beneath the right costal arch, checking for Murphy's sign or pain on deep inspiration.
F. Pelvic examination:
1. Consider evaluation to rule out gynecological sources of the abdominal pain.
G. Rectal examination:
1. Evaluate for hemorrhoids, masses, fissures, fistulas, inflammation, and stool in the ampulla.

Diagnostic Tests
The diagnosis of acute diverticulitis can often be made following a focused history and physician examination, especially in clients with recurrent diverticulitis whose diagnosis has been previously confirmed.
A. The diagnosis of diverticular colitis is made endoscopically and histologically.
B. CT scan of the abdomen and pelvis is the optimal method of investigation for suspected acute diverticulitis.
C. CBC with differential: WBC may show leukocytosis with a shift to the left; Hgb and Hct may be low with chronic or acute bleeding.
D. CRP: Greater than 50 in the client with LLQ pain and no vomiting is highly suggestive of diverticulitis.
E. Radiography: Flat plate and upright films of abdomen to evaluate ileus or obstruction, free air, and perforation.
F. Proctosigmoidoscopy/colonoscopy: Endoscopy is not performed in clients with acute diverticulitis due to the risk of perforation or worsening of disease. After the acute episode subsides, colonoscopy can be performed to evaluate the extent of the disease or to rule out a malignancy.
G. BE after infection subsides. Caution: A BE during the acute phase may increase intraluminal pressure and cause bowel perforation.
H. Hemoccult: Stool
I. Pregnancy test if there is a possibility of pregnancy
J. Urinalysis (excludes UTIs)

Differential Diagnoses
A. Diverticulitis
B. Diverticulosis
C. Acute appendicitis
D. Bowel obstruction
E. Ischemic colitis
F. Colon cancer
G. Hemorrhoids
H. Constipation or impaction
I. IBD
J. Urological disorder: Pyelonephritis
K. Tubo-ovarian abscess/ PID
L. Torsion (testicular or ovarian)
M. Ectopic pregnancy
N. Cholecystitis
O. Hernia
P. Renal colic
Q. UTI
R. Mesenteric artery ischemia

Plan
A. General interventions:
1. Stress the importance of strict adherence to the recommended diet.
B. Client teaching:
1. Nothing by mouth (NPO) status for acute treatment
2. Full-liquid diet or low-fiber diet if not on bowel rest
C. Pharmaceutical therapy:
1. Conservative management of diverticulosis: Psyllium (Metamucil) one to three teaspoons in 8 oz of liquid three times a day
2. Diverticulitis initial attack: Ciprofloxacin (Cipro) 500 mg orally twice daily and metronidazole (Flagyl) 500 mg orally three times a day for 7 to 14 days. Amoxicillin/clavulanic acid or sulfamethoxazole–trimethoprim may also be used with metronidazole. Clients with mild diverticulitis can be started on an antibiotic as an outpatient.
3. 5-ASA may be added if there is a lack of response.
4. Relapse: May repeat the same antibiotic regimen for 1 month
5. Chronic disease: Use long-term ciprofloxacin but not metronidazole.
6. Avoid laxatives, enemas, and opiates.
7. NSAIDs should be avoided due to a moderately increased risk of occurrence of diverticulitis.
D. Long-term dietary management:
1. High-fiber diet, including bran, beans, fruits, and vegetables
2. Bulk agents if unable to tolerate bran
3. Note foods to avoid, such as nuts.
E. Medical management: Acute treatments:
1. Pain management: Oral or parenteral analgesics
2. Clear liquid diet: For clients who can tolerate oral intake, a clear liquid diet is recommended for 2–3 days.
3. IV fluids: To correct volume deficits in clients requiring hospitalization; continued until oral intake is tolerated
F. Surgical management:
1. Surgical intervention is required for abscess, peritonitis, obstruction, fistula, or failure to improve after several days of medical management, or recurrence after successful medical management

Follow-Up
A. Follow up in 2 to 3 days. Continue conservative management if the client has no signs of complications.
B. A colonoscopy should be performed from 6 to 8 weeks after recovery to evaluate the extent of the diverticulosis and/or rule out other manifestations.

Consultation/Referral

A. Consult a physician if the client has mild diverticulitis: Temperature less than 101°F; WBC less than 13,000 to 15,000

B. Arrange for prompt hospitalization and surgical consultation if the client's temperature rises above 101.0°F, his or her pain worsens, peritoneal signs develop, or WBC continues to rise. Surgery consultation is required for abscess, peritonitis, obstruction, fistula, or failure to improve after several days of medical management.

Individual Considerations

A. Immunocompromised and elderly clients may have a normal WBC without a left shift (indicating presence of immature neutrophils that suggest inflammation/disease) and still have a severe infection.

Bibliography

Feingold, D., Steele, S. R., Lee, S., Kaiser, A., Boushey, R., Buie, W. D., & Frederick Rafferty, J. (2014). Practice parameters for the treatment of sigmoid diverticulitis. *Diseases of the Colon & Rectum, 57*, 284–294. doi:10.1097/DCR.0000000000000075

Ghoulam, E. M. (2018, October 18). Diverticulitis workup. *Medscape*. Retrieved from https://emedicine.medscape.com/article/173388-workup#c6

Natesan, A., & Bury, C. (2015, April). *Diverticulitis: Evaluation and management*. Retrieved from http://www.ahcmedia.com/articles/135320-diverticulitis-evaluation-and-management

Nettina, S. (2010). *The Lippincott manual of nursing practice* (9th ed.). Philadelphia, PA: Wolters Kluwer Lippincott Williams & Wilkins.

Pemberton, J. H. (2018, August 23). Acute colonic diverticulitis: Medical management. *UpToDate*. Retrieved from https://www.uptodate.com/contents/acute-colonic-diverticulitis-medical-management#H5

Pemberton, J. H. (2019, April 18). Acute colonic diverticulitis: Surgical management. *UpToDate*. Retrieved from https://www.uptodate.com/contents/acute-colonic-diverticulitis-surgical-management

Elevated Liver Enzymes

Cheryl A. Glass, Audra Malone, and Doncy Eapen

Definition

Many of the liver function tests (LFTs) determine the health of the liver but are not direct measures of its function. The liver has excretory, metabolic, protective, detoxification, hematological, and circulatory functions. LFTs may be abnormal even in clients with a healthy liver. Normal laboratory chemistry values may vary according to age, gender, ethnicity, blood group, and postprandial state, as well as other factors such as exercise and pregnancy. Common rationales for ordering liver chemistry tests (see Table 11.8) include the following:

A. Making a differential diagnosis of the different types of jaundice

B. Assessing the severity of hepatocellular injury

C. Following the trend of the disease

D. Diagnosing of the presence of latent liver disease (i.e., differential diagnosis of ascites or hematemesis)

E. Screening the suspected case during outbreaks of infective hepatitis

F. Screening those persons exposed to hepatotoxic drugs

G. Evaluating cholestatic problems

Incidence

A. The incidence of elevated liver enzymes is undetermined. Abnormal elevations of serum liver chemistries may occur in 1% to 4% of the asymptomatic population.

Pathogenesis

A. Pathogenesis varies by diagnosis.

Predisposing Factors

A. Predisposing factors depend on the suspected or known medical diagnosis.

Common Complaints

A. Asymptomatic
B. Pruritus
C. Jaundice
D. Ascites
E. Fatigue
F. Weight loss
G. Change in the color of urine (dark) or stools (clay colored)
H. Loss of appetite

Subjective Data

A complete medical history is the single most important part of the evaluation of the client with elevated LFTs.

A. Review use of medications, including prescription medications, statins, and OTC medications, as well as herbal therapies.

B. Determine the duration of LFT abnormalities (if known).

C. Review the presence of accompanying symptoms, including arthralgias, myalgias, rash, abdominal pain, fever, pruritus, and changes in the color of urine or stool.

D. Has the client experienced any anorexia or weight loss? Over what period did weight loss occur?

E. Review parenteral exposures, including transfusions, IV and intranasal drug use, tattoos, and sexual history.

F. Review the client's recent travel history and possible exposure to contaminated foods.

G. Review the client's exposure to people with jaundice.

H. Review the client's occupational history and exposure to hepatotoxins.

I. Review the client's history of alcohol consumption, including when started, amount, type of alcohol (beer, liquor, and moonshine), and frequency.

J. Evaluate the gestational age of pregnancy. HELLP syndrome is generally present in the third trimester of pregnancy.

Physical Examination

A. Check temperature (if indicated), pulse, respirations, and BP.

B. Inspect:
   1. Observe for temporal and proximal muscle wasting.
   2. Perform an eye and mouth (mucous membranes) examination for icterus.

TABLE 11.8 LIVER CHEMISTRY TESTS AND IMPLICATIONS

Liver Chemistry Test	Clinical Implication of Abnormality
ALT (8–20 U/L)	Mild elevation: Nonalcoholic/alcoholic fatty liver or medications (statins, Tylenol). If ALT/AST > ALP, it suggests hepatocellular damage.
AST (8–20 U/L)	Mild elevation: Nonalcoholic/alcoholic fatty liver or medications (statins, Tylenol). If ALT/AST > ALP, it suggests hepatocellular damage. Ratio of AST to ALT ≥ 2:1 suggests alcoholic liver disease; a ratio > 3 strongly indicates alcoholic hepatitis.
ALP (20–70 U/L)	If ALP > ALT/AST, it is cholestatic. If ALP is high and ALT/AST is near normal, it suggests infiltrative disease or biliary obstruction. Differentiation would require CT/MRI.
Albumin (3.5–5.5 g/dL)	Synthetic function: Low levels suggest malnutrition, hepatic disease, or inflammation. Higher levels suggest acute infections, burns, stress from trauma/surgery, or MI.
Alpha-fetoprotein (0–20 ng/mL)	Cancer marker when elevated.
Bile acids: Urine bile salts, bile pigments, and *urobilinogen* (<1 mg/dL)	Abnormal levels: Cholestasis or biliary obstruction, impaired hepatic uptake or secretion, or portal–systemic shunting; intrahepatic cholestasis of pregnancy. Elevated levels indicate RBC lysis, cirrhosis, or poisoning.
Bilirubin: Serum total (0.1–1.0 mg/dL) Direct (0.0–0.3 mg/dL) Indirect (0.2–0.7 mg/dL)	Elevated levels indicate the liver is not clearing bilirubin appropriately and suggests cholestasis, impaired conjugation, or biliary obstruction
Cholesterol (< 200 mg/dL) Triglycerides (35–160 mg/dL)	Elevated levels could lead to nonalcoholic fatty liver disease, which results in long-term liver damage, increased lipoprotein production and metabolism, chronic cholestasis, and increased risk for stroke and diabetes
Fibrinogen (150–350 mg/dL)	Abnormal levels reflect poor hepatic synthesis: decreased clotting and inhibitor factors, platelet defects, and hyperfibrinolysis, which suggest liver damage/cirrhosis, acute liver insufficiency, or poisoning.
GGT (0–30 U/L)	Sensitive for cholestasis or biliary obstruction or malignant hepatocellular disease. Often used in conjunction with ALP: Both GGT and ALP are increased in hepatocellular damage, whereas an elevated ALP with a normal GGT would suggest bone disease. Distinguish between acute alcohol (ETOH) use or chronic ETOH (binge/abuse) use: Minimal increase in GGT with small amounts of ETOH; yet a much higher increase with > 2–3 ETOH drinks per day.
Hepatitis surface antigen, IgM, antibody, RNA, genotype, viral load	Differentiation of type of hepatitis (see Table 11.9)
LDH (45–90 U/L)	Elevated levels suggest hepatocellular damage, anemia, cancers, MI, muscle trauma, or bone fractures
Total proteins (6.0–7.8 g/dL) Albumin (3.5–5.5 g/dL) Globulin (2.3–3.5 g/dL) (A/C ratio)	Abnormal ratio suggests hepatitis or advanced liver disease
PT (11–15 seconds)	Synthesis function: Elevated levels indicate slow coagulability, hepatocellular disease, or fulminate hepatitis
Plasma ammonia (40–80 mcg/dL)	Elevated levels suggest CNS dysfunction/toxicity, Reye syndrome, kidney failure, or end-stage liver disease
5NT (2–15 U/L)	Elevated levels suggest cholestasis, primary biliary cirrhosis, or biliary obstruction. A deficiency suggests an autosomal recessive disorder or hemolytic anemia.
Urea (blood urea nitrogen) (7–18 mg/dL)	Elevated levels indicate nonalcoholic fatty liver disease, or end-stage liver disease when correlated with renal failure

ALP, alkaline phosphatase; ALT, alanine transaminase; AST, aspartate transaminase; CNS, central nervous system; 5NT, 5′-nucleotidase; GGT, gamma-glutamyl transpeptidase; IgM, immunoglobulin M; LDH, lactate dehydrogenase; PT, prothrombin time.

Hepatocellular—primary injury to hepatocytes; cholestatic—primary injury to bile ducts; infiltrative—liver invaded by non-hepatic substances.

Sources: Data from National Board of Medical Examiners. (2019). *Laboratory values*. Retrieved from www.nbme.org; American College of Physicians. (2019). *Laboratory values*. Retrieved from https://annualmeeting.acponline.org/sites/default/files/shared/documents/for-meeting-attendees/normal-lab-values.pdf; LabCorp, American Association for Clinical Chemistry. (2019). *Test information*. Retrieved from www.labcorp.com.

3. Perform a dermal examination for icterus, spider nevi, palmar erythema, and caput medusae (the presence of dilated veins seen on the abdomen; noted with cirrhosis of the liver and portal hypertension).

4. Evaluate the presence of gynecomastia.

5. Observe for the presence of jugular venous distention (JVD), a sign of right-sided HF that suggests hepatic congestion.

C. Auscultate:
  1. Heart
  2. Lungs
D. Percuss:
  1. Abdomen (liver and spleen aspects)
E. Palpate:
  1. Abdominal examination:
      a. Evaluate the presence of hepatomegaly; focus on the size and consistency of the liver
      b. Evaluate the presence of splenomegaly; focus on the size of the spleen. An enlarged spleen is most easily appreciated with the client in the right lateral decubitus position.
      c. Assess for ascites: Note the presence of a fluid wave or shifting dullness.
      d. Assess for an abdominal mass.
F. Lymph nodes examination:
  1. Evaluate for lymphadenopathy.
G. Testicular examination:
  1. Evaluate for testicular atrophy (increased estrogen/reduced testosterone).

Diagnostic Tests

A. The particular LFT tests ordered are related to the suspected or identified medical diagnosis. Table 11.9 shows common serologic tests for viral hepatitis.

Differential Diagnoses

A. Table 11.10 shows differential diagnoses for elevated liver enzymes.

Plan

A. General interventions:
  1. **The clinical significance of any liver chemistry test abnormality must be interpreted in the context of the clinical situation.**
B. Client teaching:
  1. The plan of care depends on the suspected or identified medical diagnosis. Lifestyle modifications, including discontinuance of medications and alcohol, weight loss, and dietary changes, can be recommended as appropriate.
C. Pharmaceutical therapy:
  1. Clients with marked abnormalities of liver tests, or with signs and symptoms of chronic liver disease or hepatic decompensation (i.e., ascites, encephalopathy, coagulopathy, or portal hypertension), should be evaluated and treated in a more expeditious manner than asymptomatic clients.

Follow-Up

A. Follow-up testing for elevated LFTs, including abdominal/liver ultrasonography, CT, MRI, and liver biopsy,

TABLE 11.9   SEROLOGIC TESTS FOR HEPATITIS

Virologic Test	Usual Clinical Implication of a Positive Test
Hepatitis A-IgM	Positive in acute hepatitis A
Hepatitis A-IgG	Positive in response to previous hepatitis A infection or vaccination
HBsAg	Positive during active hepatitis B infection
HBsAg	Positive in response to previous hepatitis B infection or vaccination
Hepatitis B core antibody-IgM	Positive during active hepatitis B infection
Hepatitis B core antibody-IgG	Positive in response to current or prior hepatitis B infection
HBV DNA	Positive during active hepatitis B infection
Hepatitis B e antigen	Positive test indicates replicative state of wild-type hepatitis B infection
Hepatitis B e antibody	Positive after replicative state of wild-type hepatitis B infection
HBV viral load	Assesses hepatitis B virology
HCV antibody ELISA	Positive during or after hepatitis C infection
HCV-immunoblot assay (RIBA)	Positive during or after hepatitis C infection
HCV RNA	Positive during hepatitis C infection
HCV viral load	Assesses hepatitis C virology
HCV genotype	Genotyping is used for evaluation of the appropriate medication and length of therapy

ELISA, enzyme-linked immunosorbent assay; HBV, hepatitis B virus; HCV, hepatitis C virus; HBsAg, hepatitis B surface antigen; IgG, immunoglobulin G; IgM, immunoglobulin M, RIBA, recombinant immunoblot assay.

TABLE 11.10   DIFFERENTIAL DIAGNOSIS WITH ELEVATED LIVER ENZYMES

Infiltrating Diseases of the Liver	
• Sarcoidosis • Tuberculosis • Fungal infection • Amyloidosis • Lymphoma • Metastatic malignancy • Hepatocellular carcinoma	
Autoimmune hepatitis	
Acute viral hepatitis (A–E, EBV, CMV, herpes)	Wilson's disease (genetic disorder of biliary copper excretion)
Cholestasis disease	Acute bile duct obstruction
Chronic hepatitis B, C	Hemolysis
Steatosis/nonalcoholic steatohepatitis	Myopathy
Hereditary hemochromatosis	Thyroid disorders
Medication/herbal induced	Strenuous exercise-induced changes
Alpha-1-antitrypsin deficiency	Pregnancy—HELLP syndrome
Cirrhosis	Toxin(s) exposure
Celiac disease	Acute Budd–Chiari syndrome
Alcohol-related liver injury	Anorexia nervosa
Nonalcoholic fatty liver disease	Adrenal insufficiency

CMV, cytomegalovirus; EBV, Epstein–Barr virus; HELLP, hemolysis, elevated liver enzymes, and low platelets.

depends on the risk factors for disease, symptoms and history, and physical findings of the suspected or identified medical diagnosis. A liver chemistry test that is normal does not ensure that the client is free of liver disease. If a laboratory error is suspected, the laboratory test should be repeated.

Consultation/Referral
A. Consider a consultation or referral to a hepatologist, gastroenterologist, or infectious disease specialist.

Individual Considerations
A. Pregnancy:
1. HELLP syndrome is a severe form of pregnancy-induced hypertension (PIH or preeclampsia). It may occur anywhere from the mid-second trimester to immediately postpartum. This syndrome occurs in 0.1% to 0.8% of pregnancies. Its etiology is unknown. The presence of laboratory abnormalities confirms the diagnosis. Treatment of HELLP syndrome will not be covered here. However, the laboratory abnormalities noted include the following:
   a. Hemolytic anemia
   b. Proteinuria
   c. Serum AST level > 70 IU/L
   d. Low platelet count < 10,000 cells/mL
   e. Serum lactate dehydrogenase (LDH) level > 600 IU/L
   f. Total bilirubin level > 1.2 mg/dL

Bibliography
Nettina, S. (2010). *The Lippincott manual of nursing practice* (9th ed.). Philadelphia, PA: Wolters Kluwer Lippincott Williams & Wilkins.
Utah Library of Medicine. (n.d.). *Hepatitic pathology: Caput medusae.* Retrieved from http://library.med.utah.edu/WebPath/LIVEHTML/LIVER061.html

Gastroenteritis, Bacterial and Viral

Cheryl A. Glass, Audra Malone, and Doncy Eapen

Definition
A. Bacterial and viral gastroenteritis is an acute inflammation of the GI mucosa of the middle or lower intestine. It is primarily an acute, self-limiting illness. Immunocompromised clients can develop unremitting or fatal symptoms from gastroenteritis.

Incidence
A. Gastroenteritis is very common, occurring in all age groups. Epidemic outbreaks of bacterial gastroenteritis occur in groups who have ingested contaminated food. Viral excretion can begin before symptoms. Gastroenteritis is responsible for an estimated 8 million healthcare visits and 250,000 hospitalizations a year.
B. Rotavirus is most common in young children, with peak incidence at 3 to 15 months of age.
C. Norovirus most commonly infects older children and adults.
D. Astrovirus usually infects infants and young children; however, it can infect people of all ages.
E. Adenoviruses primarily affect children younger than 2 years.

Pathogenesis
A. Gastroenteritis is commonly caused by infectious agents—viruses, bacteria, and parasites (see Table 11.11). There are four viral agents: rotavirus, norovirus, enteric adenovirus, and astrovirus (Lee et al., 2013). Rotavirus is the most common cause of severe diarrhea in children. Exotoxins produced by some organisms induce

TABLE 11.11 INFECTIOUS AGENTS CAUSING GASTROENTERITIS

Causative Agent	Incubation Period
Noroviruses	12 hours–2 days
E. coli	24–72 hours
Campylobacter	2–5 days
Staphylococcus	1–6 hours
Shigella	8–24 hours
Botulism	12–36 hours
Giardia lamblia	7–21 days
Salmonella	6–72 hours
Rotaviruses	1–3 days
Astrovirus	1–5 days
Adenoviruses	5–8 days
Clostridium perfringens	10–12 hours
Clostridium difficile	Variable
Listeria species	20 hours

hypersecretion or increased peristalsis, resulting in diarrhea or vomiting. Bacteria, such as *E. coli* and *Salmonella*, penetrate and invade the gastric mucosa and lead to diarrhea accompanied by fever and fecal leukocytes. Viruses destroy enterocytes of the upper jejunal villi, often producing secondary lactose intolerance.

Predisposing Factors
A. Travel to areas where cholera or *Giardia* is epidemic:
   1. Ingestion of raw or undercooked seafood or drinks containing cholera-contaminated ice or water
   2. Ingestion of *Giardia*-contaminated water supplies
B. Ingestion of food contaminated with *Salmonella* or *Shigella*. Foods that are often implicated are domestic fowl and eggs, custard-filled pastries, processed meats, foods warmed on steam tables, poultry, red meat, raw seafood, raw milk, rice, and bean sprouts due to the following:
   1. Inadequate cooking time and temperatures
   2. Poor hygiene, lack of handwashing
   3. Improper storage of food
   4. Ingestion of fruits and vegetables contaminated by an infected person or by animal products
C. Infection by person-to-person spread:
   1. Day-care centers: Rotavirus can be found on toys and hard surfaces.
   2. Overcrowded environments, inadequate healthcare or education
   3. Schools and dormitories
   4. Nursing homes
   5. Banquet halls and cruise ships
   6. Schools and community centers
   7. Natural disasters
   8. Prisons
D. Contact with *Salmonella*-infected turtles, iguanas, and other reptiles

E. Seasonal outbreaks:
   1. Rotavirus and astrovirus outbreaks occur from October to April.
   2. Adenovirus outbreaks occur throughout the year.
   3. Norovirus outbreaks occur throughout the year but tend to increase in cooler months (November to April).
   4. Astrovirus outbreaks are most common in the winter.

Common Complaints
A. Abrupt onset of nausea and vomiting
B. Abrupt onset of diarrhea (with or without blood and mucus)
C. Abdominal pain
D. Fever occurs in approximately half of the cases.

Other Signs and Symptoms
A. Explosive flatulence
B. Cramping abdominal pain
C. Abdominal tenderness
D. Frequent watery diarrhea
E. Mucoid stools with or without blood
F. Tenesmus
G. Myalgia
H. Headache
I. Weakness
J. Malaise
K. Potential for seizures in children with high fever or electrolyte abnormalities

Subjective Data
A. Review the onset, duration, and course of symptoms, including the presence of abdominal pain and frequency of BMs. Ask the client if anyone else in the family has the same symptoms.
B. Ask the client about travel history, including travel by cruise ships or travel to foreign countries and camping with ingestion of water from streams, springs, or untreated wells.
C. Ask the client about crowded or unsanitary living conditions, use of day-care centers, and institutional living.
D. Take a 24-hour diet history, including ingestion of prunes or beans.
E. Review diarrhea history:
   1. How many stools?
   2. How frequent are the diarrheal stools?
   3. What color is the stool?
   4. Does the stool contain mucus?
   5. Has there been blood in the stool?
   6. Does the client have tenesmus (constant feeling of the need to pass stool)?
F. Inquire about other symptoms, such as fever or respiratory problems.
G. If the client is an infant, ask the caregiver about activity level, irritability, sleep pattern, fluid intake, and number of wet diapers.
H. If the client is a child, ask about activity level and dietary and fluid intakes.

I. Review drug history intake, including laxatives, antacids, antibiotics, quinine, or anticancer medications.
J. Has the client been vaccinated with the rotavirus vaccine?

Physical Examination

A. Check temperature, pulse, respirations, BP, and weight:
  1. Bacterial infections: Temperatures between 101°F and 102°F
  2. Viral infections: Temperatures of 103°F and above
  3. Note hypotension and tachycardia.
B. Inspect:
  1. Inspect general appearance; note if the client is very ill.
  2. Assess hydration status. Signs of dehydration:
    a. Mild: Slightly dry buccal mucous membranes, increased thirst, and decreased urine output
    b. Moderate: Sunken eyes, sunken fontanelle in infants, loss of skin turgor, dry buccal mucous membranes, and decreased urine output
    c. Severe: Signs of moderate dehydration and one or more of the following: Rapid thready pulse, tachypnea, lethargy, and postural hypotension
  3. Assess activity level and behavior in an infant or child.
C. Auscultate:
  1. Abdomen in all quadrants for bowel sounds; note hyperactive bowel sounds, absent or hypoactive bowel sounds (common with botulism), and borborygmi.
D. Percuss:
  1. Abdomen
E. Palpate:
  1. Abdomen for diffuse tenderness, slight distention, masses, rebound tenderness, and spasm. Observe for muscle guarding during the examination.
F. Rectal examination:
  1. Check for masses, fissures, inflammation, perianal erythema, or stool in ampulla.
G. Neurological examination:
  1. Check for dizziness, difficulty swallowing, and other neurological signs.
  2. Neurological signs and symptoms indicate botulism and require emergency intervention.

Diagnostic Tests

A. No immediate laboratory tests are required if dehydration is absent or mild and the client feels well except for frequent diarrhea.
B. CBC with differential: Serologic studies can detect viral pathogens.
C. Sedimentation rate: Elevated with infections or inflammation
D. Electrolytes, sodium, chlorides, potassium, and BUN
E. Blood gases to assess acid–base balance, if indicated
F. Blood cultures, if indicated
G. Stool for guaiac, leukocytes, ova, and parasites; test specimens three times, every other day. Stool guaiac is usually negative in viral infections, and positive in invasive bacterial infections. Large numbers of white cells in stool

suggest inflammatory or invasive diarrhea, such as occurs with *Shigella*, *Salmonella*, *Campylobacter*, invasive *E. coli*, or *Entamoeba*. Mononuclear cells in stool are characteristic of salmonellosis.
H. Stool culture if blood or mucus, fever more than 24 hours, or leukocytes are present
I. Special cultures for *Campylobacter* and cholera are required.
J. Urinalysis: Excludes UTI as cause of nonspecific diarrhea; urine specific gravity to assess dehydration
K. Sigmoidoscopy: Skip bowel prep with gross blood, large numbers of leukocytes in stool, or severe illness.
L. Culture food from suspected foci for *Salmonella*.
M. Real-time reverse transcriptase–polymerase chain reaction (RT-qPCR) is the most widely used assay for detecting norovirus in stool, vomitus, and environmental specimens. The best detection is in stool specimens.

Differential Diagnoses

A. Gastroenteritis, bacterial and viral
B. Acute viral hepatitis
C. Acute appendicitis
D. Cholecystitis
E. IBD
F. PID
G. Intussusception
H. Bowel obstruction for other causes
I. *C. difficile* colitis

Plan

A. General interventions:
  1. **Meticulous handwashing is the single most important measure to decrease transmission. Hand sanitizers are an option when access to soap or clean water is limited.**
  2. Advise the client to begin bed rest with progression to regular activities.
  3. If the client is diapered and/or incontinent, tell the client or caregiver to adhere strictly to contact precautions. Alcohol-based handwashing may decrease the spread.
  4. Diaper changing areas should be separate from food preparation areas.
  5. Chlorine-based disinfectants inactivate rotavirus and may prevent disease transmission from contact with environmental surfaces.
B. Client teaching:
  1. *See Section III: Client Teaching Guide for this chapter, "Diarrhea."* ◀
C. Pharmaceutical therapy:
  1. The primary treatment for viral gastroenteritis is fluid replacement. There are no specific antiviral pharmaceutical therapies. IV rehydration of fluids and electrolytes may be required in severe dehydration.
  2. Antibiotics may or may not be prescribed according to the bacterial source. Antimicrobial therapy is not indicated for uncomplicated (noninvasive) gastroenteritis because therapy does not shorten duration of the disease and can prolong duration of excretion of *Salmonella* organisms.

3. Antidiarrheal therapy delays transit time and can reduce the severity and duration of abdominal cramping; however, it may prolong the course of some bacterial diarrhea such as that caused by *Shigella* and *E. coli*. Bismuth subsalicylate (Pepto-Bismol; OTC) is not recommended for young children with gastroenteritis due to the potential toxicity from salicylate absorption.

4. Stop other medications that may be triggering diarrhea.

5. Vaccinate children with rotavirus live vaccine. Both vaccinations are oral.

   a. RotaTeq is given in three doses at ages 2, 4, and 6 months. The third dose should not be given after 32 weeks of age.

   b. Rotarix is given in two doses at ages 2 months and 4 months and before 24 weeks of age.

   c. The rotavirus vaccine can be administered together with the diphtheria, tetanus, and acellular pertussis (DTaP) vaccine; *Haemophilus influenzae* type b (Hib) vaccine; inactivated polio vaccine (IPV); hepatitis B vaccine; and pneumococcal conjugate vaccine.

   d. In March 2010, the Centers for Disease Control and Prevention (CDC) learned that a virus (or parts of a virus), *Porcine circovirus* (PCV), is present in both rotavirus vaccines. There is no evidence that PCV is a safety risk or causes illness in humans. Information related to PCV and rotavirus vaccines is available on the FDA and the CDC websites.

   e. A low-level increased risk of intussusception (1 to 1.5 cases per 100,000 vaccinated infants) has been detected following rotavirus vaccination, particularly shortly after the first dose. The CDC continues to recommend both Rotarix and RotaTeq to prevent severe rotavirus disease in infants and children. The CDC continues to monitor data on intussusception.

D. Dietary management:

1. Clients should comply with nothing by mouth (NPO) restrictions and then slowly add clear liquids to maintain hydration.

2. Hydration is one of the most important factors in the prevention of complications.

3. Rehydrate with oral fluids for each diarrheal stool.

4. Administer small amounts of fluids at frequent intervals.

5. Encourage client to eat as tolerated. Smaller amounts and a bland low-residue diet may be better tolerated. No evidence shows that BRAT are useful; these are not currently recommended. See Appendix B for "Nausea and Vomiting Diet Suggestions (Children and Adults)."

Follow-Up

A. Tell the client to return if the condition worsens or if signs and symptoms have not abated in 48 to 72 hours. However, diarrhea due to *Salmonella* may be expected to persist for up to 2 weeks.

B. Renal function tests and CBC should be done in approximately 1 week after the start of symptoms in clients with *E. coli* O157:H7 to detect early-onset hemolytic–uremic syndrome.

C. If diarrhea persists for 2 weeks or more, the client should present for a secondary evaluation.

D. Reporting surveillance systems:

1. In 2009, the CDC launched the National Outbreak Reporting System (NORS) to collect information for public health agencies on outbreaks of foodborne, waterborne, and enteric diseases that are spread from person to person, animals, environmental surfaces, and other ways.

2. In 2009, the CDC developed CaliciNet for public health and food regulator laboratories to submit outbreak information to a national database.

3. New Vaccine Surveillance Network (NVSN)

4. Foodborne Disease Active Surveillance Network (FoodNet)

Consultation/Referral

A. Refer clients to a physician immediately if they have dehydration, rebound tenderness, severe abdominal pain, neurological symptoms, and intussusception.

B. Immediately refer infants younger than age 2 years with paroxysmal, severe abdominal pain, and vomiting followed by currant-jelly stool; they need immediate evaluation for intussusception.

C. Refer any client with diarrhea longer than 7 days who has had no response to usual treatment.

D. Refer an immunocompromised client.

Individual Considerations

A. Pediatrics:

1. Very young children are at a higher risk of mortality.

2. Affected children may exhibit chronic diarrhea, or more than five watery or loose stools a day, but they develop normally and show no signs of malnutrition.

3. Rotavirus is the most common cause of nosocomial diarrhea in children and an important cause of acute gastroenteritis in day-care centers. Children whose stool cannot be contained by diapers or toilet use should be excluded from day care until diarrhea stops.

4. Breastfeeding can continue during diarrhea.

5. Children should not attend day-care facilities until 24 hours or more after diarrhea ceases.

6. In cases of *Shigella*: The health department may not permit return to day-care facilities until the child has one or more stool cultures negative for *Shigella*.

7. Children should not go to water parks/swimming pools for 1 week after symptoms resolve.

B. Adults:

1. Those with concomitant chronic debilitating disease are at a higher risk of mortality.

C. Geriatrics:

1. Elderly clients are at a higher risk of mortality secondary to dehydration. Signs of dehydration include:

   a. Confusion

   b. Muscle weakness

   c. Fever

    e. Poor skin turgor
    f. Hypotension
    g. Tachycardia
  2. Diminished thirst mechanism and decreased body water exacerbate dehydration.
  3. New residents to nursing/group homes should be isolated from ill clients.

Resource

Centers for Disease Control and Prevention: www.cdc.gov

Bibliography

Alexandraki, I., & Smetana, G. W. (2019, March 1). Acute viral gastroenteritis in adults. *UpToDate*. Retrieved from https://www.uptodate.com/contents/acute-viral-gastroenteritis-in-adults?sectionName=DIFFERENTIAL%20DIAGNOSIS&topicRef=2710&anchor=H752813318&source=see_link#H752813340

Bonheur, J. L. (2015, October 13). Bacterial gastroenteritis. *Medscape*. Retrieved from http://emedicine.medscape.com/article/176400-overview

Centers for Disease Control and Prevention. (2018a, July 25) . *Rotavirus vaccination*. Celiac Disease Foundation. Retrieved https://www.cdc.gov/vaccines/vpd/rotavirus/index.html

Centers for Disease Control and Prevention. (2018b, September 20). *Rotavirus*. Immunization Action Coalition. Retrieved from http://www.immunize.org/askexperts/experts_rota.asp

Hammer, H., & Hogenauer, C. (2020). Lactose intolerance: Clinical manifestations, diagnosis, and management. *UpToDate*. Retrieved from https://www.uptodate.com/contents/lactose-intolerance-clinical-manifestations-diagnosis-and-management

McDonald, L., Gerding, D., Johnson, S., Bakken, J., Carroll, K., Coffin, S., . . . Wilcox, M. (2018, December). Clinical practice guidelines for *Clostridium difficile* infection in adults and children: 2017 update by the Infectious Diseases Society of America and Society for Healthcare Epidemiology of America. *IDSA Clinical Practice Guidelines, 2018*, 1–48. doi:10.1093/cid/ciy149. Retrieved from http://www.uphs.upenn.edu/bugdrug/antibiotic_manual/C%20difficile%20guidelines%20IDSA2017.pdf

Nettina, S. (2010). *The Lippincott manual of nursing practice* (9th ed.). Wolters Kluwer Lippincott Williams & Wilkins.

RotaTeq (rotavirus vaccine, live, oral, pentavalent). (2017). *Highlights of prescribing information*. Retrieved from http://www.fda.gov/downloads/BiologicsBloodVaccines/Vaccines/ApprovedProducts/UCM142288.pdf

Gastroesophageal Reflux Disease

Cheryl A. Glass, Audra Malone, and Doncy Eapen

Definition

A. The ACG defines GERD as symptoms or complications resulting from the reflux of gastric contents into the esophagus or beyond, into the oral cavity (including larynx) or lung.
B. Gastroesophageal reflux is considered a normal physiological process in healthy infants, children, and adults. Most episodes last less than 3 minutes, and they most often occur 30 to 60 minutes after meals and with reclining positions. GERD is present when the symptoms occur more than twice a week.
C. Complications of GERD include erosive esophagitis (EE), esophageal strictures, and Barrett's esophagus.
D. A very large population of clients will present after self-medicating with antacids, bicarbonate soda, and OTC medications. Management of GERD should be tailored to the frequency, severity, and duration of symptoms.

Incidence

A. Daily GERD (also known as heartburn) is very common; it typically occurs postprandially and has been estimated to affect 17% to 65% of the normal adult population. Reflux esophagitis affects 30% to 80% of women at some time during pregnancy. It is estimated that 30% to 90% of clients with asthma have GERD. Barrett's esophagus, which affects fewer than 1% of adults, is commonly associated with GERD.

Pathogenesis

A. Gastroesophageal reflux is relaxation or incompetence of the lower esophagus persisting beyond the newborn period. Relaxation of the lower esophageal sphincter (LES) allows reflux of gastric acid and pepsin into the distal esophagus. Heartburn occurs when reverse peristaltic waves cause regurgitation of acidic stomach contents into the esophagus. Anatomical abnormalities, such as a hiatal hernia, predispose persons to GERD. Improper diet and nervous tension are also precipitating factors.
B. As a trigger for asthma, GERD has been identified as possibly activating vagal reflexes and/or microaspiration. Asthma may promote GERD, and GERD may provoke asthma. Some asthma medications may reduce LES tone, further complicating the picture. Conversely, a client with GERD may experience pulmonary disease as a response to the esophageal acid exposure.

Predisposing Factors

A. Obesity
B. Consuming large meals
C. Pregnancy
D. Immature, weak sphincter in newborns
E. Emotional stress
F. Increased abdominal pressure from tight clothes, straining to lift or defecate, or swallowing air
G. Ingesting drugs and foods that promote LES relaxation:
  1. NSAIDs
  2. Benzodiazepines
  3. Calcium-channel blockers
  4. Theophylline
  5. Nitrates
  6. Anticholinergics
  7. Alcohol
  8. Chocolate and peppermint
H. Smoking: Increases stomach acid and LES pressure
I. Ingestion of caustic agents such as lye
J. Infection by agents, such as *Candida*, herpes simplex, or CMV, which directly attack the esophageal mucosa, causing esophagitis that leads to/aggravates GERD
K. Compromised immunity, from AIDS, diabetes, or chemotherapy
L. Asthma

Common Complaints

A. Heartburn
B. Regurgitation of fluid or food
C. Chest pain

Alarm Symptoms

A. Dysphagia (difficulty swallowing)
B. Unintentional weight loss
C. Predominant upper abdominal pain
D. Hematemesis (vomiting blood)
E. Melena (black feces/blood stool)
F. Odynophagia (painful swallowing)
G. Severe symptoms

Other Signs and Symptoms

A. Retrosternal aching or burning
B. Nocturnal aspiration, water or "acid" brash
C. Harsh taste in the mouth upon awakening
D. Chronic cough, especially at bedtime
E. Hoarseness
F. Globus sensation
G. Nausea
H. Dental erosion
I. Infants: FTT, vomiting

Subjective Data

A. Review the onset, duration, and course of heartburn or other symptoms.
B. Review the client's medication history, including OTC medication and herbals:
   1. Has the client been taking OTC antacids, H_2 blockers, or OTC proton pump inhibitors (PPIs)?
   2. How long has the client been using these OTC agents?
   3. Is the client taking drugs that induce esophagitis?
      a. Antibiotics
      b. Alendronate
      c. NSAIDs
      d. Ascorbic acid
      e. Potassium chloride
      f. Quinidine
      g. Iron
C. Ask the client about alleviating and aggravating factors.
D. Review the client's habits, including smoking and alcohol intake.
E. Inquire about other symptoms, such as weight loss, dysphagia, blood loss, regurgitation, and diarrhea.
F. Establish the client's usual weight to determine the extent of the problem.
G. Ask the client about any history of asthma and CD.
H. Rule out ingestion of caustic agents, especially in the pediatric population.
I. Review the client's dietary history for bulimia.

Physical Examination

A. Check pulse, respirations, BP, and weight.
B. Inspect:
   1. Examine the throat and evaluate the mouth for dental erosion.
   2. Assess swallowing ability.
C. Auscultate:
   1. Evaluate the presence of wheezing in the lungs.
   2. General observation of respiratory distress, including stridor
   3. Auscultate the heart.
   4. Evaluate the abdomen in all four quadrants.
D. Percuss:
   1. Abdomen
E. Palpate:
   1. Palpate the abdomen for the presence of hepato-splenomegaly and masses.
   2. Assess the abdomen for tenderness or distention.
F. Rectal examination:
   1. Perform this exam if indicated for any history of hematemesis.

Diagnostic Tests

A. Clinical examination and history alone usually confirm the diagnosis in the vast majority of clients with reflux.
B. Rule out cardiac/noncardiac chest pain before institution of therapy (see the Chapter 10 discussion of chest pain).
C. Endoscopy is not required for the presence of typical GERD symptoms, but is recommended for the presence of alarm symptoms or for screening clients at high risk for complications.
D. Endoscopy with biopsy is usually the first diagnostic tool in cases of caustic ingestion or suspected infectious etiology. The ACG does not recommend an endoscopy to establish the diagnosis of GERD-related asthma, chronic cough, or laryngitis.
E. Ambulatory 24-hour pH monitoring: Prolonged monitoring is the best clinical tool for diagnosing GERD in clients with asthma. However, it is very expensive and not universally available.
F. Upper GI series or barium contrast radiography is not used to diagnose GERD but rules out anatomical abnormalities of the upper digestive tract.
G. Esophageal manometry is not used for the diagnosis of GERD, but is used to evaluate clients who have failed to respond to an empirical trial of PPIs.
H. Guaiac test for occult blood: Bleeding may accompany reflux esophagitis and be slow and chronic, resulting in iron-deficiency anemia, or brisk, resulting in hematemesis. GERD may not be obvious to the clinician when obtaining a client history, especially in a client with asthma and confounding respiratory symptoms.
I. Consider *H. pylori* testing.

Differential Diagnoses

A. GERD
B. MI/angina
C. Esophageal spasm
D. Gallbladder disease
E. Cancer—gastric or esophageal
F. Infections: CMV, herpes simplex virus, and *Candida*
G. Peptic ulcer
H. Ingestion of caustic substance
I. Self-induced vomiting/bulimia
J. Pyloric stenosis
K. Food allergy
L. Eosinophilic esophagitis
M. Autoimmune skin disorders affecting the esophagus
N. Esophageal motility disorder
O. Hiatal hernia
P. Esophagitis
Q. Achalasia

Plan

A. General interventions:

1. Management depends on the cause and severity of symptoms.

B. Client teaching:

1. *See Section III: Client Teaching Guide for this chapter, "Gastroesophageal Reflux Disease."*

C. Pharmaceutical therapy:

1. The potentially adverse effects of acid suppression include increased risk of community-acquired pneumonia and GI infections, including *C. difficile*–associated diarrhea.

2. Long-term use of acid suppression therapy without a diagnosis is not advised.

3. The target of pharmaceutical therapy is improvement in quality of life through the reduction/relief of symptoms and healing of EE.

4. On-demand or self-directed therapy has been shown to be effective; however, the client's use and response should be evaluated.

5. Histamine-2 receptor antagonists (H$_2$ blockers) are effective in managing milder, infrequent GI symptoms. Tolerance occurs with chronic use of H$_2$ blockers. Several H$_2$ blockers are currently available by prescription or OTC: nizatidine (Axid), famotidine (Pepcid), cimetidine (Tagamet), and ranitidine (Zantac).

6. PPIs are used for both GERD and EE and are considered the "gold standard" of treatment:

   a. Initially a PPI should be prescribed once a day, before the first meal of the day. For maximal pH control, the traditional delayed-release PPI should be administered 30 to 60 minutes before a meal.

   b. Avoid the concomitant use of clopidogrel (Plavix) with omeprazole or esomeprazole because of the significant reduction of the antiplatelet activity of clopidogrel. This is an FDA safety labeling change.

   c. Dosages are age and weight based.

   d. Long-term therapy should be titrated down to the lowest effective dose based on symptom control.

   e. Clients may experience a relapse in their GERD symptoms after discontinuance, and therefore may need to be tapered off or use a step-down approach with an antacid or an H$_2$ blocker.

   f. No PPI is approved for use in infants younger than 1 year.

   g. PPIs are currently available by prescription and OTC (see Table 11.12).

   h. Clients with known osteoporosis can remain on PPI therapy except for long-term use in clients with other risks for hip fracture.

   i. PPI therapy can be a risk factor for *C. difficile* infection and should be used with care for clients at risk.

7. Antacids: Used for relief of mild GERD symptoms

8. Surface agents: Sucralfate adheres to mucosal surface and promotes healing.

D. Dietary management:

1. Weight loss is advised for overweight or obese clients with GERD symptoms.

2. At present, there are no supporting data for special dietary precautions; however, dietary elimination of foods (fatty foods, caffeine, chocolate, spicy foods, food with high fat content, carbonated beverages, and peppermint) helps identify triggers.

E. Surgical management:

1. Nissen fundoplication is a surgical procedure used to treat GERD in clients with asthma. It improves

TABLE 11.12 PROTON PUMP INHIBITORS

PPI	Available Dosages	Over the Counter
Omeprazole (Prilosec, Losec, Omesec)	Capsules: 10, 20, and 40 mg	Tablet 20 mg
Lansoprazole (Prevacid)	Capsules: 15 and 30 mg	Capsules: 15 mg
	Oral suspension and SoluTab: 15 and 30 mg	
	IV: 30 mg	
Rabeprazole (Aciphex)	Capsules: 20 mg	Not available
Pantoprazole (Protonix)	Capsules: 20 and 40 mg	Not available
	Oral suspension: 30 mg	
	IV: 40 mg	
Esomeprazole (Nexium)	Capsules: 20 and 40 mg	Not available
	Oral suspension: 20 and 40 mg	
	IV: 20 and 40 mg	
Dexlansoprazole (Dexilant)	Capsules: 30 and 60 mg	Not available
Omeprazole + sodium bicarbonate (Zegerid)	Capsules: omeprazole 20 and 20 mg plus 300 mg Na$^+$	Capsules: 20 mg
	Oral suspension: omeprazole 20 and 40 mg plus 460 mg Na$^+$	

IV, intravenous; PPI, proton pump inhibitor.

the anti-reflux barrier and provides a lasting solution. Because it is not always successful, it is reserved for severe cases. The Nissen operation is often performed as a laparoscopic procedure. Achalasia or severe hypomotility (scleroderma-like esophagus) are conditions that would be contraindications to Nissen fundoplication.

2. Surgical therapy is not recommended for clients who do not respond to PPI therapy.

3. The ACG guidelines note that surgical therapy is as effective as medical therapy for carefully selected clients with chronic GERD when performed by an experienced surgeon.

4. Clients on NSAIDs who experience upper gastric pain, including reflux, need to be referred for endoscopy as soon as possible.

Follow-Up

A. Noncardiac chest pain due to GERD should have a diagnostic evaluation before institution of therapy.

B. Empirical treatment with a PPI may be attempted for a short period except for clients presenting with any alarm symptoms. Schedule a return visit in 1 to 2 weeks to evaluate the relief of symptoms.

C. Some clients have frequent relapses; failure to adequately respond or long-term OTC H_2 blockers and PPI use warrants an endoscopic evaluation.

D. The need for prescribed long-term PPI treatment or the presence of alarm symptoms requires a gastroenterology consultation.

E. Consider bone density studies for clients with long-term PPI use.

Consultation/Referral

A. A GERD diagnosis should not be made without a full evaluation in infants with vomiting or poor weight gain; refer the client to a pediatric gastroenterologist for evaluation.

B. Referral is necessary if the client fails to improve after trying two different medications, or if the client has dysphagia, recent weight loss, or blood loss.

C. PPI nonresponders need to be referred for evaluation.

Individual Considerations

A. Pregnancy:

1. The diagnosis of heartburn during pregnancy is usually made by taking a thorough history. Underlying causes of GERD in pregnancy are diminished gastric motility and displacement of the stomach by the enlarging uterus.

2. Sodium bicarbonate–containing antacids should be avoided as they may lead to metabolic alkalosis and fluid overload in both the fetus and the mother.

3. To rule out PIH, evaluate the client immediately for signs and symptoms of sudden-onset discomfort with no relief from antacids (PIH or HELLP syndrome).

B. Pediatrics:

1. Some regurgitation is normal in neonates because the cardiac sphincter is immature and weak. However, vomiting is an abnormal sign associated with overfeeding, sepsis, metabolic disorders such as galactosemia, increased intracranial pressure (ICP), and intestinal atresia and stenosis. Regurgitation and vomiting must be differentiated.

a. Regurgitation most frequently occurs within the first hour after feeding in conjunction with burping or spontaneous eructation of air.

b. Infants may exhibit refusal to eat, irritability, or arching of their back during or immediately after feeding.

c. Vomiting, often projectile in nature, can occur at any time and results in the loss of significant amounts of body fluids and electrolytes.

2. Milk protein sensitivity should be ruled out.

3. There is no evidence for eliminating specific foods in children and adolescents as a means to manage GERD.

4. The major agents used in children are gastric acid buffering agents, mucosal surface barriers, and gastric antisecretory agents.

C. Geriatrics:

1. GERD prevalence increases with age and may be associated with a hiatal hernia.

2. Prolonged reflux results in esophagitis and may lead to stricture development. Chronic recurrence may develop into Barrett's syndrome.

3. Treatment of GERD in geriatric clients is the same as that for general adults; however, diagnostic testing should be performed in a short time sequence secondary to stricture and cancer in the elderly.

Resources

American Gastroenterological Association: www.gastro.org

Rome Foundation: https://theromefoundation.org

2013 guidelines for the diagnosis and management of gastroesophageal reflux disease: https://journals.lww.com/ajg/Fulltext/2013/03000/Guidelines_for_the_Diagnosis_and_Management_of.6.aspx

Bibliography

Kahrilas, P. (2018, March 28). Medical management of gastroesophageal reflux disease in adults. *UpToDate*. Retrieved from https://www.uptodate.com/contents/medical-management-of-gastroesophageal-reflux-disease-in-adults#H1576013433

Katz, P. O., Gerson, L. B., & Vela, M. F. (2013, February). Guidelines for the diagnosis and management of gastroesophageal reflux disease. *American Journal of Gastroenterology, 108*, 308–328. doi:10.1038/ajg.2012.444

McDonald, L., Gerding, D., Johnson, S., Bakken, J., Carroll, K., Coffin, S., . . . Wilcox, M. (2018, December). Clinical practice guidelines for *Clostridium difficile* infection in adults and children: 2017 update by the Infectious Diseases Society of America and Society for Healthcare Epidemiology of America. *IDSA Clinical Practice Guidelines, 2018*, 1–48. doi:10.1093/cid/ciy149. Retrieved from http://www.uphs.upenn.edu/bugdrug/antibiotic_manual/C%20difficile%20guidelines%20IDSA2017.pdf

Nettina, S. (2010). *The Lippincott manual of nursing practice* (9th ed.). Philadelphia, PA: Wolters Kluwer Lippincott Williams & Wilkins.

Patti, M. G. (2017, October 17). Gastroesophageal reflux disease. *Medscape*. Retrieved from https://emedicine.medscape.com/article/176595-differential

Saad, R. J., & Chey, W. D. (2015, June 23). First-line treatment strategies for *Helicobacter pylori* infection. *Gastroenterology & Endoscopy News, 6*, 1–8. Retrieved from https://www.gastroendonews.com/Review-Articles/Article/06-15/First-Line-Treatment-Strategies-for-Helicobacter-nbsp-pylori-Infection/32678/ses=ogst

Giardiasis Intestinalis

Cheryl A. Glass, Audra Malone, and Doncy Eapen

Definition

A. *Giardiasis intestinalis* (formerly *Giardia lamblia*) is the leading parasitic cause of diarrhea. Infestation can lead to malabsorption by coating large areas of the small bowel, particularly the lower duodenum and upper jejunum. Most people infected with *G. intestinalis* remain asymptomatic, and most infections are self-limited.

Incidence

A. Giardiasis has a worldwide distribution. It is common in areas where water supplies are contaminated by human sewage. The age-specific prevalence of giardiasis is highest in children 1 to 9 years and adults 35 to 44 years of age. The peak onset occurs annually during early summer through early fall.

Pathogenesis

A. *G. intestinalis* is a flagellated protozoan. The infective form is the cyst. Humans are the principal reservoir of infection, but *Giardia* can also infect dogs, cats, beavers, and other animals, which may then contaminate water with feces containing cysts.

B. People become infected either directly, by hand-to-mouth transfer of cysts from feces of an infected person (e.g., child care), or indirectly, by ingestion of fecal-contaminated water or food. Most community-wide epidemics result from contaminated water supplies.

C. The incubation period is 1 to 3 weeks, with an average of 7 to 10 days. The infective form is the cyst, with infection limited to the small intestine and the biliary tract. Disease is communicable for as long as the infected person excretes cysts.

Predisposing Factors

A. About 50% to 75% of outbreaks occur in child-care settings

B. Travel to endemic areas

C. Subjection to unsanitary food handling

D. Exposure to contaminated water supplies

E. Male homosexuality

F. CF

G. Immunocompromised individuals are at high risk.

Common Complaints

Asymptomatic infection: About half of all infected individuals clear the infection in the absence of clinical symptoms, and approximately 15% shed cysts asymptomatically.

Acute Complaints

A. Explosive, foul-smelling diarrhea

B. Mucus in stools, bulky stools

C. Upper abdominal pain or discomfort

D. Flatulence

E. Nausea

F. Anorexia

G. Weight loss

H. Fever

Other Signs and Symptoms

Chronic Complaints

A. Intermittent loose stools (but not diarrhea)

B. Steatorrhea

C. Increased flatulence or distention

D. Vague abdominal discomfort

E. Fatigue related to anemia

F. Profound weight loss (10%–20% of body weight)

G. Malabsorption

H. Urticaria

I. Dehydration

Subjective Data

A. Review the onset, duration, and course of symptoms. Is diarrhea acute or chronic?

B. Ask the client about travel to areas known for giardiasis.

C. Review the client's intake of medications and other substances that can cause diarrhea, especially antibiotics, laxatives, quinidine, magnesium-containing antacids, excess alcohol, caffeine, herbal teas, digitalis, loop diuretics, antihypertensive agents, and sorbitol-containing (sugar-free) gums and mints.

D. Review the nature of the client's BMs, including frequency; consistency; volume; and presence of blood, pus, or mucus.

E. Does diarrhea have any relationship to meals? Onset of diarrhea within hours of ingesting a potentially contaminated food is suggestive of bacterial infection with a pathogen such as *E. coli*; this is confirmed by checking if others were similarly affected.

F. Ask the client about associated symptoms that need evaluation, such as fever, abdominal pain, or rash.

G. Ask the client if other family members or sexual contacts are also ill.

H. Establish the client's normal weight, and, if any weight has recently been lost, review the amount and over what period of time.

Physical Examination

The physical examination may reveal no specific finding.

A. Check temperature (if indicated), pulse, respirations, BP, and weight.

B. Inspect:

1. General appearance for signs of dehydration include evaluation of mucous membranes and infants' fontanelles

C. Auscultate:

1. Abdomen for bowel sounds in all quadrants

D. Percuss:

1. Abdomen for dullness or shifting dullness

E. Palpate:

1. Abdomen for masses, tenderness, guarding, and rebound. Clients with periumbilical or RLQ pain and copious volumes of watery stool are likely to have a small-bowel etiology.

2. Lymph nodes for enlargement

F. Rectal examination

Diagnostic Tests

A. EIA and DFA are becoming the standard for diagnosis of giardiasis in the United States.

B. Stool bacteria culture and sensitivity

C. Mucous stool for leukocytes: Mucus free of leukocytes is the hallmark of IBS; a large number of white blood cells suggests inflammatory or invasive diarrhea.

D. Stool for ova and parasites; test three times on alternate days. Parasites are passed intermittently, so examine stools on alternating days.

E. Stool for occult blood

F. Endoscopy to identify cysts in duodenal fluid or small-bowel tissue

Differential Diagnoses

A. Giardiasis

B. Malabsorption

C. *E. coli* infection

D. IBS

E. Viral diarrhea

F. Lactose intolerance

G. Other bacterial infections, such as *Shigella*, *Salmonella*, and *Campylobacter*

H. CD

I. Sprue

Plan

A. General interventions:

1. Advise children and adult workers with diarrhea to stay away from day-care centers until they become asymptomatic.

2. Advise the client's household and sexual contacts to seek medical examination and treatment.

B. Client teaching:

▶ 1. *See Section III: Client Teaching Guide for this chapter, "Diarrhea."*

2. Discuss safe sexual practices. Avoiding oral–anal and oral–genital sex can decrease venereal transmission.

3. Recommend contact precautions for the duration of illness for diapered and/or incontinent children.

4. People with diarrhea caused by *Giardia* should not use recreational water venues, including swimming pools and water slides, for 2 weeks after symptoms resolve.

C. Pharmaceutical therapy:

1. Treatment of asymptomatic carriers is not generally recommended.

2. Fluid and electrolyte management is critical in clients with large-volume diarrheal losses.

3. Treat children with acute or chronic diarrhea who manifest FTT, malabsorption, or other GI tract symptoms when *Giardia* has been identified.

4. Metronidazole, tinidazole, and nitazoxanide are the drugs of choice for treatment.

a. Metronidazole (Flagyl) is the principal agent used to treat giardiasis in the United States.

i. Adults: 250 mg orally three times daily for 5 to 7 days

ii. Pediatric: 5 mg/kg/d orally divided in three times daily dosing for 5 to 7 days; not to exceed 750 mg/d

b. Tinidazole (Tindamax) is a one-time dose for children 3 years of age and older; it has fewer side effects than metronidazole.

i. Adults: 2 g single dose

ii. Pediatrics: 50 mg/kg single dose (maximum 2 g)

c. Nitazoxanide (Alinia) oral suspension has similar efficacy to metronidazole and has the advantage of treating other intestinal parasites; it has been approved for children 1 year of age and older.

i. Age 1 to 3 years: 5 mL (100 mg) oral suspension every 12 hours with food for 3 days

ii. Age 4 to 11 years: 10 mL (200 mg) oral suspension every 12 hours with food for 3 days

iii. Age 12 years and older: 500 mg tablet every 12 hours or 25 mL oral suspension every 12 hours with food for 3 days

5. Paromomycin (Humatin), a nonabsorbable aminoglycoside, is recommended for treatment of symptomatic infection in pregnant women in the second and third trimesters.

a. Adults: 100 mg three times daily for 5 to 7 days

b. Pediatrics: 20 mg/kg/d three times daily with meals for 5 to 7 days

D. Dietary management:

1. Tell the client or caregiver to prevent dehydration from diarrhea by increasing fluids.

2. Advise restricting milk products to rule out lactose intolerance. Post-giardiasis lactose intolerance occurs in 20% to 40% of clients.

3. Tell backpackers, campers, and people likely to be exposed to contaminated water to avoid drinking directly from streams. To make water for safe drinking, boil water or use chemical disinfection or filtration. Boiling water is the most reliable method to make water safe for drinking.

Follow-Up

A. Relapses after treatment are common, especially in immunocompromised clients.

B. Schedule follow-ups at 6 weeks and 6 months after treatment, as indicated.

C. If diarrhea persists for 2 weeks or more, secondary evaluation is indicated. Stools should be examined again for blood, leukocytes, and parasites.

D. Clients who remain undiagnosed after an extensive evaluation and trial of metronidazole (Flagyl) often turn out to have IBS or surreptitious laxative abuse.

Consultation/Referral

A. Severely dehydrated or malnourished clients should be admitted for further care.

B. Consult a physician if the client has no relief of symptoms after completion of therapies.

C. Consultations with a pediatric infectious disease specialist and pediatric gastroenterologist are recommended.

Individual Considerations

A. Pregnancy:

1. Treatment of clients during pregnancy is recommended. Giardiasis in pregnancy is associated with dehydration, malabsorption, and severe symptoms.

2. Malabsorptive symptoms may persist, as regeneration of functioning intestinal mucosa requires time.

3. Breastfeeding appears to protect infants from *G. intestinalis.*

B. Pediatrics:

1. **When an outbreak is suspected in a child-care setting, the local health department should be notified to investigate.**

2. Children who are carriers do not have to be excluded from child care; however, personal hygiene/universal precautions should be followed.

Bibliography

Hammer, H., & Hogenauer, C. (2020). Lactose intolerance: Clinical manifestations, diagnosis, and management. *UpToDate.* Retrieved from https://www.uptodate.com/contents/lactose-intolerance-clinical-manifestations-diagnosis-and-management

Leder, K., & Weller, P. F. (2018, January 26). Giardiasis: Epidemiology, clinical manifestations and diagnosis. *UpToDate.* Retrieved from https://www.uptodate.com/contents/giardiasis-epidemiology-clinical-manifestations-and-diagnosis#H8

Nazer, H. (2016, February 15). Giardiasis. *Medscape.* Retrieved from http://emedicine.medscape.com/article/176718-overview

Nettina, S. (2010). *The Lippincott manual of nursing practice* (9th ed.). Philadelphia, PA: Wolters Kluwer Lippincott Williams & Wilkins.

Sharma, G. D. (2019, May 2). Cystic fibrosis. *Medscape.* Retrieved from http://emedicine.medscape.com/article/1001602-overview

Weller, P. F., & Kaplan, S. L. (2015, June 16). Treatment and prevention of giardiasis. *UpToDate.* Retrieved from http://www.uptodate.com/contents/treatment-and-prevention-of-giardiasis

Hemorrhoids

Cheryl A. Glass, Audra Malone, and Doncy Eapen

Definition

A. Hemorrhoids are clusters of vascular tissues, smooth muscle, and connective tissue of the anal canal.

B. Internal hemorrhoids are above the anorectal line, covered by rectal mucosa, and can be found at any position in the rectum. Hemorrhoids can be found at any position of the rectum. Internal hemorrhoids are graded by severity (see Table 11.13).

C. External hemorrhoids are below the anorectal line, covered by anal skin, and appear as painless, flaccid skin tags (see Figure 11.2).

Internal hemorrhoid   External hemorrhoid

FIGURE 11.2   Internal and external hemorrhoids.

A. Internal hemorrhoid: Covered by a thin sheet of tissue called mucous membrane, an internal hemorrhoid bulges into the rectal opening and may sink a bit during bowel movements.

B. External hemorrhoid: Covered by skin, an external hemorrhoid protrudes from the rectum.

D. When blood within the hemorrhoid becomes clotted due to obstruction, the hemorrhoids are referred to as thrombosed and appear as blue, shiny masses.

E. Although rectal bleeding is commonly associated with hemorrhoids, it may be a symptom of other disease processes, such as CRC, IBD, other colitides, diverticular disease, and angiodysplasia.

Incidence

A. In the United States, the self-reported incidence of hemorrhoids is 10 million per years, corresponding to a 4.4% prevalence. Clients tend to present after utilization and failure of OTC treatments. Hemorrhoids are common in people older than 20 years of age. They are uncommon in people younger than age 20 years except secondary to pregnancy.

Pathogenesis

A. The underlying mechanism is unknown. Prolapse may be initiated by shearing force from passage of large firm stool, by increased venous pressure from HF or pregnancy, or by straining that occurs with lifting or defecation.

Predisposing Factors

A. Increased abdominal pressure (constipation, pelvic congestion, pregnancy, portal hypertension, cirrhosis)

B. Altered bowel function (constipation, diarrhea)

C. Poor muscle tone

D. Low-fiber diet

E. Sedentary jobs, such as driving trucks, piloting planes

F. Loss of muscle tone due to advanced age

G. Anal intercourse

H. Obesity

TABLE 11.13   SEVERITY OF HEMORRHOIDS TO GUIDE TREATMENT OPTIONS

Grade	Severity
I	The hemorrhoids bleed but do not prolapse
II	The hemorrhoids prolapse upon defecation but reduce spontaneously
III	The hemorrhoids prolapse upon defecation and must be reduced manually
IV	The hemorrhoids are prolapsed and cannot be reduced manually

I. Colon malignancy
J. Rectal surgery
K. IBD

Common Complaints
A. Cardinal features:
1. Bleeding: Painless, bright red bleeding with defecation (internal)
2. Anal pruritus
3. Prolapse
4. Pain related to thrombosis

Other Signs and Symptoms
A. Visible prolapsed mass
B. Incomplete defecation
C. Leakage of feces (internal hemorrhoids)
D. Excessive moisture
E. Weakness or fatigue, with anemia
F. External hemorrhoid: Covered by skin, an external hemorrhoid protrudes from the rectum

Subjective Data
A. Review the onset and duration of symptoms, especially the history of rectal bleeding, prolapse, and issues of hygiene and pain.
B. Review the client's history of hemorrhoids and treatments, including surgery.
C. Ask the client about recent pregnancy, liver disease, and constipation.
D. Inquire about the client's job and level of daily activity.
E. Review the client's sexual practices for anal intercourse.
F. Review the client's dietary history for fluid intake and sources/amount of fiber.
G. Ask about bowel habits, including frequency, consistency, and ease of evacuation.
H. Review a detailed family history, with emphasis on intestinal disease.

Physical Examination
A. Check temperature (if indicated), pulse, respirations, BP, and weight.
B. Inspect:
1. Observe the rectal area for skin tags, prolapse, irritation, fissures, and condyloma.
   a. Internal hemorrhoids are usually not visible unless prolapsed.
   b. External hemorrhoids protrude with straining or standing.
2. Using anoscopy: Visualize internal rectum for hemorrhoids, fissures, or masses.
C. Palpate:
1. Palpate abdomen for masses.
D. Rectal examination:
1. Internal hemorrhoids are usually not palpable unless thrombosed.
2. Digital rectal evaluation

Diagnostic Tests
A. Hct and Hgb, if bleeding present
B. Anoscopy: Reveals internal hemorrhoids as bright red to purplish bulges. Digital rectal examination alone can neither diagnose nor exclude internal hemorrhoids; anoscopy is required.
C. Endoscopic evaluation: In clients older than 40 years, flexible sigmoidoscopy or colonoscopy is performed if there are risk factors for CRC.
D. Stool for guaiac testing
E. Air-contrast BE for atypical bleeding

Differential Diagnoses
A. Hemorrhoids
B. Condyloma acuminata
C. Rectal prolapse
D. Rectal bleeding due to one of the following:
1. CRC
2. Polyps
3. Anal fissure
4. Fistula
5. Perianal abscess
6. IBD, including UC and CD
7. Diverticulitis
8. Pelvic tumor
E. Proctitis

Plan
A. General interventions:
1. No treatment is necessary if the client is asymptomatic except for maintaining regular bowel habits and performing comfort measures.
B. Client teaching:
1. *See Section III: Client Teaching Guide for this chapter,* ◀ *"Hemorrhoids."*
C. Pharmaceutical therapy:
1. Drug of choice: Bulk-forming agents such as psyllium seed (Metamucil), methylcellulose (Citrucel), or calcium polycarbophil (Fibercon), 1 to 3 teaspoons in 8 oz of liquid three times a day. Maintenance dose is 1 to 3 teaspoons after dinner.
2. Stool softener: Docusate sodium (Colace) or docusate calcium (Doxidan) 100 mg three times daily
3. For irritation and pruritus, topical creams and anesthetics are found in OTC products such as Anusol, pramoxine HCl (Tronolane Cream), Preparation H, and topical hydrocortisone preparations.
4. NSAIDs supplemented with narcotics: An oral analgesic such as codeine may be prescribed for thrombosed hemorrhoids. However, codeine causes constipation.
D. Dietary management:
1. High-fiber diet and an adequate fluid intake should be continued indefinitely to maintain a soft bulky stool that can be passed without straining (see Appendix B, Table B.6).
E. Medical management:
1. Use warm sitz baths up to three times a day for irritation and pruritus.
2. Conservative treatment for thrombosed hemorrhoids includes lying prone and applying an ice pack to the area.
3. Incision and evacuation of thrombosis or clot may be performed under local anesthesia. Other treatments

for thrombosed hemorrhoids noted in clinical trials have included the following:

    a. Topical nitroglycerin 0.2% topical ointment for temporary analgesia. The most common side effect was headache.

    b. Topical nifedipine

    c. In a small study, one intrasphincter injection of botulinum toxin relieved pain within 24 hours.

F. Surgical management:

  1. Symptomatic Grade I, Grade II, and some Grade III hemorrhoids may be treated by the following:

    a. Rubber band ligation is the treatment of choice for Grades I and II hemorrhoids. Rubber band ligation is the most widely used procedure and is associated with fewer complications than surgery.

    b. Bipolar, infrared, and laser coagulation (may require more than one treatment)

    c. Sclerotherapy

    d. Stapled hemorrhoidopexy can be performed in clients with Grade III hemorrhoids.

  2. External hemorrhoids usually do not require surgical therapy except in cases of thrombosis. For selective Grade III and Grade IV internal and strangulated hemorrhoids that fail to respond to medical and nonoperative therapies, surgical treatment is required. **Stapled hemorrhoidopexy has a faster recovery but a higher recurrence rate. Hemorrhoidectomy is the treatment of last choice because it requires hospitalization and an extended recovery period, and it risks compromising competence of the anal sphincter.** Hemorrhoidectomy complications include:

    a. Urinary retention

    b. UTI

    c. Fecal impaction

    d. Pain

    e. Hemorrhage

    f. Stricture formation (1%) or sphincter damage (rare)

    g. Nonhealing wound

    h. Fistula formation

    i. Anal leakage

Follow-Up

A. None is necessary if resolution occurs and the client is asymptomatic.

B. Reevaluate the client in 2 weeks for further treatment if symptoms persist.

C. Evaluate the client with an intervention in 7 to 10 days.

Consultation/Referral

A. The onset of urinary retention and fever immediately after an office-based procedure may be the initial sign of perianal sepsis and mandates emergent client evaluation.

B. Clients with family history of CRC, familial polyposis, constitutional symptoms such as anemia, weight loss, and changes in the consistency of stools that are suggestive of malignancy should be referred to a gastroenterologist for endoscopic evaluation.

C. Refer the client with an acute thrombosed external hemorrhoid to a GI specialist if client is experiencing severe pain, or if the pain does not resolve after 48 hours with conservative measures.

D. Refer the client to a surgeon if hemorrhoids bleed repeatedly, prolapse, produce intractable pain, or are thrombosed, and if three to five consecutive days of treatment do not provide relief.

Individual Considerations

A. Pregnancy:

  1. Labor, which results in pressure on the pelvic floor by the presenting part of the fetus and the expulsive efforts of the woman, may aggravate hemorrhoids, causing protrusion and inflammation during the puerperium. Hemorrhoids may be pushed back after delivery to prevent them from becoming swollen and painful.

  2. Surgical treatment is contraindicated in pregnancy because of the risk of inducing labor.

  3. Conservative treatment is recommended, with excision of thrombosed external hemorrhoids if necessary.

B. Pediatrics:

  1. Rectal prolapse in children is associated with CF.

Prolapse looks like a pink doughnut or rosette; complete prolapse involving the muscular wall is larger and red, and has circular folds.

C. Geriatrics:

  1. Prolapse of rectal mucosa is more common in the elderly.

  2. Colonoscopy is recommended in the geriatric population to exclude malignancy or other underlying disease.

Bibliography

Bleday, R., & Breen, E. (2019, April 3). Hemorrhoids: Clinical manifestations and diagnosis. *UpToDate*. Retrieved from https://www.uptodate.com/contents/hemorrhoids-clinical-manifestations-and-diagnosis#H909159015

Lohsiriwat, V. (2015). Treatment of hemorrhoids: A coloproctologist's view. *World of Gastroenterology*, 21(31), 9245–9252. doi:10.3748/wjg.v21.i31.9245

Nettina, S. (2010). *The Lippincott manual of nursing practice* (9th ed.). Philadelphia, PA: Wolters Kluwer Lippincott Williams & Wilkins.

Sharma, G. D. (2019, May 2). Cystic fibrosis. *Medscape*. Retrieved from http://emedicine.medscape.com/article/1001602-overview

Sun, Z., & Miglay, J. (2016). Review of hemorrhoid disease: Presentation and management. *Clinics in Colon and Rectal Surgery*, 29(1), 22–29. doi:10.1055/s-0035-1568144

Hepatitis A

Cheryl A. Glass, Audra Malone, and Doncy Eapen

Definition

A. Hepatitis A is an acute self-limited illness with inflammation of the liver caused by a viral infection. Hepatitis A virus (HAV) is spread by viral shedding. All cases of hepatitis A are reportable to the public health department.

B. The highest titers of HAV in the stool of infected clients occur 1 to 2 weeks before the onset of illness (jaundice or elevation of liver enzymes), during which time clients are most likely to transmit infection. Risk subsequently diminishes and is minimal in the week after the onset of jaundice. Few children younger than 6 years have concomitant jaundice, whereas up to 70% of older children and adults will have jaundice. Fulminant hepatitis is rare, and chronic infectious and carrier states do not occur.

C. Duration of HAV infection is typically 8 weeks, but prolonged disease, as long as 6 months, can occur in 10% to 15% of symptomatic clients, especially in neonates and young children.

D. Fulminant hepatic failure occurs in less than 1% of cases.

E. The major methods of prevention include improved sanitation of water sources, improved hygiene practice prior to food preparation and diaper changes, immunization with the hepatitis A vaccine, and administration of immune globulin (IG).

Incidence

A. Approximately 30% to 35% of acute hepatitis cases in the United States are due to HAV. In developing countries, where infection is endemic, most people are infected during the first decade of life. In the United States, the incidence of HAV has declined since 1995 due to the administration of the HAV vaccine.

B. Outbreaks in custodial institutions account for about 10% to 15% of reported HAV in the United States. No appreciable seasonal variation in incidence has been noted.

C. Mortality from HAV ranges from 0% to 1%. The single most important determinant of illness severity is age; increasing age directly correlates with the likelihood of adverse events.

Pathogenesis

A. HAV is a small RNA enterovirus classified as a member of the picornavirus group. Viral replication depends on hepatocyte uptake and synthesis, and assembly occurs exclusively in liver cells. Transmission of HAV is person-to-person, primarily by the fecal–oral route and parenterally. The incubation period is 15 to 50 days, with an average of 25 to 30 days. HAV does not cause chronic infection.

B. Common-source, foodborne, and waterborne epidemics have occurred, including several caused by shellfish contaminated with human sewage. Nosocomial outbreaks have occurred as a result of shedding of HAV from infected asymptomatic neonates, children, or adults.

Predisposing Factors

A. Ingestion of infected water, food, and shellfish:
1. Undercooked HAV-contaminated foods are a source of outbreaks.
2. Cooked foods also can transmit HAV if the temperature during food preparation is inadequate to kill the virus.
3. Food contaminated after cooking is associated with infected food handlers.

B. Close personal contact with an HAV-infected person:
1. Contact with a child who attends a child-care center (especially with children in diapers)
2. Male homosexual activity

3. Vertical transmission from mother to fetus (limited)
4. Personal contact with a newly arriving international adoptee

C. Poor sanitation or personal hygiene

D. Crowded living conditions

E. International travel

F. IV drug abuse

G. Persons with clotting factor disorders

H. Persons working with nonhuman primates

Common Complaints

A. Asymptomatic, particularly in young children

B. Malaise

C. Anorexia

D. Nausea with/without vomiting

E. Low-grade fever

F. Jaundice—icteric phase (70% of older children and adults):
1. Tea-colored urine
2. Clay-colored stool
3. Abdominal pain
4. Pruritus
5. Enlarged liver

Other Signs and Symptoms

A. Infants and children: Mild, nonspecific, flu-like symptoms without jaundice

B. Adults: Severe, prolonged course with fatigue, headache, vomiting, and symptoms noted earlier

C. Relapsing hepatitis A is more common in the elderly. This variant generally involves a protracted course of symptoms, then a relapse of symptoms following an apparent resolution.

Subjective Data

A. Review the duration, onset, and severity of symptoms, including specifics about urine or stool color changes.

B. Ask the client about family members and sexual contacts with similar symptoms.

C. Review the client's history of blood transfusions, IV drug use, and alcohol abuse.

D. Inquire about occupational exposure.

E. Ask the client about recent international travel or exposure to newly arrived international adoptees.

F. Review the client's immunization status.

G. Review the client's medications for a possible Tylenol overdose or Ecstasy use as a cause for acute drug-induced liver injury.

Physical Examination

A. Check temperature (acute illness), pulse, respirations, BP, and weight.

B. Inspect:
1. Note general appearance.
2. Inspect the skin for slight jaundice or rash.
3. Inspect the mucous membranes and nail beds.
4. Inspect the eyes for yellow sclera.

C. Auscultate:
1. Lung fields
2. All quadrants of the abdomen
3. Heart

D. Percuss:
1. Abdomen
E. Palpate:
1. Palpate all quadrants of the abdomen for masses, liver tenderness, hepatomegaly (80% of cases) and splenomegaly (less common).

Diagnostic Tests

A. Viral serology for typing HAV, IgG, and immunoglobulin M (IgM). Serum IgM presents at the onset of illness and disappears within 4 months, generally indicating current or recent infection. However, it may persist for 6 months or longer. Presence of IgG anti-HAV antibodies without virus-specific IgM indicates past infection and lifelong immunity.
B. Liver function studies, including ALT, AST, LDH, and ALP
C. Bilirubin, direct and indirect
D. CBC
E. PT
F. Urinalysis: Reveals proteinuria and bilirubinuria
G. Imaging studies are usually not indicated for hepatitis A infection. An ultrasound may be used to exclude other pathology.

Differential Diagnoses

A. Hepatitis A
B. Mononucleosis
C. Cancer
D. Obstructive jaundice
E. Alcoholic hepatitis or cirrhosis
F. Hepatotoxic drug use:
1. Drug-induced liver injury (e.g., Tylenol, Ecstasy)
2. Drug-induced hypersensitivity reaction (e.g., sulfasalazine hypersensitivity)
G. Food poisoning
H. Exclusion of other hepatitis types
I. CMV
J. Acute HIV infection
K. Autoimmune hepatitis, Budd–Chiari syndrome, Wilson's disease
L. Hepatitis B, C, D, or E virus

Plan

A. General interventions:
1. Contact precautions are recommended for diapered and/or incontinent clients for 1 week after the onset of symptoms.
2. Children and adults with acute HAV infection should be excluded from school, work, and child-care centers for 1 week after the onset of illness.
3. Hepatitis is self-limiting and does not require therapy. Treatment is supportive:
   a. Limit activities secondary to malaise.
   b. OCPs and HRT should be stopped to avoid cholestasis.
   c. Alcohol consumption is not advised.
   d. Adults who work as food handlers should not work for 1 week after the onset of the illness.
   e. Discontinue Tylenol until fully recovered from infection.
4. Encourage strict handwashing.
B. Client teaching:
1. *See Section III: Client Teaching Guide for this chapter, "Jaundice and Hepatitis."*
2. Teach the client that major methods for prevention are improved sanitation (e.g., of water sources and in food preparation) and personal hygiene.
3. Food and travel precautions:
   a. Avoid use of uncontrolled water resources: Use bottled water, boil water, or add iodine to inactivate the virus.
   b. Avoid raw shellfish.
   c. Avoid uncooked foods.
   d. All fruit should be washed and peeled.
C. Pharmaceutical therapy:
1. IG (Gamastan, Gammar-P): Preexposure administration is 0.02 mL/kg, two doses intramuscularly (IM). HAV vaccine preexposure is preferred in all populations unless contraindicated.
2. Postexposure IG administration given IM within 2 weeks of HAV exposure is 80% to 90% effective in preventing symptomatic infection:
   a. Time of exposure: 2 weeks or less:
      i. Younger than 12 months: 0.02 mL/kg of IG given IM into a large muscle. No more than 3 mL in one site should be given to small children and infants.
      ii. 12 months to 40 years: Hepatitis A vaccine
      iii. 41 years and older: 0.02 mL/kg IG is given IM into a large muscle. No more than 5 mL should be administered into one site for an adult or large child.
   b. Postexposure prophylaxis with IG is recommended for the following:
      i. Household and sexual contacts of infected persons
      ii. Newborn infants of HAV-infected mothers
      iii. Child-care center staff, children, and their household contacts
      iv. Students when transmission within school is documented
      v. Staff in institutions and hospitals
      vi. People who ingested HAV-contaminated food or water, within 2 weeks of last exposure
3. Vaccines:
   a. Two inactivated HAV vaccines, Havrix and Vaqta, are available in the United States.
   b. TWINRIX is a combination of hepatitis A (Havrix) and hepatitis B (Engerix-B) vaccine available in the United States for those aged 18 years or older (see Table 11.14).
4. Hepatitis A vaccine is recommended for the following:
   a. Children 1 year and older in defined and circumscribed communities with high endemic rates and/or periodic outbreaks of HAV infection.

TABLE 11.14 LICENSED DOSAGES AND SCHEDULES FOR HEPATITIS A VACCINES

A. HAVRIX[a]

Age	Dose (ELISA units)[b]	Volume (mL)	Number of Doses	Schedule (mo)[c]
12 months to 18 years	720	0.5	2	0, 6–12
≥19 years	1,440	1.0	2	0, 6–12

B. VAQTA[d]

Age	Dose (U)[e]	Volume (mL)	Number of Doses	Schedule (mo)[f]
12 months to 18 years	25	0.5	2	0, 6–18
≥19 years	50	1.0	2	0, 6–18

C. TWINRIX[g, h]

Age	Dose (ELISA units)[b]	Volume (mL)	Number of Doses	Schedule[i]
≥18 years	720	1.0	3	0, 1, 6 mo
≥18 years	720	1.0	4	0, 7, 21–30 d + 12 mo[b]

[a]Hepatitis A vaccine, inactivated, GlaxoSmithKline.

[b]Enzyme-linked immunosorbent assay units.

[c]0 months represents timing of the initial dose; subsequent numbers represent months after the initial dose.

[d]Hepatitis A vaccine, inactivated, Merck & Co.

[e]Units.

[f]0 months represents timing of the initial dose; subsequent numbers represent months after the initial dose.

[g]Combined hepatitis A and hepatitis B vaccine, inactivated, GlaxoSmithKline.

[h]Not recommended for postexposure prophylaxis.

[i]This four-dose schedule enables clients to receive three doses in 21 days; this schedule is used before planned exposure with short notice and requires a fourth dose at 12 months.

Source: Centers for Disease Control and Prevention: www.cdc.gov/hepatitis/hav/havfaq.htm#B1

Children who have not been vaccinated by age 2 can be vaccinated at subsequent visits.

b. Children and adolescents ages 2 to 18 years who live in states or communities where routine hepatitis A vaccination has been implemented because of high disease incidence

c. Clients with chronic liver disease

d. Homosexual and bisexual men (both adolescents and adults)

e. Users of illegal injected and noninjected drugs

f. Those with occupational risk of exposure, such as handlers of nonhuman primates and persons working with HAV in a laboratory setting

g. Travelers who need preexposure immunoprophylaxis: The first dose of hepatitis A vaccine should be administered as soon as travel is considered

h. Clients with clotting-factor disorders such as hemophilia

5. Routine HAV vaccination is *not* indicated for the following groups:

a. Child-care center staff and children

b. Clients and staff in custodial care institutions

c. Hospital personnel; if a client with hepatitis A is admitted to the hospital, routine infection-control precautions will prevent transmission to hospital staff.

d. Food service workers

e. Clients with hemophilia

f. Sewage workers

6. HAV vaccine may be administered simultaneously with other vaccines, including hepatitis B, diphtheria, poliovirus (oral and inactivated), tetanus, oral and IM typhoid, cholera, Japanese encephalitis, rabies, and yellow fever. The HAV vaccine should be given in a separate syringe and at a separate site.

7. The need for an additional hepatitis A booster beyond the two-dose primary immunization has not been established; however, the CDC reports that extra doses of HAV vaccine are not harmful.

8. Immune response in immunocompromised clients, such as those with HIV or on hemodialysis, may be suboptimal. The vaccine is inactivated; therefore, no special precautions are needed when vaccinating immunocompromised clients.

9. Vaccine side effects are generally mild:

a. Local pain at the immunization site

b. Localized induration at the injection site

10. Tylenol may be administered for fever and arthralgia but is strictly limited to a maximum dose of 3 to 4 g/d in adults

D. Dietary management:

1. Encourage optimal nutrition

Follow-Up

A. Dehydration may require hospital admission.

B. Follow up in 2 weeks for reevaluation.

C. Check for hepatitis B immunity and vaccinate if necessary.

D. Hepatitis A is reportable to the public health department.

Consultation/Referral

A. Consult a gastroenterologist/infectious disease specialist if necessary.

Individual Considerations

A. Pregnancy:

1. Pregnant women recently exposed to HAV should receive prophylactic gamma-globulin.

2. HAV is an inactivated vaccine and is considered safe during pregnancy.

3. HAV infection during pregnancy is associated with an increased risk of premature labor and delivery.

B. Pediatrics:

1. In the United States, the highest rates for symptomatic HAV infection occur in children 5 to 14 years of age, and the lowest rates occur in children from birth to 4 years.

2. Children who have received HAV vaccine rarely have detectable anti-HAV IgM titers.

3. Risk of outbreak in child-care centers increases with the number of children younger than age 2 years who wear diapers.

4. Immunization is recommended routinely for children 12 through 23 months of age (follow the childhood immunization schedule).

5. The hepatitis A vaccine is not currently licensed for children younger than 12 months.

C. Adults:

1. In the United States, the lowest rate of HAV infection is in people older than 40 years.

D. Geriatrics:

1. The elderly have greater numbers of HAV antibodies, resulting in fewer cases in this population.

2. Symptoms are usually vague. Fatigue, pruritus, and the classic symptoms of jaundice, hepatomegaly, and liver tenderness are commonly absent in the elderly.

3. Diagnostic test results in the elderly include elevated bilirubin, lower or normal transaminase and ALP, and normal ultrasonography.

4. Treatment is supportive. Corticosteroids may relieve symptoms but prolong the disease state due to prolonged viral replication.

E. Special populations:

1. People with chronic liver disease are at risk of fulminant hepatitis and should be immunized.

2. People who are awaiting or have received liver transplants should be immunized.

Bibliography

Centers for Disease Control and Prevention. (2016b, July 13). *Viral hepatitis: Hepatitis A information*. Retrieved from https://www.cdc.gov/hepatitis/HAV/index.htm

Gilroy, K. R. (2017, October 16). Hepatitis A differential diagnosis. *Medscape*. Retrieved from https://emedicine.medscape.com/article/177484-differential

Lai, M., & Chopra, S. (2018, December 7). Hepatitis A virus infection in adults: Epidemiology, clinical manifestations, and diagnosis. *UpToDate*. Retrieved from https://www.uptodate.com/contents/hepatitis-a-virus-infection-in-adults-epidemiology-clinical-manifestations-and-diagnosis#H3024115574

Nettina, S. (2010). *The Lippincott manual of nursing practice* (9th ed.). Philadelphia, PA: Wolters Kluwer Lippincott Williams & Wilkins.

Hepatitis B

Cheryl A. Glass, Audra Malone, and Doncy Eapen

Definition

A. Hepatitis B is inflammation of the liver caused by the hepatitis B virus (HBV). Acute HBV infection cannot be distinguished from other forms of acute viral hepatitis on the basis of clinical signs and symptoms or nonspecific laboratory findings. Acutely infected clients may be asymptomatic or symptomatic. The likelihood of developing symptoms of acute hepatitis is age dependent.

B. Chronic HBV infection is defined as the presence of hepatitis B surface antigen (HBsAg) in serum for at least 6 months or as the presence of HBsAg in a person who tests negative for antibodies of the immunoglobulin (Ig) M subclass to hepatitis B core antigen (IgM antihepatitis B core antigen)

C. HBV is the main cause of cirrhosis and hepatocellular carcinoma (HCC) worldwide. For selected candidates, liver transplantation currently seems to be the only viable treatment for the latest stages of hepatitis B.

D. Antiviral treatment may be effective in approximately one-third of clients who receive it. Ten different genotypes (A through J) have been identified. The progression of the disease seems to be more accelerated, and the response to treatment with antiviral agents is less favorable, for clients infected by genotype C compared with those infected by genotype B. Clients infected with genotypes A and B have a better response to interferon (IFN) treatment compared with clients infected with genotypes C and D.

E. Acute HBV is undistinguishable from other forms of hepatitis in the acute viral stage on the basis of clinical symptoms.

F. In 2012, the CDC recommended HBV testing for the following groups:

1. All pregnant women

2. Persons born in regions with intermediate or high rates of hepatitis B (HBsAg prevalence ≥ 2%)

3. U.S.-born persons not vaccinated as infants whose parents were born in regions with high rates of hepatitis B (HBsAg prevalence ≥ 8%)

4. Infants born to HBsAg-positive mothers

5. Household, needle-sharing, or sex contacts of HBsAg-positive persons

6. Men who have sex with men (MSM)

7. Injection-drug users

8. Clients with elevated liver enzymes (ALT/AST) of unknown etiology

9. Clients receiving hemodialysis

10. Persons needing immunosuppressive or cytotoxic therapy

11. HIV-infected persons

12. Donors of blood, plasma, organs, tissues, or semen

13. Adults with diabetes mellitus are at an increased risk of acquiring HBV infection if they share diabetes care equipment such as blood glucose meters, finger-stick devices, syringes, and/or insulin pens. Adults with diabetes aged less than 60 years are, therefore, recommended by the CDC to receive hepatitis B vaccination, and those aged greater than 60 years are to be considered for vaccination.

Incidence

A. An estimated one-third of the global population has been infected with HBV. Approximately 257 million people are chronically infected, and only 2% spontaneously seroconvert annually. Of chronically infected clients, 15% to 40% will develop cirrhosis, progressing to liver failure and/or HCC.

B. In 2014, rates were highest for persons aged 30 to 39 years (2.23 cases per 100,000 population); the lowest rates were among children and adolescents aged less than 19 years (0.02 cases per 100,000 population).

C. Acute hepatitis B occurs in 1 to 2 out of every 1,000 pregnancies in the United States, and chronic infection occurs in 5 to 15 out of every 1,000 pregnancies. The course of maternal HBV infection does not seem to be affected by coexistent pregnancy. However, rates of premature labor and delivery are increased.

D. Chronic HBV infections with persistence of HBsAg occur in as many as 90% of infants infected by perinatal transmission; in 30% of children 1 to 5 years old infected after birth; and in 5% to 10% of older children, adolescents, and adults with HBV infection.

Pathogenesis

A. HBV is a hepadnavirus. HBV-related liver injury is largely caused by immune-mediated mechanisms mediated via cytotoxic T-lymphocyte lysis of infected hepatocytes. The virus is transmitted through blood or body fluids, such as wound exudates, semen, cervical secretions, and saliva that are HBsAg positive. It is not transmitted by the fecal–oral route or by water. Blood and serum contain the highest concentration of virus; saliva contains the lowest.

B. The incubation period is 45 to 160 days (2–5 months), with an average of 120 days. An infected person can infect others 4 to 6 weeks before symptoms appear and for an unpredictable time thereafter.

C. The production of antibodies against HBsAg confers protective immunity and can be detected in clients who have recovered from HBV or in those clients who have been vaccinated. The IgM subtype indicates an acute infection or reactivation. The IgG subtype indicates chronic infection.

Predisposing Factors

A. Higher prevalence in non-Hispanic Blacks and other populations:
   1. Asian origin
   2. American Indians/Alaskan Eskimos
   3. Asia Pacific islanders

B. Sexual contact is the major mode of transmission:
   1. High number of sexual partners
   2. Early age of first intercourse
   3. Homosexuality/bisexuality

C. IV drug use, sharing needles

D. Occupational exposure

E. Household exposure

F. Perinatal exposure, by vertical infection

G. Receiving blood transfusions or blood products for hemophilia and hemodialysis

H. Breastfeeding, by transmission in breast milk

I. Staffing or residing in institutions

J. International travel

K. Incarceration in long-term correctional facilities

L. Percutaneous contact with inanimate objects contaminated with HBV; virus can survive 1 week or longer

M. Diabetics

N. Recipient of dialysis or kidney transplant

Common Complaints

A. The following symptoms occur in the acute phase of HBV:
   1. Anicteric hepatitis: Subclinical (approximately 70% of clients)
   2. Icteric hepatitis: Associated with a prodromal period. Around 30% of clients progress to the icteric phase:
      a. Anorexia
      b. Nausea and vomiting
      c. Low-grade fever
      d. Headache
      e. Diarrhea
      f. Myalgia
      g. Fatigue
      h. Aversion to food and cigarettes
      i. Intermittent, mild to moderate RUQ and epigastric pain
   3. Hyperacute, acute, and subacute hepatitis symptoms:
      a. Hepatic encephalopathy
      b. Somnolence
      c. Disturbances in sleep pattern
      d. Mental confusion
      e. Coma

B. The following symptoms occur in the chronic phase of HBV:
   1. Asymptomatic: May be healthy carriers without any evidence of active disease
   2. During the replicative state, common symptoms are:
      a. Fatigue
      b. Anorexia
      c. Nausea
      d. Mild upper quadrant pain or discomfort
      e. Hepatic decompensation

Other Signs and Symptoms

A. In young children:
   1. Jaundice and other symptoms may not be present.
   2. Symptoms may be prolonged and insidious compared with HAV infection.

B. Icteric phase: 10 days after the appearance of constitutional symptoms and lasts for 1–3 months:
   1. Jaundice of sclera and skin
   2. Tea-colored urine
   3. Clay-colored stools, often precede jaundice
   4. RUQ tenderness
   5. Enlarged liver

Subjective Data

A. Review the onset, duration, course, and severity of symptoms. Ask the client for specifics about urine and stool color:
   1. Ask whether the client has ever been treated for any type of hepatitis.
B. How long ago was her or she treated?
   1. Did the client complete the therapy? If not, why?
   2. What was the client's response to therapy (i.e., non-responder, responder)?
C. Review vaccination status.
D. Review the family history for HCC.
E. Ask the client about other family members and sexual contacts with similar symptoms.
F. Discuss the client's history of blood transfusions, IV drug use, and alcohol abuse.
G. Review the client's occupational exposure.
H. Inquire about recent international travel.
I. Review the client's history for variceal bleeding.
J. Is the client coinfected with hepatitis C virus (HCV) or HIV?

Physical Examination

A. Check temperature (if indicated), pulse, respirations, BP, and weight. Establish the client's usual weight; note the amount of any weight lost and over what length of time.
B. Inspect:
   1. Observe general appearance, muscle wasting, ascites, and peripheral edema.
   2. Inspect the skin for jaundice, palmar erythema, rash, spider nevi, spider angioma, and dehydration.
   3. Inspect the eyes for yellow sclera.
   4. Inspect the mucous membranes and nail beds.
   5. Evaluate for the presence of gynecomastia.
C. Auscultate:
   1. Lung fields and the heart
   2. All quadrants of the abdomen
D. Percuss:
   1. Abdomen
E. Palpate:
   1. All quadrants of the abdomen for masses, liver enlargement or tenderness, hepatomegaly, and splenomegaly
   2. The lymph nodes for lymphadenopathy
   3. For testicular atrophy

Diagnostic Tests

A. Diagnostic tests for HBV antigens and antibodies (Table 11.15)
B. CBC with differential
C. Complete liver panel:
   1. AST/ALT
   2. Total bilirubin
   3. INR
   4. Albumin
   5. ALP
D. Other viral infection markers: HCV and hepatitis delta virus (HDV)
E. ALP
F. Serum iron levels
G. Gamma-glutamyl transpeptidase (GGT; rule out other causes of chronic liver disease)
H. Alpha-fetoprotein (AFP; rule out other causes of liver disease)
I. HBV genotype

TABLE 11.15 DIAGNOSTIC TESTS FOR HBV ANTIGENS AND ANTIBODIES

Factors to Be Tested	HBV Antigen or Antibody	Indication
HBsAg	HBsAg	Detects acute or chronic infection; antigen used in hepatitis B vaccine
Anti-HBs	Antibody to HBsAg	Identifies resolved HBV infections; determines immunity after immunization
HBeAg	HBeAg	Identifies clients at risk of transmitting HBV
Anti-HBe	Antibody to HBeAg	Identifies clients with a lower risk of transmitting HBV
Anti-HBc	Antibody to hepatitis B core antigen; IgM (HBcAg)	Identifies acute, resolved, or chronic HBV infection. Anti-HBc is not present after immunization.
IgM anti-HBc Anti-HAV	IgM antibody to HBcAg	Identifies acute or recent HBV infection (includes HBsAg-negative client during the window phase of infection) Determines need for vaccination

HAV, hepatitis A virus; HBcAg, hepatitis B core antigen; HBeAg, hepatitis B envelope antigen; HBsAg, hepatitis B surface antigen; HBV, hepatitis B virus; IgM, immunoglobulin M.

J. HBV DNA viral load quantitation

K. Serum fibrosis panel:

1. APRI: Aspartate aminotransferase (AST)-to-platelet ratio index used for estimating hepatic fibrosis; online calculator can be found at www.hepatitisc.uw.edu/page/clinical-calculators/apri

2. Fibrosis-4 (FIB-4): An index for estimating hepatic fibrosis based on a calculation derived from AST, ALT, platelet concentrations, and age; online calculator can be found at www.hepatitisc.uw.edu/page/clinical-calculators/fib-4

3. FibroTest (FibroSure): Commercial biomarker test that uses the results of six blood markers to estimate hepatic fibrosis

L. Imaging:

1. Abdominal ultrasound

2. FibroScan: Transient shear-wave elastography measures liver stiffness as a surrogate for fibrosis

3. CT or MRI to help exclude biliary obstruction

M. Liver biopsy to assess the severity of disease

N. Pregnancy testing before antiviral therapy

O. Before oral antiviral therapy is introduced, all clients should be screened for HIV.

P. HCV and HIV testing to rule out coinfection

Differential Diagnoses

A. Hepatitis B

B. Exclusion of other types of hepatitis (A, C, D, E, viral, or autoimmune hepatitis)

C. Infectious mononucleosis

D. Hepatotoxic drug ingestion—for example, chloramphenicol, acetaminophen, or methyldopa

E. Metastatic cancer to the liver

F. Alcoholic hepatitis

G. Alcoholic cirrhosis

H. Hemochromatosis

I. Wilson's disease

Plan

A. General interventions:

1. No specific therapy for acute HBV infection is available.

2. Before any form of HBV therapy is started, and optimally at the first presentation, the client needs to be provided with information about the natural history of chronic hepatitis B infection and the fact that most infections remain entirely without symptoms even in those persons with severe disease, so that there is a need for regular lifelong monitoring.

3. Hepatitis B immune globulin (HBIG) and corticosteroids are not effective treatment.

B. Client teaching:

1. *See Section III: Client Teaching Guide for this chapter, "Jaundice and Hepatitis."*

2. Tell the client to avoid sexual activity until he or she is free of HBsAg.

3. History of anaphylactic reaction to common baker's yeast is a contraindication to HBV vaccination.

4. There are no dietary restrictions with acute and chronic hepatitis (without cirrhosis). Clients with decompensated cirrhosis, portal hypertension, or encephalopathy are prescribed the following diets:

a. Low-sodium diet: 1.5 g/d

b. High-protein diet: White-meat protein, such as pork, turkey, and fish

c. Fluid restriction of 1.5 L/d in the presence of hyponatremia

C. Pharmaceutical therapy:

1. The goal of treatment is to prevent progression to cirrhosis, hepatic failure, and hepatocellular cancer.

2. Primary prevention includes vaccination of high-risk individuals, including teens. Vaccination is up to 95% effective.

3. HBV vaccine is the recommended preexposure measure for the following groups:

a. Prevention of perinatal HBV infection through routine screening of all pregnant women for HBV infection and provision of hepatitis B vaccine and immunoprophylaxis to infants born to HBsAg-positive mothers

b. All infants: All major authorities recommend that all children receive a complete series of HBV immunizations during the first 18 months of life. **Universal immunization of infants begins at birth.**

c. Routine vaccination of previously unvaccinated children and adolescents

d. Children at risk of acquiring HBV by person-to-person (horizontal) transmission

e. All adolescents

f. IV drug users

g. Sexually active individuals with more than one sex partner in the previous 6 months or those who have an STI, MSM, and persons who inject drugs (PWID)

h. Healthcare workers and others at occupational risk

i. Residents and staff of institutions for developmentally disabled persons

j. Staff of nonresidential child-care centers

k. Clients undergoing hemodialysis

l. Clients with bleeding disorders who receive clotting factor concentrates

m. Household contacts and sexual partners of HBV carriers

n. Members of households with adoptees who are HBsAg positive

o. International travelers to areas of high or intermediate endemicity

p. Inmates of long-term correctional facilities

4. Hepatitis B vaccine can be given concurrently with other vaccines.

5. Early prophylaxis is paramount after an HBsAg needle stick. HBIG should be administered immediately, no later than 48 hours, after exposure. Postexposure prophylaxis with HBV vaccine is recommended.

6. The length of therapy depends on the genotype, any previous treatment, and/or coinfection with hepatitis C (HCV):

a. Treatment: Naïve—not previously treated for HCV

b. Relapser: Reappearance of HCV occurs after therapy is discontinued

c. Partial responder: HCV declines at week 12 of therapy but client is still positive at week 24 after completion of treatment

7. Antiviral therapy: Indicated in clients with compensated cirrhosis, decompensated cirrhosis, liver failure, or HCC; and clients on immunosuppressive therapy and coinfected with HCV:

a. IFN is used in young clients with compensated liver disease who do not wish to be on long-term treatment.

b. Nucleotide analogues: Entecavir, Tenofovir, Lamivudine, Adefovir, and Telbivudine. Most clients require 4 to 5 years of treatment, and some requires indefinite treatment.

8. Management of side effects with therapeutic agents is targeted to the symptoms.

9. Multiple drug–drug interactions are possible; consult with a pharmaceutical reference before instituting of drug therapy.

10. Dose adjustment is required in the presence of renal impairment and dialysis, and is used with caution in clients with a history of pancreatitis.

D. Surgical management:

1. Orthotopic liver transplantation (OLT) is the treatment of choice for clients with fulminant hepatic failure who do not recover and for clients with end-stage liver disease.

2. The guidelines for treatment are rapidly changing. The most current guideline recommendations are available from the American Association for the Study of Liver Diseases (AASLD) at www.aasld.org/publications/practice-guidelines-0. Guidelines include:

a. Acute liver failure management
b. Ascites due to cirrhosis management
c. Gastroesophageal varices and variceal hemorrhage in cirrhosis management
d. Hepatic encephalopathy
e. Hepatitis B, guidance
f. Hepatitis C, guidance
g. HCC management
h. Liver biopsy
i. Several chapters in the AASLD guideline recommendations are related to liver transplantation

3. The World Health Organization's (WHO) current *Guidelines for the Prevention, Care, and Treatment of Persons With Chronic Hepatitis B Infection* is located at www.who.int/hiv/pub/hepatitis/hepatitis-b-guidelines/en.

Follow-Up

A. Laboratory monitoring:

1. Monitor liver function (ALT) every 3 to 6 months for active disease.

2. Monitor hepatitis B envelope antigen (HBeAg) every 3 to 6 months, depending on ALT levels.

3. Monitor CBC and creatinine every month (1–2 days before treatment).

4. Monitor HBV DNA every 3 to 6 months when the client is receiving treatment in the reactivation phase.

B. Risk of exposure to HBsAg ceases when antigen disappears from the bloodstream, usually within 6 to 8 weeks of infection. Repeated serum determinations of HBsAg can help define when precautions may be relaxed.

C. Laboratory, physical examination, and psychosocial evaluation are required for antiviral therapy.

D. The AASLD recommends HCC surveillance using ultrasound in the following types of clients with chronic HBV:

1. Asian men older than 40 years and Asian women older than 50 years

2. All clients with cirrhosis, regardless of age

3. Clients with a family history of HCC, regardless of age

4. Africans older than age 20 years and any carriers older than age 40 years with persistent or intermittent ALT evaluation and/or HBV DNA level greater than 2,000 IU/mL should be screened with an ultrasound every 6 to 12 months

5. Any individual with HBV/HIV coinfection

E. Routine booster doses of hepatitis B vaccine are not recommended for children or adults with normal immune status.

Consultation/Referral

A. Clients with persistently elevated serum transaminase concentrations (exceeding twice the upper limits of normal), as well as those with elevated serum AFP concentrations or abnormal ultrasounds, should be referred to a gastroenterologist for further management.

Individual Considerations

A. Pregnancy:

1. No adverse effect on the developing fetus has been observed when pregnant women are vaccinated against HBV.

2. There are insufficient data to recommend delivery by cesarean section.

3. The AASLD suggests antiviral therapy to reduce the risk of perinatal transmission of hepatitis B in HBsAg-positive pregnant women with an HBV DNA level greater than 200,000 IU/mL.

4. The only antiviral agents studied in pregnant women are lamivudine, telbivudine, and tenofovir.

5. Antiviral therapy has been most often started at 28 to 32 weeks' gestation and discontinued at birth to 3 months postpartum.

6. Pregnancy and lactation are not a contraindication to vaccination.

7. Prenatal HBsAg testing of all pregnant women is recommended to identify newborns who require immediate postexposure prophylaxis.

8. Breastfeeding by an HBsAg-positive mother poses no additional risk for acquisition of HBV infection by the infant.

B. Pediatrics:

1. Infants born to HBsAg-positive mothers need no special precautions for spread of infectious disease other than removal of maternal blood by a gloved attendant and standard universal precautions.

2. Infants of all HBsAg-positive women should receive immunoprophylaxis (HBV vaccination ± HBIG) per WHO and the CDC recommendations.

3. All infants, including those who are premature, born to HbsAg-positive mothers need HBIG within 12 hours of birth.

4. More than 90% of infants infected perinatally will develop chronic HBV infection.

5. Adoptees from countries where HBV infection is endemic should be screened for HBsAg. If a child is HBsAg positive, previously unimmunized family members and other household contacts should be vaccinated, preferably before adoption.

6. Persons infected as infants or young children are at higher risk of death due to liver disease than are those infected as adults. Children with chronic HBV should be screened periodically for hepatic complications using serum liver transaminase tests, AFP concentration, and abdominal ultrasound.

7. All children 11 to 12 years should have their immunization records reviewed and should complete the vaccine series if they have not received the vaccine or did not complete the immunization series.

8. Children who stop antiviral therapy should be monitored every 3 months for at least 1 year for recurrent viremia, ALT flares, and clinical decompensation.

C. Adults:

1. Most HBV infections are acquired in adolescence or adulthood, largely as a result of IV drug use, sexual contact, or occupational or household exposure. HBV infection is associated with other sexually transmitted diseases, including syphilis.

2. Clients who have received a blood transfusion should refrain from blood donation for 6 months, the incubation period for HBV. Blood should never be donated if the client is a hepatitis B carrier or was infected with hepatitis C.

D. Geriatrics:

1. The elderly have fewer cases of HBV due to diminished immune response; however, they tend to be asymptomatic HBV carriers.

2. The disease has a greater tendency to deteriorate into chronic liver failure or chronic hepatitis in older adults.

Resources

American Association for the Study of Liver Diseases: www.aasld.org

American Liver Foundation: www.liverfoundation.org

Centers for Disease Control and Prevention: www.cdc .gov/hepatitis

Hepatitis B Foundation: www.hepb.org

Hepatitis Foundation International: www.hepfi.org

Immunization Action Coalition: www.immunize.org

National Institute of Diabetes and Digestive and Kidney Diseases: www2.niddk.nih.gov

United Network for Organ Sharing: www.unos.org

World Health Organization: who.int/en

Bibliography

Lok, A. S. F. (2017, September 29). Hepatitis B virus: Overview of management. *UpToDate*. Retrieved from https://www.uptodate.com/contents/hepatitis-b-virus-overview-of-management#H2130204242

Nettina, S. (2010). *The Lippincott manual of nursing practice* (9th ed.). Philadelphia, PA: Wolters Kluwer Lippincott Williams & Wilkins.

World Health Organization. (2019). *Hepatitis B*. Retrieved from https://www.who.int/en/news-room/fact-sheets/detail/hepatitis-b

Hepatitis C

Doncy Eapen and Cheryl A. Glass

Definition

A. Hepatitis C is an inflammation of the liver caused by HCV. HCV infection has signs and symptoms often undistinguishable from those of HAV or HBV infection. The disease tends to be asymptomatic to mild in severity and has an insidious onset. Acute fulminate infection is rare. The major feature of HCV infection is its propensity to become chronic. Persistent infection occurs in at least 75% to 85% of clients, even in the absence of biochemical evidence of liver disease. Approximately 60% to 70% of clients develop chronic hepatitis, and 5% to 20% develop cirrhosis.

B. Six HCV genotypes and subtypes exist. The genotype is a major factor in determining the effectiveness of the client's response to therapy. Approximately 50% of clients infected with genotype 1 and approximately 80% of clients infected with genotypes 2 and 3 achieve a sustained virologic response (SVR). SVR is defined as undetectable HCV RNA 12 months or more after treatment cessation.

C. The development of chronic hepatitis and its complications increase with several factors, including older age at acquisition, HIV infection, excessive alcohol consumption, and male gender. Among children, liver disease progression appears to be accelerated with comorbid conditions, including cancer, iron overload, thalassemia, or coinfection with HIV.

D. Hepatitis C is the leading cause of nonalcoholic hepatic failure and cirrhosis, and the cause of 90% of all cases of posttransfusion hepatitis. Primary HCC also occurs in these clients.

Incidence

A. Worldwide, more than 177.5 million individuals are chronically infected with HCV.

B. The "emerging epidemic" of acute HCV infection resulted from people who have transitioned from oral prescription opioid abuse to injection of these opioids and heroin.

C. Seroprevalence rates among individuals vary according to their associated risk factors. The highest rates occur in persons with large or repeated direct percutaneous exposure to blood or blood products, such as IV drug users and clients with hemophilia who have received multiple blood transfusions.

D. Seroprevalence among pregnant women in the United States has been estimated at 1% to 2%. Maternal–fetal (vertical) transmission is only 5% from women who are HCV RNA positive at the time of delivery. Maternal coinfection with HIV has been associated with increased risk of perinatal transmission of HCV RNA.

E. Serum anti-HCV antibody and HCV RNA have been detected in colostrum. However, although only a limited number of clients have been studied, the rate of transmission among breastfed infants is the same as that among bottle-fed infants.

F. More than 20% of adults with chronic infection progress to cirrhosis an average of 20 years after their initial infection. Clients with cirrhosis have a secondary risk of portal hypertension, liver failure, and other complications. HCV is the leading indication for liver transplantation among adults in the United States.

G. HCC is diagnosed an average of 30 years after initial HCV infection in 1% to 5% of clients, most of whom have underlying cirrhosis.

Pathogenesis

A. HCV is a small, single-stranded RNA virus with a lipid envelope and is a member of the Flavivirus family. Infection is spread primarily by parenteral exposure to blood and blood products from HCV-infected persons. In the United States, the current risk of HCV infection following blood transfusion is estimated at 0.1% or less because of exclusion of high-risk individuals from the blood donor pool and screening for HCV. Sexual transmission of HCV is uncommon except with high-risk behavior.

B. The incubation period averages 6 to 7 weeks, with a range of 2 weeks to 6 months. The time from exposure to the development of viremia generally is 1 to 2 weeks.

Predisposing Factors

All people with HCV RNA in their blood are considered to be infectious. The following groups are at high risk of HCV infection and should be tested:

A. IV drug users who have shared needles
B. Intranasal cocaine users, presumably resulting from epistaxis and shared equipment
C. Individuals with hemophilia, those undergoing hemodialysis, and those who received blood transfusions before 1992
D. Recipients of solid-organ transplants before 1992
E. Healthcare workers with percutaneous exposures
F. Individuals with multiple sexual partners
G. Transmission among contacts living with infected persons may occur with percutaneous or mucosal exposure to blood.
H. Infants of infected mothers, by vertical transmission
I. More common in males than in females
J. Tattooing, body piercing, and acupuncture with unsterile equipment
K. HIV infection

Common Complaints

A. Most clients with acute HCV infection are asymptomatic. Clients with chronic HCV infection may have nonspecific symptoms from progressive inflammation and complications from cirrhosis.
B. Malaise
C. Anorexia
D. Nausea
E. Myalgia
F. Fever
G. Abdominal pain

Other Signs and Symptoms

A. Jaundice (occurs in fewer than 20% of clients)
B. Hepatomegaly is present in one-third of clients with an acute infection
C. Ascites
D. Spider nevi
E. Dark urine

Subjective Data

A. Review the onset, duration, course, and severity of symptoms. Ask the client for specifics about urine and stool color.
B. Ask the client about other family members and sexual contacts with similar symptoms.
C. Review the client's history of blood transfusions, tattoos, incarnation, IV drug use, and alcohol abuse.
D. Ask the client about occupational exposure.
E. Ask about high-risk sexual practices.
F. Review family history of hepatocellular carcinoma (HCC).
G. When was HCV infection diagnosed?
H. Has the client had a liver biopsy? when?
I. Ask if the client has ever been treated for any type of hepatitis:
   1. How long ago the client treated?
   2. Did the client complete therapy? If not, why?
   3. What was the client's response to therapy (i.e., nonresponder, relapser)?
J. Review the client's history of variceal bleeding.

Physical Examination

A. Check temperature (acute infection), pulse, respirations, BP, and weight.
B. Inspect:
   1. Observe general appearance, muscle wasting, edema, and demeanor. **Administer a depression self-assessment tool at each visit when the client is on HCV therapy.**
   2. Inspect the skin for jaundice, rash, dehydration, palmar erythema, excoriations, spider nevi, and tattoos/piercings.
   3. Inspect the eyes for yellow sclera.
   4. Inspect the mucous membranes and nail beds for clubbing and cyanosis.
   5. Inspect for gynecomastia and small testes.
C. Auscultate:
   1. Lung fields and heart
   2. All quadrants of the abdomen and evaluate for abdominal bruit

D. Percuss:
1. Abdomen
E. Palpate:
1. All quadrants of the abdomen for masses; liver enlargement or tenderness; characteristics of cirrhosis; and hepatosplenomegaly, which occurs in about 10% of cases
2. Lymph node examination:
   a. Evaluate the lymph nodes for lymphadenopathy and enlarged parotid.

Diagnostic Tests
A. Laboratory tests:
1. IgG antibody EIAs for HCV and nucleic acid amplification (NAA) tests to detect HCV RNA
2. HCV genotyping
3. HCV viral load: Quantitative assay used as a prognostic indicator for clients undergoing antiviral therapy
4. ALT and AST
5. Hepatitis A IgM and IgG
6. HBsAg and antibody, core antibody
7. CMV immunoglobulin (IgM) and IgG (and/or CMV in urine culture)
8. Epstein–Barr virus IgM and IgG
9. HIV IgG enzyme-linked immunoassay (ELISA)
10. AFP
B. Ultrasonography is used for monitoring HCV-related complications. FibroScan—transient shear wave elastography—measures liver stiffness as a surrogate for fibrosis.
C. Serum fibrosis panel:
1. APRI = AST-to-platelet ratio index used for estimating hepatic fibrosis; online calculator can be found at www.hepatitisc.uw.edu/page/clinical-calculators/apri
2. FIB-4: An index for estimating hepatic fibrosis based on a calculation derived from AST, ALT, platelet concentrations, and age; online calculator can be found at www.hepatitisc.uw.edu/page/clinical-calculators/fib-4
3. FibroTest (FibroSure): Commercial biomarker test that uses the results of six blood markers to estimate hepatic fibrosis
D. Liver biopsy is the most accurate method of evaluating the extent of HCV-related liver disease. Liver biopsy is the gold standard for determining the histological grade and stage of fibrosis/cirrhosis. The *absolute* requirement for a liver biopsy prior to the institution of medication therapy is currently under discussion. For clients with genotypes 2 and 3, the likelihood of response to therapy is so high that the benefits of treatment may outweigh the risk of biopsy and histological considerations.
E. Prior to the institution/during antiviral therapy, perform the following tests:
1. CBC with platelets
2. Viral load
3. Liver function (ALT/AST)
4. Pregnancy test
5. Thyroid profile
6. Blood glucose/A1C

7. Consider a dilated retinal examination.
8. Consider a stress test.
9. Screen for alcohol abuse, drug abuse, and/or depression

Differential Diagnoses
A. Hepatitis C
B. Hepatitis A
C. Hepatitis B
D. Alcoholic liver disease
E. Drug toxicities
F. Opportunistic infections associated with HIV infection
G. Cholangitis
H. Autoimmune hepatitis

Plan
A. General interventions:
1. **Clients and their spouses should be counseled to not become pregnant while on therapy and for 6 months after the completion of treatment. Pregnancy tests should be done prior to institution of HCV therapy and monthly thereafter.**
B. Client teaching:
1. *See Section III: Client Teaching Guide for this chapter, "Jaundice and Hepatitis."* ◀
2. Warn the client of the possibility of transmission to others, and tell the client to refrain from donating blood, organs, tissues, or semen and from sharing toothbrushes and razors.
3. All clients with chronic HCV infection should be immunized against hepatitis A and hepatitis B.
4. Counsel the client to avoid hepatotoxic medications and alcohol.
5. Immunoprophylaxis for postexposure prophylaxis with IG is not recommended.
6. The CDC recommends anyone born between 1945 and 1965 be tested for HCV.
C. Pharmaceutical therapy:
1. The primary aim is inhibiting HCV replication, eradicating infection, preventing progression of fibrosis, and preventing development of HCC.
2. Direct-acting antiviral therapy (DAA): Eradicates HCV RNA and is predicted by attainment of SVR
3. The length of therapy depends on the genotype and previous treatment:
   a. Treatment-naïve: Clients who have never received any treatment for HCV
   b. Treatment-experienced: Clients who have failed prior treatment for HCV:
      i. Peginterferon and ribavirin failure: Clients who did not respond to or relapsed after treatment with peginterferon and ribavirin (without direct-acting antiviral exposure)
      ii. Protease inhibitor failures: Clients who did not respond to or relapsed after treatment with boceprevir, telaprevir, or simeprevir in combination with peginterferon and ribavirin
      iii. Sofosbuvir failures: Clients who did not respond to or relapsed after treatment with a

regimen that contained sofosbuvir (but did not contain an NS5A inhibitor)

iv. NS5A inhibitor failures: Clients who did not respond to or relapsed after treatment with a regimen containing an NS5A inhibitor (such as ledipasvir, daclatasvir, elbasvir, or ombitasvir)

c. Relapser: Reappearance of HCV after therapy is discontinued

d. Partial responder: HCV declines at week 12 of therapy but is still positive at week 24 after completion of treatment:

i. Manage side effects with therapeutic agents related to symptoms.

ii. If there are multiple drug–drug interactions, consult with a pharmaceutical reference before instituting drug therapy.

iii. The guidelines for treatment are changing rapidly. The most current guideline recommendations are available from the AASLD and the IDSA at www.aasld.org/publications/practice-guidelines-0. Guidelines break down therapy in detail by genotype, length of therapy, and medications. The AASLD guidelines also include:

1) Acute liver failure management

2) Ascites due to cirrhosis management

3) Gastroesophageal varices and variceal hemorrhage in cirrhosis management

4) Hepatic encephalopathy

5) Hepatitis B guidance

6) Hepatitis C guidance

7) HCC management

8) Liver biopsy

9) Several chapters in the AASLD guideline recommendations are related to liver transplantation.

4. WHO's *Guidelines for the Screening, Care, and Treatment of Persons With Hepatitis C Infection* is available at https://apps.who.int/iris/bitstream/handle/10665/273174/9789241550345-eng.pdf?ua=1.

Follow-Up

A. Test the client within 5 to 6 weeks after the onset of hepatitis; 80% of clients are positive for serum anti-HCV antibody.

B. Persons with chronic HCV infections should be vaccinated against hepatitis A and B, unless they have previously been demonstrated to be nonsusceptible.

C. Children with chronic infection should be screened periodically for chronic hepatitis with serum LFTs because of their potential long-term risk for chronic liver disease. Definitive recommendations on frequency of screening have not been established.

D. Monitor for mental dysfunction related to IFN, including depression, psychosis, aggressive behavior, hallucinations, violent behavior, suicidal ideation, suicide attempt, and homicidal ideation (rare), even without previous history of psychiatric illness.

Consultation/Referral

A. Referrals include a gastroenterologist, psychiatrist, endocrinologist, neurologist, hematologist, dietitian, and social worker.

B. Clients who are coinfected with HBV or HIV or have end-stage renal disease should be referred for treatment.

C. Children with severe disease or histologically advanced pathology (bridging necrosis or active cirrhosis) should be referred to a specialist in the management of chronic HCV infection.

D. Children with persistently elevated serum transaminase concentrations, or those with concentrations exceeding twice the upper limits of normal, should be referred to a gastroenterologist for further management.

Individual Considerations

A. Pregnancy:

1. No data currently exist to support counseling a woman against pregnancy (unless she is under active treatment)

2. Routine serologic testing of pregnant women for HCV infection is not recommended. Women with significant risk factors for HCV should be offered antibody screening.

3. According to the current guidelines offered by the U.S. Public Health Service and the American Academy of Pediatrics, maternal HCV infection is not a contraindication to breastfeeding. HCV-positive mothers should consider abstaining from breastfeeding if their nipples are cracked or bleeding.

4. **Ribavirin (RBV) is a pregnancy category X drug with abortifacient potential.**

5. IFN is a pregnancy category C drug and should be used only if the benefits outweigh the risk to the fetus. **IFN is a pregnancy category X drug when combined with RBV.**

6. The method of delivery has not been shown to increase the risk of vertical transmission of HCV. Cesarean delivery is reserved for obstetrical indications.

B. Pediatrics:

1. Serologic testing for anti-HCV antibodies in children born to women previously identified to be HCV infected is recommended because approximately 5% acquire the infection. The duration of the passive maternal antibody in infants is unknown. Testing for anti-HCV antibodies should not be performed until after 12 months of age.

2. Exclusion of children with HCV infections from out-of-home child-care centers is not indicated.

3. In 2017, the FDA approved the DAA combination of Sovaldi (sofosbuvir) plus ribavirin and Harvoni (ledipasvir and sofosbuvir) to treat HCV infection in children ages 12 to 17.

4. The need for testing for AFP concentration and for abdominal ultrasonography in children has not been determined.

5. Routine serologic testing of adoptees, either domestic or international, is not recommended.

C. Adults:

1. The CDC recommends that anyone born between 1945 and 1965 be tested for HCV.

2. Infected persons with steady partners do not need to change their sexual practices. However, they should be informed of the possible risk of transmission and the precautions that can prevent transmission.

3. Persons with multiple sexual partners should be advised to reduce the number of partners and to use condoms to prevent transmission.

4. The best means of limiting transfusion-associated HCV is to rely exclusively on volunteer rather than commercial blood donors and to screen donors for anti-HCV antibodies.

D. Geriatrics:

1. There are fewer cases of HCV infection in the elderly than in other age groups. However, they tend to develop chronic hepatitis or hepatic failure.

Resources

American Association for the Study of Liver Diseases: www.aasld.org

American Liver Foundation: www.liverfoundation.org

Centers for Disease Control and Prevention: www.cdc .gov/hepatitis

Hepatitis Foundation International: www.hepfi.org

Immunization Action Coalition: www.immunize.org

National Institute of Diabetes and Digestive and Kidney Diseases: www.niddk.nih.gov

United Network for Organ Sharing: www.unos.org

World Health Organization: www.who.int/en

Bibliography

Chopra, S., & Pockros, P. J. (2018, June 5). Overview of the management of chronic hepatitis C virus infection. *UpToDate*. Retrieved from https:// www.uptodate.com/contents/overview-of-the-management-of-chronic -hepatitis-c-virus-infection#H9644102

Chou, R., & Wasson, N. (2013, June 4). Blood tests to diagnose fibrosis or cirrhosis in patients with chronic hepatitis C infection. *Annals of Internal Medicine, 158*, 807–820, W328–W330. doi:10.7326/0003-4819-158- 11-201306040-00005

Nettina, S. (2010). *The Lippincott manual of nursing practice* (9th ed.). Philadelphia, PA: Wolters Kluwer Lippincott Williams & Wilkins.

U.S. Food and Drug Administration. (2017, April 7). *FDA approves two hepatitis C drugs for pediatric patients*. Retrieved from https://www.fda .gov/newsevents/newsroom/pressannouncements/ucm551407.htm

Hernias, Abdominal

Doncy Eapen and Cheryl A. Glass

Definition

A hernia is the protrusion of a peritoneum-lined sac through a defect in the abdominal wall. Abdominal wall hernias are the most common indication addressed by surgical procedures. Hernias are a leading cause of disability and work loss. Abdominal hernias can be congenital or acquired. Types include the following:

A. Umbilical hernia: Occurs when the intestinal muscles fail to close around the umbilicus, allowing the omentum and/or intestines to protrude into the weaker area

B. Incisional hernia: Caused by a defect in the abdominal musculature that develops after a surgical incision

C. Epigastric hernia: Protrusion of fat or omentum through the linea alba between the umbilicus and the xiphoid. Epigastric hernias are generally less than 2 cm in diameter.

D. Diastasis recti: Acquired hernia most often due to pregnancy and obesity. The right and left rectus muscles separate, but there is no facial defect.

E. Obturator hernia: Follows the path of the obturator nerves and muscles

Incidence

A. Umbilical hernias are more common in African American infants, women, and the elderly. This type of hernia has a higher risk of incarceration and strangulation, and, therefore, a greater mortality because the large bowel is frequently entrapped.

B. Epigastric hernias are most common in men 20 to 50 years old.

C. Incisional hernias typically are noted in the early postoperative period; however, there is an increase in incisional hernias during pregnancy. These iatrogenic hernias occur in 2% to 10% of abdominal surgeries. In addition to hernias, separation of the recti abdominis muscles (diastasis recti) is often caused by pregnancy or obesity.

D. Obturator hernias occur more commonly in females. Females have a larger canal diameter, which is noted predominantly in thin elderly women.

Pathogenesis

A. Incisional hernias are due to failure of fascial tissues to heal and close.

B. Epigastric hernias are defects in the abdominal midline between the umbilicus and the xiphoid process. They are usually related to a congenital weakness, increased intra-abdominal pressure, surrounding muscle weakness, or chronic abdominal wall strain.

C. An umbilical hernia is caused by failure of the umbilical ring to obliterate after birth. In the infant, the umbilical ring often closes spontaneously within the first 1 to 2 years of life. Increased abdominal pressure or congenital defects cause abdominal hernias that allow abdominal contents to protrude through the opening defect. In adults with an umbilical hernia, obesity increases the danger of incarceration.

D. Parastomal hernia is caused by the bowel intrusion into the defect in the abdominal wall when the ileostomy or colostomy was created.

Predisposing Factors

A. Congenital predisposition

B. Gender

C. Obesity

D. Multiparity

E. Cirrhosis and ascites

F. Trauma or straining

G. African American ancestry and infancy

H. Chronic cough; can precipitate or worsen herniation

I. Previous abdominal surgery

J. Straining, coughing, and sneezing in infancy

K. Straining with chronic constipation

L. Incisional hernia factors:
1. Smoking
2. Connective tissue disorder
3. Infection
4. Malnutrition
5. Immunosuppressive medications

M. Age: Obturator hernias occur predominately in the elderly.

N. Maternal smoking is associated with an increased prevalence of omphalocele and gastroschisis.

Common Complaints
A. Bulge of the abdomen or of a previous scar
B. Symptoms aggravated by cough and straining
C. Small hernias may be asymptomatic or, as the hernia progresses, varying degrees of discomfort and pain may occur.
D. The only sign of a hernia may be increased irritability.

Other Signs and Symptoms
A. Incisional: Bulge through the incision wall (may be intermittent)
B. Epigastric: Small, usually painless subcutaneous mass
C. Umbilical:
1. Adult: Vague, intermittent pain; palpable mass
2. Infant: Vomiting and irritability
D. Reducible or irreducible: Signs and symptoms are related to the degree of pressure of their contents rather than to size. Most clients are asymptomatic or complain of only mild pain.
E. Strangulated: Colicky abdominal pain, nausea, vomiting, abdominal distention, hyperperistalsis

Subjective Data
A. Review the onset, duration, and course of symptoms.
B. Ask the client about previous abdominal surgeries, wound infection, and pregnancies.
C. Review the history of straining, trauma, or physical labor.
D. Determine if the client has signs and symptoms of strangulation of entrapped bowel: Pain, nausea, vomiting, distention, and fever.
E. Determine if the client can reduce the hernia.
F. Ask the client whether the hernia is enlarging and uncomfortable.
G. Review the client's bowel history, specifically constipation.
H. Review the client's history for chronic obstructive pulmonary disease (COPD)/chronic cough.
I. Review the client's history for symptoms of obstructive uropathy.
J. Review how the hernia affects the client's activities of daily living (ADLs).

Physical Examination
Examination is the same for all types of abdominal hernias. Perform the examination while the client is standing and supine. History and physical examination are the best means of diagnosing hernias.
A. Check temperature (if indicated), pulse, respirations, and BP.

B. Inspect:
1. Inspect the contour and symmetry of the abdomen for bulges or masses. The bulge may be asymmetric.
2. Inspect irreducible hernias for discoloration, edema, and ascites.
3. Assess:
a. Have the client perform the Valsalva maneuver while standing.
b. Have the client lie supine, lift the head from the examination table, and then bear down to tense the abdomen.
C. Auscultate:
1. All quadrants of the abdomen for bowel sounds
D. Percuss:
1. Liver
2. Spleen
3. Abdomen
E. Palpate:
1. The entire abdomen for masses, hepatomegaly, and ascites. Umbilical hernias may be obscured by subcutaneous fat.
2. The groin
3. The hernia, to try to gently reduce it

Diagnostic Tests
A. None is required if the hernia is easily reducible (depending on the type of hernia).
B. CBC: WBC increased, Hct increased
C. Electrolytes: Na$^+$ increased or decreased
D. Abdominal radiography: Limited use
E. Ultrasonography: Helpful in detecting a scrotal mass or a mass below the inguinal ligament
F. CT scan of the abdomen and pelvis is the best imaging study in clients with suspected abdominal wall hernia that cannot be diagnosed on physical examination.

Differential Diagnoses
A. Abdominal hernia
B. Diastasis recti
C. Ascites
D. Abdominal wall tumor or cyst
E. Bowel obstruction
F. Abdominal wall cellulitis
G. Rectus sheath hematoma

Plan
A. General interventions:
1. Difficult reduction of the abdominal hernia must be promptly referred for repair.
B. Client teaching:
1. Discuss the hernia and available options for treatment.
2. Teach the client signs and symptoms of strangulation.
3. Instruct the client to refrain from heavy lifting.
4. Advise the client to wear a support garment.
C. Pharmaceutical therapy:
1. Broad-spectrum antibiotics are administered if bowel ischemia or strangulated hernias are suspected. Collaborate with a gastroenterologist for these clients.

D. Surgical management:
1. Gastroenterologists and general surgeons for management

> Reduction should not be attempted if there are signs of inflammation or obstruction.

1. Try to reduce the hernia unless strangulated. See Section II: Procedure, "Hernia Reduction (Inguinal/Groin)."
    a. Easily reducible: Abdominal contents can be easily returned to their original compartment. Allows symptomatic relief
    b. Incarcerated: Cannot be returned to its original compartment. The incarcerated tissue may be bowel, omentum, or other abdominal contents.
    c. Strangulated: Surgical emergency—blood supply to the herniated tissue is compromised.
2. Do not try to reduce strangulated hernias because reduction can cause gangrenous bowel to enter the peritoneal cavity.
3. A truss fits snugly over a hernia to prevent abdominal contents from entering the hernial sac. It does not cure a hernia and is used only when the client is not a surgical candidate.
4. Umbilical hernia repair is best performed under general anesthesia in children.
5. Surgery may be done laparoscopically or through an open procedure and by sutured or mesh repair, depending on the age of the person, the type and size of the hernia, and the presence of strangulation.

Follow-Up
A. Instruct the client to call the office if fever or severe pain occurs. Otherwise, no follow-up is required unless for postoperative repair. Postoperative follow-up is with the physician who performed the surgery.

Consultation/Referral
Consult a physician if the client has abdominal tenderness, discoloration, or edema at the site; fever; or signs of bowel obstruction.

Individual Considerations
A. Pregnancy:
1. Incisional hernias are more common during pregnancy because of increased intra-abdominal pressure.
2. Bowel obstruction secondary to previous scarring may also be seen and is most common when the uterus emerges from the pelvis early in the second trimester, when the uterus is maximally distended at term, and in immediate puerperium when the uterus promptly decreases in size.
B. Pediatrics:
1. Infants with umbilical hernias require no special treatment because the majority of these hernias close by the fifth year.
2. The infant's abdomen should be soft. Masses may be due to enlargement of tumors or liver. The liver is normally felt 1 to 3 cm below the right costal margin.
3. Tell caregivers that the umbilicus normally everts when a baby cries. However, they should report if the lump becomes large or irreducible, particularly if the baby is vomiting. These signs indicate strangulation and the need for urgent surgery.
4. Genetic testing should be considered in infants with an omphalocele. An omphalocele is associated with chromosomal abnormalities, including trisomy 13, trisomy 18, trisomy 21, and Klinefelter syndrome.
C. Geriatrics:
1. Because of the anatomical position of the obturator hernia, the presentation in elderly clients more commonly takes the form of a bowel obstruction rather than a protrusion of bowel contents:
    1. The geriatric population is more prone to develop electrolyte and acid–base imbalances from obstruction.
2. The geriatric population has a higher rate of ventral hernias attributed to the loss of muscle strength in the anterior abdominal wall and the prevalence of comorbidities that lead to an increased intra-abdominal pressure.

Bibliography
Brooks, D. C. (2018, October 30). Overview of abdominal wall hernias in adults. *UpToDate*. Retrieved from https://www.uptodate.com/contents/overview-of-abdominal-wall-hernias-in-adults#H1829942152
Nettina, S. (2010). *The Lippincott manual of nursing practice* (9th ed.). Philadelphia, PA: Wolters Kluwer Lippincott Williams & Wilkins.
Rather, A. A. (2018, October 3). Abdominal hernias workup. *Medscape*. Retrieved from https://emedicine.medscape.com/article/189563-workup#c9

Hernias, Pelvic

Doncy Eapen and Cheryl A. Glass

Definition
A hernia is the protrusion of a peritoneum-lined sac through some defect from one anatomical space to another. As shown in Figure 11.3, there are three types of pelvic (inguinal) hernias distinguished by presentation:
A. Indirect: Protrudes through the internal inguinal ring; can remain in the canal, exit the external ring, or pass into the scrotum; unilateral or bilateral
B. Direct: Protrudes through the external inguinal ring; located in the region of Hesselbach's triangle; rarely enters the scrotum
C. Femoral: Protrudes through the femoral ring, femoral canal, and fossa ovalis

Incidence
A. Indirect inguinal hernias are the most common type of hernia. They affect both sexes, but most often are seen in children and young males (7:1 male-to-female ratio). Incidence increases with age.
B. Direct inguinal hernias are less common than indirect inguinal hernias. They occur more often in males and are more common in individuals older than age 40. Primary inguinal hernias occur in 1% to 5% of infants and in 9% to 10% of those born prematurely.
C. Femoral hernias are the least common type of hernias. They are rarely seen in children and occur more often in

A

B

Internal
ring
External
ring

Femoral
canal

C

FIGURE 11.3 Pelvic hernias. A. Indirect hernia comes down the canal and touches the fingertip on examination. B. Direct hernia bulges anteriorly and pushes against the side of the finger on examination. C. Femoral hernia protrudes through the femoral ring, femoral canal, and fossa ovalis, so the inguinal canal is empty on examination.

females (1.8:1 female-to-male ratio). Right-side presentation is more common than left-side presentation.

D. Among inguinal hernias, a sliding component is found in 3%; they are overwhelmingly on the left side (4.5:1 left-to-right ratio). Sliding hernias are much more common in men than in women, and the predominance increases with age. Female infants have a high incidence of sliding tube, ovary, or broad ligament hernias.

E. Primary perineal hernias occur most often in elderly multiparous women.

Pathogenesis

Pelvic hernias occur because there is a potential space for protrusion—commonly of the bowel but occasionally of the omentum.

A. Indirect and direct hernias arise along the course that the testicle travels as it exits the abdomen and enters the scrotum during intrauterine life. Indirect hernias may be due to a congenital defect in which the processus vaginalis remains patent.

B. Femoral hernias occur at the fossa ovalis, where the femoral artery exits the abdomen.

Predisposing Factors

A. Pregnancy
B. Straining
C. Age
D. Obesity
E. Gender
F. Repetitive stress/hard physical labor
G. Congenital defect
H. Premature birth
I. Chronic cough
J. Chronic constipation
K. Family history of hernia
L. History of an AAA

Common Complaints

A. Bulging or swelling localized in the groin or scrotum
B. Dull ache in the lower abdomen or groin
C. Swelling of the labia majora in women
D. Children with inguinal hernias have minimal symptoms and may present with a history of an intermittent mass noted when straining or crying.
E. Bowel obstruction

Other Signs and Symptoms

A. Ability to reduce hernia

B. Exacerbation on standing, straining, or coughing

C. Strangulation:
   1. Colicky abdominal pain
   2. Nausea or vomiting
   3. Hyperperistalsis
   4. Fever
   5. Edema
   6. Discoloration
   7. Tenderness

D. Infants:
   1. Distress
   2. Vomiting
   3. Poor feeding
   4. Irritable and crying

Subjective Data

A. Review the time of onset, duration, and course of hernia and swelling.

B. Review any symptoms and quality of pain. Outright pain with hernias is unusual, and its presence should raise the suspicion for incarceration or strangulation.

C. Ask the client about history of straining, trauma, physical labor, and pregnancy.

D. Inquire about symptoms of obstruction or strangulation of entrapped bowel, including pain, nausea, and vomiting. Groin pain and tenderness are generally absent in strangulated femoral hernias.

E. Determine if the client can reduce the hernia.

F. Review irritating (e.g., exercise, straining, cough) and alleviating factors.

G. Review bowel habits, particularly constipation.

H. Evaluate history of COPD and cough.

Physical Examination

Physical examination is the same for all types of hernias and is directed at determining the type of hernia and whether it is reducible, incarcerated, or strangulated. Perform the examination while the client is standing or supine. Palpation is best done with the client standing.

A. Check temperature (if indicated), pulse, respirations, and BP.

B. Inspect:
   1. Inspect for discoloration and edema of the herniated area.
   2. Inspect for visible hernia. Instruct the client to perform a Valsalva maneuver to increase intra-abdominal pressure.
   3. Transillumination of the scrotum is performed to evaluate any bowel contents.
   4. Inspect for the presence of ascites.

C. Auscultate:
   1. Abdomen for bowel sounds

D. Palpate:
   1. Palpate the groin for lymphadenopathy, masses, and tenderness. *The right side is more commonly affected in both genders.*
      a. Males: Using the second or third finger, invaginate the scrotal skin, with and without cough and strain. There will be some degree of pressure with this maneuver, but a true hernia can typically be felt as a "silky" impulse tapping against the finger. Palpate the scrotum: A scrotal lump is either soft or unusually firm.
      b. Females: Visually examine for a bulge, and then place two or three fingers across the inguinal canal and ask the client to bear down or cough to elicit the characteristic bulge or impulse. Palpate the labia for swelling, either soft or unusually firm.

Diagnostic Tests

A. History and physical examination remain the best means of diagnosing hernias.

B. Ultrasonography helps identify occult inguinal hernia in clients with suggestive symptoms but in whom the hernia is not detectable on physical examination.

C. MRI appears to be able to differentiate inguinal and femoral hernias with a high sensitivity.

D. CT of the groin can help differentiate femoral from inguinal hernias.

E. Sigmoidoscopy is not recommended as a screening test.

F. Plain abdominal x-rays are of limited value in the evaluation of an incarcerated hernia.

G. Karyotyping should be considered when a testicle is palpable in the inguinal canal or found at herniorrhaphy in phenotypic females.

H. Routine laboratory work is not recommended.

Differential Diagnoses

A. Inguinal or pelvic hernia

B. Acute conditions:
   1. Testicular torsion causes sudden, excruciating pain in or around the testicle, which may spread to the lower abdomen; the pain may get worse with standing. Other signs and symptoms include swelling, rising of the affected testicle, nausea, vomiting, fever, and fainting or lightheadedness.
   2. Epididymitis

C. Nonacute conditions:
   1. Testicular tumor
   2. Muscle strain
   3. Hip arthritis
   4. Undescended testicle
   5. Hydrocele
   6. Varicocele
   7. Spermatocele

D. Bowel obstruction

Plan

A. General interventions:
   1. Gently reduce a groin hernia while the client lies supine with hips slightly flexed to relax the abdominal muscles.

B. Client teaching:
   1. Tell the client to call the office right away if he finds a lump or swelling in the scrotum, even if it is small or painless. Testicular tumors are usually painless.
   2. Discuss the condition and treatment options with the client:

a. Surgery is the only effective treatment. Open hernia repair and laparoscopic repair are the two types of herniorrhaphy.

b. Watchful waiting rather than surgical repair is an option if the client is asymptomatic as long as he is aware of the risk and understands the need for prompt attention should symptoms of complication occur.

c. Nonsurgical therapy for groin hernias is the use of a truss. There are insufficient data to determine the efficacy of trusses in controlling symptoms. A truss has the potential risk of bowel constriction; prolonged use of a truss can lead to atrophy of the spermatic cord or fusion to the hernial sac.

3. Teach the client signs of strangulation.

4. Instruct the client to avoid heavy lifting.

C. Pharmaceutical therapy:

1. Treat any underlying acute conditions such as nausea/vomiting or fever/pain. Collaborate with the gastroenterologist or general surgeon regarding medications prescribed prior to and after surgery.

Follow-Up

A. Tell the client to return to the office if fever, severe pain, or strangulation occurs.

B. Postoperative evaluation for hernia recurrences as needed:

1. Immediately from repair

2. Greater than 6 months and up to 5 years from repair

3. Late recurrences beyond 5 years from the repair

Consultation/Referral

A. Refer clients with femoral hernias to a surgeon. These hernias need to be repaired as soon as possible because of increased risk of incarceration and strangulation.

B. Contemporary practice triages surgical repair versus watchful waiting according to the severity of symptoms, type of hernia, and gender:

1. Females should undergo inguinal herniorrhaphy once a diagnosis is established instead of watchful waiting.

2. Surgical repair is indicated for males with moderate to severe symptoms from an inguinal hernia.

3. Surgical repair is indicated in men with scrotal or recurrent hernias, even if they are asymptomatic or have only minimal symptoms.

4. Strangulated hernias are nonreducible, and blood supply to protruded tissue is compromised. Refer clients for immediate surgical intervention.

Individual Considerations

A. Pregnancy:

1. Preexisting groin hernias may become more symptomatic during the first trimester of pregnancy. The symptoms must be differentiated from round ligament pain.

2. Surgical repair of a groin hernia during a pregnancy is generally contraindicated. Typically, elective repair is deferred until 4 weeks postpartum.

B. Pediatrics:

1. A high incidence (16%–25%) of inguinal hernias occurs in premature infants. The incidence is inversely related to weight.

2. In infants, the only symptom of a hernia may be increased irritability.

C. Geriatrics:

1. Groin hernias are one of the most frequently encountered pathologies occurring in old age, secondary to the presence of constipation, coughing, abdominal fat deposits, and loss of strength of the abdominal wall.

2. Signs and symptoms of prostatism are frequently present in men with hernias and may require relief before herniorrhaphy.

3. Excessive waiting time for elective repair increases the risk of strangulation, bowel resection, and mortality, especially with older clients.

Bibliography

Brooks, D. C. (2016, May 3). Overview of treatment for inguinal and femoral hernia in adults. *UpToDate*. Retrieved from http://www.uptodate.com/contents/overview-of-treatment-for-inguinal-and-femoral-hernia-in-adults

Brooks, D. C., & Hawn, M. (2018, January 4). Classification, clinical features, and diagnosis of inguinal and femoral hernias in adults. *UpToDate*. Retrieved from https://www.uptodate.com/contents/classification-clinical-features-and-diagnosis-of-inguinal-and-femoral-hernias-in-adults?search=inguinal%20hernia&sectionRank=1&usage_type=default&anchor=H14&source=machineLearning&selectedTitle=2-122&display_rank=2#H14

National Institute of Diabetes and Digestive and Kidney Diseases. (2014, June). *Inguinal hernia*. Retrieved from https://www.niddk.nih.gov/health-information/digestive-diseases/inguinal-hernia

Nettina, S. (2010). *The Lippincott manual of nursing practice* (9th ed.). Philadelphia, PA: Wolters Kluwer Lippincott Williams & Wilkins.

Hirschsprung's Disease or Congenital Aganglionic Megacolon

Doncy Eapen and Cheryl A. Glass

Definition

A. HD is the major cause of intestinal obstruction in newborns. It is congenital or present at birth and presents as a motor disorder of the gut. The aganglionic segment is aperistaltic and remains in a state of contraction, causing a functional obstruction. The majority of clients with HD are diagnosed in the neonatal period. Although infants appear normal at birth, more than half do not pass meconium for more than 48 hours. Absence of peristalsis causes feces to accumulate proximal to the defect and leads to intestinal obstruction. Bacterial enterocolitis is the most severe complication of untreated HD, and mortality from the complications may be as great as 25% to 30%.

Incidence

A. HD occurs in one in every 5,400 to 7,200 live births. It is uncommon in premature infants.

B. Occurrence is more common in males; however, incidence of long-segment disease is increased in females.

The incidence is roughly three times more common among Asian Americans.

C. About 10% to 50% of cases have familial incidence. Approximately eight genetic mutations have been identified. One in 100 children with Down syndrome also has HD.

D. Other chromosomal abnormalities and syndromes associated with HD:

1. Trisomy 21 (Down syndrome)
2. Cardiac disease (septal defects)
3. Bardet–Biedl syndrome (BBS)
4. Congenital central hypoventilation syndrome (CCHS)
5. Waardenburg's syndrome
6. Smith–Lemli–Opitz syndrome
7. Multiple endocrine neoplasia type 2
8. Shprintzen–Goldberg syndrome
9. Piebaldism
10. Yemenite deaf–blind syndrome
11. Neurocristopathy syndromes

E. Approximately 80% of affected clients have the disorder limited to the rectum or rectosigmoid region.

F. Approximately 3% to 5% of affected clients have aganglionosis of the entire colon.

G. The disease is three times more common in people of European ancestry.

H. Approximately 25% of affected clients have associated congenital anomalies of the kidney and urinary tract (hydronephrosis and renal hypoplasia).

Pathogenesis

A. HD is due to congenital absence of ganglion cells in both Meissner's (submucosal) and Auerbach's (myenteric) plexus. It occurs secondary to the failure of migration of ganglia from the neural crest, which normally occurs before the 12th week of gestation. The disorder starts in the distal rectum and extends proximally to involve a varying amount of the bowel.

Predisposing Factors

A. Full-term infant of normal weight
B. European ancestry
C. Male gender
D. Family history of disorder
E. Down syndrome

Common Complaints

A. Newborns: Failure to pass meconium for more than 48 hours
B. Blast sign: Explosive expulsion of gas and stool after the use of a digital rectal examination
C. Children: Failure to grow
D. Constipation
E. Abdominal distention

Other Signs and Symptoms

A. Newborns:
1. Overflow-type diarrhea
2. Bile- or feces-stained vomitus
3. FTT

4. Anorexia due to early satiety, abdominal discomfort, and distention
5. Temporary relief with enema

B. Older infants and children (nearly all children with HD are diagnosed during the first 2 years of life):
1. Constipation since birth; may have a history of requiring a daily enema
2. Older presentation is more common in breastfed infants; constipation will typically develop around the time of weaning
3. Intestinal obstruction
4. Progressive abdominal distention with visible peristaltic activity
5. Temporary relief with enema
6. Ribbon-like, fluid-like, or pellet stools
7. FTT
8. Anemia

Subjective Data

A. In newborns, review the onset, duration, and course of symptoms, including number of BMs, passage of first stool, and expulsion of flatus.
B. Ask the client or caregiver about family history of HD.
C. Review the infant's weight and growth parameters.
D. Inquire about other symptoms of bowel obstruction, such as vomiting and diarrhea.
E. Ask about other complications such as blood in stool.
F. Review the history of BMs and feeding habits, including onset of constipation, character of stools (ribbon-like or fluid-filled), frequency of BMs, and use of enemas.

Physical Examination

A. Check temperature (if indicated), pulse, respirations, BP, weight, and growth parameters, including length and head circumference.
B. Inspect:
1. Note the client's general appearance, level of activity, abdominal distention, and signs of malnutrition.
2. Inspect the fontanelles for signs of dehydration.
3. Inspect the lower back for evidence of spinal cord involvement such as a hairy or hyperpigmented patch, gluteal fold asymmetry, cutaneous dimples, sinus tracts, and lipomas.
C. Auscultate:
1. Abdomen for bowel sounds in all quadrants
D. Percuss:
1. Abdomen for organomegaly
E. Palpate:
1. Abdomen for distention and masses. Specifically examine the left quadrant for the presence of stool.
F. Neurological examination:
1. Evaluate other systemic disease related to constipation.
G. Rectal examination:
1. Check for a "tight" anal sphincter and absence of stool in the rectal ampulla.
2. Many infants have relief of symptoms and pass large amounts of stool and flatus after examination (blast sign).

3. Test the perineal sensation and the anocutaneous "wink" reflex by stroking the skin around the anus using a cotton-tipped swab.

Diagnostic Tests
A. Full-thickness rectal biopsy is considered the gold standard for diagnosis of HD. Absence of ganglion cells confirms the diagnosis of HD.
B. Suction rectal biopsy: Obtained by mucosal suction and can be performed at the bedside
C. Contrast BE: 25% of cases appear normal
D. Anorectal manometry
E. Ultrasonography
F. Plain abdominal x-ray (distended bowel loops and air in the rectum)
G. Chemistry panel to evaluate fluid and electrolyte management

Differential Diagnoses
A. HD
B. Meconium peritonitis
C. Meconium plug syndrome
D. Meconium ileus
E. Intestinal obstruction
F. Enterocolitis
G. Megacolon (acute, chronic, or toxic)
H. Hypothyroidism
I. Constipation
J. IBS

Plan
A. General interventions:
   1. Prepare caregivers or the client for referral or consultation.
B. Client teaching:
   1. Teach caregivers or the client about HD and treatment therapy.
   2. Signs and symptoms in newborns with HD typically occur within 24 hours; however, some may appear later in life. Assure parents that this condition is congenital. The American Pediatric Surgical Association has the following link for clients and families: https://eapsa.org/parents/learn-about-a-condition/f-o/hirschsprung-disease/
C. Pharmaceutical therapy:
   1. The first priority is hydration and antibiotics if enterocolitis is associated with HD. Collaborate with the gastroenterologist or general surgeon regarding medications prescribed prior to and after surgery.
D. Surgical management:
   1. Treatment consists of colostomy performed proximal to aganglionic segment with biopsies taken at the time of surgery to identify level of involvement. Definitive repair can then be performed when the infant is 6 to 12 months old.
      1. There are two types of surgical procedures:
         i. Pull-through procedure involves removal of the affected part of the large intestine and anastomosis to the healthy part of the anus.
         ii. Ostomy surgery reroutes the intestine through the abdominal wall, forming a stoma.

2. The mainstay of treatment is surgery. However, in older children when symptoms are chronic, but not severe, treatment may consist of isotonic enemas, stool softeners, and low-residue diet.

Follow-Up
A. Pediatric surgeons and gastroenterologists should generally care for children with HD.

Consultation/Referral
A. Consult or refer the client to a physician if HD is suspected in an infant:
   1. Bloody mucoid diarrhea in an infant with a history of constipation could be an indication of enterocolitis complicating HD
   2. An empty contracted anal canal in a constipated child may suggest HD
B. Consider genetic testing.

Individual Considerations
A. Pediatrics:
   1. Recurrence risk is proportional to the length of aganglionic segment of the colon.
   2. Infants who have symptom relief after rectal examination and pass large amounts of stool and gas (blast sign) can have recurrence of symptoms, often fail to grow normally, can have constipation or diarrhea, and may have protein loss in their stool.

Bibliography
National Institute of Diabetes and Digestive and Kidney Diseases. (2015, September). *Hirschsprung disease.* Retrieved from https://www.niddk.nih.gov/health-information/digestive-diseases/hirschsprung-disease
Nettina, S. (2010). *The Lippincott manual of nursing practice* (9th ed.). Philadelphia, PA: Wolters Kluwer Lippincott Williams & Wilkins.
Neville, H. L. (2012, May 8). Pediatric Hirschsprung disease. *Medscape.* Retrieved from http://emedicine.medscape.com/article/929733-overview
Wagner, J. P. (2018, August 1). Hirschsprung disease workup. *Medscape.* Retrieved from https://emedicine.medscape.com/article/178493-workup#c6

Hookworm

Doncy Eapen and Cheryl A. Glass

Definition
A. Hookworm is a chronic, debilitating parasitic disease with vague symptoms that vary in proportion to the degree of iron-deficiency anemia and hypoproteinemia of the host. The adult hookworm attaches to the small intestinal wall and ingests the host's blood and nutrients. Chronic infection in children may lead to physical growth delay, cognitive deficits, and developmental delay. Anemia and hypoproteinemia are produced by the blood-clotting activity of adult nematodes in the intestines.

Incidence
A. Incidence in the United States is unknown. Globally, more than 500 million people are infected with hookworms.

Pathogenesis
A. Disease is caused by infection with *Ancylostoma duodenale*, *Ancylostoma ceylonicum*, or *Necator americanus* (soil-transmitted helminths) intestinal parasites. Mixed infections are common. Humans are the major reservoir.

A. duodenale may be ingested. Eggs of the nematode hatch into larvae that penetrate the soles of feet and palms of hands from contact with contaminated soil. Contact for 5 to 10 minutes results in skin penetration. Larvae are carried by circulation to the lungs and eventually to their final habitat, the small intestines. Eggs are passed in stools of infected persons. Although hookworms are not transmitted from person to person, infected persons can contaminate soil by defecation as long as they are untreated.

B. Incubation period, or the time from exposure to eggs excreted in stool to the development of noncutaneous symptoms, is 4 to 12 weeks. The appearance of parasites in the blood is 4 to 6 weeks. Adult worms or larvae are rarely seen.

Predisposing Factors

A. Living in or traveling to rural, tropical, or subtropical areas where soil contamination with human feces is common
B. Exposure to loose, sandy, moist, shady, well-aerated, warm soil where larvae and eggs thrive
C. Agricultural workers
D. Tourists with bare feet or open footwear that exposes skin to contaminated soil
E. Military troops in endemic areas
F. Children

Common Complaints

A. Intense stinging or burning at the penetration site, followed by pruritus and a papulovesicular rash that persists for 1 to 2 weeks
B. Fatigue
C. Weight loss
D. Vague abdominal discomfort
E. Loss of appetite

Other Signs and Symptoms

A. **Anemia is the principal manifestation of hookworm infestation; it occurs secondary to blood loss.** *Severe anemia affects children and pregnant women disproportionately due to their preexisting iron stores.* **Severe anemia symptoms include:**
    1. Fatigue
    2. Syncope
    3. Exertional dyspnea
    4. Tachycardia
    5. Pallor
B. Pharyngeal itching after oral ingestion
C. Hoarseness
D. Nausea or vomiting
E. Cough or wheeze from pulmonary infiltration due to heavy infestation
F. Colicky abdominal pain or diarrhea: Late sign, occurring with marked eosinophilia 29 to 38 days after exposure
G. Edema
H. Mild diarrhea
I. Chronic nutritional impairment occurs in endemic areas with limited access to adequate nourishment.

Subjective Data

A. Review the onset, duration, and course of symptoms, including recent episodes of intense itching of feet, palms of hands, or buttocks.
B. Establish the client's normal weight, the amount of weight lost, and the length of time over which the loss occurred.
C. Inquire about abdominal symptoms, including onset and intensity.
D. Review other GI symptoms such as diarrhea.
E. Review any transitory chest symptoms, such as cough or wheezing. Is there a history of asthma?
F. Ask the client if any other family members are exhibiting the same symptoms.

Physical Examination

A. Check temperature (if indicated), pulse, respirations, BP, and weight.
B. Inspect:
    1. Skin on the entire body, especially the soles of both feet. Erythematous, papular vesicular lesions may be excoriated from scratching. Rash persists for 1 to 2 weeks.
C. Auscultate:
    1. Abdomen
    2. Lungs
D. Palpate:
    1. Abdomen for masses and tenderness

Diagnostic Tests

A. Identification of hookworm eggs in feces is diagnostic. Fecal egg excretion does not become detectable until around 2 months after dermal exposure. Repeated stool samples may be needed for diagnosis.
B. Hgb and Hct for anemia
C. CBC with differential: May have mild eosinophilia
D. Beaver direct smear, Stoll egg-counting, or Kato–Katz techniques quantify infection
E. Endoscopic examination may reveal the adult worms

Differential Diagnoses

A. Hookworm
B. Acute or chronic anemia
C. Asthma
D. Poor nutrition
E. Giardiasis
F. Amebiasis
G. Ascariasis
H. Gastroenteritis
I. Growth failure/ FTT

Plan

A. General interventions:
    1. Biopsy of affected areas in the epidermis: Results give evidence of larvae surrounded by eosinophilic infiltrates.
B. Client teaching:
    1. Discuss the dangers of going barefoot outdoors with the client.

2. Explain that good handwashing is critical, especially after defecation.

3. There is no direct person-to-person transmission.

4. Use good sanitary practices to prevent soil contamination.

C. Pharmaceutical therapy:

The dosage is the same for children as for adults:

1. Mebendazole (Vermox) 100 mg orally twice a day for 3 days *or* a one-time single dose of 500 mg is the drug of choice

 a. Mebendazole is available in the United States only through compounding pharmacies.

 b. WHO recommends that 1-year-old children be given half of the dose (50 mg) prescribed for older children and adults.

2. Albendazole (Albenza) 400 mg, one-time dose, is also a drug of choice.

3. Pyrantel pamoate (Pyrantel) 11 mg/kg/d for 3 days; do not exceed 1 g/d

4. Thiabendazole applied topically

5. Iron replacement therapy and nutritional supplements (proteins and vitamins including folate) may be needed to correct anemia.

6. At the present time, there is no hookworm vaccine.

7. Ivermectin (Stromectol) is ineffective against hookworms.

D. Dietary management:

1. Teach the client how to correct anemia through good nutrition.

Follow-Up

A. Stool should be examined again 2 weeks after therapy is completed. If results are positive, repeat therapy is indicated.

B. Reinfection is common.

C. Iron supplement should be continued even after Hgb values return to normal.

Consultation/Referral

A. Refer pregnant clients to a physician.

B. Refer children to a physician if Hgb is less than 6 g/dL. Cardiac decompensation occasionally develops in children with Hgb concentrations of less than 6 g/dL.

Individual Considerations

A. Pregnancy:

1. Anthelmintics are in pregnancy category C; however, the potential risks to the fetus versus benefits should be considered.

2. WHO has determined that the benefit of pharmaceutical treatment outweighs its risk:

 a. WHO allows the use of albendazole in the second and third trimesters of pregnancy.

 b. WHO allows the use of pyrantel pamoate in the second and third trimesters of pregnancy.

3. Adequate protein and iron nutrition should be maintained throughout pregnancy.

4. Consider delaying treatment until after delivery if necessary.

B. Pediatrics:

1. All medications are appropriate for children:

 a. WHO guidelines for mass prevention campaigns indicate albendazole can be used in children as young as 1 year.

 b. Mebendazole and pyrantel pamoate are on WHO's Model List of Essential Medicines for Children; they are intended for the use in children up to 12 years of age.

2. Severely affected children may require a blood transfusion.

3. Children's physical and cognitive growth can be affected.

Bibliography

Haburchak, D. R. (2016, February 24). Hookworm disease treatment & management. *Medscape reference*. Retrieved from http://emedicine.medscape.com/article/218805

Nettina, S. (2010). *The Lippincott manual of nursing practice* (9th ed.). Philadelphia, PA: Wolters Kluwer Lippincott Williams & Wilkins.

Weller, P. F., & Leder, K. (2018, January 26). Hookworm infection. *UpToDate*. Retrieved from https://www.uptodate.com/contents/hookworm-infection

Irritable Bowel Syndrome

Doncy Eapen and Cheryl A. Glass

Definition

IBS is a functional disorder of the GI tract characterized by chronic pain and altered bowel habits, and is responsible for significant direct and indirect healthcare costs. It is a relapsing functional disturbance of intestinal motility marked by a common symptom complex that includes bloating and abdominal pain or discomfort associated with defecation. It is defined by symptom-based diagnostic criteria, in the absence of detectable organic causes. The Rome III criteria for IBS are related to stool characteristics. The Rome IV criteria require recurrent abdominal pain (on average) at least once a week for three consecutive months, and associated with two or more of the following: related to defecation (increase/unchanged); change in stool frequency; or change in stool form/appearance.

A. When IBS diarrhea (IBS-D) is predominant: Loose stools (small volume, pasty/mushy or watery) more than 25% of the time and hard stools less than 25% of the time

B. When IBS constipation (IBS-C) is predominant: Hard, small, pellet-like stools more than 25% of the time and loose stools less than 25% of the time

C. When IBS mixed/cyclic pattern (IBS-M) occurs with alternating bouts of constipation and diarrhea: Both hard and soft stools more than 25% of the time

D. On clinical grounds, other subclassifications are used:

1. Based on symptoms:

 a. IBS with predominant bowel dysfunction

 b. IBS with predominant pain

 c. IBS with predominant bloating

2. Based on precipitating factors:
   a. Postinfectious (PI-IBS)
   b. Food induced (meal induced)
   c. Stress related

Incidence

A. IBS is common, accounting for about 50% of GI complaints seen by healthcare professionals, and is a major cause of morbidity in the United States. Nearly 20% of all adults suffer from some form of the condition; however, only a fraction seek medical help. In children, IBS is recognized; symptoms consistent with IBS are reported in 16% of students aged 11 to 17 years. IBS is not described in preschool-aged children.

B. IBS-D: More common in men

C. IBS-C: More common in women

D. The ACG has recognized IBS as a key component of Gulf War syndrome.

Pathogenesis

A. There is an absence of detectable IBS pathology, and laboratory tests are unrevealing. The understanding of IBS has evolved from a disturbance in bowel motor activity to a more integrated understanding of visceral hypersensitivity and brain–gut interaction. It is thought to be both a normal response to severe stress and a learned visceral response to stress.

   1. Nonpropulsive colonic contractions lead to IBS-C predominant.
   2. Increased contractions in the small bowel and proximal colon with diminished activity in the distal colon lead to IBS-D predominant.

B. Most clients with functional disorders appear to have inappropriate perception of physiological events and altered reflex responses in different gut regions.

C. The brain–gut transmitters act at different sites in the brain and gut and lead to varied effects on GI motility, pain control, emotional behavior, and immunity. Serotonin plays a critical role in the regulation of GI motility, secretion, and sensation. There is evidence that IBS may be related to an imbalance in mucosal serotonin and 5-hydroxytryptamine (5-HT) availability caused by defects in 5-HT production, serotonin receptors, or serotonin transport.

Predisposing Factors

A. Age:
   1. IBS mainly occurs between the ages of 15 and 65 years.
      a. About 50% of IBS cases occur before age 35 years.
      b. About 40% of IBS cases occur between ages 35 and 50 years.

B. Gender:
   1. Women are two to three times more likely to have IBS compared to men.
   2. In pediatric clients, both sexes are equally affected.

C. Emotional factors and situational stress

D. Prior GI infection-induced IBS

E. Genetics is considered a factor.

F. Carbohydrate intolerance may produce significant symptoms.

Common Complaints

A. Chronic relapsing stool pattern:
   1. Diarrhea: More than three loose stools per day, *or*
   2. Alternation of diarrhea with constipation. Diarrhea is typically small in volume, has visible mucus, and may follow a hard movement by a few hours, *or*
   3. Constipation: Fewer than three BMs per week

B. Feeling of incomplete evacuation

C. Abdominal distention and bloating

D. Straining with BMs

E. Aching or cramps in periumbilical or lower abdominal region

F. Pain relief with BM

Other Signs and Symptoms

A. Change in bowel function

B. Clear mucous stool

C. Pain may be precipitated by meals

D. Pain radiates to the left chest or arm, from gas in splenic flexure. Nocturnal pain is unusual and is considered a warning sign.

E. Flatulence

F. Nausea

G. Anxiety

H. Depression

I. Preoccupation with bowel symptoms

J. Extraintestinal symptoms:
   1. Dysmenorrhea
   2. Urinary frequency, urgency, and incomplete bladder emptying
   3. Impaired sexual function and dyspareunia
   4. Fibromyalgia

K. Menses may exacerbate IBS symptoms.

L. Red-flag symptoms and differential diagnoses for IBS (see Table 11.16)

Subjective Data

A. Review the pattern of main symptoms, including the onset, duration, and usual course.

B. Ask the client about the predominant symptoms: Abdominal pain, diarrhea, or constipation.

C. Review the client's history for stress factors, and ask whether recurrent symptoms occur in relation to them.

D. Ask the client what other symptoms occur with the pain, diarrhea, or constipation, such as bloating, blood in stool, or nighttime BMs. **Bleeding, weight loss, and nocturnal diarrhea are not characteristic of IBS. Symptoms of IBS disappear during sleep.**

E. Establish the client's normal weight history, and determine the amount of weight loss, if any, and over what time period.

F. Review the client's diet:
   1. Response to milk or lactose products
   2. Artificial sweeteners
   3. Alcohol intake

TABLE 11.16   COMMON AND RED-FLAG DIFFERENTIAL DIAGNOSES FOR IBS

Disorder	Signs and Symptoms	Diagnostic Tests
UC	Peaks at ages 15–35 years	Sigmoidoscopy, colonoscopy, BE
	Bloody diarrhea with mucus, fever, abdominal pain, tenesmus, weight loss	
CD	Onset at ages 15–35 or 70–80 years Fever, abdominal pain, diarrhea, fatigue, weight loss, anorectal fissures, fistulae, abscesses	Sigmoidoscopy, colonoscopy, BE
Infectious diarrhea	Chronic diarrhea with cramps with or without blood and mucus	Microscopy, stool studies, sigmoidoscopy
Diverticulitis	Lower left abdominal pain, fever, altered bowel habits	CBC, CT, BE
Colorectal malignancy	Age 50 years or older Rectal bleeding, altered bowel habits, abdominal or back pain, anemia, occult blood in stool, weight loss	Colonoscopy
Medication side effects	Antacids, laxatives, SSRIs, thyroid hormones, metformin, narcotics, calcium-channel blockers, anticholinergics	History of concordance of symptoms with medication initiation, trial of drug holiday or reducing dosage, rechallenge

BE, barium enema; CBC, complete blood count; CD, Crohn's disease; IBS, irritable bowel syndrome; SSRIs, selective serotonin reuptake inhibitors; UC, ulcerative colitis.

4. Irregular or inadequate meals
5. Insufficient fluid intake
6. Excessive fiber intake
7. Obsession with dietary hygiene
8. Response to gluten (wheat, barley, rye) ingestion

G. Inquire about the client's prescription, herbal, and OTC medications. Ask specifically about the use of laxatives.

H. Review travel and food history for dominant history of diarrhea.

I. Ask the client if there is a family history of colon cancer, UC, CD, or malabsorption.

J. Is there any fever accompanying lower abdominal pain?

K. What is the relation of symptoms to menstruation?

Physical Examination

A. Check temperature (if indicated), pulse, respirations, BP, and weight.

B. Inspect:
   1. Observe the client's general appearance. Does the client appear anxious or depressed?
   2. Inspect the abdominal contour for masses and bulges.

C. Auscultate:
   1. All quadrants of the abdomen for bowel sounds; note whether they are normal or mildly hyperactive.

D. Percuss:
   1. Abdomen for tympany or dullness

E. Palpate:
   1. Abdomen for mild tenderness, rigidity, guarding, and masses.
   2. Evaluate for hepatosplenomegaly.
   3. Evaluate for lymphadenopathy.

F. Rectal examination:
   1. Check for masses and tenderness.
   2. Obtain stool for diagnostic tests.
   3. Rectal examination is normal with IBS.

Diagnostic Tests

A. **The AGA Task Force on IBS recommendations state that clients younger than 50 years who do not have alarm features need not undergo routine colonic imaging. Clients with IBS symptoms who have alarm features, such as anemia or weight loss, or those who are older than 60 years, should undergo colonic imaging to exclude organic disease.**

B. Diagnosis of IBS is usually suspected on the basis of the client's history and physical examination without additional tests (see Box 11.1).

C. Diagnostic tests are performed to exclude organic disease that may masquerade as IBS:
   1. CBC
   2. Sedimentation rate or CRP
   3. Serum potassium if the client is on diuretics; hypokalemia may reduce bowel contractility and produce an ileus.
   4. Blood glucose if diarrhea predominates; rule out diabetes mellitus, which may present as diarrhea resulting from diabetic gastroenteropathy.
   5. Thyroid function study
   6. Stool specimen: Culture for leukocytes and fat, ova and parasites, and occult blood; leukocyte-free mucus is a hallmark of IBS.
   7. Stool cultures for *C. difficile* toxin assay if clinically indicated
   8. BE and/or proctosigmoidoscopy for severe signs and symptoms, after consultation or referral

BOX 11.1 Rome III Diagnostic Criteria for IBS

Onset of symptoms at least 6 months before diagnosis
Recurrent abdominal pain or discomfort for more than 3 days per month during the past 3 months
At least two of the following features: A. Improvement with defecation B. Association with a change in frequency of stool C. Association with a change in stool form

IBS, irritable bowel syndrome.

9. Celiac serology, if appropriate

10. A mucosal biopsy is appropriate if a colonoscopy or sigmoidoscopy is performed.

11. Esophagogastroduodenoscopy (EGD) and distal duodenal biopsy in clients with diarrhea should be considered to rule out celiac disease, tropical sprue, and giardiasis, and for clients in whom abdominal pain and discomfort are located more in the upper abdomen.

12. Hydrogen breath test to evaluate lactose intolerance and small-intestinal bacterial overgrowth (SIBO)

Differential Diagnoses

A. IBS

B. IBD (CD/UC)

C. Viral or bacterial gastroenteritis

D. GI neoplasm

E. Acute diarrhea caused by protozoa or bacteria

F. Lactose insufficiency/deficiency

G. Laxative abuse

H. Drug side effect

I. Diabetes

J. Celiac spruce/gluten etiology

K. Diverticulitis

L. FTT in children

M. Endometriosis/PID

N. Zollinger–Ellison's syndrome

O. Diverticulitis

P. Microscopic colitis

Q. SIBO

Plan

A. General interventions:

1. Advise the client to keep a diary of events of BMs and precipitating factors.

2. Encourage the client to quit smoking: Nicotine may aggravate symptoms.

3. Recommend daily exercise to reduce stress.

4. Stress management should be encouraged, including counseling, tapes, meditation, and yoga.

B. Client teaching:

1. *See Section III: Client Teaching Guide for this chapter, "Irritable Bowel Syndrome."*

C. Pharmaceutical therapy:

1. Tell the client to stop all nonessential medications that may affect bowel function, especially irritant laxatives. Avoid narcotics, depressants, and other long-term drug use if possible.

2. Recommend eliminating sorbitol-containing candy and restricting lactose-containing milk products.

3. Drug of choice: Psyllium hydrophilic mucilloid (Metamucil) 1 tablespoon per day in 8 oz of juice or water, followed with another 8 oz of liquid. This treats both diarrhea and constipation.

4. Pain relief:

   a. Opiates should be avoided due to the risk of dependence and addiction in clients with chronic conditions.

   b. NSAIDs have an undesirable side effect on the GI tract.

   c. Antispasmodics and anticholinergic agents (IBS-D predominant):

   i. Hyoscyamine (Levsin, Levbid):

   1) Levsin 0.125 to 0.25 mg (1–2 tablets) orally or sublingual every 4 hours; not to exceed 12 tablets a day

   2) Levbid tablets for adults and pediatric clients 12 years or older: Take 2 tablets every 12 hours. Do not crush or chew tablets; not to exceed 4 tablets in 24 hours.

   3) Pediatric doses are dependent on age and weight.

   4) Hyoscyamine is available in immediate-release, extended-release, time capsules, biphasic tablets, elixir, and drop formulations.

   ii. Dicyclomine (Bentyl) 20 to 40 mg four times a day; discontinue if not effective within 2 weeks or if 80 mg daily is associated with adverse effects. Also available in IM formulation.

   d. Tricyclic antidepressants for IBS-D predominant. Tricyclics should be avoided for constipated clients:

   i. Amitriptyline (Elavil) 10 mg at bedtime initially; titrate up slowly to 75 mg/d at bedtime as needed.

   ii. Desipramine (Norpramin) 10 mg at bedtime initially; titrate up slowly up to 75 mg/d.

   iii. Imipramine (Tofranil) 10 to 50 mg orally at bedtime

5. Selective serotonin reuptake inhibitors (SSRIs):

   a. Paroxetine (Paxil) 10 to 60 mg/d

   b. Citalopram (Celexa) 5 to 60 mg/d

6. Antidiarrheals:

a. Opiate-derived medications are reserved for very severe cases secondary to the potential for abuse.

b. Loperamide (Imodium):

i. Adults: 2 to 12 mg orally in divided twice daily/three times daily doses; doses differ greatly among individuals.

ii. Pediatrics older than 2 years: 0.08 mg to 0.24 mg/kg/d orally divided in twice daily/three times daily doses; not to exceed 2 mg/dose

c. Alosetron (Lotronex), a 5-HT$_3$ receptor antagonist, is indicated only for women with severe IBS-D predominant. Starting dose is 0.5 mg twice a day; may increase to 1 mg twice a day (bid) after 4 weeks of starting dose. Discontinue if no relief after 4 weeks of 1 mg dosing.

7. Laxatives and stool softeners (IBS-C predominant) along with dietary measures and fiber supplements:

a. Mineral oil 15 to 45 mL orally daily or in divided three times daily dosing

b. Stimulant laxatives may be necessary intermittently for short periods, but prolonged use of stimulant laxatives should be avoided.

c. Lactulose is a colonic acidifier that promotes laxation. Transit time through the colon may be slow; 24 to 48 hours may be required to produce a BM. The usual dose is 1 to 2 tablespoons daily. Lactulose contains galactose and lactose and should be used with caution in clients with diabetes. Safety in pediatric clients has not been established.

8. Lubiprostone (Amitiza), a selective C-2 chloride-channel activator, is indicated for women 18 years and over with IBS-C predominant; 8 mcg twice a day with food and water

9. Probiotics

10. Linaclotide (LINZESS), guanylate cyclase-C (GC-C) agonist, is used for both IBS-C and CIC

11. Eluxadoline (Viberzi), a mu-opioid receptor agonist, is indicated for IBS-D predominant. There are two recommended dosing regimens:

a. Dosing is 100 mg tablet twice a day taken with food

b. Alternative dosing is 75 mg twice a day taken with food for clients with the following conditions:

i. Do not have a gallbladder

ii. Unable to tolerate 100 mg twice a day

iii. Are receiving a concomitant OATP1B1 inhibitor, such as the lipid-lowering drug gemfibrozil and its metabolite gemfibrozil 1Oβ

iv. Have mild or moderate hepatic impairment

c. If a dose is missed, clients should not compensate by taking two doses at once.

12. Antibiotic: Two-week trial of rifaximin may be used in clients who fail to respond to other therapies.

13. Probiotics have been associated with improvement of symptoms in some clients.

D. Dietary management:

1. Increasing fiber intake may improve symptoms. However, some clients experience worsening of symptoms with increased fiber intake.

2. Tell the client to avoid foods that aggravate the bowel, including gas-producing foods, such as broccoli, beans, onions, garlic, and so forth. Advise the client to follow a low-fermentable oligosaccharides, disaccharides, monosaccharides, and polyols (FODMAP) diet. See Appendix B for the FODMAP diet. When diarrhea predominates, dietary review is essential for clues of intolerance to lactose or sorbitol.

Follow-Up

A. Reevaluate the effectiveness of treatment in 2 weeks. Treatment may be challenging for symptom management; numerous tests are inconclusive but rule out pathology.

B. If symptoms persist without relief, have the client return as needed.

C. Return if diarrhea/constipation lasts more than 2 weeks on medication therapy.

Consultation/Referral

A. Refer to a gastroenterologist for red-flag symptoms.

B. Refer to a pediatric gastroenterologist if findings from the client's history, physical examination, or screening laboratory tests are suggestive of organic disease.

C. Alosetron (Lotronex) is prescribed under a restricted distribution program through a gastroenterologist.

D. Consult a physician if all treatment options fail.

E. Consider a psychiatric consultation if indicated for anxiety, depression, somatization, and symptom-related fears.

Individual Considerations

A. Pediatrics:

1. In children, IBS is recognized, and many clients trace the onset of symptoms to childhood

2. Children who have a history of recurrent abdominal pain are at increased risk of IBS during adolescence and young adulthood.

3. The recommended daily intake of fiber (in grams) for children is estimated by adding four to their age in years.

B. Adults:

1. Annual rectal examination and sigmoidoscopy are recommended after age 50 years.

2. When constipation predominates, rule out malignancy, particularly in clients older than age 40 years who have weight loss or a family history of colon cancer.

Resource

Rome Foundation: https://theromefoundation.org

Bibliography

Ford, A. C., Moayyedi, P., Lacy, B. E., Lembo, A. J., Saito, Y. A., Schiller, L. R., . . . Quigley, E. M. (2018). >American College of Gastroenterology monograph on management of irritable bowel syndrome and chronic idiopathic constipation. *American Journal of Gastroenterology*, *113*(suppl 2), S1–S18. doi: 10.1038/s41395-018-0084-x

Lehrer, J. K. (2018, February 6). Irritable bowel syndrome treatment and management. *UpToDate*. Retrieved from https://emedicine.medscape.com/article/180389-treatment#d10

McDonald, L., Gerding, D., Johnson, S., Bakken, J., Carroll, K., Coffin, S., . . . Wilcox, M. (2018, December). Clinical practice guidelines for *Clostridium difficile* infection in adults and children: 2017 update by the Infectious Diseases Society of America and Society for Healthcare Epidemiology of America. *IDSA Clinical Practice Guidelines, 2018*, 1–48. Retrieved from http://www.uphs.upenn.edu/bugdrug/antibiotic_manual/C%20difficile%20guidelines%20IDSA2017.pdf

National Institute of Diabetes and Digestive and Kidney Diseases, National Institutes of Health. (2019). *Irritable bowel syndrome*. Retrieved from https://www.niddk.nih.gov/health-information/digestive-diseases/irritable-bowel-syndrome

Nettina, S. (2010). *The Lippincott manual of nursing practice* (9th ed.). Philadelphia, PA: Wolters Kluwer Lippincott Williams & Wilkins.

Sartor, R. B. (2015, July 6). Antibiotics for treatment of inflammatory bowel diseases. *UpToDate*. Retrieved from http://www.uptodate.com/contents/antibiotics-for-treatment-of-inflammatory-bowel-diseases

Wald, A. (2017, September 11). Clinical manifestations and diagnosis of irritable bowel syndrome in adults. *UpToDate*. Retrieved from https://www.uptodate.com/contents/clinical-manifestations-and-diagnosis-of-irritable-bowel-syndrome-in-adults

Wald, A. (2018a, April 27). Patient education: Irritable bowel syndrome (beyond the basics). *UpToDate*. Retrieved from https://www.uptodate.com/contents/irritable-bowel-syndrome-beyond-the-basics

Wald, A. (2018b, December 12). Treatment of irritable bowel syndrome in adults. *UpToDate*. Retrieved from https://www.uptodate.com/contents/treatment-of-irritable-bowel-syndrome-in-adults#H2957204

World Gastroenterology Organisation Global Guidelines. (2015, September). *Irritable bowel syndrome: A global perspective*. Retrieved from http://www.worldgastroenterology.org/guidelines/global-guidelines/irritable-bowel-syndrome-ibs/irritable-bowel-syndrome-ibs-english

Jaundice

Doncy Eapen and Cheryl A. Glass

Definition

A. Jaundice is a yellow tinge to the skin or mucous membranes. It is a symptom, not a disease. The diagnostic approach begins with gathering a comprehensive history, physical examination, and screening laboratory tests. The differential diagnosis is formulated, and further testing may be warranted. The onset of jaundice usually prompts the client or family to seek medical attention. Jaundice can reflect a medical emergency secondary to massive hemolysis, ascending cholangitis, unconjugated hyperbilirubinemia in the neonatal period, and fulminant liver failure.

Incidence

A. Incidence is variable according to pathogenesis, age, and population.

Pathogenesis

The mechanism responsible for jaundice includes excess bilirubin production, decreased hepatic uptake, impaired conjugation, intrahepatic cholestasis, extrahepatic obstruction, and hepatocellular injury (see Table 11.17). However, it is important to recognize that more than one mechanism can be operating in a given case (i.e., sickle cell anemia and HIV).

A. Excess bilirubin production results from accelerated red cell destruction. The excessive amounts of Hgb and resultant bilirubin released into the bloodstream overwhelm the liver's normal capacity for uptake, and an unconjugated hyperbilirubinemia ensues.

B. With decreased uptake and conjugation, there is often a concurrent, acquired illness such as infection, cardiac disease, or cancer. Hereditary conditions, such as Gilbert and Crigler–Najjar syndromes, are responsible.

C. Intrahepatic cholestasis may occur at a number of levels: Intracellularly (e.g., hepatitis), at the canalicular level (when estrogen is induced), at the ductule (phenothiazine exposure), at the septal ducts (primary biliary cirrhosis), and at the intralobular ducts (cholangiocarcinoma).

D. Extrahepatic obstruction occurs when a stone, stricture, or tumor blocks the flow of bile within the extrahepatic biliary tree. A history of gallstones, biliary tract surgery, or malignancy may be elicited.

Predisposing Factors

A. Previous blood transfusion
B. Travel to an area endemic for hepatitis
C. Raw shellfish consumption
D. IV drug abuse
E. High-risk sexual practices
F. Family history of episodic jaundice
G. History of gallstones
H. Biliary obstruction/previous biliary tract surgery
I. Alcoholism
J. Chemical exposure
K. Working in the healthcare profession
L. Sickle cell disease
M. Pregnancy (intrahepatic cholestasis)
N. Liver, gallbladder, and biliary tract cancer
O. Sepsis and hypoperfusion states

Common Complaints

A. Pruritus
B. Dark, tea-colored urine, from conjugated bilirubinuria
C. Light, clay-colored stools, from absence of bile
D. Fatigue
E. RUQ pain

Other Signs and Symptoms

A. Enlarged liver
B. Splenomegaly

TABLE 11.17   CLASSIFICATION OF JAUNDICE ACCORDING TO BILE PIGMENT AND BY MECHANISM

Unconjugated Hyperbilirubinemia	Conjugated Hyperbilirubinemia
Increased/overproduction of bilirubin	Hepatocellular injury/disease
Impaired/decreased hepatic uptake of bilirubin	Intrahepatic cholestasis
Impaired/decreased conjugation	Extrahepatic cholestasis (biliary obstruction)

C. Fever
D. Chills
E. GI: Appetite loss, weight loss, abdominal pain, nausea, or vomiting
F. Ascites
G. Shortness of breath
H. Palpitations
I. Ecchymosis
J. Steatorrhea, severe
K. Asterixis (tremor)
L. Myalgias
M. Malaise

Subjective Data

A. Review the onset, duration, and course of symptoms.
B. Review the client's medication history for drugs/herbal products that may induce jaundice (see Box 11.2).
C. Inquire about recent blood transfusions. Are there any known blood disorders in the client's family history?
D. Ask about contact with a person who has an infection, such as infectious hepatitis.
E. Ask about unprotected sexual activity/HIV status.
F. Review ingestion of potentially contaminated food or water, including *Amanita* mushrooms, milk, or shellfish.

G. Ask about the client's exposure to any toxic chemicals, such as carbon tetrachloride, chloroform, phosphorus, arsenic, ethanol, or halothane (Fluothane).
H. Review the client's history of nonsterile needle punctures.
I. Review the client's medical/surgical history for gallstones, hepatitis, tumor, pancreatitis, Wilson's disease, Budd–Chiari syndrome, liver surgery, or transplantation. Is there a family history of gallstones?
J. Ask how much alcohol the client has ingested over the years.
K. Ask about dark urine or white or clay-colored stool.
L. Inquire about dyspepsia, anorexia, nausea, vomiting, RUQ or epigastric pain, or pain radiating to back or shoulder blade. Ask about the relationship of pain to eating.
M. Inquire about fever, fatigue, malaise, loss of vigor and strength, easy bruising, and weight loss.
N. Review travel history.

Physical Examination

A. Check temperature (if indicated), pulse, respirations, BP, and weight. Marked weight loss accompanied by jaundice suggests carcinoma of the head of the pancreas

---

BOX 11.2   Drugs and Herbal Products Associated With Jaundice

Angiotensin-converting enzyme (ACE) inhibitors
Acetaminophen (Tylenol)
Alkylated steroids
Aminobenzoic acid
Antibiotics
Antidiabetic drugs
Arsenic
Chloramphenicol
Chlorpromazine
Ethinyl estradiol/oral contraceptives/hormone replacement
Herbal medications (e.g., Jamaican bush tea)
Isoniazid (INH)
Mercaptopurine (Purinethol)
Methyldopa (Aldomet)
Monoamine oxidase inhibitors Nitrofurantoin
Perphenazine (Trilafon)
Phenothiazine derivatives
Probenecid Propylthiouracil (PTU)
Rifampin
Sulfonamides
Tamoxifen
Total parenteral nutrition (TPN)

or metastatic disease obstructing the common duct. Note breath odor for fetor hepaticus (breath of the dead).

B. Inspect:
1. Skin, mouth, palms, and sclera for yellow tinge. Severe jaundice may cause greenish tinge from oxidation of bilirubin to biliverdin:
   a. In fair-skinned people, discoloration is most evident on the face, trunk, and sclera (sclera icterus).
   b. In dark-skinned people, discoloration is most evident in the sclera and the roof of the mouth.
   c. In newborns, jaundice first appears over the face or upper body, then progresses over larger areas; it can also be seen in conjunctivae of the eyes.
   d. Jaundice is most noticeable in natural sunlight. In artificial or poor light, it may be hard to detect.
2. The skin for spider angiomata, rashes or scratches from severe itching due to pruritus, and bruising or petechiae
3. The palms for erythema or overt bleeding
4. The chest for gynecomastia

C. Auscultate:
1. Heart
2. Lungs
3. Abdomen for bowel sounds

D. Percuss:
1. Abdomen

E. Palpate:
1. Abdomen for tenderness, masses, liver enlargement in RUQ, and ascites:
   a. Extrahepatic obstruction and intrahepatic cholestasis may be identical in presentation
   b. Tenderness is minimal unless cholangitis or rapid distention occur
   c. Splenomegaly is unlikely except in primary biliary cirrhosis
   d. Gallbladder may be palpable (Courvoisier sign). A sudden onset of pain results from passage of a stone that becomes wedged into a common duct; fever and sepsis shortly thereafter indicate cholangitis.
   e. Malignancy usually presents as a rock-hard mass
   f. Absence of abdominal pain does not rule out obstruction, especially when it develops slowly from tumor growth or primary biliary cirrhosis
   g. Advanced hepatocellular disease is indicated by a small liver, signs of portal hypertension (ascites, splenomegaly, prominent abdominal venous pattern), asterixis, peripheral edema (from hypoalbuminemia), spider angiomata, gynecomastia, palmar erythema, and testicular atrophy
   h. Palpate the liver for hepatomegaly

F. Neurological examination:
1. Note the client's level of consciousness.
2. The asterixis test can be used to test for peripheral neuritis caused by impaired liver function. Screen for a flapping tremor occurring with the wrist dorsiflexed.

G. Rectal examination:
1. Check for masses and occult blood.

Diagnostic Tests

The diagnostic approach begins with a careful history, physical examination, and screening laboratory studies. A differential diagnosis is formulated, and appropriate further testing is performed to narrow the diagnosis.

A. Initial laboratory tests:
1. Serum bilirubin: Direct, indirect (unconjugated), and total; clinically, jaundice becomes noticeable when levels reach 2.0 to 2.5 mg/dL:
   a. Intrahepatic cholestasis and extrahepatic obstruction: Elevated conjugated bilirubin, elevated serum ALP, mild to moderate rise in transaminase
   b. Gilbert syndrome is the most common cause of decreased uptake and unconjugated hyperbilirubinemia. This benign disorder produces recurrent self-limited episodes of mild jaundice. Typically, the unconjugated fraction rises to no more than 1.5 to 3.0 mg/100 mL. In Gilbert syndrome, fasting and minor illness can precipitate jaundice.
2. ALP
3. AST/ALT:
   a. Elevation of ALT and AST may indicate liver cell damage or may be caused by opiates and aspirin.
   b. Aspirin use may also decrease AST and ALT.
4. PT:
   a. PT may be prolonged due to malabsorption, but this effect is reversible by vitamin K injection.
   b. Prolonged PT unresponsive to parenteral vitamin K strongly suggests hepatocellular failure.
   c. Cholestasis and obstruction may also produce prolongation of PT but can be reversed by vitamin K.
   d. Phenazopyridine (Pyridium) may cause a false-positive bilirubin result.

B. Other laboratory testing as needed:
1. Total serum protein
2. Serum albumin and globulin:
   a. Albumin decreases with cirrhosis and chronic hepatitis.
   b. Globulin increases with cirrhosis, chronic obstructive jaundice, and viral hepatitis.
   c. To interpret the albumin level, consider the client's dietary intake and sources of possible protein loss.
3. Cholesterol
4. LDH
5. GGT
6. Serum ammonia
7. Bile acid radioimmunoassay: Elevated levels indicate hepatic disease
8. Serologic tests for viral hepatitis
9. Serum iron, transferrin, and ferritin to evaluate hemochromatosis
10. Serum ceruloplasmin levels to evaluate for Wilson's disease
11. Alpha-1 antitrypsin activity to evaluate for alpha-1 antitrypsin deficiency

12. Urine for bilirubin: Bilirubinuria may be an early sign of liver disease:
    a. Collect specimens over a 2-hour period after lunch.
    b. Place the specimen in a dark brown container and send it to the laboratory immediately to prevent decomposition.

C. Abdominal ultrasound is considered the screening procedure of choice. More selective imaging procedures are ordered based on clinical evaluation.

D. Other imaging procedures:
    1. Endoscopic ultrasound (EUS)
    2. Hepatobiliary iminodiacetic acid (HIDA) scan: Uses radioactive isotopes to create a picture of the liver, gallbladder, biliary tract, and small intestines
    3. Oral cholecystography
    4. ERCP
    5. Percutaneous transhepatic cholangiography (PTC)
    6. Helical CT
    7. MRCP is an alternative to ERCP
    8. Liver biopsy may be indicated for definitive diagnosis

Differential Diagnoses

A. Jaundice is a symptom, not a diagnosis
B. Cancer of the pancreas
C. Obstruction of the biliary tract
D. Icteric phase of hepatitis
E. Cirrhosis
F. Right-sided HF
G. Chronic hemolysis from a prosthetic heart valve

Plan

A. General interventions
    1. Management depends on the primary diagnosis. Most clients can be managed on an ambulatory basis, unless they are unable to maintain hydration or begin to show evidence of severe hepatocellular failure.

B. Client teaching:
    1. Explain that jaundice is secondary to the client's disorder, and that a multidisciplinary team will be managing treatment (primary care provider, gastroenterologist, pathologist, general surgeon, and radiologist).

C. Pharmaceutical therapy:
    1. Cholestyramine 2 to 8 g orally twice a day may be used to help relieve itching. Cholestyramine is ineffective with complete biliary obstruction.
    2. OTC antihistamines could be used at bedtime (not recommended for geriatric clients).
    3. Generally, collaborate with the gastroenterologist or general surgeon regarding medications specific to the underlying etiology.

Follow-Up

A. See the client 2 to 4 weeks after initial diagnosis and referral.
B. Subsequent routine evaluations are related to the primary diagnosis.

Consultation/Referral

A. Consult with a gastroenterologist or hepatologist when hepatocellular disease is suspected; when there is evidence of hepatic failure, portal hypertension, or encephalopathy; or when jaundice persists longer than 3 months.

B. Consultation with a gastroenterologist, surgeon, or radiologist experienced in evaluation of jaundice can be very useful when there is clinical suspicion of extrahepatic obstruction.

C. Admission is mandatory when jaundice is complicated by a fever and peritoneal signs indicative of cholangitis. IV antibiotics and prompt surgical consultation are required.

Individual Considerations

A. Pregnancy:
    1. Viral hepatitis is the most frequent cause of jaundice in pregnancy.
    2. Intrahepatic cholestasis in pregnancy is associated with modest maternal risks, including increased risk of peripartum bleeding and increased likelihood of subsequent cholelithiasis.
    3. Cholestyramine resin, generally 4 g every 4 to 6 hours, has been reported to afford some relief of pruritus in 50% of affected women, presumably by removing a portion of the bile acids by irreversible binding in the gut.
    4. Pregnant women who take cholestyramine are at increased risk for depletion of vitamin K–dependent coagulation factors and should be followed with serial PT times. Such women should also receive prophylactic vitamin K supplementation. If PT becomes prolonged, medication should be discontinued.
    5. Liver dysfunction and jaundice are common in clients with hyperemesis gravidarum.

B. Pediatrics:
    1. Hepatitis predominates as a cause of jaundice.
    2. Neonatal jaundice is more common when the mother has insulin-dependent diabetes, probably resulting from a higher Hct developed in utero, especially if oxygen availability is decreased. Newborn jaundice due to liver immaturity is common. It begins on day 2, peaks at 1 week, and disappears in 2 to 3 weeks. About half of all full-term newborns and 90% of premature newborns have some degree of jaundice. Jaundice is usually mild and can be treated with hydration and UV lamp exposure.
    3. Intense, persistent jaundice suggests liver disease or severe, overwhelming infection.
    4. In infants with Rh isoimmunization who do not receive appropriate treatment (exchange transfusion), progressive jaundice leads to brain damage (kernicterus), death, or severe handicap (deafness, spasticity, and choreoathetosis).
    5. Acute jaundice in young, healthy individuals suggests acute viral hepatitis.
    6. An overdose of acetaminophen is a common cause of jaundice in the young adult.

C. Geriatrics:

1. The most frequent cause of jaundice in clients older than 65 years is choledocholithiasis (the presence of one or more gallstones in the common bile duct).

2. The second most frequent cause of jaundice for clients 65 years and older is cancer, especially of the gallbladder.

3. Painless jaundice in the elderly with weight loss and a mass, but with minimal pruritus, suggests biliary obstruction caused by cancer.

Bibliography

Herrine, S. K. (2016, May). Jaundice. *Merck manual: Professional version.* Retrieved from http://www.merckmanuals.com/professional/hepatic-and-biliary-disorders/approach-to-the-patient-with-liver-disease/jaundice

Nettina, S. (2010). *The Lippincott manual of nursing practice* (9th ed.). Philadelphia, PA: Wolters Kluwer Lippincott Williams & Wilkins.

Zakko, S. F. (2018, February 21). Patient education: Gallstones (beyond the basics). *UpToDate.* Retrieved from https://www.uptodate.com/contents/gallstones-beyond-the-basics

Malabsorption

Doncy Eapen and Cheryl A. Glass

Definition

A. Malabsorption syndrome is a group of signs and symptoms that occur as a result of digestive problems and problems with absorption of nutrients. There may be a resultant decrease in absorption of fat-soluble vitamins A, D, E, and K. Poor absorption of carbohydrates, minerals, and proteins may also occur.

B. The presentation of malabsorption varies from severe overt symptoms with weight loss to discrete oligosymptomatic changes in hematological/laboratory tests that are found incidentally. Malabsorption can result from congenital defects or from acquired defects, such as bariatric surgery, and may be either global or partial. The degree of nutrient malabsorption from bariatric surgery depends on the type of bariatric procedure.

Incidence

A. Incidence is unknown.

Pathogenesis

A. Deficiency of intestinal enzymes: Lactase deficiency

B. Inadequate digestion caused by disease of the pancreas (such as CF), pancreatic cancer, gallbladder, or liver)

C. Change in the bacteria that normally live in the intestinal tract

D. Disease of the intestinal walls, such as helminths (worms) or parasites, tropical sprue, or celiac disease

E. Surgery that reduces the intestinal tract, decreasing the area for absorption, such as bariatric surgery

F. Intolerance to gluten or celiac sprue

G. Atrophic gastritis results in hypochlorhydria and achlorhydria. The body does not produce enough pepsin and hydrochloric acid to release the food-bound vitamin B_{12} from protein.

Predisposing Factors

A. Lactase deficiency:

1. Incidence is increased in African Americans, Indians, and Asians.

2. Jews typically have onset in adulthood

B. Family history of malabsorption or CF

C. Use of drugs, such as mineral oil or other laxatives

D. Excess alcohol consumption

E. Travel to foreign countries

F. Intestinal surgery:

1. Partial or total gastrectomy

2. Small-bowel resections (jejunum, ileum, ileocecal)

3. Partial or total resection of the pancreas

G. Chronic pancreatitis

H. Advanced age (increased risk for malabsorption and malnutrition)

I. Long-term adherence to a strict vegetarian or vegan diet (exclusion of all forms of animal protein, including eggs and dairy products)

J. HIV infection

Common Complaints

A. Diarrheal stools that are pale, greasy, and copious

B. Foul-smelling stools, frequently with mucus

C. Weight loss despite adequate food intake

D. Gas or vague abdominal discomfort

E. Anorexia

Other Signs and Symptoms

A. Early malabsorption:

1. Minimal weight loss

2. Softer, more frequent stools

3. Steatorrhea; stools "float" because of increased trapped gas

4. Abdominal discomfort

5. Bloating

B. Later signs: Aforementioned symptoms plus the following:

1. Marked weight loss

2. Foul-smelling, bulky, greasy stools

C. Malabsorption of fats and carbohydrates: Previous symptoms plus the following:

1. Foul-smelling, bulky, greasy, "sticky" stools that may be difficult to flush down the toilet

2. Ecchymosis

3. Bone pain

4. Glossitis

5. Muscle tenderness

6. Cramping in the lower abdomen after BMs

D. Malabsorption of lactose:

1. Nausea and bloating

2. Cramps

3. Diarrhea after ingesting more than customary intake of milk products

4. Absent or mild weight loss and steatorrhea

5. Good appetite

E. Edema: With severe protein depletion

F. Ecchymosis and bleeding disorders secondary to vitamin K malabsorption

G. Vitamin malabsorption:
1. Generalized motor weakness (pantothenic acid, vitamin D)
2. Peripheral neuropathy (thiamine)
3. Sense of loss for vibration and position, anemia (cobalamin)
4. Night blindness, follicular hyperkeratosis (vitamin A)
5. Seizures (biotin)
6. Hematoma, bleeding disorders (vitamin K)
H. Malabsorption of calcium: Tetany, paresthesia, pathological fractures

Subjective Data

A. Review the onset, duration, and course of symptoms. Are there any other family members with the same history/symptoms?
B. Ask the client about dietary intake history.
C. Review any changes in BMs and stool characteristics.
D. Inquire about recent travel to areas known for giardiasis or other parasites.
E. Document weight loss, including how much and over what period of time.
F. Review previous GI surgery, including the bariatric procedures and reversals, small-bowel resections, and partial or total resection of the pancreas.
G. Ask the client about signs and symptoms of IBD, such as easy bruising, paresthesia, and sore tongue.
H. Ask about any irradiation treatment.

Physical Examination

A. Check temperature, pulse, respirations, BP (may have orthostatic hypotension), and weight. Follow serial weight loss, and plot on growth charts.
B. Inspect:
1. Observe the client's general appearance, noting wasting and an apathetic appearance.
2. If the client experiences a BM after the examination, observe the stool for volume, appearance, and presence of blood, mucus, and gross worms/parasites.
3. Inspect the skin for ecchymosis, jaundice, pallor, surgical scars, stigmata of hyperthyroidism or hepatocellular failure, or signs of Kaposi's sarcoma. Alopecia or seborrheic dermatitis may be present.
4. Inspect the ears, nose, and throat for glossitis, stomatitis, aphthous ulcers, poor dentition, and goiter.
C. Auscultate:
1. Heart for tachycardia
2. Abdomen in all four quadrants for bowel sounds, noting borborygmi
D. Percuss:
1. Abdomen
E. Palpate:
1. All lymph nodes; look for lymphadenopathy.
2. Abdomen for organomegaly, focal tenderness, masses, distention, and ascites
F. Neurological examination:
1. Assess for signs of vitamin B_{12} deficiency, including motor weakness, peripheral neuropathy, or ataxia.

G. Rectal examination:
1. Evaluate tenderness, discharge, blood, and stool.

Diagnostic Tests

A. Assessment of stool fat: Qualitative assessment on a single specimen
B. Quantitative assessment of a 72-hour stool collection while the client is following a 100 g fat/d diet
C. Increased fecal fat: Test for celiac disease
D. Abdominal ultrasound
E. Colonoscopy to evaluate and obtain biopsies
F. Upper endoscopy to evaluate and obtain biopsies
G. Barium studies
H. Consider CT of the abdomen
I. MRCP to evaluate the pancreas and bile ducts
J. Breath tests for carbohydrate malabsorption
K. CBC and electrolytes
L. Serum iron, vitamin B_{12}, and folate concentrations
M. PT: May be prolonged due to vitamin K deficiency
N. Vitamin levels: Vitamins A, D, E, and K may be decreased
O. Total protein: May be decreased
P. Albumin: May be decreased
Q. Serum amylase
R. Stool for ova and parasites; obtain on alternate days for three or more specimens because parasites are passed intermittently.
S. Serum IgA: Used to rule out IgA deficiency
T. Three-stage Schilling test: Vitamin B_{12} deficiency
U. EUS to detect the cause of malabsorption due to pancreatic diseases such as chronic pancreatitis or pancreatic malignancy

Differential Diagnoses

A. Malabsorption
B. AIDS
C. Alcoholism
D. Worms or parasites
E. CF
F. FTT
G. CD
H. Tropical sprue
I. Side effect from bariatric surgery
J. Disaccharidase deficiencies (lactase)
K. Fructose intolerance
L. Milk or protein allergy
M. Whipple disease
N. Zollinger–Ellison syndrome
O. Chronic pancreatitis
P. Cirrhosis
Q. Pancreatic insufficiency

Plan

A. General interventions:
1. Treatment depends on the underlying cause.
B. Client teaching:
1. *See Section III: Client Teaching Guide for this chapter,* ◀ *"Lactose Intolerance and Malabsorption."*

C. Pharmaceutical therapy:

1. Vitamin supplements: Fat-soluble vitamins A, D, and K are most likely to be depleted. Supplements help prevent malnutrition, even though caloric intake may be replenished:

   a. Vitamin A: 25,000 to 50,000 U/d orally
   b. Vitamin D: 30,000 U/d orally
   c. Vitamin K: 4 to 12 mg/d orally
   d. Vitamin B_{12}: 1,000 g/mo by IM injection

2. Enzyme replacements: These replace endogenous exocrine pancreatic enzymes and aid in digestion of starches, fat, and proteins. Pancreatic supplements are typically expressed in U.S. Pharmacopeia Convention (USP) units: 1 international unit (IU) is equivalent to approximately 2 to 3 USP units.

   a. Pancreatin, adults and children: Doses vary with the condition being treated. Oral doses are given before or with meals or each snack. They may also be given in divided doses at 1- to 2-hour intervals throughout the day. **Use with extreme caution in clients with a known hypersensitivity to pork products.**

      i. Malabsorption syndrome: 8,000 to 24,000 USP units of lipase activity; occasionally up to 36,000 units of lipase activity may be required. Considerable dosage variation exists, partly due to the susceptibility of pancreatin to acid–peptic inactivity in the upper GI tract.

      ii. Functional indigestion: 1,200 to 2,400 USP of lipase activity

   b. Pancrelipase (Creon, Pancrease, Zenpep, Viokase): This must be given with each meal or snack

      i. Adults and children older than 4 years: Dosage for pancreatic exocrine dysfunction or for CF is 400 to 2,500 units/kg with meals; titrate dose to desired clinical response. Total daily dose should not exceed 10,000 units/kg body weight/d.

      ii. Children aged 1 to 4 years: Dosages for pancreatic exocrine dysfunction or for CF: 1,000 U of lipase/kg/meal orally; dosage should be individualized to the client's response. Adjust dose according to stool fat and nitrogen content. Dosage range: 1,000 to 25,000 units/kg/meal.

3. Antispasmodics:

   a. Anticholinergic agents are used to reduce the cholinergic stimulation of colonic activity that occurs in response to a meal.

   b. Drug of choice: Dicyclomine hydrochloride (Antispas), 10 to 20 mg orally before meals

4. Iron and folic acid supplementation are usually required for celiac disease.

5. Calcium and magnesium supplementation are required after extensive small-intestine resection.

6. Antibiotic therapy for bacterial overgrowth

7. Corticosteroids and anti-inflammatory agents to treat regional enteritis

D. Dietary management:

1. In most clients, diet modification, such as a gluten-free diet for celiac disease, or dietary supplements will restore health.

2. A lactose-free diet is recommended for clients with lactose intolerance.

3. A low-fat diet is recommended for clients with malabsorption due to short bowel syndrome.

Follow-Up

A. If the examination is normal, observe the client for 1 month and have the client keep a diary of food intake and weight.

B. For persistent malabsorption, monitor for osteoporosis/bone mass with a dual-energy x-ray absorptiometry (DEXA) scan.

Consultation/Referral

A. Any client with weight loss of 15 kg is likely to have a life-threatening condition and requires prompt consultation and hospitalization.

B. Consult a gastroenterologist when malabsorption is documented by a 72-hour stool fat assessment.

C. Consider a dietary consultation.

D. Refer the client back to the bariatric surgeon/center, depending on surgical complications from bariatric surgery.

E. Consider a referral for allergy testing for milk and proteins.

Individual Considerations

A. Geriatrics:

1. To identify impediments to adequate food intake, question the client about social isolation, depression, bereavement, physical impairment, poor dentition/edentulism, inability to fix meals, and poverty.

2. Loss of taste is sometimes responsible for poor intake and should be checked.

Bibliography

Hammami, M. B. (2019, January 24). Malabsorption work up. *Medscape.* Retrieved from https://emedicine.medscape.com/article/180785-workup#c4

Harreiter, J., Schindler, K., Bancher-Todesca, D., Gobel, C., Langer, F., Prager, G., . . . Krebs, M. (2018, June). Management of pregnant women after bariatric surgery. *Journal of Obesity, 2018,* 1–14. doi: https://doi.org/10.1155/2018/4587064

Mason, J. B. (2019, April 9). Approach to the adult patient with suspected malabsorption. *UpToDate.* Retrieved from https://www.uptodate.com/contents/approach-to-the-adult-patient-with-suspected-malabsorption#H1338969811

Mason, J. B., & Milovic, V. (2018, September 12). Overview of the treatment of malabsorption. *UpToDate.* Retrieved from https://www.uptodate.com/contents/overview-of-the-treatment-of-malabsorption

Nettina, S. (2010). *The Lippincott manual of nursing practice* (9th ed.). Philadelphia, PA: Wolters Kluwer Lippincott Williams & Wilkins.

Ren, C. J., & Fielding, G. A. (2003). Laparoscopic adjustable gastric banding: Surgical technique. *Journal of Laparoendoscopic & Advanced Surgical Techniques, 13,* 257–263. doi:10.1089/109264203322333584

Ruiz, A. R. (2014, May). Overview of malabsorption. *The Merck manual for health care professionals.* Retrieved from http://www.merckmanuals.com/professional/gastrointestinal_disorders/malabsorption_syndromes/overview_of_malabsorption.html

Sharma, G. D. (2019, May 2). Cystic fibrosis. *Medscape.* Retrieved from http://emedicine.medscape.com/article/1001602-overview

Nausea and Vomiting

Doncy Eapen and Cheryl A. Glass

Definition
Nausea and vomiting are common symptoms of many conditions and diseases, and several terms are used to describe these symptoms (see Table 11.18).
A. Hyperemesis gravidarum is a condition of persistent, uncontrollable vomiting that begins in the first weeks of pregnancy and improves by the end of the first trimester; however, it may persist throughout pregnancy.
B. Chronic nausea and vomiting is defined as lasting at least 1 month in duration.
C. Complications of nausea and vomiting include fluid depletion, hypokalemia, and metabolic alkalosis.
D. Vomiting is also considered a protective mechanism to remove harmful ingested substances.

Incidence
A. Nausea and vomiting are very common, and the etiology depends on the disease/condition.
B. During pregnancy, 50% to 90% of women experience nausea and/or vomiting; 50% have both nausea and vomiting. Onset after the initial 9 weeks of pregnancy should direct especially careful evaluation for another cause within the differential diagnoses of nausea and vomiting in nonpregnant clients.
C. Hyperemesis gravidarum occurs in as much as 2% of all pregnancies.
D. Severe hyperemesis requires hospitalization in 0.3% to 2% of pregnancies.
E. Approximately one-third of surgical clients have nausea and/or vomiting after general anesthesia.
F. The incidence of nausea and/or vomiting subsequent to cancer treatment is high.

Pathogenesis
A. Protective mechanisms are activated by numerous GI and non-GI causes. Normal function of the upper GI tract involves an interaction between the gut and the central nervous system (CNS).
B. Nausea and vomiting in pregnancy are related to increased hormones, including HCG, estrogen, and progesterone, as well as decreased gastric motility and relative hypoglycemia that results from a night-long fast.

Predisposing Factors
A. Acute nausea and vomiting:
  1. Medications: Digitalis toxicity, opiate use, chemotherapy agents, drug withdrawal, nicotine/nicotine patches, antibiotics, hormones, and antivirals
  2. Ketoacidosis
  3. Pregnancy or hormones
  4. Binge drinking
  5. Hepatitis
B. Recurrent or chronic nausea and vomiting:
  1. Psychogenic vomiting
  2. Metabolic disturbances
  3. Gastric retention
  4. Bile reflux
  5. Pregnancy
  6. Radiation
  7. Gastroparesis
C. Nausea and vomiting with abdominal pain:
  1. Viral gastroenteritis
  2. Acute gastritis
  3. Food poisoning
  4. PUD
  5. Acute pancreatitis
  6. Small-bowel obstruction
  7. Acute appendicitis
  8. Acute cholecystitis
  9. Acute cholangitis
  10. Acute pyelonephritis
  11. Inferior MI
D. Nausea and vomiting with neurological symptoms:
  1. Increased ICP
  2. Midline cerebellar hemorrhage
  3. Vestibular disturbances
  4. Migraine headaches
  5. Autonomic dysfunction
  6. Head trauma
  7. Multiple sclerosis

TABLE 11.18 DEFINITIONS OF TERMS USED TO DESCRIBE NAUSEA AND VOMITING

Term	Definition
Vomiting	Forceful oral expulsion of gastric contents associated with contraction of the abdominal and chest wall musculature
Nausea	The unpleasant sensation of the imminent need to vomit, usually referred to the throat or epigastrium; a sensation that may or may not ultimately lead to vomiting
Regurgitation	The act by which food is brought back into the mouth without the abdominal and diaphragmatic muscular activity that characterizes vomiting
Anorexia	Loss of desire to eat; a true loss of appetite
Sitophobia	Fear of eating because of subsequent or associated discomfort
Early satiety	Feeling full after eating an unusually small quantity of food
Retching	Spasmodic respiratory movements against a closed glottis with contraction of the abdominal musculature without expulsion of any gastric contents, referred to as "dry heaves"
Rumination	Chewing and swallowing of regurgitated food that has come back into the mouth through voluntary increase in abdominal pressure within minutes of eating or during eating; rumination may be accompanied by weight loss and bulimia

Common Complaints
A. Food aversion
B. Inability to retain food or liquids
C. "Queasy" sensation

Other Signs and Symptoms
A. Increased salivation
B. Bitter taste, "acid brash": Indicates ulcer or small-bowel obstruction
C. Weight loss
D. Dehydration
E. Sweating
F. Fast pulse
G. Pale skin
H. Rapid breathing
I. Lightheadedness

Subjective Data
A. Review the onset, duration (acute or chronic problem?), and course of symptoms, including the quality (projectile?) and quantity of emesis. What was the color, taste, and consistency of the emesis? Was blood present?
  1. Vomiting bright red blood indicates a hemorrhage: Peptic ulcer
  2. Dark red blood indicates a hemorrhage: Esophageal or gastric varices
  3. Coffee-ground material is indicative of digested blood from a slowly bleeding gastric or DU.
  4. Vomiting fecal material is a sign of distal small-bowel obstruction and blind-loop syndrome.
B. Ask the client about other symptoms, including pain, fever, diarrhea, and headache.
C. Inquire if other family members are also ill and what their symptoms are.
D. Review the timing of vomiting in relation to meals, time of day, odors, and activity. Does vomiting occur before or after food intake?
E. Ask the client about medication intake, such as antibiotics, chemotherapy, herbals, digitalis, opiates, and birth control pills.
F. Ask about self-image, binge eating, and self-induced emesis.
G. Review any exposure to hepatitis or travel to places with poor sanitation and outbreaks of cholera.
H. Review the client's medical history for vertigo, head injury, jaundice, diabetes, hypertension, and pregnancy.
I. Inquire about the first day of the client's last period and the birth control method used.
J. Establish usual weight. Has there been any recent weight change, how many pounds, and over what period of time?
K. Ask about the client's history of diabetes, gallbladder disease, ulcer disease, or cancer.

Physical Examination
A. Check temperature (if indicated), BP, and pulse (which should be evaluated both standing and lying down), respirations, and weight.
B. Inspect:
  1. Observe the general overall appearance of the skin for pallor and signs of dehydration. Tenting of skin when it is rolled between the clinician's thumb and index finger may indicate dehydration.
  2. Inspect for signs of autonomic insufficiency. Postural hypotension, lack of sweat, or blunted pulse and BP responses to Valsalva maneuver suggest autonomic dysfunction and a bowel motility problem as the underlying etiology of nausea and vomiting. Postural hypotension indicates marked volume depletion or circulatory collapse.
  3. Oral examination: Inspect the mouth, teeth, and gums.
  4. Inspect the fontanelles in infants.
C. Auscultate:
  1. Abdomen for bowel sounds in all quadrants
  2. Heart
  3. Lungs
D. Percuss:
  1. Abdomen
E. Palpate:
  1. Abdomen for masses, distention, tenderness, signs of peritonitis, and organomegaly
  2. The back; note CVAT
F. Rectal examination (if indicated)
G. Neurological examination (if indicated)

Diagnostic Tests
The cause of an acute episode of nausea and vomiting is typically determined through a detailed history and physical examination. Only if the cause is unclear should further testing be performed.
A. Urine: Urinalysis, pregnancy test, culture, and sensitivity if indicated
B. Urinalysis for ketones and specific gravity
C. Serum labs: Multiple chemistry profile, including amylase, electrolytes, BUN, creatinine, glucose, bilirubin, and transaminase
D. Hepatitis panel
E. Drug screen
F. Upper GI series?
G. Ultrasonography:
  1. Obstetrical ultrasound to rule out multiple gestations or molar pregnancy if persistent nausea and vomiting, especially after 16 weeks' gestation
  2. Upper abdominal ultrasound, if clinically indicated, to evaluate the pancreas and/or biliary tree
H. Stool for occult blood
I. Upper endoscopy or esophagcogastroduodenoscopy (EGD)
J. CT scan:
  1. Head CT scan, if indicated
  2. Abdominal CT if appendicitis is suspected
K. Gastric scintigraphy, to rule out gastroparesis if indicated
L. EKG if chest pain/MI is suspected

Differential Diagnoses

A. See the "Predisposing Factors" section.

Plan

A. General interventions:
1. Assess hydration status. Provide IV hydration and antiemetics until ketones are clear.
B. Client teaching:
1. Dietary management: See Appendix B, "Nausea and Vomiting Diet Suggestions (Children and Adults)."
C. Pharmaceutical therapy (not an exhaustive list):

Antiemetics should not be used in vomiting of unknown etiology in children and adolescents.

---

1. Antiemetics:
a. Dextrose/fructose/phosphoric acid solution (Emetrol); available OTC:
i. Adults: 15 to 30 mL by mouth at 15-minute intervals (not to exceed five doses)
ii. Children older than 2 years: 5 to 10 mL by mouth at 15-minute intervals (not to exceed five doses)
iii. Children younger than 2 years or less than 30 lb: Dose is not available
iv. Tell the client not to dilute the drug or take fluids 15 minutes before or after taking the medication
v. Clients with diabetes should be instructed not to use Emetrol without consulting their provider
vi. If nausea continues despite use of medication, contact the healthcare provider
b. Promethazine (Phenergan):
i. Drug of choice for gastroenteritis
ii. Adults: 25 to 50 mg by mouth or per rectum every 4 to 6 hours
iii. Children older than 2 years: 12.5 to 25 mg by mouth every 12 hours (usual dose 0.5 mg/lb of body weight, adjusted to age and weight)
iv. Children younger than 2 years or less than 30 lb: Not recommended
c. Trimethobenzamide (Tigan):
i. Used for gastroenteritis and motion sickness
ii. Adults: 300 mg orally three or four times daily
iii. Adults: 200 mg IM three or four times daily
iv. Children: Rectal suppositories and oral forms for pediatrics are no longer commercially available in the United States
v. Dose adjustment should be considered in elderly clients and clients with renal impairment (creatinine clearance ≤ 70 mL/min/1.73 m^2)
d. Prochlorperazine (Compazine is no longer available in the United States):
i. Adults: 5 to 10 mg three or four times daily; spansules 15 mg every 12 hours; suppositories 25 mg twice daily. Do not use more than 20 mg/d or for longer than 12 weeks, as high doses and long intervals of use may cause persistent (irreversible) tardive dyskinesia.
ii. Children 40 to 85 lb: 2.5 mg twice daily, up to a maximum of 15 mg/d
iii. Children 30 to 39 lb: 2.5 mg two or three times a day up to a maximum of 10 mg/d
iv. Children younger than 2 years, 20 to 39 lb: 2.5 mg one to two times a day, up to a maximum of 7.5 mg/d
v. Children younger than 2 years or less than 20 lb: Not recommended
2. Outpatient IV hydration in pregnancy: 1 L lactated Ringer's solution to correct dehydration and restore electrolyte balance. Check urine ketones after administration of the first liter to determine if an additional liter is necessary to clear ketones.
3. 5-Hydroxytryptamine-3 (5-HT$_3$) antagonists are utilized for nausea related to chemotherapy and postoperative nausea and vomiting. 5-HT$_3$ drugs are available in oral, IV, and transdermal formulations. Consult a prescribing reference for current dosing/formulations:
a. Ondansetron (Zofran)
b. Granisetron (Sancuso, Kytril)
c. Palonosetron (Aloxi)
d. Dolasetron mesylate (Anzemet)
4. Dronabinol (Marinol), cannabinoid 2.5, 5, and 10 mg capsules are indicated for refractory nausea and vomiting associated with chemotherapy. Therapy is individualized before and after chemotherapy.
5. Metoclopramide: Used for nausea and vomiting secondary to gastroparesis or chemotherapy. It should not be used continuously for more than 12 weeks to decrease the risk of extrapyramidal symptoms (EPS). Discontinue use immediately if EPS develop.

Follow-Up

A. Tell the client to call or visit the office in 24 hours to check the client's response and nutritional intake.
B. Tell parents who are giving simple treatment at home to call the office promptly if projectile or prolonged vomiting occurs.

Consultation/Referral

A. ***If overdose is suspected: Contact 1-800-222-1222, the American Association of Poison Control Centers, the local poison control center, or the ED immediately.***
B. Hyperemesis gravidarum is the most severe form of nausea and vomiting in pregnancy. This condition may require hospitalization to correct fluid and electrolyte imbalances and nutritional deficiencies.

C. Consult a specialist and hospitalize the client promptly if there is evidence of bowel obstruction; increased ICP; or another GI, neurological, or metabolic emergency. **The first priority is to rule out an acute surgical etiology such as bowel obstruction or peritonitis.**

D. Call for a pediatric consultation immediately for vomiting lasting more than 24 hours, projectile vomiting, vomiting after a fall or head injury, or prolonged vomiting coupled with diarrhea.

E. Call for a psychiatric consultation for suspected psychogenic nausea and vomiting.

F. If postural hypotension occurs, especially in elderly clients, hospital admission for parenteral fluid and electrolyte replacement is indicated.

G. Endocrinologist, gastroenterologist, and surgical consultations for treatment, consideration, and placement of a gastric stimulator for diabetes gastroparesis.

Individual Considerations

A. Pregnancy:
1. Determine whether the woman is ingesting non-food substances, such as starch, clay, or toothpaste, which would indicate pica.
2. Intractable nausea and vomiting require ultrasonography to rule out hydatidiform mole.
3. The only FDA-approved drug for treating nausea and vomiting in pregnancy is doxylamine/pyridoxine. Antihistamines, promotility agents (e.g., metoclopramide), Emetrol, promethazine (Phenergan), and prochlorperazine (Compazine) may be used during pregnancy. In cases refractory to standard therapy, ondansetron and steroids may be considered.
4. Uncorrected hyperemesis gravidarum can result in severe electrolyte imbalances and possible hepatic and renal damage. The major concern for fetal well-being is uncorrected ketosis, which may result in fetal abnormalities or death in early pregnancy.
5. Tell the client to eat toast or dry crackers; to eat small, frequent meals and snacks; to drink fluids separately from meals; and to avoid fatty, fried, greasy, or spicy foods and foods with strong odors.

B. Pediatrics:
1. The differential diagnosis of vomiting is age dependent.
2. For neonates and young infants, the most frequent diagnostic considerations are the following:
   a. GERD
   b. Excessive feeding volume
   c. Increased ICP/meningitis
   d. Food allergy
   e. Intestinal obstruction:
      i. Malrotation without volvulus
      ii. HD
      iii. Intussusception
      iv. Intestinal atresia
      v. Pyloric stenosis
3. Differential diagnoses for older infants and children include:
   a. Gastroenteritis
   b. GERD
   c. Gastroparesis
   d. Mechanical obstruction
   e. Munchausen syndrome by proxy
4. Adolescent disorders include the disorders affecting children as well as:
   a. Appendicitis
   b. IBD
   c. Pregnancy
   d. Bulimia or psychogenic vomiting
5. Question caregivers regarding the infant's feeding, activity level, irritability, lethargy, and number of wet diapers.
6. Otitis media, pharyngitis, and UTIs may present with nausea and/or vomiting in the pediatric population.
7. Rumination syndrome is a behavioral disorder that is most commonly identified among mentally disadvantaged children and adolescents with cognitive disabilities. The behavior consists of daily, effortless regurgitation of undigested food within minutes of starting or completing ingestion of a meal.

C. Geriatrics:
1. Use of the lower dose ranges of an antiemetic is sufficient for most elderly clients due to their susceptibility to hypotension and neuromuscular reactions.
2. Dosages should be increased more gradually in the elderly.

There should be a low threshold for hospitalization of the elderly to treat dehydration and to correct fluid and electrolyte imbalances.

Resources

American Cancer Society: www.cancer.org
Rome Foundation: https://theromefoundation.org

Bibliography

Feinleib, J., Kwan, L., & Yamani, A. (2019, May 30). Postoperative nausea and vomiting. *UpToDate*. Retrieved from https://www.uptodate.com/contents/postoperative-nausea-and-vomiting?search=metoclopramide%20drug%20information&source=search_result&selectedTitle=3-150&usage_type=default&display_rank=3

National Board of Medical Examiners. (2019). *Laboratory values (Biochemical Profile SMA-12)*. Retrieved from https://www.nbme.org

Nettina, S. (2010). *The Lippincott manual of nursing practice* (9th ed.). Philadelphia, PA: Wolters Kluwer Lippincott Williams & Wilkins.

Ogunyemi, D. A. (2015, November 14). Hyperemesis gravidarum. *Medscape*. Retrieved from http://emedicine.medscape.com/article/254751-overview#a4

Vege, S. S. (2019, January 9). Etiology of acute pancreatitis. *UpToDate*. Retrieved from https://www.uptodate.com/contents/etiology-of-acute-pancreatitis

Peptic Ulcer Disease

Doncy Eapen and Cheryl A. Glass

Definition

A. PUD is circumscribed ulceration of the GI mucosa occurring in areas exposed to acid and pepsin. The client's prior ulcer history tends to predict future behavior and risk of future complications. Complications include bleeding ulcer, perforation, and obstruction.

B. The stomach is divided on the basis of its physiological functions into two main portions. The proximal two-thirds, the fundic gland area, acts as a receptable for ingested food and secretes acid and pepsin. The distal third, the pyloric gland area, mixes and propels food into the duodenum and produces the hormone gastrin. "Peptic" lesions may occur in the esophagus (esophagitis), stomach (gastritis), or duodenum (duodenitis).

C. There is often no correlation between the presence of an active ulcer, noted by endoscopy, and symptoms. The disappearance of symptoms does not guarantee ulcer healing.

Incidence

A. The annual incidence of peptic ulcer is estimated to range from 0.1% to 1.8%. The ulcer incidence in *H. pylori*–infected individuals is about 1% per year. The recurrence rate is 50% to 80% during the 6 to 12 months following the initial ulcer healing, although relapses are not always symptomatic. Some peptic ulcers heal spontaneously, and 2% to 20% of clients have multiple simultaneous ulcers.

B. From 16% to 31% of ulcers are caused by NSAIDs. Risks of peptic ulcer and death are three to six times higher among people who take NSAIDs.

C. Cigarette smokers are twice as likely to develop ulcers as are nonsmokers.

Pathogenesis

A. Although the precise mechanisms of ulcer formation remain incompletely understood, the process appears to involve the interplay of acid production, pepsin secretion, *H. pylori* bacterial infection, and mucosal defense mechanisms. Excess acid production is the hallmark of DU disease. Pepsin secretion is also elevated in DU disease.

B. The relation of aspirin and other NSAIDs to ulcer disease is due largely to the drugs' potent inhibition of gastric mucosal prostaglandin synthesis. In addition to prostaglandin inhibition, many NSAID preparations produce acute diffuse mucosal injury by means of a direct erosive effect.

Predisposing Factors

A. *H. pylori* infection is the most common cause of ulceration.

B. Use of NSAIDs, especially aspirin, ibuprofen, and naproxen, is associated with acute erosive gastritis

C. Smoking

D. Genetic factors: Family history of ulcer disease

E. Age:
   1. DU occurs between ages 25 and 75 years.
   2. Gastric ulcer (GU) occurs between ages 55 and 65 years.

F. Gender:
   1. The ratio of males to females with gastritis is 1:1.
   2. The ratio of males to females with peptic ulcers is 2:1.

G. Excessive alcohol consumption, which stimulates acid secretion

H. Medications:
   1. Corticosteroids potentiate ulcer risk in clients who use NSAIDs concurrently.

   2. Anticoagulants
   3. Bisphosphonates
   4. Spironolactone
   5. SSRIs

I. Improper diet, irregular meals, and skipped meals

J. Severe physiological stress:
   1. Burns
   2. CNS trauma
   3. Surgery
   4. Severe medical illness:
      a. Cirrhosis
      b. COPD
      c. Renal failure
      d. Organ transplantation
      e. Celiac disease
      f. CD

K. Other causes:
   1. Radiation-induced ulcer
   2. Chemotherapy-induced ulcer
   3. Vascular insufficiency
   4. Duodenal obstruction

L. Zollinger–Ellison syndrome

M. Bile reflux

N. Illicit drugs: Crack cocaine

Common Complaints

A. Pain described as an aching, boring, gnawing, or burning feeling

B. Epigastric pain in the RUQ and LUQ of the abdomen or occasionally below the breast

C. Pain that awakens the client at night or in the early morning

D. Perforated peptic ulcer presents with a sudden onset of severe sharp abdominal pain.

Other Signs and Symptoms

A. Asymptomatic

B. GI distress 1 to 3 hours after a meal, on an empty stomach

C. Pain relieved by food, antacids, or vomiting

D. Nausea and vomiting

E. Hematemesis

F. Chest discomfort

G. Blood in stools, "grape jelly" or maroon-colored stools

H. Loss of appetite or weight

I. Weight gain; clients with DU may eat more to ease the pain.

J. Anemia

Signs and Symptoms of Bleeding

A. Massive bleeding:
   1. Acute, bright red hematemesis or a large amount of melena with clots in the stool, or "grape jelly" stool
   2. Rapid pulse, drop in BP, hypovolemia, and shock

B. Subacute bleeding:
   1. Intermittent melena or coffee-ground emesis
   2. Hypotension
   3. Weakness and dizziness

C. Chronic bleeding:
  1. Intermittent appearance of blood
  2. Increased weakness, paleness, or shortness of breath
  3. Occult blood

Subjective Data

A. Ask the client to describe the onset, duration, type, and location of pain. Does it occur at any special time—for example, before meals, after meals, or during the night?

B. Has the client had a previous ulcer? What was the treatment? If oral treatment was prescribed, did the client complete the therapy?

C. Have the client describe what alleviates pain, such as taking antacids, and what worsens pain, such as use of aspirin, oral steroids, or NSAIDs

D. Review associated symptoms, such as nausea, vomiting, and heartburn.

E. Ask the client if any first-degree relatives have ulcers.

F. Inquire whether the client is a smoker. If so, how much and for how long?

G. Ask the client about alcohol consumption: How much and for how long?

H. Inquire whether any blood has ever been vomited or passed in stool. If so, have the client describe it.

I. Take the client's dietary history, including time of meals, frequency of skipped meals, weight loss, and so forth.

J. Review all medications, including a review of OTC and herbal products such as ginkgo biloba.

K. Obtain the client's past medical history of associated diseases, such as cirrhosis, pancreatitis, arthritis, COPD, and hyperparathyroidism.

L. If the client suspects blood in stool, ask if there has been a change in bowel pattern, presence of abdominal pain or tenderness, and whether the client recently ingested food such as red beets.

Physical Examination

A. Check temperature (if indicated), pulse, respirations, BP, and weight.

B. Inspect:
  1. Abdominal distention, client crossing arms over abdomen, flatulence
  2. Physical signs of anemia

C. Auscultate:
  1. Abdomen for bowel sounds in all quadrants

D. Percuss:
  1. Abdomen for hepatosplenomegaly

E. Palpate:
  1. Abdomen for tenderness, guarding, rigidity, masses, and liver or spleen enlargement

F. Rectal examination:
  1. Check for tenderness and masses.
  2. Take stool specimen.

Diagnostic Tests

A. CBC
B. Stool for occult blood
C. Coagulation studies
D. Testing for *H. pylori*:
  1. **Endoscopy with biopsy is the most accurate test.**
  2. **Rapid urease test is the diagnostic test of choice.**
  3. Urea breath test (UBT)
  4. Serum test for *H. pylori* antibodies
  5. Stool *H. pylori* antigen testing: More accurate and less expensive than antibody testing

E. Radiography with barium meal
F. Mucosal biopsy, after GI consultation, to rule out cancer
G. Fasting gastrin level: Screen for Zollinger–Ellison syndrome

Differential Diagnoses

A. PUD
B. GERD
C. Zollinger–Ellison syndrome: Fasting serum gastrin level 500 pg/mL in the presence of acid hypersecretion is diagnostic.
D. Cancer:
  1. Gastric lymphoma
  2. Gastric cancer
  3. Pancreatic cancer
E. Pancreatitis (acute or chronic)
F. Myocardial ischemia
G. Abdominal aneurysm
H. Diverticulitis
I. Drug-induced dyspepsia:
  1. Theophylline
  2. Digitalis
J. CD involving the stomach or duodenum
K. Gastric infections
L. Cholelithiasis
M. Acute gastritis

Plan

A. General interventions:
  1. Goals are to alleviate pain, promote healing, limit complications, and prevent recurrences while minimizing costs and side effects of treatment.
  2. Encourage the client to stop taking NSAIDs, unless medically indicated:
    1. If NSAID use is unavoidable, the lowest possible dose and duration and co-therapy with a PPI based on triple therapy is recommended.
  3. Smoking cessation should be highly encouraged at each visit.

B. Client teaching:
  1. *See Section III: Client Teaching Guide for this chapter, "Ulcer Management."* ◀

C. Pharmaceutical therapy:
  1. The treatment of peptic ulcer begins with the eradication of *H. pylori* in infected individuals. Empirical therapy for the infection is reasonable for uncomplicated cases in the absence of NSAID use. Documenting infection, even in clients with known ulcers, is an essential step prior to initiating antimicrobial therapy.

a. Triple therapy anti–*H. pylori* regimen: PPI + amoxicillin + clarithromycin:

  i. PPI-based regimen (choose one):

    1) Rabeprazole (Aciphex) 20 mg twice a day—total treatment duration: 7 days

    2) Esomeprazole (Nexium) 40 mg once a day—total treatment duration: 10 days

    3) Lansoprazole (Prevacid) 30 mg twice a day—total treatment duration: 10 to 14 days

    4) Omeprazole (Prilosec) 20 mg twice a day—total treatment duration: 14 days

  ii. Amoxicillin 1,000 mg twice a day

  iii. Clarithromycin 500 mg twice a day

b. Quadruple therapy—14 days

  i. Choose standard-dose PPI, or ranitidine 150 mg, two times daily

  ii. Metronidazole (Flagyl) 500 mg four times daily

  iii. Tetracycline 500 mg four times daily

  iv. Bismuth subsalicylate 525 mg (two chewable tablets) four times daily

2. Antisecretory therapy is the mainstay of therapy in uninfected clients and is used for maintenance therapy in selected cases. Full doses of an H_2 receptor antagonist provide effective initial therapy; however, PPIs are more effective.

3. Clients with uncomplicated, small (less than 1 cm) DU or GU who have received adequate treatment for *H. pylori* probably are asymptomatic and do not need any further therapy directed at ulcer healing. Maintenance acid suppression with a PPI for 1 year following *H. pyloric* eradication is recommended for clients with a complicated DU. If the ulcer is giant (greater than 2 cm), showing densely fibrosed ulcer beds, or if the client is a high-risk individual with a protracted prior history, then the client should be kept on a PPI until a follow-up endoscopy is performed.

a. H_2 receptor antagonists: Split-dose, evening, and nighttime therapy are all effective. In the United States, cimetidine, ranitidine, and famotidine are approved for GU healing. H2 receptor antagonist–based regimens are not FDA-approved treatment regimens.

  i. Cimetidine (Tagamet) 400 mg orally twice a day or 800 mg at bedtime for 6 to 8 weeks

  ii. Ranitidine (Zantac) 150 mg orally twice a day or 300 mg at bedtime

  iii. Famotidine (Pepsid) 20 mg orally twice a day or 40 mg at bedtime

  iv. Nizatidine (Axid) 150 mg orally twice a day or 300 mg at bedtime

b. PPIs are effective in inducing ulcer healing and are the most potent inhibitors of gastric acid secretion. Once-daily dosing is generally sufficient for acid inhibition; however, a second dose may be necessary and should be given before the evening meal. Once-daily PPI dosing inhibits acid output by 66% after 5 days. Optimal dosing is immediately before breakfast.

  i. Omeprazole (Prilosec/Zegerid) 20 to 40 mg every morning for 4 weeks

  ii. Esomeprazole (Nexium) 20 to 40 mg every morning for 4 to 8 weeks

  iii. Lansoprazole (Prevacid) 15 to 30 mg every morning for 4 weeks

  iv. Dexlansoprazole (Kapidex) 30 to 60 mg every morning for 4 to 8 weeks

  v. Pantoprazole (Protonix) 20 to 40 mg every morning for 4 weeks

  vi. Rabeprazole (Aciphex) 20 mg every morning for 4 weeks

  vii. Dexlansoprazole (Dexilant) 60 mg every morning for 8 weeks

c. PPIs should not be given concomitantly with prostaglandins, or other antisecretory agents, because of the marked reduction in their effects. An H_2 antagonist can be used with a PPI if given after a sufficient interval between their administrations; the minimal times have not been established. The H_2 antagonist could be given at bedtime for breakthrough symptoms after a morning dose of a PPI.

d. Combination products currently on the market:

  i. Omeclamox-Pak: Omeprazole 20 mg (2 caps), amoxicillin 500 mg (4 caps), and clarithromycin 500 mg (2 tabs) per pack. Take omeprazole 20 mg, amoxicillin 100 mg, and clarithromycin 500 mg twice a day. Treatment is 10 days.

  ii. Prevpac: Lansoprazole 30 mg (2 caps), amoxicillin 500 mg (4 caps), and clarithromycin 500 mg (2 caps) per pack. Take lansoprazole 30 mg, amoxicillin 1,000 mg, and clarithromycin 500 mg twice daily. Treatment is 10 or 14 days.

4. Sucralfate (Carafate) 1 g orally four times daily, 1 hour before meals and at bedtime; maintenance therapy is 1 g twice daily. Sucralfate is not recommended for *H. pylori* or NSAID ulcers.

5. Misoprostol (Cytotec, a prostaglandin analog) is effective for peptic ulcers caused by NSAID use; peptic ulcers respond well to misoprostol 100 to 200 mcg orally four times a day

D. Dietary management:

1. Advise the client to avoid alcohol, coffee (including decaffeinated), and other caffeine-containing beverages, because they stimulate acid secretion (see Appendix B, Table B.8).

E. Medical management:

1. Test for *H. pylori*:

a. A single negative *H. pylori* test should be interpreted cautiously, especially in the face of active bleeding. Blood in the stomach can alter the pH indicator in the rapid urease test. False negatives are likely, and additional testing for *H. pylori* is essential.

   b. Concurrent use of a PPI, antibiotics, or bismuth will cause a false negative test.

F. Surgical management:

1. Diagnostic evaluation of the ulcer is by means of endoscopy.

2. Surgery remains an option for treatment of refractory disease and complications. The most serious indications for surgery include brisk bleeding of 6 to 8 units of blood in 24 hours, recurrent bleeding episodes, perforation, gastric outlet obstruction refractory to medical therapy, and failure of a benign GU to heal after 15 weeks. Emergency intervention may be required, such as withholding food and oral fluids, starting an IV, placing a nasogastric (NG) tube, oxygen therapy, or blood transfusion. If life-threatening bleeding occurs, treat the client for shock.

Follow-Up

A. Therapeutic trial of lifestyle changes combined with an H_2 receptor antagonist, sucralfate, or omeprazole for 1 to 2 weeks should provide relief. Reevaluate the client after 2 weeks, and if symptoms are improved, prescribe a full course of 6 to 8 weeks.

B. Reevaluate the client again at 8 weeks, after the full course of therapy is completed.

C. Consider repeating the breath test to confirm eradication of *H. pylori*.

D. Repeat endoscopy is not recommended for DU unless symptoms persist or recur.

E. For refractory GU—that is, persistent pain after 8 weeks despite a full medical regimen or unresponsive to treatment for *H. pylori*—endoscopic examination and biopsy are needed after 12 weeks of therapy, especially in clients older than age 40 who are at increased risk of gastric cancer. Barium study is not sufficient, because even malignant ulcers may shrink in size in response to therapy.

F. Evaluate refractory cases for Zollinger–Ellison syndrome, especially when there are multiple ulcers, occurrences in unusual places, marked abdominal pain, or secretory diarrhea.

G. There is an increased risk of osteoporotic fracture from the long-term use of PPIs.

H. Clients beginning long-term NSAID therapy should first be tested for *H. pylori*.

Consultation/Referral

A. Consult both a surgeon and a gastroenterologist, and admit the client to a hospital when symptoms of hemorrhage, penetration, perforation, or gastric outlet obstruction are present.

B. Refer clients with recurrences or refractory disease to a physician for evaluation for *H. pylori* infection by endoscopy or breath test. If present, eradicate with a 2-week course of triple therapy.

Individual Considerations

A. Pregnancy:

1. The drugs misoprostol and ranitidine are abortifacients. They cross the placental barrier and are excreted in breast milk and are contraindicated in pregnancy or suspected pregnancy. Use in sexually active women of childbearing age should be done with proper warning and detailed client education.

B. Adults:

1. DUs are more common in people between ages 45 and 54 years; GUs are more common in people between 55 and 64 years.

2. Clients older than age 40 years are at greater risk of gastric cancer and should undergo either an upper GI series or endoscopy to document the nature and location of lesions when there is strong clinical suspicion of ulcer disease.

3. Gastritis not associated with reflux is present in 75% of people older than age 50 years.

C. Geriatrics:

1. Silent disease is particularly common among the elderly and those using NSAIDs.

2. Lethargy, confusion, slurred speech, agitation, and visual hallucinations have been reported with use of cimetidine, particularly in the elderly.

3. In the elderly, DU symptoms match the classic form—early-morning awakening to pain, then quick relief by food or antacids. GU symptoms are less obvious, with burning or gnawing pain experienced by fewer than 50% of elderly clients.

4. Anemia may be the only symptom of gastric cancer. Cancer must always be considered and confirmed by endoscopy with biopsy.

5. When prescribing an NSAID to the elderly, use the lowest dose, for the shortest period of time, and avoid prescribing a long-acting NSAID, such as indomethacin (Indocin) and piroxicam (Feldene).

6. Due to other medications taken for comorbid health conditions, the elderly are especially at risk with the combination of NSAIDs and the following:

   a. Aspirin
   b. Clopidogrel (Plavix)
   c. Dabigatran (Pradaxa)
   d. Dipyridamole (Persantine)
   e. Prasugrel (Effient)
   f. Ticlopidine (Ticlid)
   g. Warfarin (Coumadin)

Bibliography

American Gastroenterological Association.(2016, July). *Peptic ulcer disease*. Retrieved from https://www.gastro.org/patient-care/conditions-diseases/peptic-ulcer-disease

Anand, B. S. (2015, January 9). Peptic ulcer disease. *Medscape*. Retrieved from http://emedicine.medscape.com/article/181753-overview

Crowe, S. E. (2018, April 23). Patient education: Peptic ulcer disease (beyond the basics). *UpToDate*. Retrieved from https://www.uptodate.com/contents/peptic-ulcer-disease-beyond-the-basics#H1053244020

Feldman, M.& Shounak, D. (2019, April 3). NSAIDs (including aspirin): Primary prevention of gastroduodenal toxicity. *UpToDate*. Retrieved from https://www.uptodate.com/contents/nsaids-including-aspirin-primary-prevention-of-gastroduodenal-toxicity

Nettina, S. (2010). *The Lippincott manual of nursing practice* (9th ed.). Philadelphia, PA: Wolters Kluwer Lippincott Williams & Wilkins.

Saad, R. J., & Chey, W. D. (2015, June 23). First-line treatment strategies for *Helicobacter pylori* infection. *Gastroenterology & Endoscopy News*, 1–8. Retrieved from http://www.gastroendonews.com/Review-Articles/Article/06-15/First-Line-Treatment-Strategies-for-Helicobacter-nbsp-pylori-Infection/32678/ses=ogst

Vakil, N. B. (2017, September 5). Peptic ulcer disease: Management. *UpToDate*. Retrieved from https://www.uptodate.com/contents/peptic-ulcer-disease-management#H15

Vakil, N. B. (2018). *Overview of the complications of peptic ulcer disease.* Retrieved from https://www.uptodate.com/contents/overview-of-the-complications-of-peptic-ulcer-disease?search=perforated%20duodenal%20ulcer&sectionRank=2&usage_type=default&anchor=H66923600&source=machineLearning&selectedTitle=1~96&display_rank=1#H66923600

Pinworm

Cheryl A. Glass, Audra Malone, and Doncy Eapen

Definition

A. Pinworm, *Enterobius vermicularis*, is the most common helminth infection. It is characterized by a white, threadlike worm infestation.

Incidence

A. Pinworm infection is very common. *Enterobius* is found worldwide, and infection with this organism commonly occurs in family clusters. It has a high incidence of reinfection. Exact data are not available because helminth infestations are not reportable to the CDC.

Pathogenesis

A. The *E. vermicularis* adult nematode, or pinworm, lives in the human rectum or colon and emerges onto the perianal skin to lay eggs. It is transmissible by direct transfer of infective eggs to the mouth, or indirectly through clothing, bedding, food, or other articles contaminated with eggs of the parasite. The period of communicability is as long as female nematodes continue discharging eggs on the perianal skin. Eggs remain infective in an indoor environment for usually 2 to 3 weeks. Humans are the only known hosts; dogs and cats do not harbor *E. vermicularis.*

B. The incubation period is 1 to 2 months or longer, from ingestion of an egg until an adult gravid female migrates to the perianal region.

Predisposing Factors

A. Preschool and school age
B. Member of a family with an infected person
C. Institutional residence
D. Overcrowded living conditions

Common Complaints

A. Intense nighttime anal pruritus
B. Irritability in infants and children

Other Signs and Symptoms

A. Disturbed sleep or insomnia
B. Pruritus vulvae
C. Urethritis
D. Vaginitis
E. Local irritation
F. Secondary infections from scratching
G. Loss of appetite or weight loss
H. Grinding teeth at night

Subjective Data

A. Review the onset, duration, course, and time of symptoms, especially anal itching.
B. Ask the client about symptoms in other family members.
C. Inquire about genital irritation symptoms in female children.

Physical Examination

A. Check temperature (if indicated), pulse, respirations, BP, and weight.
B. Inspect:
    1. Anus and female genitals for irritation and skin abrasions

Diagnostic Tests

A. Press the sticky side of transparent (not translucent) cellulose tape against the perianal folds, and then press the tape on a glass slide. Eggs will be visible under a microscope.
    1. The "tape method" should be conducted on three consecutive mornings.
    2. Eggs are most likely to be present on awakening and before the person bathes or uses the toilet.
B. Pinworm eggs may be obtained from a scraping sample from under the fingernails.
C. Order urinalysis to rule out UTI.
D. Obtain a stool specimen for ova and parasite; adult worms in feces are diagnostic.
E. Serologic tests are not available for diagnosing pinworm infections.

Differential Diagnoses

A. Pinworms
B. UTI
C. Poor hygiene
D. Chemical irritants, soaps, and bubble baths
E. Proctitis

Plan

A. General interventions:
    1. All household members should be treated as a group when there are multiple instances of infection.
B. Client teaching:
    1. *See Section III: Client Teaching Guide for this chapter,* ◄ *"Roundworms and Pinworms."*
    2. Teach the mother how to obtain a specimen from a child.
    3. Infected people should bathe or shower in the morning to remove eggs.
        a. Showering is better than taking a bath. Showering avoids potentially contaminating the bath water with pinworm eggs.

b. Infected people should not co-bathe with others during their time of infection.

4. Use good handwashing habits after using the toilet and before eating or preparing food.

5. Keep fingernails short and avoid nail biting.

6. Thoroughly launder bedding and clothing to destroy any eggs.

C. Pharmaceutical therapy:

1. Albendazole (Albenza): 400 mg one-time dose and then another single dose 2 weeks later to prevent reinfection. Albendazole is the most commonly used drug for treatment of pinworms.

2. Mebendazole (Vermox): 500 mg one-time dose and then another single dose 2 weeks later to prevent reinfection

a. Mebendazole is available in the United States only through compounding pharmacies.

b. WHO recommends that 1-year-old children be given half of the dose (50 mg) for older children and adults.

3. Pyrantel pamoate (Pyrantel): 11 mg/kg/d for 3 days; do not exceed 1 g/d.

4. It is recommended that all household members be treated at the same time.

Follow-Up

A. If single-dose therapy is not effective, a second course of medication is advised in 2 weeks.

B. Reinfection is common.

Consultation/Referral

A. Consult a physician if the client is pregnant.

Individual Considerations

A. Pregnancy:

1. Anthelmintic drugs are in pregnancy category C; however, the potential risks to the fetus versus the benefits should be considered.

2. Breastfeeding should not be withheld during mebendazole therapy.

3. WHO has determined that the benefit of pharmaceutical treatment outweighs the risk.

a. WHO allows the use of albendazole in the second and third trimesters of pregnancy.

b. WHO allows the use of pyrantel pamoate in the second and third trimesters of pregnancy.

B. Pediatrics:

1. All medications are advised for children.

a. In WHO guidelines for mass prevention campaigns, albendazole can be used in children as young as 1 year.

b. Mebendazole and pyrantel pamoate are on WHO's Model List of Essential Medicines for Children intended for use in children up to 12 years of age.

2. Pinworms may predispose children to developing UTIs.

3. No unusual cleansing other than basic hygiene measures should be undertaken. Excessive zeal in this regard can induce guilt and is counterproductive.

4. The best time to examine a child is 2 to 3 hours after he or she falls asleep.

C. Adults:

1. Lowest incidence of pinworms

Bibliography

Centers for Disease Control and Prevention. (2016, February 3). *Parasites: Enterobiasis (also known as pinworm infection).* Retrieved from https://www.cdc.gov/parasites/pinworm/health_professionals/index.html

Nettina, S. (2010). *The Lippincott manual of nursing practice* (9th ed.). Philadelphia, PA: Wolters Kluwer Lippincott Williams & Wilkins.

Roundworm

Cheryl A. Glass and Audra Malone

Definition

A. Roundworm, *Ascaris lumbricoides*, is a helminthic parasitic infection of the lumen of the small intestines and sometimes the lungs. Most infections with *A. lumbricoides* are asymptomatic. Roundworms are brownish, are the size and shape of earthworms, and can be seen easily without a microscope. The majority of worms are noted in the jejunum but can be found from the esophagus to the rectum. Ova can survive for prolonged periods, up to 10 years. The eggs are resistant to normal water purification but can be removed by boiling and water filtration.

Incidence

A. *A. lumbricoides* is very common. Approximately 25% to 33% of the world's population, more than 1.4 billion people, are infected with these human intestinal nematodes. *A. lumbricoides* is the third most frequent helminth infection; only hookworms and whipworms exceed its rate of infection. It occurs worldwide, especially in tropical and warm climates. Roundworm infection affects people of all ages but is most common in young children between 3 and 8 years of age.

B. Individuals can be asymptomatic and continue to shed eggs for years. The parasitic eggs are extremely durable in various environments, and each roundworm produces a large number of eggs. Rates of complications secondary to *A. lumbricoides* infection range from 11% to 67% of infected individuals, with intestinal and biliary tract obstruction being the most common serious sequelae. Rates of bowel obstruction or perforation are highest in children.

C. Many individuals infected with *A. lumbricoides* are also coinfected with other intestinal parasites, including trichuriasis (*Trichuris trichiura*) and hookworm (*N. americanus* and *A. duodenale*).

Pathogenesis

A. *A. lumbricoides* is a large roundworm that infects humans. The nematode measures 15 to 35 cm in length in adulthood. It is contracted by ingesting eggs in contaminated soil through eating the soil (pica), children playing in contaminated soil, eating unwashed fruits and raw vegetables, drinking water contaminated with feces, or touching food with soil-contaminated hands. Occasionally, transplacental migration of larvae has been reported.

B. The life cycle of *A. lumbricoides* is 4 to 8 weeks, and feces contain eggs about 2 months after ingestion of embryonated eggs. Female roundworms produce 200,000 eggs per day, which are excreted in stool and must incubate in soil for 2 to 3 weeks for the embryo to form and become infectious (second-stage larvae). The interval between ingestion of egg and development of egg-laying adults is approximately 8 weeks. If infection is untreated, adult worms can live 6 to 24 months, resulting in daily excretion of large numbers of ova.

C. The ingested ova hatch in the small intestine (jejunum or ileum) and release larvae. They then may migrate via blood or via the lymphatic system to the heart, lungs, and biliary tree, and occasionally to the kidney or brain. It takes approximately 4 days for the larvae to reach the lungs. After maturation, they are passed through the bronchi and the trachea and are subsequently swallowed.

D. Eggs are not shed in the stool until roughly 40 days after the development of pulmonary symptoms.

Predisposing Factors
A. Crowded or unsanitary living conditions
B. Tropical or warm climates, including the southern United States
C. Preschool or early school age (2–10 years)
D. Tend to cluster in families
E. Residence in areas where human feces is used as fertilizer
F. Travelers to endemic areas (Asia, Africa, and South America)
G. Recent immigrants (especially from Latin America and Asia)
H. International adoptees

Common Complaints
A. Asymptomatic
B. Restlessness at night
C. Colicky abdominal pain
D. Frequent fatigue
E. Worms found in BMs or in bed

Other Signs and Symptoms
A. Transient respiratory symptoms during migration
B. Nausea and vomiting
C. Anorexia and erratic or poor appetite
D. Fever
E. Irritability
F. Diarrhea or constipation
G. Weight loss or gain
H. Dry cough, dyspnea, wheezing, substernal discomfort, or blood-tinged sputum from larvae in lungs
I. Parasites regurgitated or passed through the nares of febrile clients
J. Acute transient pneumonitis
K. Acute obstructive jaundice
L. Appendicitis
M. Urticaria
N. Impaired absorption of protein, lactose, and vitamin A
O. Burning chest pain

Subjective Data
A. Review the onset, duration, and course of symptoms.
B. Ask about any problems with pica.
C. Inquire about worms in stool or emesis.
D. Review any history of pets treated for worms.
E. Establish the client's normal weight for evaluation.

Physical Examination
A. Check temperature (as indicated), pulse, respirations, BP, and weight. Plot the child's height and weight on a growth curve.
B. Inspect:
    1. Skin to rule out jaundice and evaluate urticaria
C. Auscultate:
    1. Lungs to evaluate the presence of rales, wheezes, diminished breath sounds, and tachypnea
    2. Heart
    3. Abdomen
D. Percuss:
    1. Abdomen to evaluate dullness
E. Palpate:
    1. Abdomen for distention, tenderness, and masses (worm bolus); upper right quadrant, lower right quadrant, or hypogastrium tenderness may suggest complications of ascariasis

Diagnostic Tests
A. None, if the worm is visualized; they are occasionally passed from the rectum and nose, and are seen in vomitus.
B. Stool for occult blood, ova, and parasites, and culture
C. CBC: Eosinophilia may be noted particularly during the migration of larvae through the lungs
D. Plain abdominal radiograph
E. Ultrasound or CT to diagnose hepatobiliary or pancreatic ascariasis. ERCP is used for diagnosis and removal.
F. Chest radiography is rarely needed.
G. Microscopic wet prep of sputum may be helpful with respiratory symptoms.

Differential Diagnoses
A. Roundworm
B. Asthma
C. Pneumonia
D. Poor nutrition
E. Giardiasis
F. Pancreatitis from other causes
G. Impaired growth/FTT
H. Iron-deficiency anemia
I. Appendicitis
J. Bowel obstruction (large or small)
K. Intussusception
L. Acute cholangitis

Plan
A. General interventions:
    1. All family members must be treated with medication.
B. Client teaching:
    1. *See Section III: Client Teaching Guide for this chapter,* ◀ *"Roundworms and Pinworms."*

2. Stress the importance of maintaining a clean play area for children.

3. Stress sanitary disposal of feces.

4. Explain that household bleach is ineffective in killing eggs *and* worms.

5. There is no direct person-to-person transmission.

C. Pharmaceutical therapy:

1. Treatment of symptomatic and asymptomatic infections may be achieved by a single dose of the following agents:

    a. A single dose of albendazole 400 mg orally is effective in achieving cure in almost 100% of ascariasis cases.

    b. Pyrantel pamoate (Antiminth) 11 mg/kg up to a maximum of 1 g given in a single dose. The single dose is 90% effective.

    c. Mebendazole (Vermox) 100 mg twice daily for 3 days or 500 mg as a single dose. Both the 1- and 3-day treatments are about 95% effective.

        1. WHO recommends that 1-year-old children be given half of the dose (50 mg) for older children and adults.

2. Administer the drug to all family members to decrease the risk of spreading infection.

3. Consider a vitamin A supplement if growth is retarded.

4. Inhaled beta-agonists may be indicated for respiratory symptoms.

Follow-Up

A. Reexamine a stool specimen in 2 weeks to determine if the therapy was successful in eliminating the worms. If the client is not cured, give a second course of medication.

B. Therapy is effective for adult worms only. Reevaluate in 2 to 3 months for detectable eggs.

C. Endoscopy or laparoscopic extraction of worms may be required with hepatobiliary infestations.

Consultation/Referral

A. Consult with a physician if the client is pregnant or is considered a surgical risk.

B. Bowel or hepatobiliary obstruction may require surgical or gastroenterological consultation.

Individual Considerations

A. Pregnancy:

1. Anthelmintics are pregnancy category C; however, the potential risks to the fetus versus the benefits should be considered.

2. WHO has determined that the benefit of pharmaceutical treatment outweighs the risk.

    a. WHO allows the use of albendazole in the second and third trimesters of pregnancy.

    b. WHO allows the use of pyrantel pamoate in the second and third trimesters of pregnancy.

B. Pediatrics:

1. All medications are advised for children.

    a. WHO guidelines for mass prevention campaigns: Albendazole can be used in children as young as 1 year old.

    b. Mebendazole and pyrantel pamoate are on WHO's Model List of Essential Medicines for Children intended for use in children up to 12 years of age.

2. Children are more prone to acute intestinal obstruction because they have smaller diameters of the intestinal lumen and often have large numbers of worms.

C. Adults:

1. Acute intestinal obstruction may develop with heavy infestation.

Bibliography

Dora-Laskey, A. (2016, May 18). *Ascaris lumbricoides. Medscape.* Retrieved from http://emedicine.medscape.com/article/788398-overview

Leder, K., & Weller, P.F. (2019, February 5). Ascariasis. *UpToDate.* Retrieved from https://www.uptodate.com/contents/ascariasis#H1108088292

Nettina, S. (2010). *The Lippincott manual of nursing practice* (9th ed.). Philadelphia, PA: Wolters Kluwer Lippincott Williams & Wilkins.

Vege, S. S. (2019, January 9). Etiology of acute pancreatitis. *UpToDate.* Retrieved from https://www.uptodate.com/contents/etiology-of-acute-pancreatitis

Ulcerative Colitis

Doncy Eapen and Cheryl A. Glass

Definition

A. UC is one of the two forms of IBD, along with CD, and is limited to the colon. It extends proximally from the anal verge in an uninterrupted pattern to a part of or the entire colon. Extracolonic manifestations also include uveitis, pyoderma gangrenosum, pleuritis, erythema nodosum, ankylosing spondylitis, and spondyloarthropathies (Table 11.19).

B. Neither UC nor CD should be confused with IBS, which affects the motility of the colon. Smoking is negatively associated with UC; the relationship is reversed in CD. The general course of UC is intermittent exacerbations and remissions. In severe cases, surgery may result in a cure. The choice of treatment depends on disease activity and extent of pathology, client acceptability, and mode of drug delivery.

C. Histologically, most of the pathology of UC is limited to the mucosa and submucosa. The extent of UC is defined as follows:

1. Pan-ulcerative (total colitis): Extensive disease with evidence of UC proximal to the splenic flexure. Massive dilation of the colon (toxic megacolon) may lead to bowel perforation.

2. Left-sided disease: Continuous UC that is present from the rectum and the descending colon up to, but not proximal to, the splenic flexure

3. Proctosigmoiditis: Disease limited to the rectum and sigmoid colon involvement

4. Ulcerative proctitis: Disease limited to the rectum—usually less than the full rectum

D. In 2015, the Toronto Consensus Clinical Practice Guidelines for the Management of Nonhospitalized UC provided 34 recommendations, including statements on 5-ASA, corticosteroids, immunosuppressants, anti-TNF

TABLE 11.19 DEFINITION OF SEVERITY OF ULCERATIVE COLITIS

Mild UC	• ≤4 bloody stools/d with or without blood
	• No systemic toxicity
	• Normal ESR
	• Mild abdominal pain or cramping
Moderate UC	• >4 bloody stools/d
	• No signs of systemic toxicity
	• Pulse < 90 beats per minute
	• Temperature < 37.5°C (99.5°F)
	• Hgb > 10.5 g/dL
	• ESR < 30 mm/hr
	• Moderate abdominal pain
Acute severe UC[a]	• ≥6 bloody stools/d or observable massive and significant blood BM *and*
	• One or more symptoms of systemic toxicity
	• Tachycardia > 90 beats per minute
	• Temperature > 37.8°C (100.4°F)
	• Hgb > 10.5 g/dL
	• Increased ESR (>30 mm/hr)
Fulminant UC	• >10 stools/d
	• Continuous rectal bleeding
	• Systemic toxicity
	• Tachycardia > 90 beats per minute
	• Fever > 37.8°C (100.4°F)
	• Anemia requiring blood transfusions
	• Abdominal tenderness and distention
	• Colonic dilation on radiography
	• May lead to toxic megacolon or colonic perforation

[a]Acute severe colitis is defined by Truelove and Witt's Criteria (1955).

ESR, erythrocyte sedimentation rate; UC, ulcerative colitis.

therapy, and other agents, including probiotics. The guidelines are available at www.gastrojournal.org/article/S0016-5085(15)00303-0/abstract and www.gastrojournal.org/article/S0016-5085(18)35407-6/pdf.
E. The 2015 Toronto Consensus Guidelines defined remission and response with UC as:
 1. Complete remission: Both symptomatic remission and endoscopic healing defined as follows:
  a. Endoscopic healing: Normal mucosa, vascular blurring, or chronic changes (e.g., inflammatory polyps, scarring) without friability
  b. **Symptomatic remission: Normal stool frequency (less than or equal to 3/d) and no blood in the stool**

2. **Symptomatic response: Meaningful improvement in symptoms as judged by both the client and the physician in the absence of remission; response should not be considered a desirable final outcome but is useful to assess early response to treatment.**

Incidence
A. The annual incidence of UC is 10.4 to 12 per 100,000, depending on the country.
B. UC is three times more common than CD.
C. The most common cause of death in clients with UC is toxic megacolon.
D. Adenocarcinoma of the colon develops in 3% to 5% of clients with UC; the risk increases with the duration of the disease.
E. **Approximately 6.2% of clients with IBD have a major extraintestinal manifestation:**
 1. **Uveitis is the most common: 3.8%**
 2. **Primary sclerosing cholangitis (PSC): 3%**
 3. **Ankylosing spondylitis: 2.7%**
 4. **Erythema nodosum: 1.9%**
 5. **Pyoderma gangrenosum: 1.2%**

Pathogenesis
A. The exact etiology is unknown.
B. UC may be considered an autoimmune disease. Persons with UC often have p-antineutrophil cytoplasmic antibodies (p-ANCAs). Abnormalities of humoral and cell-mediated immunity and/or generalized enhanced reactivity against intestinal bacterial antigen may also be causes of UC.

Predisposing Factors
A. Caucasian
B. Jewish descent
C. Affects 30% more females than males
D. Genetic susceptibility: Family history is associated with a higher risk of developing the disease.

Common Complaints
A. Frequent small-volume diarrhea
B. Bloody diarrhea with or without mucus
C. Severe bowel urgency
D. Abdominal cramps and pain with BM
E. Constipation in clients with distal disease
F. Anorexia
G. Anemia
H. Nocturnal BMs

Other Signs and Symptoms
A. Tenesmus (rectal urgency/constant feeling of need to pass stool)
B. Abdominal tenderness
C. Arthralgias
D. Fatigue secondary to anemia
E. FTT in children
F. Severe UC:
 1. Fever
 2. Tachycardia
 3. Significant abdominal tenderness
 4. Signs of volume depletion

Subjective Data

A. Review the onset, duration, signs, and symptoms (number of stools, presence/absence of blood in the stool, fever, and abdominal pain).

B. Review the client's recent history of travel or camping trips for the presence of intestinal infection.

C. Review the client's medication history including antibiotics and NSAIDs: One-third of clients with exacerbation of UC report recent NSAID use).

D. Review family history for IBD, celiac disease, and CRC.

E. Review the client's smoking status.

F. Review the client's history or contact related to TB (testing required before biological therapy).

G. Evaluate if the client has symptoms of uveitis including light sensitivity, floaters, blurry vision, or pain/tenderness to touch.

Physical Examination

A. Check temperature (if indicated), pulse, BP, and weight. Follow serial weights.

B. Inspect:
1. Observe the client's general overall appearance for nutritional status, cachexia, and pallor.
2. Observe the perianal region for the presence of tags, fissures, fistulas, and abscess.
3. Observe the abdomen for distention and presence of surgical scars.
4. Examine the eyes for redness, irritation, and ocular complications (episcleritis, scleritis, and uveitis).
5. Evaluate for the presence of dermatological findings, including erythema nodosum and pyoderma gangrenosum.

C. Auscultate:
1. Heart
2. Lungs
3. Abdomen: All four quadrants

D. Percuss:
1. Abdomen for organomegaly, masses, ascites, and hepatic tenderness

E. Palpate:
1. Palpate all four quadrants of the abdomen, observing for tenderness, rebound, and guarding.
2. Evaluate for the presence of hepatomegaly.
3. Perform a digital rectal examination to assess for anal strictures and rectal masses.
4. Palpate the joints for warmth, tenderness, and range of motion.

Diagnostic Tests

A. **Diagnosis is best made with endoscopy and biopsy.**

B. Laboratory tests:
1. CBC with electrolytes
2. Platelet count
3. Sedimentation rate
4. CRP
5. CMV (chronic immunosuppressive steroids)
6. HIV

C. Stool testing:
1. Evaluate bacterial, viral, or parasitic causes of diarrhea.
2. Occult blood
3. Fecal leukocytes

D. Plain abdominal radiograph

E. CT scan

F. MRI

G. Ultrasound

H. DCBE

I. Celiac antibody testing should be considered.

J. Intestinal TB testing should be considered.

Differential Diagnoses

A. UC

B. Ischemic colitis (especially in the elderly)

C. Toxic megacolon

D. Colon cancer

E. Adenocarcinoma

F. Rectal cancer

G. Radiation colitis

H. Intestinal infections

I. Intestinal lymphoma

J. Chronic diverticulitis

K. Amebiasis

L. CD

Plan

A. General interventions:
1. See Table 11.19 for the definition of severity of UC.
2. Severe UC should be managed jointly by a gastroenterologist in conjunction with a colorectal surgeon (Table 11.20).
3. Stress reduction and stress management may improve symptoms.
4. Pretreatment screening for TB, using Mantoux (a PPD) skin testing, is needed before initiation of immunomodulators and thiopurines.
5. Immunization status:
   a. Immunizations with inactivated vaccine should be brought up to date and rigorously maintained during treatment, including influenza, meningococcal, and pneumococcal immunizations.
   b. Check varicella titers prior to treatment with immunomodulators and reimmunize if titers are low.

TABLE 11.20 MANAGEMENT OF MILD-TO-MODERATE DISTAL ULCERATIVE COLITIS WITH TOPICAL AGENTS

Topical agent	Proximal extent/distribution of agent
Suppository	10 cm
Hydrocortisone foam	15–20 cm
Enema	As far as the splenic flexure

Source: Adapted from AGA Clinical Practice Guidelines of Management of Mild-to-Moderate Ulcerative Colitis (2019).

c. The risk of administering live vaccines (polio, rubella, and yellow fever) to clients on immuno-modulators has not been established; however, most experts avoid live vaccines during treatment.

B. Client teaching:

▶ 1. *See Section III: Client Teaching Guide for this chapter, "Crohn's Disease."*

C. Pharmaceutical therapy:

1. Refer to the ACG Practice Guidelines for full treatment algorithms at s3.gi.org/physicians/guide-lines/UlcerativeColitis.pdf or the 2015 Toronto Consensus Guidelines for the Management of UC algorithms at www.cag-acg.org/images/publications/cpg_toronto_consensus_on_uc_may2015.pdf.

2. The choice of topical agents is guided by the proximal distribution of UC into the bowel, as well as client preference (see Table 11.20).

3. Stepwise medication approach (see Table 11.6): The 5-ASA class of anti-inflammatory drugs is the most common treatment for clients with mild (less than four bloody stools per day) or moderate active disease (more than four bloody stools a day without systemic toxicity):

a. Sulfasalazine (Azulfidine) for mild-to-moder-ate UC and remission maintenance:

i. Pediatrics: 50 to 75 mg/kg each 24 hours, divided into three to four doses

ii. **Reduced absorption of folic acid and digoxin has been reported when they are administered with sulfasalazine.**

b. Balsalazide (Colazal) for mild-to-moderate UC and remission maintenance:

i. Induction: 6.75 g/d, three times daily dosing

ii. Maintenance: 2 to 6.75 g/d, twice daily dosing

iii. Pediatric dose: 5 years or older: 750 mg, three times daily dosing for up to 8 weeks

4. Mesalamine for mild-to-moderate UC and remis-sion maintenance:

a. Asacol:

i. Pediatrics: For clients 5 years or older, dosage is weight based (up to a maximum of 2.4 g/d), divided into two daily doses for a duration of 6 weeks.

ii. **Two Asacol 400 mg tablets are not inter-changeable or substitutable with one mesa-lamine delayed-release 800 mg tablet.**

b. Apriso: 1.5 mg/d orally in the morning

c. Salofalk: 1 to 4 g/d in one or two divided doses:

1. Also available as a suppository, rectal sus-pension, and enema

d. Pentasa: 1 g/d orally, four times daily dosing for up to 8 weeks:

1. Also available as a suppository

e. MMX marketed as Lialda: Active to moder-ate UC:

i. Induction: 2.4 to 4.8 g/d for up to 8 weeks

ii. Maintenance: 2.4 g/d

iii. *Lialda is not recommended for children younger than 18 years.*

f. Rowasa enema: 4 g/60 mL rectally at bedtime; retain for approximately 8 hours.

g. Mesalamine (Canasa) suppository 1 g/d at bedtime; retain in the rectum for at least 1 to 3 hours. Treat active proctitis for 3 to 6 weeks.

5. Corticosteroids suppress the immune system and are used for moderate-to-severe UC.

a. Prednisone (Deltasone, Orasone):

i. Induction: 40 to 60 mg/d by mouth for 7 to 14 days, followed by gradual taper by 5 mg/wk

ii. Maintenance: 2.5 to 5 mg/wk

b. Budesonide (Entocort EC):

1. Pediatric: For clients 8 to 17 years old who weigh more than 25 kg: 9 mg orally for up to 8 weeks, followed by 6 mg once a day for 2 weeks

6. Immune modifiers are used to decrease cortico-steroid dosage.

a. Azathioprine (AZA; Imuran) 2 to 3 mg/kg/d orally:

i. Monitoring includes CBC, including platelet counts weekly during the first month, twice monthly for the second and third months of therapy, then monthly or more fre-quently if dosage alteration is necessary.

ii. TPMT testing: Testing is recommended for either genotype- or phenotype-identified clients for TPMT.

b. 6-MP (Purinethol) 1 to 1.5 mg/kg/d orally:

i. Clients with little or no inherited TPMT activity are at increased risk for severe Purinethol toxicity and generally require sub-stantial dose reduction.

ii. Pediatrics: 1.0 to 2.0 mg/kg/d orally (maximum of 150 mg/d)

c. Cyclosporine (Neoral, Sandimmune):

i. IV infusion: 2 to 4 mg/kg/d

ii. Can be switched to a doubled oral dose for outpatient therapy; used only short term

7. Antibiotics:

a. Ciprofloxacin (Cipro) 500 mg orally twice a day

b. Metronidazole (Flagyl)

8. Biological therapy (anti-TNF agents) for mod-erate-to-severe UC. **A tuberculin skin test is rec-ommended before therapy. Clients started on infliximab should also be screened for hepatitis B before initiating therapy.**

a. Infliximab (Remicade) infusion therapy has a half-life of approximately 10 days.

b. Adalimumab (Humira) for the treatment of moderate-to-severe UC:

1. *Pediatrics: Not recommended for those younger than 18 years*

c. Golimumab (Simponi):

i. Initial dosage: 200 mg subcutaneously at week 0

ii. Second dose (week 2): 100 mg

iii. Maintenance dose: 100 mg every 4 weeks

d. Vedolizumab (Entyvio):

i. Initial dose: 300 mg IV at weeks 0, 2, and 6

ii. Maintenance dose: 300 mg IV every 8 weeks of therapy

iii. **Discontinue if no evidence of therapeutic benefit by week 14**

D. Dietary management:

1. Adequate nutrition is critical to promotion of healing. Sufficient protein and calories limit the stress on an inflamed bowel.

2. Many clients with UC have concurrent lactose intolerance. (See Appendix B for lactose-intolerance dietary recommendations.)

3. Decrease dietary fiber during increased disease activity.

4. A low-residue diet may decrease the frequency of BMs.

5. A high-residue diet may be helpful in ulcerative proctitis when constipation is the dominant symptom (see Appendix B, Table B.6).

E. Surgical management:

1. Indications for considering a total colectomy:

a. Failed medical therapy: Refractory UC

b. Severe hemorrhage

c. Fulminate colitis not responsive to treatment

d. Toxic megacolon

e. Obstruction or stricture

f. FTT in children

2. Indications for considering elective surgery:

a. Long-term steroid dependence

b. Dysplasia or adenocarcinoma found on screening biopsy

c. Disease present 7 to 10 years

Follow-Up

A. Screening colonoscopy is recommended for all clients with UC for 8 years after the onset of symptoms due to the increase in colonic neoplasia; it should be repeated every 5 years if they do not have any intermediate or high risk factors.

B. Clients with extensive UC or left-sided colitis with negative findings on the screening colonoscopy should begin surveillance colonoscopy in 1 to 2 years.

C. Clients with mild-to-moderate inflammation and a first-degree relative with CRC are considered intermediate risk; screening colonoscopy is recommended every 3 years.

D. Annual screening colonoscopy is recommended for clients with high risk factors including presence of PSC, moderate-to-severe active inflammation sustained over time, first-degree relative with CRC at an age younger than 50 years, or stenosis or dysplasia detected during the previous 5 years.

E. Steroids should not be used as maintenance therapy. Clients who require long-term steroids are at increased risk of osteoporosis.

F. Subsequent laboratory monitoring tests depend on the prescribed therapy.

G. Rates of anxiety and depression are higher in clients with IBD. Screen for depression at each visit.

Consultation/Referral

A. Gastroenterologist for confirmatory diagnosis with a colonoscopy

B. Surgeon for severe or fulminant colitis. Toxic megacolon is a life-threatening complication and requires urgent surgical intervention.

C. Clients with ocular complications require an urgent consultation.

D. Clients who have had UC for 8 to 10 years are at risk of colon cancer; therefore, colonoscopy for surveillance is recommended.

Individual Considerations

A. Pediatrics:

1. UC is uncommon in persons younger than 10 years.

2. Fulminant disease occurs more in children than in adults.

3. Children may present with systemic complaints, including fatigue, arthritis, failure to gain weight, and delayed puberty.

B. Adults:

1. Live vaccinations should not be administered to immunocompromised clients. If required, vaccines should be administered at the time of UC diagnosis.

a. The flu and pneumonia vaccines should be routinely administered.

b. Consider administering the human papillomavirus vaccine.

2. Women with IBD have reported to have a high incidence of abnormal Pap smears. Adherence to Pap smear guidelines are recommended by the ACG.

3. Abnormal sperm counts, motility, and morphology are seen with sulfasalazine.

Resources

American College of Gastroenterology: gi.org

Crohn's and Colitis Foundation of America: www.ccfa .org

Bibliography

Basson, M. D. (2015, November 18). Ulcerative colitis. *Medscape*. Retrieved from http://emedicine.medscape.com/article/183084-overview

Bressler, B., Marshall, J. K., Berstein, C. N., Bitton, A., Jones, J., Leontiadis, G. I., & Fegan, B. (2015). Clinical practice guidelines for the medical management of nonhospitalized ulcerative colitis: The Toronto consensus. *Gastroenterology, 148*, 1035–1058. doi:10.1053/ j.gastro.2015.03.001

Crohn's and Colitis Foundation of America. (n.d.). *Types of ulcerative colitis*. Retrieved from http://www.ccfa.org/what-are-crohns-and-colitis/what -is-ulcerative-colitis/types-of-ulcerative-colitis.html

Ko, C., Singh, S., Feuerstein, J., Falck-Yttr, C., Falck-Yttr, Y., & Cross, R. (2019). AGA clinical practice guidelines of management of mild-to -moderate ulcerative colitis. American Gastroenterological Association Institute Clinical Guidelines Committee. *Journal of Gastroenterology, 156*(3), 748–764. doi:10.1053/j.gastro.2o18.12.009

Nettina, S. (2010). *The Lippincott manual of nursing practice* (9th ed.). Philadelphia, PA: Wolters Kluwer Lippincott Williams & Wilkins.

12 Genitourinary Guidelines

Benign Prostatic Hypertrophy

Cheryl A. Glass and Debbie Gunter

Definition

A. Benign prostatic hypertrophy (BPH) is enlargement of the prostate gland that constricts the urethra, causing urinary symptoms. BPH is not believed to be a risk factor for prostate cancer. BPH occurs primarily in the central or transitional zone of the prostate, whereas prostate cancer originates primarily in the peripheral part of the prostate (see Figure 12.1).

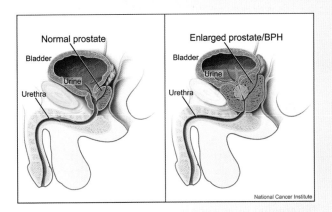

FIGURE 12.1 Benign prostatic hyperplasia (BPH). Flow of urine with a normal prostate (A) and with an enlarged prostate/ BPH (B).

B. The voiding dysfunction that results from prostate enlargement and bladder outlet obstruction (BOO) is termed lower urinary tract symptoms (LUTS).

Incidence

A. BPH increases progressively with age. The prevalence of prostatic hyperplasia increases from 8% in men aged 31 to 40 years to 60% at age 60 and 80% in men 80 years and older.

Pathogenesis

A. The exact cause is unknown; BPH may be a response to the androgen hormone. The process of aging and the presence of circulating androgens lead to the development of BPH. Hyperplasia, in which the normally thin and fibrous outer capsule of the prostate becomes spongy and thick, and the contraction of muscle fibers cause pressure on the urethra. This condition requires the bladder musculature to work harder to empty urine.

Predisposing Factors

A. Advancing age
B. Race: African American men younger than 65 years may need treatment more often than Caucasian men.
C. Genetic predisposition: Increases with a positive family history of BPH having moderate to severe LUTS
D. Obesity
E. Diabetes
F. High levels of alcohol consumption
G. Physical inactivity

Common Complaints

The clinical manifestations of BPH are LUTS that typically appear slowly and progress gradually over a period of years.
A. Difficulty starting urine flow
B. Dribbling at end of urination
C. Bladder does not feel like it completely empties
D. Frequent urination
E. Nocturia

Other Signs and Symptoms

A. Obstructive symptoms:
  1. Hesitancy
  2. Diminution in size and force of urinary stream
  3. Stream interruption (double voiding)
  4. Urinary retention
  5. Straining/Valsalva maneuver to fully empty the bladder
B. Irritative voiding symptoms:
  1. Urgency
  2. Frequency
  3. Nocturia
  4. Painless hematuria: an early symptom; may also indicate malignancy
C. Severe late symptoms with untreated BPH:
  1. Acute urinary retention
  2. Recurrent urinary tract infections (UTIs)
  3. Hydronephrosis

4. Loss of renal concentrating ability
5. Systemic acidosis and renal failure

Subjective Data

A. Have the client complete the American Urological Association Symptom Score (AUASS) assessment tool at each visit to track symptoms. The AUASS (see Table 12.1) is used to assess the severity of symptoms of BPH.

B. Review the onset, duration, and course of symptoms. The AUASS assessment tool can be used to quantitatively assess BPH symptoms over time.

C. Does the client have signs of a UTI?

D. Is there any blood in the urine or pain in the bladder region? (Evaluate bladder tumor or calculi.)

E. Does the client have new symptoms such as bone or back pain, loss of appetite, or weight loss (rule out cancer)?

F. Review the client's history for medical illness, including diabetes and neurologic problems.

G. Review previous urinary problems, surgeries, infections, treatments, success of treatments, and testing.

H. Review the client's history of sexual dysfunction, any new sexual partners, and sexually transmitted infections (STIs).

I. Review the client's history of urethral trauma, urethritis, or urethral instrumentation that could have led to urethral stricture.

J. Review medications, both prescription and over-the-counter (OTC) drugs, including sinus or cold products, anticholinergic drugs (impair bladder function), and sympathomimetic drugs (increase outflow resistance).

K. Review family history of BPH and prostate cancer.

L. Review fluid intake, especially caffeinated/carbonated drinks.

M. Evaluate how bothersome the symptoms are to the client's quality of life:
1. How often does he have interrupted sleep to get up to go to the bathroom?
2. How often does he urinate?
3. Does he have to wear an absorptive underwear pad?

Physical Examination

A. Check temperature (if indicated), blood pressure (BP), and weight (if indicated).

B. Inspect:
1. Inspect general appearance for discomfort or acute discomfort with urinary retention.
2. Consider having the client void: Normal urination for a man is the ability to empty the bladder of 300 mL of urine in 12 to 15 seconds.
3. Examine the urethral meatus for discharge.
4. Retract foreskin (if present) and assess for hygiene and smegma.
5. Check the shaft of the penis, glans, and prepuce for lesions.
6. Check inguinal and femoral areas for bulges or hernias; have the client bear down and cough, and reexamine him.
7. Perform a neurologic examination (evaluate sensory and motor deficits).

C. Palpate:
1. Palpate the abdomen for masses or bladder distension.
2. Palpate lymph nodes in the groin for enlargement.
3. Check costovertebral angle (CVA) tenderness.
4. Palpate the testes and epididymides for inflammation, tenderness, and masses.
5. Palpate the scrotum for hydrocele or varicocele.

D. Digital rectal examination (DRE): use the index finger of the dominant hand for the DRE.
1. Note sphincter tone, nodules or masses, and tenderness. Decreased anal sphincter tone or the lack of muscle reflex may indicate an underlying neurologic disorder.
2. Palpate the two lateral lobes of the prostate gland and its median sulcus for irregularities, nodules, induration, swelling, or tenderness just above the prostate anteriorly; determine whether the rectum lies adjacent to the peritoneal cavity. If possible, palpate this region for peritoneal masses and tenderness.

Diagnostic Tests

A. Urinalysis: evaluate for infection and hematuria.

B. Urine culture if indicated (clients with BPH are more susceptible to UTIs)

C. Optional studies:
1. Prostate-specific antigen (PSA): Reference ranges vary by age and ethnicity and may be elevated with BPH. Recommended in men with at least a 10-year life expectancy
2. Urodynamic testing, including maximal urinary flow rate
3. Postvoid residual (PVR; as shown by in–out catheterization, radiography, or ultrasound)
4. Cystourethroscopy: Not recommended in the initial routine evaluation visit (may be needed later depending on workup for planning for surgical therapy)

D. The American Urological Association (AUA) holds that the routine measurement of serum creatinine levels is *not* indicated in the initial evaluation.

Differential Diagnoses

A. Other obstructive causes: prostate cancer, urethral obstruction, urethral stricture, and vesical neck obstruction

B. Neurogenic bladder

C. Cystitis

D. Prostatitis

E. Bladder calculi

Plan

A. General interventions:
1. Have the client complete a 24-hour voiding chart with assessment of frequency and volume.
2. Any client with other than mild symptoms needs referral to a urologist to discuss treatment options (surgery or drugs).
3. Monitor the client with mild symptoms every 3 to 6 months to determine the progression of symptoms. Imaging studies are not routinely necessary in typical

TABLE 12.1   AMERICAN UROLOGICAL ASSOCIATION SYMPTOM SCORE FOR BENIGN PROSTATIC HYPERTROPHY (BPH)

CLIENT NAME: _____

TODAY'S DATE: _____

(Circle One Number on Each Line)	Not at All	Less Than One Time in Five	Less Than Half the Time	About Half the Time	More Than Half the Time	Almost Always
Over the past month or so, how often have you had a sensation of not emptying your bladder completely after you finished urinating?	0	1	2	3	4	5
During the past month or so, how often have you had to urinate again less than 2 hours after you finished urinating?	0	1	2	3	4	5
During the past month or so, how often have you found you stopped and started again several times when you urinated?	0	1	2	3	4	5
During the past month or so, how often have you found it difficult to postpone urination?	0	1	2	3	4	5
During the past month or so, how often have you had a weak urinary stream?	0	1	2	3	4	5
During the past month or so, how often have you had to push or strain to begin urination?	0	1	2	3	4	5
	None	Once	Two Times	Three Times	Four Times	Five or More Times

CLIENT NAME: _____

TODAY'S DATE: _____

(Circle One Number on Each Line)	Not at All	Less Than One Time in Five	Less Than Half the Time	About Half the Time	More Than Half the Time	Almost Always
Over the past month, how many times per night did you most typically get up to urinate from the time you went to bed at night until the time you got up in the morning?	0	1	2	3	4	5

Add the score for each number above and write the total in the space to the right.   **TOTAL:** _____

SYMPTOM SCORE: 1–7 (Mild);   8–19 (Moderate);   20–35 (Severe)

Quality of Life (QOL)						
	Delighted	Pleased	Mostly Satisfied	Mixed	Mostly Dissatisfied	Unhappy	Terrible
How would you feel if you had to live with your urinary condition the way it is now, no better, no worse, for the rest of your life?	0	1	2	3	4	5	6

Source: American Urological Association (AUA) Education and Research Inc.

▶

cases of BPH unless there is hematuria, an elevated creatinine, or another indication.

4. Treat concurrent UTI and STIs.

B. Client teaching:

1. Client teaching: *See Section III: Client Teaching Guide for this chapter, "Prostatic Hypertrophy/Benign."*

2. Client should be instructed about the hypotensive effect, asthenia, nasal congestion, and effect on ejaculation of the long-acting alpha-1 antagonists. The hypotensive effects can be potentiated by concomitant use of phosphodiesterase-5 (PDE-5) inhibitors sildenafil (Viagra), tadalafil (Cialis), or vardenafil (Levitra).

3. Alpha-1 antagonists have been associated with intraoperative floppy iris syndrome. Clients need to discuss using these medicines with their ophthalmologist before eye surgery (i.e., cataract).

C. Pharmaceutical therapy:

1. Five long-acting alpha-1 antagonists are Food and Drug Administration (FDA) approved for the treatment of BPH. Two are selective alpha-1 blockers and three are nonselective alpha-1 blockers.

   a. Terazosin (Hytrin) 1 to 20 mg/d; side effect increases hypotensive effect with PDE-5 inhibitor. Terazosin requires dose titration to minimize side effects (nonselective).

   b. Doxazosin (Cardura) 1 to 8 mg/d; side effect increases hypotensive effect with PDE-5 inhibitor. Doxazosin requires dose titration to minimize side effects (nonselective).

   c. Tamsulosin (Flomax) 0.4 to 0.8 mg/d; side effect decreases ejaculate volume (selective).

   d. Alfuzosin (Uroxatral) 10 mg/d; generally does not cause ejaculation problems.

   e. Silodosin (Rapaflo) 8 mg/d; side effect may produce retrograde ejaculation (selective).

2. Prazosin (Minipress), a short-acting alpha-1 antagonist, is approved for the treatment of HTN. It improves urine flow rates and may be considered for a client with HTN and urinary symptoms.

3. Two 5-alpha-reductase inhibitors (ARI) are FDA approved for BPH with an enlarged prostate and bothersome LUTS. These medications help reduce the risk of acute urinary retention and the need for surgical interventions. The major side effects of these drugs are decreased libido and ejaculatory or erectile dysfunction.

   a. The FDA has issued safety information for the use of the 5-alpha-reductase inhibitors because of an increased risk of being diagnosed with a more serious form of prostate cancer (high-grade prostate cancer).

   b. Women who are, or may become, pregnant should not handle the 5-alpha-reductase inhibitors. The inhibitors are pregnancy category X drugs known to cause birth defects.

   c. Finasteride (Proscar) 5 mg/d

   d. Dutasteride (Avodart) 0.5 mg/d

   e. Dutasteride–tamsulosin (Jalyn): Each capsule contains 0.5 mg dutasteride and 0.4 mg tamsulosin.

4. Dual-drug combination with an alpha blocker and a 5-alpha-reductase inhibitor can be used if a single agent is not effective.

5. There are no herbal supplements that have been approved by the FDA for the treatment of BPH; however, clients may report taking saw palmetto. The AUA does not endorse supplements.

Follow-Up

A. See the client in 2 to 3 weeks to monitor symptoms after specialty referral.

B. The concept of "watchful waiting" may be appropriate for clients with mild symptoms. The client should be seen yearly for evaluation and an examination.

C. PSA detects BPH more commonly than cancer, and the U.S. Preventive Services Task Force (USPSTF) current recommendations suggest the screening be implemented as a shared decision between client and the healthcare provider. The USPSTF advises to routinely discuss the client's desire for screening for men that are between the ages of 55 to 69, have a family history of prostate cancer, African descent, or lower socioeconomic status. The Task Force does not recommend screening for men above 70 years old.

Consultation/Referral

A. Refer to a urologist for any complicated LUTS, including:

1. History of prostate cancer
2. Elevated PSA
3. Urethral stricture
4. Spinal cord injury
5. Stroke
6. Recurrent/persistent UTI

B. The presence of microscopic hematuria requires an evaluation of the complete urinary system and needs a referral to a urologist.

C. Refer for procedures after failed medication therapy:

1. Minimally invasive surgical therapies (MIST) should be used in a select client group, particularly those that place importance on preserved sexual and continence function, rather than urinary improvement.

   a. Transurethral microwave therapy (TUMT)

   b. Transurethral incision of the prostate (TUIP)

   c. Transurethral vaporization of the prostate (TUVP)

   d. Laser enucleation

   e. Laser therapies

   f. Prostatic urethral life (PUL)

   g. Water vapor thermal therapy (WVTT)

   h. Photoselective vaporization of the prostate (PVP)

2. Surgical therapies:

   a. Transurethral resection of the prostate (TURP) is considered the gold standard of surgical treatment of BPH. Sexual dysfunction may occur after a TURP, including decreased libido, impotence, and ejaculatory difficulties. Balloon dilation may be used to reduce symptoms; however, relapse is common.

   b. Open prostatectomy

   c. Simple prostatectomy

Individual Consideration

A. Geriatrics: Elderly men require special attention because their symptoms may be poorly expressed or confusing.

Resources

Adult Pediatric Urology & Urogynecology: www.adult pediatricuro.com

American Urological Association (AUA): www.auanet.org

National Kidney Urologic Diseases Information Clearing-house (KNUDIC): kidney.niddk.nih.gov

Bibliography

American Urological Association. (2010, revised 2018). *American Urological Association guideline: Surgical management of lower urinary tract symptoms attributed to benign prostatic hyperplasia.* Retrieved from https://www.auanet.org/guidelines/benign-prostatic-hyperplasia-(bph)-guideline#x8215

American Urological Association. (2010, revised 2018). *American Urological Association guideline: Management of benign prostatic hyperplasia (BPH).* Retrieved from https://www.auanet.org/guidelines/benign-prostatic-hyperplasia-(bph)-guideline

American Urological Association. (2016, July). *Education and research Inc. American urologic association symptom score.* Retrieved from https://www.auanet.org

Associates in Urology. (n.d.). *Patient questionnaire: AUA symptom score (AUASS).* Retrieved from https://bsci-prod2-origin.adobecqms.net/content/dam/bostonscientific-anz/patients/downloads/Enlarged_Prostate_Symptom_Score_Questionnaire.pdf

Christidis, D., McGrath, S., Perera, M. (2017). Minimally invasive surgical therapies for benign prostatic hypertrophy: The rise in minimally invasive surgical therapies. *Prostate International, 5*(2), 41–46. doi:10.1016/j.prnil.2017.01.007

Deters, L. A. (2019, January 15). Benign prostatic hypertrophy. *Medscape.* Retrieved from emedicine.medscape.com/article/437359-overview

Chronic Kidney Disease in Adults

Angelito Tacderas and Debbie Gunter

Definition

Chronic kidney disease (CKD) is specifically defined as follows:

A. The persistent and usually progressive reduction in glomerular filtration rate (GFR) less than 60 mL/min/1.73 m^2 and/or

B. Albuminuria: more than 30 mg of urinary albumin per gram of urinary creatinine

CKD is a disorder that leads to progressive kidney damage from a variety of causes, including diabetes, HTN, cardiovascular (CV) disease, urinary obstructions, prolonged use of nephrotoxic medications, and inherited diseases such as polycystic kidney disease. Associated comorbidities of CKD include renal osteodystrophy, anemia, metabolic acidosis, and malnutrition. Early recognition of CKD as well as treatment of complications can improve long-term outcomes.

Stages of CKD

A. Stage 1 disease is defined by a normal GFR (>90 mL/min/1.73 m^2) and persistent albuminuria.

B. Stage 2 disease is a GFR between 60 and 89 mL/min/1.73 m^2 and persistent albuminuria.

C. Stage 3 disease is a GFR between 30 and 59 mL/min/1.73 m^2.

D. Stage 4 disease is a GFR between 15 and 29 mL/min/1.73 m^2.

E. Stage 5 disease is a GFR of less than 15 mL/min/1.73 m^2 or end-stage renal disease (ESRD).

Incidence

A. Kidney disease is the ninth leading cause of death in the United States. It is estimated that 15% of Americans are living with CKD. It is estimated that 80,000 new cases of nondialysis-dependent CKD are diagnosed annually; the incidence of CKD and ESRD has doubled every decade since 1980. The number of clients enrolled in the ESRD Medicare-funded program has increased from approximately 10,000 beneficiaries in 1973 to 517,776 as of December 31, 2016. Those who live with ESRD are 1% of the U.S. Medicare population but account for 7% of the Medicare budget. More than 100,000 clients in the United States are on the kidney transplant list, yet in 2017 there were just over 21,000 donor organs available for transplant. The need for donor kidneys in the United States is rising at 8% per year.

B. By age group, CKD is more prevalent among persons older than 65 years (38%) than among persons aged 40 to 65 years (13%) or persons aged 18 to 44 years (7%). CKD is more common in women (15%) than men (12%). CKD prevalence is greater among persons with diabetes than among those without diabetes (40.2% vs. 15.4%) and among persons with CV disease than among those without CV disease (28.2% vs. 15.4%). CKD is higher among persons with HTN than among those without HTN (24.6% vs. 12.5%). In addition, CKD prevalence is greater among non-Hispanic Blacks (16%) and Mexican Americans (14%) than among non-Hispanic Whites (13%).

Pathogenesis

Blood from the renal arteries and their subdivisions is delivered to the glomeruli. The glomeruli form an ultrafiltrate, nearly free of protein and blood elements, which subsequently flows into the renal tubules. The tubules reabsorb and secrete solute and/or water from the ultrafiltrate. The final tubular fluid, the urine, leaves the kidney, draining sequentially into the renal pelvis, ureter, and bladder, from which it is excreted through the urethra. The causes of CKD are traditionally classified by which portion of the renal anatomy is most affected by the disorder.

A. Vascular disease: Vascular disorders of the kidneys may involve partial or complete occlusion of large, medium, or small renal vessels. Examples of macrovascular or large renal vessel disease are renal artery stenosis and atherosclerotic disease. Benign hypertensive arteriolar nephrosclerosis results when chronic HTN damages small blood vessels, glomeruli, renal tubules, and interstitial tissues. Glomerulosclerosis is a severe microvascular or small vessel kidney disease caused by diabetes and uncontrolled HTN in which glomerular function of blood filtration is lost as fibrous scar tissue replaces the glomeruli. Loss of glomerular function leads to proteinuria, hematuria,

HTN, and nephrosis, with variable progression to ESRD. Proteinuria occurs because of changes to capillary endothelial cells, the glomerular basement membrane (GBM), or podocytes, which normally filter serum protein selectively by size and charge.

B. Tubular and interstitial disease: As with vascular disease, chronic tubulointerstitial nephritis (CTIN) can be primary or secondary to glomerular damage and renovascular disease. CTIN arises when chronic tubular insults cause gradual interstitial infiltration and fibrosis, tubular atrophy and dysfunction, and a gradual deterioration of renal function, usually over years. Causes of CTIN are immune disorders, infections, reflux or obstructive nephropathy, and drugs. Analgesic abuse nephropathy (AAN) is a type of CTIN caused by cumulative lifetime use of large amounts of certain analgesics such as nonsteroidal anti-inflammatory drugs (NSAIDs).

Predisposing Factors

A. Diabetes
B. HTN
C. CV disease
D. Chronic use of analgesics such as NSAIDs
E. Autoimmune disorder
F. Polycystic kidney disease
G. Urinary tract obstructions such as BPH or kidney stones
H. Recurrent UTIs
I. Older than 60 years
J. African American, Native American, or Hispanic ethnicity
K. Smoking
L. Exposure to toxins
M. Family history of kidney disease

Common Complaints

A. In CKD Stages 1 and 2 there are usually no presenting complaints; however, HTN is usually present. CKD is usually identified through routine screening of kidney function and urine tests for microalbumin.

Other Signs and Symptoms

A. In CKD Stage 3, the person will develop CKD complications but will usually still not have identifiable signs/symptoms:
  1. HTN
  2. Decreased dietary calcium absorption
  3. Reduced renal phosphate excretion
  4. Elevation of parathyroid hormone
  5. Altered lipoprotein metabolism
  6. Reduced spontaneous protein intake
  7. Anemia
  8. Left ventricular hypertrophy
  9. Salt and water retention
  10. Decreased renal potassium excretion
B. These complications gradually worsen as the person moves to Stage 4 CKD. The person will begin to display signs and symptoms of complications:
  1. Changes in bone density
  2. Fatigue and pallor related to anemia
  3. Edema
  4. Decrease in muscle mass
C. As the CKD progresses to Stage 5, in addition to gradual worsening of the signs/symptoms noted in Stages 3 and 4, the person will experience symptoms indicating chronic uremia:
  1. Impaired sleep
  2. Nocturia
  3. Fatigue
  4. Anorexia, nausea, vomiting, and weight change
  5. Decreased mental acuity
  6. Pruritus
  7. Edema
  8. Respiratory symptoms, including orthopnea and dyspnea
  9. Muscle cramps, twitching, and restless legs
  10. Peripheral neuropathy

Subjective Data

A. Review the client's medical history to identify risk factors for CKD (previously noted in "Predisposing Factors" section).
B. Elicit information about how well risk factors such as diabetes mellitus (DM) and HTN are controlled.
C. Review the onset and duration of signs/symptoms of CKD complications and uremia.
D. Review all medications—including all OTC medications, especially NSAIDs, and supplements. Obtain specific information about dosing and length of time the drug was used.
E. Elicit smoking history.

Physical Examination

A. Observe general demeanor, attentiveness, and signs of fatigue.
B. Measure:
  1. Height, weight, and body mass index (BMI)
  2. Vital signs, including orthostatic BP and pulse
C. Inspect:
  1. Skin for color, moisture, turgor, and signs of scratching because of chronic pruritus
  2. Neck for jugular venous distension
  3. Abdomen for distension
  4. Extremities for edema, muscle mass, and signs of pain disorders such as arthritis
D. Auscultate:
  1. Lungs for crackles
  2. Heart for cardiac heave, gallop, or rub
  3. Abdomen for bruit
E. Palpate:
  1. Abdomen for masses, distension
  2. Bladder and assess for flank tenderness
F. Neurologic examination:
  1. Assess for sensation and vibratory sense on both feet.

Diagnostic Tests

Laboratory testing is critical in ascertaining the stage, course, chronicity, and complications (and associated comorbid conditions) of CKD.

A. Routine kidney function tests:
  1. Serum creatinine
  2. Blood urea nitrogen (BUN)
  3. Urinalysis
  4. Measuring GFR: The severity of CKD should be classified based on the level of the estimated GFR (eGFR). Serum creatinine alone should *not* be used as a measure of kidney function. Kidney function in clients with CKD should be assessed by formula-based estimation of GFR (eGFR), preferably using the four-variable Modification of Diet in Renal Disease (MDRD) equation. Clinicians who do not have access to an automated tool may use a web-based tool which is available at https://www.niddk.nih.gov/health-information/communication-programs/nkdep/laboratory-evaluation/glomerular-filtration-rate-calculators.

Calculate eGFRs using the actual MDRD equation:
  eGFR = 186 × (SCr) – 1.154 × (age) – 0.203 × (0.742 if female) × (1.210 if Black)
  (SCr, serum creatinine concentration)

B. Assess proteinuria:
  1. When screening adults at increased risk for CKD, albumin in the urine should be measured in a spot urine sample using:
    a. Albumin-specific dipstick
    b. Albumin-to-creatinine ratio (ACR):
      i. It is usually not necessary to obtain a timed urine collection (overnight or 24 hours).
      ii. First-morning specimens are preferred, but random specimens are acceptable if first-morning specimens are not available.
      iii. In most cases, screening with urine dipsticks is acceptable for detecting proteinuria.
      iv. Standard urine dipsticks are acceptable for detecting increased total urine protein.
      v. Albumin-specific dipsticks are acceptable for detecting albuminuria.
  2. Clients with a positive dipstick test (1 or greater) should undergo confirmation of proteinuria by a quantitative measurement (protein-to-creatinine ratio [PCR] or ACR) within 3 months.
  3. Clients with two or more positive quantitative tests spaced apart by 1 to 2 weeks should be diagnosed as having persistent proteinuria and undergo further evaluation and management for CKD.

Other Tests to Determine CKD Complications

A. Complete blood count (CBC)
B. Hemoglobin (Hgb): If Hgb level is less than 12 g/dL in females and less than 13.5 g/dL in adult males, also do blood cell indices, absolute reticulocyte count, serum iron, total iron-binding capacity, percent transferrin saturation, serum ferritin, white blood cell (WBC) count and differential, platelet count, and testing for blood in stool.
C. Lipid profile and triglycerides
D. Comprehensive metabolic profile (serum total protein, serum albumin, glucose, calcium, sodium, potassium, chloride, bicarbonate, BUN, creatinine, alkaline phosphatase, alanine aminotransferase [ALT], aspartate aminotransferase [AST], bilirubin)
E. Prealbumin
F. Phosphorus
G. Parathyroid hormone
H. Urine immunofixation study
I. Antinuclear antibody (ANA), antineutrophil cytoplasmic autoantibody (ANCA), complement 3 and complement 4 (C3–C4):
  1. Test is done to rule out autoimmune disorder, lupus, vasculitis, and cancer.
  2. No fasting is needed.
J. Hepatitis B surface antigen (HBsAg) and hepatitis C antibody
K. Anti-GBM antibody
L. Renal ultrasound to rule out postobstructive uropathy
M. Renal Doppler to rule out renal artery stenosis

Differential Diagnoses

Evaluation is meant to determine whether kidney disease is acute or chronic and to determine prerenal, intrarenal, or postrenal causation.
A. Acute kidney disease

Plan

The treatment plan focuses on clients in earlier stages of CKD—Stages 1, 2, and 3. Persons with Stages 4 and 5 CKD need specialized interventions provided by nephrologists and should be referred immediately.
A. General interventions:
  1. Provide support to the client.
  2. Initiate appropriate referrals for a nephrologist, client education, and social and financial support as soon as possible.
  3. For Stage 4 or 5 CKD, access devices for hemodialysis, such as a primary arteriovenous fistula or graft, require months to mature and should be in place for 6 months before the start of dialysis.
B. Client teaching: *See Section III: Client Teaching Guide for this chapter, "Kidney Disease: Chronic."* ◄
  1. Instruct the client how the kidneys work and how his or her body is affected by the CKD.
  2. Emphasize the importance of following instructions to prevent further kidney damage:
    a. Follow medication management instructions as carefully as possible.
    b. No OTC medications should be taken that are not approved by the provider.
    c. Keep diabetes and HTN under control to maintain kidney function.
    d. Prevent cardiovascular complications by lowering cholesterol and BP.
    e. Smoking cessation is an important way to prevent worsening kidney function.
    f. Routine follow-ups with provider are necessary to monitor kidney function. Client should be educated and encouraged to keep all appointments.
    g. Follow dietary instructions regarding protein, fats, sodium, and minerals.

h. Dietary intake of protein is usually restricted to 0.8 to 1.0 g/kg/d of high biologic value protein.

i. Dietary sodium should be restricted to no more than 2 g daily.

j. Potassium should be restricted to 40 to 70 meq/d.

k. Calories should be restricted to 35 kcal/kg/d. If the body weight is greater than 120% of normal or the client is older than 60 years, a lower amount may be prescribed.

l. Fat intake should be between 30% and 40% of total daily caloric intake.

m. Phosphorus should be restricted to 600 to 800 mg/d.

n. Calcium should be restricted to 1,400 to 1,600 mg/d.

o. Magnesium should be restricted to 200 to 300 mg/d.

3. Instruct when to notify the provider with urgent signs/symptoms or changes in kidney function.

a. Changes in urine volume

b. Anorexia, nausea, and vomiting

c. Increased edema

d. Shortness of breath (SOB)

e. Increased fatigue

f. Difficulty concentrating

g. Muscle weakness, cramping, or twitching

h. Fever

i. Chest pain

C. Pharmaceutical therapy:

D. General principles of medications used to prevent progression of CKD and to manage symptoms of complications of CKD:

1. Always prescribe the smallest effective dose of any medication.

2. Start with a low dose and gradually increase. Dosage intervals may need to be extended.

3. Monitor the effect of any new medication on kidney function with appropriate follow-up with appropriate laboratory follow-up.

4. Educate the client of signs/symptoms to report to the provider immediately regarding drug therapy.

5. Avoid use of nephrotoxic drugs such as radiographic contrast materials, aminoglycoside antibiotics, and NSAIDs to prevent nephrogenic systemic fibrosis. If radiocontrast material use cannot be avoided because the benefit outweighs the risks, protect the kidney with acetylcysteine (Mucomyst) 600 mg orally twice daily on the day of intravenous (IV) contrast.

6. Immunizations: Some vaccines in usual doses provide protection, while other vaccines require more frequent dosing or larger doses to achieve and maintain protective antibodies. Protective antibody titers may fall and booster doses should be given if appropriate. In general, the recommendations are:

a. Annual influenza vaccination

b. Pneumococcal vaccine with both Prevnar 13 and Pneumovax 23 as recommended by the CDC

c. Hepatitis B vaccine series for clients before starting dialysis

d. All other inactivated vaccines and toxoids according to CDC schedule

7. HTN control and kidney protection: It is recommended that BP goal of 130/80 mmHg or less should be achieved. Use of an angiotensin-converting enzyme (ACE) inhibitor or angiotensin II receptor blocker (ARB) therapy in early stages of CKD with persons who have proteinuria can preserve kidney function. The clinician should monitor serum potassium on initiation of the therapy. It is common for the serum potassium to initially rise and then return to normal levels in 2 to 3 months. Follow-up serum potassium levels are recommended. In the early stages of CKD, with no proteinuria, the ACE inhibitors and ARBs have not been shown to be effective in protecting kidney function. HTN control can still be achieved with the ACE/ARB drugs, but other antihypertensive drugs can be used as well.

8. Fluid overload: Occurs when sodium intake exceeds sodium excretion. The combination of sodium restrictions and a loop diuretic, such as furosemide (Lasix), can lower intraglomerular pressure and provide some kidney protection.

9. Hyperkalemia: Hyperkalemia is managed with a low potassium diet in combination with prescribing a loop diuretic such as furosemide. If a client is on an ACE or ARB, the addition of the loop diuretic will compensate for the elevation of serum potassium related to the ACE/ARB treatment.

10. Metabolic acidosis: Buildup of hydrogen ions causes bicarbonate levels to fall below acceptable levels. Sodium bicarbonate in a daily dose of 0.5 to 1 meq/kg/d is often given. This medication prevents the symptoms of metabolic acidosis, which can increase muscle mass loss and worsen bone disease.

11. Renal osteodystrophy: The development of renal osteodystrophy is caused by hyperphosphatemia and hypocalcemia that are secondary to decreased kidney function. In order to compensate, the client develops secondary hyperparathyroidism. Dietary restriction of phosphate to 800 mg/d is recommended. In Stage 3 CKD, the client will usually require an oral phosphate binder like calcium carbonate or calcium acetate to prevent hyperphosphatemia. Oral phosphate binders must be taken with meals to be effective. It is imperative to avoid phosphate binders that contain aluminum or magnesium. To suppress parathyroid hormone secretion, the client is given calcitriol, a vitamin D analog.

12. Anemia: Use of elemental iron 200 mg, such as ferrous sulfate 325 mg three times daily (65 mg elemental iron per dose), is recommended to maintain the percent transferrin saturation greater than 20% and the serum ferritin level greater than 100 ng/mL.

Although primarily used in clients with ESRD, erythropoietic agents (EPO), such as epoetin alfa (Procrit, Epogen) and darbepoetin alfa (Aranesp), are used to correct anemia in those with CKD who do not yet require dialysis. Dosages of the EPO agents should be prescribed in order to maintain Hgb levels in the range of 11 to 12 g/dL in predialysis clients with CKD.

13. Dyslipidemia: Management of dyslipidemia has been shown to slow progression of CKD. Statins and fibrates are commonly prescribed to lower total cholesterol and low-density lipoprotein (LDL) and triglycerides. The incidence of untoward side effects with statins and fibrates is increased in persons with CKD; therefore, lower dosages and careful monitoring are required.

Follow-Up

A. Regular, consistent follow-up appointments to monitor progression of CKD, management of complications of CKD, and management of comorbidities such as DM and HTN are recommended.

Consultation/Referral

A. Early referral to a nephrologist is recommended for anyone who has CKD. The benefits of early referral to a nephrologist are well known, and early referral can improve client survival and quality of life as well as reduce hospitalization, length of hospital stay, and medical costs. Referral to a nephrologist must be done as quickly as possible for symptomatic clients with Stage 4 or 5 CKD. Consultation with an endocrinologist or HTN specialist may be helpful in cases in which DM and HTN continue to be poorly controlled.

B. After the client is evaluated as a candidate for kidney transplantation, counseling on renal transplantation should be completed by a nephrologist on what types of transplant are available and how the transplant process works.

C. Referral to a dietitian for nutritional counseling and education to assist the client to understand and follow complex dietary instructions is recommended.

D. Clients with Stage 4 or 5 CKD need counseling regarding the psychosocial and financial impact of progressive renal disease. Referral to a renal social worker or case manager can help the client understand his or her health insurance benefits, how the transition to Medicare occurs after the health insurance benefit changes, and to help the client deal with concerns about work or family life.

E. Clients should be referred to educational and support organizations for further education regarding CKD.

F. Websites:

1. National Kidney Foundation: www.kidney.org
2. National Kidney Disease Education Program: www.nkdep.nih.gov

Individual Consideration

A. Geriatrics:

1. Debilitated elderly clients will need education and counseling about renal replacement therapy and the lack of efficacy in clients over the age of 80, or in those 70 and older with concurrent CHF or other chronic diseases.

2. Referral to a palliative care specialist can be helpful in identifying goals and assisting with advance care planning discussions.

Bibliography

Aora, P. (2018, July). Chronic kidney disease. *Medscape*. Retrieved from http://emedicine.medscape.com/article/238798-overview

Carrero, J. J., Burrowes, J., & Wanner, C. (2016). A long road to travel: Adherence to dietary recommendations and adequate dietary phosphorus control. *Journal of Renal Nutrition, 26*(3), 133–135. doi:10.1053/j.jrn.2016.03.004

Centers for Disease Control and Prevention. (2019). *Chronic kidney disease in the United States, 2019*. Atlanta, GA: U.S. Department of Health and Human Services, Centers for Disease Control and Prevention.

Demircioglu, K., Akbalik, K., Buyukcelik, M., & Balat, A. (2018). Pediatric post-streptococcal glomerulonephritis: Clinical and laboratory data. *Pediatric International, 60*(7), 645–650. doi:10.1111/ped.13587

Inker, L. A., Astor, B. C., Fox, C. H., Isakova, T., Lash, J. P., Peralta, C. A., & Feldman, H. I. (2014). KDOQI U.S. commentary on the 2012 KDIGO clinical practice guideline for the evaluation and management of CKD. *American Journal of Kidney Disease, 63*(5), 713–735. doi:10.1053/j.ajkd.2014.01.416

Lee, J., Lee, L., An, J. (2016). Factors affecting the referral time to nephrologists in patients with chronic kidney disease: A prospective cohort study in Korea. *Medicine, 95*(19), e3648. doi:10.1097/MD.0000000000003648

National Kidney and Urologic Diseases Information Clearinghouse, National Institutes of Health. (n.d.). *Kidney disease*. Retrieved from https://www.niddk.nih.gov/health-information/kidney-disease

National Kidney Disease Education Program. (n.d.). *Glomerular filtration rate (GFR) calculators*. Retrieved from https://www.niddk.nih.gov/healthinformation/healthcommunicationprograms/nkdep/labevaluation/gfr-calculators/Pages/gfrcalculators.aspx

National Kidney Disease Education Program. (n.d.). *Manage patients with CKD*. Retrieved from https://www.niddk.nih.gov/healthinformation/health-communication-programs/nkdep/identify-manage/manage-patients/Pages/manage-patients.aspx

National Kidney Foundation. (2014). KDOQI U.S. commentary on the 2012 KDIGO clinical practice guideline for the evaluation and management of CKD. *American Journal of Kidney Diseases, 63*(5), 713–735. doi:10.1053/j.ajkd.2014.01.416

Rak, A., Raina, R., Suh, T. (2017). Palliative care for patients with end-stage renal disease: Approach to treatment that aims to improve quality of life and relieve suffering for patients (and families) with chronic illnesses. *Clinical Kidney Journal, 10*(1), 68–73.

Stephen, R., Jolly, S. (2014). Albuminuria: When urine predicts kidney and cardiovascular disease. *Cleveland Clinic Journal of Medicine, 81*(1), 41–50. https://doi.org/10.3949/ccjm.81a.13040

U.S. Renal Data System. (2018). *2018 USRDS annual data report: Atlas of end-stage renal disease in the United States (Vol. 2)*. Bethesda, MD: National Institutes of Health, National Institute of Diabetes and Digestive and Kidney Diseases.

Epididymitis

Cheryl A. Glass and Debbie Gunter

Definition

Epididymitis is acute infection of the epididymis, the coiled segment of the spermatic duct that connects the efferent duct from the posterior aspect of the testicle to the vas deferens. Epididymitis is commonly found to develop during strenuous exertion in conjunction with a full bladder. **Testicular torsion should be considered in all cases—this is a surgical emergency.**

A. Acute epididymitis: duration of symptoms lasts less than 6 weeks:

1. Acute epididymitis often involves the testis (epididymo-orchitis).

B. Chronic epididymitis: duration of symptoms lasts more than 6 weeks:
1. Inflammation chronic
2. Obstructive chronic
3. Chronic epididymalgia

Incidence

A. Epididymitis is the fifth most common urologic diagnosis in men aged 20 to 40 years. There are more than 600,000 medical visits per year related to epididymitis. Chronic epididymitis may account for up to 80% of scrotal pain noted in the outpatient setting. The mumps, measles, and rubella (MMR) vaccine has markedly reduced the incidence of mumps orchitis.

Pathogenesis

A. The exact pathophysiology is unclear. The cause may be the retrograde passage of infected urine from the prostatic urethra to the epididymis from the ejaculatory ducts and vas deferens. Reflux may be induced by having the client perform the Valsalva maneuver or may be from strenuous exertion. Pathogens include *Chlamydia trachomatis, Neisseria gonorrhoeae, Escherichia coli, Proteus* species, *Klebsiella* species, *Pseudomonas, Mycoplasma* species, and *Treponema pallidum*.

Predisposing Factors

A. Age:
1. Age less than 35 years is generally associated with urethritis with the following organisms:
   a. *C. trachomatis* (chlamydia)
   b. *N. gonorrhoeae* (gonorrhea)
2. Benign prostatic hyperplasia (BPH) is more common for men older than 35 years and common organisms include:
   a. *E. coli*
   b. *Pseudomonas* species
   c. *Proteus* species
   d. *Klebsiella* species
3. The older populations of men usually have nonsexual epididymitis related to urinary tract instrumentation, surgery, and immunosuppression.
4. Boys prior to sexual maturity may experience epididymitis as a result of an inflammatory process induced from repetitive activities such as running and jumping.
B. Men having sex with men (MSM) who are the insertive partner during anal intercourse have epididymitis with the following organisms:
1. *E. coli*
2. *Pseudomonas*
3. Coliform bacteria
C. UTIs
D. Tuberculosis (TB; should be considered if there is a history of or recent exposure to TB)
E. Vasectomy
F. Indwelling urethral catheter
G. Urethral stricture
H. Amiodarone—high drug concentrations (dose dependent)
I. Prolonged sitting (sedentary job, travel)
J. Mumps

Common Complaints

A. Swelling and tenderness of the scrotum (usually located on one side)
B. Fever
C. Chronic epididymitis:
1. Epididymal pain and inflammation that last more than 6 weeks
2. May be accompanied by scrotal induration

Other Signs and Symptoms

A. Gradual onset of localized, unilateral testicular pain. The client may get relief with elevation of the scrotum, which *is* a positive Prehn's sign.
B. Urethral discharge
C. Dysuria, frequency, urgency
D. Hematuria
E. Fever and chills (found in only 25% of adults with acute epididymitis but in up to 71% of children with the condition)

Subjective Data

A. Elicit the onset, duration, and course of the client's symptoms.
B. Review the client's history for vasectomy or trauma to the groin.
C. Are there any other symptoms, including fever, dysuria, or discharge?
D. What makes the pain better? Ask about elevating the scrotum.
E. Does the client's sexual partner(s) have any symptoms or discharge?
F. Has there been any recent instrumentation or catheterization?
G. Is the pain unilateral or bilateral?
H. Review medication history for amiodarone.
I. Does the client have a recent TB exposure?

Physical Examination

A. Check temperature, BP, and pulse
B. Inspect:
1. Examine the client generally for discomfort before and during examination.
2. Check the urethral meatus for discharge. Retract foreskin (if present) and assess for hygiene and smegma. Check the shaft of the penis, glans, and prepuce for lesions.
3. Check the inguinal and femoral areas for bulges and hernias; have the client bear down and cough and reexamine him.
C. Palpate:
1. Palpate testes and epididymides for inflammation, tenderness, and masses. In chronic cases, the epididymis feels firm and lumpy. Vas deferens may be beaded.
2. Check Prehn's sign by elevating the affected hemiscrotum. This action relieves the pain of epididymitis but exacerbates the pain of torsion.
3. Elicit a cremasteric reflex. Stroking the inner thigh should result in rise of the testicle and scrotum on the affected side. A normal cremasteric reflex indicates that testicular torsion is less likely.
4. Palpate the scrotum for hydrocele or varicocele.

5. Check for CVA tenderness.
6. Examine the abdomen for masses, urinary distension, tenderness, and organomegaly.
7. Palpate lymph nodes in the groin.
8. Evaluate for an inguinal hernia.

D. Rectal examination: check for symmetry, swelling, tenderness, and enlarged prostate.

Diagnostic Tests

A. Gram stain of urethral secretions
B. Urinalysis and urine cultures
C. Urethra swab (before void, after prostate massage) for gonorrhea and chlamydia culture
D. In clients older than 40 years: express prostatic secretions
E. TB skin test to rule out TB
F. CBC

Differential Diagnoses

A. Testicular torsion (surgical emergency)
B. Testicular tumor
C. Prostatitis
D. Incarcerated inguinal hernia
E. Orchitis (occurs with parotitis)
F. Trauma
G. Vasectomy side effect
H. Folliculitis
I. Herpes outbreak

Plan

A. General interventions:
1. Encourage and stress the importance of adequate fluid intake.
2. Stress importance of taking all antibiotics as directed.
B. Client teaching:
1. Offer supportive therapy: Client teaching: *See Section III: Client Teaching Guide for this chapter, "Epididymitis."*
C. Pharmaceutical therapy:
1. Antibiotic therapy (both partners must be treated for STI): Treat empirically until laboratory test results are available.

2. Current CDC guidelines (2015) for acute epididymitis recommends treatment with antibiotics for 10 days (see Table 12.2).
3. Chronic epididymitis should be treated for 4 to 6 weeks for bacterial pathogens, especially chlamydia.
4. NSAIDs for pain management
5. Antitubercular triple therapy consists of rifampin, isoniazid, and pyrazinamide for 6 months.
a. Rifampin (Rifadin) 450 mg orally every day for 2 months, then 900 mg orally every day for an additional 4 months
b. Isoniazid (Laniazid) 300 mg orally every day for 2 months, then 600 mg orally every day for an additional 4 months
c. Pyrazinamide 25 mg/kg/d orally for 2 months only
6. Amiodarone epididymitis usually responds to a dosage reduction or discontinuation.

Follow-Up

A. See the client in 2 to 7 days depending on severity of infection:
1. Pain typically improves within 1 to 3 days, but may take up to 2 to 4 weeks.
2. Inadequate treatment can result in abscess formation and decreased fertility.
B. Culture urine at end of treatment (test of cure)
C. Failure to recognize and treat both partners for STIs is a potential legal pitfall; test for all STIs and do not just focus on chlamydia and gonorrhea
D. Consider testing for HIV
E. Tuberculous epididymitis should be suspected if clinical signs worsen despite appropriate antibiotic therapy
F. Men older than 50 years should be evaluated for urethral obstruction secondary to prostatic enlargement.

Consultation/Referral

A. Obtain an immediate consultation with a urologist if testicular torsion, scrotal abscess, or failed medical treatment is suspected.

TABLE 12.2 THE 2015 CENTERS FOR DISEASE CONTROL AND PREVENTION (CDC) RECOMMENDATION REGIMENS FOR ACUTE EPIDIDYMITIS

For acute epididymitis all clients should receive: Ceftriaxone 250 mg intramuscular (IM) in a single dose *PLUS* Doxycycline 100 mg orally twice a day for 10 days.
For acute epididymitis most likely caused by enteric organisms, additional therapy can include: Levofloxacin 500 mg orally once a day for 10 days *OR* Ofloxacin 300 mg orally twice a day for 10 days.
For MSM who report insertive anal intercourse and are at risk of both STI and enteric organisms: Ceftriaxone 250 mg IM in single dose *PLUS* Levofloxacin 500 mg once a day × 10 days *OR* Ofloxacin 300 mg orally twice a day × 10 days.

MSM, men having sex with men; STI, sexually transmitted infection.

B. Consult physician for the following:
  1. Intravenous pyelography (IVP)
  2. Doppler ultrasonography
  3. Scrotal ultrasonography
  4. Radionuclide scrotal imaging
C. Refer for evaluation of pediatric clients for an underlying congenital anomaly.

Individual Considerations

A. Partner: treat sexual partners for STI; consider testing for HIV.
B. Pediatric: Epididymitis is rare prepubertally, and testicular torsion is more common in this age group.
C. Geriatrics:
  1. Epididymitis in the elderly is often caused by an enlarged prostate gland.
  2. Trouble voiding can be an early finding.

Bibliography

Centers for Disease Control and Prevention. (2015, June 15). *2015 sexually transmitted diseases treatment guidelines: Epididymitis*. Retrieved from https://www.cdc.gov/std/tg2015/epididymitis.htm

Centers for Disease Control and Prevention. (2015). *Epididymitis*. Retrieved from https://www.cdc.gov/std/tg2015/epididymitis.htm

Ching, C. B. (2015, December 20). Epididymitis treatment and management. *Medscape*. Retrieved from http://emedicine.medscape.com/article/436154-treatment

National Kidney Foundation. (2015). KDOQI clinical practice guideline for hemodialysis adequacy 2015 update. *American Journal of Kidney Diseases, 66*(5), 884–930. doi:10.1053/j.ajkd.2015.07.015. Retrieved from www.kidney.org/professionals/guidelines/hemodialysis2015

Rupp, T., & Leslie, S. (2018). Epididymitis. *StatPearls [Internet] National Institute of Health*. Retrieved from https://www.ncbi.nlm.nih.gov/books/NBK430814/

Hematuria

Cheryl A. Glass and Debbie Gunter

Definition

A. Hematuria is blood in the urine. Hematuria is a symptom of an underlying disease/condition; however, routine screening is not recommended. Microscopic hematuria is defined as three or more red blood cells (RBCs) per high-power microscope field (HPF) in urinary sediment from two of three properly collected clean-catch midstream urine specimens.
B. Asymptomatic microscopic hematuria can range from minor findings that do not require treatment to highly significant, life-threatening lesions. Microscopic hematuria is an incidental finding. The AUA recommends an appropriate renal or urologic evaluation with asymptomatic microscopic hematuria for clients who are at risk of urologic disease or primary renal disease.
C. If the excretion rate exceeds 1 million RBCs, macroscopic or gross hematuria is noted. Gross hematuria (macroscopic hematuria) is suspected when red or brown urine is present. Glomerulonephritis is associated with brown urine, while bleeding from the lower urinary tract is suggested by pink or red urine. Gross hematuria with passage of clots almost always indicates a lower urinary tract source.

Incidence

A. The prevalence of asymptomatic hematuria is from 1% to 20% of the general population. Less than 3% excrete 10 RBC/HPF. Every disease of the genitourinary (GU) tract can produce hematuria.

Pathogenesis

A. Prerenal pathology:
  1. Coagulopathy: hemophilia or idiopathic thrombocytopenia purpura (ITP)
  2. Drugs: anticoagulants, aspirin
  3. Sickle cell disease or trait
  4. Collagen vascular disease; lupus
  5. Wilms' tumor
B. Renal pathology:
  1. Nonglomerular pathology
    a. Pyelonephritis
    b. Polycystic kidney disease
    c. Granulomatous disease; TB
    d. Malignant neoplasm
    e. Congenital and vascular anomalies
  2. Glomerular pathology:
    a. Glomerulonephritis
    b. Berger's disease
    c. Lupus nephritis
    d. Benign familial hematuria
    e. Vascular abnormalities; vasculitis
    f. Alport syndrome; familial nephritis
C. Postrenal pathology:
  1. Renal calculi
  2. Ureteritis
  3. Cystitis
  4. Prostatitis
  5. BPH
  6. Epididymitis
  7. Urethritis
  8. Malignant neoplasm
D. False hematuria:
  1. Vaginal bleeding
  2. Recent circumcision
  3. Pigmentation:
    a. Food: beets, blackberries
    b. Medications: quinine sulfate, phenazopyridine, and rifampin
E. Other causes:
  1. Trauma
  2. Strenuous exercise (marathons)
  3. Fever

Predisposing Factors

A. See "Pathogenesis" section.
B. Risk factors for malignancy:
  1. Age greater than 35 years
  2. Smoking (current use or past history)
  3. Chemical exposure (cyclophosphamide, benzenes, aromatic amines)
  4. History of pelvic irradiation
  5. Prior urologic disease or treatment
  6. Chronic UTIs

Common Complaint

A. Pink or red urine (clots may be present) or brown, cola-colored urine on toilet tissue is the common complaint.

Other Signs and Symptoms

A. Pain may or may not be present. Colicky flank pain radiating to the groin suggests a kidney stone. Significant flank pain of renal colic is usually secondary to renal calculi, but may occasionally be associated with passage of clots.

B. Frequency, dysuria, urgency, and suprapubic pain occur with cystitis and inflammatory lesions of the lower urinary tract.

C. Dull flank pain with fever and chills may accompany pyelonephritis.

D. Hesitancy and dribbling of urine suggest BPH.

Subjective Data

A. Elicit the onset, duration, and occurrence (beginning, ending, or during voiding) of hematuria. Describe the color and amount: Is it "pink on tissue" or bright red in the toilet and tissue?

B. Question the client regarding past medical history of renal disease, systemic disease such as lupus, or sickle cell disease.

C. Review all medications including OTC and herbal products. Evaluate specifically for the use of aspirin, ibuprofen, anticoagulants, especially warfarin (Coumadin), and laxatives containing phenolphthalein. Rifampin and phenazopyridine HCl (Pyridium) can change the color of urine to orange or red.

D. Review other symptoms, such as dysuria, fever, chills, pain, and hesitancy with voiding.

E. Female clients:
1. Establish whether the blood was urinary or vaginal (after intercourse or during menstruation)
2. Is the client postpartum?
3. Is there a history of endometriosis?

F. Does the client bruise easily? Does the client have bleeding when flossing or brushing teeth?

G. Has the client had a recent bout of pharyngitis with a rash, hematuria, edema, or hypertension (HTN [glomerulonephritis])?

H. Has he or she had any recent trauma, car accident, or strenuous exercise (i.e., running a marathon)?

I. Does the client know if there was any exposure to TB?

J. Is there any family history of kidney disease, stones, and familial nephritis?

K. Does the client have any current outbreaks of herpes or other STIs?

L. Review the client's smoking history.

M. Review occupational exposure to chemicals or dyes (benzenes or aromatic amines).

N. Review food intake of foods such as beets and blackberries.

O. Does the male client have any hesitancy and dribbling (signs of prostatic obstruction)?

P. Evaluate if there is rectal bleeding from hemorrhoids from straining with a bowel movement (BM).

Physical Examination

A. Check temperature, BP, and weight in the presence of recent weight gain or edema.

B. Male or female clients:
1. Inspect:
   a. Inspect mouth: check tonsils for enlargement and gums for petechiae.
   b. Examine skin for signs of bleeding or bruises and pallor.
   c. Examine for edema.
2. Palpate:
   a. Check the back and abdomen for CVA tenderness.
   b. Check the abdomen for masses, urinary distension, tenderness, and organomegaly.
   c. Palpate groin lymph nodes for enlargement.
3. Auscultate:
   a. The heart and lungs
   b. For abdominal bruits

C. Female clients:
1. Inspect:
   a. Direct visualization of the external genitalia for inflammation, ulcerations, nodules, lesions, and hemorrhoids
   b. Ask the client to bear down to check for cystocele and rectocele.
   c. Speculum examination: observe for atrophic vaginitis, torn tissue, discharge, and friable cervix.
2. Palpate:
   a. Milk urethra for discharge
   b. Bimanual examination: check for cervical motion tenderness (CMT) and adnexal masses
   c. Rectal examination: check for the presence of hemorrhoids

D. Male clients:
1. Inspect:
   a. Direct visualization of the genitals; check the urethral meatus for discharge
   b. Retract the foreskin (if present) and assess for hygiene and smegma. Check the shaft of the penis, glans, and prepuce for lesions or urethral meatal erosion.
2. Palpate:
   a. Palpate the testes and epididymides for inflammation, tenderness, and masses; palpate the scrotum for hydrocele or varicocele.
   b. Check the inguinal and femoral areas for bulges and hernias; have the client bear down and cough and reexamine him.
   c. Rectal examination:
      i. Check for swollen or tender prostate.
      ii. Check for the presence of hemorrhoids.

Diagnostic Tests

A. Urinalysis: An efficient specimen would consist of a random midstream clean-catch after discarding the first 10 mL. Urine specimens that should not be examined to assess for microhematuria are first void in morning or the first voiding after vigorous physical or sexual activity.

1. Centrifuge the urine specimen to see if the red or brown color is in the urine sediment or supernatant.

2. If the supernatant is red to brown, test for heme (Hgb or myoglobin) with a urine dipstick. Semen is in urine after ejaculation and may cause a positive heme reaction on the dipstick.

3. A positive dipstick must always be confirmed with a microscopic examination.

4. Urine culture and sensitivity

5. Urine cytology

6. CBC with differential

7. BUN/creatinine

8. Prothrombin time (PT), partial thromboplastin time (PTT), platelet count, and bleeding time (if indicated)

9. Sickle cell testing (if indicated)

10. CT urography (CTU) is considered the preferred initial imaging in most clients for any unexplained persistent hematuria. CT is considered the best imaging modality for the evaluation of urinary stones, renal and perirenal infections, and associated complications. IVP and ultrasound are not as sensitive in the evaluation.

11. Cystoscopy (the combination of a CTU and cystoscopy) provides a complete evaluation.

12. A CT scan of the abdomen or pelvis should be considered with a history of trauma to determine the source of blood.

B. Based on history, consider the following tests:

1. Strep testing to detect poststreptococcal glomerulonephritis

2. Antinuclear antibody to detect lupus nephritis

C. Urologic referral testing includes:

1. CTU and cystoscopy

2. MRI if a mass is suspected

3. Renal biopsy

Differential Diagnoses

A. See "Pathogenesis" section for differential diagnoses.

Plan

A. General interventions:

1. Investigate and diagnose cause(s). Only a limited workup (electrolytes, CBC) is needed in clients younger than 35 years with normal physical examination.

2. Clients older than 35 years need detailed investigation and referral.

3. Microhematuria with clients on an anticoagulant requires a urologic/nephrology workup regardless of the type or level of anticoagulation.

4. Repeat urinalysis in 2 weeks.

B. Client teaching:

1. There is no one specific treatment for all cases of hematuria.

2. Treatment is aimed at the specific underlying cause, if a cause can be identified.

C. Pharmaceutical therapy: None is recommended for hematuria unless an infection is diagnosed.

Follow-Up

A. For clients at risk of malignancy who have a negative workup:

1. Evaluate in 1 year.

2. After two consecutive negative urinalyses tests, discontinue the follow-up.

3. If gross hematuria occurs after the initial negative urinalysis, repeat a full evaluation.

B. For clients with HTN, proteinuria and/or an increase in creatinine needs to be reevaluated for renal disease.

C. For persistent asymptomatic microhematuria, after a negative workup by the urologist, a yearly urinalysis is needed.

D. For persistent or recurrent asymptomatic microhematuria after the initial negative workup, consider repeating the evaluation within 3 to 5 years.

E. Culture urine for acid-fast bacillus if sterile pyuria and hematuria persist.

Consultation/Referral

A. If all benign causes for hematuria have been ruled out, found conditions treated, and it persists, referral to a urologist or a nephrologist should be made.

B. The presence of significant proteinuria (excretion of more than 1,000 mg per 24 hours), red cell cast or renal insufficiency, or a predominance of dysmorphic RBCs in the urine should prompt an evaluation for renal parenchymal disease by a nephrologist. Red cell casts are considered virtually pathognomonic for glomerular bleeding.

C. New gross hematuria should be promptly reevaluated.

Individual Considerations

A. Women:

1. Nonpregnant: rule out menstruation and sexual activity

2. Pregnant: rule out vaginal bleeding such as threatened abortion, abruptio placentae, or placenta previa.

3. Ultrasound can be used to evaluate the pregnant woman. CTU should not be used secondary to the radiation exposure.

B. Pediatrics:

1. UTI is the most common cause for hematuria in children. Irritation or ulceration of the perineum or urethral meatus is the next most common cause, followed by trauma.

2. The majority of children who present with gross hematuria have an easily recognizable and apparent cause. The underlying etiology is generally easy to establish by a complete history, physical examination, and urinalysis.

3. Renal ultrasound is the preferred modality for evaluation in children.

4. Cystoscopy is rarely indicated for hematuria in children. It is usually reserved for the child with a bladder mass noted on ultrasound and the child with urethral abnormalities because of trauma.

5. Hematuria might develop after streptococcal infection (strep throat or impetigo), which could indicate post-streptococcal glomerulonephritis.

C. Geriatrics: The risk of malignancy increases among older individuals with a significant history of smoking or analgesic abuse. The use of anticoagulants increases in this population, so a careful review of medications is imperative.

Bibliography

American Urological Association. (2012, revised 2016). *Diagnosis, evaluation and follow-up of asymptomatic microhematuria (AMH) in adults: AUA guideline.* Retrieved from https://www.auanet.org/education/guidelines/asymptomatic-microhematuria.cfm

Bignall, O., & Dixon, B. (2018). Management of hematuria in children. *Current Treatment Options in Pediatrics, 4*(3), 333–349. doi:10.1007/s40746-018-0134-z

Feldman, A. (2018, July 20). Etiology and evaluation of hematuria in adults. *UpToDate.* Retrieved from https://www.uptodate.com/contents/etiology-and-evaluation-of-hematuria-in-adults

Gulati, S. (2019, January 3). Hematuria. *Medscape.* Retrieved from emedicine.medscape.com/article/981898-overview

Hydrocele

Cheryl A. Glass and Debbie Gunter

Definition

A. Hydrocele is the collection of fluid between layers of the processus vaginalis producing swelling in the scrotum or inguinal area. Cystic masses containing fluid or sperm often develop spontaneously. Inguinal hernia and hydrocele share a similar etiology and pathophysiology and may coexist (see Figure 12.2).

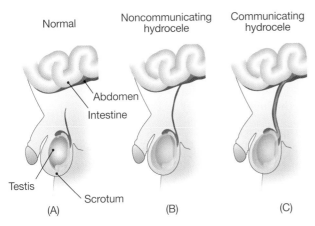

FIGURE 12.2 Hydrocele. (A) Normal scrotum. Hydrocele. (A) Normal scrotum. (B) Noncommunicating hydrocele. (C) Communicating hydrocele.

Incidence

A. Incidence is unknown; hydrocele occurs in 6% of the male pediatric population at birth or in the neonatal period. It occurs infrequently in adulthood.

B. Parasitic infection, filariasis, caused by *Wuchereria bancrofti*, is the cause in more than 120 million people worldwide.

Pathogenesis

A. Congenital: patent processus vaginalis (PPV)

B. Reactive: inflammatory condition in the scrotum (e.g., trauma, torsion, infection)

C. Idiopathic: arises over a long period (most common)

D. Hydroceles are believed to arise from an imbalance of secretion and reabsorption of fluid from the tunica vaginalis.

Predisposing Factors

A. Males; most commonly seen in childhood

B. *W. bancrofti* parasite

C. Viral illness

D. Chronic increased intra-abdominal pressure

E. Increased abdominal fluid production

Common Complaint

A. Swollen scrotum is the common indication.

Other Signs and Symptoms

A. Painless swollen scrotum; pain increases with the size of the mass.

B. Rarely does a hydrocele become infected and cause pain.

Subjective Data

A. Elicit the onset, duration, and course of swelling: Is scrotal sac full all day, or does the client have a flat scrotum in the morning and a gradual increase in fluid during the day?

B. Was the hydrocele noted in the neonatal period?

C. How old is the client? Has this ever occurred before? If so, what happened, and how was it treated?

D. Review the client's history for injury to the scrotum.

E. Is there any pain or other symptoms related to hernia with the swelling?

F. Review other symptoms such as discharge, dysuria, fever, or backaches.

G. Review birth control method (vasectomy).

Physical Examination

A. Check temperature (if indicated) and BP.

B. Inspect:

1. Careful examination is necessary to rule out masses and tumor. Examine in the supine and standing positions.

2. Genital examination: note amount of swelling, symmetry, lesions, discharge, hernias, varices, and color of scrotum.

3. Transilluminate the scrotum to determine if the lesion is cystic, solid, or a varicocele. In a dark room, transillumination light appears as a red glow with serous fluid. If normal, blood and tissue do not transilluminate; however, the bowel may transilluminate.

C. Auscultate:

1. Scrotum for bowel sounds to rule out hernia

D. Palpate:

1. Check warmth, tenderness, swelling, and any nodularity. If mass is present, check if it has a solid versus cystic feel.

2. Palpate lymph nodes: supraclavicular, chest, abdomen, and groin

3. Check for inguinal hernia.

4. Palpate the abdomen for masses, rebound, and tenderness

Diagnostic Tests

A. Laboratory evaluation is not required for the evaluation of hydroceles.

B. Scrotal ultrasonography

Differential Diagnoses

A. Varicocele: feels like a "bag of worms"

B. Hernia: Herniated bowel makes gurgling sounds upon auscultation of the scrotum.

C. Testicular tumors tend to occur in young men and are the most common tumors in males from ages 15 to 30 years. Consider a tumor if the onset is acute. Tumors feel firm, nontender, and fixed and do not transilluminate. Inguinal lymphadenopathy may also be seen. The client may complain of heaviness with a tumor.

D. Testicular torsion

E. Orchitis: rare except with mumps. Orchitis is usually unilateral and is associated with fever, swelling, pain, and tenderness. On occasion, parotitis is absent.

F. Epididymitis: Inflammation is often concurrent with a UTI. Epididymis is very tender; scrotal elevation may relieve the pain.

G. Spermatocele: cystic swelling of the epididymis. It is not as large as a hydrocele, but it also transilluminates.

Plan

A. General interventions:

1. Monitor children every 3 months until resolution or until a decision is made to refer to a specialist for evaluation.

2. Factors that indicate surgical repair:

   a. Failure to resolve by age 2 years

   b. Continued discomfort

   c. Enlargement or waxing and waning in volume

   d. Unsightly appearance

   e. Secondary infection

B. Client teaching:

1. Most hydroceles are painless.

2. In adults, if there are no symptoms, it can be left alone and monitored.

C. Pharmaceutical therapy: none recommended

Follow-Up

A. Monitor every 3 months.

Consultation/Referral

A. Refer to a urologist for evaluation, as needed.

B. A persistent hydrocele or the association of discomfort may indicate the need for a surgical referral.

Individual Considerations

A. Pediatrics:

1. An infant testicle usually measures 1 cm. The parent may notice a hydrocele that fluctuates slightly in size and usually resolves on its own by 6 months of age.

B. Adults:

1. If an adult experiences a hydrocele, he should be instructed to return for evaluation if the hydrocele becomes larger or uncomfortable, or if it interferes with sexual intercourse.

Bibliography

Parke, J. (2018, July 26). Hydrocele. *Medscape*. Retrieved from https://emedicine.medscape.com/article/438724-overview

Interstitial Cystitis

Cheryl A. Glass and Debbie Gunter

Definition

A. Interstitial cystitis (IC) is a chronic condition that is defined as a recurring pelvic discomfort, or suprapubic pain related to bladder filling, or chronic pelvic pain and pressure accompanied by frequency. IC is also commonly known as painful bladder syndrome (PBS). IC/PBS includes all cases of urinary pain with persistent urge to void or urinary frequency that cannot be attributed to other causes (e.g., infection, stones, or other pathology).

B. The persistent urge to void helps to distinguish the symptoms of IC/PBS from those of overactive bladder (OAB). IC/PBS affects quality of life related to social activities, lost work productivity, sleep deprivation because of urinary frequency, fatigue, and even depression.

C. The Society for Urodynamics and Female Urology (SUFU) has stated that the symptoms should last more than 6 weeks in order for therapy to begin.

D. IC/PBS clients void to avoid or relieve pain, whereas clients with OAB void to avoid incontinence.

Incidence

A. Actual prevalence is unknown because of the variability of diagnostic criteria. It is not uncommon for clients to experience a lag time of 5 to 7 years before diagnosis. It is estimated that in the United States 3.3 to 7.9 million women older than 18 years are affected by symptoms of IC/PBS. Of these women, however, only 9.7% report being assigned a diagnosis of IC/PBS. The majority of the affected persons are women (10:1 rated over males). The symptom complex is the same for males. IC also occurs in children.

Pathogenesis

A. The pathophysiology of IC/PBS remains unclear. It is not established whether IC/PBS is a localized condition just involving the bladder or whether it is a systemic disease that affects the bladder.

Predisposing Factors

A. In both genders, with a higher prevalence in females

B. Mean age of diagnosis 42 to 45 years

C. UTI

D. Prostatitis

E. Chronic yeast infections

F. Posthysterectomy or other pelvic surgery

G. Medications:

1. Calcium channel blockers

2. Cardiac glycosides

H. Other hypersensitivity conditions that coexist with IC:

1. Fibromyalgia

2. Irritable bowel syndrome (IBS)

3. Chronic headaches

4. Vulvodynia

5. Sjögren's syndrome

Common Complaints

A. Mild discomfort to intense pain with bladder filling and/or emptying is the hallmark symptom. The pain is not limited to the bladder/suprapubic area but includes symptoms throughout the pelvic area, lower abdomen, and back.
B. Persistent urge to void/frequency
C. Frequency
D. Urgency
E. Nocturia

Other Signs and Symptoms

A. Combination of urgency and frequency
B. Pressure
C. Increase in symptoms during menstruation
D. Pain during vaginal intercourse
E. Low back pain with bladder filling

Subjective Data

A. Review the onset, frequency, duration, and severity of symptoms.
B. Evaluate if the pain of bladder filling is partially or completely relieved by voiding.
C. Does the client void frequently in order to maintain a low bladder volume and avoid discomfort versus voiding frequently to avoid urge incontinence (OAB)?
D. Are there any OAB triggers (e.g., citrus, beer, coffee) that exacerbate symptoms?
E. Are symptoms increased after stress, exercise, intercourse, being seated for a long period, or during the menstrual cycle?
F. How much do the symptoms affect the client's quality of life (e.g., sleep disturbance, loss of work, avoiding activities)?
G. Does the client have any other chronic pain syndromes such as IBS, chronic fatigue, dyspareunia, or fibromyalgia?
H. Review the client's surgical history and history of GU cancers
I. Any GU trauma or falls onto the coccyx?
J. Review the client's history of UTIs, urinary retention, and urinary tract stones
K. Review all medications including OTC and herbal products
L. Administer a pain/symptom evaluation tool at each visit:
  1. The Pelvic Pain and Urgency/Frequency Patient Symptom Scale (PUF) is available at https://www.ichelp.org/wp-content/uploads/2015/06/PUF_Questionnaire.pdf.
  2. The Interstitial Cystitis Symptom Index (ICSI) is available at file:///C:/Users/npdeb/AppData/Local/Microsoft/Windows/INetCache/IE/TC92HYH6/021908-140925.pdf.

Physical Examination

A. Temperature (if indicated to rule out infection; fever is not associated with IC) and BP.
B. Inspect:
  1. Note general appearance for signs of depression and discomfort before and during examination.
  2. Inspect the male external genitalia for redness, edema, lesions, and discharge.
  3. Inspect female genitalia for discharge, lesions, fissures; inspect cervix for cervicitis.
C. Auscultate:
  1. The heart and lungs
  2. Bowel sounds in all four quadrants
D. Palpate:
  1. Palpate back; note CVA tenderness.
  2. Palpate the abdomen for suprapubic tenderness, rebound masses, or pain.
  3. Perform bimanual examination to rule out other infections and pelvic inflammatory disease (PID; tenderness of the cervix, uterus, and adnexa should be absent). During the pelvic examination, evaluate locations of tenderness and trigger points.
  4. Males: complete palpation of external genitalia, prostate, and rectal examination
E. Percuss:
  1. Bladder
  2. Back for CVA tenderness
F. Neurologic:
  1. Perform a limited neurologic examination to rule out an occult problem.

Diagnostic Tests

A. Urinalysis with microscopy to exclude hematuria
B. Urine culture and sensitivity may be ordered even with a negative urinalysis to evaluate low levels of bacteria.
C. PVR volume by straight catheter or ultrasound
D. Urodynamic testing is not currently considered to have a role in the diagnosis of IC/PBS; however, urodynamic testing should be used for complex presentations.
E. Cystoscopy is usually reserved for gross or microscopic hematuria.
F. Hydrodistension is not required for diagnosis or treatment.
G. Bladder biopsy is not required for diagnosis; however, it is used for exclusion of other disorders.
H. The potassium sensitivity test is not recommended for routine use as results are nonspecific for IC/PBS.

Differential Diagnoses

A. UTI
B. IBS
C. Females:
  1. Endometriosis
  2. Vulvodynia
D. Males:
  1. Chronic prostatitis
  2. BPH

Plan

A. General interventions:
  1. Behavior modifications are recommended. Restrict fluids to 64 oz/d, divided into 16 oz per meal and 8 oz between meals.

2. Progressively timed voiding on a 2- to 3-hour schedule. If the client is unable to hold urine for this interval, progressively increase urine storage time between void by 15 minutes per week until the goal of a 2- to 3-hour interval is reached.

3. Kegel exercises should be avoided with IC.

4. Psychosocial support is an integral part of chronic pain disorders.

B. Client teaching:

1. Several foods have been identified as bladder irritants, including foods rich in potassium. Clients may try to eliminate foods/drinks and reintroduce them one at a time to identify any items that make their symptoms worse. Examples:
   a. Alcohol
   b. Tomatoes
   c. Spices/spicy foods
   d. Chocolate
   e. Caffeinated beverages
   f. Coffee
   g. Artificial sweeteners
   h. Citrus: lemons, limes, and oranges (including citrus-flavored beverages)
   i. Cranberries/cranberry juice

C. Pharmaceutical therapies:

1. Pentosan polysulfate sodium (Elmiron) is the only oral medication approved by the FDA for the treatment of IC.
   a. Dosage: 100 mg orally three times daily

2. Amitriptyline (Elavil) is used in the treatment of other pain syndromes, including IC. May use a self-titrated dose of 25 mg orally every night and increase in increments of 25 mg every week to a maximum dose of 100 mg orally per day.

3. Bladder instillation:
   a. Intravesical dimethyl sulfoxide (DMSO) (Rimso-50) is the only drug approved by the FDA for bladder instillation.
   b. Heparin instillation
   c. Lidocaine instillation
   d. "Bladder cocktail" combination of sodium bicarbonate, heparin, lidocaine, and/or triamcinolone. There are various formulas/combinations.

4. Medications may be instituted for treating any comorbid depression.

5. Medications for treating any comorbid infections (e.g., UTIs, STIs), inflammatory bowel disease, or endometriosis

6. Other medications that have been used for symptomatic relief:
   a. Hydroxyzine hydrochloride (Vistaril, Atarax) 25 to 75 mg orally at bedtime
   b. Gabapentin 300 mg up to 2,400 mg in divided doses. Gabapentin requires careful dose titration because of sedation.
   c. Uro-Blue medications for short-term bladder spasms
   d. NSAIDs

7. Cyclosporine A has been used when other treatments have not provided relief or control of symptoms.

D. Intradetrusor botulinum toxin A (BTX-A)—this therapy may require posttreatment intermittent self-catheterization.

E. Laser or electrocautery if Hunner's ulcers are present

F. Surgical options are available if all other therapies have failed.

G. Therapies that are not recommended/should not be offered include:
   1. Long-term antibiotics
   2. High-pressure, long-duration hydrodistention
   3. Systemic steroids
   4. Intravesical resiniferatoxin (ultrapotent capsaicin analog)
   5. Intravesical bacillus Calmette–Guérin (BCG)
   6. Potassium sensitivity test—not recommended for routine use. It is nonspecific and is a painful test.

Follow-Up

A. Allodynia, the perception of nonnoxious stimuli, such as touch being noxious or painful, may be present; therefore, an adequate pelvic examination may not be possible. Consider empiric treatment and have the client return for a pelvic examination to finish evaluation.

B. Have the client keep a 1-day bladder diary before visits to evaluate a pattern of low urine volume frequency characteristic of IC/PBS

C. As with all medications, start at the lowest dose and titrate/increase doses if there is an improvement in symptoms

Consultation/Referral

A. Refer to a urologist for more thorough workup and testing

B. Refer to a pain management specialist if indicated

C. Electrical stimulation therapy may be considered. The implanted sacral neuromodulation device is FDA approved for the treatment of urinary urgency and frequency but not specifically for the treatment of IC/PBS.

Individual Considerations

A. Pediatrics:
   1. The evaluation for IC is essentially the same in children as it is for adults.
   2. Treatment options are similar to those discussed, including dietary modifications and self-help strategies.

Resources

Adult Pediatric Urology & Urogynecology: www.adultpe-diatricuro.com
American Urological Association (AUA): www.auanet.org
International Painful Bladder Foundation: www.painful-bladder.org
Interstitial Cystitis Association (ICA): www.ichelp.org
Interstitial Cystitis Network: www.ic-network.com
Pelvic Pain and Urgency/Frequency Patient Symptom Scale: https://www.ichelp.org/wp-content/uploads/2015/06/PUF_Questionnaire.pdf
Society of Urodynamics, Female Pelvic Medicine & Urogenital Reconstruction: www.sufuorg.com

Bibliography

American Urological Association. (2014). *Diagnosis and treatment of interstitial cystitis/bladder pain syndrome*. Retrieved from https://www.auanet.org/education/guidelines/ic-bladder-pain-syndrome.cfm

Clemens, J. Q. (2017, October 17). Pathogenesis, clinical features, and diagnosis of interstitial cystitis/bladder pain syndrome. *UpToDate.* Retrieved from https://www.uptodate.com/contents/pathogenesis-clinical-features-and-diagnosis-of-interstitial-cystitis-bladder-pain-syndrome

Patolia, S. (2017, June 28). Cystitis empiric therapy. *Medscape.* Retrieved from http://emedicine.medscape.com/article/1976451-overview

Rovner, E. S. (2018, November 14). Interstitial cystitis. *Medscape.* Retrieved from emedicine.medscape.com/article/2055505-overview

Prostatitis

Cheryl A. Glass and Debbie Gunter

Definition

Prostatitis is acute or chronic infection of the prostate gland. Prostatitis is the most important cause of urinary infection in men. Prostatitis constitutes about 2 million outpatient visits a year to urologists and primary care providers. There are four types of prostatitis according to the National Institutes of Health (NIH):

A. Acute bacterial prostatitis (least common)
B. Chronic bacterial prostatitis
C. Chronic prostatitis/chronic pelvic pain syndrome (CP/CPPS) (common in men of any age):
    1. Inflammatory (presence of white blood cells [WBCs] in the semen, expressed prostatic secretions [EPSs], or voided bladder urine postprostatic massage)
    2. Noninflammatory (absence of white cells)
D. Asymptomatic inflammatory prostatitis

Incidence

A. About 50% of adult men in the United States will be treated for prostate conditions during their lifetime.
B. Acute and chronic bacterial prostatitis occurs in about 1 in 10 men. About 5% of acute prostatitis cases progress to chronic prostatitis.
C. Nonbacterial prostatitis occurs in about six in 10 men.
D. Prostatodynia occurs in about three in 10 men.

Pathogenesis

A. Nonbacterial prostatitis is an inflammatory condition with an unknown etiology. Infection results in prostatitis in four ways:
    1. Ascending infection of urethra
    2. Reflux of infected urine into the prostate through ejaculatory and prostatic ducts that empty into the prostatic urethra
    3. Hematogenous spread, causing bacterial prostatitis
    4. Invasion by rectal bacteria by direct extension or lymph system spread
B. Causative organisms: *E. coli, Klebsiella, Pseudomonas, Enterococcus, Ureaplasma, Gardnerella vaginalis, Trichomonas vaginalis, C. trachomatis, Chlamydia, Mycoplasma,* or *N. gonorrhoeae;* cytomegalovirus (CMV), *Mycobacterium tuberculosis,* and fungi have all been associated with prostatitis in HIV-infected clients.
C. Incubation period depends on pathogen

Predisposing Factors

A. More common in younger and middle-aged men
B. Sexual transmission of bacteria
C. Neuromuscular dysfunction
D. Structural voiding dysfunction
E. BPH
F. History of allergies and asthma (increase in nonbacterial prostatitis)

Common Complaints

A. Dysuria
B. Perineal, rectal, or suprapubic pain (chronic pain syndrome)
C. Less urine flow
D. Spiking fever
E. Back pain
F. Sexual dysfunction

Other Signs and Symptoms

A. Acute bacterial prostatitis:
    1. Fever and chills, malaise
    2. Acute onset of dysuria
    3. Hesitancy
    4. Urinary frequency and low back pain
    5. Pain with intercourse and with defecation
    6. Initial or terminal hematuria and edema with acute urinary retention
    7. Arthralgia or myalgia
    8. Nocturia
B. Chronic bacterial prostatitis:
    1. Usually presents with recurrent UTI
    2. May be asymptomatic between acute episodes; some men have large fluctuation in symptom severity.
    3. Perineal, inguinal, or suprapubic pain, or irritative symptoms on voiding, such as frequency and urgency
    4. Hematuria, hematospermia, or painful ejaculations
    5. Prostatic calculi
C. Nonbacterial prostatitis (most common):
    1. Vague discomfort or increasing pain: Prostatic, lower back, perineum, groin, scrotum, or suprapubic pain; ejaculatory pain
    2. Dysuria, urinary frequency, urgency, hesitancy, and decreased urine flow
    3. Penile discharge, especially noted during the first BM of the day
    4. Sexual difficulty
    5. Low sperm count
    6. Blood or urine in ejaculate
D. Asymptomatic inflammatory prostatitis is found when looking for causes of infertility and testing for prostate cancer.
E. Prostatodynia (cause is unknown):
    1. Prostate irritation
    2. Pain and discomfort in the prostate, testicles, penis, and urethra
    3. Difficulty urinating

Subjective Data

A. Ask the client to complete the National Institutes of Health Chronic Prostatitis Symptom Index (NIH-CPSI) self-evaluation form (see Table 12.3). The assessment tool

TABLE 12.3 **NATIONAL INSTITUTES OF HEALTH CHRONIC PROSTATITIS SYMPTOMS INDEX (NIH-CPSI)**

Pain or Discomfort

1. In the past week, have you experienced any pain or discomfort in the following areas?		
	Yes	**No**
a. Area between rectum and testicles (perineum)	☐ 1	☐ 0
b. Testicles	☐ 1	☐ 0
c. Tip of the penis (not related to urination)	☐ 1	☐ 0
d. Below your waist, in your pubic or bladder area	☐ 1	☐ 0
2. In the past week, have you experienced:		
	Yes	**No**
a. Pain or burning during urination?	☐ 1	☐ 0
b. Pain or discomfort during or after sexual climax (ejaculation)?	☐ 1	☐ 0
3. How often have you had pain or discomfort in any of these areas over the past week?		
☐ 0 Never		
☐ 1 Rarely		
☐ 2 Sometimes		
☐ 3 Often		
☐ 4 Usually		
☐ 5 Always		
4. Which number best describes your *average* pain or discomfort on the days that you had it, over the past week?		
☐ 0 No pain ☐ 1 ☐ 2 ☐ 3 ☐ 4 ☐ 5 ☐ 6 ☐ 7 ☐ 8 ☐ 9 ☐ 10 Pain as bad as you can imagine		

Urination

5. How often have you had a sensation of not emptying your bladder completely after you finished urinating, over the past week?		
☐ 0 Not at all		
☐ 1 Less than one time in five		
☐ 2 Less than half the time		
☐ 3 About half the time		
☐ 4 More than half the time		
☐ 5 Almost always		
6. How often have you had to urinate again less than 2 hours after you finished urinating, over the past week?		
☐ 0 Not at all		
☐ 1 Less than one time in five		
☐ 2 Less than half the time		
☐ 3 About half the time		
☐ 4 More than half the time		
☐ 5 Almost always		

Impact of Symptoms

7. How much have your symptoms kept you from doing the kinds of things you would usually do, over the past week?		
☐ 0 None		
☐ 1 Only a little		

(*continued*)

TABLE 12.3   NATIONAL INSTITUTES OF HEALTH CHRONIC PROSTATITIS SYMPTOMS INDEX (NIH-CPSI) *(continued)*

☐ 2 Some		
☐ 3 A lot		
8. How much did you think about your symptoms, over the past week?		
☐ 0 None		
☐ 1 Only a little		
☐ 2 Some		
☐ 3 A lot		
Quality of Life		
9. If you were to spend the rest of your life with your symptoms just the way they have been during the past week, how would you feel about that?		
☐ 0 Delighted		
☐ 1 Pleased		
☐ 2 Mostly satisfied		
☐ 3 Mixed (about equally satisfied and dissatisfied)		
☐ 4 Mostly dissatisfied		
☐ 5 Unhappy		
☐ 6 Terrible		
Scoring the NIH-CPSI Domains *Pain:* Total of items 1a, 1b, 1c, 1d, 2a, 2b, 3, and 4 = _____ *Urinary symptoms:* Total of items 5 and 6 = _____ *Quality-of-life impact:* Total of items 7, 8, and 9 = _____		
Calculate and report three separate scores (pain, urinary symptoms, and quality of life).		
Calculate and report a pain and urinary score (range 0–31), referred to as the "symptom scale score": mild = 0–9; moderate = 10–18; severe = 19–31.		
Calculate and report total score (range 0–43).		

Source: Adapted from NIDDK-funded Chronic Prostatitis Research Network. National Institutes of Health. (www.prostatitis.org/symptomindex.html)

evaluates pain, urinary symptoms, and the impact on quality of life.

1. Mild = 0 to 14 total score
2. Moderate = 15 to 29 total score
3. Severe = 30 to 43 total score

   An online NIH symptom index that self-scores is available at www.prostatitis.org/symptomindex.html.

B. Review the onset, duration, and course of symptoms
C. Are there any other symptoms such as discharge, pain, hematuria, hesitancy, back pain, or weight loss?
D. Has the client ever had the same symptoms? If so, how were they treated?
E. Does any sexual partner(s) have any symptoms, lesions, or known STIs?
F. Does the client engage in anal intercourse?
G. Has the client noted any impaired urinary flow?
H. Has the client required any recent urethral catheterization or instrumentation?

Physical Examination
A. Check temperature and BP.
B. Inspect:
   1. Examine the client generally for discomfort before and during examination.
   2. Check the urethral meatus for discharge.
   3. Retract foreskin (if present) and assess for hygiene and smegma.
   4. Check the shaft of the penis, glans, and prepuce for lesions.
C. Palpate:
   1. Palpate testes and epididymides for inflammation, tenderness, and masses; palpate scrotum for hydrocele or varicocele.
   2. Check back for CVA tenderness.
   3. Evaluate for an enlarged tender bladder because of urinary retention.
   4. Palpate the abdomen for masses, urinary distension, suprapubic tenderness, and organomegaly.
   5. Palpate inguinal lymph nodes; check the inguinal and femoral areas for bulges and hernias; have the client bear down and cough, and reexamine him.
   6. Rectal examination:
      a. Before the rectal examination, have the client obtain a clean-catch urine specimen for culture. Check for symmetry, swelling, tenderness, and enlarged prostate.
      b. In acute prostatitis, rectal examination reveals the prostate gland to be exquisitely tender and boggy.

c. A fluctuant prostatic mass suggests an abscess that may require surgical intervention.

d. Perform prostate massage for postmassage urine sample (see Section II: Procedure, "Prostatic Massage Technique: 2-Glass Test").

Diagnostic Tests

A. Acute infection:
1. CBC with differential
2. Urinalysis and urine culture
3. Culture for STIs
4. Gram stain, culture of EPS
   a. Avoid vigorous massage when obtaining specimen because of the risk of inducing bacteremia
   b. Gram stain of EPS demonstrates infectious organisms or WBCs typical of an immune response (>10 WBC/HPF is abnormal). Clients with abnormal WBC but no bacterial growth may have chlamydial or *Ureaplasma* infection and need to be tested or treated empirically.
B. Chronic infection:
1. BUN
2. CBC with differential
3. Creatinine
C. Chronic bacterial prostatitis:
1. If recurrent infections are confirmed, evaluate for structural or functional abnormality with CT scan.
2. Measure residual urine after voiding.
3. If no urologic abnormalities are found and repeated cultures indicate the same bacterial strain, chronic bacterial prostatitis is likely.
D. Other tests, such as ultrasound, MRI, and biopsies are used as required to rule out other pathology.

Differential Diagnoses

A. Prostatitis:
1. Acute: readily evident by clinical presentation and examination
2. Chronic: more difficult to diagnose. The hallmark symptom is recurrent UTI. It often resembles prostatic hypertrophy, strictures, and prostatic carcinoma.
3. Chronic pelvic pain syndrome
B. Pyelonephritis
C. Epididymitis
D. Anal fistulas and fissures
E. BPH causes urinary retention due to obstruction.
F. Urethral stricture or stone
G. Chronic pain syndromes/back pain

Plan

A. General interventions: Treatment should be directed toward symptom support and culture findings.
1. Clients with acute prostatitis may need hospitalization and IV therapy for severe infection (high fever, increased WBC, dehydration). Less toxic clients may be treated on an outpatient basis.
2. Older men without evidence of infection with lower tract symptoms should have urine cytology to rule out malignancy.

B. Client teaching:
1. Client teaching: *See Section III: Client Teaching Guide for this chapter, "Prostatitis."* ◄
2. Having the client self-massage to reduce symptoms is questionable; the massage of an acutely infected gland is contraindicated because of the risk of bacteremia.
3. Recommend sitz baths two to three times daily.
C. Dietary management:
1. Increase fluid intake.
2. Decrease caffeine and alcohol, which can irritate the urethra.
D. Pharmaceutical therapy:
Full treatment guideline for the "Diagnosis and treatment of chronic bacterial prostatitis and chronic prostatitis/chronic pelvic pain syndrome: A consensus guideline" is available with open access through the Wiley Online Library at onlinelibrary.wiley.com/doi/abs/10.1111/bju.13101.
1. Pain relief:
   a. Analgesics:
      i. NSAIDs should be offered only for short-term treatment of pain to clients with early-stage CBP or chronic prostatitis/chronic pelvic pain syndrome whose symptoms are suspected to be caused by an inflammatory process/flare. NSAIDs should be stopped within 4 to 6 weeks of treatment if they do not reduce symptoms.
      ii. Opioids should not be used in clients with early-stage CBP or CP/CPPS because of the risk of dependency.
      iii. If pain is considered neuropathic in origin, treatment may include a gabapentinoid (e.g., pregabalin or gabapentin), a tricyclic antidepressant (e.g., amitriptyline, nortriptyline, or trimipramine), or a selective serotonin and norepinephrine reuptake inhibitor (SNRI; e.g., duloxetine).
      iv. When pain is severe and refractory to the treatments or is significantly impairing the client's quality of life in daily activities, referral to a pain specialist should be considered.
2. Alpha-adrenergic antagonists:
   a. Because of the adverse side effect profiles, consider offering uroselective α-adrenergic antagonists (e.g., tamsulosin, alfuzosin, and silodosin) as first-line treatment in clients with CBP and CP/CPPS who present with voiding lower urinary tract symptoms (LUTS).
3. Antibiotics: Antimicrobial therapy should be guided by bacterial cultures and sensitivities, taking into consideration drug interactions and/or contraindications. Dose and duration should be sufficient to eradicate the infection. Treatment typically consists of 4 to 8 weeks of antibiotic therapy but may need to be extended to 12 weeks.
   a. First-line therapy for early-stage CBP and CP/CPPS is a quinolone:
      i. Ciprofloxacin 500 mg bid × 4 weeks
      ii. Ofloxacin 400 mg bid × 4 to 6 weeks
      iii. Levofloxacin 500 to 750 mg daily × 4 weeks

b. Second-line therapy:
   i. Trimethoprim/sulfamethoxazole (TMP/SMX): 1 double strength (DS) bid × 14 days or 2 to 3 months if chronic infection
   ii. Tetracyclines: doxycycline 100 mg bid × 4 weeks
c. Macrolides are reserved for special indications, based on advice from microbiological findings.
4. There is insufficient evidence to warrant recommending 5-alpha-reductase inhibitors as monotherapy in CP/CPPS, unless coexisting BPH is present.

Follow-Up
A. See the client in 2 to 10 days depending on the client's symptoms and course
B. Culture urine at completion of drug therapy. Test of cure for antibiotics requires elimination of bacteria from prostatic fluid to prevent chronic flares. Some clients may not achieve cure even after 6 to 12 weeks of therapy.
C. Clients who achieve a partial response may be given a second course of antibiotics. Those failing to demonstrate an organism may benefit from a course of doxycycline or erythromycin for *Chlamydia* and/or *Ureaplasma* coverage.
D. Notify the health department for reportable STIs.

Consultation/Referral
A. Obtain a referral to a urologist for recurrent acute bacterial prostatic infections or infections that persist.
B. Cystoscopy may be required to rule out IC.
C. Urinary retention concomitant with acute prostatitis may require hospitalization.

Individual Considerations
A. Adults:
   1. Prostatitis is the most common prostate infection in men younger than 50 years.

Resources
American Urological Association (AUA): www.auanet.org
National Institute of Diabetes and Digestive and Kidney Diseases (NIDDK): www.niddk.nih.gov
The Prostatitis Foundation: www.prostatitis.org

Bibliography
Ahuja, S. (2016, February 20). Nonbacterial prostatitis. *Medscape*. Retrieved from https://emedicine.medscape.com/article/456165-overview
American Urological Association. (2013, revised 2018). *Early detection of prostate cancer: AUA guideline*. Retrieved from https://www.auanet.org/guidelines/prostate-cancer-early-detection-guideline
Associates in Urology. (n.d.[c]). *Quality of life questionnaire*. Retrieved from http://www.njurology.com/_forms/qualityoflife.php
Deem, S. (2017, September 7). Acute bacterial prostatitis. *Medscape*. Retrieved from emedicine.medscape.com/article/2002872-overview
Kreamer, S. (2019, January 15). Chronic Bacterial Prostatitis. *Medscape*. Retrieved from https://emedicine.medscape.com/article/458391-overview
Turek, P. J. (2018, December 6). Prostatitis. *Medscape*. Retrieved from http://emedicine.medscape.com/article/785418-overview
U.S. Preventive Services Task Force. (2019). *Final update summary: Prostate cancer screening*. Retrieved from https://www.uspreventiveservicestask-force.org/Page/Document/UpdateSummaryFinal/prostate-cancer-screening1?ds=1&s=prostate
Watson, R. (2017, May 22). Chronic pelvic pain in men. *Medscape*. Retrieved from https://emedicine.medscape.com/article/437745-overview

Proteinuria

Cheryl A. Glass and Debbie Gunter

Definition
A. Proteinuria is excess protein (albumin) in urine. Proteinuria may be an incidental finding and have no symptoms. Use of a urine dipstick for screening is acceptable for first detecting proteinuria (see Table 12.4); however, the dipstick should not be used to quantify the amount of urinary protein. Protein concentration is a function of urine volume as well as the quantity of protein present.
B. The measurement of protein excretion is used to establish the diagnosis and to follow the course of glomerular disease. The normal rate of albumin excretion is less than 20 mg/d; the rate is about 4 to 7 mg/d in healthy young adults and increases with age and an increase in body weight. Persistent albumin excretion between 30 and 300 mg/d is called microalbuminuria. Values of 300 mg/d or higher of protein are considered overt proteinuria or macroalbuminuria. Levels over 300 mg/d which persist for 3 months are considered CKD.
C. **When proteinuria coexists with hematuria, the likelihood of clinically significant renal disease is high**. In clients with diabetes, microalbuminuria usually indicates incipient diabetic nephropathy. In nondiabetics, the presence of microalbuminuria is associated with CV disease. Protein is also the cardinal sign of pregnancy-induced hypertension (PIH).
D. Functional/transient proteinuria is associated with fever, exercise, dehydration, cold exposure, and stress and is not associated with underlying renal disease. Orthostatic proteinuria, a transient proteinuria condition, is related to postural changes that affect the glomerular hemodynamics. Orthostatic proteinuria rarely exceeds 1 g/d. Significant renal disease is not usually found upon further testing and workup.
E. Persistent proteinuria is defined as greater than 4 mg/m^2/hr of protein in a 24-hour urine collection or greater than 0.02 mg/mg of PCR on a spot urine. Persistent proteinuria requires further evaluation to rule out underlying renal pathology.
   1. Glomerular proteinuria (albuminuria): Associated with pathological damage to the glomerulus and increased filtration of macromolecules across the

TABLE 12.4 DIPSTICK ANALYSIS—DETECTING AND QUANTIFYING PROTEINURIA

Dipstick Grade	Quantity of Protein (mg/dL)
Negative	<10
Trace	10–20
1+	30
2+	100
3+	300
4+	1,000

There are three types of mechanisms of persistent proteinuria.

glomerular capillary wall. The standard urine dipstick is able to detect glomerular proteinuria. Some causes of glomerular proteinuria include diabetes, HTN, nephrotic syndrome, infections including hepatitis, HIV, CMV, malaria, syphilis, and streptococcal infections, chemotherapeutic agents, Alport syndrome, and hemolytic uremic syndrome.

2. Tubular proteinuria: related to interference with proximal tubular reabsorption. A urinary dipstick is often unable to detect tubular proteinuria. Some causes of tubular proteinuria include toxins, pyelonephritis, NSAIDs, antibiotics, and inherited causes such as Lowe syndrome and Wilson disease.

3. Secretory (overflow) proteinuria: increased excretion from the tubules secondary to an overproduction of a particular protein (light chains in multiple myeloma, myoglobin in rhabdomyolysis) or commonly noted in interstitial nephritis. A urinary dipstick is unable to detect overflow protein.

4. It is currently recommended that a diagnosis of kidney damage can only be made if at least two measurements are elevated.

Incidence

A. Approximately 6% of males and 9.7% of females have proteinuria detected by a single routine dipstick test.

B. The incidence of proteinuria found on a urine dipstick in school-age children is approximately 10%. When repeat testing is done, the incidence decreases to 0.1% of school-age children.

C. The prevalence of orthostatic proteinuria is 2% to 5% and is noted more commonly in older children and adolescents.

D. The prevalence of proteinuria is higher in the elderly and in clients with comorbidities.

Pathogenesis

A. Pathogenesis depends on the underlying etiology. An alteration in glomerular filtration that increases excretion (filtration) of plasma proteins occurs. Increased glomerular permeability, increased production of abnormal proteins (Bence Jones protein), decreased tubular reabsorption, surgical traumas, and infections may increase urinary protein. Urinary protein may also be affected by dietary protein intake.

Predisposing Factors

A. Fever
B. Increased exercise
C. UTI/pyelonephritis
D. Medications:
   1. Penicillamine
   2. NSAIDs
   3. ACE inhibitors
   4. Aminoglycosides
   5. Cisplatin
   6. Amphotericin B
   7. Quinolones
   8. Sulfonamides
   9. Cimetidine (Tagamet)
   10. Allopurinol (Zyloprim)
   11. Antiretroviral drugs can be nephrotoxic.
E. Heavy metal exposure:
   1. Gold
   2. Cadmium
   3. Mercury
   4. Lead
   5. Copper
F. Collagen vascular disease or vasculitis
G. Family history of proteinuria or pyelonephritis
H. HTN
I. Renal disease
J. Congestive heart failure (CHF) or endocarditis
K. Diabetes
L. Lupus
M. Infections:
   1. HIV
   2. Syphilis
   3. Hepatitis B and C
   4. Group A beta-hemolytic *Streptococcus*
   5. Viral infection (e.g., mononucleosis)
   6. Malaria
N. Malignancy:
   1. Lymphoma
   2. Hodgkin's disease
   3. Breast tumor
   4. Lung tumor
   5. Colon tumor
O. Heroin use
P. PIH
Q. Radiocontrast media

Common Complaints

A. Asymptomatic
B. Increased weight
C. Decreased urine output
D. Pediatrics:
   1. Growth failure
   2. Deafness or visual impairment suggests hereditary nephritis

Other Signs and Symptoms

A. Edema: periorbital, presacral, genital, or ankle
B. Nephrotic syndrome: hypercholesterolemia and hypertriglyceridemia
C. Protein malnutrition: anorexia and vomiting
D. "Frothy" urine

Subjective Data

A. Review the onset, course, and duration of presenting complaints.
B. Question the client concerning urinary output, thirst or fluid intake, edema, increase in weight. Establish usual weight history.
C. If a woman, establish the first day of the client's last period. Is she pregnant? If so, what is the fetus's gestational age? Is there edema, HTN, headache, visual changes (scotoma), hyperreflexia, and/or right upper quadrant pain?
D. Review the client's past medical history for renal disease, diabetes, CHF, systemic disorders such as lupus, and substance abuse.

E. Does the client have signs or symptoms of a UTI or pyelonephritis?
F. Review the client's recent history for exertion, emotional stress, surgical trauma, fever, and any acute illness.
G. When was the client's last evaluation for cholesterol? Is he or she on any special diet?
H. Review medication list, including prescribed and OTC medications and herbal products.
I. Review the client's occupational exposure, smoking history, and risk factors for infectious diseases.

Physical Examination

The client's physical examination may have few abnormalities unless there are features of multisystem disease.
A. Check temperature (if indicated), BP, pulse, respiration, and weight.
B. Inspect:
    1. Inspect overall general appearance for edema (pedal, hand, facial, or periorbital edema), butterfly rash (lupus), or ascites.
    2. Evaluate for protein wasting.
    3. Evaluate for jugular vein distension.
    4. Funduscopic examination: evaluate for retinopathy.
    5. Inspect for pharyngitis.
C. Auscultate:
    1. The heart and lungs
D. Palpate:
    1. Examine the abdomen; evaluate bladder distension, suprapubic tenderness, masses or ascites, abdominal tenderness
    2. Palpate for CVA tenderness.
    3. Check deep tendon reflexes, especially in pregnant women.

Diagnostic Tests

A. Urine dipstick is a good screening tool in the outpatient setting.
B. Single-void "spot" urine testing:
    1. The first urine specimen of the morning is optimal and is guideline recommended. Evaluation of the first morning specimen excludes any postural effect on the protein component.
    2. The gold standard for measurement of protein excretion is a 24-hour urine collection, but is now being replaced by the easier-to-obtain and less-complicated spot test. The 24-hour urine is considered impractical for generalized testing, especially in the pediatric population. The normal amount of protein in the urine is < 150 mg/d.
C. Polymerase chain reaction (PCR) test or ACR test on a first-morning or a random spot specimen. The PCR or ACR is useful in following trends in the client's proteinuria.
D. CBC and serum electrolytes
E. Serum creatinine (if renal disease is suspected)
F. Lipid profile
G. BUN: serves as an index of renal excretory capacity. Urea is the nitrogenous end product of protein metabolism.
H. Urinalysis, urine culture, and sensitivity (if indicated)
I. Ultrasound of the full urinary tract

J. Screen for diabetes and other testing related to physical findings
K. Renal biopsy is required to establish the diagnosis in most cases.

Differential Diagnoses

A. See "Predisposing Factors" section.

Plan

A. General interventions:
    1. Current guidelines for screening for evaluation of albuminuria/proteinuria vary by country, but recommendations include at-risk individuals with diabetes, HTN, obesity, smokers, indigenous populations, family history of CKD, age greater than 50 years, structural renal tract disease, renal calculi, prostatic hypertrophy, vascular disease, and autoimmune disease.
    2. Management for nephrotic syndrome includes diet with sodium and protein restriction, loop and distal-acting diuretics, control of cholesterol (low-saturated-fat, low-cholesterol diet), lipid-lowering agents, pneumococcal and influenza vaccines to prevent infections, and use of steroids and immunosuppressive agents as necessary.
    3. Clients with hematuria and proteinuria need a 24-hour urine collection for protein and creatinine clearance.
B. Client teaching:
    1. Encourage low-fat/low-cholesterol diet if hyperlipidemia is present
    2. Encourage sodium- and protein-restricted diet for nephrotic syndrome.
C. Pharmaceutical therapy:
    1. There is no specific drug therapy for excess protein.
    2. Use drug therapy appropriate to the underlying medical disease causing proteinuria.
    3. In clients with CKD, the administration of ACE inhibitors and/or ARBs is aimed at reducing the degree of proteinuria.
    4. The Advisory Committee on Immunization Practices (ACIP) recommends immunization with 13-valent pneumococcal conjugate vaccine (PCV13), followed by a dose of 23-valent pneumococcal polysaccharide vaccine (PPSV23) at least 8 weeks later, in clients with nephrotic syndrome.

Follow-Up

A. If proteinuria is found on a dipstick and the first-morning test results are trace or negative for protein, repeat a first-morning test in 1 year.
B. There is no consensus on how often to screen for proteinuria. Guidelines include annual screening, every 5 years for clients older than 50 years or smokers, and every 3 years for clients who have HTN, obesity, a family history of kidney disease, or are indigenous. Monitoring should always include BP, quantitative testing by PCR or ACR, and a serum creatinine.
C. Client should be assessed at routine examination appointments for vasculitic skin changes, rashes,

retinopathy, lymphadenopathy, signs of heart failure, abdominal masses, organomegaly, guaiac stools, prostatic enlargement, and joint inflammation.

Consultation/Referral

A. Consider client referral to nephrologist if kidney damage is progressing from medical disease (systemic lupus erythematosus, HTN, diabetes).

B. Refer the client as necessary; HTN is a poor prognostic sign for significant renal impairment.

C. Consultation for diagnostic tests to be considered: kidney, ureter, and bladder (KUB); IVP; renal ultrasonography; renal biopsy

D. Referral to a pediatric nephrologist should be considered if a definitive diagnosis is required or a renal biopsy is considered.

Individual Considerations

A. Pregnancy:

1. Protein excretion is considered abnormal in pregnancy when it exceeds 300 mg/24 hr or greater than 0.3 g of protein per gram of creatinine in a random urine specimen. A urine specimen with 1+ protein is considered the cutoff for proteinuria.

2. The gestational age at which proteinuria is first documented is important in establishing the likelihood of PIH versus other renal diseases. Proteinuria before or early in pregnancy suggests preexisting renal disease.

3. Monitor urine protein and BP at each prenatal visit and refer the client if urinary protein remains elevated.

4. Monitor for intrauterine growth restriction (IUGR).

5. Proteinuria (or HTN) that persists longer than 3 months after delivery should be followed closely.

B. Pediatrics:

1. The American Academy of Pediatrics recommends that children be screened on two occasions during childhood:

   a. Before entrance into school

   b. During adolescence

2. Although there are no set guidelines for children, a child with persistent proteinuria should be initially worked up with a physical examination, BP, urinalysis, serum creatinine, and BUN every 6 to 12 months.

3. When the child is stable, the follow-up should be done annually.

4. There are no dietary or physical activity limitations.

C. Geriatrics:

1. Renal function deteriorates in the elderly who may also have coexisting medical conditions (HTN, diabetes) that may cause nephropathy.

Bibliography

American College of Obstetricians and Gynecologists. (2019). *Hypertension in pregnancy*. Retrieved from https://www.acog.org/Clinical-Guidance-and-Publications/Practice-Guidelines-and-Reports-Search?Keyword=hypertension%20in%20pregnancy

Ekiz, A., Kaya, B., & Polat, I. (2016). The outcome of pregnancy with new onset proteinuria without hypertension: Retrospective observational study. *Journal of Maternal-Fetal & Neonatal Medicine, 29*(11), 1765–1769.

Gagnadoux, M. (2016, May 31). Evaluation of proteinuria in children. *UpToDate*. Retrieved from www.uptodate.com/contents/evaluation-of-proteinuria-in-children

Lane, J. (2018, October 24). Pediatric nephrotic syndrome. *Medscape*. Retrieved from http://emedicine.medscape.com/article/982920-overview

Rovin, B. (2019, January 11). Assessment of urinary protein excretion and evaluation of isolated non-nephrotic proteinuria in adults. *UpToDate*. Retrieved from www.uptodate.com/contents/assessment-of-urinary-protein-excretion-and-evaluation-of-isolated-non-nephrotic-proteinuria-in-adults

Stephen, R., & Jolly, S. (2014). Albuminuria: When urine predicts kidney and cardiovascular disease. *Cleveland Clinic Journal of Medicine, 81*(1), 41–50. https://doi.org/10.3949/ccjm.81a.13040

Thadhani, R. (2019, February 11). Proteinuria in pregnancy: Evaluation and management. *UpToDate*. Retrieved from www.uptodate.com/contents/proteinuria-in-pregnancy-evaluation-and-management

Thomas, B. (2018, April 28). Proteinuria. *Medscape*. Retrieved from https://emedicine.medscape.com/article/238158-overview

Pyelonephritis

Cheryl A. Glass and Debbie Gunter

Definition

A. Pyelonephritis is an acute infection and inflammatory disease of the upper urinary tract (renal pelvis, tubules, and interstitial tissue) of one or both kidneys. Acute pyelonephritis is an ascending UTI that has progressed from the lower urinary tract.

B. Fever has been strongly correlated with the diagnosis of acute pyelonephritis; therefore, clients with clinical symptoms of pyelonephritis in the absence of fever should be evaluated for alternative diagnoses.

C. Acute pyelonephritis characteristically causes some scarring to the kidney and may lead to significant damage, kidney failure, abscess formation, and sepsis. Antibiotic therapy is essential to prevent the progression of pyelonephritis.

Incidence

A. Thirty percent of the female population have at least one UTI in their lifetime.

B. Annual rates of pyelonephritis in women are 15 to 17 cases per 10,000 and three to four cases per 10,000 for men.

C. Acute pyelonephritis develops in 20%–30% of pregnant women who have untreated asymptomatic bacteriuria (ABU) (2%–9.5%). This infection occurs most often during the late second and early third trimesters.

D. Upper UTIs are less common and more serious than lower UTIs. After puberty, the prevalence of UTIs increases slightly in females, but remains low in males.

E. After age 65 years, UTIs are more common with an equal incidence in both sexes.

Pathogenesis

A. Pyelonephritis is caused by ascending infection from the bladder, usually caused by *E. coli* (75%–90%) and other gram-negative bacteria including *Proteus mirabilis* (5%), *Klebsiella pneumoniae* (5%), *Enterobacter* (3%), and group B *Streptococcus* (GBS: 1%). Gram-positive causative agents are less common; 10% to 15% of cases are caused by *Staphylococcus saprophyticus*.

B. Bacteria can also reach the kidneys through the bloodstream from IV drug abuse and endocarditis.
C. In women, the short urethra in close proximity to the perirectal area makes colonization possible. In pregnancy, the increased glycosuria, increase in urinary amino acids, urinary stasis, and the presence of vesicoureteral reflux facilitate bacterial growth.
D. In children, vesicoureteric reflux is the most common pathology.
E. In men, BPH causing bladder obstruction is a common pathology.
F. Indwelling catheters increase ascending infections and pyelonephritis.

Predisposing Factors
A. Previous UTI, cystitis, and pyelonephritis
B. Sickle cell disease
C. Diabetes
D. Urinary catheterization
E. Obstruction: calculi, tumors, and urethral strictures
F. Neurogenic bladder disease: strokes, multiple sclerosis, and spinal cord injuries
G. Urinary reflux
H. HIV
I. Trauma
J. Chronic constipation (children)
K. Incomplete bladder emptying related to medications (e.g., anticholinergics)
L. Gender:
  1. Females:
    a. Increased sexual activity, failure to void after intercourse, diaphragms, and spermicides
    b. Pregnancy
    c. Atrophic vaginal mucosa predisposes to the colonization of pathogens and UTIs
  2. Males:
    a. Homosexuality
    b. Sexual partner with colonization
    c. Obstruction: prostatic hypertrophy
    d. Age 50 years or older
    e. Acute or chronic bacterial prostatitis

Common Complaints
A. Shaking, chills, and fever
B. Flank pain or tenderness
C. Urinary frequency or urgency
D. CVA tenderness
E. Guarding
F. Urinary frequency, nocturia, hematuria, and dysuria (not always present in upper tract infections)
G. Blood in urine secondary to hemorrhagic cystitis (unusual in males with pyelonephritis)

Other Signs and Symptoms
A. Adults (particularly the elderly): may be asymptomatic with cystitis
B. Abdominal pain and suprapubic heaviness
C. Pregnancy: uterine contractions
D. SOB
E. Anorexia

F. Children:
  1. Fever may be a child's only presenting symptom.
  2. Nausea and vomiting
  3. Irritability
  4. Diarrhea
  5. Abdominal pain/tenderness
  6. Feeding difficulty
  7. Failure to thrive
G. Elderly:
  1. Mental status change
  2. Generalized deterioration with loss of function

Subjective Data
A. Review the onset, course, and duration of symptoms.
B. Are there any problems with voiding such as frequency, urgency, and dysuria?
C. Review the client's history of fever and any treatment.
D. Are there any other symptoms, odor, and nausea?
E. Have the client point to the area of the backache. Is it unilateral or bilateral? What makes the backache better?
F. In women, rule out pregnancy; review first day of last menses.
G. Rule out sickle cell disease, diabetes, and multiple sclerosis.
H. Review the client's previous history of GU tract problems, stones, UTIs, previous pyelonephritis, any previous testing, and any previous anomalies.
I. Review the strength and character of the urinary stream, especially in older men. Ask if the client has ever been diagnosed with BPH.
J. Review the client's history for active herpes lesion. Does urine flow hurt when urine stream begins? Or is the pain noted when urine passes over the lesion?
K. Review drug allergies.
L. Review all medications, including OTC and herbal products. Review medications for a recent history of an incomplete course of antibiotics and current use of anticholinergics.

Physical Examination
A. Check temperature, pulse, and BP; note orthostatic hypotension. Tachycardia may or may not be present, depending on associated fever, dehydration, and sepsis.
B. Inspect:
  1. Note general appearance for respiratory distress and dehydration.
  2. Inspect the male external genitalia for redness, edema, lesions, and discharge.
  3. Inspect the female genitalia for discharge, lesions, and fissures; inspect cervix for cervicitis.
C. Palpate:
  1. Palpate the back; check CVA tenderness (usually unilateral over the involved kidney).
  2. Palpate the abdomen for suprapubic tenderness, rebound masses, or pain.
  3. Perform a pelvic examination to rule out other infections and PID (tenderness of the cervix, uterus, and adnexa should be absent).

D. Auscultate:
  1. The lungs and heart
E. Pregnancy:
  1. Check fetal heart rate; fetal tachycardia may be present with fever.
  2. Palpate for uterine tenderness and contractions.
  3. Pelvic examination for cervical dilation, if indicated for increased risk of preterm labor
F. Males:
  1. Complete palpation of external genitalia, prostate, and rectal examination

Diagnostic Tests

A. Urine culture and sensitivity should always be performed before initial empiric treatment with antibiotics.
B. Urinalysis for evaluation of pyuria. Pyuria is present in almost all women with acute cystitis and pyelonephritis; its absence strongly suggests an alternative diagnosis.
  1. Leukocyte esterase on dipstick detects pyuria or WBCs.
  2. Significant pyuria is greater than two to five leukocytes per HPF.
  3. Urine may need to be obtained from straight in-and-out catheterization if the client is incontinent or has altered mental status.
  4. White cell casts are indicative of pyelonephritis.
C. CBC with differential or WBC, especially with systemic symptoms
D. Blood culture, if indicated
E. Arterial blood gases (ABGs), if indicated
F. Consider sedimentation rate, especially with severe illness and in the elderly
G. Culture for gonorrhea and chlamydia, if symptoms are associated with STIs
H. Wet prep, if symptoms are associated with STI
I. Imaging studies are not routinely required for the diagnosis of acute pyelonephritis but can be helpful.
  1. CT scan to identify altered parenchymal perfusion, hemorrhage, nonrenal disease, inflammatory masses, and obstruction. CT with contrast medium is considered the imaging modality of choice for nonpregnant women.
  2. MRI to rule out masses or obstruction
  3. Renal ultrasonography
  4. Scintigraphy to detect focal renal abnormalities
  5. Voiding cystourethrogram
  6. IVP, if indicated
  7. CT and magnetic resonance (MR) urography used in the evaluation of hematuria

Differential Diagnoses

A. Appendicitis/acute abdomen
B. Cholecystitis
C. Pancreatitis
D. Diverticulitis
E. Pneumonia
F. Prostatitis
G. Epididymitis
H. PID
I. Nephrolithiasis

Plan

A. General interventions:
  1. Optimal therapy for acute uncomplicated pyelonephritis depends on the severity of the illness at presentation.
  2. Many severe infections (increased WBC, dehydration or vomiting, high fever) may need hospital admission for IV therapy. Risk factors include older adult, coexisting illness, pregnancy, and uncontrolled vomiting.
B. Client teaching:
  1. Give instruction on early recognition of UTIs.
  2. Client teaching: *See Section III: Client Teaching Guide for "Urinary Tract Infection (Acute Cystitis)."* ◄
C. Dietary management:
  1. Increase fluids: Have the client drink at least one large glass of water every hour while awake.
  2. Encourage the client to drink cranberry juice to help fight and prevent UTIs. If the taste is objectionable, he or she may mix cranberry juice 1:1 with another juice such as grape juice.
  3. There are no dietary restrictions with pyelonephritis.
D. Pharmaceutical therapy:
  1. Acetaminophen (Tylenol) for fever
  2. Urinary analgesic as needed to relieve dysuria. Dysuria is usually diminished fairly quickly after the start of antibiotics.
  3. Antiemetics as needed; however, if the client is not able to tolerate oral fluids, he or she should be hospitalized.
  4. Antibiotics: Empiric antibiotic selection should be guided by local antibiotic resistance patterns, allergies, and culture results. Clients with delayed response to therapy should also receive a longer course of antibiotics of 14 to 21 days. Oral versus IV therapy remains controversial. In order to use oral antibiotics, the client must be able to take oral medication, food and fluids, have no indication for hospital admission, and have close monitoring nearby.
    a. Adults:
      i. First-line therapy: ciprofloxacin (Cipro) 500 mg twice daily for 7 days, *or* extended-release Cipro XR 1,000 mg once a day for 7 days
      ii. First-line therapy: levofloxacin (Levaquin) 750 mg once daily for 5 to 7 days
      iii. Second-line therapy: trimethoprim and sulfamethoxazole (TMP-SMX; Septra DS, Bactrim DS) 160 mg and 800 mg, respectively, one tablet twice daily for 7 to 10 days. Because of the high rate of resistance of *E. coli*, the empirical use of TMP-SMX should be avoided in clients who require hospitalization.

iv. Alternative therapy: amoxicillin-clavulanate (Augmentin) 500 mg/125 mg orally twice a day for 14 days *or* Augmentin 250 mg/125 mg orally three times a day for 3 to 7 days

b. Children younger than 2 years are usually treated for 7 to 14 days. Children older than 2 years who are afebrile and without abnormalities of the urinary tract or have previous episodes of UTIs are usually treated for 5 days.

   i. Amoxicillin–clavulanate (Augmentin) 20 to 40 mg/kg orally per day in three doses for 7 to 14 days

   ii. Sulfonamide–trimethoprim–sulfamethoxazole (TMP-SMX) 6 to 12 mg/kg trimethoprim and 30 to 60 mg/kg sulfamethoxazole per day orally in two doses for 7 to 14 days

   iii. Cephalosporin–cefuroxime (Ceftin) 8 mg/kg/d in one dose for 7 to 14 days

c. Antibiotics that should not be used for pyelonephritis:

   i. Nitrofurantoin (Macrodantin) and fosfomycin (Monurol) should not be used to treat pyelonephritis in adults or children; they are excreted in the urine but do not achieve therapeutic serum levels.

   ii. Fluoroquinolones are not used in children because of potential concerns about sustained injury to developing joints.

   iii. Tetracyclines should not be used in children because of tooth staining.

   iv. Fluoroquinolones are not used in pregnancy because of the risk of auditory and vestibular toxicity in the fetus.

   v. Aminoglycosides are contraindicated in pregnancy because of the risk of permanent ototoxicity to the fetus.

Follow-Up

A. Follow up with the client in 24 to 48 hours depending on the evaluation of the initial severity of symptoms.

  1. Clients with persistent fever or clinical symptoms after 48 to 72 hours of appropriate antibiotic therapy should undergo initiation of another class of antibiotics and consider radiologic evaluation.

  2. If the client feels that he or she is not progressing well or is getting worse, evaluate the client emergently and consider hospital admission and IV antibiotics.

B. Follow-up urine cultures are not needed for clients with acute cystitis or pyelonephritis if symptoms resolved on antibiotics; however, repeat cultures for clients with recurrent symptoms or any complicated course of illness.

C. Women with recurrence of pyelonephritis need further urologic investigation.

Consultation/Referral

A. Consult physician and consider hospitalization for infants with both lower and upper infections, children with pyelonephritis, and children with recurrent infections.

B. Consult or refer the client to a physician if he or she requires IVP, cystoscopy, or renal biopsy.

C. IV therapy and hospitalization are needed in all cases suggestive of bacteremia in children who are vomiting, children younger than 2 years, and children with documented parenchymal damage.

D. Males with persistent bladder infections need a urologic consultation.

E. Pyelonephritis in men suggests structural problems and needs hospitalization and further evaluation (IVP).

F. Consult an infectious disease specialist for clients with unusual or resistant pathogens.

G. For pregnant clients, consultation with an obstetrician is required.

Individual Considerations

A. Pregnancy:

  1. Pyelonephritis is the most common urinary tract complication in pregnancy.

  2. Untreated ASB is a risk factor for acute cystitis and pyelonephritis in pregnancy.

  3. Based on the higher risk of complications in pregnancy, pyelonephritis has traditionally been treated with hospitalization and IV antibiotics until the woman is afebrile for 48 hours and symptoms improve.

  4. Once the pregnant client is discharged from the hospital, oral antibiotics should continue for 10 to 14 days of treatment.

  5. A urine culture should be obtained 1 to 2 weeks after completion of therapy and monthly thereafter to monitor for recurrent infection.

  6. Aminoglycosides should be avoided because of the potential risk of ototoxicity following prolonged fetal exposure.

  7. Fluoroquinolones are contraindicated during pregnancy because of the risk of auditory and vestibular toxicity in the fetus.

B. Pediatrics:

  1. Always order a urine culture and sensitivity on children suspected of UTI.

  2. Suprapubic aspiration of the bladder should be considered in young infants.

  3. A voiding cystogram should be considered in all children younger than 16 years with a documented UTI.

  4. Indications for hospitalization:

    a. Age less than 2 months

    b. Clinical urosepsis or potential bacteremia

    c. Immunocompromised client

    d. Vomiting or inability to tolerate oral medication

    e. Lack of adequate outpatient follow-up (e.g., no phone, lives far from hospital)

    f. Failure to respond to outpatient therapy

  5. Vesicoureteric reflux is responsible for up to 50% of pyelonephritis in children younger than 6 years.

  6. Assess the child for chronic constipation as a potential cause for urinary obstruction.

C. Males:
1. Consider ordering renal function tests (BUN and creatinine).
2. Men older than 50 years: consider urologic consultation and IVP.
D. Geriatrics:
1. Clients may need hospitalization for IV antibiotics and hydration.
2. Bladder or kidney infections may be common in clients with long-term urinary catheters and can lead to septicemia if untreated or unrecognized.
3. Fluoroquinolone use in the elderly has the potential to cause neuropsychiatric symptoms, including seizures to worsening dementia.

Bibliography

Fulop, T. (2018, December 12). Acute pyelonephritis. *Medscape*. Retrieved from emedicine.medscape.com/article/245559-overview

Hooton, T. M. (2018, July 27). Acute simple cystitis in men. *UpToDate*. Retrieved from https://www.uptodate.com/contents/acute-simple-cystitis-in-men

Hooton, T. M. (2019, April 1). Acute complicated urinary tract infection (including pyelonephritis) in adults. *UpToDate*. Retrieved from https://www.uptodate.com/contents/acute-complicated-urinary-tract-infection-including-pyelonephritis-in-adults

Hooton, T. M., & Gupta, K. (2019, March 13). Acute simple cystitis in women. *UpToDate*. Retrieved from https://www.uptodate.com/contents/acute-simple-cystitis-in-women

Renal Calculi or Kidney Stones (Nephrolithiasis)

Cheryl A. Glass and Debbie Gunter

Definition

A. Renal calculi, or kidney stones, are caused by the formation of crystals in the urinary system from the kidneys to the bladder. *Nephrolithiasis* refers to renal stone disease; *urolithiasis* refers to the presence of stones in the urinary system. The majority of stones (80%) consist of calcium, usually as calcium oxalate, but they can contain uric acid, struvite (magnesium, ammonium, and phosphate), oxalic acid, phosphate salts, or the amino acid cysteine. Spontaneous passage of a stone is related to the stone size and location. Approximately one half of symptomatic clients require intervention for stone removal. An untreated staghorn (branch shaped) with persistent renal obstruction can destroy renal tissue with potential for life-threatening sepsis.

Incidence

A. Renal calculi are very common in the United States, with a higher incidence noted in males. The overall incidence is rising. At least 12% of men and 7% of women have one symptomatic stone by age 70 years. Having a family member with a history of stones doubles these rates. Initial cases typically occur between ages 20 and 49 years, with peak incidence between 35 and 45 and prevalence continuing to increase with age. Idiopathic nephrolithiasis is common in males, whereas primary hyperparathyroidism is more common in females.

B. Most kidney stones pass spontaneously; however, 10% to 30% do not pass and can cause continuing pain, infection, or obstruction.
C. Nephrolithiasis is uncommon in children.
D. Stones because of infection (struvite) are more common in women.
E. The incidence of stones in pregnancy is one in every 1,500 to 3,000 pregnancies.
F. The recurrence rate for calculi is 14% at 1 year, 35% at 5 years, and 52% at 10 years.

Pathogenesis

A. The formation of uric acid stones requires continued and excessive oversaturation of urine with stone-forming constituents, uric acid, calcium, and oxalate. Dehydration, hyperuricosuria, and significantly acidic urine contribute to uric acid supersaturation and stone formation. Struvite stones form only when the urinary tract is infected with urea-splitting organisms such as *Proteus* species.
B. Hydroureteronephrosis is the most significant renal alteration in pregnancy. Dilatation is greater on the right side than the left because of pressure because of physiological engorgement of the right ovarian vein and dextrorotation of the uterus.

Predisposing Factors

A. Male
B. Dehydration (poor intake and immobility)
C. Chronic obstruction with stasis of urine
D. Hypercalcemia caused by hyperparathyroidism; renal tubular acidosis; multiple myeloma; or excessive intake of vitamin D, milk, and alkali
E. Diet high in purines and abnormal purine metabolism (gout)
F. Pregnancy (1 per 1,500)
G. Chronic infections
H. Foreign bodies
I. Excessive oxalate absorption in inflammatory bowel disease, bowel resection, or ileostomy
J. Previous stone formation
K. Family history of nephrolithiasis
L. Medications:
1. Vitamins A, C, and D
2. Loop diuretics
3. Acetazolamide
4. Ammonium chloride
5. Calcium-containing medications, including alkali and antacids
6. Indinavir
7. Sulfadiazine
8. Atazanavir
9. Guaifenesin
10. Sulfa drugs
11. Topiramate
12. Acyclovir
M. Obesity
N. Gastric bypass/bariatric surgical procedures
O. Diabetes

Common Complaints
A. Severe flank pain
B. Pelvic pain
C. Groin pain
D. Blood in urine
E. Asymptomatic (dependent on the size of the stone)

Other Signs and Symptoms
A. Unilateral flank pain that radiates to the groin
B. Sudden onset of colicky pain
C. Hematuria

> The timing and appearance of hematuria are important. Hematuria seen at the beginning of the urine stream may indicate bleeding in the urethra. Terminal hematuria, or blood in the end of the urine stream, denotes bladder neck or the prostate as the source. Finally, blood throughout the entire urine stream suggests a lesion.

D. Nausea and vomiting
E. Restlessness
F. Symptoms common with cystitis or inflammatory lesions of the lower tract are usually absent, such as frequency, dysuria, urgency, and suprapubic pain.

Subjective Data
A. Review the onset, duration, and course of symptoms.
B. Review other signs and symptoms of UTI or pyelonephritis: frequency, dysuria, and fever.
C. Have the client describe pain (colicky). Note intensity (use a 1- to 10-point scale, 10 being the worst pain) and the characteristics of pain (constant, intermittent).
D. Has the client ever had a stone before? How was it treated? What tests were performed? Has the client ever seen a urologist?
E. Review dietary intake of high animal protein in the diet, milk, and other calcium-containing products for excessive intake.
F. Review the client's medication history including excessive vitamin C or D supplements, antacids that contain calcium, and other medications noted in the predisposing factors.
G. Ask the client to describe any hematuria or blood clots passed.
H. Ask about recent trauma to the back or abdomen.
I. Is there a family history of stone formation?
J. Is the client pregnant?

Physical Examination
A. Check temperature, BP, and pulse (may have tachycardia). Children: check growth measurements to evaluate poor weight gain and/or failure to thrive (congenital and chronic conditions).
B. Inspect:
  1. Inspect general appearance for discomfort before and during examination. Clients with renal colic are extremely restless and exhibit active movement on presentation.
  2. During the examination evaluate voluntary guarding of the abdominal musculature.
  3. Inspect external genitalia (male or female) for lesions, discharge, inflammation, and ulcerations.
  4. Assess for peripheral edema.
C. Auscultate:
  1. The abdomen, noting bruits if present
  2. Bowel sounds
D. Palpate:
  1. "Milk" the urethra for discharge.
  2. Palpate the abdomen for masses and tenderness, organomegaly, and suprapubic tenderness.
  3. Palpate the groin; check lymph nodes.
  4. Palpate the back and abdomen.
  5. Check for the presence of CVA tenderness.
E. Perform pelvic or bimanual examination, if indicated, to rule out PID.

Diagnostic Tests
The diagnosis of nephrolithiasis can be made on the basis of clinical symptoms alone, but diagnostic testing is needed to confirm.
A. Laboratory tests:
  1. Serum BUN
  2. Creatinine
  3. Calcium
  4. Uric acid
  5. Serum electrolytes; consider fasting serum calcium and phosphorus and parathyroid hormone
  6. Pregnancy test (if indicated) to rule out an ectopic pregnancy
B. Stone for analysis
C. Urinalysis:
  1. Urine dipstick for a gross screen
  2. pH determination (pH greater than 7.5 is compatible with infection lithiasis, and a pH less than 5.5 favors uric acid lithiasis)
  3. Red cell casts strongly suggest glomerulonephritis.
  4. Evaluate urine sediment for crystalluria.
D. Urine culture, if indicated
E. 24-hour urine for creatinine, calcium, uric acid, oxalate, pH, and sodium measurement:
  1. Client should be on his or her usual diet before taking 24-hour specimen.
  2. Collection should be 1 to 2 months after any interventions, including shock-wave lithotripsy, ureteroscopy, or percutaneous stone removal.
F. Noncontrast helical CT scan is the imaging standard to assess the urinary tract in acute renal colic.
G. Renal ultrasound is the procedure of choice for pregnancy.
H. X-ray of the KUB is often ordered with the pelvic CT or ultrasound.
I. IVP
J. Nuclear renal scan

Differential Diagnoses
A. UTI: Passage of large, bulky blood clots implicates the bladder as the source, whereas long, shoestring-shaped specks or thin, stringy clots suggest an upper urinary tract or ureteral origin.
B. Acute abdomen/appendicitis

C. Cholecystitis

D. Pyelonephritis: associated with dull flank pain with fever and chills. In evaluating urine sediment, the presence of WBCs and bacteria favors a diagnosis of pyelonephritis or interstitial nephritis.

E. PID

F. Inflammatory bowel disease

G. Urinary tract obstruction

H. Constipation

I. Ectopic pregnancy

Plan

A. General interventions:

    1. Increase fluids to allow passage of stone. Strain all urine to recover stone for analysis.

    2. Reduce possibility of recurrence with dietary modifications.

    3. The client is usually referred for imaging after evaluation of creatinine.

    4. Clients can be managed on an outpatient basis with close follow-up if stones are small (less than 6 mm).

B. Client teaching/dietary management:

    1. Force fluids to maintain a daily output of 2 to 3 L of urine. Fluid intake that increases urinary production of at least 2 L of urine per day increases the flow rate and lowers the urine solute concentration.

    2. Dietary consultation may be needed secondary to stone analysis.

C. Pharmaceutical therapy:

    1. Pain medication (narcotic and nonnarcotic) is a priority.

        a. NSAIDs should be discontinued 3 days before shock-wave lithotripsy to decrease the risk of bleeding.

    2. Antibiotics should be given for infection.

    3. Antiemetics if needed

    4. Other medical/pharmaceutical management depends on the etiology of the stone.

D. Surgical options are dependent on stone size and location.

    1. Percutaneous nephrolithotomy is the first treatment option for most clients and is considered the treatment of choice for clients with staghorn calculi.

    2. Extracorporeal shock-wave lithotripsy is the least invasive of the surgical methods.

    3. Percutaneous nephrostomy should be the last procedure for most clients.

    4. Open nephrostomy may also be used.

Follow-Up

A. Reevaluate the client in 24 hours by phone or in the clinic.

B. Evaluate sooner if pain increases, because of the potential to progress to complete obstruction.

C. Recurrent stone formation is a manifestation of a systemic disease; evaluate for the management of the metabolic abnormality.

Consultation/Referral

A. Clients with severe pain, nausea, and vomiting need hospitalization for IV hydration and pain control. Consult with a physician.

B. Clients with severe symptoms and persistent obstruction beyond 3 to 4 days should be referred for urologic evaluation.

C. Refer to urology for surgical interventions: Lithotripsy, urethroscope interventions, extracorporeal shock-wave lithotripsy, and percutaneous ultrasonic lithotripsy may be indicated. Treatment varies based on the location and size of the stone. Laparoscopy may be indicated for the removal of large or severely impacted ureteral calculi.

Individual Considerations

A. Pregnancy:

    1. Urolithiasis is the most common cause of nonobstetrical abdominal pain that requires hospitalization in pregnancy.

    2. Approximately 80% to 90% are diagnosed in the first trimester.

    3. Renal ultrasound is the first-line screening test for pregnant clients. A transvaginal ultrasound may also be performed.

    4. Low-dose CT is reserved for complex cases in the second and third trimesters.

    5. Conservative treatment is used: bed rest, hydration, and analgesia.

    6. Invasive measures include stent placement, ureteroscopy, and percutaneous nephrostomy.

    7. Upon presentation, rule out:

        a. Ectopic pregnancy

        b. Abruptio placentae

        c. Preterm labor

B. Pediatrics:

    1. Young children generally do not present with the classic acute onset of flank pain; instead, they may present with abdominal pain. Stone may be detected when abdominal imaging is performed.

    2. Hematuria can present as the sole symptom or in conjunction with abdominal pain.

    3. Ten percent of children present with symptoms of dysuria and urgency.

    4. Shock-wave lithotripsy and percutaneous-based therapy may be considered in children.

Bibliography

American Urological Association. (2014). *Medical management of kidney stones.* Retrieved from https://www.auanet.org/guidelines/kidney-stones-medical-mangement-guideline

American Urological Association. (2016, April). *Surgical management of stones: American Urological Association/Endourological Society guideline.* Retrieved from www.auanet.org/education/guidelines/surgical-manage-ment-of-stones.cfm

Curhan, G. C., Aronson, M. D., & Preminger, G. M. (2018, September 21). Diagnosis and acute management of suspected nephrolithiasis in adults. *UpToDate.* Retrieved from https://www.uptodate.com/contents/diagnosis-and-acute-management-of-suspected-nephrolithiasis-in-adults

Dave, C. (2018, June 21). Nephrolithiasis. *Medscape*. Retrieved from https://emedicine.medscape.com/article/437096-overview

Preminger, G. M., & Curhan, G. C. (2017, August 29). Nephrolithiasis during pregnancy. *UpToDate*. Retrieved from https://www.uptodate.com/contents/nephrolithiasis-during-pregnancy

Smith, J., & Stapleton, F. B. (2018, August 29). Clinical features and diagnosis of nephrolithiasis in children. *UpToDate*. Retrieved from https://www.uptodate.com/contents/clinical-features-and-diagnosis-of-nephrolithiasis-in-children

Wayment, R. O. (2018, July 23). Pregnancy and urolithiasis. *Medscape*. Retrieved from http://emedicine.medscape.com/article/455830-overview

Sexual Dysfunction Male: Erectile Dysfunction

Debbie Gunter and Nancy Pesta Walsh

Definition

A. Erectile dysfunction, also known as impotence, is the persistent inability to achieve or maintain penile erection sufficient for satisfactory sexual performance. Erectile dysfunction occurs with reduced blood flow to the penis or nerve damage as well as psychological triggers. Low self-esteem, performance anxiety, depression, stress, and effects to quality of life occur secondary to erectile dysfunction. Erectile dysfunction is noted to be a precursor to symptomatic coronary artery disease (CAD).

B. Age-associated changes in sexual function in men include delay in erection, diminished intensity and duration of orgasm, and decreased force of seminal emission. Erectile dysfunction lasting 3 months or longer should have further evaluation and consideration of treatment.

C. Multiple male sexual dysfunction questionnaires are available for order through the website www.pfizerpatientreportedoutcomes.com/order-measures sponsored by Pfizer, Inc. The website notes the questionnaires may be ordered free of charge and are available in several translations. Questionnaires include:

1. Erectile Dysfunction Inventory of Treatment Satisfaction (EDITS) used in the evaluation of satisfaction with medical treatment modalities for erectile dysfunction

2. Erectile Hardness Scale (EHS)

3. International Index of Erectile Function (IIEF) is available in two versions. Version 1 is applicable to heterosexual men. Version 2 is edited so that it is applicable to heterosexual and homosexual men. The IIEF assesses five dimensions relevant to sexual function:

   a. Erectile function (six items)

   b. Orgasmic function (two items)

   c. Sexual desire (two items)

   d. Intercourse satisfaction (three items)

   e. Overall satisfaction (two items)

4. Index of Premature Ejaculation (IPE) assesses control over ejaculation, sexual satisfaction, and distress.

5. Premature Ejaculation Diagnostic (PED) tool was developed to screen for premature ejaculation (PE), including control, frequency, minimal sexual stimulation, distress, and interpersonal difficulty.

6. Quality of Erection Questionnaire (QEQ) evaluates satisfaction with the quality of erections, including hardness, onset, and duration.

7. Self-Esteem and Relationship (SEAR) Questionnaire assesses confidence, self-esteem, and relationships.

8. Sexual Health Inventory for Men (SHIM) is a five-item abridged version of the 15-item IIEF.

9. Sexual Quality of Life–Men (SQOL-M) was developed to assess sexual confidence, emotional well-being, and relationship issues. This questionnaire has been validated for men with erectile dysfunction and PE.

Incidence

A. Erectile dysfunction can occur at any age; however, it is more common in men older than 60 years.

B. It is estimated that 18 to 30 million American men have erectile dysfunction, that is, approximately 52% of males aged 40 to 70 years.

C. By 2025, it is estimated that 322 million men worldwide will have ED.

D. Men with erectile dysfunction have a 65% to 85% increased risk of subsequent CAD.

E. Reduced libido is estimated as affecting 5% to 15% of men.

Pathogenesis

A. Normal pathology: The dorsal nerve of the penis provides innervation, the dorsal somatic nerve provides sensation, and the autonomic nervous system, via the cavernosal nerves, regulates blood flow to the penis, allowing for erection to occur. The ability to maintain an erection relies on the dorsal nerve, the peripheral nerves, penile vasculature, and biochemical releases within the corpora.

B. Multiple factors may contribute to erectile dysfunction:

1. Vascular (most common):

   a. This system is responsible for delivering and trapping the blood in the corporal sinusoids. Usually, the blood flowing in is not the problem; rather, the erectile dysfunction is the result of venous leaking from the corporal sinusoids.

   b. Arterial insufficiency contributes to decreased blood flow to the cavernosal sinuses, which prevents an effective enlargement and rigidity of the penis. The dysfunction of the corporal bodies might cause leakage of blood from the expanded sinusoids, which interrupts the retention of blood in the penis. These impairments result in the client's inability to attain and/or maintain an erection long enough to complete the sexual act.

   c. Other causes of erectile dysfunction:

     i. Chronic diseases such as CV disease, HTN, dyslipidemia, and obesity can cause ED.

     ii. Certain medications can contribute to this physiological effect.

     iii. Smoking is also a contributing factor, especially in the presence of existing CV disease, because of the vasoconstrictive effects it causes.

2. Psychological:
   a. Direct inhibition of the spinal erection center and/or excessive sympathetic nervous system biochemical release occurs, which increases the smooth muscle tone of the penis, preventing erection
      i. Age-related decline
      ii. Lack of sexual response
      iii. Personal intimacy-related issues
      iv. Partner-specific intimacy issues
      v. Performance anxiety
      vi. Depression or life stress related
3. Neurologic:
   a. Any disease affecting the brain, spinal cord, and cavernous and penile nerves can impair the ability to achieve erection, such as spinal cord injury, stroke, or diabetes.
   b. Surgery in the pelvic region, including prostatectomy, perineal resection, and sphincterotome
4. Endocrine:
   a. Decreased testosterone level
   b. Increased prolactin level
   c. Hyperthyroidism
   d. Hypothyroidism

Predisposing Factors
A. CV disease
B. Diabetes (neurologic and vascular problems)
C. HTN
D. Hyperlipidemia
E. Advanced age (greater than 60 years)
F. Peripheral neuropathy
G. Obesity
H. Neurologic disorders:
   1. Spinal cord injuries
   2. Brain injuries
   3. Multiple sclerosis
   4. Parkinson's disease
I. Alcohol/tobacco abuse
J. Drug abuse:
   1. Heroin
   2. Cocaine
   3. Marijuana
K. Side effect of medication (e.g., serotonin reuptake inhibitors, antihypertensives, antihistamines, diuretics, nonsteroidal anti-inflammatories, muscle relaxants)
L. Surgical/radiation therapy for cancers of the pelvis or pelvic trauma
M. Hypogonadism
N. Psychological and psychiatric disorders
O. Peyronie's disease (deformity of the penis)
P. Obstructive sleep apnea
Q. Physical inactivity

Common Complaints
A. Inability to achieve or sustain an erection
B. Erection is not firm enough for penetration
C. Absent or delayed ejaculation
D. Inability to control the timing of ejaculation
E. Lack of interest or desire (most common)
F. Pain with intercourse

Other Signs and Symptoms
A. Diminished self-esteem
B. Depression
C. Anxiety
D. Reduced libido
E. Relationship difficulties
F. PE

Subjective Data
A. Sexual history:

> History taking for erectile dysfunction includes sexual, medical, surgical, emotional, and medication evaluations.

1. Did the onset of erectile dysfunction coincide with a specific event?
2. How long has the client had trouble attaining or maintaining an erection?
3. Is he able to obtain an erection in order to penetrate? On a scale of 0 to 10, how hard is the erection?
4. Is the erectile dysfunction getting worse?
5. Is he about to achieve orgasm and ejaculate?
6. How long is the client able to have intercourse before ejaculation?
7. Is there pain or discomfort with ejaculation?
8. Does the client have nocturnal or morning erections?
9. How frequently does the client have sexual activity?
   a. Is the activity planned or does it occur spontaneously?
   b. How much foreplay occurs?
   c. Do the client and partner agree on the frequency of intercourse?
   d. Is the client's partner satisfied?
10. Has the client tried any treatment(s) for erectile dysfunction?
    a. What treatments have been tried?
    b. Inquire about his desire to try any particular therapy. Is he opposed to try any particular therapy?
B. Medical history:
1. Does the client have HTN? When was HTN diagnosed? What is his usual BP?
2. Does the client have diabetes?
   a. Is he insulin dependent?
   b. Does he have any peripheral neuropathy?
3. Does the client have heart disease? When was his heart disease diagnosed?
4. Has the client ever had cancer, including any surgery, chemotherapy, and radiation?
5. Does the client have dyslipidemia? What were the results of his last laboratory tests?
6. Does the client smoke? How much, including the number of pack-years?

7. Does the client drink? How much, how often?

8. Does the client have penile curvature (Peyronie's disease)?

9. Does the client have any neurologic disorders?

C. Surgical history:

1. Has the client had any prior surgeries, including pelvic, prostate, or trauma?

2. Has the client had any invasive cardiac procedures or surgery?

D. Emotional history:

1. Has the client ever had a traumatic sexual experience?

2. Has the client had a loss of libido?

3. Does the client have a history of depression or mood disorders?

4. Is the client experiencing any problems related to work and/or family?

5. Does the client have any intrapartner problems such as separation or divorce?

E. Medication history: ask the client to list all medications currently being taken, particularly substances not prescribed, including herbal products and illicit drugs. Multiple drug classifications have medications that contribute to erectile dysfunction. Review medications from these drug classes:

1. Nitrates

2. Antihypertensives (particularly alpha blockers)

3. Anti-ulcer medications

4. Lipid-lowering medications

5. 5-alpha-reductase inhibitors (e.g., finasteride or dutasteride)

6. Antidepressants

7. Herbal products

8. Illicit drugs

9. Caffeine

Physical Examination

A. Vital signs: check BP, height, and weight. Calculate BMI.

B. Inspect:

1. Inspect general appearance, noting dyspnea and weakness.

2. Inspect skin for jaundice, pallor, and diaphoresis.

3. Inspect legs for edema, cyanosis, and venous stasis.

4. Perform a funduscopic examination.

5. Evaluate visual field defects (present in hypogonadal men with pituitary tumors).

6. Inspect for penile plaques (indicates Peyronie's disease).

7. Inspect the testicles:

   a. Check for presence of atrophy.

   b. Assess asymmetry.

   c. Evaluate the cremasteric reflex by stroking the inner thighs and observe ipsilateral contraction of the scrotum.

C. Palpate:

1. Palpate abdomen for masses, tenderness, bounding pulses, and organomegaly.

2. Palpate peripheral pulses in legs.

3. Palpate femoral pulses.

4. Examine breasts to detect gynecomastia.

5. Palpate the testicles for masses.

6. Perform a rectal examination to evaluate the prostate.

D. Auscultate:

1. Carotid arteries for bruits

2. Abdomen for bruits and bowel sounds

3. Heart for murmurs, rubs, clicks, irregularities, or extra sounds

4. Femoral bruits (possible pelvic blood occlusion)

5. All lung fields

E. Observe ipsilateral contraction of the scrotum.

F. Mental status: Assess for depression.

G. Perform a neurologic examination if neurologic etiology is suspected.

Diagnostic Tests

Hormonal testing and treatment of erectile dysfunction should be individualized based on clinical presentation, including libido, PE, fatigue, testicular atrophy, and muscle atrophy that suggests a hormonal abnormality.

A. Serum laboratory tests:

1. Lipid profile

2. Triglycerides

3. Glucose or hemoglobin A1C (Hgb A1C)

4. PSA testing (if on testosterone replacement)

5. Hematocrit (if on testosterone replacement)

6. Testosterone (performed in the morning) and other hormone levels, such as prolactin level, if high index of suspicion for prolactinoma, including visual disturbances or headache

7. Urinalysis for protein and glucose

B. Duplex ultrasound of the cavernous arteries and other vascular testing as indicated. Penile perfusion ultrasound may be done to evaluate arterial perfusion of the penis (not commonly used).

C. Nocturnal penile tumescence (NPT) as indicated. This determines the quality and number of nighttime erections. This test is not routinely used and is typically used in younger, more complicated clients.

D. Other tests as indicated for abnormal findings on physical examination

Differential Diagnoses

A. Testosterone deficiency

B. Decreased libido

C. Anorgasmia

D. Peyronie's disease

Plan

A. General interventions:

1. A prolonged erection (priapism) lasting more than 4 hours is a medical emergency often requiring immediate urologic attention.

2. Lifestyle modifications to include weight loss, increased physical activity, limited alcohol consumption, and smoking cessation

3. Control of comorbidities, including CV disease, diabetes, and HTN, is desired.

B. Client teaching:

1. Educate client about modifying controllable risk factors such as keeping diabetes and HTN under control, diet, exercise, and smoking cessation.

2. Failure to respond to phosphodiesterase-5 (PDE-5) inhibitor treatment may result from improper instructions or an inadequate dosage of medication. (See Table 12.5 for dosing and side effects.)

TABLE 12.5 DOSING AND SIDE EFFECTS OF ORAL PDE-5 INHIBITORS

Dosing Instructions	Sildenafil Citrate (Viagra)	Vardenafil HCl (Levitra)	Tadalafil (Cialis)
Doses	25, 50, and 100 mg doses	5, 10, and 20 mg doses	2.5 and 5 mg—available for continuous daily use 10 and 20 mg doses
Instructions	• Recommended starting dose is 50 mg • Take on an empty stomach • Maximum dosing once a day • Titrate according to client response/side effects • Effective 30–60 minutes from administration • A heavy fatty meal may reduce or prolong absorption	• Recommended starting dose is 10 mg (5 mg initial dose for the elderly) • Take on an empty stomach • Titrate according to client response/side effects • Effective 60 minutes from administration • A fatty meal reduces its effect	• Recommended starting dose is 10 mg • Titrated according to client response • Maximum dosing once a day • Effective 30–60 minutes from administration • Peak efficacy occurs after 2 hours; efficacy is maintained for up to 36 hours • Not affected by food • Has been approved for continuous, daily use in 2.5 and 5 mg doses • Also prescribed for BPH
Common Side Effects	**Sildenafil Citrate (Viagra)**	**Vardenafil HCl (Levitra)**	**Tadalafil (Cialis)**
Headache	×	×	×
Flushing	×	×	×
Nasal congestion/rhinitis	×	×	×
Dyspepsia	×	×	×
Priapism	×	Rare	Rare
Myalgia			×
Sinusitis		×	
Backache			×
Limb pain			×
Prolonged erection	×		
Tachycardia		×	
Visual disturbance	Blue-green color tinge to vision, light sensitivity, and blurred vision (lasts 2–3 hours)		
Hypotension with alpha blockers	Should be stable on alpha blocker before initiating a PDE-5 inhibitor; use lowest recommended PDE-5 inhibitor dose	Should be stable on alpha blocker before initiating a PDE-5 inhibitor; use lowest recommended PDE-5 inhibitor dose	Should be stable on alpha blocker before initiating a PDE-5 inhibitor; use lowest recommended PDE-5 inhibitor dose
Sudden vision loss	Discontinue if vision loss occurs	Discontinue if vision loss occurs	Discontinue if vision loss occurs
Sudden hearing loss	Discontinue if hearing loss occurs	Discontinue if hearing loss occurs	Discontinue if hearing loss occurs
Use with nitrates (includes nitroglycerin, isosorbide dinitrate, amyl nitrate, and sodium nitroprusside)	Contraindicated because of hypotension	Contraindicated because of hypotension	Contraindicated because of hypotension

BPH, benign prostatic hyperplasia; PDE-5, phosphodiesterase-5.

3. The initial administration of an alprostadil intraurethral suppository should be done in the office in order to demonstrate correct administration.

4. The initial intrapenile administration of alprostadil should be done in the office in order to demonstrate correct administration.

5. Stepwise therapy for erectile dysfunction includes pharmaceuticals and surgery.

C. Pharmaceutical therapy:

1. **First-line therapy**: Treatment with PDE-5 inhibitors is the first-line therapy for the treatment of erectile dysfunction. PDE-5 inhibitors are not initiators of erection and require sexual stimulation for an erection to occur. The evidence shows that PDE-5 inhibitors improve erections and successful intercourse, with approximately 80% success rate. The use of PDE-5 inhibitors has been extensively studied; however, they are not without side effects. (See Table 12.5 for dosing and side effects.)

a. Contraindications to PDE-5 inhibitors include high-risk conditions and the concomitant use of nitrites. If the client develops angina while using a PDE-5 inhibitor, other antianginal agents should be used instead of nitroglycerin.

b. High-risk clients/conditions are defined as:

i. Unstable or refractory angina

ii. Refractory angina

iii. Uncontrolled HTN

iv. CHF (New York Heart Association classes III and IV)

v. Myocardial infarction (MI) or a CV accident within the previous 2 weeks

vi. High-risk arrhythmias

vii. Hypertrophic obstructive and other cardiomyopathies

c. Before proceeding to other erectile dysfunction therapies, clients reporting failure of PDE-5 inhibitors should be evaluated to determine whether the medication trial was adequate. Evaluate:

i. Food/drug interactions

ii. Timing and frequency of dosing

iii. Lack of adequate sexual stimulation

iv. Heavy alcohol use

v. Relationship issues

vi. Using a licensed PDE-5 inhibitor medication

d. After evaluation and reeducation and counseling on the medications and partner–partner expectations, titrate to the maximum dosing or prescribe different PDE-5 inhibitor.

e. Discuss other options for erectile dysfunction if the client has a contraindication to, or an unsuccessful trial of, PDE-5 inhibitors.

2. **Second-line therapy:** Pharmaceutical therapy with intracavernous injection is the second-line therapy for the treatment of erectile dysfunction. Penile injection therapy involves injection of alprostadil, a vasoactive drug, into the corpora cavernosa of the penis to expand the blood vessels and increase the blood flow to produce an erection. The most common side effect of alprostadil is burning and a prolonged erection lasting over 4 hours. Hypotension is also a potential side effect. Prolonged erections require medical intervention to reverse the erection.

a. Alprostadil intercavernal injections are titrated according to client erection response, within the healthcare clinic setting. Precise dosing requirements exist for intracavernosal therapy and are specific to the brand name. Adverse effects include penile pain, hematoma, penile fibrosis, and a high potential for priapism.

b. Alprostadil MUSE pellet (alprostadil urethral suppository) urethral pellet: 125 to 250 mcg is to be used before intercourse. Duration of 30 to 60 minutes is followed; use only twice in each 24-hour period.

D. Surgical alternatives:

1. Penile implant is the third-line therapy for the treatment of erectile dysfunction. Penile prostheses (implants) are surgically implanted items, semirigid rods or a hydraulic device, to ensure a rigid erection. The prosthesis does not usually affect urination, sex drive, orgasm, or ejaculation. Pain and/or reduced sensation, infection, or mechanical failure may occur from the prosthesis.

2. Vacuum erection devices are external cylinders used to pump the penis into the cylinder and produce an erection by drawing blood into the penis. An occluding band is then placed at the base of the penis in order to prevent the blood from leaving, with subsequent loss of the erection. **Only vacuum constrictor devices containing a vacuum limiter should be used. The occluding band to maintain the erection should be limited to 30 minutes.**

3. Penile arterial revascularization is indicated for young men (younger than 45 years) with no known risk factors for atherosclerosis. The goal of the surgery is to correct injury by rerouting the blood vessel around a blockage or injured blood vessel. Men with insulin-dependent diabetes or widespread atherosclerosis are not candidates for this surgery.

4. Venous ligation surgery is rarely used. Men with insulin-dependent diabetes or widespread atherosclerosis are also not candidates for venous surgery.

Follow-Up

A. Follow up in 1 to 3 weeks after treatments are initiated to monitor client satisfaction and the quality of erections.

B. At the time of prescription renewal, clients prescribed PDE-5 inhibitors should have a review of the effectiveness, side effects, and any significant change in health status, including all medications.

Consultation/Referral

A. Client should be directed to go to the ED if an erection lasts for more than 4 hours.

B. Clients whose CV risk is indeterminant for PDE-5 inhibitors should undergo further evaluation by a cardiologist before receiving therapies for sexual dysfunction.

C. Surgical consultation: Men with penile deformities may require surgical correction.

D. Urologist consultation should be considered for surgical therapies, including implantation of penile prosthesis.

E. Endocrinology consultation for complex endocrine disorders

F. Psychosexual counseling may be considered for the client and/or couple.

G. Psychotherapy is recommended when erectile dysfunction is related to anxiety and/or depression.

Individual Considerations

A. Adults:

1. A mild prolongation of the QT interval has been observed with vardenafil. The product labeling for vardenafil recommends that caution be used in clients with known history of QT prolongation or in clients who are on current medications that prolong the QT interval.

2. Testosterone therapy is not indicated in the treatment of erectile dysfunction if the client has a normal serum testosterone level.

3. Men who present with sleep disorders should also be questioned about the presence of erectile dysfunction.

4. In clients with diabetes, PDE-5 inhibitors may fail.

5. PDE-5 inhibitors are contraindicated in clients with high CV risk and for clients on nitrates.

6. Men with erectile dysfunction are associated with a higher incidence of CV events.

B. Geriatrics:

1. Dose medications on the lower end for elderly clients:

   a. Sildenafil: dose at 25 mg for age greater than 65 years. Renal and hepatic dosing required

   b. Vardenafil: dose at 5 mg for age greater than 65 years. Renal and hepatic dosing required

   c. Tadalafil: renal and hepatic dosing required

Resources

American Association of Sex Educators, Counselors, and Therapists
I Street, NW, Suite 700
Washington, DC 20005
(202) 449–1099
info@aasect.org
www.aasect.org

American Society for Reproductive Medicine
Montgomery Highway
Birmingham, AL 35216
205-978-5000
https://connect.asrm.org/home?ssopc=1

American Urological Association
Corporate Boulevard
Linthicum, MD 21090
866-746-4282
aua@AUAnet.org

International Society for Sexual Medicine
PO Box 94
AB Wormerveer, The Netherlands

Secretariat@issm.info
https://www.issm.info

Society for Sex Therapy and Research
(847)-647–8832
https://sstarnet.org

Bibliography

Akre, C., Berchtold, A., Gmel, G., & Suris, J. (2014). The evolution of sexual dysfunction in young men aged 18–25 years. *Journal of Adolescent Health, 55*(6), 736–743. doi:10.1016/j.jadohealth.2014.05.014

American Urological Association. (2011, revised 2018). *The management of erectile dysfunction: An update.* Retrieved from https://www.auanet.org/guidelines/erectile-dysfunction-(ed)-guideline

Annam, K., Voznesensky, M., & Kreder, K. J. (2016). Understanding and managing erectile dysfunction in patients treated for cancer. *Journal of Oncology Practice, 12*(4), 297–305. doi:10.1200/JOP.2016.010678

Associates in Urology. (n.d.[b]). *Sexual health inventory for men (SHIM).* Retrieved from http://rohbaltimore.com/SHIM.pdf

Cunningham, G. R., & Rosen, R. C. (2019, April 18). Overview of male sexual dysfunction. *UpToDate.* Retrieved from http://www.uptodate.com/contents/overview-of-male-sexual-dysfunction

Hilz, M. (2015). Assessment and treatment of male and female sexual dysfunction. *Journal of the Neurological Sciences, 357*(1), 498–499. doi:10.1016/j.jns.2015.09.295

Kim, E. D. (2018, August 8). Erectile dysfunction. *Medscape.* Retrieved from https://emedicine.medscape.com/article/444220-overview

McCabe, M. P., & Connaughton, C. (2014). Psychosocial factors associated with male sexual difficulties. *Journal of Sex Research, 51*(1), 31–42. doi:10.1080/00224499.2013.789820

Urology Care Foundation. (2016a). *ED: Non-surgical management (erectile dysfunction).* Retrieved from http://www.urologyhealth.org/urology/index.cfm?article=60

Urology Care Foundation. (2016b). *ED: Surgical management (erectile dysfunction).* Retrieved from http://www.urologyhealth.org/urology/index.cfm?article=28

Walsh, T. J., Hotaling, J. M., Smith, A., Saigal, C., & Wessells, H. (2014). Men with diabetes may require more aggressive treatment for erectile dysfunction. *International Journal of Impotence Research, 26*(3), 112–115. doi:10.1038/ijir.2013.46

Weinberg, A. E., Eisenberg, M., Patel, C. J., Chertow, G. M., & Leppert, J. T. (2013). Diabetes severity, metabolic syndrome, and the risk of erectile dysfunction. *Journal of Sexual Medicine, 10*(12), 3102–3109. doi:10.1111/jsm.12318

Sexual Dysfunction Male: Premature Ejaculation

Debbie Gunter and Nancy Pesta Walsh

Definition

A. Premature ejaculation (PE) is defined as the inability to control or delay ejaculation, which causes personal distress for the male. Two subtypes exist, based on intravaginal ejaculation latency time (IELT):

1. Lifelong PE is an IELT of less than 1 minute. Onset is typically from the first sexual encounter. Males have no ability to control the ejaculation.

2. Acquired PE is an IELT of less than 3 minutes. Onset is at any point in sexual history. The ability to delay ejaculation is decreased or absent.

   Two subtypes exist based on personal experience; neither is a true sexual dysfunction.

3. Variable PE is irregular and not the result of psychogenic cause. Onset is at any point in sexual history. The ability to delay ejaculation is decreased or absent.

4. Subjective PE is self-reported rapid ejaculation despite normal ejaculation time. Onset is at any point in sexual history. The ability to delay ejaculation is decreased or absent.

Incidence

A. PE is reported in approximately 21% to 31% of males. It is the most common type of sexual dysfunction. Erectile dysfunction commonly coexists.

B. Approximately 31% of men report problems with sexual function.

Pathogenesis

A. The exact cause is unknown.

B. Organic: chronic prostatitis, hyperthyroidism, genetic disorders

C. Psychogenic: relationship problems, psychological preoccupation with performance

   1. Iatrogenic: nerve damage from surgery or trauma

Predisposing Factors

A. Depression

B. Consumption of alcohol

C. Obesity

D. High BP

E. High cholesterol

F. Diabetes

G. Obesity

H. Smoking

I. Depression and anxiety medication use

Common Complaints

A. Men:

   1. Inability to achieve or sustain erection

   2. Absent or delayed ejaculation

   3. Inability to control the timing of ejaculation

B. Both sexes:

   1. Lack of interest or desire (most common)

   2. Inability to become aroused

   3. Pain with intercourse

Other Signs and Symptoms

A. Diminished self-esteem

B. Depression

C. Anxiety

D. Erectile dysfunction

E. Reduced libido

F. Relationship difficulties

Subjective Data

A. Include full medical history, sexual history, and psychological, social, and drug history using open-ended questions.

B. Ask:

   1. Partner(s)' sexual history

   2. Perceived ejaculatory control

   3. Estimated IELT

   4. Previous interventions used to correct the issue

   5. Impact on personal life and relationships

   6. If the issue has been lifelong or acquired

   7. If a loss of erection occurs before ejaculation, to distinguish erectile dysfunction from PE

C. Screening tools:

   1. PE Diagnostic Tool available at www.sexhealth-matters.org/resources/premature-ejaculation-diagnostic-tool

   2. Index of PE available at www.pfizerpatientreport-edoutcomes.com/therapeutic-areas/sexual-health/male-sexual-dysfunction

Physical Examination

A. Vital signs: check BP, pulse, and respiration

B. Inspect:

   1. Thyroid for nodules

   2. Abdomen for surgical scars

   3. Neurologic examination for deficiencies

   4. Lower extremities for hair distribution pattern, lesions, or trauma

   5. Genitalia for abnormalities

   6. Any additional examination should be based on history and previous examination findings

C. Palpate:

   1. Thyroid for nodules

   2. Abdomen for masses or tenderness

   3. Lower extremities for pain and pulses

   4. Neurologic examination of lower extremities

   5. Genitalia for lesions, masses, or pain

Diagnostic Tests

A. Should be based on individual history and physical findings

Differential Diagnoses

A. Erectile dysfunction

B. Testosterone deficiency

Plan

A. General interventions:

   1. The treatment plan should include the client and sexual partner.

   2. The client and partner should be educated about the possible interventions.

      a. Both should be educated in treatment options.

      b. Client and partner satisfaction is the desired outcome.

B. Client teaching:

   1. Consider the impact of the severity of the issue on the client, any treatable causes, and client wishes.

   2. Effectiveness of psychotherapy may diminish over time.

   3. Behavioral therapy: "stop-and-start" method of ceasing genital stimulation until arousal sensation diminishes or the "squeeze" method of squeezing the glans prepuce at heightened arousal

C. Psychotherapy: recommended for lifelong, acquired, or variable PE and is the first-line treatment for subjective PE.

D. Pharmaceutical therapy: Off-label medications include selective serotonin reuptake inhibitors (SSRIs) and eutectic mixture of local anesthetics (EMLA).

   1. Paroxetine 10, 20, or 40 mg/d *or* 20 mg 3 to 4 hours preintercourse

      a. Typically most effective for the indication of PE

2. Fluoxetine 5 to 20 mg/d
3. Sertraline 25 to 200 mg/d *or* 50 mg 4 to 8 hours preintercourse
4. EMLA (lidocaine 2.5%/prilocaine 2.5%) cream: apply to glans penis 20 to 30 minutes preintercourse

Follow-Up
A. The client should be seen in 2 to 4 weeks if medication was started to assess for efficacy. SSRIs typically achieve maximum effect after 1 to 2 weeks.

Consultation/Referral
A. May refer to urologist or sexual health specialist/counselor, particularly if there is provider discomfort with this topic
B. Psychotherapy: recommended for lifelong, acquired, or variable PE and is the first-line treatment for subjective PE. Referral to a practitioner who specializes in sexual therapy is recommended.

Individual Considerations
A. Adults:
1. Off-label SSRIs should be used with caution due to the increased risk of serotonin syndrome.
2. Off-label EMLA cream used without a condom may result in vaginal wall numbness in the sexual partner.
3. Prolonged application of EMLA may result in loss of erection if used for 30 to 45 minutes.
B. Geriatrics:
1. Renal and hepatic dosing of paroxetine is required.
2. Hepatic dosing of fluoxetine and sertraline is required.
3. Taper to discontinue any SSRIs is required.

Bibliography
American Urological Association. (2010). *Pharmacologic management of premature ejaculation*. Retrieved from https://www.auanet.org/guidelines/premature-ejaculation-guideline

Chung, E., Gilbert, B., Perera, M., & Roberts, M. J. (2015). Premature ejaculation: A clinical review for the general physician. *Australian Family Physician, 44*(10), 737–743.

International Society for Sexual Medicine. (2015, January). *ISSM patient information sheet on premature ejaculation*. Retrieved from http://www.issm.info/images/uploads/ISSM_Patient_Information_Sheet_on_PE_-_website_JAN_2015.pdf

Ogunyemi, O. (2018, August 31). Testicular torsion. *Medscape*. Retrieved from http://emedicine.medscape.com/article/2036003-overview

Paco, J. S., & Pereira, B. J. (2016). New therapeutic perspectives in premature ejaculation. *Urology, 88*, 87–92. doi:10.1016/j.urology.2015.11.003

Testicular Torsion

Cheryl A. Glass and Debbie Gunter

Definition
A. Testicular torsion is twisting of the testicle around the vas deferens, with compromise in the blood supply and possible necrosis to the testicles. Testicular torsion is a urologic emergency and is the most frequent cause of testicle loss in the adolescent male population. Approximately 40% of all cases of acute scrotal pain and swelling are diagnosed with testicular torsion. There is often a history of recurrent episodes of testicular pain before torsion (see Figure 12.3).

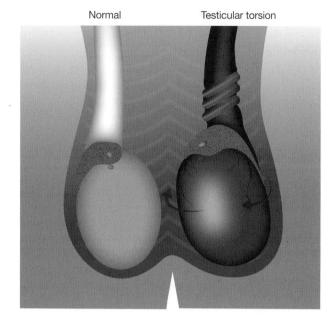

Normal   Testicular torsion

FIGURE 12.3 Testicular torsion.

B. Testicular torsion is most commonly misdiagnosed as epididymitis.
1. Epididymitis usually presents with gradual onset of pain that is localized posterior to the testes that gradually radiates to the lower abdomen.
2. Gradual onset of testicular pain that radiates to the abdomen is rare with torsion.

Incidence
A. Incidence in males younger than 25 years is approximately one in 4,000. Although torsion can occur at any age, the largest number of cases occur during adolescence.
B. The bell clapper congenital anomaly is present in approximately 12% of males, and 40% have the abnormality in the contralateral testicle.

Pathogenesis
A. Testicular torsion and torsion of the spermatic cord occur because of abnormal fixation of the testicle to the scrotum, allowing free rotation. The bell clapper deformity allows the testicle to twist spontaneously on the spermatic cord. Venous occlusion and engorgement cause arterial ischemia and infarction of the testicle.

Predisposing Factors
A. Age: more common in adolescence
B. Trauma to testicle
C. Spontaneous occurrence
D. Congenital bell clapper anomaly
E. Exercise
F. Undescended testicle
G. Active cremasteric reflex

Common Complaints
A. Sudden onset of severe unilateral scrotal pain (less than 24 hours)
B. Swelling of scrotal sac

C. High position of the testicle
D. Abnormal cremasteric reflex

Other Signs and Symptoms

A. Sudden onset of testicular pain, may radiate to groin
B. Possible edema
C. Abdominal pain (22%–30%)
D. Nausea and vomiting (50% of cases)
E. Fever (16%)
F. Urinary frequency (4%)

Subjective Data

A. Review the onset, duration, and course of symptoms
B. Review for a history of prior episodes of intermittent testicular pain that resolved spontaneously
C. Review abdominal symptoms such as pain, nausea and vomiting, and fever
D. Review urethral discharge (possible STI) and dysuria
E. Review the client's history for trauma to the scrotum or testicle

Physical Examination

A. Check temperature, BP, pulse, and respiration
B. Inspect:
  1. Observe the client generally for pain before and during examination.
  2. Visualize the scrotal sac for edema, symmetry, lesions, discharge, color (especially for blue dot superior to the affected testicle). Testis is located high in the scrotum as a result of shortening of the cord by twisting.
  3. Check the inguinal and femoral areas for bulges and hernias.
C. Auscultate:
  1. Auscultate all four quadrants of the abdomen; note bowel sounds.
D. Palpate:
  1. Palpate the abdomen for masses, rebound, and tenderness or guarding.
  2. Palpate the groin; check the lymph nodes.
  3. Examine for an inguinal hernia.
  4. Genital examination:
     a. Check warmth, tenderness, swelling, and any nodularity; if a mass is present, check if it is solid or cystic. The testes should be sensitive to gentle compression, but not tender. They should feel smooth, rubbery, and free of nodules.
     b. Elicit a cremasteric reflex by stroking the inner thigh with a blunt object (reflex hammer or ink pen). The testicle and scrotum should rise on the stroked side. Cremasteric reflex is usually absent in testicular torsion.
     c. Elevate the scrotum; there is usually no relief in pain with torsion. Elevation of the scrotum may improve the pain of epididymitis (Prehn's sign).

Diagnostic Tests

A. Urinalysis: normal in 90% of cases of testicular torsion
B. Doppler ultrasonography for blood flow and scrotal ultrasonography

Differential Diagnoses

A. Epididymitis
B. Orchitis
C. Hydrocele
D. Testicular tumor: usually a hard, enlarged, painless testicle
E. Acute appendicitis
F. Scrotal/testicular trauma
G. Varicocele

Plan

A. General interventions:
  1. Testicular torsion is a urologic emergency requiring surgery.
  2. Immediately refer the client to a urologist and/or ED.
  3. Symptoms for more than 6 hours can indicate testicular necrosis.
  4. The opposite testicle is usually stabilized during the same surgery.
B. Pharmaceutical therapy:
  1. None

Follow-Up

A. Client should follow up with the urologist as directed.

Consultation/Referral

A. All clients with suspected testicular torsion need to be immediately evaluated by a physician and referred to a urologist.

Individual Considerations

A. Pediatrics: Neonatal testicular torsion is rare. The exact mechanism is unknown. The torsion may occur prenatal (at or within 24 hours of delivery) or postnatal (within first 30 days of delivery). On physical examination, a hardened, fixed nontender scrotal mass with a discolored scrotum is noted. Management is controversial because of the lack of data on whether the testis can be salvaged and the risk for concomitant or subsequent torsion of the contralateral side.
B. Geriatrics: In older males, rule out epididymitis, especially with new sexual partners or with symptoms of dysuria and urethral discharge.

Bibliography

Govindarajan, K. (2017, April). Pediatric testicular torsion clinical presentation. *Medscape*. Retrieved from https://emedicine.medscape.com/article/2035074-clinical
Ogunyemi, O. (2018, August 31). Testicular torsion. *Medscape*. Retrieved from http://emedicine.medscape.com/article/2036003-overview

Undescended Testes or Cryptorchidism

Cheryl A. Glass and Debbie Gunter

Definition

A. Undescended testicle(s) or cryptorchidism is a testicle that is not within the scrotum and cannot be manipulated from the inguinal canal into the scrotum or is absent. Spontaneous descent of testes usually happens at the end of the first year. Bilaterally absent testicles is anorchia (see Figure 12.4).

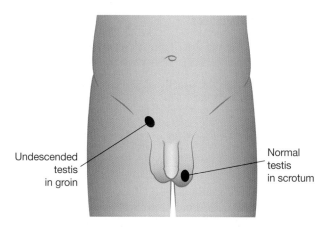

Undescended testis in groin

Normal testis in scrotum

FIGURE 12.4 Undescended testicle and normal testicle.

Incidence

A. Approximately 10% of males have bilateral cryptorchidism.
B. In unilateral cases, left-side predominance is noted.
C. Between 2% and 5% of full-term and 30% of premature male infants are born with an undescended testicle.
D. 20% to 30% of boys have at least one nonpalpable testis.

Pathogenesis

A. An absent testicle may occur because of agenesis or an intrauterine vascular problem such as torsion. It may also be related to the lack of gonadotropic and androgenic hormones during fetal development. Most undescended testes are a result of a mechanical factor, a hernia sac, or a shortened spermatic artery that impedes the testes' descent into the scrotum.

Predisposing Factors

A. Prematurity; the testes descend into the scrotum at approximately 36 weeks gestation. Most testicles will complete their descent within the first few months of life.
B. Birth weight is the principal determining factor for undescended testes from birth to 1 year of age.
C. Twinning
D. Maternal exposure to estrogen during the first trimester of pregnancy
E. Family history
F. Congenital disorder of testosterone secretion or testosterone action:
  1. Kallmann syndrome
  2. Abdominal wall defects
  3. Neural tube defects
  4. Cerebral palsy
  5. Genetic syndromes:
    a. Trisomy 18
    b. Trisomy 13
    c. Noonan syndrome
    d. Prader–Willi syndrome
G. Exposure to dibutyl phthalate (endocrine-disrupting chemical)

Common Complaints

A. Empty scrotum
B. Small, flat, undeveloped scrotum
C. Inguinal hernia

Other Signs and Symptoms

A. Absence of testicle noted on newborn examination or by parents during a bath or diaper change

Subjective Data

A. Review the course, duration, and symptoms. Have the testes ever been noticed in the scrotum during a bath or while the baby has been relaxed?
B. Note gestational age and birth weight at delivery (term vs. preterm).
C. Has any healthcare provider ever noted that the testis was not descended or was absent on examination?
D. Review the maternal history for evidence of an endocrine disturbance during pregnancy.
E. Review family history of congenital abnormalities, genital anomalies, and abnormal pubertal development.
F. Review if the client has undergone prior inguinal surgery.

Physical Examination

A. Temperature, BP, pulse, and respiration
B. Inspect:
  1. Check the scrotum for size, shape, rugae, and any anomaly, particularly hypospadias.
  2. Look for a bulge in the inguinal area.
  3. Transilluminate the scrotum to look for testes and note fluid (if present).
    a. To locate the testis, darken the room and shine a bright light from behind the scrotum. In a normal male, the testis stands out as the darker area.
C. Palpate:
  1. Before you palpate the scrotum, place the thumb and index finger of one hand over the inguinal canals at the upper part of the scrotal sac. This maneuver helps prevent retraction of the testes into the inguinal canal or abdomen.
  2. Check each side of the scrotum to detect the presence of the testes and other masses. If either of the testicles is not palpable, place a finger over the upper inguinal ring and gently push toward the scrotum. You may feel a soft mass in the inguinal canal. Try to push it toward the scrotum and palpate it with your thumb and index finger. The testicle of a newborn is approximately 1 cm in diameter.
  3. When any mass other than the testicle or spermatic cord is palpated in the scrotum, determine if it is filled with fluid, gas, or solid material. It is most likely to be a hernia or hydrocele. If it is reducible, then transilluminate to differentiate a hydrocele from a hernia.
  4. Check the cremasteric reflex: scrotal sac retracts in response to cold hands and/or abrupt handling (yo-yo reflux).
  5. Bimanual DRE may be used to evaluate the nonpalpable testis.

Diagnostic Tests

A. For a unilateral undescended testis without hypospadias, no laboratory studies are needed.
B. Hormone levels (testosterone) may be obtained if both testes are nonpalpable.

C. Karyotype to rule out chromosomal abnormalities
D. Ultrasonography of the abdomen
E. Possible CT of the abdomen

Differential Diagnoses

A. Anorchia (complete absence)
B. Retractile testis
C. Ectopic testis
D. Ambiguous genitalia: In male-appearing genitals, at least one testis must be palpated; if not, ambiguous genitalia cannot be eliminated. A deep cleft in the scrotum (bifid scrotum) is usually associated with other GU anomalies or ambiguous genitalia.
E. Tumor: A hard, enlarged, painless testicle may indicate a tumor.

Plan

A. General interventions:
1. Refer all children with cryptorchidism by 6 months of age to a surgeon for evaluation.
2. Surgery (orchiopexy) is usually indicated before 18 months, and no later than 2 years of age, secondary to the increased risks of malignancy, infertility, testicular torsion, trauma, and hernia. After orchiopexy, the rate of fertility in these children is about 80% to 90%.
B. Pharmaceutical therapy: Hormonal therapy is carried out only by a specialist.

Follow-Up

A. Follow up with surgeon as recommended per surgeon.
B. Monitor the client's testicles at each well-child visit.

Consultation/Referral

A. A mass that does not transilluminate or reduce with gentle pressure is likely to be an incarcerated hernia. This condition is a surgical emergency.
B. Refer the client for urologic recommendations regarding surgery.

Individual Considerations

A. Pediatrics:
1. Testicular cancer screening should be done during and after puberty.
2. Examine a child in the tailor's position or with the child sitting on a chair or examination table with legs in "frog position," kneeling, or standing. Note: If the child sits cross-legged, it abolishes the reflex of the cremaster muscle.
3. Examine adolescents while standing and straining.
4. Examination of an adolescent includes evaluation of maturation described by Tanner.
B. Adults:
1. Males who have undescended testicles may have an increased risk of developing breast cancer and developing testicular germ cell cancers.
2. Men with a history of undescended testes have an increased incidence of infertility (lower sperm counts, sperm of lower quality, and low fertility rates).
3. Testicular torsion is 10 times higher in undescended testes. Torsion of an intra-abdominal testis can present as acute abdominal pain related to incarcerated hernia or inguinal lymphadenitis.

Bibliography

American Urological Association. (2014, April). *Evaluation and treatment of cryptorchidism: AUA guideline*. Retrieved from https://www.auanet.org/education/guidelines/cryptorchidism.cfm
Govindarajan, K. (2017, April). Pediatric testicular torsion clinical presentation. *Medscape*. Retrieved from https://emedicine.medscape.com/article/2035074-clinical
Ogunyemi, O. (2018, August 31). Testicular torsion. *Medscape*. Retrieved from http://emedicine.medscape.com/article/2036003-overview
Sachdeva, K. (2018, December 18). Testicular cancer. *Medscape*. Retrieved from emedicine.medscape.com/article/279007-overview
Shrourou, A. (2018, August 29). Boys with undescended testes may have increased risk for testicular cancer, infertility in adulthood. *The Lancet Child & Adolescent Health*.

Urinary Incontinence (UI)

Cheryl A. Glass and Debbie Gunter

Definition

A. Urinary incontinence (UI) is the involuntary loss of urine severe enough to have unpleasant social or hygienic consequences. UI is diagnosed primarily on history; inquire about UI at every interview. UI is a symptom of an underlying disease process in most cases; some cases are reversible with appropriate treatment.
B. Incontinence is not considered a part of normal aging. Morbidity related to incontinence includes UTIs, indwelling catheters, falls/fractures, sleep interruption, social withdrawal, and depression.
C. Successful toileting depends on ready access to facilities, motivation to remain dry, mobility and manual dexterity, and the cognitive ability to recognize/react to the urge to void.
D. UI can be divided into the following categories: functional, urge, overflow, stress, and mixed. Each category has a unique etiology, pathophysiology, symptoms, and management.

Incidence

A. The exact incidence of UI is unknown. The prevalence of incontinence increases with age.
B. UI is common in children. Daytime urinary continence normally occurs by age 4 years. Successful day-and-night continence is generally achieved by age 5 or 7 years.
1. Up to 20% of children aged 4 to 6 years have an occasional daytime wetting. Three percent have urinary accidents more than two times per week.
2. Daytime incontinence, a wetting accident at least once every 2 weeks, decreases with age in the pediatric population.
3. OAB in children has also been associated with other symptoms, including nocturnal enuresis, constipation, fecal incontinence, a history of UTIs, and poor toilet facilities.
C. The incidence of women identified with the definition of any leakage at least once in the past year ranges from 25% to 51%. The incidence is reported to be 10% when identified with weekly urinary leakage.
D. The prevalence of UI in men is approximately half that of women. The incidence of UI is affected by treatment of prostate disease. Men with incontinence have a higher risk of institutionalization compared with men without UI.

E. The elderly are more frequently affected with UI; 6% to 10% of admissions to long-term care facilities are related to incontinence.

Pathogenesis

UI can be caused by pathologic, anatomic, or physiological factors and differs by type of incontinence.

A. Functional incontinence: loss of urine because of the inability to get to the bathroom, either caused by problems of mobility or cognition

B. Urge incontinence/OAB: inability to delay voiding after the sensation of fullness is perceived. Common causes are detrusor hyperactivity or hyperreflexia associated with disorders of the lower urinary tract, tumors, stones, uterine prolapse, cystitis, urethritis, or impaired bladder contractility. Central nervous system disorders, such as stroke, dementia, parkinsonism, or spinal cord injury, also can be causative factors.

C. Overflow incontinence: loss of urine associated with an overdistension of the bladder. Common causes are anatomic obstruction by an enlarged prostate, a prolapsed cystocele, acontractile bladder caused by diabetes, spinal cord injury, multiple sclerosis, or suprasacral cord lesions.

D. Stress incontinence: involuntary loss of urine during coughing, sneezing, laughing, bending over, or other physical activity that increases intra-abdominal pressure. Prostate surgery is the most common cause of stress incontinence in men.

E. Mixed incontinence: combination of stress and urge incontinence in which the bladder outlet is weak and the detrusor is overactive

Predisposing Factors

A. Age for both males and females
B. Female: 85% of cases are in women
C. Increased parity
D. Previous GU surgeries (e.g., prostate surgery, hysterectomy)
E. Restricted mobility
F. Menopause
G. Infections
H. Chronic illnesses (e.g., diabetes)
I. Fecal impactions
J. Excessive urinary output
K. Delirium
L. Dementia
M. Neurologic disorders (e.g., stroke, spinal cord injury)
N. Variety of medications (e.g., antihypertensive medicines, diuretics, sedatives)
O. Pelvic trauma (e.g., episiotomy, forceps delivery)
P. Obesity
Q. Sleep apnea
R. Depression
S. High-impact exercise

Common Complaints

A. Urgency: sudden and compelling desire to pass urine
B. Urge incontinence: involuntary leakage accompanied by urgency with the following precipitating factors:
   1. Hearing running water
   2. Placing hands in water

   3. Trying to unlock the door when returning home
   4. Exposure to a cold environment
C. Stress incontinence: involuntary leakage with the following precipitating factors:
   1. Exertion
   2. Sneezing/coughing
   3. Little or no activity
D. OAB: Symptoms may occur with or without urge incontinence.
   1. Urgency
   2. Frequency
   3. Nocturia

Other Signs and Symptoms

A. Mixed incontinence: urge and stress leakage
B. Experiencing leakage with little or no activity
C. Continuous leakage (i.e., dribbling)
D. Daytime frequency
E. Nocturia: up one or more times a night to void
F. Slow urine stream, intermittent stream, or hesitancy
G. Need to strain to start, maintain, or improve voiding
H. Incomplete emptying sensation
I. Children exhibit holding maneuvers to postpone voiding or suppress urgency.
   1. Standing on tiptoes
   2. Forcefully crossing legs (Vincent's curtsy)
   3. Squatting with hand or heel pressed to the perineum

Subjective Data

A. Question the client regarding the onset, duration, and severity of the incontinence:
   1. Do you ever leak urine/water when you don't want to?
   2. Do you ever leak urine when you cough, laugh, or exercise?
   3. Do you ever leak urine on the way to the bathroom (urgency)?
   4. Do you ever use pads, tissue, or cloth in your underwear to catch urine?
B. Elicit situations when UI is worse, when it is improved, and what stimuli are associated with increasing UI (high fluid intake, high caffeine intake, agitation).
C. Review whether the female client is pre- or postmenopausal.
D. Review other LUTS such as nocturia.
E. Review the client's history of bowel function (e.g., fecal incontinence). If constipation is a problem, abdominal pressure from a large retained stool can cause symptoms, including retention.
F. Review medications, including OTC drugs and herbals.
   1. Do not prescribe a muscarinic medication for clients who are currently on other medications with anticholinergic properties.
G. Review previous continence therapy including surgical treatments.
H. Review the impact of incontinence on quality of life, including work impairment, sexual dysfunction, activities of daily living, sleep, recreational activity, social interaction, and depression.

I. Assess whether the elderly client has incontinence despite toileting.
J. Review sexual function.
K. Review history and previous treatment for prostate disease.
L. Review other comorbid medical diagnoses such as neurologic disabilities, narrow-angle glaucoma, and diabetes:
    1. Do not prescribe a muscarinic medication in a client with narrow-angle glaucoma unless approved by the treating ophthalmologist.
    2. Use caution when prescribing antimuscarinic for OAB with a frail client.
M. What is the diabetic client's blood glucose average?

Physical Examination

Both sexes:
A. Check temperature (if an infection is suspected), pulse, BP, and respiration.
B. Inspect:
    1. Look for evidence of cardiac overload: pedal edema.
C. Auscultate:
    1. Lungs for evidence of fluid overload: rales
D. Palpate:
    1. Abdomen for masses, fullness over bladder, and tenderness
E. Neurologic examination:
    1. Assess cognitive and functional status, including mobility, transfers, manual dexterity, and ability to toilet in the elderly.
    2. Screen for depression.
    3. Assess for any change in sensation of the perineal area.
        a. Ask the client if he or she feels pressure in the bladder or rectal area when he or she needs to urinate or defecate.
        b. To assess for neuropathy, ask the client if she or he can feel the texture of the tissue or hand when wiping after urination.
        c. During the physical exam, assess for perineal sensation.

Females

A. Inspect:
    1. Assess perineal skin for irritation, thinning, vaginal atrophy, and vaginal discharge.
B. Palpate:
    1. Perform a bimanual pelvic examination for prolapse, masses, or tenderness.
    2. Perform rectal examination for sphincter tone, masses, and fecal impaction.
C. Perform pelvic examination when appropriate:
    1. Remove the top blade of the speculum and evaluate the vaginal wall support.
    2. Ask the woman to cough to reevaluate the vaginal wall support.

Males

A. Inspect:
    1. Inspect the glans penis for abnormalities in urethral meatus. (Hypospadias may cause postvoid dribbling.)
    2. Uncircumcised men should be evaluated for phimosis and balanitis.

B. Palpate:
    1. Perform rectal examination for sphincter tone, masses, fecal impaction, prostate size, and contour.
    2. Palpate the scrotum to evaluate masses.
    3. Evaluate the presence of an inguinal hernia because straining with a partial urinary obstruction can worsen an inguinal hernia.

Diagnostic Tests

The history, physical examination, and urinalysis are sufficient to guide initial therapy. Other tests include the following:
A. Urine culture and sensitivity if infection is suspected
B. Urine cytology if hematuria or pelvic pain is present
C. Cystometry: see Section II: Procedure, "Cystometry: Bedside."
D. PVR by catheterization or ultrasound. A PVR of less than 50 mL is considered adequate emptying and greater than 200 mL is considered inadequate, suggesting either detrusor weakness or obstruction. Indications for PVR:
    1. Men with mild to moderate lower urinary symptoms
    2. Men with OAB (urgency)
    3. Persons with spinal cord injury or Parkinson's disease
    4. Persons with prior episodes of urinary retention
    5. Persons with severe constipation
E. A serum PSA should be considered.
F. Routine urodynamic testing is not recommended.
G. Cystoscopy is not required for incontinence; however, it is indicated for hematuria.

Differential Diagnoses

Eight reversible causes of transient incontinence can be remembered by using the mnemonic: DIAPPERS

Delirium
Infection (urinary)
Atrophic urethritis and vaginitis
Pharmaceuticals
Psychological disorders, especially depression
Excessive urine output
Restricted mobility
Stool impaction

Plan

A. General interventions:
    1. Functional UI: Therapy is directed at the cause of the condition, such as overdiuresis, inability to go to the toilet, or poor access to toilet facilities.
    2. Behavioral interventions should be reviewed.
        a. A bladder diary (see Table 12.6) may provide information on usual timing and circumstances of UI.
        b. Timed scheduled voiding and/or prompted caregiver scheduled toileting
        c. Bladder training by systematic ability to delay voiding through the use of urge of inhibition
        d. Stress incontinence: Kegel perineal exercises may improve UI by 30% to 90%. Exercises using graduated vaginal cones or weights induce pelvic muscle tone and strength, reducing UI.

TABLE 12.6   BLADDER CONTROL DIARY

Your Daily Bladder Diary

This diary will help you and your healthcare team figure out the causes of your bladder control trouble. The "sample" line shows you how to use the diary. Use this sheet as a master for making copies that you can use as a bladder diary for as many days as you need.

Your name: _____

Date: _____

Time	Drinks		Trips to the Bathroom		Accidental Leaks	Did You Feel a Strong Urge to Go?	What Were You Doing at the Time?
	What kind?	*How much?*	*How many times?*	*How much urine? (circle one)*	*How much? (circle one)*	*Circle one*	*Sneezing, exercising, having sex, lifting, etc.*
Sample	Coffee	2 cups	✓ ✓	⬤ ◯ ◯ sm med lg	◯ ⬤ ◯ sm med lg	Yes (No)	Running
6–7 a.m.				◯ ◯ ◯	◯ ◯ ◯	Yes No	
7–8 a.m.				◯ ◯ ◯	◯ ◯ ◯	Yes No	
8–9 a.m.				◯ ◯ ◯	◯ ◯ ◯	Yes No	
9–10 a.m.				◯ ◯ ◯	◯ ◯ ◯	Yes No	
10–11 a.m.				◯ ◯ ◯	◯ ◯ ◯	Yes No	
11–12 noon				◯ ◯ ◯	◯ ◯ ◯	Yes No	
12–1 p.m.				◯ ◯ ◯	◯ ◯ ◯	Yes No	
1–2 p.m.				◯ ◯ ◯	◯ ◯ ◯	Yes No	
2–3 p.m.				◯ ◯ ◯	◯ ◯ ◯	Yes No	
3–4 p.m.				◯ ◯ ◯	◯ ◯ ◯	Yes No	
4–5 p.m.				◯ ◯ ◯	◯ ◯ ◯	Yes No	
5–6 p.m.				◯ ◯ ◯	◯ ◯ ◯	Yes No	
6–7 p.m.				◯ ◯ ◯	◯ ◯ ◯	Yes No	
7–8 p.m.				◯ ◯ ◯	◯ ◯ ◯	Yes No	
8–9 p.m.				◯ ◯ ◯	◯ ◯ ◯	Yes No	
9–10 p.m.				◯ ◯ ◯	◯ ◯ ◯	Yes No	
10–11 p.m.				◯ ◯ ◯	◯ ◯ ◯	Yes No	
11–12 midnight				◯ ◯ ◯	◯ ◯ ◯	Yes No	
12–1 a.m.				◯ ◯ ◯	◯ ◯ ◯	Yes No	
1–2 a.m.				◯ ◯ ◯	◯ ◯ ◯	Yes No	
2–3 a.m.				◯ ◯ ◯	◯ ◯ ◯	Yes No	
3–4 a.m.				◯ ◯ ◯	◯ ◯ ◯	Yes No	
4–5 a.m.				◯ ◯ ◯	◯ ◯ ◯	Yes No	
5–6 a.m.				◯ ◯ ◯	◯ ◯ ◯	Yes No	

(continued)

TABLE 12.6   BLADDER CONTROL DIARY (*continued*)

I used _____ pads today. I used _____ diapers today (write number).
Questions to ask my healthcare team: _____
_____
_____
_____
_____

Let's Talk About Bladder Control for Women is a public health awareness campaign conducted by the National Kidney and Urologic Diseases Information Clearinghouse (NKUDIC), an information dissemination service of the National Institute of Diabetes and Digestive and Kidney Diseases (NIDDK), National Institutes of Health.

Source: Adapted from NKUDIC, National Institutes of Health (NIH). (www.niddk.nih.gov/health-information/health-topics/urologic-disease/urinary-incontinencewomen/pages/insertb.aspx)

e. Overflow UI: Crede's method is used for expressing the bladder, by applying pressure with the hands placed in the suprapubic area after voiding to assist in emptying.

f. Intermittent catheterization is an option frequently used after other measures have failed for overflow UI.

g. Weight loss is suggested for obese clients.

h. Dietary changes including elimination of bladder irritants: caffeine, citrus/acidic foods, alcohol, and carbonated drinks

i. Avoid constipation. Discuss measures to prevent constipation.

j. Reduce excessive fluid intake, with no fluid intake 3 to 4 hours before bedtime if nocturia is a problem

B. Client teaching: *See Section III: Client Teaching Guide for this chapter, "Urinary Incontinence: Women."*

C. Other alternatives:

1. Surgical treatment is based on the cause of incontinence.

2. Continence pessaries may benefit women with stress UI.

3. Electrical stimulation may be prescribed to inhibit bladder instability and improve striated and levator contractility and efficiency.

4. Treatment of concomitant constipation is an important step in the treatment of incontinence.

5. Treatment of vaginal atrophy is another important step in the treatment of incontinence.

6. Injection of BTX is an option for treatment of urge incontinence in selected clients.

7. Transurethral bulking agents injected into the submucosal tissues of the urethra or bladder neck are an option for women and men with UI caused by BPH.

8. Indwelling catheters are not recommended as a management strategy for OAB. Please see Table 12.6 for a copy of the Bladder Control Diary to hand out to clients.

D. Pharmaceutical therapy:

1. Use of anticholinergic and antispasmodic drugs to decrease reflex bladder contractions and increase bladder capacity (contraindicated in uncontrolled narrow-angle glaucoma, urinary retention, or gastric retention) are indicated for urge or mixed incontinence.

a. Oxybutynin chloride (Ditropan): tablets and syrup formulation:

i. Adults: 5 mg orally two to three times per day (maximum of 20 mg/d)

ii. Pediatrics: indicated for children 5 years of age and older; 5 mg twice a day (maximum of 15 mg/d)

b. Oxybutynin chloride (Ditropan XL): extended release tablets:

i. Adults: initially 5 to 10 mg once a day; may increase the dosage weekly in 5 mg increments (maximum of 30 mg/d)

ii. Pediatrics: indicated for children 6 years of age and older. Initially 5 mg once a day; may increase weekly in 5 mg increments (maximum of 20 mg/d)

c. Oxybutynin chloride (Gelnique): topical gel:

i. Apply 1 g gel sachet once a day to intact skin

ii. Not recommended for children

d. Tolterodine tartrate (Detrol LA):

i. 2 to 4 mg orally per day

ii. Not recommended for children

e. Fesoterodine (Toviaz): extended release capsule:

i. 4 mg once a day (maximum of 8 mg/d)

ii. Not recommended for children

f. Trospium (Sanctura XR): extended release capsule:

i. Taken on an empty stomach, 60 mg orally every morning

ii. Not recommended for children

g. Darifenacin (Enablex):

i. 7.5 mg orally once a day

ii. May increase to 15 mg once a day

iii. Not recommended for children

h. Solifenacin (Vesicare):

i. Initially 5 mg orally once a day

ii. May increase to 10 mg daily

iii. Not recommended for children

2. Alpha-adrenergic antagonists stimulate urethral smooth muscle contraction.

  a. Imipramine (Tofranil): used for childhood enuresis:

    i. Children younger than 6 years: not recommended

    ii. Children older than 6 years: 25 mg initially 1 hour before bedtime

    iii. Children 6 to 12 years: 25 mg initially 1 hour before bedtime; increase up to 50 mg after 1 week

    iv. Children older than 12 years: 25 mg initially 1 hour before bedtime; may increase up to 75 mg as needed

3. Beta-3 adrenergic agonist: mirabegron (Myrbetriq):

  a. Initially 25 mg once a day

  b. May increase to 50 mg once a day

  c. Not recommended for children

4. The FDA has not approved any medication for stress incontinence.

5. For postmenopausal women, vaginal estrogen may restore urethral mucosa; use the same type, dosage, and client selection criteria as with estrogen therapy (ET). Systemic estrogen should not be prescribed for UI.

Follow-Up

A. Follow-up is based on the type and cause of UI.

Consultation/Referral

A. When to consult a physician for UI depends on the type and cause of UI. UI is a problem that can often be successfully treated or severity at least reduced.

B. Refer to a specialist for incontinence with abdominal and/or pelvic pain or hematuria in the absence of a UTI, or when surgical treatment is desired.

C. Refer for urodynamic testing, which is considered the gold standard. Testing requires special equipment and training.

D. Refer to a gynecologist or urology clinic practitioner experienced in fitting a continence pessary.

E. Refer to a urologist for hematuria and/or risk factors of bladder cancer.

Individual Considerations

A. Pregnancy: Stress incontinence is frequently associated with pregnancy and is treated with pelvic exercises.

B. Pediatrics:

1. UI is most often experienced as enuresis.

2. UI in previously bladder-controlled children requires a thorough workup and referral to a pediatrician.

3. Any child with a suspected neurologic abnormality should be evaluated for an occult neurologic lesion.

4. Dysfunctional voiding is often associated with a psychological comorbidity or behavioral issues.

C. Geriatrics:

1. Incontinence in the elderly is a risk factor for falls. Many falls occur en route to the bathroom, especially at night.

2. Incontinence increases social isolation and depression.

3. Functional incontinence is common in older adults with arthritis or Parkinson's or dementing diseases. Clients are unable to hold their urine until they reach the bathroom and undress. A timed toileting program usually assists in this situation.

4. Durable medical equipment, such as a bedside commode, should be considered.

5. Antimuscarinic medications may increase confusion due to anticholinergic side effects and are often ineffective in dementing diseases.

Bibliography

American Urological Association. (2017). *Surgical treatment of female stress urinary incontinence: AUA/SUFU Guideline.* Retrieved from https://www.auanet.org/guidelines/stress-urinary-incontinence-(sui)-guideline

American Urological Association. (2014). *Diagnosis and treatment of non-neurogenic overactive bladder (OAB) in adults: AUA/SUFU guideline.* Retrieved from https://www.auanet.org/guidelines/overactive-bladder-(oab)-guideline

Clemens, J. Q. (2018, August 19). Urinary incontinence in men. *UpToDate.* Retrieved from https://www.uptodate.com/contents/urinary-incontinence-in-men

Lukacz, E. (2017, December 12). Patient education: Urinary incontinence in women (Beyond the Basics). *UpToDate.* Retrieved from https://www.uptodate.com/contents/urinary-incontinence-in-women-beyond-the-basics

Nepple, K. G., & Cooper, C. S. (2018, January 5). Etiology and clinical features of bladder dysfunction in children. *UpToDate.* Retrieved from https://www.uptodate.com/contents/etiology-and-clinical-features-of-bladder-dysfunction-in-children

Vasavada, S. (2019, March 19). Urinary incontinence. *Medscape.* Retrieved from http://emedicine.medscape.com/article/452289-overview

Urinary Tract Infection (UTI; Acute Cystitis)

Cheryl A. Glass and Debbie Gunter

Definition

A. UTI is an infection of the urinary bladder. UTI is defined as the presence of at least 100,000 organisms per mL of urine in an asymptomatic client or more than 100 organisms per mL of urine with accompanying pyuria (> 7 WBCs/mL) in a symptomatic client. ASB when left untreated is a risk factor for acute cystitis (40%) and pyelonephritis in 25% to 30% in pregnancy.

B. UTIs can be divided anatomically into upper and lower tract (cystitis) infections. For a discussion of upper tract infection, see the section in this chapter, "Pyelonephritis."

C. UTIs may be considered uncomplicated or complicated.

1. An uncomplicated UTI is noted in a healthy person with a normal urinary tract system and may be treated with oral antibiotics.

2. A UTI noted in a person with a structural or functional urinary tract system or in a person who is immunocompromised is considered complicated. It may require parental therapy until afebrile.

Incidence

A. Incidence depends on age and gender. The prevalence of UTI in males varies according to age.

1. Young men aged 15 to 50 years rarely develop a UTI.

2. The incidence of a UTI in geriatric males may be as high as in geriatric females (up to 15%).

B. In children, the incidence varies by age and gender. In neonates, boys are slightly more likely than girls to present with UTI as part of a gram negative sepsis syndrome. A UTI is the most common cause of fever of unknown origin in pediatrics.

C. More than 50% of women will have one UTI in their lifetime.

1. Prevalence for females increases by 1% per decade and 2% to 4% throughout childbearing years.

2. The incidence of UTIs in pregnancy ranges from 4% to 7%. In pregnancy, the increased incidence is related to both hormonal influence and anatomic changes that increase the risk of urinary stasis and vesicoureteral reflux.

3. By age 30 years, approximately 50% of women have experienced symptoms of a UTI; almost 25% of these women have spontaneous resolution of symptoms, and the other 25% become infected.

Pathogenesis

A. Bacteria ascend from the perineum through the urethra. The greater susceptibility of younger women and girls is related to a shorter urethra. In older women, it is related to estrogen-mediated dilation of the urethra.

B. The normal male urinary tract has many natural defenses to infection. The greater susceptibility of elderly males is related to problems with the prostate and other urologic disease and can be linked to the instrumentation required for therapy.

C. Gram-negative bacilli are the most common pathogens; 80% to 90% of cases are related to coliform bacteria (*E. coli*). It originates from fecal floras that colonize the periurethral area.

D. Other gram-negative bacteria include *K. pneumoniae* or *P. mirabilis*. *S. saprophyticus* (gram-positive coccus) accounts for about 10% to 15% of UTIs.

E. Other pathogens include *Enterobacter*, *Pseudomonas*, *Enterococci*, and *Staphylococci*.

F. The incubation period depends on the pathogen.

Predisposing Factors

A. Female (until elderly, then equal frequency in males and females)

B. Pregnancy

C. Poor hygiene

D. Trauma

E. Instrumentation

F. Sexual intercourse

G. Oral contraceptive or diaphragm use

H. Female client diagnosed with diabetes (there is no increased risk for diabetic males)

I. Anomalies of the GU tract

J. Neurologic factors

K. Vesicourethral reflux

L. Obstruction: stones

M. Foreign bodies

N. Bubble baths and hot tubs

O. Douching

P. Anal intercourse

Q. HIV

R. Uncircumcised penis

S. Catheterization

T. Nosocomial infection

U. Phimosis

Common Complaints

A. Burning on urination

B. Frequency

C. Cloudy or bloody urine

D. Urgency

E. UTI in infants and children:

1. Vague symptoms with or without fever

2. Gastrointestinal symptoms (vomiting and diarrhea)

3. Frequent voiding

4. Incontinence

5. Dysuria

6. Suprapubic, abdominal, or lumbar pain

F. Geriatrics:

1. May not present with classic symptoms

2. Fever

3. Incontinence

4. Mental confusion

Other Signs and Symptoms

A. Asymptomatic

B. Frequency, dysuria, bladder spasms, suprapubic discomfort, urgency, and nocturia

C. Suprapubic pain

D. Fever

E. CVA tenderness

F. Hematuria

Subjective Data

A. Review the onset, course, and duration of symptoms

B. Does the client have fever and chills or back or flank pain (unilateral or bilateral)?

C. Are there any other genital problems such as herpes lesions or vaginal discharge?

D. Review the associated factors: sexual intercourse (specifically review for anal intercourse), douching, or bubble bath

E. Ask female clients if they use appropriate hygiene practices after urination and BMs:

1. Wiping from front to back

2. Frequent changes of hygienic products

3. Handwashing

F. Is the client pregnant? If not, what type of birth control does she use?

G. Is there any history of previous UTIs? How often, and how were they treated? Were any tests performed in a workup by a urologist?

H. How much liquid or water does the client drink every day? Note the amount of caffeine.

I. In older men, review the strength of the urinary flow, dribbling, hesitancy, and so forth

J. In the postmenopausal woman, review whether she has a known prolapse and/or vaginal atrophy. Does she use any systemic or local estrogen medications?

K. Is there any history of other medical diseases including diabetes or sickle cell disease?

L. Review for the presence of neurologic disorders including spinal cord injury or multiple sclerosis

M. Does the client require self-catheterization?

Physical Examination

A. Check temperature, BP, pulse, and respiration. The absence of a fever does not exclude the presence of an infective process.

B. Inspect:
1. General observation of general appearance for discomfort before and during examination

C. Auscultate:
1. Heart and all lung fields

D. Percuss:
1. The bladder and the CVA area for tenderness

E. Palpate:
1. Palpate the abdomen: kidneys, masses; assess for suprapubic tenderness.
2. Palpate the back; note CVA tenderness.
3. Check for inguinal lymph node enlargement.
4. Palpate the suprapubic area.

F. Females:
1. Pelvic examination:
   a. Inspect external genitalia for lesions, Bartholin's gland cysts, irritation, and discharge.
   b. Milk urethra for discharge.
   c. Assess rectal area.
   d. Speculum examination: evaluate vaginal vault for discharge, cervicitis, and inflammation; evaluate for atrophic vaginal changes and torn tissue.
   e. Bimanual examination: check for cervical motion, tenderness, and masses.

G. Males:
1. Inspect the penis/urinary meatus for phimosis, lesions, signs of inflammation, and discharge. Retract the foreskin (if present) and assess for hygiene and smegma.
2. Palpate the testes and epididymides for inflammation, tenderness, and masses.
3. Rectal examination is mandatory in males: check for swollen and tender prostate. In clients with suspected acute bacterial prostatitis, palpation should be very gentle because of the potential for bacteremia.

Diagnostic Tests

The diagnosis of a UTI can often be made based on a focused history and the presenting symptoms.

A. Urinalysis: Clean-catch urinalysis may be performed. However, catheterization or suprapubic aspiration may be necessary depending on the client's age and condition. Examples include pediatrics, elderly, obese, microscopic hematuria or for functionally impaired clients. Catheterization should be reserved for clients with an obstruction or for those who cannot cooperate or collect a clean-catch urine specimen. The percutaneous bladder aspiration is used for young children and infants.

A. Urinalysis dipstick findings:
1. Appearance: should be clear. Cloudy urine may indicate presence of pyuria, pus, blood, cells, phosphate, or lymph fluid.
2. Odor: usually faint aromatic odor; ammonia odor indicates *Proteus*, related to food changes; offensive odor indicates bacterial infection.
3. pH: normal is around 6 (acid); may normally vary from 4.6 to 7.5. Greater than 7.5 may indicate infection.
4. Specific gravity: reflects the kidney's ability to concentrate urine and the body's hydration or dehydration status. Normal is 1.005 to 1.025.
5. Color: shows concentration; usually yellow or amber:
   a. Straw color = dilute urine
   b. Dark color = concentrated (dehydrated)
   c. Red or red-brown to bloody = transfusion reaction, drugs, and bleeding lesions
   d. Yellow brown = bile duct disease, jaundice
   e. Dark brown or black = melanoma or leukemia
6. Positive leukocyte esterase and nitrates indicate infection.
   A negative urine dipstick does not rule out an infection.

B. Microscopic examination of urine findings: WBCs greater than 2 to 5; WBC/HPF; bacteria; positive Gram stain for cocci or rods, yeast, and blood indicate infection.

C. Urine culture and sensitivity:
1. Positive culture standard 10^5 colony-forming units; symptomatic female 10^2; symptomatic males 10^3
2. Screening for asymptomatic bacteria is recommended for clients in pregnancy, for elderly males with documented prostatic or urologic abnormalities, for clients with a recent catheterization, and for clients with known stones or documented structural abnormalities.

D. Culture for STIs if suspected

E. Wet prep for female, if indicated

F. Imaging:
1. Ultrasound (especially useful in children)
2. Conventional voiding cystourethrography
3. Urodynamic evaluation

Differential Diagnoses

A. Vaginal or pelvic infection

B. Prostatitis or epididymitis: tender, enlarged prostate; tender testicle or scrotum

C. Bladder tumor

D. IC

E. Urinary calculi

F. BPH: changes in urinary stream and nocturia

G. OAB/urge incontinence

H. Pelvic organ prolapse

I. Irritant urethritis

J. Consider the possibility that chronic, asymptomatic infections are a potential source of disseminated infection, such as endocarditis. This possibility is particularly likely in the male client with prostate disease and infection requiring instrumentation.

Plan

A. General interventions:

1. Treatment of acute cystitis is aimed at identifying the underlying cause and initiating treatment as soon as possible.

2. If antibiotic therapy is initiated, stress the importance of taking all medication as directed, even if symptoms improve before the end of treatment.

B. Client teaching:

1. Provide client teaching sheet. Client teaching: See *Section III: Client Teaching Guide for this chapter, "Urinary Tract Infection (Acute Cystitis)."*

C. Dietary management:

1. Instruct the client to increase fluids and drink at least one large glass of liquid every hour.

2. Instruct the client to avoid foods that irritate the bladder: caffeine, alcohol, tomatoes, citrus, and spicy foods.

3. Encourage the client to drink cranberry juice to help fight bladder infections. If the client dislikes the taste of plain cranberry juice, have him or her mix it 1:1 with another juice, such as orange juice.

D. Pharmaceutical therapy:

1. Antibiotics: 3-day course may be efficacious and is less expensive than the traditional 7- to 10-day course of therapy for uncomplicated infections.

2. The antibiotic of choice depends on the specific bacteria found on culture. Empiric antimicrobial therapy should cover all likely pathogens.

3. First-line therapy:

a. Nitrofurantoin monohydrate/macrocrystals (Macrobid) 100 mg orally twice a day for 5 days *or*

b. Trimethoprim/sulfamethoxazole 160 mg/800 mg (Bactrim DS, Septra DS) 1 tablet orally twice a day for 3 days (use when bacterial resistance is less than 20% and client has no allergy) *or*

c. Fosfomycin (Monurol) 3 g orally in a single dose with 3 to 4 oz of water

4. Second-line therapy:

a. Ciprofloxacin (Cipro) 250 mg orally twice a day for 3 days *or*

b. Ciprofloxacin extended-release (Cipro XR) 500 mg orally twice a day for 3 days *or*

c. Levofloxacin (Levaquin) 250 mg orally twice a day for 3 days

5. Alternative therapy:

a. Amoxicillin–clavulanate (Augmentin) 875 mg/125 mg orally twice a day for 7 days *or*

b. Amoxicillin–clavulanate (Augmentin) 500 mg/125 mg orally three times per day for 7 days

6. Urinary analgesic, if needed:

a. Phenazopyridine HCl (Pyridium): 100 to 200 mg tid for 1 to 2 days only when given with an antibiotic. Educate the client that this drug turns urine orange.

b. Multiple Uro Blue medications are available; take one orally four times a day. Educate the client that this drug turns the urine blue/green.

7. Drugs of choice for UTI or pyelonephritis in pregnancy:

a. Nitrofurantoin (Macrobid) 100 mg: One tablet orally every 12 hours for 5 days

b. Amoxicillin: 500 mg orally every 12 hours for 3 to 7 days

c. Amoxicillin–clavulanate (Augmentin): 500 mg orally every 12 hours for 3 to 7 days

d. Cephalexin (Keflex): 500 mg orally four times a day for 3 to 5 days

e. Cefpodoxime (Vantin) 100 mg twice a day for 5 to 7 days *or*

f. Fosfomycin (Monurol) 3 g orally in a single dose with 3 to 4 oz of water

g. If dysuria is present: phenazopyridine HCl (Pyridium) 200 mg orally three times daily for 2 days when given with an antibiotic

8. Children younger than 2 years are usually treated for 7 to 14 days; children older than 2 years who are afebrile and without abnormalities of the urinary tract or have previous episodes of UTIs are usually treated for 5 days.

a. Amoxicillin–clavulanate (Augmentin): 20 to 45 mg/kg orally per day every 12 hours

b. Sulfonamide–trimethoprim–sulfamethoxazole (Bactrim, Septra): 6 to 12 mg/kg trimethoprim and 30 to 60 mg/kg sulfamethoxazole per day orally in two doses

c. Cephalosporin–cefixime (Suprax): 8 mg/kg/d in one dose or in divided doses every 12 hours

9. Antibiotics that should not be used in pediatrics or pregnancy include the following:

a. Fluoroquinolones are not used in children because of potential concerns about sustained injury to developing joints.

b. Fluoroquinolones (Mirabegron) are contraindicated during pregnancy because of auditory and vestibular toxicity in the fetus.

c. Tetracyclines should not be used in pregnancy (Category D) or in children because of tooth staining.

d. Nitrofurantoin is contraindicated in pregnant clients at term, during labor, and during delivery.

10. Consider prophylactic therapy for clients with chronic conditions/recurrent infections:

a. Low-dose antibiotics daily for 3 to 6 months

b. Self-start antibiotics

c. Postcoital antibiotics

11. Quinolones, cephalosporins, and macrolides should be reserved for complicated or resistant infections.

12. Vaginal estrogen should be considered in postmenopausal women with urogenital atrophic changes.

Follow-Up

A. Routine posttreatment urinalysis/culture is not indicated in asymptomatic clients.

B. Have the client return if symptoms do not resolve at the end of treatment.

C. Have the client return if the symptoms reoccur within 2 weeks of treatment for a urine culture. Retreatment with a 7-day course of antibiotics using a different agent should be considered.

D. Two UTIs in girls and one UTI in boys should trigger an evaluation to rule out an obstruction, vesicoureteric reflux, and dysfunctional voiding. UTI in children who are severely ill with vomiting and dehydration requires hospitalization and IV antibiotics.

Consultation/Referral

A. Refer all children with more than one UTI to a physician.

B. Young men do not have UTIs very often; a urologic workup may be needed if etiology, such as an STI, cannot be determined.

C. Clients with bacteriuria are also more likely to have identifiable abnormalities on an IVP, including small kidneys, delayed excretion, calyceal dilation and blunting, ureteral reflux, stones, and obstructive lesions.

D. Consultation with a urologist is essential in all forms of prostatitis or in all but the most clear-cut cases of acute scrotum.

Individual Considerations

A. Women:
1. Recurrent infections are common in females.
2. Repeat urine culture and sensitivity after an antibiotic course is complete (approximately 2–4 weeks after therapy is completed).
3. If the client is perimenopausal and has two or fewer UTIs a year, consider client-initiated therapy to start when symptomatic. Consider topical estradiol cream for atrophic vaginitis. If the client has three UTIs a year, prescribe a prophylactic single-dose regimen after intercourse. If infections are not related to intercourse, consider urine cultures every 2 months, with extended antibiotic therapy.

B. Pregnancy:
1. The incidence of pyelonephritis in pregnancy is 1% to 2%. Most cases develop as a consequence of undiagnosed or inadequately treated lower UTI.
    a. In the presumptive diagnosis of pyelonephritis in pregnancy, ultrasound of the kidneys and urinary tract should be considered.
2. Approximately 75% to 80% of pyelonephritis cases occur on the right side, with a 10% to 15% incidence on the left side. A small percentage of cases are bilateral.
3. GBS colonization has important implications during pregnancy, contributing to maternal pyelonephritis and preterm birth. Intrapartum transmission may lead to neonatal GBS infection.
    a. Women with documented GBS bacteriuria in the current pregnancy should be treated at the time of labor or rupture of membranes with appropriate IV antibiotics for the prevention of early-onset neonatal GBS disease.
    b. Asymptomatic women with urinary GBS in pregnancy should not be treated with antibiotics for the prevention of adverse maternal and perinatal outcomes.
    c. Women with documented GBS bacteriuria should not be rescreened by genital tract culture or urinary culture in the third trimester, as they are presumed to be GBS colonized.
4. Current guidelines recommend universal vaginal and rectal screening in all pregnant women at 35 to 37 weeks gestation rather than treatment based on risk factors.
5. A urine culture screening is recommended for all pregnant women at their first prenatal visit.
6. Suppressive antibiotic therapy should be instituted in pregnant clients who develop acute cystitis, recurrent or persistent ASB, or pyelonephritis.
7. Clients with sickle cell hemoglobinopathies are at increased risk of UTI and should be screened more aggressively. They may possibly benefit from antibiotic prophylaxis.
8. Antibiotics that should not be used during pregnancy include:
    a. Tetracyclines (adverse effects on fetal teeth/bones and congenital defects)
    b. Quinolones (congenital defects)
    c. Trimethoprim in the first trimester (facial defects and cardiac abnormalities)
    d. Sulfonamides in the last trimester (kernicterus)
    e. Aminoglycosides (permanent ototoxicity in the fetus)

C. Pediatrics:
1. Tetracyclines should not be given to children because of tooth staining.
2. Fluorinated quinolones may produce cartilage toxicity.
3. Antibiotic therapy includes amoxicillin, cephalosporins, trimethoprim, and nitrofurantoin.
4. Children diagnosed with recurrent UTIs should be referred and assessed for sexual abuse.

D. Geriatrics:
1. Clients may not have classic symptoms. Consider UTI if the client presents with increased UI, fever, and mental confusion.

Bibliography

American Academy of Pediatrics. (reaffirmed in November 2016). Urinary tract infection: Clinical practice guideline for the diagnosis and management of the initial UTI in febrile infants and children 2 to 24 months. *Pediatrics, 128*, 595–610. doi:10.1542/peds.2011-1330

American Urological Association. (2014). *Diagnosis and treatment of non-neurogenic overactive bladder (OAB) in adults: AUA/SUFU guideline.* Retrieved from https://www.auanet.org/guidelines/overactive-bladder-(oab)-guideline

Brusch, J. (2019, August 27). Urinary tract infection (UTI) and cystitis (bladder infection) in females treatment & management. *Medscape*. Retrieved from https://emedicine.medscape.com/article/233101-treatment

Grabe, M., Bjerklund-Johansen, T. E., Botto, H., Cek, M., Naber, K. G., Pickard, R. S., & Wullt, B. (2015). Guidelines on urological infections. *European Association of Urology.* Retrieved from www.uroweb.org/guidelines/online-guidelines

Hooton, T. M. (2018). Patient education: Urinary tract infections in adolescents and adults (Beyond the Basics). *UpToDate.* Retrieved from https://www.uptodate.com/contents/urinary-tract-infections-in-adolescents-and-adults-beyond-the-basics#H1

Hooton, T. M. (2018, July 27). Acute simple cystitis in men. *UpToDate*. Retrieved from https://www.uptodate.com/contents/acute-simple-cystitis -in-men

Hooton, T. M., & Gupta, K. (2019, March 13). Acute simple cystitis in women. *UpToDate*. Retrieved from https://www.uptodate.com/contents/ acute-simple-cystitis-in-women

Johnson, E. (2018, October 27). Urinary tract infections in pregnancy. *Medscape*. Retrieved from http://emedicine.medscape.com/article/ 452604-overview

Varicocele

Cheryl A. Glass and Debbie Gunter

Definition

A. Varicocele is engorgement of the internal spermatic veins above the testes. This vascular abnormality is a cause of decreased testicular function. Some varicoceles are easy to identify and may be surgically corrected. The presence of a varicocele does not mean that surgical correction is a necessity (see Figure 12.5).

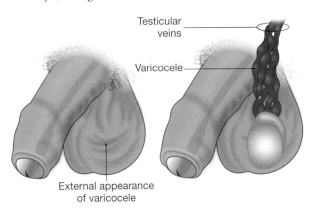

FIGURE 12.5 Varicocele.

Incidence

A. Varicocele may occur in 15% to 20% of normal males; 80% to 90% of cases occur on the left side. Up to 35% to 40% of men with a palpable left-sided varicocele may actually have bilateral varicoceles that are identified on physical examination.

B. Right-sided varicocele is uncommon and can indicate retroperitoneal malignancy. Varicocele is the leading known cause of male infertility (40%). Decreased sperm counts, infertility, and testicular atrophy occur in 65% to 75% of varicocele cases. There is no correlation between the size of the varicocele and the degree of infertility.

Pathogenesis

A. The exact pathophysiologic mechanisms for varicoceles are not fully identified. Varicoceles may be because of valvular incompetence or elevated hydrostatic pressure in the spermatic veins. Testicular temperature elevation also appears to play a role in varicocele-induced dysfunction. New varicoceles in older men may be secondary to renal tumors.

Predisposing Factor

A. Varicoceles generally manifest at the time of puberty.

Common Complaints

A. Asymptomatic

B. Infertility

C. Pain or discomfort in the scrotum

Other Signs and Symptoms

A. Pain or aching and heaviness in the scrotum

B. Feels like "worms"; scrotum may have bluish discoloration

Subjective Data

A. Note the onset, course, and duration of symptoms. When was the varicocele first noted?

B. Has the scrotum enlarged? If there is enlargement, over what time span? Does the varicocele collapse with lying or sitting down?

C. Is there any pain or discomfort?

D. Has there been any history of infertility?

Physical Examination

A. Check vital signs and temperature as indicated.

B. Inspect:
1. The examination should be done when the client is lying or standing in a warm room. Warm temperature promotes relaxation of the scrotum.
2. Examine the general appearance of the penis; note scrotal size, shape, and rugae. Varicocele tends to collapse with the client sitting or supine.
3. Transilluminate the scrotum to visualize the varicocele
4. A large varicocele can easily be identified by inspection.

C. Auscultate: listen over the scrotum to assess bowel sounds to rule out hernia.

D. Palpate:
1. Palpate each side of the scrotum for testicular size, presence of varicocele (Valsalva maneuver performed while the client stands helps to reveal a small varicocele), and absence of vas deferens.
   a. A moderate-size varicocele can be identified by palpation without having the client perform the Valsalva maneuver.
2. Palpate the spermatic cord between the thumb and forefinger while the client performs a Valsalva maneuver.
   a. A small varicocele is identified only when the client bears down, increasing the intra-abdominal pressure.
   b. A varicocele should significantly diminish in size when the client assumes the supine position.
3. Evaluate whether the varicocele can be reduced while the client is supine.
4. Palpate the abdomen for hernias, masses, and tenderness.
5. Rectal examination: palpate the prostate and seminal vesicles for tenderness and other signs of infection.

Diagnostic Tests

A. Scrotal ultrasound with a high-resolution color-flow Doppler is the diagnostic method of choice when clinical examinations are equivocal, but are not indicated for standard evaluation.

B. Semen analysis times two, if indicated

C. CT to evaluate retroperitoneal pathology (e.g., renal cell carcinoma) for:
  1. Sudden onset of varicocele
  2. Single right-sided varicocele
  3. Any varicocele that is not reducible in the supine position

Differential Diagnoses

A. Varicocele classifications
  1. Grade I (small): palpable only on Valsalva maneuver, which increases intra-abdominal pressure and therefore impedes drainage and increases the varicocele size
  2. Grade II (medium): palpable when standing and bearing down (Valsalva maneuver)
  3. Grade III (large): visible on inspection alone
  4. Subclinical: not palpable, vein larger than 3 mm on ultrasound; Doppler reflux on Valsalva maneuver

B. Hernia

C. Epididymitis

D. Hydrocele

E. Testicular tumor: consider retroperitoneal tumor, especially if presenting symptoms have a sudden onset.

Plan

A. General interventions:
  1. Urologic consultation for diagnosis and possible surgery. Surgery should be considered when all of the following conditions are met:
    a. Palpable varicocele on physical examination
    b. Couples with known infertility
    c. Female has normal fertility or potential treatable cause of infertility
    d. Male partner has abnormal semen parameters or abnormal results from sperm function tests

B. Client teaching:
  1. If discomfort is present, an athletic supporter should be tried.
  2. If surgery is not indicated, no other interventions are needed.

C. Pharmaceutical therapy: None is recommended.

Follow-Up

A. After surgery, no follow-up is necessary if the client is taught scrotal self-examination.

B. If no surgery is performed, the client should be taught self-examination and instructed to return for pain or change in size and shape.

C. Adolescents with varicoceles should be followed with annual objective measurements of testis size and/or semen analyses in order to detect the earliest sign of varicocele-related testicular injury.

Consultation/Referral

A. Refer the client to a urologist for surgical evaluation. Varicocelectomy is recommended in cases of pain and infertility, and it may be offered in the preadolescent to ensure proper testicular development.

Individual Considerations

A. Adults:
  1. New onset varicocele in an older male may indicate a renal tumor.

B. Pediatrics:
  1. The young client with a varicocele should be followed every 6 months or yearly to see how the testis is growing.

Bibliography

Rovito, M. J., Cavayero, C., Leone, J. E., & Harlin, S. (2015). Interventions promoting testicular self-examination (TSE) performance: A systematic review. *American Journal of Men's Health*, 9(6), 506–518. doi:10.1177/1557988314555360

The Testicular Cancer Resource Center. (2018, March 28). How to do a testicular self examination. Retrieved from http://thetcrc.org/tcexam.html

White, W. M. (2019, January 2). Varicocele. *Medscape*. Retrieved from http://emedicine.medscape.com/article/438591-overview

13 Obstetrics Guidelines

Preconception Counseling: Identifying Clients at Risk

Jill C. Cash, Susan Drummond, and Christina C. Reed

Anemia

A woman's health before conception influences her ability not only to conceive but also to maintain pregnancy and to achieve a healthy outcome. Some women are unaware that their medical conditions, medications, occupational exposure, or social practices may have negative consequences in the earliest weeks of pregnancy, before the pregnancy test is positive. They don't know that organogenesis begins around 17 days after fertilization. Steps to provide the ideal environment for the developing fetus are most likely to be effective if they precede the traditional initiation of prenatal care.

The goal of preconceptional care is to reduce perinatal mortality and morbidity. Targeting only self-referred women who are planning their next conception or women referred with risk factors can result in a significant number of missed opportunities for primary prevention. Nurses working with women of childbearing age and their families have a responsibility to promote reproductive health during every health encounter. Even among married women in the United States, the unintended pregnancy rate is nearly 45%; 85% of teen pregnancies are unintended.

During the antepartum period, assessment for routine screening exams should be performed to promote a healthy pregnancy. Topics of discussion should include status on current immunizations, including Tdap (tetanus, diphtheria, and pertussis), assessing rubella immunity, determining hepatitis status, doing Pap smears and cultures for sexually transmitted infections (STIs), and reviewing her and her partner's family history for chronic diseases, such as diabetes, hypertension, lupus, and so forth.

When discussing preconception plans, the client's history, as well as that of her partner, should be evaluated for poor health habits (alcohol, smoking, drug use), exposure to toxic substances (radiation and chemicals), multiple sexual partners (risk of HIV, hepatitis, and STIs), and racial or ethnic origin. Preconceptional evaluation should include the following:

A. Maternal age: Pregnancy-induced hypertension (PIH) occurs at the extreme of ages; insulin-dependent diabetes, the risks of Down syndrome, and other chromosomal abnormalities increase with maternal age. Advanced maternal age (AMA) is defined as 35 years of age at delivery. The American College of Obstetricians and Gynecologists (ACOG) requires counseling on genetic screening/testing options for women of AMA.

B. Universal carrier screening is available for women who desire to know if they are carriers for an autosomal recessive disorder, such as Tay–Sachs disease, sickle cell anemia, alpha and beta thalassemias, cystic fibrosis, and spinal muscular atrophy. Ideally, this blood test should be done preconceptionally, but it can be performed at any time during the pregnancy. If the screening test is positive, the woman's partner can then be tested.

C. Social issues: Screen every woman for intimate partner violence. Research indicates that most abused women continue to be victimized during pregnancy and that the violence may escalate. Child abuse is also common in homes where there is abuse of adults. This assessment should be done only if the partner is not present. Information should be given to the client concerning available community, social, and legal resources, and her immediate safety, the safety of her children, and an escape plan should be assessed. Report child abuse to the state's mandatory reporting agency.

D. Financial: Discuss insurance, maternity benefits, work–leave policy, and contingency plans for lost wages because of pregnancy complications with the client.

E. Environmental and occupational considerations: Routine assessment of hobbies and home and employment environments may identify exposures that have been associated with adverse reproductive consequences that can be minimized in the preconceptual period.

F. Adverse fetal effects are dose-dependent and gestational age at exposure related to the following:

   1. Radiation: Fetal effects include microcephaly, mental retardation, eye anomalies, intrauterine

growth retardation (IUGR), and visceral malformations. Lead aprons should be used to protect the client from any radiation exposures.

2. Heavy metals: Mercury exposure is related to brain damage and neuromuscular defects. Lead exposure is related to increased spontaneous abortion, low birth weight, brain damage, and increased premature rupture of membranes (PROM). Cadmium is retained by the fetal liver and kidney and is also associated with fetal craniofacial defects. Nickel is associated with neonatal deaths.

3. Pesticides: Occupations at risk for pesticide exposure include, but are not limited to, the following: ranch and farm workers (including migrant workers); gardeners (home and professional); groundskeepers; florists; structural pest control workers; hunting and fishing guides; healthcare workers who deal with contamination; and people employed in pesticide production, mixing, and application. Dioxin is associated with an increased rate of spontaneous abortion, myelomeningocele, and limb defects. The pesticides DDT and dichlorodiphenyldichloroethylene (DDE) are associated with increased abortion, prematurity, low birth weight, PIH, and early weaning.

4. Other: Carbon monoxide is associated with increased stillbirths, neurologic deficits, seizures, spasticity, and retarded psychomotor development. Ozone is associated with increased spontaneous abortion and increased structural defects. Anesthetic gases are associated with increased abortion, birth defects, low birth weight, and infertility.

G. Infectious diseases: See Chapters 15 (Sexually Transmitted Infections) and 16 (Infectious Diseases).

H. Medications: Assess and minimize the risk of exposure to medications by reviewing the client's use of prescription and nonprescription drugs, including herbal supplements. Provide the client with information on the safest choices and avoiding drugs associated with fetal risks. Identify all prescription and nonprescription medications taken by the mother and partner to assess for risks to the fetus associated with current medications. Teratogenic defects linked to certain medications may include cleft lip and palate, congenital heart disease, microcephaly, caudal dysplasia, and caudal regression syndrome.

I. Medical problems: Health assessment of potential risk not only to the fetus but also to the woman should she become pregnant should be discussed. Care must be taken to identify and counsel all women whose life expectancy could be markedly reduced by pregnancy or whose fetus would have a high likelihood of complications. For example, women with known cardiac problems, epilepsy, transplanted organs, or uncontrolled diabetes and hypertension should be told of the risks associated with pregnancy.

1. Diabetes: Researchers have demonstrated a dose-related response between glycosylated hemoglobin (HgbA1c) during the first trimester of pregnancy and the incidence of congenital defects: the better the glycemic control, the lower the risk for birth defects.

The preconceptional plan for diabetes includes the following:

a. Change all clients on oral agents to insulin therapy before pregnancy is attempted.

b. Achieve strict plasma glucose control. The ACOG recommends self-monitoring of blood glucose during pregnancy with the following glucose levels to be met:

i. Fasting: Less than or equal to 95 mg/dL

ii. Preprandial glucose values less than 100 mg/dL

iii. 1-hour postprandial glucose levels less than 140 mg/dL

iv. 2-hour postprandial glucose levels less than 120 mg/dL

v. Nighttime glucose levels should not drop below 60 mg/dL. Care should be taken to avoid hypoglycemia during pregnancy.

c. Reduce the HgbA1c to 6% or less.

d. Assess the client for vasculopathy, neuropathy, nephropathy, and retinopathy.

e. Refer the client for genetic and nutritional counseling.

f. Enhance the woman's knowledge of diabetes during pregnancy.

J. Nutrition: Dietary evaluation and recommendations of alternatives that may benefit the fetus's development are important components of preconceptional counseling. Evaluation of nutritional status should include assessment of the appropriate weight for the client's height as well as a discussion of eating habits, such as vegetarianism, fasting for religious or personal reasons, eating disorders, the use of megavitamins, and herbal supplements.

1. Neural tube defects (NTDs): In about 90% of the cases, NTDs are not expected on the basis of past history. NTDs are associated with multifactorial causes, including environmental factors, undernutrition (lack of folic acid), chromosomal defects, maternal hyperthermia, diabetes, clomiphene citrate (Clomid) induction, and maternal obesity. In 1996, the Food and Drug Administration (FDA) approved a population-based strategy, effective January 1998, to fortify grain food sources with folic acid. The recurrence risk of NTD is 2% to 3% without the use of preconceptional doses of folic acid. Even with the FDA strategy, folic acid supplement of 0.4 mg (400 mcg) per day at least 1 month before conception and during the first trimester of pregnancy is recommended. Women who have had a child with an NTD require higher doses of folic acid, 4 mg daily.

K. Obstetric considerations: Preconceptional reproductive history is an important tool for identifying factors that may be amenable to intervention. Review term, preterm, aborted (elective, spontaneous, and therapeutic) pregnancies, as well as a short history on living children. Review the gestational age at delivery of each neonate and any pregnancy and delivery complications. Preterm labor (PTL) has a 30% recurrence risk, and preeclampsia has a 5% to 70% recurrence rate in subsequent pregnancies.

Women who developed severe features of preeclampsia and were delivered before 30 weeks' gestation have the highest risk of preeclampsia in future pregnancies. In some instances, after preconceptual and genetic counseling, the couple may decide to forgo pregnancy or to use assisted reproductive technologies such as donor eggs and/or sperm.

L. Genetic screening: Recommended for all women. Genetic counseling for discussion of testing options is recommended if the mother is 35 years or older at the time of delivery, or if she has a family history of any abnormal genetic disorders, such as Down syndrome. The parents choose whether they would like to have genetic testing performed to evaluate the fetus for abnormal chromosomes. The following tests can be performed for genetic screening:

1. Noninvasive prenatal screening: Cell-free DNA from the fetus is found in maternal serum and can lead to prenatal identification of pregnancies at high risk for trisomy 13, 18, and 21, as well as detection of gender. This screen is a maternal blood test and can be done as early as 10 weeks. A positive screen should be confirmed with a diagnostic test such as chorionic villus sampling (CVS) or amniocentesis.

2. CVS: Performed at 10 to 12 weeks gestation

3. Amniocentesis: Performed at 15 to 18 weeks gestation, ideally, but can be performed later in pregnancy

   a. Amniocentesis can also be performed to assess for spinal cord defects. Amniocentesis can detect elevated protein levels (alpha-fetoprotein and the presence of acetyl cholinesterase) in the amniotic fluid that is present in the event of a spinal cord defect. Therefore, if performing an amniocentesis, information regarding both genetic makeup and spinal cord defects can be determined during the single procedure of the amniocentesis.

M. Recurrent loss: The workup and counseling for recurrent losses include evaluation for a uterine defect (septal or bicornuate uterus or uterus didelphys), endocrine problems (luteal phase defect or hypothyroidism), chromosomal defects, or presence of antiphospholipid syndrome. Antiphospholipid syndrome is defined as the presence of maternal anticardiolipin antibodies and/or lupus anticoagulant in association with recurrent pregnancy loss, thrombotic events, and/or thrombocytopenia. Testing for anticardiolipin antibodies and lupus anticoagulant should be considered for women who have a history of three or more unexplained consecutive pregnancy losses before 10 weeks, or have a history of one or more unexplained pregnancy losses after 10 weeks with a morphologically normal fetus. In the nonpregnant client, thrombosis of a single vessel is the most common complication associated with antiphospholipid syndrome.

N. Lifestyle: Queries regarding a woman's social lifestyle history should seek to identify behaviors and exposures that may compromise reproductive outcome. While environmental exposures are a frequent concern of couples considering pregnancy, women should be informed that, in general, maternal use of alcohol, tobacco, and other mood-altering drugs is more hazardous for a fetus than most other lifestyle choices.

1. Alcohol: Alcohol is a known teratogen. There is no safe limit of alcohol use during pregnancy. Women should be informed that prenatal alcohol consumption is a preventable cause of birth defects including neurodevelopmental deficits and intellectual disability. Research indicates that as many as 73% of 12- to 34-year-old women expose their fetuses to alcohol at some time during pregnancy.

2. Smoking: Fetal effects of smoking are also related to the dose–response effect. Smoking is associated with an increase in bleeding in pregnancy (abruption and placenta previa), IUGR, preterm birth (PTB), low birth weight, stillbirth, respiratory distress in the neonate, and sudden infant death syndrome. Counsel the client on smoking cessation. Suggestions of ways to quit include tapering the use of nicotine (tapering and brand switching to lower tar and nicotine), monitoring smoking behavior, setting a contract to quit smoking, identifying social support or a buddy, and restricting area(s) such as a no smoking zone. Give the client positive reinforcement for behavior change and cessation of the use of tobacco. Nicotine replacement therapy may be considered but only under close supervision with careful discussions with the client, as the U.S. Preventive Services Task Force (USPSTF) has concluded that nicotine replacement products during pregnancy have not been sufficiently evaluated for safety or efficacy.

3. Substance use: If substance exposure is complicated by addiction, structured recovery programs are usually needed to effect behavioral change. Substance use/abuse is teratogenic to the fetus, and cessation of all substances is imperative before, during, and after pregnancy.

O. Exercise: Exercise and recreational activities should be reviewed and discussed relative to safety, including the use of bike helmets, avoiding strenuous exercise, and hyperthermia. The ACOG recommends that maternal heart rate (for pregnant women) not exceed 140 beats per minute (bpm). If the woman is not currently exercising, walking and swimming can be suggested. Heat exposure appears to be teratogenic. Use of saunas or hot tubs and high fevers in the first trimester have been associated with an increased risk of NTDs.

P. Preconceptual counseling helps to identify high-risk clients who need intensive care during pregnancy and delivery, and it identifies women who need referral for medical management, nutritional counseling, genetic counseling, or behavior modification. Prescribe a prenatal vitamin with the recommended 800 to 1,000 mcg daily of folic acid for any woman less than 35 years of age, and 4,000 mcg daily of folic acid for women 35 years and older considering pregnancy.

Bibliography

American College of Obstetricians and Gynecologists. (2012). ACOG Practice Bulletin No. 130: Prediction and prevention of preterm birth (Reaffirmed 2018). *Obstetrics and Gynecology, 120,* 964–973. doi:10.1097/AOG.0b013e3182723b1b

American College of Obstetricians and Gynecologists. (2014). Preconception and interconception care. In *Guidelines for women's health care: A resource manual*. Washington, DC: Author.

de Weerd, S., Thomas, C., Cikot, R., Steegers-Theunissen, R., de Boo, T., & Steegers, E. (2002). Preconception counseling improves folate status of women planning pregnancy. *Obstetrics and Gynecology, 99*(1), 45–50. doi:10.1016/S0029-7844(01)01573-3

Levy, B., Sigurjonsson, S., Pettersen, B., Maisenbacher, M. K., Hall, M. P., Demko, Z., . . . Rabinowitz, M. (2014, August). Genomic imbalance in products of conception: Single-nucleotide polymorphism chromosomal microarray analysis. *Obstetrics and Gynecology, 124*(2 Pt 1), 202–209. doi:10.1097/AOG.0000000000000325

Prenatal Care: Initial Prenatal Visit

Jill C. Cash, Susan Drummond, and Christina C. Reed

The initial prenatal visit is a very important visit. Ideally, all clients should start prenatal care in the first trimester; however, clients may not initiate or have access to prenatal care until the second or third trimester. Therefore, each client's plan of care needs to be adaptive to his or her gestational age on entry of care. During the initial visit, a comprehensive health history is obtained, blood is drawn and urine is collected for baseline prenatal laboratory values to be established, and depending on the time, the physical examination may also be performed. Prescribe a prenatal vitamin if the client is not currently taking them. For women less than 35 years old, prescribe a prenatal vitamin with the recommended 800 to 1,000 mcg daily of folic acid. For women 35 years or older, prescribe a prenatal vitamin and increase their folic acid to 4,000 mcg daily. Many practitioners have the client return in 1 to 2 weeks to perform the physical exam and to review the blood and urine results from the initial visit.

The initial visit is also a time for teaching the pregnant client: literature and brochures on health promotion (i.e., breast self-exam, dietary recommendations, exercise, and smoking cessation) and information regarding the normal changes, discomforts, and concerns during pregnancy should be provided. The after-hours contact information should also be provided, along with contact information for the labor and delivery unit at the hospital or birth center. Reassure the client that as the pregnancy progresses you will answer questions she may have; however, outside resources may also be beneficial for the client and her family. Encourage the client to enroll in childbirth education, sibling classes (if applicable), breastfeeding classes, and any other classes of interest to her and her partner.

Review the client's medical and surgical history (including previous obstetric history), family genetic history, psychiatric disorders, contraception history, medications taken since the last menstrual period, menstrual history, social habits (smoking, substance abuse, alcohol), environmental exposures (job, hobbies, pets in the home, travel history, and so on), exposure to abuse (mental, physical, sexual), and sources of social support and health promotion (immunizations up to date, enrolled in Women, Infants, and Children [WIC], etc.).

Bibliography

American College of Obstetricians and Gynecologists. (2010). ACOG Committee Opinion No. 462: Moderate caffeine consumption during pregnancy (Reaffirmed 2018). *Obstetrics and Gynecology, 116*, 467–468. doi:10.1097/AOG.0b013e3181eeb2a1

American College of Obstetricians and Gynecologists. (2011). ACOG Committee Opinion No. 495: Vitamin D: Screening and supplementation during pregnancy (Reaffirmed 2017). *Obstetrics and Gynecology, 118*, 197–198. doi:10.1097/AOG.0b013e318227f06b

American College of Obstetricians and Gynecologists. (2015). ACOG Committee Opinion, No. 650: Physical activity and exercise during pregnancy and the postpartum period (Reaffirmed 2017). *Obstetrics and Gynecology, 126*, e135–e142. doi:10.1097/AOG.0000000000001214

Cash, J. C. (2014). Assessing childbearing women. In J. Weber & J. Kelley (Eds.), *Health assessment in nursing* (5th ed., pp. 665–692). Philadelphia, PA: Lippincott Williams & Wilkins.

Epocrates. (2018, October 9). *Routine prenatal care*. Retrieved from https://online.epocrates.com/u/2911493/Routine+prenatal+care

Kilpatrick, S. J., Papile, L-A., & Macones, G. A. (Eds.). (2017). *Guidelines for perinatal care* (8th ed.). Elk Grove Village, IL: American Academy of Pediatrics.

Prenatal Care: First Trimester Overview

Jill C. Cash, Susan Drummond, and Christina C. Reed

Physical Examination

A. General assessment:
   1. Vital signs
   2. Weight and height
   3. Fetal heart tones (FHT) (120–160 bpm), usually heard at 13 weeks or higher
   4. Fetal movement, usually first felt between 18 and 22 weeks
B. General appearance
C. Thyroid:
   1. Enlarged/goiter—thyroid-stimulating hormone (TSH) and free T4 and T3 labs, thyroid ultrasound (US) needed
   2. Nodules palpated—TSH and free T4 and T3 labs, thyroid US needed
D. Breasts:
   1. Symmetry
   2. Pain—breast US needed
   3. Masses—breast US needed
   4. Nipple discharge:
      a. Bloody discharge—breast US needed
E. Heart:
   1. Normal auscultatory changes start in the first trimester and end 1 week after delivery:
      a. Higher basal heart rate
      b. Louder heart sounds
      c. Wide splitting of S1
      d. Splitting of S2 in third trimester
      e. Systolic ejection murmur—pulmonary and tricuspid
      f. Third heart sound—most women
      g. Fourth heart sound—rare
      h. Venous hum
      i. Mammary souffle (systolic or continuous) in third trimester and postpartum in breastfeeding women
      j. Diastolic murmurs are not normal in pregnant women—consult cardiology

F. Lungs:
   1. Clients with history of asthma need high-risk consultation.
G. Abdomen:
   1. Measure the fundal height after 12 weeks' gestation.
H. Skin:
   1. Dermatitis is common.
   2. Scarring
I. Extremities
J. External genitalia:
   1. Herpes outbreak present
   2. Bartholin gland enlargement
   3. Condyloma present
K. Adnexa:
   1. Enlarged—transvaginal US needed
   2. Pain—transvaginal US needed
L. Cervix:
   1. Chadwick's sign—the cervix has a bluish hue from 6 to 8 weeks.
M. Vagina:
   1. Increased vaginal discharge—white and clear are normal.
N. Rectum:
   1. Hemorrhoid present

Common Diagnostic Tests
A. Complete blood count (CBC) with platelets
B. Rubella titer
C. HIV fourth generation (with the client's consent)
D. Syphilis with reflex to TP-PA or FTA-ABS or TP-EIA (treponemal test; rapid plasma reagin [RPR] or VDRL—nontreponemal tests)
E. Hepatitis B surface antigen
F. Blood type and Rh factor
G. Antibody screen
H. Urine culture and sensitivity
I. Hemoglobin fractionation
J. Hemoglobin A1c
K. Cystic fibrosis and spinal muscular atrophy genetic carrier screening (with client's consent)
L. Tuberculosis testing, if client has exposure to tuberculosis or is symptomatic
M. Chest x-ray, if the client has a history of tuberculosis and/or positive purified protein derivative (PPD) or QuantiFERON TB Gold blood test
N. Early 1-hour glucose challenge test (GCT), if client has a prior history of gestational diabetes, family history of diabetes, obese (body mass index [BMI] 30 or higher), history of fetal macrosomia, or advanced maternal age (AMA)
O. Thyroid panel, including TSH and free T4, if client has a thyroid disorder or family history of a thyroid disorder
P. Vaginal infection testing, including chlamydia, gonorrhea, trichomonas, bacterial vaginosis, and candida
Q. Pap smears performed on women 21 years and older
   1. Human papillomavirus (HPV) testing on all women 30 years and older
R. Dating US before 14 weeks' gestation

Plan
A. Pharmaceutical therapy:
   1. Prescribe a prenatal vitamin if the client is not currently taking one.
      a. Women less than 35 years old: prescribe a prenatal vitamin with the recommended 800 to 1,000 mcg daily of folic acid.
      b. Women 35 years or older: prescribe a prenatal vitamin and increase their folic acid to 4,000 mcg daily.
   2. Iron supplement:
      a. Prophylaxis: Prenatal vitamins contain the recommended dose of iron.
      b. Anemia: Increase elemental iron by 30 to 120 mg/d and instruct the client to take the iron with orange juice to increase the absorption in the stomach.
B. Client teaching:
   1. Nutrition
   2. Recommended weight gain based on prepregnancy BMI
   3. Prenatal classes
   4. Substance abuse (alcohol, smoking, drugs)
   5. Environmental exposures
   6. Domestic violence (history, type of injuries)
   7. Over-the-counter (OTC) and herbal supplement medication use
   8. Activity (work, exercise)
   9. Travel
   10. Personal hygiene
   11. Sexual activity
   12. Common discomforts/treatments in pregnancy
   13. Symptoms to report immediately

Complications
A. Ectopic pregnancy
B. Spontaneous abortion
C. Missed abortion
D. Blighted ovum
E. Threatened abortion
F. Urinary tract infection (UTI)
G. Pyelonephritis
H. Anemia

Consultations
A. WIC
B. History of asthma—needs high-risk consultation
C. History of cardiac abnormalities—needs high-risk consultation

Emergent Issues/Instructions
A. Nausea and vomiting are normal; however, if client is unable to eat or drink without vomiting she needs to be sent to the ED because of dehydration and abnormal electrolyte levels. Vitamin B6 and Unisom are used as the drugs of choice to prevent nausea and ondansetron is used in more severe cases.
B. Abdominal pain and/or cramping, backache, pelvic pressure, or other pain need to be evaluated and sent to the ED.
C. Vaginal bleeding with or without pain needs to be evaluated and sent to the ED.

Bibliography

American College of Obstetricians and Gynecologists. (2005, September). ACOG Committee Opinion No. 313: The importance of preconception care in the continuum of women's health care (Reaffirmed 2017). *Obstetrics and Gynecology, 106,* 665–666. doi:10.1097/00006250-200509000-00052

American College of Obstetricians and Gynecologists. (2018). ACOG Practice Bulletin No. 189: Nausea and vomiting of pregnancy. *Obstetrics and Gynecology, 131,* e15–e30. doi:10.1097/AOG.0000000000002456

Catalano, P. (2007). Management of obesity in pregnancy. *Obstetrics and Gynecology, 109*(2 Pt 1), 419–433. doi:10.1097/01.AOG.0000253311.44696.85

Centers for Disease Control and Prevention. (2010, November 19). Prevention of perinatal group B streptococcal disease: Revised guidelines from CDC, 2010. *MMWR Recommendations and Reports, 59*(RR-10), 1–36. Retrieved from https://www.cdc.gov/mmwr/pdf/rr/rr5910.pdf

Epocrates. (2018, October 9). *Routine prenatal care.* Retrieved from https://online.epocrates.com/u/2911493/Routine+prenatal+care

Kilpatrick, S. J., Papile, L.- A., & Macones, G. A. (Eds.). (2017). *Guidelines for perinatal care* (8th ed.). Elk Grove Village, IL: American Academy of Pediatrics.

Worcester, S. (2019). 2019 Update: Contraceptives and unintended pregnancy rates. *Ob.Gyn.News.* Parsippany, NJ: Frontline Medical Communications, Inc.

Prenatal Care: Second Trimester Overview

Jill C. Cash, Susan Drummond, and Christina C. Reed

Include components of the first trimester evaluation (see previous text) at the client's initial visit.

Physical Examination

A. General assessment:
  1. Vital signs
  2. Weight
  3. Blood pressure (BP)
  4. FHT (120–160 bpm)
  5. Fetal movement, usually first felt between 18 and 22 weeks
  6. Fundal height
B. Abdomen:
  1. Measure the fundal height
C. Skin:
  1. Striae distensae (stretch marks)
  2. Varicose veins
D. Extremities:
  1. Edema

Common Diagnostic Tests

A. Test of cure for UTIs and STIs previously treated
B. Genetic testing offered to all women: Maternal serum multiple marker screening (quad screen) between 15 weeks, 6 days and 21 weeks, 6 days. Genetic testing offered to women who are of AMA, have history of genetic abnormalities, history of prior fetal abnormalities, and positive quad screen: noninvasive prenatal testing (NIPT). Patient consent is needed:
  1. Amniocentesis/CVS, if applicable
C. Fetal anatomy US at 20 weeks' gestation
D. Gestational diabetes screening with 1-hour GCT between 24 and 28 weeks. If the 1-hour 50-g GCT is above or equal to 135, the client needs to complete the 3-hour 100-g glucose tolerance test (GTT). Gestational diabetes is diagnosed when two or more out of four values from the 3-hour 100-g GTT are equal or higher than the cutoffs.

Plan

A. Pharmaceutical therapy:
  1. Influenza vaccine (seasonal)
  2. Anemia: Increase elemental iron by 30 to 120 mg/d and instruct the client to take the iron with orange juice to increase the absorption in the stomach.
B. Client teaching:
  1. Physiological changes during pregnancy
  2. Fetal development
  3. Father's role during pregnancy
  4. Genetic testing in pregnancy
  5. Review symptoms to report immediately.

Complications

A. UTIs
B. Pyelonephritis
C. Preeclampsia and eclampsia
D. Gestational diabetes
E. Anemia
F. Fetal abnormalities
G. Abnormal genetic screening results
H. STIs

Consultations

A. Genetic consultation is needed with abnormal genetic testing, AMA, and abnormal US findings.
B. High-risk consultation is needed with gestational diabetes, thyroid disorder, asthma exacerbation in pregnancy, severe anemia unresponsive to treatment, HIV positive, acute tuberculosis infection, congenital syphilis, positive antibody, fetal abnormalities, and maternal cardiac complications.

Emergent Issues/Instructions

A. **Abdominal pain, contractions, backache, pelvic pressure, or other pain needs to be evaluated and sent to the ED.**
B. **Vaginal bleeding with or without pain needs to be evaluated and sent to the ED.**
C. **Fever greater than 100.4°F**
D. **Evaluate fetal movement, noting when movement was first felt (quickening). If client reports decreased fetal movement, send to the ED to have biophysical profile (BPP) and nonstress test (NST) to evaluate fetal well-being.**
E. **Headaches with or without blurry vision need to be addressed. BP should be monitored, and if client has elevated BP, with or without headaches and blurry vision, she needs to be sent to the ED.**
F. **Leaking of clear fluid from the vagina needs to be assessed, and if client has unexplained fluid from the vagina she needs to go to the ED.**

Bibliography

Epocrates. (2018, October 9). *Routine prenatal care.* Retrieved from https://online.epocrates.com/u/2911493/Routine+prenatal+care

Kilpatrick, S. J., Papile, L.- A., & Macones, G. A.. (Eds.). (2017). *Guidelines for perinatal care* (8th ed.). Elk Grove Village, IL: American Academy of Pediatrics.

Lockwood, C. J., & Magriples, U. (2018, October 25). Prenatal care: Second and third trimesters. In V. A. Barss (Ed.), *UpToDate*. Retrieved from https://www.uptodate.com/contents/prenatal-care-second-and-third -trimesters

Prenatal Care: Third Trimester Overview

Jill C. Cash, Susan Drummond, and Christina C. Reed

If the client presents for entry for prenatal care in the third trimester, complete all of the first and second trimester evaluations at the initial visit.

Physical Examination

A. General assessment:
1. Vital signs
2. Weight and height
3. BP
4. FHT (120–160 bpm)
5. Fetal movement (fetal kick counts)
6. Fundal height
7. Maternal heart rate
B. Abdomen:
1. Fetal presentation
C. Skin:
1. Striae distensae
2. Varicose veins
D. Extremities:
1. Bishop
E. Cervix-Bishop score:
1. Dilation
2. Effacement
3. Station
4. Position
5. Consistency

Common Diagnostic Tests

A. Vaginal and rectal culture to identify the presence of group B *Streptococcus* (GBS) infection at 35 to 36 weeks; repeat the culture every 5 weeks, if indicated
B. Fetal growth US, if indicated
C. Antenatal testing consisting of BPP and NST, if indicated
D. CBC with platelets
E. HIV
F. RPR with reflex to TP-PA or FTA-ABS or TP-EIA (treponemal test)

Plan

A. Pharmaceutical therapy:
1. Tdap vaccine given to all pregnant women during each pregnancy. Advise all family members who will be in contact with newborn to also have the Tdap vaccine.
2. Anemia: Increase elemental iron by 30 to 120 mg/d and instruct the client to take the iron with orange juice to increase the absorption in the stomach.
3. Rho(D) immune globulin (RhoGAM) is given to pregnant clients who are Rh negative at 28 weeks' gestational age.

B. Client teaching:
1. Fetal kick counts
2. Breastfeeding/bottle-feeding
3. Circumcision
4. Infant–sibling preparation
5. Safety/car seat
6. Birth plan
7. Postpartum birth control options
8. Labor and delivery expectations
9. Choosing a pediatrician
10. Symptoms to report immediately and/or to go to the hospital to labor and delivery

Complications

A. IUGR
B. Preeclampsia and eclampsia
C. Gestational diabetes
D. Fetal demise
E. Oligohydramnios
F. Polyhydramnios
G. Fetal abnormality
H. Pruritic urticarial papules and plaques of pregnancy (PUPPP)
I. Cholestasis
J. PTL
K. Placenta previa
L. Placenta accreta
M. Placenta abruption
N. Anemia
O. GBS

Consultations

A. Genetic consultation is needed with abnormal genetic testing, AMA, and abnormal US findings.
B. High-risk consultation is needed with gestational diabetes, thyroid disorder, asthma exacerbation in pregnancy, severe anemia, HIV positive, acute tuberculosis infection, congenital syphilis, positive antibody, fetal abnormalities, and maternal cardiac complications.
C. Vaginal birth after Cesarean section counseling, if the client wants to attempt a vaginal delivery after having one to two prior Cesarean sections

Emergent Issues/Instructions

A. **Abdominal pain, contractions, backache, pelvic pressure, or other pain needs to be evaluated and sent to the ED if PTL needs to be ruled out.**
B. **Vaginal bleeding with or without pain needs to be evaluated and sent to the ED.**
C. **Fever greater than 100.4°F**
D. **Evaluate fetal movement and daily fetal kick counts. If client reports decreased fetal movement, send to the ED to have BPP and NST to evaluate fetal well-being.**
E. **Headaches with or without blurry vision need to be addressed. BP should be monitored; if client has elevated BP with or without headaches and blurry vision, she needs to be sent to the ED.**

F. Leaking of clear fluid from the vagina needs to be assessed; if client has unexplained fluid from the vagina, she needs to go to ED.

G. Pruritis on hands and feet causing client to wake up at night needs to be evaluated and client sent to the ED.

Bibliography

Epocrates. (2018, October 9). *Routine prenatal care*. Retrieved from https://online.epocrates.com/u/2911493/Routine+prenatal+care

Kilpatrick, S. J., Papile, L.- A., & Macones, G. A. (Eds.). (2017). *Guidelines for perinatal care* (8th ed.). Elk Grove Village, IL: American Academy of Pediatrics.

Lockwood, C. J., & Magriples, U. (2018, October 25). Prenatal care: Second and third trimesters. In V. A. Barss (Ed.), *UpToDate*. Retrieved from https://www.uptodate.com/contents/prenatal-care-second-and-third-trimesters

Postpartum Overview

Jill C. Cash, Susan Drummond, and Christina C. Reed

The ACOG recommendations for postpartum care include developing a postpartum care plan prenatally; scheduling an initial postpartum contact in the first 3 weeks to address acute issues, followed by a comprehensive visit no later than 12 weeks after delivery; and counseling women who had gestational diabetes, pregnancy-related hypertension, or a PTB about their increased risk for cardiovascular disease. ACOG also advises documenting pregnancy complications in the electronic medical record to inform future providers regarding screening for diabetes and risk assessment for cardiovascular disease.

Physical Examination

A. General assessment:
1. Vital signs
2. Weight
B. Breasts:
1. Issues with breastfeeding: Discomfort or pain associated with breastfeeding; adequate breast milk production; comfort and confidence with breastfeeding
2. Engorgement: Breast fullness and firmness, which is accompanied by pain and tenderness. Primary engorgement is caused by interstitial edema and onset of copious milk production. It typically occurs between 24 and 72 hours postpartum, with a normal range of 1 to 7 days; peak symptomatology averages 3 to 5 days postpartum. Secondary engorgement typically occurs later if the mother's milk supply exceeds the amount of milk removed by her infant. Breast engorgement usually resolves spontaneously over a few days, but supportive care (warm compresses or a warm shower before feeding to enhance let-down and facilitate milk removal, cool compresses after or between feedings, mild analgesics such as acetaminophen or ibuprofen) is appropriate. In women who are not breastfeeding, the use of a tight brassiere and avoidance of breast stimulation suppresses lactation in 60% to 70% of clients and is the recommended treatment.
3. Mastitis: Lactation mastitis typically presents as a firm, red, and tender area of one breast with a maternal temperature that exceeds 38.5°C. A tender, fluctuant area is more indicative of an abscess. Systemic complaints may be present and include myalgia, chills, malaise, and flu-like symptoms. Differential diagnosis includes plugged ducts, galactocele, and, in rare cases, inflammatory breast cancer.

C. Heart:
1. Postpartum physiologic changes in the cardiovascular system are particularly important in women with underlying cardiac disease. The cardiac output and stroke volume increase by approximately 50% and 70%, while the heart rate decreases by 15% and BP remains unchanged. The increases in stroke volume and cardiac output most likely result from improved cardiac preload from auto transfusion of uteroplacental blood to the intravascular space. As the uterus decompresses following delivery, a reduction in the mechanical compression of the vena cava allows for further increases in cardiac preload.

D. Abdomen:
1. Uterine involution: The uterus recedes by approximately 1 cm/d to lie midway between the symphysis pubis and umbilicus by the end of the first postpartum week. It is not palpable abdominally by 2 weeks postpartum and attains its normal nonpregnant size by 6 to 8 weeks postpartum.
2. Abdominal wall: The abdominal wall is lax postpartum and will regain its normal muscular tone over several weeks; however, separation (diastasis) of the rectus abdominis muscles may persist.

E. Skin:
1. Linea nigra will fade gradually, but may never completely disappear.
2. Striae fade from red to silvery by 6 to 12 months postpartum, but are permanent.
3. Abdominal skin may remain lax if extensive rupture of elastic fibers occurred during pregnancy.
4. Melasma gravidarum resolves spontaneously over a period of months.

F. Extremities:
1. Edema and varicose veins: Varicose veins may appear during the antepartum or postpartum period. Leg elevation, exercise, and compression therapy improve oxygen transport to the skin and subcutaneous tissues, decrease edema, reduce inflammation, and compress dilated veins.
2. Deep vein thrombosis (DVT) is more common in postpartum women than in antepartum and nonpregnant women. The risk is highest in the first few weeks postpartum and then gradually declines to baseline by 12 weeks postpartum. Risk factors include a previous DVT, thrombophilia, sickle cell disease, obesity, smoking, Cesarean delivery, and postpartum hemorrhage.

G. Vagina:
1. The vagina slowly contracts and decreases in size postpartum, but never completely returns to its nulligravid size.

2. The vaginal walls appear smooth immediately postdelivery; rugae are restored in the third week as edema and vascularity subside.

3. Pelvic floor stretching and trauma during childbirth result in pelvic muscle relaxation, which may not return to the pregravid state.

4. Persistent vaginal bleeding: Vaginal bleeding that persists for more than approximately 8 weeks after delivery is unusual and may be caused by infection, retained products of conception, a bleeding diathesis, or, rarely, choriocarcinoma or a uterine vascular anomaly. A temporary increase in bleeding at this time may represent menses; in such cases, bleeding should stop within a few days.

5. Vaginal dryness: Symptoms of vaginal dryness can be managed by regular use of vaginal moisturizing agents with supplemental use of vaginal lubricants for sexual intercourse.

6. Surgical site infection (episiotomy, laceration, abdominal incision): Perineal infections, and subsequent breakdown of previously repaired lacerations or episiotomies, are usually localized to the skin and subcutaneous tissue. On examination, the area appears swollen and erythematous with a purulent exudate. Treatment consists of opening the wound, drainage, irrigation, and debridement of foreign material and necrotic tissue. Antibiotics are not necessary unless there is accompanying cellulitis. The area will heal by granulation, but large defects may be resutured when the wound surface is free from exudate and covered by pink granulation tissue.

H. Cervix:

1. The cervix remains 2 to 3 cm dilated for the first few postpartum days and is less than 1 cm dilated at 1 week.

2. The external os never resumes its pregravid shape; the small, smooth, regular circular opening of the nulligravida becomes a transverse, stellate slit after childbirth.

3. Histologically, the cervix does not return to baseline for up to 3 to 4 months postpartum.

I. Lochia:

1. Lochia rubra: Normal shedding of blood and decidua is a red/red-brown vaginal discharge that lasts 3 to 5 days following delivery.

2. Lochia serosa: A watery, pinkish brown discharge that lasts for 2 to 3 weeks

3. Lochia alba: In the final stage, the discharge turns yellowish white and may last 4 to 6 weeks.

J. Rectal:

1. Symptomatic hemorrhoids are common postpartum, occurring in approximately one third of women. The treatment approach depends on the specific symptoms—pruritus, bleeding, pain, or prolapse.

2. Postpartum incontinence of urine, flatus, or feces is common in the immediate postpartum period and generally improves over the subsequent weeks but may persist long term. Women should be asked about incontinence as they may not bring the issue up themselves.

Common Diagnostic Tests

A. CBC with platelets

B. 2-hour postload glucose (clients with gestational diabetes mellitus [GDM])

Plan

A. Pharmaceutical therapy:

1. All household members in the newborn's home should have up-to-date immunizations to create a protective "cocoon" around the infant and thus minimize newborn exposure to infection; Tdap and influenza vaccines are particularly important in this respect. Whooping cough immunization is recommended for all family members whose immunization is not up to date.

B. Client teaching:

1. Weight loss:

a. The mean weight loss from delivery of the fetus, placenta, and amniotic fluid is 13 pounds.

b. Contraction of the uterus and loss of fluid (lochia) and excess intra- and extracellular fluid leads to an additional loss of 5 to 15 pounds in the first 6 weeks postdelivery.

c. Approximately one half of gestational weight gain is lost in the first 6 weeks after delivery, with a slower rate of loss through the first 6 months postpartum.

2. Activity:

a. There are no evidence-based data on which to base recommendations regarding postpartum physical activity. In particular, there are no high-quality data on which to base restrictions on lifting, climbing stairs, bathing, swimming, driving, or resuming vaginal intercourse, exercise, or work after delivery.

3. Depression: Screen all women for postpartum depression, as recommended by the ACOG, the American Academy of Pediatrics, and the USPSTF Recommendation Statement. The validated questionnaire most commonly used for screening pregnant and postpartum women is the Edinburgh Postnatal Depression Scale (EPDS), but other validated tools can be used. Screening is important because postpartum depression is common, the combination of screening and adequate support improves clinical outcomes, and treatment (especially with cognitive behavioral therapy) is associated with symptom remission. Depression screening is performed at the routine postpartum visit, but consideration should be given to additional earlier screening and follow-up in clients at high risk for depression.

4. Intimate partner violence: Screen all postpartum women for intimate partner violence. Ideally, screening should be performed at the initial prenatal visit, at least once per trimester, and again during postpartum care. Screening should be routinely performed for women who have not accessed prenatal care or who have concerning signs or symptoms. See Chapter 22, "Psychiatric Guidelines."

5. Screen for tobacco use; counsel regarding relapse risk in the postpartum period.

6. Screen for substance use disorder and refer as indicated.

Complications
A. Postpartum depression

B. Diabetes: Approximately 6 to 8 weeks after delivery, women with GDM should undergo an oral glucose tolerance test (OGTT). They should be counseled about the increased risk of future diabetes, even when the postpartum GTT is normal. These women may benefit from lifestyle changes, such as weight loss if they are obese.

C. Complications that occurred during the pregnancy or postpartum should be reviewed in terms of the cause, risk of recurrence, and prevention.

Consultations
A. Behavioral health counseling for postpartum depression

B. Any underlying medical conditions that were present prior to or during the pregnancy should be addressed at the postpartum visit.

C. Cardiovascular risk: Women with gestational diabetes, pregnancy-related hypertension, or PTB are at increased risk of future cardiovascular disease, even if postpartum BP and glucose tolerance testing are normal.

D. The ACOG recommends that clinicians make women with these complications of pregnancy aware of their increased risk for developing cardiovascular disease. Including this information in their health record can facilitate ongoing monitoring and risk assessment. For women with preeclampsia, this may include yearly assessment of BP, lipids, fasting blood glucose, and BMI. Increased awareness about her cardiovascular risk may increase the woman's motivation to reduce modifiable risk factors, if present, by adopting a healthy lifestyle.

Emergent Issues/Instructions
A. **Severe abdominal pain and/or afebrile with temperature above 100.4°F needs to be evaluated in the ED.**

B. **Excessive vaginal bleeding soaking one pad per hour after the first 3 to 5 days after delivery needs to be evaluated in the clinic. If the client complains of weakness, cold intolerance, dizziness, nausea, and rapid heart rate, she needs to go to the ED.**

C. **Foul-smelling drainage from the vagina and/or incision needs to be evaluated in the clinic.**

D. **Separation of wound or incision needs to be evaluated in the ED.**

E. **Elevated BP with complaints of headaches and/or blurry vision need to be evaluated for preeclampsia in the ED.**

Bibliography
American College of Obstetricians and Gynecologists. (2018). ACOG Practice Bulletin No. 198: Prevention and management of obstetric lacerations at vaginal delivery. *Obstetrics and Gynecology, 132*(3), e87–e102. doi:10.1097/AOG.0000000000002841

Anemia, Iron Deficiency

Jill C. Cash, Susan Drummond, and Christina C. Reed

Definition
A. Anemia in pregnancy results from decreased serum iron. The iron-binding capacity is increased. Red blood cells (RBCs) are microcytic and hypochromic. The Centers for Disease Control and Prevention (CDC) and the ACOG define first- and third-trimester anemia as a hemoglobin (Hgb) of less than 11.0 g/dL and hematocrit (Hct) of less than 33%, and second-trimester anemia as an Hgb of less than 10.5 g/dL and Hct of less than 32%.

Incidence
A. Anemia is a common medical complication of pregnancy. Iron-deficiency anemia constitutes 75% to 95% of pregnancy-related anemias.

Pathogenesis
A. Increased demand for iron during pregnancy occurs because of increased maternal blood volume. Hgb and Hct decrease during the first and second trimesters because of a greater expansion of plasma volume relative to the increase in RBC mass and usually increase during the third trimester when plasma expansion has ceased.

B. During most pregnancies, diet alone does not provide the necessary iron; however, in lactation less elemental iron is needed. In women 19 years and older, 9 mg/d is needed and in adolescents 10 mg/d is recommended.

Predisposing Factors
A. Failure to take oral iron, often because of inability to tolerate oral iron supplements

B. Multiple gestation increases iron requirement and may contribute to increased blood loss at delivery

C. Diet high in phosphorus or food and beverages such as tea, coffee, milk, or soy

D. Low iron and protein diet, eating nonfood items (pica)

E. Not eating foods that help with absorption of iron (orange juice, broccoli, strawberries)

F. History of gastrointestinal surgery causing iron malabsorption (i.e., gastrectomy)

G. Chronic bleeding during pregnancy (i.e., placenta previa, marginal sinus separation of placenta, hemorrhoidal bleeding)

H. Short intervals between pregnancies

I. Race: non-Hispanic Black females

J. Age: teenage girls

Common Complaints
A. Tiredness

B. Inability to take prenatal vitamins because of nausea

C. Bleeding problems (see section "Predisposing Factors")

D. Pica

Other Signs and Symptoms
A. Fatigue

B. Pale mucous membranes and skin

C. Tachycardia

Subjective Data

A. Elicit the onset, duration, and course of presenting symptoms.

B. Elicit information about the client's "typical" dietary intake for meals and snacks and review pica (eating clay, starch, ice, and other nonnutritive substances).

C. Review the client's intake of prenatal vitamins and supplemental iron. How often does she take iron? Elicit the reason for skipping the supplemental iron (nausea, constipation), if applicable.

D. Review the client's history of gastrointestinal surgeries, irritable bowel syndrome (IBS), and Crohn's disease.

E. Review the client's history for any type of anemia and previous treatment, including blood transfusions.

F. Review pregnancy history for closely spaced pregnancies (two in a calendar year) and multiple gestation.

G. Review the client's intake of medications for the use of aspirin and other nonsteroidal anti-inflammatory drugs (NSAIDs).

Physical Examination

A. Check pulse and BP: Note postural hypotension and tachycardia.

B. Inspect:
1. Inspect the skin, mucous membranes, and conjunctivae for pallor.
2. Observe the mouth and tongue: Note atrophy of papillae and smooth, beefy red appearance of tongue with anemia.
3. Note dryness of skin. Inspect texture of nails (brittle, spoon-shaped, concave); inspect the hair for brittleness.

C. Auscultate:
1. Heart for systolic flow murmurs
2. Lungs

D. Palpate:
1. Abdomen for masses; assess fundal height.

Diagnostic Tests

A. Blood work: Hgb and Hct:
1. First trimester: Less than 11 g/dL Hgb or less than 33% Hct
2. Second trimester: Less than 10.5 g/dL Hgb or less than 32% Hct
3. Third trimester: Less than 11 g/dL Hgb or less than 33% Hct

B. Peripheral blood smear: Note microcytic and hypochromic RBCs on peripheral smear.

C. Sickle cell screen, if applicable

D. Serum iron: Low with anemia

E. Iron-binding capacity: High iron-binding capacity with anemia

F. Transferrin: Saturation less than 15%

G. Stool for occult blood, if applicable

H. Emesis for presence of blood, if applicable

Differential Diagnoses

A. Iron-deficiency anemia

B. Normal physiologic anemia of pregnancy: During normal pregnancy, concentrations of erythrocytes and Hgb usually fall because of the greater increase in plasma volume (increased by 45%) relative to the increase in erythrocyte volume (increased by 25%).

C. Megaloblastic anemia: Commonly associated with iron-deficiency anemia and is rarely seen alone

D. Hemolytic anemia: Sickle cell anemia, thalassemia, hereditary spherocytosis, and erythrocyte enzyme deficiency

E. Aplastic anemia: Bone marrow failure

F. Hematologic malignancies: Leukemia and lymphoma

G. Clotting factor or other hemostatic deficiencies: Von Willebrand's disease, idiopathic thrombocytopenia (ITP), and disseminated intravascular coagulation (DIC)

Plan

A. General interventions:
1. Perform initial evaluation of Hgb and Hct at first prenatal visit; repeat at 24- to 28-week blood draw with diabetes testing.
2. Diet counseling and nutrition consultation
3. The client may be eligible for the WIC program that provides supplemental foods for pregnant women and young children. Ask your local health department for information available in your community.
   a. Advise the client to take supplemental iron in addition to prenatal vitamins. If she is unable to tolerate prenatal vitamins, suggest a children's chewable vitamin, two tablets daily.
   b. Encourage the client to continue iron supplementation through the first month postpartum and throughout breastfeeding

B. Client teaching: *See Section III: Client Teaching Guide "Anemia, Iron Deficiency."* ◄

C. Pharmaceutical therapy:
1. Prophylaxis: Increase daily elemental oral iron supplements from 15 to 30 mg/d in pregnancy to prevent iron-deficiency anemia.
2. Most prenatal vitamin formulations contain 30 mg of elemental iron per day; however, if the woman has iron-deficiency anemia she needs to increase her elemental iron by 30 to 120 mg/d. Nausea and vomiting occur in 20% to 25% of clients. These side effects are dose-related. Have the client alter times of administration of the iron supplement to determine when the iron is best tolerated.
3. Treatment: With iron-deficiency anemia, three times the prophylactic dose of iron should be given. Instruct the client to take the iron concurrently with orange juice as vitamin C increases the absorption of iron.
4. Intramuscular (IM) or intravenous (IV) iron may be ordered for the small proportion of clients who do not tolerate oral iron because of gastrointestinal complaints, malabsorption syndrome, or noncompliance with the oral iron regimen.
5. Blood transfusion may be needed per institute guidelines.

Follow-Up

A. Carry out routine prenatal and postpartum follow-up care. When the client begins taking the recommended

dose of supplemental iron, the RBC response can be measured in 2 weeks by an elevation in her reticulocyte count.
B. Repeat Hct after 4 to 6 weeks of therapy.
C. If no improvement is seen in reticulocyte count or Hct after 4 weeks of therapy and the client has been compliant, another cause of anemia should be investigated.

Consultation/Referral
A. Consider consult with a physician if Hgb is less than 9 g/dL or Hct is less than or equal to 27% and does not improve with the previously noted treatments.

Bibliography
American College of Obstetricians and Gynecologists. (2008). ACOG Practice Bulletin, No. 95: Anemia in pregnancy (Reaffirmed 2017). *Obstetrics and Gynecology*, *112*, 201–207. doi:10.1097/AOG.0b013e3181809c0d

American College of Obstetricians and Gynecologists. (2018). ACOG Committee Opinion No. 743: Low-dose aspirin use during pregnancy. *Obstetrics and Gynecology*, *132*(1), e44–e52. doi:10.1097/AOG.0000000000002708

Auerbach, M., & Landy, H. (2018, October 23). Anemia in pregnancy. In Tirnauer J. S. & V. A. Barss (Eds.), *UpToDate*. Retrieved from https://www.uptodate.com/contents/maternal-adaptations-to-pregnancy-hematologic-changes

Bauer, K. (2018, July 23). Maternal adaptations to pregnancy: Hematologic changes. In K. Eckler & J. S. Tirnauer (Eds.), *UpToDate*. Retrieved from https://www.uptodate.com/contents/maternal-adaptations-to-pregnancy-hematologic-changes

Gestational Diabetes Mellitus

Jill C. Cash, Susan Drummond, and Christina C. Reed

Definition
A. Gestational diabetes mellitus (GDM) is a carbohydrate intolerance with onset or recognition during pregnancy.

Incidence
A. It is estimated that up to 6% to 7% of pregnancies are complicated by diabetes mellitus (DM) and approximately 90% of these cases represent women with GDM. It usually resolves after pregnancy.

Pathogenesis
A. Insulin antagonism caused by the placental hormones leads to gestational diabetes. As greater amounts of these hormones are produced with advancing gestation, the diabetogenic effect of pregnancy becomes more pronounced, reaching significant levels in the second trimester. Women with GDM are at risk for later development of type 1 and type 2 diabetes, metabolic syndrome, and cardiovascular disease. GDM may actually be the expression of pregnancy-induced stresses on carbohydrate metabolism in the genetically predisposed client. It is estimated that 50% to 70% of women with GDM will develop DM within approximately 15 to 25 years of the pregnancy. Some women have undiagnosed type 1 or type 2 diabetes prior to pregnancy.

Predisposing Factors
A. Members of any of the following ethnic groups:
1. Hispanic American
2. African American
3. Native American
4. South or East Asian
5. Pacific Islander
B. Maternal age older than 25 years
C. Obesity (BMI > 30)
D. Family history of diabetes, first-degree relatives
E. Previous birth of a macrosomic, malformed, or stillborn baby
F. Comorbidity: Metabolic syndrome, hypertension, polycystic ovarian syndrome, use of glucocorticoids
G. Glycosuria at prenatal visit
H. Gestational diabetes in a previous pregnancy
I. Multiple gestation

Common Complaints
A. Common complaints of hyperglycemia include polydipsia, polyuria, nocturia, fatigue, and blurred vision. However, gestational diabetes is often asymptomatic.

Other Signs and Symptoms
A. Glycosuria
B. Fundal height measurement greater than gestational age in weeks
C. Frequent candidal infections
D. Rapid weight gain

Potential Complications
A. Ketoacidosis:
1. May develop in GDM
2. More common in insulin-dependent diabetes
3. May develop with glucose levels as low as 200 mg/dL
4. May be present in an undiagnosed diabetic woman receiving beta-mimetic agents (such as terbutaline) for tocolysis or steroids to enhance fetal lung maturity. **Fetal mortality rate is 10% in women who come to the hospital in diabetic ketoacidosis (DKA): glucose and ketones cross the placenta.**
5. Therapy hinges on timely, aggressive volume resuscitation, insulin administration, and correction of maternal electrolyte imbalance.
B. Polyhydramnios
C. Increased risk for neonatal morbidity such as hypoglycemia, hyperbilirubinemia, polycythemia, respiratory distress caused by delayed lung maturity, and/or traumatic birth injury related to shoulder dystocia, which is associated with macrosomia
D. Increased risk for stillbirth—risk is related primarily to poor glycemic control.
E. Preeclampsia
F. Operative delivery
G. Fetal organomegaly
H. Long-term sequelae for the offspring: Abnormal glucose tolerance, metabolic syndrome, and obesity

Subjective Data
A. Review previous pregnancy history for two or more spontaneous abortions, previous stillbirths, or unexplained neonatal deaths.

B. Review birth weight (macrosomia) and gestational age of previous children.

C. Review previous pregnancy history for polyhydramnios and/or congenital anomalies.

D. Review the client's history for a predisposition to infections, especially UTIs and candidal vaginitis, and for family history of diabetes.

E. Review previous pregnancy history for gestational diabetes, diet restrictions, and need for insulin therapy.

Physical Examination

A. Check BP, pulse, and weight.

B. Inspect:
1. Perform speculum exam to rule out STIs, bacterial vaginosis, and candidal vaginitis, if indicated.

C. Auscultate:
1. FHT after 10 to 12 weeks' gestation

D. Palpate:
1. Check the client's fundal height each visit after 20 weeks.

Screening/Diagnostic Tests

Women who have risk factors for type 2 diabetes should be screened at the initial prenatal visit.

A. Perform "one-step" 2-hour 75-g (fasting) OGTT or "two-step" 1-hour 50-g (nonfasting) followed by a 3-hour 100-g (fasting) OGTT for positive results.

B. Blood glucose measurements (fasting blood sugar [FBS] and 2-hour postprandial blood glucose values)

C. HgbA1c

D. Urine dipstick for glucose: Early glycosuria needs further evaluation (i.e., HgbA1c, urine culture, random glucose "finger stick")

E. Ultrasonography, if fetal size is greater than average for gestational date to rule out twins, congenital anomaly such as atresia, and polyhydramnios

Differential Diagnoses

A. Gestational diabetes:
1. A1: diet-controlled gestational diabetes (A1 GDM)
2. A2: insulin-treated gestational diabetes (A2 GDM)

Plan

A. General interventions:
1. American Diabetes Association (ADA) recommended screening for all pregnant women:
   a. Diabetes mellitus screen (DMS): "two-step" 1-hour 50-g (nonfasting) OGCT followed by a 3-hour 100-g OGTT for positive results:
      i. Administer 50 g oral glucose load (fasting not required; however, no food/nonwater beverages for 2 hours prior to the test).
      ii. Draw blood for glucose assessment 1 hour after glucose load is given.
      iii. Typically performed between 24 and 28 weeks' gestation; performed earlier if the client has glycosuria, predisposing risk factors, or AMA, or if fetal size is greater than

average for gestational date by fundal height measurement.
      iv. Abnormal result of the 1-hour 50-g OGCT is a glucose level of 130 to 140 mg/dL (use your institutional limits).
      v. If the result of the 1-hour 50-g OGCT is greater than or equal to 200 mg/dL, the client skips the 3-hour 100-g OGTT and begins dietary modifications and glucose evaluation for insulin needs.
      vi. Follow up all abnormal 1-hour OGCT with a 3-hour OGTT.
   b. 3-hour OGTT:
      i. Draw fasting blood glucose first.
      ii. Administer 100 g glucose load.
      iii. Draw blood for glucose assessment after 1 hour, 2 hours, and 3 hours from the time the glucose load is given.
      iv. Plasma or serum glucose results (Carpenter-Coustan criteria or use institutional limits):
         - Fasting = 95 mg/dL
         - 1 hour = 180 mg/dL
         - 2 hours = 155 mg/dL
         - 3 hours = 140 mg/dL
      v. If two or more values of 3-hour GTT are elevated:
         - Refer the client for nutritional counseling for dietary modifications.
         - Educate client on glucose evaluation for insulin needs: daily blood sugar log to record fasting and 2-hour postprandial blood glucose measurements.
   c. "One-step" 2-hour 75 mg (fasting) OGTT may be performed instead of the "two-step" approach.

2. Antepartum testing:
   a. For women with well-controlled A1 GDM on nutritional therapy and no other pregnancy complication, there is no national consensus with respect to criteria for initiation and timing of testing. Options include weekly or twice weekly NSTs and BPPs beginning at 32 weeks. Use institutional guidelines.
   b. Women with insulin-dependent diabetes or using oral hyperglycemic agents, or with poorly controlled A2 GDM, need twice weekly NSTs and BPPs beginning at 32 weeks or sooner depending on if other pregnancy complications exist. If a client's diabetes is poorly controlled, consider fetal assessment earlier and more frequently.

3. Serial ultrasonography:
   a. Evaluate fetal growth, estimate fetal weight, and detect polyhydramnios and malformations.
   b. There is no national consensus with respect to criteria for initiation and timing to assess growth; however, practice agrees on one single US at 36 weeks or starting USs at 28 weeks and repeating them thereafter, every 4 weeks (28, 32, 36 weeks).

c. Macrosomia is a leading risk factor for shoulder dystocia at vaginal delivery and cephalopelvic disproportion. Women with GDM should be counseled regarding the option of a scheduled Cesarean delivery when the fetus is more than or equal to 4,500 g.

4. Neonate evaluation:

1. Monitor neonate carefully for hypoglycemia, especially if the client has a history of insulin-dependent diabetes.

5. Postpartum:

a. Testing:

i. Two-hour GTT between 6 and 12 weeks postpartum (fasting):
■ Administer 75 g glucose load.
■ Draw blood for glucose assessment at 2 hours after the glucose load is given.
■ Results less than or equal to 200: diabetes management is needed.

ii. Consider serial measurement of total cholesterol, low-density lipoprotein, high-density lipoprotein, and triglycerides.

b. Contraception:

i. Low-dose oral contraceptives (OCs) may be used in women with GDM who do not have other risk factors.

ii. Rate of subsequent diabetes in OC users is not significantly different from those who do not use OCs.

B. Client teaching:

1. *See Section III: Client Teaching Guide "Gestational Diabetes Mellitus."*

2. GDM requires intensive client and family education to maintain glucose targets to help reduce perinatal complications.

a. Exercise:

i. If the client had an active lifestyle prior to pregnancy, encourage her to continue a program of exercise approved for pregnancy, such as walking or swimming for 20 minutes per day.

ii. Upper extremity exercise and walking in previously sedentary women with GDM may improve glycemic control.

b. Instruct the client in self-monitoring blood glucose and encourage her to record each blood glucose measurement.

i. Have her take measurements, fasting and 2 hours postprandially, every day and record the measurements. Postprandial blood sugar values are recommended over preprandial values because of better glycemic control and better maternal/fetal outcomes. FBS should be less than 95 mg/dL. The 1-hour postprandial values should be less than 140 mg/L and the 2-hour postprandial values should be less than 120 mg/L. The HgbA1c goal is less than 6%. Nighttime levels should not decrease lower than 60 mg/dL.

ii. If the client is taking multiple doses of insulin, she may need to take measurements more frequently.

C. Pharmaceutical therapy:

1. Insulin therapy is the drug of choice if medical nutritional therapy does not consistently maintain fasting glucose levels of less than 95 mg/dL. One-hour postprandial values should be less than 140 mg/dL. Two-hour postprandial values should be less than 120 mg/dL (see Figure 13.1).

2. Oral antihyperglycemic medications (glyburide and metformin) are being increasingly used in women with GDM, although they are not yet approved by the U.S. FDA for this indication. Glyburide results in increased insulin secretion and insulin sensitivity at the tissue level. Metformin inhibits hepatic gluconeogenesis and glucose absorption and stimulates glucose uptake in peripheral tissues.

3. In general, insulin therapy in pregnancy is no different than from vigorous management of diabetes with insulin in nonpregnant women. Insulin does not cross the placenta.

4. Therapy must respond to the changing insulin requirements during pregnancy; typical starting dosage is 0.7 to 2.0 units/kg/d in divided doses based on current pregnancy weight.

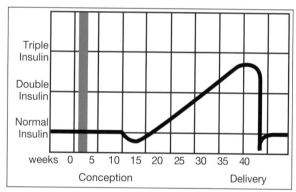

FIGURE 13.1 Insulin requirements during pregnancy.

a. Women with relatively simple insulin programs may require more complex regimens as the pregnancy progresses.

5. Intensive insulin therapy (as opposed to conventional therapy) is often required in pregnancy.

6. Human insulin (Humulin) is preferred to animal or synthetic insulin.

7. Instruct clients to report glucose values on at least a weekly basis. Secure client portals can be used to upload values, which will be sent to their provider. Alternatively, clients may opt to fax or telephone in their values.

8. The blood glucose values should be evaluated at least weekly to adjust to the client's changing needs.

D. Dietary management: place the client on a diet that is prescribed for preexisting diabetes in pregnancy, such as the ADA diet, in the following amounts:

1. Current weight less than 80% ideal body weight (IBW): 35 to 40 kcal/kg/d

2. Current weight 80% to 120% IBW: 30 kcal/kg/d

3. Current weight 120% to 150% IBW: 22 to 25 kcal/kg/d

4. Current weight more than 150% IBW: 12 to 14 kcal/kg/d (minimum of 1,800 cal/d to prevent ketosis)

5. Dietary consumption:

   a. Total calories: 1,800 to 2,500 kcal/d based on IBW

   b. Trimester specific recommendations:

      i. First trimester: no increase in calories

      ii. Second trimester: 340 kcal/d increase above prepregnancy levels

      iii. Third trimester: 452 kcal/d increase above prepregnancy levels

   c. Nutrition distribution:

      i. Carbohydrate 40% to 50% (minimum 175 g/d)

      ii. Protein 20% (71 g/d)

      iii. Fat 30% to 40%

      iv. Fiber 28 g/d

Follow-Up

A. Weekly evaluation of blood glucose values

B. Antepartum testing consisting of NSTs and BPPs

C. Fetal growth USs

D. For women who develop diabetes during pregnancy, give the client 75 g glucose load to evaluate for the development of type 2 diabetes at the return postpartum visit at 6 weeks after delivery. These women should be screened at least every 3 years from then on. Encourage lifestyle changes to prevent the development of diabetes.

E. Contraception

Consultation/Referral

A. Consult or comanage the client with a maternal fetal medicine physician as indicated and if GDM is not controlled by diet and exercise.

B. Refer to a dietician for nutritional consult for carbohydrate counting and teaching the client dietary and lifestyle changes needed for tight glucose control.

Bibliography

American College of Obstetricians and Gynecologists. (2018a). ACOG Practice Bulletin No 190: Gestational diabetes mellitus. *Obstetrics and Gynecology, 131*(2), e49–e64. doi:10.1097/AOG.0000000000002501

American College of Obstetricians and Gynecologists. (2018b, February). ACOG Practice Bulletin No. 190 summary: Gestational diabetes mellitus. *Obstetrics and Gynecology, 131*(2), 406–408. doi:10.1097/AOG.0000000000002498

American Diabetes Association. (2014a). Correction to American Diabetes Association (2014). *Diabetes Care, 37*(3), 887. doi:10.2337/dc14-er03

American Diabetes Association. (2014b). Standards of medical care in diabetes—2014. *Diabetes Care, 37*(Suppl. 1), s18–s20. doi:10.2337/dc14-S014

Bell, R., Glinianaia, S. V., Tennant, P. W., Rankin, J., & Bilous, R. W. (2012). Peri-conception hyperglycaemia and nephropathy are associated with risk of congenital anomaly in women with pre-existing diabetes: A population-based cohort study. *Diabetologia, 55,* 936–947. doi:10.1007/s00125-012-2455-y

Catalano, P. (2007). Management of obesity in pregnancy. *Obstetrics and Gynecology, 109*(2 Pt 1), 419–433. doi:10.1097/01.AOG.0000253311.44696.85

Caughey, A. (2018, October 31). Gestational diabetes mellitus: Obstetrical issues and management. In Barss V. A. (Ed.), *UpToDate*. Retrieved from https://www.uptodate.com/contents/gestational-diabetes-mellitus-obstetrical-issues-and-management

Centers for Disease Control and Prevention. (2015). Gestational diabetes and pregnancy. Retrieved from https://www.cdc.gov/pregnancy/diabetes-gestational.html

Durnwald, C. (2018a, October 31). Gestational diabetes mellitus: Glycemic control and maternal prognosis. In Barss V. A. (Ed.), *UpToDate*. Retrieved from http://uptodate.com/home/index.html

Durnwald, C. (2018b, November 1). Diabetes mellitus in pregnancy: Screening and diagnosis. In Barss V. A. (Ed.), *UpToDate*. Retrieved from https://www.uptodate.com/contents/diabetes-mellitus-in-pregnancy-screening-and-diagnosis

Mathiesen, E. R., Ringholm, L., & Damm, P. (2011). Pregnancy management of women with pregestational diabetes. *Endocrinology and Metabolism Clinics of North America, 40,* 727–738. doi:10.1016/j.ecl.2011.08.005

McCance, D. R.. (2011a). Diabetes management in pregnancy. In J. A. H. Wass, P. M. Stewart, S. A. Amiel, & M. J. Davies (Eds.), *Oxford textbook of endocrinology and diabetes* (2nd ed.). doi:10.1093/med/9780199235292.003.1499

McCance, D. R.. (2011b). Pregnancy and diabetes. *Best Practice & Research: Clinical Endocrinology & Metabolism, 25,* 945–958. doi:10.1016/j.beem.2011.07.009

Roman, M. (2011). Preconception care for women with preexisting type 2 diabetes. *Clinical Diabetes, 29*(1), 10–16. doi:10.2337/diaclin.29.1.10

Uma, R., Bhavadharini, B., Ranjani, H., Mahalakshmi, M. M., Anjana, R. M., Unnikrishnan, R., . . . Mohan, V. (2017). Pregnancy outcome of gestational diabetes mellitus using a structured model of care: WINGS project (WINGS-10). *Journal of Obstetrics & Gynaecology Research, 43*(3), 468–475.

Preeclampsia

Jill C. Cash, Susan Drummond, and Merita O'Sullivan

Definition

A. Preeclampsia, also called PIH (antiquated term *toxemia*), is the new onset of hypertension with proteinuria that develops after 20 weeks' gestation in pregnancy or develops up to 6 weeks postpartum in a previously normotensive woman. In the absence of proteinuria, any of the following can establish the diagnosis: new-onset thrombocytopenia, impaired liver function, renal insufficiency, pulmonary edema, or visual or cerebral disturbances.

B. Preeclampsia with severe features. In 2013, the ACOG replaced the term "severe preeclampsia" with the term "preeclampsia with severe features." In a client with preeclampsia, the presence of one or more of the following indicates a diagnosis of "preeclampsia with severe features":

1. Symptoms of central nervous system (CNS) dysfunction:

   a. New-onset cerebral or visual disturbances, such as:

      i. Photopsia, scotomata, cortical blindness, retinal vasospasm

      ii. Severe incapacitating headache ("the worst headache in my life") or a headache that persists and progresses despite analgesic therapy

      iii. Altered mental status

2. Hepatic abnormality:

a. Severe persistent right upper quadrant (RUQ) or epigastric pain unresponsive to medication and not accounted for by an alternative diagnosis or a serum transaminase concentration greater than two times the upper limit of the upper range, or both.

3. Severe BP elevation:

a. Systolic BP greater than 160 mmHg or diastolic BP greater than 110 mmHg on two or more occasions at least 4 hours apart. Antihypertensive therapy may be initiated upon confirmation of severe hypertension in which case criteria for severe BP elevation can be satisfied without waiting until 4 hours have elapsed.

4. Thrombocytopenia:

a. Platelets less than 100,000 per microliter

5. Renal abnormality:

a. Progressive renal insufficiency (serum creatinine > 1.1 mg/dL [97.2 micromol/L] or a doubling of the serum creatinine concentration in the absence of other renal disease)

6. Pulmonary edema

C. Hypertension. The 2017 changes in the definition for elevated BP and hypertension in nonpregnant adults do not affect diagnostic criteria for pregnancy-related hypertensive disorders:

1. Either a systolic BP more than 140 mmHg or a diastolic BP more than 90 mmHg, or both. The values must be elevated on at least two separate occasions at least 4 hours apart. **Severity of hypertension is not necessarily associated with the severity of preeclampsia.**

2. Eclampsia is the development of grand mal seizures in a client with preeclampsia in the absence of other neurologic conditions that could account for the seizures.

3. HELLP (hemolysis, elevated liver enzymes, and low platelets) syndrome: It probably represents a severe form of preeclampsia, but this relationship is controversial; HELLP may be an independent disorder.

4. Chronic hypertension in pregnancy is often complicated by superimposed preeclampsia.

5. Gestational hypertension (GHTN) is hypertension without proteinuria or other signs and symptoms of preeclampsia or related end-organ dysfunction that develops after 20 weeks' gestation and resolves by 12 weeks postpartum. Between 10% and 25% of women with GHTN may develop signs and symptoms of preeclampsia.

Incidence

A. Hypertensive disorders are the most common medical complication of pregnancy, with a reported incidence of up to 10% worldwide. Incidence varies among different regions and countries. The incidence of preeclampsia has increased by 25% in the United States during the past two decades, and 4.6% of all pregnancies worldwide are complicated by preeclampsia. The risk of recurrent preeclampsia is between 5% and 70%. Women who develop severe features of preeclampsia prior to 30 weeks' gestation have the highest risk of preeclampsia in future pregnancies.

B. Prognosis:

1. Women with preeclampsia are at an increased risk for life-threatening obstetric or medical complications. Worldwide, 10% to 15% of direct maternal deaths (resulting from obstetric complications of pregnancy) are associated with preeclampsia/eclampsia. In the United States, preeclampsia/eclampsia is one of the four leading causes of maternal death, along with hemorrhage, cardiovascular conditions, and thromboembolism. There is approximately one maternal death caused by preeclampsia/eclampsia per 100,000 live births, with a case-fatality rate of 6.4 deaths per 10,000 cases.

2. Fetal implications: Preeclampsia can lead to IUGR and oligohydramnios, as well as medically or obstetrically indicated PTB. As a result, perinatal morbidity and mortality are increased.

C. Prevention

1. Low-dose aspirin: This drug reduces the frequency of preeclampsia, as well as related adverse pregnancy outcomes (PTB, growth restriction), by about 10% to 20% when given to women at moderate to high risk of the disease; it has an excellent maternal/fetal safety profile in pregnancy.

2. Candidates: There is no consensus on the criteria that confer high risk for developing preeclampsia.

3. USPSTF criteria for high risk include one or more of the following (the incidence of preeclampsia is estimated to be at least 8% in a pregnant woman with one of these risk factors):

a. Previous pregnancy with preeclampsia, especially early onset and with an adverse outcome

b. Multifetal gestation

c. Chronic hypertension

d. Type 1 or type 2 DM

e. Chronic kidney disease

f. Autoimmune disease (antiphospholipid syndrome, systemic lupus erythematosus)

4. USPSTF criteria for moderate risk include the following (the incidence of preeclampsia is estimated to be less than 8% in a pregnant woman with only one of these risk factors):

a. Nulliparity

b. Obesity (BMI > 30)

c. Family history of preeclampsia in mother or sister

d. Age ≥ 35 years

e. Sociodemographic characteristics (African American race, low socioeconomic level)

f. Personal risk factors (previous pregnancy with low birth weight or small-for-gestational-age infant, previous adverse pregnancy outcome [fetal demise], interval > 10 years between pregnancies)

D. The following summaries represent the recommendations of some national organizations:

1. The American Heart Association and American Stroke Association recommend low-dose aspirin for women with chronic primary or secondary hypertension or previous pregnancy-related hypertension for prevention of preeclampsia-related stroke.

2. The USPSTF recommends the use of low-dose aspirin (81 mg/d) in women at high risk of developing preeclampsia to reduce the risk for preeclampsia, PTB, and fetal growth restriction. Women with ≥1 high-risk factor should receive low-dose aspirin. For women with multiple moderate risk factors, the benefit of aspirin therapy is less clear, so clinicians should use clinical judgment and talk with their clients about the benefits and harms of low-dose aspirin use. Aspirin should be initiated between 12 and 28 weeks of gestation.

3. In July 2016, the ACOG endorsed the USPSTF recommendation for use of low-dose aspirin (81 mg/d) in women at high risk of developing preeclampsia based on the same high-risk factors designated by the USPSTF. Prior to July 2016, the ACOG defined high risk more narrowly: history of early-onset preeclampsia and preterm delivery less than 34 0/7 weeks of gestation or more than one prior pregnancy complicated by preeclampsia.

4. The World Health Organization recommends the use of low-dose aspirin (75 mg/d) for high-risk women (history of preeclampsia, diabetes, chronic hypertension, renal or autoimmune disease, or multifetal pregnancies).

Pathogenesis

A. The etiology of preeclampsia is unknown, although several theories exist. Generalized vascular endothelial damage is a hallmark of the pathophysiologic responses.

Predisposing Factors

A. Nulliparity
B. Chronic hypertension
C. Age extreme (< 18 years and > 35 years old)
D. Race (African American women are at higher risk)
E. Pregestational and gestational diabetes
F. Renal disease
G. Family history of preeclampsia in a sister or mother
H. Previous pregnancy with PIH
I. Multiple gestation
J. Hydatidiform mole
K. Obesity (BMI > 30)
L. Autoimmune disease (systemic lupus erythematosus or antiphospholipid syndrome)
M. Hydrops fetalis
N. Vascular disease
O. IUGR, abruptio placenta, or fetal demise in a previous pregnancy
P. Prolonged interpregnancy interval if previous pregnancy was normotensive
Q. Short interpregnancy interval if previous pregnancy was preeclamptic

Common Complaints

A. Persistent and/or severe headache unrelieved by analgesics
B. RUQ epigastric pain
C. Severe heartburn unrelieved by antacids
D. Nausea and vomiting
E. Edema: peripheral and/or facial
F. Visual disturbances (photophobia, scotomata, ametropia)

Other Signs and Symptoms

A. Hypertension (BP of 140 mmHg systolic or greater, or 90 mmHg diastolic or greater that occurs after 20 weeks' gestation in a woman without a previous history of hypertension)
B. First-trimester signs of PIH need ultrasonographic evaluation for the presence of a gestational trophoblastic disease (molar pregnancy) as well as the other differential diagnoses.
C. Proteinuria:
   1. Random urine protein: creatinine ratio of greater than 0.3 mg protein/mg creatinine
   2. Timed excretion of greater than 0.3 g protein in a 24-hour urine collection specimen. The completeness of the 24-hour collection can be estimated from the creatinine excretion, which should be 15 to 20 mg/kg of lean body weight in women
D. Brisk deep tendon reflexes (DTRs; hyperreflexia) or ankle clonus

Potential Complications

A. Multiple organ involvement
B. HELLP syndrome
C. Eclampsia, which may lead to maternal demise
D. Fetal complications: IUGR, oligohydramnios, abruptio placenta

Subjective Data

A. Elicit information about headaches, their onset and duration, the progression of headache, and/or other symptoms.
B. What part of the head hurts? Differentiate headache from sinus headache. Note severity and any relief measure tried (acetaminophen, massage, sleep).
C. Is the headache "new"? Does the client have a previous history of migraines? Is this like a previous migraine?
D. What are other concurrent symptoms? Nausea, vomiting, RUQ pain, and visual changes?
E. Question the client about edema. If edema is present, has it significantly worsened over the past few days? Has she been able to wear rings up to this point? Has she had to wear different shoes because of pedal edema?
F. What are her usual weight and today's weight (on the same scales)? Has she gained more than 2 pounds in 1 week?
G. Ask specifics about RUQ pain, sometimes identified as "severe heartburn." Note the duration, severity, and relief measures tried. Have the client point to the area of discomfort (midsternum or under right breast).
H. Are there any visual disturbances, such as black dots she can't see through?

I. Review other gastrointestinal symptoms such as diarrhea, abdominal pain, and gallbladder attack.

J. Review for signs of fever and thyroid storm.

K. Review the client's history for seizures.

L. Review for signs of pulmonary edema: dyspnea, chest pain, and/or decreased (≤93%) oxygen saturation by pulse oximetry.

Physical Examination

A. Check BP, pulse, respirations, oxygen saturation via pulse oximetry, weight, and FHT.

B. Inspect:
1. Check pedal, hand, and facial edema.
2. Check fundal height.

C. Auscultate:
1. Heart and lungs
2. FHT

D. Percuss:
1. Gently check for liver enlargement or pain. Hepatic tenderness is caused by stretching of Glisson capsule from hepatic swelling or bleeding.
2. Perform neurologic exam for hyperreflexia: check lower extremities for DTR and ankle clonus.

E. Palpate:
1. Palpate the abdomen, noting any hepatosplenomegaly and RUQ tenderness to the palpation.
2. Palpate the lower extremities for pitting edema. Peripheral edema may be related to capillary leaking or "overfill" edema.

Diagnostic Tests

A. CBC and platelets

B. Liver profile (alanine aminotransferase [ALT] and aspartate aminotransferase [AST])

C. Renal workup:
1. Uric acid and serum creatinine
2. Urine protein:
   a. ≥ 0.3 g protein in a 24-hour urine specimen
   b. Random urine protein: creatinine ratio ≥ 0.3 mg protein/mg creatinine
   c. Protein ≥ 1 + (30 mg/dL) on a paper test strip dipped into a fresh, clean voided midstream urine specimen (only if one of the previous quantitative methods is not available)
3. Urine culture if proteinuria is present to rule out UTI

D. Coagulation studies: Prothrombin time (PT), partial thromboplastin time (PTT), and fibrinogen are indicated in clients with additional complications such as abruptio placenta, severe bleeding, severe liver dysfunction, or severe thrombocytopenia.

E. Ultrasonography to evaluate the amniotic fluid index and the estimated fetal weight, because of the increased risk for oligohydramnios and IUGR with preeclampsia

Differential Diagnoses

A. Hyperemesis gravidarum

B. Infection: appendicitis, gastroenteritis, pyelonephritis, glomerulonephritis, hepatitis, and pancreatitis

C. Acute fatty liver of pregnancy

D. Exacerbation of systemic lupus erythematosus

E. Hemolytic uremic syndrome

F. Hepatic encephalopathy

G. Gastrointestinal disorder: peptic ulcer and heartburn

H. Thrombotic or idiopathic thrombocytopenia (ITP) purpura

I. Gallbladder disease

J. Chronic hypertension

K. Thyroid storm

L. GHTN

M. Migraine headache

N. Antiphospholipid syndrome

O. Superimposed preeclampsia

P. Pheochromocytoma

Q. Mirror syndrome (also called Ballantyne syndrome)

Plan

A. General interventions:

1. Any client with an elevated BP should be reassessed, using proper cuff size, after the client is allowed to relax for several minutes prior to repeat BP measurement

2. BP is repeated after 5 minutes of rest, with the client sitting with feet on the ground and legs uncrossed or in a semi-reclining position with her back supported. Whether sitting or in semi-Fowler, the arm should be supported and at heart level. Measurement of BP in left lateral recumbency, on the left arm, does not differ substantially from BP that is recorded in the sitting position, and may be used if a seated BP is not feasible.

3. If client's BP begins to rise above baseline values:
   a. Advise the client to maintain a modified bed rest schedule (stop working).
   b. Recommend frequent BP evaluation at home with documentation in a BP log.
   c. See the client weekly to review her home BP log and further maternal and neonatal assessment; administer NST and take BPP, if appropriate.

4. If hypertension and proteinuria are present, refer the client to an obstetrician, the hospital's OB triage unit, or a perinatologist for further assessment and management. She may need immediate admission to the hospital for inpatient management or delivery.

5. Women with preeclampsia with severe features are usually delivered promptly to prevent maternal and fetal complications. Since the disease is progressive and there is no medical treatment, delivery is always in the best interest of the mother. However, preterm delivery is not always in the best interest of the fetus; therefore, a decision to delay delivery can be considered under certain circumstances. The rationale for delaying delivery in these pregnancies is to reduce perinatal morbidity and mortality by delivery of a more mature fetus and, to a lesser degree, to achieve a more favorable cervix for vaginal birth. The risks of prolonging pregnancy are worsening maternal endothelial dysfunction and continued poor perfusion of major maternal organs with the potential for severe end-organ damage to the brain, liver, kidneys, placenta/fetus, and hematologic and vascular systems.

6. If the client has a grand mal seizure, the primary consideration is to protect her. Monitor seizure type and duration. Call for immediate transport to the hospital labor and delivery unit. Place the client in the lateral recumbent position following the seizure.

7. Immediately transfer the client to a hospital for eclampsia after stabilization.

B. Client teaching:

1. Educate the client and family about the concerns of high BP during pregnancy.

2. Discuss risks of having high BP during pregnancy for the mother and fetus.

C. Pharmaceutical therapy:

1. Diuretics are *not* prescribed during pregnancy for edema.

2. Angiotensin-converting enzyme (ACE) inhibitors, angiotensin II receptor blockers (ARBs), and direct renin inhibitors are *not* recommended during pregnancy because of the teratogenic effects on the fetus that may occur, such as renal dysgenesis and/or fetal death.

3. Aldomet (methyldopa), labetalol, or nifedipine are commonly used during pregnancy to control severe acute-onset hypertension, severe chronic hypertension, or superimposed hypertension during pregnancy. These antihypertensives are recommended as first-line therapy by the ACOG Task Force on Hypertension in Pregnancy when the systolic BP is greater than 160 mmHg or diastolic BP is greater than 105 mmHg. The ACOG Task Force also suggests avoiding antihypertensive therapy in pregnant women below this level if no evidence of end-organ damage. The goal of management is the maintenance of BP between 120/80 and 160/105 mmHg.

4. Daily low-dose aspirin is recommended as a preventative measure for women with known risk factors associated with preeclampsia.

5. Inpatient therapy is determined by a physician and may include the following:

  a. Magnesium sulfate for seizure prophylaxis

  b. Hydralazine or labetalol if the client's systolic BP is greater than 160 mmHg and/or diastolic BP is greater than 105 mmHg

  c. Corticosteroids, which may be given to enhance fetal lung maturity prior to delivery in clients between 24 and 34 weeks' gestation

  d. In severe preeclampsia, therapy may include cervical ripening agents, such as prostaglandins or misoprostol and/or oxytocin induction of labor.

  e. Narcotics may be used for severe headaches.

  f. Diazepam (Valium) and phenytoin (Dilantin) are not recommended for seizures in pregnancy; there is increased risk of recurrent seizures.

D. Dietary management:

1. Salt restriction does not stop swelling and high BP problems in pregnancy.

Follow-Up

A. The only "cure" for preeclampsia is delivery. See the client in 1 week after delivery for BP assessment, or sooner if symptoms persist.

Consultation/Referral

A. If the client is diagnosed with preeclampsia, refer her to a physician for continued care and delivery.

Bibliography

Abdul Sultan, A., West, J., Tata, L. J., Fleming, K. M., Nelson-Piercy, C., & Grainge, M. J. (2013). Risk of first venous thromboembolism in pregnant women in hospital: Population-based cohort study from England. *British Medical Journal, 347*, f6099. doi:10.1136/bmj.f6099

American College of Obstetricians and Gynecologists. (2012). ACOG Practice Bulletin, No 125: Chronic hypertension in pregnancy. *Obstetrics and Gynecology, 119*, 396–407 doi:10.1097/AOG.0b013e318249ff06

American College of Obstetricians and Gynecologists. (2013). Hypertension in pregnancy: Executive summary. *Obstetrics and Gynecology, 122*(5), 1122–1131. doi:10.1097/01.AOG.0000437382.03963.88

American College of Obstetricians and Gynecologists. (2017). Committee Opinion No. 692: Emergent therapy for acute-onset, severe hypertension during pregnancy and the postpartum period. *Obstetrics and Gynecology, 129*(4), e90–e95. doi:10.1097/AOG.0000000000002019

American College of Obstetricians and Gynecologists. (2018). ACOG Committee Opinion No. 743: Low-dose aspirin use during pregnancy. *Obstetrics and Gynecology, 132*(1), e44–e52. doi:10.1097/AOG.0000000000002708

Booker, W. A., Wright, J. D., Siddiq, Z., D'Alton, M. E., Cleary, K. L., Goffman, D., . . . Ananth, C. V. (2019). Trends in comorbidity, acuity, and maternal risk associated with preeclampsia across obstetric volume settings. *Journal of Maternal-Fetal & Neonatal Medicine, 32*(16), 2680–2687.

Catalano, P. (2007). Management of obesity in pregnancy. *Obstetrics and Gynecology, 109*(2 Pt 1), 419–433. doi:10.1097/01.AOG.0000253311.44696.85

Duley, L. (2009). The global impact of pre-eclampsia and eclampsia. *Seminars in Perinatology, 33*, 130–137. doi:10.1053/j.semperi.2009.02.010

LeFevre, M. L. (2014). Low-dose aspirin use for the prevention of morbidity and mortality from preeclampsia: U.S. preventative services task force recommendation statement. *Annals of Internal Medicine, 161*(11), 819–826. doi:10.7326/M14-1884

Sovio, U., & Smith, G. (2019). Evaluation of a simple risk score to predict preterm pre-eclampsia using maternal characteristics: A prospective cohort study. *BJOG: An International Journal of Obstetrics & Gynaecology, 126*(8), 963–970. https://doi-org.proxy.library.vanderbilt.edu/10.1111/1471-0528.15664

Syngelaki, A., Sequeira Campos, M., Roberge, S., Andrade, W., & Nicolaides, K. H. (2019). Diet and exercise for preeclampsia prevention in overweight and obese pregnant women: Systematic review and meta-analysis. *Journal of Maternal-Fetal & Neonatal Medicine, 32*(20), 3495–3501.

Preterm Labor

Jill C. Cash, Susan Drummond, and Merita O'Sullivan

Definition

A. Preterm labor (PTL) is defined as regular uterine contractions that produce documented cervical changes after 20 weeks and prior to 37 completed weeks of gestation. Cervical changes may include dilation, effacement, softening, or movement of the cervix to a more anterior position.

Incidence

A. PTL occurs in approximately 10% of the live births in the United States and precedes 50% of the PTBs. It also accounts for more than 70% of neonatal mortality.

Pathogenesis

A. Infection, inflammation, decidual hemorrhage, and ischemia are common causes of PTL. Infection may originate from several sites, including the bladder, kidney(s), cervix, uterus, gastrointestinal tract, and upper respiratory tract. Ischemia may be caused by decreased oxygen delivery to the uterus because of maternal hypoxia, hypovolemia, or vena caval compression. Pathologic overdistension of the uterus in the presence of polyhydramnios or multiple gestation may cause PTL symptoms. Vaginal bleeding from a decidual hemorrhage (placental abruption) is associated with a high risk of PTL. The bleeding originates in damaged decidual blood vessels and presents clinically as vaginal bleeding or a retroplacental hematoma formation. However, in most cases, the cause is unknown.

B. Paternal risk factors: No paternal risk factors for the development of PTB in their partners have been identified. PTB risk is not increased by the father's history of preterm children with other women or PTBs to members of the father's family.

Prevention

A. Progesterone supplementation decreases the risk of PTB by approximately 30% in women with a singleton pregnancy and a history of a spontaneous single preterm delivery.

B. Women with a singleton pregnancy and a previous history of spontaneous PTB should be offered hydroxy-progesterone caproate 250 mg given via IM route once weekly, starting at 16 to 24 weeks' gestation and continuing through 36 6/7 weeks' gestation to reduce the risk of recurrent spontaneous PTB.

C. In asymptomatic women with a singleton gestation without a prior PTB with an incidentally identified very short cervix (< 20 mm) before or at 24 weeks' gestation, vaginal progesterone is recommended as a management option to reduce the risk of PTB. Vaginal micronized progesterone, 200 mg daily, is associated with a 44% decrease in spontaneous PTB at less than 34 weeks' gestation, and vaginal progesterone gel, 90 mg daily, has shown a 45% decrease in spontaneous PTB at less than 33 weeks' gestation in asymptomatic women with a very short cervix.

Predisposing Factors

A. Previous PTL or preterm delivery is the major risk factor for recurrence.

B. Preterm premature rupture of membranes (PPROM)

C. Uterine anomalies, surgery, and fibroids

D. Multiple gestations

E. History of second-trimester abortion(s)

F. Incompetent cervix

G. History of cervical surgery (cone biopsy or loop electrosurgical excision procedure [LEEP] for the treatment of cervical dysplasia)

H. Recurrent urinary tract and kidney infections, asymptomatic bacteriuria

I. Polyhydramnios

J. Fetal macrosomia

K. Maternal age extremes (< 18 or > 40 years old)

L. Placenta previa

M. Abruptio placentae

N. Poor nutritional status and low prepregnancy weight

O. Maternal dehydration

P. Maternal race (occurs more frequently in African American population)

Q. Low socioeconomic status

R. Inadequate prenatal care

S. Anemia (Hgb < 10 g/dL)

T. Substance use/abuse (smoking, drug, alcohol)

U. Vaginal infection

V. Presence of fetal fibronectin, a protein produced by the trophoblast and other fetal tissues, has been noted in cervical–vaginal secretions between 24 and 34 weeks' gestation in a subgroup of women who are at increased risk for PTB.

W. Short cervical length

X. Short interpregnancy interval

Y. Abdominal surgery during pregnancy

Z. Episodes of vaginal bleeding in more than one trimester

AA. Maternal first-degree family history of PTB, especially if the woman herself was born preterm

AB. Fetal anomaly or fetal growth restriction

AC. Intrauterine fetal demise

Common Complaints

A. Abdominal pain or menstrual-like cramping

B. Low backache

C. Increase or change in vaginal discharge, "gush" of fluid, loss of mucus plug, and bloody show or vaginal spotting

D. Diarrhea

E. "Something's not right"

Other Signs and Symptoms

A. Pelvic pressure (vaginal and/or rectal)

B. Contractions or period-like cramps

Subjective Data

A. **Review the client's past medical history and obstetric history, including risk factors for PTL.**

B. Elicit information about the onset, frequency, duration, and course of abdominal pain or cramping; presence or absence of backache; the duration and frequency of these symptoms; and whether symptoms began subsequent to a certain event or activity. What, if anything, makes these symptoms better or worse?

C. Question the client about color, odor, consistency, and amount of vaginal discharge or bleeding. Is the discharge clear, pink, blood-tinged, or bright red vaginal bleeding? Was there a spot the size of a quarter or a half-dollar? Has she been wearing a perineal pad? How often does she have to change the pad? Is the pad soaked with blood when she changes it?

D. For fetuses older than 18 weeks' gestation, question the client about frequency of fetal movements.

E. Question the client about urinary frequency, presence of urgency, or dysuria. Is the urine discolored, blood-tinged, or malodorous?

F. Question the client about recent sexual activity (i.e., has there been recent intercourse?)

G. If the client complains of diarrhea, ask her if she has a fever and if anyone else in the family is ill.

Physical Examination

A. Check temperature, BP, pulse, respiratory rate, and FHT.

B. Inspect:
1. Note general appearance of discomfort.

C. Auscultate:
1. Heart
2. Lungs (especially if the client is on tocolytics)

D. Palpate:
1. Abdomen: note presence, frequency, and intensity of uterine contractions; resting tone; and the presence of uterine tenderness or suprapubic pain.
2. Measure fundal height and gently assess fetal lie, position, and estimated fetal weight via Leopold's maneuvers (typically reliable after 24 weeks' gestation). It may be difficult to palpate fetal parts in the presence of maternal obesity or polyhydramnios.
3. Back: check for costovertebral angle (CVA) tenderness

E. Pelvic exam:
1. Sterile speculum exam: visualize the cervix for an estimate of dilation. Evaluate rupture of membranes and vaginal discharge or bleeding. **If meconium-stained amniotic fluid is noted, immediately consult a physician and transfer the client to a hospital. Note if meconium is thin or thick (thick meconium may be associated with breech presentation).**
2. Bimanual exam: After rupture of membranes and placenta previa have been excluded by the client history, sterile speculum exam, physical exam, laboratory testing, and US evaluation, as appropriate, perform a gentle bimanual examination. Note cervical dilation, effacement, station, cervical position, and softness of cervix
3. Cervical exam during pregnancy: *See Section II: Procedure "Bimanual Examination: Cervical Evaluation During Pregnancy."* **Do not perform a digital examination of the cervix if PROM is present without active labor or before a US has been performed to confirm placental location.**

Diagnostic Tests

A. White blood cell (WBC), if indicated

B. Urine dipstick for ketones, leukocyte, esterase, protein, and nitrite

C. Evaluate vaginal discharge for pH with phenaphthazine (nitrazine) tape.

Note: False-positive and false-negative nitrazine test results occur in approximately 5% of cases.

False-negative test results can occur when leaking of amniotic fluid is intermittent or is diluted by other vaginal fluids. False-positive results can be caused by alkaline fluids in the vagina such as blood, seminal fluid, or soap.

D. Check ferning if discharge is nitrazine positive or PPROM is suspected. When viewed under a microscope, amniotic fluid produces a delicate ferning pattern in contrast to the thick, wide branching pattern seen with cervical mucus.

Note: A false-positive fern test can be caused by well-estrogenized cervical mucus or a fingerprint on the microscope slide. A false-negative result can be caused by inadequate amniotic fluid collection on the vaginal swab or if the sample collected is heavily contaminated by other vaginal fluids or blood.

E. Wet prep, if indicated

F. Cervical cultures for STIs (gonorrhea and chlamydia)

G. Cervical and rectal culture for GBS (if not performed in the previous 5 weeks)

H. Fetal fibronectin, where available. Candidates for fetal fibronectin testing must meet the following criteria:
1. Intact fetal membranes
2. Cervical dilatation less than 3 cm
3. Gestational age 24 0/7 weeks to 34 6/7 weeks
4. No sexual intercourse in preceding 24 hours
5. No gross vaginal bleeding

A positive fetal fibronectin result correlates with an increased risk of preterm delivery within 7 days.

Note: False-positive results can occur because of ejaculate from coitus within the previous 24 hours, a grossly bloody specimen, or a digital cervical exam. A digital cervical exam can also produce a false-negative result. Administration of intravaginal substances, such as lubricants, medications, or douching, may also interfere with the assay.

Urine culture: Asymptomatic bacteriuria is associated with an increased risk of PTL.

I. Urine drug screen: in clients with risk factors for substance abuse, because of the link between cocaine use and placental abruption

J. Ultrasonography: fetal biometry and dating, cervical length, amniotic fluid volume, BPP, placental location, fetal presentation, and ruling out fetal, placental, and maternal anatomic anomalies

K. Electronic fetal monitoring (EFM) for contractions and fetal heart rate (FHR)

Differential Diagnoses

A. Preterm (or Braxton Hicks) contractions, with no cervical change

B. Incompetent cervix

C. PPROM

D. Low back muscle strain

E. Pyelonephritis or UTI

F. Placenta previa

G. Abruptio placentae

H. Gastroenteritis

I. Vaginal infection

J. Maternal dehydration

K. Ketoacidosis

L. Round ligament pain

Plan

A. General interventions:
1. Regular uterine contractions with cervical dilation or effacement, with pressure on the lower uterine segment, strongly indicate PTL.

2. If the cervix is dilated more than 3 cm with contractions upon presentation, the client is probably having PTL. Consult with a physician for hospital admission and tocolytic candidacy.

3. If the client is symptomatic with a positive fetal fibronectin test, consult with a physician for maternal transfer to a hospital equipped to care for preterm infants.

4. Second trimester: If the client shows signs and symptoms of PTL, consider diagnosis of incompetent cervix. Refer the client to a physician for ultrasonography for cervical length and possible cerclage placement.

B. Outpatient management:

1. *See Section III: Client Teaching Guide "Preterm Labor."*

2. Outpatient bed rest is not beneficial. While bed rest improves uteroplacental blood flow and can lead to a slight increase in fetal birthweight, there is no evidence that it decreases the incidence of PTB. Additionally, prolonged immobility increases the risk of thrombolytic events, has clear negative psychosocial effects on clients and families, and leads to musculoskeletal deconditioning.

3. Limit physical activity: Women at high risk for PTL should reduce their level of physical activity/exercise, particularly strength training, and occupational activities that require heavy lifting.

4. Prophylactic treatment against infection is not recommended. There is no clear evidence of benefit from prophylactic antibiotic therapy in women with PTL with intact membranes and no evidence of infection.

5. Sexual activity: Patients should consider avoiding sexual activity if they experience an increased frequency or intensity of contractions after sexual intercourse.

6. Administer corticosteroids to enhance fetal lung maturity if less than 34 weeks' gestation. Observe the client for contractions in the office

7. Fetal fibronectin testing, where available, using the ACOG guidelines

C. Inpatient management of PTL:

1. Observation, possibly with IV hydration

2. Cervical cerclage

3. Antibiotic treatment against infection (GBS) until urine and cervical culture results are available

4. Parenteral tocolysis either to stop PTL or delay delivery long enough to allow transfer to a facility with the ability to care for preterm infants. According to numerous clinical studies, predelivery administration of magnesium sulfate offers fetal neuroprotection, which reduces the occurrence and severity of cerebral palsy and, therefore, may be the drug of choice for parenteral tocolysis in the hospital setting.

5. Administer corticosteroids to enhance fetal lung maturity if less than 34 weeks. Predelivery of betamethasone reduces the risk of neonatal death,

respiratory distress syndrome, intraventricular hemorrhage, and necrotizing enterocolitis in premature neonates.

6. Transport the client to a perinatal center for neonatal care

D. Pharmaceutical therapy:

1. Tocolytics may be utilized between 24 and 34 weeks' gestation. Maintenance therapy with tocolytics is generally ineffective, while short-term use is recommended mainly to allow for the administration of antenatal steroids. The FDA cautions against the use of maintenance oral terbutaline during pregnancy because of lack of efficacy and potential maternal cardiac risks and death; it should not be prescribed on an outpatient basis. Injectable terbutaline may be used on a short-term basis (48–72 hours) in a hospital setting.

2. Corticosteroids:

a. Steroids are given to enhance lung maturity in the fetus.

b. A single rescue course may be considered if the antecedent treatment was given more than 2 weeks prior, and the client is judged to be likely to deliver within the next week.

Follow-Up

A. Depending on the clinical scenario, the client may need to be seen weekly or biweekly. Fetal fibronectin test may be repeated every 2 weeks, but positive results alone should not be used to exclusively direct management. Repeat cultures as indicated, discontinuing antibiotics if cultures are negative. Encourage close phone contact with the client regarding questions or concerns.

Bibliography

American College of Obstetricians and Gynecologists. (2012). ACOG Practice Bulletin No. 130: Prediction and prevention of preterm birth (Reaffirmed 2018). *Obstetrics and Gynecology, 120*, 964–973. doi:10.1097/AOG.0b013e3182723b1b

American College of Obstetricians and Gynecologists. (2016). ACOG Practice Bulletin No. 171: Management of preterm labor. *Obstetrics and Gynecology, 128*(4), e155–e164. doi:10.1097/AOG.0000000000001711

American College of Obstetricians and Gynecologists. (2017). ACOG Committee Opinion No. 713: Antenatal corticosteroid therapy for fetal maturation (Reaffirmed 2018). *Obstetrics and Gynecology, 130*, e102–e109. doi:10.1097/AOG.0000000000002237

American College of Obstetricians and Gynecologists. (2018). ACOG Practice Bulletin No. 199: Use of prophylactic antibiotics in labor and delivery. *Obstetrics and Gynecology, 132*(3), e103–e119. doi:10.1097/AOG.0000000000002833

Centers for Disease Control and Prevention. (2010, November 19). Prevention of perinatal group B streptococcal disease: Revised guidelines from CDC, 2010. *MMWR Recommendations and Reports, 59*(RR-10), 1–36. Retrieved from https://www.cdc.gov/mmwr/pdf/rr/rr5910.pdf

Hooton, T., & Gupta, K. (2017, August 24). Urinary tract infections and asymptomatic bacteriuria in pregnancy. In A. Bloom (Ed.), *UpToDate*. Retrieved from https://www.uptodate.com/contents/urinary-tract-infections-and-asymptomatic-bacteriuria-in-pregnancy

Iams, J. D. (2014). Identification of candidates for progesterone: Why, who, how, and when? *Obstetrics and Gynecology, 123*(6), 1317–1326. doi:10.1097/AOG.0000000000000276

Janevic, T., Zeitlin, J., Auger, N., Egorova, N. N., Hebert, P., Balbierz, A., & Howell, E. A. (2018). Association of race/ethnicity with very preterm neonatal morbidities. *JAMA Pediatrics, 172*(11), 1061–1069.

Keeler, S. M., Roman, A. S., Coletta, J. M., Kiefer, D. G., Feuerman, M., & Rust, O. A. (2009). Fetal fibronectin testing in patients with short cervix in the midtrimester: Can it identify optimal candidates for ultrasound-indicated cerclage? *American Journal of Obstetrics and Gynecology*, 200, 158.e1–158e6. doi:10.1016/j.ajog.2008.08.050

Levin, H. I., Sciscione, A., Ananth, C. V., Drassinower, D., Obican, S. G., & Wapner, R. J. (2018). Activity restriction and risk of preterm delivery. *Journal of Maternal-Fetal & Neonatal Medicine*, 31(16), 2136–2140.

Mourgues, C., Rossi, A., Favre, N., Delabaere, A., Roszyk, L., Sapin, V., Debost-Legrand, A., & Gallot, D. (2019). Fetal fibronectin test for threatened preterm delivery 48 h after admission: Cost-effectiveness study. *European Journal of Obstetrics & Gynecology & Reproductive Biology*, 234, 75–78.

Oh, K. J., Romero, R., Park, J. Y., Kang, J., Hong, J. -S., & Yoon, B. H. (2019). A high concentration of fetal fibronectin in cervical secretions increases the risk of intra-amniotic infection and inflammation in patients with preterm labor and intact membranes. *Journal of Perinatal Medicine*, 47(3), 288–303.

Society for Maternal-Fetal Medicine Publications Committee. (2016). Implementation of the use of antenatal corticosteroids in the late preterm birth period in women at high risk for preterm delivery. *American Journal of Obstetrics and Gynecology*, 215(2), B12–B15. doi:10.1016/j.ajog.2016.03.013

Sosa, C. G., Althabe, F., Belizán, J. M., & Bergel, E. (2015). Bed rest in singleton pregnancies for preventing preterm birth. *Cochrane Database of Systematic Reviews, 2015*, (3), CD003581. doi:10.1002/14651858.CD003581.pub3

Sperling, J. D., Dahlke, J. D., & Gonzalez, J. M. (2017). Cerclage Use: A Review of 3 National Guidelines. *Obstetrical & Gynecological Survey*, 72(4), 235–241. https://doi-org.proxy.library.vanderbilt.edu/10.1097/OGX.0000000000000422

Wong, T. T. C., Tung, J. S. Z., Lau, H. C. Q., & Tagore, S. (2018). Antenatal corticosteroids administration: Are we giving them at the right time? *Archives of Gynecology & Obstetrics*, 297(2), 373–379. https://doi-org.proxy.library.vanderbilt.edu/10.1007/s00404-017-4577-4

Pyelonephritis in Pregnancy

Jill C. Cash, Susan Drummond, and Christina C. Reed

Definition

A. Pyelonephritis is an infection in one or both kidneys, usually involving the entire urinary tract.

Pyelonephritis may evolve into acute respiratory distress syndrome (ARDS) in pregnancy.

Incidence

A. The incidence of pyelonephritis in pregnancy is 1% to 2%. Most cases develop as a consequence of undiagnosed or inadequately treated lower UTI. Approximately 75% to 80% of pyelonephritis cases occur on the right side, with a 10% to 15% incidence on the left side. A small percentage of cases are bilateral.

Pathogenesis

A. *Escherichia coli* is the main pathogen in pyelonephritis, though *Klebsiella pneumoniae* and *Proteus* species are also important causes of infection. Occasionally highly virulent Gram-negative bacilli, such as *Pseudomonas, Enterobacter*, and *Serratia*, are responsible (more commonly noted in immunocompromised clients). Gram-positive GBS may also be responsible. Anaerobes also are unlikely pathogens in pyelonephritis except in cases of chronic obstruction or instrumentation.

Predisposing Factors

A. Pregnancy-related anatomic changes in the urinary tract, such as dilated ureters caused by smooth muscle relaxation and pressure on the bladder from the enlarging uterus. The immunosuppression of pregnancy may also contribute.

B. History of UTI, cystitis, and pyelonephritis

C. Sickle cell disease

Common Complaints

A. Fever

B. Chills

C. Flank pain or tenderness

D. Urinary frequency or urgency

E. Hematuria and dysuria

Other Signs and Symptoms

A. UTI is associated with urinary frequency, urgency, and dysuria; hematuria; and suprapubic pain.

   1. Chemical reactions to deodorant or douches can affect urination.

   2. Patients with frequent pyelonephritis do *not* complain of frequency and dysuria.

B. Pyelonephritis is associated with fever, palpitations, dizziness, backache, and urinary frequency.

   1. Hematuria may be present, especially if the client has a history of a previous kidney stone.

   2. Dysuria is not always present in upper tract infections.

C. Abdominal pain and uterine contractions, risk of preterm labor (PTL) and birth

D. Shortness of breath

Potential Complications

A. Sepsis and septic shock

B. Adult respiratory distress syndrome: mortality rate 50% to 70%

C. Pulmonary embolus, usually presents as sudden-onset costovertebral angle (CVA) tenderness

Subjective Data

A. Elicit information on the onset, duration, and progression of symptoms.

B. Elicit problems with voiding. Ask the client about urinary frequency, urgency, and dysuria.

C. Ask the client if she has experienced preterm contractions.

D. Ask if the client is complaining of fever or chills.

E. Ask the client if her urine has a bad odor.

F. Ask the client if she has felt more tired than usual.

G. Ask the client if she has felt more nauseated than usual or if she has been vomiting.

H. Does client have a backache? Note location (unilateral or bilateral) and what, if anything, makes the backache better or worse.

I. Review the client's history for sickle cell disease, if appropriate. Has she been tested?

J. Review prenatal history for recurrent UTIs, previous pyelonephritis, and any abnormalities of the genitourinary (GU) tract.

Physical Examination

A. Check temperature, pulse, respirations, and BP: fever more than 100.4°F, tachycardia, tachypnea, hypotension associated with sepsis, septic shock, and ARDS.

B. Inspect:
1. Note general appearance for respiratory distress.

C. Auscultate:
1. Lungs and heart
2. FHT

D. Palpate:
1. Back: check CVA tenderness (right CVA tenderness is more common in pregnancy).
2. Abdomen:
   a. Palpate for uterine tenderness and contractions.
   b. Palpate for suprapubic tenderness.

E. Bimanual exam: check for cervical dilation.

Diagnostic Tests

A. CBC with differential or WBC: leukocytosis with left shift on differential seen

B. Blood culture, if indicated

C. Respiratory function:
1. Arterial blood gases (ABGs), if indicated
2. Pulse oximetry, if indicated

D. Renal function:
1. Urinalysis:
   a. Check urinalysis for WBCs, RBCs, leukocyte esterase, and/or nitrites.
   b. Glucosuria may be normal in pregnancy because of decreased tubular capacity to reabsorb glucose. If it is consistently noted, further testing is needed.
   c. Proteinuria is *not* normal during pregnancy. All cases warrant further investigation.
2. Urine culture and sensitivity: Bacterial count greater than 100,000 colonies/mL indicates a UTI and should be treated. The consensus is unclear whether GBS bacteriuria less than 100,000 colonies/mL should be treated prior to 35 weeks to prevent pyelonephritis, preterm delivery, and postpartum endometritis. Currently the ACOG recommends treating GBS bacteriuria greater than 100,000 colonies/mL even if the client is asymptomatic.
3. Intravenous pyelogram (IVP), if indicated
4. Renal ultrasonography, if indicated

Differential Diagnoses

A. Cystitis
B. Urethritis
C. Urethral stricture
D. Urolithiasis
E. Genital infection
F. Chorioamnionitis
G. Septic abortion
H. Postpartum endometritis
I. Muscular strain
J. Pulmonary embolus
K. Severe upper respiratory tract infection
L. Postprocedural dysuria or urinary frequency (i.e., following bladder catheterization or cystoscopy)
M. Chemical irritants
N. Postpartum septic pelvic thrombophlebitis
O. Renal calculi

Plan

A. General interventions:
1. Rule out other sources of infection.
2. Assess for PTL.

B. Client teaching: *See Section III: Client Teaching Guide "Pyelonephritis in Pregnancy."* ◄

C. Pharmaceutical therapy:
1. Broad-spectrum antibiotic coverage until cultures and sensitivity results are back.
2. Drug of choice:
   a. Nitrofurantoin (Macrobid) 100 mg orally every 12 hours for 7 days
   b. Amoxicillin 500 mg orally every 12 hours for 10 days or 250 mg orally every 8 hours for 10 days
   c. Augmentin 500 mg orally every 8 hours for 7 days or 875 mg orally every 12 hours for 7 days
3. If dysuria is present: phenazopyridine (Pyridium) 200 mg orally three times daily after meals for 3 days. Warn the client that phenazopyridine (Pyridium) turns urine orange.
4. Alternative medications:
   1. Cephalexin (Keflex) 500 mg orally every 12 hours for 7 days

D. Dietary management:
1. Advise the client to eat a regular diet as tolerated.
2. Encourage her to drink eight to 10 glasses of water a day.
3. Warn the client to avoid beverages with caffeine. One hundred percent cranberry juice and cranberry and blueberry capsules are good for urinary tract problems.

Follow-Up

A. Once antibiotic therapy is initiated, most clients have a decrease in symptoms within 48 hours. By the end of 72 hours, almost 95% of clients are afebrile and asymptomatic. Stress to clients the importance of completing the course of antibiotics regardless of the absence of symptoms.

B. The most likely causes of treatment failure are a resistant microorganism or obstruction; common causes of obstruction in pregnancy are urolithiasis or compression of the ureter by the gravid uterus.

C. Repeat a urine culture at a 2-week follow-up visit.

D. Recurrence rates are very high. After the initial antibiotic therapy course is completed, start a prophylactic dose of an antibiotic that is to be taken daily till delivery, such as nitrofurantoin (Macrodantin) 50 to 100 mg by mouth at bedtime for recurrent infections.

E. Patients receiving prophylactic antibiotics should have their urine screened for bacteria at each subsequent office visit and be questioned about the recurrence of symptoms.

F. If no prophylactic treatment is undertaken, obtain a urine culture if symptoms recur or if urine dipstick is positive for leukocyte esterase or nitrites.

Bibliography

Centers for Disease Control and Prevention. (2010, November 19). Prevention of perinatal group B streptococcal disease: Revised guidelines from CDC, 2010. *MMWR Recommendations and Reports, 59*(RR-10), 1–36. Retrieved from https://www.cdc.gov/mmwr/pdf/rr/rr5910.pdf

Vaginal Bleeding: First Trimester

Jill C. Cash, Susan Drummond, and Merita O'Sullivan

Definition

Vaginal bleeding is common during the first trimester of pregnancy, occurring in 20% to 40% of all pregnancies. It may range from spotting to massive hemorrhage and be intermittent or constant, with or without pain. Types of abortion are:

A. Threatened abortion: vaginal bleeding with absent or minimal pain *and* a closed, long, thick cervix

B. Inevitable abortion: vaginal bleeding with pain and cervical dilation and/or effacement

C. Spontaneous abortion: nonviable products of conception are expelled from the uterus spontaneously. This process may be complete or incomplete.

D. Missed abortion: in utero death of the fetus before 20 weeks' gestation, with retention of the pregnancy. Vaginal bleeding may occur but the cervix usually remains closed. US reveals an intrauterine gestational sac with or without an embryonic/fetal pole but no cardiac activity.

E. Vanishing twin: a single pregnancy that results from very early loss of one embryo of a multiple gestation; may be associated with vaginal bleeding

F. Vaginal bleeding may also be related to ectopic pregnancy, implantation of the pregnancy, postcoital bleeding, cervical inflammation/infection, or cervical, vaginal, or uterine pathology.

Incidence

A. Vaginal bleeding is a common event in pregnancy. Spontaneous abortion, a primary concern in the first trimester, occurs in about 30% of all pregnancies; most occur before the 16th week. Ectopic pregnancy is much less common, occurring in one of every 200 pregnancies; 75% of pregnancies occurring after failure of tubal sterilization are likely to be ectopic. Rupture of an extrauterine pregnancy is life threatening and must be excluded in every pregnant woman with vaginal bleeding.

Pathogenesis

A. Spontaneous abortion: pathogenesis varies according to cause. In most cases, it is caused by embryonic death, with resultant decrease in hormone levels and subsequent sloughing of the uterine decidua. Many of the embryonic deaths occur because of chromosomal abnormalities that are incompatible with life.

B. Ectopic pregnancy: fertilized ovum is prevented or slowed in its progress down the fallopian tube. Pregnancy is implanted outside of the uterus, most commonly in the fallopian tube.

Predisposing Factors

A. Spontaneous abortion: In most cases, the cause is unknown.

   1. AMA (occurs more often in older women): A chromosomal abnormality in the embryo accounts for approximately 50% of cases in older women.

   2. Abnormal uterine environment: uterine septum, submucosal leiomyoma, intrauterine adhesions

   3. Systemic disease: diabetes, thyroid disease, thrombophilia

   4. Weight extremes (BMI < 18.5 or > 30)

   5. Immunologic deficiencies

   6. Substance use, including caffeine, alcohol, cigarettes, and cocaine

   7. Exposure to teratogens and infections: food contaminated with *Listeria monocytogenes,* radiation

   8. Trauma

   9. Previous spontaneous abortion (AB): history of two or more consecutive spontaneous abortions or a condition associated with spontaneous abortions such as maternal antiphospholipid syndrome or a uterine anomaly

B. Ectopic pregnancy: caused by previous damage to the fallopian tube; frequently caused by pelvic inflammatory disease, tubal surgery for infertility, or bilateral tubal ligation

Common Complaints

A. Spontaneous abortion: Vaginal bleeding occurs that may or may not be associated with cramping or uterine contractions. When a pregnancy is more than 8 weeks' gestation, the presence of uterine bleeding, uterine contractions, and/or pain are indications of a threatened abortion until proven otherwise.

B. Ectopic pregnancy: Vaginal bleeding and pelvic pain occur soon after the first missed period; the client may be unaware of pregnancy. Sudden, acute, localized abdominal pain is associated with fallopian tube rupture.

Other Signs and Symptoms

A. Threatened abortion: slight bleeding may be present over several weeks; cramping; no passage of tissue; positive pregnancy symptoms present, including nausea, vomiting, fatigue, breast tenderness, and urinary frequency

B. Inevitable abortion: moderate to profuse vaginal bleeding occurs. Tissue may or may not be passed, uterine cramps or abdominal pain are present, symptoms of pregnancy may be decreased or absent.

C. Incomplete abortion: moderate to profuse vaginal bleeding, sometimes for several weeks, occurs; reports of passage of tissue; painful uterine cramping or "contractions"; and symptoms of pregnancy often absent

D. Complete abortion: patient experiences profuse bleeding, passage of tissue and large clots, abdominal cramping, or uterine contractions

E. Ectopic pregnancy: amenorrhea or irregular vaginal bleeding; abdominal pain is usually present, may be unilateral or generalized and may be associated with vertigo and syncope; shoulder pain, with irritation of phrenic nerve, may be present. Anxiety or palpitations are often noted.

Subjective Data

A. Elicit information about the onset, duration, and progression of symptoms.

B. Ask the client about vaginal bleeding. When did it start? Is it continuous bleeding "like a period" or is it spotting? How much bleeding has occurred? How many pads have been saturated? What is the size of the blood spots? Determine amount of bleeding: How much blood is on peri-pad? (a) Scant amount: less than 1-inch diameter, (b) light amount: less than a 4-inch diameter, (c) moderate amount: less than a 6-inch diameter, (d) heavy amount: saturates the peri-pad within 1 hour. Has client passed any blood clots or tissue? Does she feel dizzy or lightheaded?

C. What is her current method of birth control? Was the birth control method used consistently? Has she had a tubal ligation, or has she recently used an intrauterine contraceptive device (IUD)?

D. Ask the client the first day of her last menstrual period to date the pregnancy. Did she have a positive pregnancy test? If so, when? Has she had an US to confirm pregnancy location and dating?

E. Does she have a history of ectopic pregnancy, adnexal surgery, or pelvic inflammatory disease?

F. Question the client regarding the presence or absence of abdominal and/or back pain. If present, is it a continuous discomfort, or is it intermittent cramping? Was the onset sudden? How severe is the pain?

G. Is the client experiencing shoulder pain? This may be referred pain from phrenic nerve irritation because of intraperitoneal bleeding.

H. Does she have a history of assisted reproductive techniques for conception with current pregnancy? This history increases the risk for a heterotopic pregnancy, a rare complication of pregnancy in which both an intrauterine and an extrauterine pregnancy occur simultaneously. This condition is also known as a combined pregnancy, multiple-sited pregnancy, or coincident pregnancy.

Physical Examination

A. Check temperature (if indicated), pulse, respirations, and BP. Note postural hypotension and tachycardia. Hemodynamic instability may be noted in cases of profuse bleeding; assess vital signs and be alert for hypotension, tachycardia, tachypnea, and/or labored breathing.

B. Inspect:
   1. Note general overall appearance of discomfort or pain and signs of shock before, during, and after examination.
   2. Examine peri-pad to determine amount and color of bleeding, if available.

C. Auscultate:
   1. Auscultate the heart, lungs, and bowel sounds to rule out other abdominal problems.
   2. If the pregnancy is beyond 10 to 12 weeks' gestation, a handheld Doppler can be used to auscultate the FHT.

D. Palpate:
   1. Perform abdominal examination for rebound tenderness, masses, softness, tenderness, or abdominal wall distension. Sudden, acute, localized abdominal pain with signs of internal hemorrhage suggests rupture of the fallopian tube.
   2. Palpate uterine size. Measure fundal height for consistency with pregnancy dates. If fundal height suggests pregnancy has advanced beyond first trimester, bleeding may be caused by abruption, placenta previa, or rupture of membranes with heavy bloody show.
   3. Check iliopsoas and obturator muscle tests.

E. Pelvic examination:
   1. Place the client in a lithotomy position to examine external genitalia to access the volume and potential source of bleeding.
   2. Perform sterile speculum examination: assess color and amount of bleeding. Tissue and the products of conception may be noted at cervical os or in vaginal vault. Assess for Chadwick's sign. The entire fetus may be noted in the vaginal vault; tissues that remain in the uterus may include portions of fetal membranes or placenta. The speculum exam may reveal a cause of bleeding unrelated to the pregnancy such as a vaginal laceration, vaginal neoplasm, condyloma acuminata, vaginitis, cervical lesions (polyps, fibroids, ectropion), acute cervicitis, or a cervical neoplasm.
   3. Bimanual examination: check Hegar's sign; elicit this sign cautiously, as a false-positive result may be related to a rough examination. Evaluate cervical dilation; cervical motion tenderness, adnexal, or abdominal tenderness. An adnexal mass and mild uterine enlargement are often present with ectopic pregnancy. A bulging cul-de-sac, represents a hemoperitoneum. Adnexal mass is present in 50% of ectopic pregnancies.

Diagnostic Tests

A. Pregnancy test: quantitative serum beta human chorionic gonadotropin (HCG); serial tests at least 48 hours apart, making sure to perform test at same lab for accurate results. 99.9% of viable pregnancies display a rise in HCG greater than 35% over 48 hours. HCG levels that plateau or rise slowly (< 35% in 48 hours) suggest an ectopic pregnancy or an abnormal intrauterine pregnancy.

B. CBC with differential and platelet

C. Blood type, Rh, antibody screen, and crossmatch if indicated

D. Prothrombin time (PT) and partial thromboplastin time (PTT)

E. Doppler ultrasonography for FHT, for fetuses older than 11 weeks

F. Ultrasonography: transvaginal and/or abdominal scan

Differential Diagnoses

A. First-trimester vaginal bleeding secondary to:
   1. Threatened abortion
   2. Inevitable abortion
   3. Incomplete abortion
   4. Complete abortion
   5. Septic abortion

6. Ectopic pregnancy: There is strong suspicion of ectopic pregnancy or fallopian tube rupture if symptoms present with history of fallopian tube damage (i.e., tubal surgery for infertility, previous ectopic pregnancy), pelvic infection, or IUD use.

7. Hydatidiform mole

8. Anovulatory bleeding with an antecedent period of amenorrhea

9. Benign or malignant genital tract lesion

10. Menstrual bleeding

11. Genital trauma

12. Advanced pregnancy with placenta previa or abruptio placentae

13. Salpingitis

14. Appendicitis

15. IUD-related symptoms

16. Pelvic inflammatory disease

17. Acute vaginitis or cervicitis

18. Physiologic/implantation bleeding

19. Postcoital bleeding

Plan

A. General interventions: Stabilize maternal condition and then determine the cause of bleeding.

1. Threatened abortion: expectant management. Bed rest is often prescribed, but multiple randomized trials have not found bed rest at home or in the hospital is beneficial in preventing fetal loss. Symptoms either subside, leading to normal gestation, or worsen, leading to inevitable abortion. If bleeding persists without leading to spontaneous abortion, the client should be evaluated frequently, usually on a weekly basis, by means of ultrasonography to assess fetal viability. The client should be placed on pelvic rest, avoiding intercourse, and should not use tampons to absorb bleeding. Treatment with progestins is the most promising treatment for threatened abortions, but its efficacy has not been established.

2. Inevitable abortion: Care may include expectant management or medical management (Misoprostol), or a surgical evacuation can be undertaken.

3. Incomplete abortion: Medical management (Misoprostol) or a surgical evacuation is generally performed.

4. Complete abortion: If abortion is complete and the products of conception are delivered with complete membranes present and cessation of bleeding has occurred, no surgical intervention is indicated. In these cases, the tissue specimens must be carefully examined for completeness. Send all specimens to the laboratory for pathologic examination. If there is any question regarding complete passing of the placenta, do serial quantitative HCGs until back to nonpregnant levels.

5. Ectopic pregnancy: consult with a physician regarding possible medical management with methotrexate (MTX) or refer the client to a physician for surgical intervention. The physician may perform culdocentesis to assess for hemoperitoneum. If the client is in shock, resuscitation with IV fluids should be started immediately by means of two large-bore angiocatheters. IV fluids such as lactated Ringer's solution or normal saline should be infused at a rapid rate. The client is taken to the operating room, where the indicated procedure is one that controls hemorrhage in the shortest period of time. Salpingectomy and/or hysterectomy may be included.

B. Client teaching: *See Section III: Client Teaching Guide "Vaginal Bleeding: First Trimester."* ◀

C. Pharmaceutical therapy:

1. RhoGAM should be administered to any Rh-negative client.

2. Acetaminophen (Tylenol) or ibuprofen as needed for discomfort.

3. Ectopic pregnancy: In current practice, pharmacologic therapy is the preferred treatment for an ectopic pregnancy, and MTX is the main agent used. MTX is a folic acid antagonist that has been used to inhibit the growth of trophoblastic cells. This chemotherapy is also the treatment of choice for ectopic pregnancy when surgery is contraindicated, or in the management of postoperative persistent trophoblast. Refer the client to a physician to evaluate her for MTX or operative intervention.

Follow-Up

A. Threatened abortion: follow the client weekly to assess for interval growth and presence of fetal cardiac motion. Instruct the client on peri-pad count.

B. Spontaneous abortion: Once the uterine contents have been evacuated, follow up with a 6-week post-abortion visit, unless the situation warrants an earlier follow-up visit. Contraception needs to be discussed with the client. Women who experience pregnancy loss may attempt conception as soon as they are medically recovered and psychologically ready. Studies do not report benefits for a delayed interval to conception.

C. Ectopic pregnancy: Once the ectopic pregnancy has been removed, the client should be seen in 2 to 6 weeks for a postoperative examination, unless the situation warrants an earlier follow-up visit. If MTX is used, do serial quantitative HCGs until they return to nonpregnant levels.

Consultation/Referral

A. Consult with a physician if the client has any frank bleeding, signs of fetal compromise, or maternal shock, or if the cause of bleeding cannot be determined.

Bibliography

American College of Obstetricians and Gynecologists. (2018). ACOG Practice Bulletin No 193: Tubal ectopic pregnancy. *Obstetrics and Gynecology*, *131*, e91–e103. doi:10.1097/AOG.0000000000002560

De Sutter, P., Bontinck, J., Schutysers, V., Van der Elst, J., Gerris, J., & Dhont, M. (2006). First-trimester bleeding and pregnancy outcome in singletons after assisted reproduction. *Human Reproduction*, *21*(7), 1907–1911. doi:10.1093/humrep/del054

Vaginal Bleeding: Second and Third Trimesters

Jill C. Cash, Susan Drummond, and Merita O'Sullivan

Definition

Bright or dark red vaginal bleeding during the second or third trimester (> 12 weeks' gestation) is less common. It may be painless, or it may be associated with uterine contractions or severe abdominal pain. Antepartum bleeding (uterine bleeding after 20 weeks' gestation that is unrelated to labor and delivery) occurs in 4% to 5% of pregnancies. Common causes of bleeding include:

A. Bloody show: associated with labor (by definition, labor occurs after 20 weeks' gestation) and vaginal discharge of mucus, which may be clear, pink, or slightly bloody

B. Cervical insufficiency: The ACOG defines cervical insufficiency as "the inability of the uterine cervix to maintain a pregnancy in the second trimester in the absence of clinical contractions, labor or both."

C. Low-lying placenta: The edge of the placenta grows into the area of the lower uterine segment located less than two centimeters from the internal cervical os.

D. Placenta previa: implantation of the blastocyst occurs in the lower uterine segment, followed by placental growth. Eventually, the placenta may partially or completely cover the cervix.

E. Abruptio placentae: partial or premature separation of a normally implanted placenta prior to delivery of the infant

F. Uterine rupture: complete uterine rupture extends through the entire uterine wall, and the uterine contents are extruded into the abdominal cavity. Incomplete rupture extends through the endometrium and myometrium, but the peritoneum remains intact. This occurs almost exclusively during labor and/or delivery.

G. Uterine dehiscence: separation of an old surgical scar

H. Vasa previa: fetal blood vessels are present in the membrane covering the internal cervical os. The membranous vessels may be associated with a velamentous umbilical cord or they may connect the lobes of a bilobed placenta or the placenta and a succenturiate lobe. Rupture of the vasa previa is an obstetric emergency and may lead to fetal death.

I. Bloody discharge is *not* normal prior to 37 weeks' gestation unless associated with recent sexual intercourse or pelvic exam. Light spotting or bleeding may be caused by recent sexual intercourse, PTL, rupture of membranes, or cervicitis. *Note:* The evaluation of vaginal bleeding prior to 20 weeks is similar to that in the first trimester.

Incidence

A. Placenta previa: approximately 1:200 pregnancies, but varies worldwide and is more common in parous women

B. Abruptio placenta: approximately 1:250 pregnancies

C. Uterine rupture: If uterus is unscarred, incidence is approximately 1:6,000 to 20,000 pregnancies. If uterus has a scar, the incidence varies depending on the type and location of the prior uterine incision. If the prior incision was low transverse, the incidence is approximately 0.7% to 2.0%, and if the prior incision was classical, the incidence is approximately 1% to 12%.

Pathogenesis

A. Placenta previa: The pathogenesis of placenta previa is unknown. One hypothesis is that the presence of areas of suboptimal endometrium in the upper uterine cavity caused by previous surgery or pregnancies promotes implantation of trophoblast in or toward the lower uterine segment. Another hypothesis is that a particularly large placental surface area, as in multiple gestation or in response to reduced uteroplacental perfusion, increases the likelihood that the placenta will cover or encroach upon the cervical os.

B. Abruptio placenta: initiated by bleeding into the decidua basalis. The decidua then splits, and the placenta is sheared off, either partially or totally. Blood may move into and through the myometrium, leading to a board-like uterus.

C. Uterine rupture: may occur from uterine injury, caused by previous surgery or trauma

Predisposing Factors

A. Placenta previa: late fertilization with delayed implantation, previous uterine scar, AMA, multiple gestation, large placenta, previous previa, and smoking

B. Abruptio placenta: a prior placental abruption is the strongest risk factor for abruption; the recurrence risk is increased 10- to 15-fold. Hypertension (chronic, gestational, or preeclampsia), cocaine use, trauma, high parity, sudden decompression of overdistended uterus (i.e., when membranes rupture), smoking, chorioamnionitis, abdominal trauma, and external cephalic version are other factors.

C. Uterine rupture: multiparity, previous uterine incision, tetanic contractions, or prolonged labor, especially with excessive use of oxytocin

Common Complaints

A. Placenta previa: painless vaginal bleeding, usually in amounts of spotting to frank hemorrhage. Bleeding occasionally is accompanied by cramping or uterine contractions. A "gush" of fluid associated with sudden onset of massive vaginal bleeding may be reported. Painless vaginal bleeding should be treated as a placenta previa until proven otherwise.

B. Abruptio placentae: Firm, tender uterus; hypertonic uterine contractions with high frequency and low amplitude are common. Typically presents with vaginal bleeding (80%), uterine tenderness (70%), and uterine contractions (35%) with or without nonreassuring FHR:

  1. Marginal abruption: Vaginal bleeding may be absent or minimal and bright red; there may be some old, dark blood. Abdominal pain is usually mild.

  Vaginal bleeding with abdominal pain should be treated as an abruption until proven otherwise.

2. Moderate abruption: Vaginal bleeding may be moderate or absent. Abdominal pain is usually significant and associated with contractions.

3. Severe abruption: Vaginal bleeding may be moderate, severe, or absent. Abdominal pain is severe. **The client may have a concealed placental abruption without vaginal bleeding.**

C. Uterine rupture: Vaginal bleeding is moderate, severe, or absent. The client may experience a sudden onset of extreme abdominal pain (commonly at the previous uterine scar site) or a cessation of uterine contractions. Recession of the fetal presenting part and maternal hypotension and tachycardia may occur.

D. Cervical insufficiency: a feeling of vaginal fullness or pressure; vaginal spotting or bleeding; an increased volume of watery, mucousy or brown vaginal discharge and vague discomfort in lower abdomen or back

Other Signs and Symptoms

A. External fetal monitor (EFM) tracings: exhibit characteristics associated with anemia or hypoxemia, such as decreased or absent variability, bradycardia, tachycardia, recurrent late or prolonged decelerations, or a sinusoidal pattern

B. Placenta previa: uterine resting tone usually relaxed. Fetal status at first exam is usually stable. Recurrence of bleeding is common. First bleeding episode in placenta previa is rarely significant. Second or third bleeding episode is often associated with significant vaginal bleeding.

C. Abruptio placentae: Rupture of membranes has bloody show with copious amounts of clear or greenish-brown fluid; the fluid is probably meconium-stained, which signifies fetal distress.

1. Marginal abruption: Uterine resting tone is usually relaxed. Fetal status on the fetal monitor at first exam is usually stable. Labor progresses rapidly with vaginal bleeding or large amounts of bloody show.

2. Moderate abruption: Uterine resting tone is hypertonic. At first exam, the fetus is usually alive. FHR may exhibit characteristics that are associated with hypoxemia or anemia such as decreased/absent variability, tachycardia, bradycardia, recurrent late or prolonged decelerations, or a sinusoidal pattern. Labor progresses rapidly with vaginal bleeding or large amounts of bloody show.

3. Severe abruption: Uterine resting tone is hypertonic or "board-like." At first exam, fetus may be dead. If fetus is alive, EFM is consistent with hypoxemia or anemia as listed above.

D. Uterine rupture: Uterine resting tone may be normal or hypertonic. At first exam, fetus may be dead or FHR pattern is consistent with hypoxemia or anemia as previously listed.

Subjective Data

A. Elicit information about onset, duration, and progression of vaginal bleeding. When did it start? Is it continuous bleeding, "like a period," or is it spotting?

B. Ask: How much bleeding has occurred? How many pads have been saturated? What is the size of the blood spots—the size of a quarter or a half dollar?

C. Elicit information regarding the presence or absence of abdominal pain. If present, review the onset, duration, and progression of pain. Is it a continuous discomfort or intermittent cramping? How severe is the pain? Did it have a sudden onset?

D. Is the client experiencing shoulder pain? This is likely to be referred pain from phrenic nerve irritation caused by intraperitoneal bleeding.

E. Elicit the first day of the client's last menstrual cycle, to date pregnancy. Has she had an US to confirm dating and placental location?

F. Ask the client if she feels the baby move and if the movement has been normal this day, if more than 18 weeks' gestation.

Physical Examination

A. Check temperature, pulse, respirations, and BP; peripheral oxygen saturation; urine output; and estimated blood loss. Continuous FHR monitoring is used for patterns suggestive of hypoxemia or anemia.

1. A pregnant client does not demonstrate signs and symptoms of hypovolemic shock until she has lost 30% of her circulating volume. Tachypnea, tachycardia, hypotension, low oxygen saturation, and air hunger are signs of hypovolemia.

2. Prepare the client for emergency transport to a hospital even if she is hemodynamically stable.

B. Inspect:

1. Inspect the client's general appearance related to discomfort and pain.

2. Observe bleeding characteristics and pooling.

C. Auscultate:

1. Auscultate the abdomen; check FHT, or EFM, for baseline and periodic FHR patterns. Verify FHR versus maternal heart rate.

2. Auscultate the maternal heart and lungs.

D. Palpate:

1. Check for palpable fetal parts on abdominal wall; note fetal movement.

2. Palpate the uterus for relaxed or hypertonic uterus. Check for contractions. If present, note frequency, duration, and intensity and resting tone to palpation.

E. **Pelvic exam:** perform sterile speculum exam to look for the source of bleeding. **Do not perform vaginal bimanual exam until placenta previa is ruled out.**

Diagnostic Tests

A. CBC and platelets

B. PT, PTT, and fibrinogen (fibrinogen levels have the best correlation with severity of bleeding)

C. Blood type, Rh status, and type and crossmatch if indicated

D. Fetal cell stain, Kleihauer–Betke test, or a flow cytometry test on a specimen of vaginal blood. Fetal cell stain can determine the amount of fetal blood in the maternal circulation.

E. Determine if RhoGAM is indicated.

F. Ultrasonography/BPP

G. NST/EFM

Differential Diagnoses

A. Placenta previa
B. Abruptio placentae
C. Uterine rupture or dehiscence
D. Ruptured vasa previa
E. Rupture of membranes
F. Normal bloody show associated with labor
G. Rectal hemorrhoidal bleeding
H. Cervical insufficiency

Plan

A. General interventions:
  1. Tocolysis may be considered if the client has no active hemorrhage and reassuring FHR pattern.
  2. If significant vaginal bleeding is present, the primary goal is to maintain oxygen delivery to the mother and fetus while preparing them for transport. Interventions include lateral maternal positioning to avoid vena caval compression; administering supplemental oxygen; initiating large-bore IV line; delivery of fluid bolus of normal saline or lactated Ringer's solution; keeping flow sheet of vital signs, assessments, actions, and responses; maintaining continuous recording of FHR and uterine activity on EFM; and providing emotional support and anticipatory guidance.
  3. If vaginal bleeding is minimal and home management is being considered, discuss risks with the client and assess her ability to modify her activity to avoid moderate or strenuous exercise, heavy lifting (greater than 20 pounds), or standing for prolonged periods (more than 4 hours). Also assess client's access to telephone and transportation in case of major bleeding episode. Consider the distance from the client's home to the nearest hospital.

▶ B. Client teaching: *See Section III: Client Teaching Guide "Vaginal Bleeding: Second and Third Trimesters."*

C. Pharmaceutical therapy:
  1. Tocolytics: In clients with contractions, tocolytics may be used while administering a course of betamethasone if bleeding is diminishing or has ceased and delivery is not otherwise mandated by the maternal or fetal condition. Tocolysis may reduce or eliminate uterine contractions which promote uterine separation and bleeding. Tocolytics should not be used in clients with active vaginal bleeding.
    a. Terbutaline sulfate (Brethine) 0.25 mg by subcutaneous injection every 15 minutes times three doses, if maternal heart rate less than 120
    b. Indomethacin is not used because of its inhibitory effect on platelet function.
    c. The client may be admitted to an inpatient antepartum unit for parenteral tocolysis such as magnesium sulfate, which has proven beneficial for fetal neuroprotection in patients with preterm (24–32 weeks' gestation) placenta previa in whom a decision has been made to deliver within 24 hours, but not emergently.
  2. Antenatal corticosteroids may be given if preterm delivery is a possibility within the next week and the estimated gestational age (EGA) is less than 34 weeks to enhance fetal pulmonary maturity. Additionally, a course of steroids may be given to women whose first bleed is at 34 0/7 to 36 6/7 weeks' gestation and who have not received a prior dose.
    a. Betamethasone 12 mg may be given by IM injection every 24 hours times two doses.
    b. Dexamethasone 6 mg IM may be given every 12 hours times four doses.
    c. A single "rescue" course of repeat antenatal steroids should be considered in women at less than 34 weeks' gestation whose prior course was administered at least 7 days previously and who remain at risk of delivering.
  3. If the client is Rh-negative, give her RhoGAM IM by injection after the initial vaginal bleeding episode. Repeat administration is not necessary if bleeding occurs within 3 weeks of the previous dose. If repeated episodes of bleeding occur, the anti-D antibody can be checked. A low titer suggests that the anti-D level is sufficient to provide ongoing protection against alloimmunization.
  4. A Cesarean delivery is always indicated with sonographic evidence of a placenta previa and a viable fetus.

Follow-Up

A. Follow-up depends on client diagnosis and on whether client hospitalization is needed.

Emergent Issues/Instructions

A. **Call 911/go to the nearest ED for frank, bright-red bleeding.**

Consultation/Referral

A. Consult a physician for all clients noted to have second- and third-trimester vaginal bleeding.
B. Consult with a physician if the client has any frank, bright red bleeding, signs of fetal compromise, or maternal shock, or if the cause of bleeding cannot be determined and/or treated by the practitioner.

Bibliography

American College of Obstetricians and Gynecologists. (2014a). ACOG Practice Bulletin No. 145: Antepartum fetal surveillance (Reaffirmed 2016). *Obstetrics and Gynecology, 124*, 182–192. doi:10.1097/01. AOG.0000451759.90082.7b

Postpartum Breast Engorgement

Jill C. Cash, Susan Drummond, and Christina C. Reed

Definition

A. Breast engorgement is swollen, tender breasts caused by overfilling of milk, increased blood flow, and fluids in the breasts.

Incidence

A. Breast engorgement may affect 40% of postpartum mothers.

Pathogenesis

A. *Primary engorgement* is the result of distension and stasis of the vascular and lymphatic circulations occurring

2 to 4 days following delivery. It is prompted by the decrease in progesterone levels after the placenta is delivered.

B. *Secondary engorgement* is caused by distension of the lobules and alveoli with milk as lactation is established. It may occur from excessive stimulation of milk production via pumping, taking medications to increase milk supply, or decreased milk extraction from not feeding the baby as often. Without stimulation by suckling and removal of milk, secretion of prolactin decreases and milk production decreases and finally ceases.

Predisposing Factors

A. Engorgement often develops if early feedings are not frequent enough, suckling is inadequate, or breastfeeding is not conducted in a relaxed atmosphere.

Common Complaints

A. Swollen, tender breasts
B. Discomfort when breastfeeding
C. A low-grade fever lasting between 4 and 16 hours

Other Signs and Symptoms

A. Pain, tenderness, and redness in one area of the breast is associated with mastitis.
B. Physical examination should not be focused just on breast symptoms but should include a general ruling out of other potential problems, such as coexistent UTI.

Subjective Data

A. Elicit onset, duration, and course of symptoms. Review the frequency of breastfeeding and/or use of breast pump. Is the client still breastfeeding, or has she stopped because of the discomfort?
B. Exclude other causes of fever, such as UTI, wound infection, and red streaks on one or both breasts, to rule out mastitis.
C. Quantify pain symptoms and relief measures, including heat packs, ice packs, breast binder, and analgesics such as Tylenol.

Physical Examination

A. Check temperature, BP, and pulse.
B. Inspect:
    1. Examine the breasts for erythemic streaks.
    2. Check episiotomy or abdominal incision, if indicated.
C. Palpate:
    1. Examine the breasts for tenderness, hardness, warmth, and lumps.
    2. Palpate axilla for lymphadenopathy.
    3. Check back for CVA tenderness.

Diagnostic Tests

A. Tests generally are not indicated for breast engorgement.
B. Urine culture or wound culture, if applicable

Differential Diagnoses

A. Mastitis
B. Cellulitis
C. Breast pain

Plan

A. General interventions:
    1. Encourage the client to take analgesics prior to breastfeeding and continue breastfeeding.
    2. Encourage ice packs for discomfort and frequent breastfeeding. There should be *no stimulation* to the breasts other than that provided by the baby when nursing, and the client should take analgesics for discomfort. Reassure her that engorgement is temporary and usually resolves within 24 to 48 hours.
B. Client teaching: *See Section III: Client Teaching Guide* ◄ *"Postpartum Breast Engorgement."*
    1. Educate the client regarding milk production.
    2. Advise the client to breastfeed frequently to reduce chances of engorgement.
    3. Provide reassurance and support for the client to continue breastfeeding through this temporary period of discomfort. Engorgement may last 2 to 3 days before milk supply meets demand; continuation of breastfeeding will resolve discomfort and problem.
C. Pharmaceutical therapy:
    1. Acetaminophen (Tylenol) two tablets 500 to 1,000 mg every 4 to 6 hours or ibuprofen 400 to 600 mg orally 30 to 45 minutes prior to breastfeeding and as needed

Follow-Up

A. Follow-up may not be required for engorgement.
B. Lactation consultation if indicated

Individual Considerations

A. Pregnancy loss: It is imperative to discuss breast care and engorgement with women who have a second-trimester termination of pregnancy, have a stillbirth, or experience a neonatal loss.

Bibliography

Breastfeeding Expert Work Group, Committee on Obstetric Practice, American College of Obstetricians and Gynecologists. (2018). ACOG Committee Opinion 756: Optimizing support for breastfeeding as part of obstetric practice. *Obstetrics & Gynecology, 132*(4), e187–e196. doi:10.1097/AOG.0000000000002890

Iams, J. D. (2014). Identification of candidates for progesterone: Why, who, how, and when? *Obstetrics and Gynecology, 123*(6), 1317–1326. doi:10.1097/AOG.0000000000000276

Endometritis

Jill C. Cash, Susan Drummond, and Christina C. Reed

Definition

A. Endometritis is an infection of the endometrium (the interior lining of the uterus) that occurs postpartum. Endometritis is the most common cause of puerperal fever in obstetrics.

Incidence

A. The incidence of endometritis has been noted to be as high as 38.5% after Cesarean section; the incidence is 1.2% after vaginal delivery.

Pathogenesis

A. During labor and delivery, indigenous cervicovaginal flora enter the uterine cavity. Onset is usually 3 to 5 days after delivery, unless it is caused by beta-hemolytic *Streptococcus*, in which case the onset is earlier and more precipitous. Infection is usually polymicrobial in nature. Undiagnosed or unsuccessfully treated infection of the endomyometrium can progress to involve the entire uterus and may spread to accessory pelvic structures. The main pathway for spread of the infection is the broad ligament. Sources of bacteria may be any one or a combination of the following:

1. Indigenous vaginal bacteria, usually pathogenic only when tissue is damaged:
   a. Beta-hemolytic *Streptococcus*
   b. *Streptococcus viridans*
   c. *Neisseria gonorrhoeae*
   d. *Gardnerella*
2. Contamination by normal bowel bacteria:
   a. *Clostridium perfringens*
   b. *E. coli*
   c. *Proteus mirabilis*
   d. *Aerobacter aerogenes*
   e. *Enterococcus*
   f. *Pseudomonas aeruginosa*
   g. *K. pneumoniae*
3. Contamination from environment; staphylococcus is a common organism.

Predisposing Factors

A. Operative delivery: Cesarean section is the major predisposing factor for pelvic infection. The most important determinant of infection for clients undergoing Cesarean delivery is the duration of labor.
B. Intrapartum: Prolonged rupture of membranes, numerous vaginal exams in labor, use of internal monitoring devices during labor, use of instruments in delivery, prolonged labor, and intrauterine manipulation such as internal rotation or manual removal of placenta can all lead to endometritis.
C. Postpartum: Retained placental fragments or membranes, improper perineal care, and host resistance also predispose a client to infection.
D. Anemia: This condition probably represents a marker for poor nutrition.
E. Obesity

Common Complaints

A. "Feeling ill" with fever or chills
B. Muscle aches
C. Headache
D. Uterine pain and tenderness
E. Foul-smelling lochia

Other Signs and Symptoms

A. Fever (100.4°F–104.0°F)
B. Subinvolution
C. Uterus may be atonic
D. Abnormalities of lochia:
   1. May be scant and odorless if anaerobic infection
   2. May be moderately heavy, foul, bloody, or seropurulent if aerobic infection
E. Tachycardia

Subjective Data

A. Elicit onset, duration, and course of symptoms.
B. Review the color, odor, and amount of lochia.
C. Review the client's pain or discomfort and the relief measures used.
D. Review other body symptoms to rule out other infections such as UTI, breast engorgement, or mastitis.
E. Review labor and delivery events for complications (see section "Predisposing Factors").

Physical Examination

A. Check temperature, pulse, and BP: The client may be tachycardic with heart rate 100 to 140 bpm.
B. Inspect:
   1. Observe color, amount, and odor of lochia.
   2. Check abdominal incision, if applicable.
   3. Check the perineum for lacerations, breakdown of incision, redness, and drainage.
C. Auscultate:
   1. Heart
   2. Lungs
D. Palpate:
   1. Abdomen: check uterine tenderness.
   2. Back: check CVA tenderness.
E. Pelvic exam:
   1. Speculum exam: inspect the cervix for lacerations, drainage, or redness
   2. Bimanual exam: check for cervical motion tenderness; palpate adnexa for masses and tenderness; note "heat" of the pelvis.

Diagnostic Tests

A. CBC with differential
B. Blood and urine cultures
C. Cervical cultures, to rule out an STI, if indicated
D. Wet mount, to rule out bacterial vaginosis and candidal vaginitis, if indicated

Differential Diagnoses

A. STIs, such as chlamydia, gonorrhea, or trichomoniasis
B. Septic pelvic thrombophlebitis
C. UTI/pyelonephritis
D. Pneumonitis
E. Extreme breast engorgement secondary to abrupt weaning causing maternal reabsorption of milk
F. Wound infection

Plan

A. General interventions:
   1. Instruct on proper hygiene. Teach the client proper techniques to prevent infection (perineal area, incision site, breast).
   2. Acetaminophen (Tylenol) for fever as needed
B. Client teaching: *See Section III: Client Teaching Guide "Endometritis."* ◄
C. Pharmaceutical therapy:
   1. Outpatient setting antibiotic therapy compatible with breastfeeding:
      a. Clindamycin 600 mg orally every 6 hours for 14 days PLUS gentamicin 4.5 mg/kg intramuscularly every 24 hours for 48 to 72 hours

b. Clindamycin 600 mg orally every 6 hours for 14 days PLUS amoxicillin-clavulanic acid 875 mg orally every 12 hours

c. Suspected clindamycin resistance per geographic region: ampicillin-sulbactam 1.5 g every 6 hours for 14 days

d. GBS colonizer in pregnancy: add ampicillin 500 mg orally every 6 hours for 14 days to the clindamycin PLUS gentamicin regimen OR use ampicillin-sulbactam 1.5 g every 6 hours for 14 days alone.

e. Penicillin allergy: use vancomycin 500 mg orally every 6 hours for 14 days instead of ampicillin.

2. Inpatient setting antibiotic therapy:

a. If uterus is boggy and/or bleeding is excessive: methylergonovine maleate (Methergine) 0.2 mg orally every 4 hours for six doses. (Do not give if the client is hypertensive.)

b. IV clindamycin 900 mg every 8 hours PLUS gentamicin 1.5 mg/kg every 8 hours OR 5 mg/kg every 24 hours till client clinical improvement and afebrile for at least 24 to 48 hours

c. Suspected clindamycin resistance and/or GBS colonizer during pregnancy: IV ampicillin-sulbactam 1.5 g every 6 hours till client clinical improvement and afebrile for at least 24 to 48 hours

Follow-Up
A. Call the client in 24 to 48 hours to evaluate her status.

Emergent Issues/Instructions
A. **Instruct the client to call immediately or go to the ED if symptoms do not resolve within 24 hours or if they worsen.**

Consultation/Referral
A. Consult with physician if symptoms do not resolve, if they worsen within 24 hours, or if the client's temperature does not go below 100.0°F after 48 hours on antibiotics. If no significant improvement is seen within 2 to 3 days, the client may need to be admitted to the hospital.

Bibliography
American College of Obstetricians and Gynecologists. (2018). ACOG Practice Bulletin No. 198: Prevention and management of obstetric lacerations at vaginal delivery. *Obstetrics and Gynecology, 132*(3), e87–e102. doi:10.1097/AOG.0000000000002841

Breastfeeding Expert Work Group, Committee on Obstetric Practice, American College of Obstetricians and Gynecologists. (2018). ACOG Committee Opinion 756: Optimizing support for breastfeeding as part of obstetric practice. *Obstetrics & Gynecology, 132*(4), e187–e196. doi:10.1097/AOG.0000000000002890

Catalano, P. (2007). Management of obesity in pregnancy. *Obstetrics and Gynecology, 109*(2 Pt 1), 419–433. doi:10.1097/01.AOG.0000253311.44696.85

Chen, K. (2018, July 24). Postpartum endometritis. In Barss V. A. (Ed.), *UpToDate*. Retrieved from https://www.uptodate.com/contents/postpartum-endometritis

Mastitis

Jill C. Cash, Susan Drummond, and Christina C. Reed

Definition
A. Mastitis is an infection of breast tissue with potential for abscess formation.

Incidence
A. Mastitis has been estimated to occur in 2% to 10% of breastfeeding mothers. Less than 1% of these require hospitalization. Symptoms seldom appear before the end of the first week postpartum and are most often seen during the first 2 months postpartum.

Pathogenesis
A. During the period of lactation, the breast changes from an essentially nonfunctioning organ to a complex functioning organ of the body. The developing multiductal system becomes a rich environment for the growth of bacteria. The most common offending organism is *Staphylococcus aureus* (95%). The immediate source of the organisms that causes mastitis is almost always the nursing infant's nose and mouth.

Predisposing Factors
Invasion of bacteria in the presence of breast injury, including:
A. Bruising from rough manipulation (pumping) or failing to break the neonate's attachment to the areola and nipple before removing from breast
B. Prolonged breast engorgement
C. Milk stasis in a duct
D. Cracking or fissures of the nipple
E. Poor handwashing

Common Complaints
A. Breast engorgement, usually bilateral
B. Pain in the breast, usually unilateral
C. Fever
D. Red streak(s)
E. Flu-like symptoms: body aches, headache, malaise, and chills

Other Signs and Symptoms
A. Fever 100.0°F to 104.0°F, rapid rise
B. Exquisitely tender breast tissue
C. Hard mass in the breast
D. Tachycardia and tachypnea
E. Axillary lymphadenopathy

Subjective Data
A. Elicit the onset, duration, and course of symptoms.
B. Note the frequency and length of time of the feeding or pumping.
C. Are there any red streaks on the breasts?
D. Are the nipples cracked and bleeding?
E. Quantify pain symptoms, relief measures tried, and results.
F. Review other symptoms to rule out other infections, such as wound infection, episiotomy breakdown, and UTI.

Physical Examination
A. Check temperature and BP, pulse, and respirations.
B. Physical exam should not be focused just on breast symptoms but should include a general ruling out of other potential problems, such as coexistent UTI or endometritis.
C. Inspect:
1. Visually inspect breasts.
2. Perform breast exam.

3. Check episiotomy or abdominal incision to rule out infection.
D. Auscultate:
  1. Heart
  2. Lungs
E. Palpate:
  1. Perform breast exam. Observe breastfeeding for adequacy of latch, suck, swallow, jaw glide, and any clicking.
  2. Palpate lymph nodes of the neck and axilla.
  3. Palpate the abdomen.
  4. Check CVA tenderness.

Diagnostic Tests

A. Treatment usually initiated based on symptoms and exam
B. CBC: leukocytosis in peripheral smear
C. WBC, culture, and sensitivity of breast milk to identify bacteria for persistent signs of infection or if antibiotic treatment is unsuccessful
D. Urine or wound cultures, if applicable
E. US considered if breast is not responding to treatment to evaluate for breast abscess

Differential Diagnoses

A. Breast engorgement: bilateral presentation of breast discomfort
B. Breast abscess: discharge of purulent exudate from nipple, masses, or reddened areas that develop a bluish hue of the skin over the area of abscess
C. Clogged milk duct
D. Viral syndrome
E. Inflammatory breast cancer

Plan

A. General interventions
  1. Encourage self-care and support. Advise the family to assist the client with self-care and infant care during this acute period. The woman may feel extremely ill for the first 24 to 48 hours of therapy and may find it difficult to continue breastfeeding, as well as perform self-care and newborn care activities.
B. Client teaching:
  1. *See Section III: Client Teaching Guide "Mastitis."*
  2. Advise the client to continue to breastfeed or pump to maintain milk supply.
  3. Stress the importance of continuation of breastfeeding or pumping despite infection.
C. Pharmaceutical therapy:
  1. Antibiotics:
    a. Nonsevere with no methicillin-resistant *S. aureus* (MRSA) risk factors: dicloxacillin 500 mg orally every 6 hours OR cephalexin 500 mg orally every 6 hours for 10 to 14 days to reduce relapse; however, 5 to 7 days can be used if rapid response occurs. If beta-lactam hypersensitive: clindamycin 300 mg orally every 8 hours
    b. Nonsevere with MRSA risk factors: clindamycin 300 mg orally every 8 hours. Trimethoprim-sulfamethoxazole (breastfeeding toxicity) one double-strength tablet orally every 12 hours

    c. Severe: vancomycin 15 to 20 mg/kg/dose every 8 to 12 hours, not to exceed 2 g per dose depending on breast milk and blood culture results
  2. Advise the client to complete the full course of antibiotics even if symptoms are improved sooner.
  3. Candidal vaginitis may develop secondary to antibiotic therapy. The client should be aware of the signs, symptoms, and treatment plan if it should occur.
  4. Acetaminophen (Tylenol) or ibuprofen for pain management
  5. The client may require pain medication if acetaminophen (Tylenol) or ibuprofen is not effective. Use acetaminophen with codeine phosphate (Tylenol No. 3) or other narcotic as needed for pain.
D. Dietary management:
  1. There are no dietary restrictions.
  2. Have the client increase fluid intake with increased temperature (at least 10–12 glasses a day).
  3. Encourage her to eliminate caffeine, if possible, or use in moderation.

Follow-Up

A. Evaluate the client in 48 hours if a breast abscess is suspected; assess need for surgical consultation.

Consultation/Referral

A. Consult a physician if a breast abscess is suspected, for persistent signs of infection, or if antibiotic treatment is unsuccessful. Treatment of a breast abscess may include surgical incision and drainage of the abscess.
B. Notify the pediatrician if mastitis is diagnosed.

Bibliography

Breastfeeding Expert Work Group, Committee on Obstetric Practice, American College of Obstetricians and Gynecologists. (2018). ACOG Committee Opinion 756: Optimizing support for breastfeeding as part of obstetric practice. *Obstetrics & Gynecology, 132*(4), e187–e196. doi:10.1097/AOG.0000000000002890

Postpartum Depression

Jill C. Cash, Susan Drummond, and Christina C. Reed

Definition

A. Postpartum depression is a mood disorder characterized by unexplained tearfulness, sadness, irritability, and disturbances in appetite and sleep patterns, as well as an inability to care for self or baby, usually presenting within 2 weeks to 3 months postpartum.

Incidence

A. Reported incidence in the United States is between 8% and 15%.

Pathogenesis

A. It is believed that postpartum depression may be related to psychological, physiologic, and cultural factors. The extreme hormonal changes that occur during the postpartum period may contribute. Postpartum thyroiditis is also a suspected factor. However, no confirmed biologic cause has been found. Some authorities have suggested that the mother's feeling of "loss of control" over her own life is the underlying precipitating factor.

Predisposing Factors

The following may make a mother more likely to experience postpartum depression:
A. Preterm infant
B. Multiple gestation
C. Maternal and/or fetal complications in pregnancy
D. History of postpartum depression or mental health conditions
E. Social stressors: dissatisfaction in the marriage, financial difficulties, and lack of support at home
F. Age younger than 20 years
G. Single parent
H. Poor relationship with the father of the baby
I. Evidence of significant emotional problems in the past
J. Having experienced separation from one or both parents during childhood or adolescence
K. Having received poor parental support and attention in childhood or having limited social support in adulthood
L. Low self-esteem

Common Complaints

A. Insomnia
B. Poor appetite
C. Tearfulness
D. Fatigue
E. Anxiety
F. Headaches
G. Difficulty concentrating or confusion
H. Feelings of excessive guilt or worthlessness
I. Possible suicidal ideations

Other Signs and Symptoms

A. Mood swings
B. Despondency, social withdrawal, and feeling of inadequacy
C. Guilt
D. Impaired memory
E. Ambivalence about motherhood and baby
F. Inability to care for self and baby
G. Poor grooming of self and/or baby

Subjective Data

A. Elicit onset, duration, and course of symptoms.
B. Review the client's medical history for predisposing factors.
C. Question the client regarding her ability to care for her infant, herself, and other family members at home.
D. Review the amount of support in the home. Is she the primary caregiver? Are there any family members or friends who help in household management, sibling child care, and newborn care?
E. Does the client get out of bed and dress herself daily?
F. Does the client have thoughts of harming the infant, herself, or others?

Physical Examination

A. Check temperature (if indicated), pulse, respirations, and BP.
B. Inspect:
  1. Note general overall appearance, including dress, makeup, neatness of hair, tearfulness, and apathy.
  2. Observe her interaction with the baby, for example, talking to the baby and tone of voice, eye contact, and so on.
C. Postpartum examination (see Exhibit 13.1)

Diagnostic Tests

A. The EPDS should be completed at every postpartum visit (see Exhibit 13.2). The EPDS is available for download at www.fresno.ucsf.edu/pediatrics/downloads/edinburghscale.pdf.
  1. Scoring:
    a. Add up the numbers associated with the answer that was underlined.
    b. If the total is above 10 then possible depression exists; advise client to seek behavior health appointment.
    c. Always look at question 10 on suicidal thoughts; if the client answers anything other than "Never," advise behavior health appointment and assess if assistance is needed immediately.
B. If depression is diagnosed, a thyroid profile should be ordered.

Differential Diagnoses

A. Baby blues: tearfulness, insomnia, fatigue, headaches, poor appetite, and so on appearing between the birth and 14 postpartum days
B. Postpartum psychosis: extreme emotional lability, agitation, delusions, hallucinations, and sleep disturbances
C. Postpartum panic disorder: extreme anxiety, fear, tightness in the chest, and increased heart rate
D. Postpartum obsessive-compulsive disorder: obsessive thoughts of harming the child, exaggerated fear of being left alone with the infant, anxiety, depression, and/or unnecessarily vigilant protectiveness of the infant
E. Bipolar disorder

Plan

A. General interventions:
  1. Assess all clients for mood disorders at all postpartum points of contact telephonic or in person.
  2. Early assessment and treatment is very important. Symptoms that are not treated for several weeks may get progressively worse. Patients with severe depression, characterized by suicidal or homicidal ideation, aggressive behavior, delusions, hallucinations, catatonia, poor judgment, or grossly impaired functioning, are typically hospitalized.
  3. Encourage involvement of the client's partner and immediate family members in the counseling sessions to assist them in learning ways to assist the client effectively.
  4. If postpartum depression is diagnosed, perform serum thyroid levels.

B. Client teaching:

1. Advise the client that she is not to blame for the condition, that it is not uncommon, and that successful treatment is likely.

2. Discuss participation in a support group, interpersonal psychotherapy, and cognitive behavioral therapy.

3. If antidepressants are prescribed, advise the client that the medication may take 4 to 6 weeks for peak effect. Review benefits/risks/side effects of the medication prescribed. The risk of suicide may increase after beginning antidepressants; therefore, a follow-up appointment in 1 to 2 weeks is recommended.

C. Pharmaceutical therapy:

1. Antidepressants may be ordered for women with moderate to severe symptoms of depression when physical and emotional functioning has been compromised. (Refer to the section "Depression" in Chapter 22, Psychiatric Guidelines.)

2. Base selection of medication on whether or not the client is breastfeeding. Selective serotonin reuptake inhibitors (SSRIs) and tricyclic antidepressants are commonly used and generally considered safe for breastfeeding infants.

a. Citalopram (Lexapro) in a single daily dose, usually taken in the morning. Initial dose 10 mg/d; dosage can be increased at intervals of 1 week to 20 mg. Excreted in breast milk; potential toxicity. Consider the risks and benefits before starting the medication while breastfeeding.

b. Sertraline (Zoloft) 50 mg in a single dose at bedtime. Dosage can be increased by 25 mg at 1 week intervals and not to exceed 200 mg/d. Enters into breast milk; potential toxicity. Use caution while breastfeeding.

c. Amitriptyline (Elavil) 75 mg/d in divided doses. Dosage can be increased up to 150 mg/d. Potential toxicity; not recommended while breastfeeding

Follow-Up

A. If the client had risk factors for depression noted prior to delivery, a follow-up office visit 3 to 4 days after hospital discharge is suggested.

EXHIBIT 13.1 Postpartum Examination

Date: _____

History: Age: _____ G _____ PT _____ P _____ A _____ L _____

Labs: Blood type and Rh: _____ If negative, was RhoGAM workup done and RhoGAM given in the hospital, if needed? _____

Rubella: _____ If nonimmune, was she immunized before hospital discharge? _____

Discharge Hct: _____

Medical and antepartum complications: _____

Intrapartum course/complications: _____

Delivery: Date: _____ Type: _____ Sex: _____ Birth weight: _____

Apgars: 1 minute: _____ 5 minutes: _____ Neonatal: Gestational age: _____

Complications: _____

Feeding: Breast/bottle: _____ Current infant status: _____

Surgery: BTL: Yes/No _____

If yes, pathology report reviewed: Postpartum complications: _____

Current status: Medical problems: _____

Sexual intercourse since delivery/problems: _____

Psychosocial/postpartum depression: _____

Medications: _____

Physical exam: BP: _____ Pulse: _____ Resp: _____ Weight: _____

Breasts: _____

Pelvic: Episiotomy or laceration: _____

Abdomen: _____

Adnexa: _____

Uterus: _____

Vagina: _____

Cervix: _____

Pap smear: Date/results: _____

Plan: Current contraception and desired contraception: _____

Referrals: Labs: _____

New prescriptions: _____

Client teaching guides: _____

Pap smear follow-up: _____

Well-woman exam with breast exam follow-up: _____

Other: _____

Signature: _____

BTL, bilateral tubal ligation; Hct, hematocrit; RhoGAM, Rho(D) immune globulin.

B. Frequent telephone contact, or several repeat visits, may be necessary during the course of the depression until the symptoms have improved.

C. The risk of suicide may increase after beginning antidepressants; therefore, a follow-up appointment in 1 to 2 weeks is recommended.

D. Assess the client for suicidal ideation and child neglect at every contact.

Consultation/Referral

A. Assess the need to refer the client to a psychiatrist, psychologist, or family counselor.

B. Refer to group therapy, interpersonal psychotherapy, and/or cognitive behavioral therapy.

C. Consult a psychiatrist about alternative treatments if no change in signs and symptoms is seen.

Resources

Pacific Post Partum Support Society: www.postpartum.org

Postpartum Support International: www.postpartum.net or 1-800-944-4773

Postpartum Support Line: (604) 255-7999

EXHIBIT 13.2 Edinburgh Postnatal Depression Scale

Name: _____   Address: _____

_____   Your Date of Birth: _____

Baby's Date of Birth: _____   Phone: _____

As you are pregnant or have recently had a baby, we would like to know how you are feeling. Please check the answer that comes closest to how you have felt **IN THE PAST 7 DAYS**, not just how you feel today.

Here is an example, already completed.

I have felt happy:

• Yes, all the time	
• Yes, most of the time	This would mean "I have felt happy most of the time" during the past week.
• No, not very often	Please complete the other questions in the same way.
• No, not at all	

In the past 7 days:

1. I have been able to laugh and see the funny side of things
   - As much as I always could
   - Not quite so much now
   - Definitely not so much now
   - Not at all

2. I have looked forward with enjoyment to things
   - As much as I ever did
   - Rather less than I used to
   - Definitely less than I used to
   - Hardly at all

3. I have blamed myself unnecessarily when things went wrong
   - Yes, most of the time
   - Yes, some of the time
   - Not very often
   - No, never

4. I have been anxious or worried for no good reason
   - No, not at all
   - Hardly ever
   - Yes, sometimes
   - Yes, very often

5. I have felt scared or panicky for no very good reason
   - Yes, quite a lot
   - Yes, sometimes
   - No, not much
   - No, not at all

6. Things have been getting on top of me
   - Yes, most of the time I haven't been able to cope at all
   - Yes, sometimes I haven't been coping as well as usual

(*continued*)

EXHIBIT 13.2 Edinburgh Postnatal Depression Scale *(continued)*

- No, most of the time I have coped quite well
- No, I have been coping as well as ever

7. I have been so unhappy that I have had difficulty sleeping
   - Yes, most of the time
   - Yes, sometimes
   - Not very often
   - No, not at all

8. I have felt sad or miserable
   - Yes, most of the time
   - Yes, quite often
   - Not very often
   - No, not at all

9. I have been so unhappy that I have been crying
   - Yes, most of the time
   - Yes, quite often
   - Only occasionally
   - No, never

10. The thought of harming myself has occurred to me
    - Yes, sometimes
    - Sometimes
    - Hardly ever
    - Never

Administered/Reviewed by: _____   Date: _____

Instructions for using the Edinburgh Postnatal Depression Scale:

A. The mother is asked to check the response that comes closest to how she has been feeling in the previous 7 days.
B. All the items must be completed.
C. Care should be taken to avoid the possibility of the mother discussing her answers with others. (Answers come from the mother or pregnant woman.)
D. The mother should complete the scale herself, unless she has limited English or has difficulty with reading.

Scoring
QUESTIONS 1, 2, and 4 (without an *) are scored 0, 1, 2, or 3, with top box scored as 0 and the bottom box scored as 3.
QUESTIONS 3, 5–10 (marked with an *) are reverse scored, with the top box scored as a 3 and the bottom box scored as 0.
• Maximum score: 30
• Possible depression: 10 or greater
• Always look at item 10 (suicidal thoughts)

EPDS, Edinburgh Postnatal Depression Scale.

Sources: Cox, J. L., Holden, J. M., & Sagovsky, R. (1987). Detection of postnatal depression: Development of the 10-item Edinburgh Postnatal Depression Scale. **British Journal of Psychiatry, 150**, 782–786. doi: 10.1192/bjp.150.6.782; Wisner, K. L., Parry, B. L., & Piontek, C. M. (2002, July 18). Postpartum depression. **New England Journal of Medicine, 347** (3), 194–199. doi: 10.1056/NEJMcp011542; Edinburgh Postnatal Depression Scale (n.d.). Retrieved from www.fresno.ucsf.edu/pediatrics/downloads/edinburghscale.pdf.

Postpartum depression is the most common complication of childbearing. The 10-question EPDS is a valuable and efficient way of identifying clients at risk for "perinatal" depression. The EPDS is easy to administer and has proven to be an effective screening tool. Mothers who score above 13 are likely to be suffering from a depressive illness of varying severity. The EPDS score should not override clinical judgment. A careful clinical assessment should be carried out to confirm the diagnosis. The scale indicates how the mother has felt *during the previous week*. In doubtful cases it may be useful to repeat the tool after 2 weeks. The scale will not detect mothers with anxiety neuroses, phobias, or personality disorders.

Women with postpartum depression need not feel alone. They may find useful information on the websites of the Office on Women's Health <www.womenshealth.gov/mental-health/mental-health-conditions/postpartum-depression>, and from groups such as Postpartum Support International <www.postpartum.net> and Postpartum Depression.org <www.postpartumdepression.org>.

Bibliography

Breastfeeding Expert Work Group, Committee on Obstetric Practice, American College of Obstetricians and Gynecologists. (2018). ACOG Committee Opinion 756: Optimizing support for breastfeeding as part of obstetric practice. *Obstetrics & Gynecology, 132*(4), e187–e196. doi:10.1097/AOG.0000000000002890

Cox, J. L., Holden, J. M., & Sagovsky, R. (1987). Detection of postnatal depression: Development of the 10-item Edinburgh postnatal depression scale. *British Journal of Psychiatry, 150*, 782–786. doi:10.1192/bjp.150.6.782

Edinburgh Postnatal Depression Scale. (n.d.). Retrieved from www.fresno.ucsf.edu/pediatrics/downloads/edinburghscale.pdf

Kennerley, H., & Gath, D. (1989). Maternity blues. I. Detection and measurement by questionnaire. *British Journal of Psychiatry*, 155, 356–362. Retrieved from http://bjp.rcpsych.org/content/155/3/356.long

Marchesi, D., Bertoni, S., & Maggini, C. (2009). Major and minor depression in pregnancy. *Obstetrics and Gynecology*, 113(6), 1292–1298. doi:10.1097/AOG.0b013e3181a45e90

Viguera, A. (2016, November 9). Postpartum unipolar major depression: Epidemiology, clinical features, assessment, and diagnosis. In D. Solomon (Ed.), *UpToDate*. Retrieved from https://www.uptodate.com/contents/postpartum-unipolar-major-depression-epidemiology-clinical-features-assessment-and-diagnosisl

Webber, E., & Benedict, J. (2019). Postpartum depression: A multidisciplinary approach to screening, management and breastfeeding support. *Archives of Psychiatric Nursing*, 33(3), 284–289. https://doi-org.proxy.library.vanderbilt.edu/10.1016/j.apnu.2019.01.008

Secondary Postpartum Hemorrhage

Jill Cash and Susan Drummond

Definition
A. Secondary postpartum hemorrhage is defined as blood loss of 500 mL or more after the first 24 hours of delivery and within 6 to 12 weeks of delivery.

Incidence
A. Incidence is approximately 0.5% to 2% of women in developed countries.

Pathogenesis
A. Hemorrhage may result from retained placental fragments, subinvolution of the uterus, intrauterine infection, or inherited coagulation defects.

Predisposing Factors
A. Abnormally adherent placenta
B. Prolonged rupture of membranes leading to infection
C. Overdistended uterus from multiple gestation and/or polyhydramnios
D. Hematoma

Common Complaints
A. Heavy red bleeding or slow reddish-brown oozing
B. Abdominal pain
C. Loss of appetite
D. Fatigue; cannot get enough rest and is unable to complete self-care and infant care activities

Other Signs and Symptoms
A. Lochia rubra is bright-red discharge immediately after delivery (1–3 days) and may contain a few small clots. A continuous trickle of bright-red blood suggests a laceration of the cervix or vagina. Saturation of one peri-pad in less than 15 minutes (two pads in 30 minutes, or rapid pooling of blood under the buttocks) is considered excessive bleeding and requires immediate attention.
B. Foul odor: Lochia should not be malodorous. Lochia usually has a "fleshy" odor.
C. Boggy uterus: Check the consistency of the uterus, whether it is firm or boggy. If atony is present, support the lower uterine segment and massage the uterus or do bimanual compression.
D. Faintness
E. Tachycardia
F. Hypotension

Subjective Data
A. Elicit onset, duration, and course of symptoms.
B. Elicit the amount and color of lochia, including size of blood clot(s).
C. Review symptoms of infection, including fever and malodorous lochia.
D. Review labor and delivery events, including the date of delivery, use of forceps or vacuum, weight of baby, manual removal of placenta, complications, and postpartum course.
E. Review pregnancy for predisposing factors such as multiple gestation and polyhydramnios (as previously noted).

Physical Examination
A. Check temperature, BP, pulse, and respirations.
B. Inspect:
   1. Note color and amount of vaginal bleeding. Lochia may appear heavier when the woman first stands up because the lochia pools in the vagina while she is recumbent. Once the pooled blood is discharged, lochial flow should return to normal.
   2. Inspect episiotomy or abdominal incision.
C. Palpate:
   1. Check for consistency of uterus, massaging uterus if boggy.
   2. Express clots, if applicable.
   3. By 2 weeks postpartum, the uterus should have involuted and once again be a "pelvic organ."
   4. Check abdominal tension.
D. Pelvic exam:
   1. Speculum exam: Assess cervical lacerations.
   2. Bimanual exam: Rule out retroperitoneal hemorrhage.

Diagnostic Tests
A. CBC with differential
B. If bleeding is not under control, type and crossmatch blood
C. Coagulation test, if DIC is suspected
D. Blood cultures to rule out infection
E. Possible evaluation for a coagulation disorder such as von Willebrand disease

Differential Diagnoses
A. Late postpartum bleeding
B. Normal postpartum bleeding
C. Postpartum infection

Plan
A. General interventions:
   1. Perform uterine massage: support the lower uterine segment during massage to prevent uterine prolapse.
   2. Give IV hydration for hypovolemic shock: hypotension, tachycardia, and faintness.
   3. Hospitalization is usually required for postpartum hemorrhage.

B. Client teaching:
1. Encourage breastfeeding (if applicable) to increase uterine contraction.
2. Advise the client to rest and increase oral fluids.
C. Pharmaceutical therapy:
1. Drug of choice: methylergonovine maleate (Methergine) 0.2 mg orally every 4 hours for six doses. **Do not give if the client is hypertensive.**
2. For severe hemorrhage:
a. Oxytocin (Pitocin) 10 to 20 units in 250 mL to 1,000 mL IV fluids
b. Methylergonovine maleate (Methergine) 0.2 mg by IM injection, if the client has no history of hypertension. Advise the client to take full course of oral Methergine even if bleeding stops
c. **Hemabate: 250 mcg; may repeat every 15 to 90 minutes as needed**
d. Misoprostol (Cytotec, PGE1): 800 to 1,000 mcg, prolonged release (PR)
e. Continue bimanual compression and notify a physician.
3. If infection is suspected or confirmed, antibiotics are prescribed.

Follow-Up
A. Reevaluate the client 1 week from the date of discharge from the hospital.
B. Repeat Hct/CBC at postpartum visit.
C. The client may need iron replacement therapy, if not already prescribed. If stable at 1-week follow-up visit, have the client return in 4 to 6 weeks postpartum for routine postpartum exam.

Consultation/Referral
A. **Immediately consult or refer the client to a physician for possible hospitalization for D&C and/or blood product replacement.**

Bibliography
American College of Obstetricians and Gynecologists. (2017). ACOG Practice Bulletin, No. 183: Postpartum hemorrhage. *Obstetrics and Gynecology, 130*, e168–e186. doi:10.1097/AOG.0000000000002351

American College of Obstetricians and Gynecologists. (2018). ACOG Practice Bulletin No. 198: Prevention and management of obstetric lacerations at vaginal delivery. *Obstetrics and Gynecology, 132*(3), e87–e102. doi:10.1097/AOG.0000000000002841

Breastfeeding Expert Work Group, Committee on Obstetric Practice, American College of Obstetricians and Gynecologists. (2018). ACOG Committee Opinion 756: Optimizing support for breastfeeding as part of obstetric practice. *Obstetrics & Gynecology, 132*(4), e187–e196. doi:10.1097/AOG.0000000000002890

Wound Infection

Jill C. Cash, Susan Drummond, and Merita O'Sullivan

Definition
A. Infection may occur at the site of the Cesarean section incision, an episiotomy, or a genital tract laceration. Most wound infections become clinically apparent 5 to 6 days after delivery.

Incidence
A. Approximately 4% of clean wounds and 35% of grossly contaminated wounds become infected. Rates of infection after Cesarean delivery range from 5 to 30 times more than vaginal delivery. To reduce this risk, a single IV dose of a narrow-spectrum antibiotic (cefazolin, ampicillin) should be given within 60 minutes to all women undergoing a Cesarean section before making the skin incision. For women with a penicillin allergy, a dose of both clindamycin 900 mg and gentamycin 5 mg/kg IV can be used for prophylaxis.

Pathogenesis
A. A variety of organisms may be responsible. Examples include *Staphylococcus* or *Streptococcus* species and Gram-negative organisms, Gram-positive cocci and *Bacteroides, Clostridium* species, or *E. coli*.
B. Early wound infections, occurring in the first 24 to 48 hours, are usually caused by group A or B beta-hemolytic *Streptococcus* and are characterized by high fever and cellulitis.
C. Delayed infections are more likely caused by *Staphylococcus epidermidis* or *aureus, E. coli, P. mirabilis*, or cervicovaginal flora.

Predisposing Factors
A. Obesity
B. Anemia
C. Malnutrition
D. Smoking
E. Diabetes
F. Substance abuse
G. Immunosuppression
H. Poor hygiene
I. Lower socioeconomic status
J. Lack of preoperative prophylactic antibiotics
K. Chorioamnionitis
L. Blood transfusion
M. Anticoagulation therapy
N. Second-stage Cesarean section
O. Subcutaneous hematoma
P. Cardiovascular disease
Q. Previous surgery
R. Prior irradiation

Common Complaints
A. Redness, heat, swelling, and tenderness at site
B. Foul-smelling drainage
C. Elevated temperature

Other Signs and Symptoms
A. Fever and chills
B. Edema
C. Foul-smelling purulent discharge
D. Leukocytosis
E. Localized erythema, induration, and warmth at the incision site
F. Pain at the incision site
G. Wound separation

Subjective Data

A. Elicit onset, duration, and course of symptoms.

B. Review medical history (see section "Predisposing Factors"); antepartum history for complications such as diabetes; intrapartum complications for prolonged rupture of membranes, fever in labor, use of internal monitoring devices, length of labor, or frequent cervical examinations.

C. Question the client regarding hygiene at wound site since delivery, including the frequency of changing peripads, use of sitz baths, and showering.

D. Question the client regarding drainage from wound or episiotomy, noting color, amount, and odor.

E. Review signs and symptoms of breast engorgement and UTI.

F. Review vaginal delivery for third- and fourth-degree episiotomy or laceration. Third- and fourth-degree vaginal lacerations/episiotomies have approximately a 25% incidence of wound breakdown and a 20% incidence of wound infection. In comparison, the incidence of infection in all types of perineal wounds is 0.1% to 5%.

Physical Examination

A. Check temperature, pulse, respirations, and BP.

B. **Examination should not be limited to the incision site. A complete physical is needed to evaluate breasts, lungs, hematomas, and concurrent UTIs.**

C. Inspect:
1. Examine the incision site (episiotomy or abdomen) for drainage, redness or edema, and intactness.

D. Auscultate:
1. Heart
2. Lungs

E. Percuss:
1. Back to assess CVA tenderness

F. Palpate:
1. Perform breast examination.
2. Palpate suture line (episiotomy or abdomen). Probe incision with cotton-tipped swab to evaluate for hematoma, cellulitis, and/or pus.
3. Palpate all abdominal quadrants.
4. Palpate the vagina to rule out concealed hematoma.

Diagnostic Tests

A. CBC with differential
B. Blood culture (optional)
C. Culture of infected area
D. Urinalysis, culture, and sensitivity, if indicated

Differential Diagnoses

A. Impending dehiscence. If serosanguinous drainage is noted after the first 24 hours, dehiscence is possible.

B. Episiotomy breakdown

Plan

A. General interventions:
1. The wound may need to be opened and cleaned.

2. For an infection at a Cesarean section site, wound irrigation and dressing changes several times a day may be necessary.

3. Home health referral may be needed.

B. Client teaching: *See Section III: Client Teaching Guide "Wound Infection."* ◄

C. Pharmaceutical therapy:

1. Topical antiseptic and antimicrobial agents (povidone-iodine, sodium hypochlorite, hydrogen peroxide) should be avoided since they may be toxic to fibroblasts and impede wound healing.

2. Empiric treatment is started using broad spectrum antibiotics with coverage of Gram-positive cocci from the skin as well as the expected flora at the wound site.

    a. Augmentin 875 mg twice a day for 7 to 10 days

    b. Clindamycin 450 mg every 6 hours for 7 to 10 days; safe for breastfeeding

    c. Cefoxitin 1 to 2 g by IM injection or IV infusion every 6 to 8 hours; safe for breastfeeding

3. Definitive antimicrobial treatment is guided by the clinical response of the client, results of the Gram stain and wound culture, and sensitivity, when available.

4. Acetaminophen (Tylenol) when required for elevated temperature

D. Dietary management:

1. No dietary restrictions are recommended; encourage the client to eat well-balanced meals. Increase protein in diet for wound healing.

2. Instruct the client to increase fluid intake; have her drink at least 10 to 12 glasses of liquid a day.

Follow-Up

A. Reevaluate the client in 48 hours to assess wound healing.

Consultation/Referral

A. **Consult a physician for evaluation and possible surgical closure.**

Bibliography

American College of Obstetricians and Gynecologists. (2018). ACOG Practice Bulletin No. 198: Prevention and management of obstetric lacerations at vaginal delivery. *Obstetrics and Gynecology, 132*(3), e87–e102. doi:10.1097/AOG.0000000000002841

Breastfeeding Expert Work Group, Committee on Obstetric Practice, American College of Obstetricians and Gynecologists. (2018). ACOG Committee Opinion 756: Optimizing support for breastfeeding as part of obstetric practice. *Obstetrics & Gynecology, 132*(4), e187–e196. doi:10.1097/AOG.0000000000002890

Catalano, P. (2007). Management of obesity in pregnancy. *Obstetrics and Gynecology, 109*(2 Pt 1), 419–433. doi:10.1097/01.AOG.0000253311.44696.85

Lewicky-Gaupp, C., Leader-Cramer, A., Johnson, L. L., Kenton, K., & Gossett, D. R. (2015, May). Wound complications after obstetric anal sphincter injuries. *Obstetrics and Gynecology, 125*(5), 1088–1093. doi:10.1097/AOG.0000000000000833

Martens, M. G., Kolrod, B. L., Faro, S., Maccato, M., & Hammill, H. (1995). Development of wound infection or separation after Cesarean delivery: Prospective evaluation of 2,431 cases. *Journal of Reproductive Medicine, 40*(3), 171–175.

Postpartum Exam

Jill C. Cash, Susan Drummond, and Christina C. Reed

History

A. Chart review:
1. Antepartum course, including prenatal laboratory data: Pap smear, cervical cultures, maternal blood type and Rh, rubella and syphilis screen, and CBC
2. Intrapartum course: length of labor, type of delivery, and any maternal complications
3. Neonatal course: gestational age, weight, length, cord gases, admission to normal or intensive care nursery, length of stay in the intensive care nursery, and any neonatal complications
4. Immediate postpartum course: postpartum recovery, any postpartum complications, laboratory data, and length of hospital stay

B. Interval history:
1. Number of weeks postpartum
2. General maternal health and well-being, including diet or appetite, bowel and bladder function, level of activity, sleep patterns, and pain or discomfort
3. Interval problems: calls to healthcare provider, visits to ED, fever, or illness
4. Adjustment and role adaptation to the baby: motherhood, fatherhood, sibling rivalry, psychosocial assessment of depression, family support, housing, or financial issues
5. Resumption of sexual activity: need to wait 40 days postdelivery, comfort measures used, and contraception use to prevent unplanned pregnancies
6. Family planning: previous method of contraception used, success of method, plans to resume contraception, and options for contraception
7. Status of infant: breastfeeding or bottle-feeding, consolability, sleep patterns, voiding, and stool patterns
8. Establishment of healthcare follow-up: pediatrician appointment, immunizations; referral to WIC, public health, and so on, if applicable, or follow-up with nurse practitioner or nurse-midwife

C. Review of relevant systems:
1. Breasts: cracked or sore nipples, clogged ducts, engorgement, mastitis; breast care practiced
2. Bladder function: stress incontinence, dysuria, urinary frequency, and flank pain
3. Bowel function: constipation; discomfort, especially if the client has a history of third- or fourth-degree laceration; relief measures used and results
4. Perineum: problems or discomfort at episiotomy site, problems with wound healing, and signs of infection
5. Lochia: duration, type, odor, presence of clots; or resumption of menses: date, duration, and amount
6. Abdomen: if Cesarean delivery, healing of wound, signs of infection; exercises initiated
7. Legs: varicosities, heat, swelling, and calf tenderness

Physical Examination

A. Weight, BP, pulse, respirations, and temperature (if indicated)
B. Inspect:
1. Breast exam: examine nipple integrity, masses, inflammation, and engorgement
2. Examine legs for varicosities and signs of thrombophlebitis.
3. Examine perineum, healing of episiotomy or lacerations, and abnormalities of Bartholin's gland.
4. Speculum exam: note lesions or lacerations of cervix and vagina, discharge, signs of infection; obtain Pap smear, if indicated.
C. Auscultate:
1. Heart
2. Lungs
D. Palpate:
1. Abdomen for tenderness, masses, involution of uterus
2. Examine Cesarean section and bilateral tubal ligation (if performed) incision for wound integrity and signs of infection.
E. Pelvic exam:
1. Check for abnormalities of cervix, uterus, adnexa; status of involution; presence of cystocele or rectocele; and vaginal muscle tone.
F. Rectovaginal exam:
1. Check for integrity of episiotomy or laceration if indicated

Diagnostic Tests

A. Pap smear, if indicated
B. CBC recommended if anemia or hemorrhage is documented or suspected
C. 75 g 2-hour GTT recommended if gestational diabetes is documented or suspected
D. Other tests as indicated if there were maternal or fetal complications

Plan

A. General interventions:
1. This visit may be the last contact the woman has with the healthcare delivery system for some time. The practitioner should evaluate any problems and provide appropriate consultations, referrals, interventions, counseling, and teaching.
2. Explain the necessity of a yearly gynecologic exam.
3. Encourage regular aerobic, abdominal, and Kegel exercises.
B. Client teaching:
1. Counsel the client on choice of contraception, including failure rates with typical use:
   a. Abstinence
   b. Tubal ligation/vasectomy
   c. Contraceptive implants
   d. IUDs
   e. Depo-Provera injection
   f. Oral contraceptives (OCs)
   g. Barrier methods: condoms, cervical caps, diaphragm

   h. Spermicides

   i.   Natural family planning, calendar method

2. Explain the benefits of a healthy diet, especially if the client is breastfeeding.

3. Discuss breastfeeding, if applicable; answer any questions and address concerns.

4. Instruct the client to communicate any breast changes to her provider, and explain the importance of yearly provider-performed breast exams during her well-woman visit.

5. Explain the benefits of an interpregnancy interval of 1 to 2 years.

C. Pharmaceutical therapy:

1. Contraception: review contraceptive methods with client, including benefits, risks, and side effects for each method. (See Chapter 14 Gynecological Guidelines for contraceptive methods and prescribing information.)

Follow-Up

A. Administer rubella vaccination if the client has non-immune status and administration of vaccine was missed in the hospital stay and she has not had unprotected intercourse since delivery.

B. If a woman's physical exam, laboratory, and Pap tests are normal, she does not require a physical for 1 year.

C. Establish a plan for the woman to obtain Pap smear results (follow-up phone call or letter with results). Adapt the Postpartum Examination sheet (Exhibit 13.1) to use for documentation in the client's chart.

Consultation/Referral

A. Schedule primary care provider appointments to address any chronic health conditions.

Bibliography

American College of Obstetricians and Gynecologists. (2018). ACOG Practice Bulletin No. 198: Prevention and management of obstetric lacerations at vaginal delivery. *Obstetrics and Gynecology, 132*(3), e87–e102. doi:10.1097/AOG.0000000000002841

Berens, P. (2018, October 25). Overview of the postpartum period: Physiology, complications, and maternal care. In V. A. Barss (Ed.), *UpToDate*. Retrieved from https://www.uptodate.com/contents/overview-of-the-postpartum-period-physiology-complications-and-maternal-care

Breastfeeding Expert Work Group, Committee on Obstetric Practice, American College of Obstetricians and Gynecologists. (2018). ACOG Committee Opinion 756: Optimizing support for breastfeeding as part of obstetric practice. *Obstetrics & Gynecology, 132*(4), e187–e196. doi:10.1097/AOG.0000000000002890

Butte, N., & Stuebe, A. (2018, October 3). Maternal nutrition during lactation. In A. G. Hoppin (Ed.), *UpToDate*. Retrieved from https://www.uptodate.com/contents/maternal-nutrition-during-lactation

Spencer, J. (2018, July 17). Common problems of breastfeeding and weaning. In A. G. Hoppin (Ed.), *UpToDate*. Retrieved from https://www.uptodate.com/contents/common-problems-of-breastfeeding-and-weaning

14 Gynecological Guidelines

Amenorrhea

Rhonda Arthur and Michelle Collins

Definition

Amenorrhea is the absence of menstruation when menses should occur. Amenorrhea is described as either primary or secondary.

A. Primary amenorrhea:
    1. No menses by age 14 years in the absence of growth or development of secondary sexual characteristics
    2. No menses by age 16 years regardless of the presence of normal growth and development with the appearance of secondary sexual characteristics

B. Secondary amenorrhea: No menses for 6 months in a woman who usually has normal menses, or for a length of time equal to three-cycle intervals in a woman with less-frequent cycles

Incidence

A. Amenorrhea, in a woman who has had menses, may occur during a woman's reproductive life. Amenorrhea that occurs as a result of agenesis of part of the reproductive system or a chromosomal anomaly is quite rare. See the following section for the incidence of each cause.

Pathogenesis

A. Physiologic: Pregnancy, breastfeeding, and menopause
B. Disorders of the central nervous system (hypothalamic): Hypothalamic amenorrhea, caused by a deficiency in pulsatile secretion of gonadotropin-releasing hormone (Gn-RH), is the most common cause of amenorrhea (28%). Common factors causing hypothalamic dysfunction include a stressful lifestyle (10%); excessive weight loss, as occurs in anorexia or bulimia (10%); extreme exercise; medications, such as hormones, as occurs sometimes in women using combined contraceptive methods, psychotropic drugs, or heroin; hypothyroidism (10%); and maladies such as Crohn's disease or systemic lupus erythematosus (SLE).
C. Disorders of the outflow tract or uterine target organ: Abnormalities of this nature are uncommon. Examples include Asherman's syndrome, which occurs as the result of the uterine lining being exposed to surgical instrumentation during surgical procedures such as dilation and curettage (D&C; the cause of 7% of amenorrhea); and agenesis or structural anomalies of the uterus, tubes, or vagina.
D. Disorders of the ovary: Examples include abnormal chromosomal syndromes such as Turner's syndrome (0.5%); conditions such as gonadal dysgenesis or agenesis, which are the cause 10% of the time; premature ovarian failure (POF); premature menopause (defined as cessation of menses before the age of 40 years); as a direct result of radiation or chemotherapy; and polycystic ovarian syndrome (PCOS)
E. Disorders of the anterior pituitary: Examples include prolactin tumors (7.5%)

Predisposing Factor

A. The disorder can affect any female between the ages of 14 and 55 years.

Common Complaints

A. "I haven't had a period in months." "I have periods only a few times each year."
B. "I have nipple discharge."
C. "I am 16 years old and have never had a period."

Other Signs and Symptoms

A. Absence of menses in a woman who has previously experienced menarche, or in a woman who has not experienced menarche.
B. Irregular, infrequent menses

Subjective Data

A. Review the client's complete menstrual history, including age of onset (menarche), duration, frequency, regularity, and history of dysmenorrhea.
B. Review the client's pregnancy history.
C. Review the client's contraception history.
D. Note other medications the client is taking, such as hormones or psychiatric medications, as well as any recreational drug use.
E. Review general medical history including treatments received, such as chemotherapy for any prior cancers.
F. Inquire about any breast discharge.

G. Review the client's weight pattern.

H. Review sources of stress in the client's life.

I. Discuss exercise pattern and history.

Physical Examination

A. Check height, weight, blood pressure (BP), and pulse.

B. Inspect:

1. Note overall appearance. Examine the thyroid. Inspect the breast/genitalia for Tanner staging (see Appendix C: Tanner's Sexual Maturity Stages).

2. Skin assessment: Check for central hair growth and hirsutism, which is androgen-responsive. Areas to inspect for coarse hair include the upper lip, chin, sideburns, neck, chest, lower abdomen, and perineum.

C. Auscultate:

1. The heart and lungs

D. Palpate:

1. The neck for thyroid enlargement

2. The abdomen for uterine enlargement compatible with pregnancy

E. Pelvic examination:

1. Inspect external genitalia. Note the pubic hair pattern for Tanner staging. Note any lesions, masses, or discharge.

2. Speculum examination: Inspect the vagina and cervix for irregularity or lesions

3. Bimanual examination: Palpate for size of the uterus and for adnexal masses

Diagnostic Tests

A. Urine: Pregnancy test

B. Serum:

1. Serum human chorionic gonadotropin (HCG), if a urine pregnancy test is negative

2. Thyroid-stimulating hormone (TSH) to rule out thyroid dysfunction

3. Prolactin: Normal is less than 20 ng/mL

4. Follicle-stimulating hormone (FSH): Greater than 40 IU/mL indicates ovarian failure

C. Pelvic ultrasound

D. Genetic testing/karyotype analysis in primary amenorrhea

Differential Diagnoses

A. Amenorrhea

B. Pregnancy

C. Constitutional delay

D. Hypothyroidism

E. POF, or early menopause

F. Perimenopause

G. Pituitary adenoma

H. Androgen insensitivity syndrome

Plan

A. General interventions:

1. If laboratory values are normal, proceed to progesterone challenge test to rule out hypothalamic amenorrhea.

2. If the client is pregnant, counsel regarding pregnancy and begin antepartum care.

3. If other laboratory information points to an underlying cause for amenorrhea, treat as appropriate.

B. Client teaching: *See Section III: Client Teaching Guide for this chapter, "Amenorrhea."*

C. Pharmaceutical therapy:

1. Progesterone challenge:

a. Micronized progesterone (Prometrium) 300 mg daily or medroxyprogesterone acetate (MPA; Provera) 10 mg each day for 10 days

b. Positive test is any vaginal bleeding. Withdrawal bleeding should occur within 7 to 10 days after finishing the medicine. A late vaginal bleed may be associated with ovulation. No response to the progesterone challenge may be associated with PCOS.

c. In the absence of galactorrhea, with a normal prolactin level, normal TSH, and positive progesterone challenge, further evaluation is unnecessary

> All anovulatory clients require therapeutic management. There is a risk of endometrial cancer with continued unopposed estrogen stimulation to the endometrium. There is a short latent period in progression from a normal endometrium to atypia to cancer, even in a young woman.

2. Progesterone therapy for hypothalamic amenorrhea

a. MPA (Provera, Cycrin) 10 mg for 10 days each month

b. Low-dose oral contraceptive pills, patch, or ring

c. Clomiphene citrate (Clomid) for women desiring pregnancy

d. Hormone replacement therapy (HRT) for perimenopausal women

Follow-Up

A. Reproductive age: The client should return after 6 months of treatment with progesterone or combined contraceptive products. Discontinue the hormones and assess for return of normal menses. If this does not occur, reinstitute progesterone or combined contraceptive therapy.

B. Perimenopausal: Maintain hormonal therapy. The client should return annually for preventive health visits.

Consultation/Referral

A. Refer the client to a physician if there is no withdrawal bleeding from the progesterone challenge. Lack of a withdrawal bleed may indicate an abnormality of the outflow tract (which is rare), ovarian production of estrogen, or hypothalamic production of gonadotropins. Any of those conditions would require the involvement of a gynecologist.

B. Refer the client to a physician (preferably one whose specialty is endocrinology) if the prolactin level is elevated (>20 mg/mL) for further workup to rule out pituitary adenoma

Individual Considerations

A. Adolescence:

1. Rule out pregnancy initially; then determine whether the client has primary or secondary amenorrhea. Refer the client to a physician for primary amenorrhea.

2. For secondary amenorrhea, complete an assessment and evaluation. Assess stress/emotional status, nutritional status, and exercise routine.

3. Refer to a physician, or a clinician specializing in gynecology, if there is no withdrawal bleeding from the progesterone challenge test.

4. Refer for evaluation and treatment as indicated for eating, exercise, or psychiatric disorders.

B. Older adults:

1. Irregular menses and amenorrhea are common during perimenopause. Provide anticipatory guidance and instructions regarding the need for contraceptive use until menopause is confirmed.

Bibliography

Gambacciani, M., Cagnacci, A., & Lello, S. (2019). Hormone replacement therapy and prevention of chronic conditions. *Climacteric, 22*, 303–306. doi:10.1080/13697137.2018.1551347

Lobo, R. A. (2017). Hormone-replacement therapy: Current thinking. *Nature Reviews Endocrinology, 13*(4), 220. doi:10.1038/nrendo.2016.164

Atrophic Vaginitis

Rhonda Arthur and Michelle Collins

Definition

A. Atrophic vaginitis describes inflammation of the vaginal epithelium due to a lack of estrogen support. Anything that lowers estrogen levels, after puberty, can result in a loss of vaginal thickness and rugosity and a decrease in the elasticity of the vaginal tissues.

Incidence

A. Atrophic vaginitis is very common, particularly at three stages of a woman's life: preadolescence, when breastfeeding a baby, and in perimenopause/postmenopause.

Pathogenesis

A. Estrogen facilitates the maintenance of vaginal pH in an acidic range. Lack of sufficient estrogen promotes an increase in vaginal pH, which in turn supports the overgrowth of bacteria that are otherwise well controlled in an acidic environment. Overgrowth of bacteria is the impetus for the development of bacterial infections. Estrogen loss also results in a decrease in vaginal glycogen and a thin-walled epithelium, promoting friability and inflammation.

Predisposing Factors

A. Preadolescence

B. Breastfeeding

C. Postmenopause

D. Ovarian failure

E. Therapy for vaginal cancer such as surgery or radiation

F. Pharmacologic therapy for breast cancer to include aromatase inhibitors

G. Use of GnRH agonists

H. Hypothalamic amenorrhea as a result of excessive physical exertion

Common Complaints

A. Vaginal dryness, irritation, and/or bleeding

B. Dyspareunia

C. Dysuria

Other Signs and Symptoms

A. Postcoital bleeding

B. Thin vaginal discharge

C. Vaginal itching

Subjective Data

A. Question the client regarding onset, duration, and course of symptoms.

B. Determine whether this is a new issue. If so, ask about the use of new soaps, laundry detergent, or hygiene products.

C. Describe the color, amount, and odor of vaginal discharge or bleeding.

D. Determine the existence of coexisting vasomotor symptoms, such as hot flashes and night sweats.

E. Ask if the client is experiencing dysuria, urinary frequency, vulvar dryness and/or itching, or dyspareunia. With dyspareunia, determine whether the discomfort is due to vaginal irritation, pain with deep penetration, or both.

F. Determine whether the client is breastfeeding and if so, how long she has been breastfeeding

G. Ask the date of her last menses and whether she is having irregular cycles. Determine whether the client has had a hysterectomy; if so, ask if oophorectomy was also done. Assess whether she has had ovarian failure.

H. Review whether client has had either any new partner or any new sexual practices.

I. Review the client's current medications, including antidepressants.

J. Explore the client's history of HRT; has she recently initiated or stopped use?

K. What measures has the client tried for relief and did they help?

L. When was the last Papanicolaou (Pap) test and/or human papillomavirus (HPV) test, if indicated by age/guidelines, and what was the result?

Physical Examination

A. Check temperature, pulse, and respirations.

B. Inspect: Observe the client generally for discomfort before, during, and after the examination.

C. Palpate:

1. Back: Check for costovertebral angle (CVA) tenderness. (CVAT)

2. Abdomen: Note suprapubic tenderness.

Pelvic Examination

A. Inspect:

1. Examine external genitalia for friability, erythema, lesions, condyloma, and amount and color of any discharge.

2. Common observations in menopausal women include sparse and brittle pubic hair, flat labia minora, and vulvar inflammation.

3. Excoriation may be present if the woman has complained of pruritus.

B. Palpate: "Milk" urethra and Skene's glands for discharge to rule out infection.

C. Speculum examination:

1. Check rugae, friability of vaginal epithelium, color and amount of any vaginal discharge; evaluate cervix for lesions, friability, and erythema.

2. Typical atrophic symptoms on inspection: Thin, friable vaginal epithelium; decreased or absent of vaginal rugae; scant vaginal discharge

D. Bimanual examination:

1. Check for cervical motion tenderness (CMT), uterine size, and position (if no hysterectomy).

2. Check adnexa for masses.

Diagnostic Tests

A. Routine hormone measurements to evaluate menopause status are not routinely indicated

B. Urine culture, if warranted, based on urinary symptoms

C. Vaginal pH: Normal pH range in premenopausal women is 4 to 4.5. Reduced levels of estrogen increase vaginal pH.

D. Pap test, if due; HPV test, if appropriate based on age/guidelines.

E. Wet prep, if applicable

1. Multiple white blood cells (WBCs) indicate inflammation; may have decreased lactobacillus, presence of bacteria

2. Prep should be negative for trichomonads. Whiff test should be negative.

F. Cultures for gonorrhea and chlamydia, if applicable. These may be obtained cervically or using a urine specimen kit.

> While atrophic vaginitis may be the cause of spotting, especially post intercourse, any bleeding in a postmenopausal woman must be thoroughly investigated to rule out the possibility of endometrial hyperplasia or endometrial cancer.

Differential Diagnoses

A. Atrophic vaginitis

B. Vaginal trauma

C. Foreign body in the vagina

D. Urinary tract infection (UTI)

E. Vaginitis from infective cause: Fungus, bacteria, or virus

F. Contact irritation: Latex (condom), spermicide, lubricant

G. Sexually transmitted infection (STI)

Plan

A. General interventions:

1. Treat any underlying infections (gonorrhea, chlamydia, vaginitis, as diagnosed).

B. Client teaching:

1. *See Section III: Client Teaching Guides for this chapter, "Atrophic Vaginitis" and "Dyspareunia (Pain With Intercourse)."*

2. Preadolescent girls have amelioration of symptoms with an increase of endogenous estrogen as puberty approaches.

3. Reassure women that this issue is physical, not psychological.

4. Discuss the benefits of regular sexual activity in decreasing issues with atrophic vaginitis. One reason

for decreased sexual activity may be lack of a partner. Masturbation also facilitates the natural resumption of the production of lubricating secretions by the body.

5. Symptomatic relief of dryness during sexual activity may be obtained with the use of water-soluble lubricants and adequate foreplay. Glycerin-containing lubricants should be avoided.

6. Vaginal moisturizer may be applied for the relief of symptoms.

7. Discuss pregnancy prevention, reinforcing that perimenopausal symptoms do not ensure lack of fertility

C. Pharmaceutical therapy:

1. Estrogen therapy (ET):

a. Vaginal hormonal therapy is the most appropriate form of HRT for women whose only symptoms are those of atrophic vaginitis. Systemically absorbed hormone products are appropriate if the client has menopausal symptoms in addition to those of atrophic vaginitis.

> Absolute contraindications for the use of ET also apply to the use of topical estrogen (i.e., breast cancer, active liver disease, history of recent thromboembolic event). Vaginal estrogen creams are systemically absorbed. As with the use of oral and transdermal estrogen, a progestin must be administered to women who have an intact uterus. However, some breast cancer survivors may be candidates for one of the vaginal ring products, as well as the vaginally administered pills, depending on their breast cancer type. The clinician should always consult with the client's oncologist prior to the prescription of such products, however.

i. Conjugated estrogen (Premarin) cream 0.625 mg/g: Use 0.5 to 1.0 g applicator inserted intravaginally at bedtime every night for 1 to 2 weeks, then every other night for 1 to 2 weeks, then as needed

ii. Estradiol (Estrace) 0.1 mg/g: Use one-half (2 g) to one (4 g) applicator inserted intravaginally at bedtime every night for 1 to 2 weeks. When vaginal mucosa is restored, maintenance dose is one-quarter applicator (1 g) one to three times weekly in a cyclic regimen.

> Vaginal estrogen creams should not be used as a lubricant before intercourse as the hormone can be absorbed through a partner's skin.
>
> Vaginal estrogen creams are systemically absorbed. As with the use of oral and transdermal estrogen, a progestin must be administered to women who have an intact uterus.

iii. Estradiol (Estring) 7.5 mcg/24 hr: Insert one ring in vagina and replace every 90 days.

iv. Estradiol hemihydrate (Vagifem) vaginal tablets 10 to 25 mcg: Insert one tablet in vagina each day for 14 days, then one tablet twice weekly after that. Women should be initiated at the 10 mcg dose, which may be increased accordingly relative to symptom relief.

b. Oral estrogen replacement therapy:

i. Conjugated estrogen (Premarin) 0.3 mg orally every day from day 1 through 25 of a month, plus conjugated estrogen (Provera) 10 mg orally on days 13 through 25. While there are various doses of oral estrogen, as with any hormonal product, it is prudent to initiate therapy at the lowest therapeutic dose, and increase from there as needed, according to symptom management.

ii. See the "Menopause" section for other HRT regimens.

Follow-Up
A. Breastfeeding women should be reevaluated following weaning, especially if symptoms persist (i.e., alternative etiology is suspected).
B. Postmenopausal women should be evaluated for additional etiologies (i.e., endometrial hyperplasia) if vaginal bleeding persists beyond initiation of therapy, and they are not on a regimen that will induce withdrawal bleeds.
C. The client should return to clinic 3 months after beginning hormonal therapy; if she is tolerating the therapy well, and symptoms of atrophic vaginitis have improved, she may revert to annual visits.
D. Perform Pap and HPV tests, and physical examination, per client health history and risks, and according to guidelines.

Consultation/Referral
A. If a postmenopausal woman presents with bleeding, the practitioner must rule out bleeding of uterine origin. If there is any doubt, the clinician should pursue exploration of bleeding with pelvic ultrasound, endometrial biopsy, or consultation for D&C.

Individual Considerations
A. Breastfeeding women:
1. Breastfeeding women have amelioration of symptoms as weaning progresses unless an alternative etiology exists
B. Postmenopausal women:
1. Evaluate the client for other risks of hypoestrogenemia, such as cardiovascular disease and osteoporosis. Continuous systemic estrogen replacement therapy may be indicated if symptoms in addition to atrophic vaginitis exist.
2. Vaginitis in the postmenopausal woman is rarely due to any of the organisms responsible for vaginitis in the premenopausal woman (unless she has new sexual partners). Candidiasis, trichomoniasis, and bacterial vaginosis (BV) are uncommon after the reproductive years.

Bibliography
Centers for Disease Control and Prevention. (2015). *2015 sexually transmitted diseases treatment guidelines*. Retrieved from http://www.cdc.gov/std/tg2015/default.htm
Gambacciani, M., Cagnacci, A., & Lello, S. (2019). Hormone replacement therapy and prevention of chronic conditions. *Climacteric, 22*, 303–306. doi:10.1080/13697137.2018.1551347
Lobo, R. A. (2017). Hormone-replacement therapy: Current thinking. *Nature Reviews Endocrinology, 13*(4), 220. doi:10.1038/nrendo.2016.164

Bacterial Vaginosis (*Gardnerella* Vaginosis)

Rhonda Arthur and Michelle Collins

Definition
A. BV is an infection of the vagina caused by an alteration in the normal flora of the vagina, with an increase in anaerobes and gram-negative bacilli as well as a decrease in the *Lactobacillus* flora.

Incidence
A. BV is the most common vaginal infection in women of reproductive age. It is not considered an STI.

Pathogenesis
A. The etiology of BV is an increase in anaerobes in the vagina. The normal vaginal pH of a woman of reproductive age is slightly acidic, and the vagina is normally colonized with lactobacilli. The vaginal lactobacilli produce lactic acid and bacteriocins, as well as hydrogen peroxide. When the normal lactobacilli of the vagina decrease, the vaginal pH is increased. The organisms present in BV cause the level of vaginal amines to be high. These amines are volatilized when the pH is increased, causing the characteristic "fishy" odor.
B. There are several risk factors associated with BV, including having multiple sexual partners or a new partner, douching, lack of condom use, race/ethnicity, and smoking. Some sources concur that BV is more common among women who have sex with women.
C. BV is primarily polymicrobial, and the pathogens seen include *Bacteroides* species, *Peptostreptococcus* species, *Eubacterium* species, *Mobiluncus* species, *Gardnerella*, and *Mycoplasma hominis*

Predisposing Factors
A. History of STIs
B. Multiple sexual partners; new sex partner
C. Factors that change the normal vaginal flora:
1. Hormonal changes (menses, pregnancy)
2. Medications: antibiotic therapy
3. Foreign bodies in the vagina (tampons), semen, and douching

Common Complaints
A. Vaginal discharge (thin, white, gray, or milky
B. Fishy vaginal odor
C. Postcoital odor and/or irritation, itching

Other Signs and Symptoms
A. Asymptomatic
B. Increase in odor after menses
C. Occasional itching and burning

Subjective Data
A. Elicit onset, duration, and course of presenting symptoms.
B. Review any changes in the characteristics and color of vaginal discharge. Does the client's partner(s) have any symptoms?
C. Review any symptoms of pruritus, perineal excoriation, or burning; signs of UTI

D. Review medications and medical history.
E. Determine whether the client is pregnant; note the first day of the last menstrual period (LMP).
F. Question the client about a history of STIs or other vaginal infections.
G. Review previous infection, treatment, compliance with treatment, and results.
H. Note the last intercourse date.
I. Elicit information about possible foreign body.
J. Review use of vaginal deodorants or sprays, scented toilet paper, tampons, pads, and douching habits.
K. Review change in laundry detergent, soaps, and fabric softeners.
L. Review use of tight restrictive clothing, tight jeans, and nylon panties.

Physical Examination

A. Check temperature, pulse, and respirations.
B. Inspect: Examine external vulva and introitus for discharge, irritation, fissures, lesions, rashes, and condyloma.
C. Palpate:
   1. Palpate the abdomen for masses or tenderness. Note enlarged or tender inguinal lymph nodes.
   2. Palpate the external perineal area for vulvar masses.
   3. "Milk" the Skene's glands for discharge.
D. Pelvic examination:
   1. Inspect:
      a. Note the color, amount, and odor of discharge.
      b. Inspect the cervix.
         i. BV is a vaginosis rather than a vaginitis. There is usually little or no inflammation of the vaginal epithelium associated with BV.
         ii. BV is associated with a pink, healthy cervix. A "strawberry cervix" is seen with cervicitis, like that due to *Trichomonas vaginalis*.
         iii. A red, edematous, friable cervix is seen with *Chlamydia trachomatis* infection.
   2. Speculum examination:
      a. Inspect sidewalls for adhering discharge.
      b. The clinical diagnosis of BV requires the presence of three of the following four signs (Amstel's criteria):
         i. Homogeneous, white, adherent vaginal discharge may be present.
         ii. Vaginal fluid pH greater than 4.5. To ensure an accurate pH measurement, take a smear for testing from the lateral walls of the vagina, not from the cervix.
         iii. A fishy, amine-like odor from vaginal fluid before or after mixing it with 10% potassium hydroxide (positive whiff test). Semen releases the vaginal amines; therefore, there is an increase in odor after intercourse.
         iv. Presence of "clue cells" (squamous vaginal epithelial cells covered with bacteria, causing a stippled or granular appearance and ragged, "moth-eaten" borders) or coccobacilli forms both in the fluid and adheres to the epithelial cells.

   3. Bimanual examination: Check for CMT and adnexal masses. BV may be a risk factor for pelvic inflammatory disease (PID).

Diagnostic Tests

A. Gram stain (considered the gold standard), though impractical for many outpatient practices to perform
B. BV can be diagnosed by the use of clinical criteria; three of the following four are needed to make a clinical diagnosis (Amsel's diagnostic criteria):
   1. Vaginal pH greater than 4.5; normal vaginal pH range is 4 to 4.5
   2. Clue cells on microscopic examination
   3. Homogeneous, thin white or gray discharge that coats the vaginal walls
   4. A fishy odor of the vaginal discharge before, or after, the addition of 10% KOH (wet prep with 10% potassium hydroxide and normal saline prep); microscopic examination of vaginal secretions should always be done
C. Herpes culture, if indicated by symptomology
D. Urinalysis and culture, if indicated by symptomology

Differential Diagnoses

A. BV
B. Vulvovaginal candidiasis
C. Trichomoniasis
D. Gonorrhea
E. Chlamydia
F. Presence of foreign body
G. Normal physiological discharge

Plan

A. General interventions:
   1. Inform the client regarding other modalities for treating BV. These methods include the following:
      a. Insertion of a tampon soaked in hydrogen peroxide in the vagina for 3 minutes, three nights in a row
      b. Supplementation of probiotics, specifically those containing *Lactobacillus acidophilus* culture
B. Client teaching:
   1. *See Section III: Client Teaching Guides for this chapter, "Bacterial Vaginosis."* ◀
   2. BV is not considered an STI.
C. Pharmaceutical therapy:
   1. Drug of choice:
      a. Metronidazole (Flagyl) 500 mg orally twice daily for 7 days *or*
      b. Metronidazole gel 0.75% one applicator (5 g) vaginally at bedtime for 5 days:
         i. Side effects of metronidazole include sharp, unpleasant metallic taste in the mouth; furry tongue; nausea/vomiting, loss of appetite, rash, itching. Advise clients to avoid alcohol while taking metronidazole and for 48 hours after completing the medication, or they will experience the severe disulfiram side effects of abdominal distress, nausea, vomiting, and headache.

ii. Metronidazole may prolong prothrombin time in clients taking oral anticoagulants.
c. Clindamycin cream 2%, one full applicator (5 g) intravaginally at bedtime for 7 days

2. Alternative regimens:
a. Tinidazole 2 g orally once daily for 2 days
b. Tinidazole 1 g orally once daily for 5 days
c. Clindamycin 300 mg by mouth twice daily for 7 days
d. Clindamycin ovules 100 mg intravaginally once at bedtime for 3 days

> Clindamycin ovules and cream have an oil base that might weaken latex or rubber products (e.g., condoms and diaphragms). Use of such products within 72 hours following treatment with clindamycin ovules is not recommended.

3. Special considerations: Pregnancy. BV has been associated with adverse pregnancy outcomes; therefore, all symptomatic pregnant women at high risk for preterm birth, who have confirmed BV, require treatment. Support in the literature for the treatment of asymptomatic pregnant women at high risk for preterm birth is inconsistent. Treatment of asymptomatic pregnant women at low risk for preterm birth also lacks consistent evidence. At this time, the evidence is insufficient to recommend routine screening for BV in asymptomatic pregnant women at either high or low risk for preterm birth.
a. Metronidazole 250 mg three times daily or 500 mg orally twice daily for 7 days or 0.75% metronidazole gel 5 g vaginally once daily for 5 days
b. Clindamycin 300 mg orally twice daily for 7 days
c. Clindamycin 300 mg orally twice daily for 7 days
d. Clindamycin ovules 100 mg intravaginally once at bedtime for 3 days

> Clinicians may be hesitant to prescribe metronidazole in the first trimester of pregnancy. However, multiple studies and meta-analyses have not demonstrated any association between metronidazole use during pregnancy and teratogenic or mutagenic effects in newborns.
>
> Some older studies suggested a possible link between the use of vaginal clindamycin during pregnancy and adverse neonatal outcomes. However, newer data demonstrate that this treatment approach is safe for pregnant women. Oral therapy has not been shown to be superior to topical therapy for treating symptomatic BV; thus, symptomatic pregnant women may be treated with either of the oral or vaginal regimens recommended for nonpregnant women.

Follow-Up
A. Nonpregnant women: No follow-up is recommended unless indicated. Recurrence is common.
B. Pregnancy: High risk for preterm birth. Pregnant women should be reevaluated 1 month after treatment.

C. Immunocompromised women: Recommendations for treatment of BV in clients infected with HIV are the same as for noninfected clients.

Consultation/Referral
A. Refer the client to an advanced practice nurse whose specialty is gynecology, or to a physician for recurrence that is unresponsive to therapies.

Individual Considerations
A. Partners:
1. Routine treatment of a client's partner(s) is not recommended at this time because it does not influence relapse or recurrence rates.

Bibliography
Centers for Disease Control and Prevention. (2015a). *2015 sexually transmitted diseases treatment guidelines*. Retrieved from http://www.cdc.gov/std/tg2015/default.htm
Centers for Disease Control and Prevention. (2015b). *Sexually transmitted diseases treatment guidelines: Bacterial vaginosis*. Retrieved from http://www.cdc.gov/std/tg2015/bv.htm

Bartholin's Cyst or Abscess

Rhonda Arthur and Michelle Collins

Definition
A. The Bartholin's glands are small, round, nonpalpable mucus-secreting organs. They are located bilaterally in the posterolateral vaginal orifice. Obstruction of the duct causes the gland to swell with mucus and form a Bartholin's cyst. The cause of obstruction is usually unknown but may be due to mechanical trauma, thickened mucus, neoplasm, stenosis of the duct, or infectious organisms not limited to STIs. The cyst may become infected, resulting in an abscess. Cysts develop more commonly in younger women, and occurrence decreases with aging; therefore, it is important to rule out neoplasm in women older than 40 years experiencing Bartholin's cysts (see Figure 14.1).

FIGURE 14.1 Infected Bartholin cyst.
Source: Centers for Disease Control and Prevention/Susan Lindsley.

B. The majority of women with Bartholin's cysts are asymptomatic, but large cysts can cause pressure and interfere with walking and sexual intercourse. Abscesses generally develop rapidly over a 2- to 3-day period and are painful. Some abscesses may spontaneously rupture and often reoccur.

Predisposing Factors

A. History of STIs
B. Local trauma
C. Prior Bartholin's cysts

Common Complaints

A. Cysts can be asymptomatic and found incidentally on physical examination.
B. Localized pain/irritation
C. Dyspareunia
D. Difficulty walking or sitting due to inflammation

Subjective Data

A. Elicit onset, duration, and course of presenting symptoms.
B. Review any changes in the characteristics and color of vaginal discharge. Does the client's partner(s) have any symptoms?
C. Review any symptoms of pruritus, perineal excoriation, burning; signs of UTI).
D. Review the client's medication and medical history.
E. Determine whether the client is pregnant; note the first day of the LMP.
F. Ask the client about history of STIs or other vaginal infections.
G. Review previous infection, treatment, compliance with treatment, and results.
H. Note last intercourse date.

Physical Examination

A. Inspect:
  1. Examine the external vulva and introitus for discharge, irritation, fissures, lesions, and rashes. Bartholin's cysts will appear as a round mass usually near the vaginal orifice causing vulvar asymmetry.
B. Palpate:
  1. Bartholin's glands: Cysts are usually unilateral, nontender, and without erythema. An abscess is usually unilateral and painful to palpation.

Diagnostic Tests

A. Culture and sensitivity of purulent abscess fluid
B. Cervical culture for STI (*Neisseria gonorrhoeae* and *C. trachomatis*)
C. Excisional biopsy in women older than 40 years

Differential Diagnoses

A. Bartholin's cyst
B. Bartholin's abscess
C. Neoplasm
D. STI
E. Sebaceous cyst

Plan

A. General interventions:
  1. Reassurance is indicated for women younger than 40 years with asymptomatic cysts. Incision and drainage (I&D) is often required for symptomatic cysts and abscesses. Because cysts and abscesses often reoccur, surgery to create a permanent opening from the duct to the exterior is often the definitive treatment. Two such surgical methods are placement of a Word catheter or marsupialization. Referral is indicated for I&D and other surgical interventions if the provider is not experienced with the procedures.
B. Client teaching:
  1. Reassure women that asymptomatic cysts do not need intervention. Rapidly enlarging cysts that are painful, or that obstruct the vaginal orifice, or recurrent cysts need to be reevaluated.
  2. Warm sitz baths three or four times a day may encourage spontaneous rupture of abscess, while also providing comfort
C. Pharmaceutical therapy:
  1. Abscesses are treated with an antibiotic that covers methicillin-resistant *Staphylococcus aureus* (MRSA) such as trimethoprim 160 mg/sulfamethoxazole 800 mg twice a day or amoxicillin/clavulanate 875 mg bid for 7 days plus clindamycin 300 mg orally four times a day for 7 days.

Follow-Up

A. Follow up with provider if symptoms are not improved in 3 to 7 days.
B. Report to care provider if symptoms recur.

Consultation/Referral

A. Refer the client to a physician for recurrence that is unresponsive to therapies.

Individual Considerations

A. Older adults:
  1. Refer women older than 40 years with cyst for excisional biopsy.
B. Pregnancy: Treatment with antibiotics is recommended due to the risk of complicated infection. Avoid the use of trimethoprim/sulfamethoxazole during the last trimester of pregnancy. Refer to an OB/GYN practitioner for recurrence.

Bibliography

McNeeley, S. G. (2014, July). *Merck manual: Bartholin gland cysts*. Rahway, NJ: Merck Publishing. Retrieved from http://www.merckmanuals.com/professional/gynecology-and-obstetrics/benign-gynecologic-lesions/bartholin-gland-cysts

Breast Pain

Rhonda Arthur and Michelle Collins

Definition

A. Benign breast disorders such as mastalgia, mastodynia, and fibrocystic breast changes are characterized by lumps or pain. The lumps may be a physiological nodularity, a ropy thickening, or distended fluid-filled cysts that are mobile. The pain may be cyclic or noncyclic, and it may be unilateral or bilateral.

Incidence

A. Breast pain is a very common problem. Fifty percent or more of menstruating women experience breast pain. Two-thirds of breast pain is cyclic and occurs in women in their 30s; one-third is noncyclic and may occur in women at any age, but it tends to occur in women closer to menopause.

Pathogenesis

A. Dysplastic, benign histologic changes occur in the breast such as hyperplasia of the breast epithelium, adenosis microcysts and macrocysts, duct ectasia, and apocrine metaplasia.

Predisposing Factors

A. Menstruation (related to hormonal changes)
B. Certain medications (combination oral contraceptives [COCs], hormone therapy, antidepressants, and others)
C. Ingesting substances containing methylxanthines (coffee, tea, chocolate, and cola drinks). Methylxanthines have been noted to contribute to breast pain by clinical observation only.
D. Pregnancy

Common Complaints

A. "My breasts are painful, particularly just before my period."
B. "I have lumps in my breasts, and they hurt."

Other Signs and Symptoms

A. Breasts tender to palpation
B. Ropelike masses, usually bilateral, with mobile, well-circumscribed masses that are cystic or rubbery

Subjective Data

A. Elicit history of pain. Note onset, duration, location, and relation to menstrual period. Ask: Is pain constant or intermittent? Is there any discharge from the nipples? If so, what are the characteristics of the discharge?
B. What has the client tried to alleviate the pain? Note what has worked, such as nonsteroidal anti-inflammatory drugs (NSAIDs).
C. Note the client's family history of breast pain, lumps, or cancer.
D. Has there been any trauma, such as being hit in the breast or having a rough experience during sex?
E. Do the client's breasts hurt during or after exercise?
F. Does the client wear a good, supportive, properly fitted bra generally, as well as for sports?
G. Has the client had any breast surgery or biopsies?
H. Note medication history.

Physical Examination

A. Inspect:
   1. Examine the breasts, noting masses or dimples, changes in the skin, and changes in the way the nipples are pointed while the client is in the sitting position with arms in neutral position in lap, above the head, and pressing in on hips.
B. Palpate:
   1. The breasts: Look for hard, fixed, or cystic masses in the breast, under the nipple, in the tail of the breast, and in the axilla. Use a standardized breast examination technique. Compress the nipple for discharge. Measure masses and describe them in the client's record. Use a clock face to describe their location.

Diagnostic Tests

A. Mammogram: May be difficult to interpret in women younger than 35 years due to the density of the breasts. If ordered, a diagnostic mammogram on the breast where the mass is palpated, rather than a screening mammogram, is appropriate.
B. Ultrasonography is a first-line method to differentiate cystic masses from solid masses.
C. Magnetic resonance imaging (MRI) is useful for detecting tissues with increased blood flow but limited by false-positive results
D. Fine-needle aspiration and biopsy
E. Excisional biopsy for solid lumps
F. Pregnancy test (as indicated)

Differential Diagnoses

A. Fibrocystic breast changes with mastalgia
B. Benign breast masses: Fibroadenoma and duct ectasia
C. Nipple discharge: Duct ectasia, prolactin-secreting pituitary tumors
D. Pain: Costal chondritis, chest wall muscle pain, neuralgia, herpes zoster infection, and fibromyalgia
E. Heart: Angina pectoris
F. Gastrointestinal (GI): Gastroesophageal reflux disease
G. Psychological: Anxiety and depression

Plan

A. General interventions:
   1. Reassure the client. Use the term *fibrocystic changes* rather than *fibrocystic disease* to stress the functional nature of the problem. Stress that the pain is real but not caused by a disease state.
B. Client teaching:
   1. See Section III: Client Teaching Guide for this chapter, "Fibrocystic Breast Changes and Breast Pain."
   2. Teach the client breast self-examination. Encourage monthly breast self-examination with the purpose of facilitating the client in becoming very familiar with the "usual" state of her own tissue so that if something new appears, she may be more likely to recognize that. Note that not all organizations that write guidelines on breast care agree that women should perform self-monthly breast exam. Continue clinical breast examinations annually.
   3. "Lumpiness" that varies with the menstrual cycle is not abnormal. Breasts may normally be of different sizes; if the change is new, then it is significant to report.
   4. Consider changing the dose, or discontinuing HRT, for women on HRT with mastalgia. Likewise, for those on combined hormonal contraceptives (pill, patch, or ring), consider lower-dosage products.
   5. Symptomatic measures to relieve discomfort:
      a. Good supportive bra that is properly fitted. Adolescents whose breasts are maturing and perimenopausal women whose bodies are changing are two groups who often wear improperly fitted bras.
      b. Local heat or ice application (whatever works best)
C. Pharmaceutical therapy:
   1. Diuretic: Spironolactone (Aldactone) 10 mg twice daily premenstrually
   2. Topical nonsteroidal anti-inflammatory gel can be used for local mastalgia.

3. Antiestrogen treatment:

a. Danazol (Danocrine) 200 mg daily for 6 months. *Note*: Doses less than 400 mg daily may not inhibit ovulation. The client must use a barrier contraceptive or intrauterine device (IUD) contraceptive measure. Although the side-effect profile is significant, long-term symptomatic relief and histologic changes may be achieved.

b. Tamoxifen citrate 10 mg/d for severe breast pain

4. Vitamins:

a. Vitamin E supplementation has support in the literature for treating mastalgia.

b. Research has demonstrated mixed results on the benefits of vitamin B_6 and vitamin A.

c. Iodine 3,000 mcg daily; violet iodine is an over-the-counter (OTC) formulation for the treatment of fibrocystic breast pain.

5. Herbs:

a. Flaxseed 25 mg daily may have some benefit in the treatment of cyclic mastalgia.

b. Evening primrose oil (EPO) 1 to 3 g daily in divided doses has had mixed results.

D. Diet:

1. Elimination of methylxanthines (i.e., caffeine-containing products) has been noted to decrease breast discomfort.

2. Reduction of dietary sodium intake has been noted anecdotally to decrease discomfort.

3. The successful use of cinnamon on cyclical breast pain has recently been noted.

Follow-Up

A. Women with mastalgia can be monitored at the annual exam for efficacy of recommended treatments.

Consultation/Referral

A. Consult or refer the client to a clinician whose specialty is breast health when breast masses are identified.

B. Consult with a physician and refer the client to a surgeon if findings include a suspicious mammographic study, an abnormal needle biopsy, or a solid mass per ultrasonogram.

Individual Considerations

A. Pregnancy:

1. Consider plugged duct or mastitis with treatment as indicated.

B. Adults:

1. Organizations that formulate guidelines for women's care disagree on breast cancer screening initiation, frequency, and discontinuation. American Cancer Society (ACS) guidelines indicate that mammography screening for women at average risk are as follows: **Women ages 40 to 44** should receive counseling on the risks and benefits of mammography and have the choice to initiate annual breast cancer screening with mammograms if they wish to do so. **Women ages 45 to 54** should be counseled to obtain annual mammograms. **Women 55 and older** can move to mammograms every

2 years, or may continue annual screening. Screening should continue as long as a woman is in good health and is expected to live 10 more years or longer. **All women** should be informed of the benefits, limitations, and potential harms linked to breast cancer screening.

2. Care should be individualized considering potential risks, benefits, and limitations of screening. High-risk women may benefit from additional screening, including earlier initiation of screening and additional screening modalities such as ultrasound, tomosynthesis, and MRI.

3. Tomosynthesis has been proven to be a valuable screening modality. The addition of tomosynthesis to digital mammography for screening has been associated with an increased cancer detection rate, with a concomitant reduction in recall rate, for women with both dense and nondense breast tissue.

4. When clinical breast examination, mammography, and needle-aspiration biopsy are used, breast cancer detection rates are 93% to 100%.

C. Geriatrics:

1. Breast pain should carry heightened suspicion for potential existing breast cancer.

D. Partners:

1. Pain may inhibit sexual activity involving the breast.

Bibliography

American Cancer Society. (2015a). *American Cancer Society guidelines for the early detection of cancer*. Retrieved from http://www.cancer.org/healthy/findcancerearly/cancerscreeningguidelines/american-cancer-society-guidelines-for-the-early-detection-of-cancer

American Cancer Society. (2015b). *American Cancer Society recommendations for early breast cancer detection in women without breast symptoms*. Retrieved from http://www.cancer.org/cancer/breastcancer/more-information/breastcancerearlydetection/breast-cancer-early-detection-acs-recs

Gharaiy, N. R., Shahnazi, M., Kia, P. Y., & Javadzadeh, Y. (2017). The effect of cinnamon on cyclical breast pain. *Iranian Red Crescent Medical Journal*, 19(6), e26442. doi:10.5812/ircmj.26442

Goyal, A., & Mansel, R. E. (2016). Mastalgia. In I. Jatoi & M. Kaufmann (Eds.), *Management of breast diseases* (pp. 73–79). Cham, Switzerland: Springer.

Gupta, P., Verma, V., Gupta, R., Kumar, A., Singh, S. P., Gupta, U. K., . . . Gupta, S. K. (2016). Role of tamoxifen and danazol in mastalgia: Prospective controlled trial. *International Surgery Journal*, 3(2), 553–556. doi:10.18203/2349-2902.isj20160703

Hafiz, S. P., Barnes, N. L., & Kirwan, C. C. (2018). Clinical management of idiopathic mastalgia: A systematic review. *Journal of Primary Health Care*, 10(4), 312–323. doi:10.1071/hc18026

Khadka, S., Adhikary, S., Rajbanshi, S., Khaniya, S., Agrawal, C. S., Niraula, S., & Srivastava, A. (2018). Effective regression of mastalgia with centchroman and tamoxifen: A randomised comparison. *Indian Journal of Surgery*, 1–6. doi:10.1007/s12262-018-1790-8

Mannu, G. S., Sudul, M., Bettencourt-Silva, J. H., Tsoti, S. M., Cunnick, G., & Ahmed, S. F. (2018). Role of tamoxifen in idiopathic gynecomastia: A 10-year prospective cohort study. *Breast Journal*, 24(6), 1043–1045. doi:10.1111/tbj.13080

Parsay, S., Olfati, F., & Nahidi, S. (2009). Therapeutic effects of vitamin E on cyclic mastalgia. *Breast Journal*, 15(5), 510–514. doi:10.1111/j.1524-4741.2009.00768.x

Pruthi, S., Wahner-Roedler, D. L., Torkelson, C. J., Cha, S. S., Thicke, L. S., Hazelton, J. H., & Bauer, B. A. (2010). Vitamin E and evening primrose oil for management of cyclical mastalgia: A randomized pilot study. *Alternative Medicine Review*, 15(1), 59–67.

Seetharam, P., & Rodrigues, G. (2015). Benign breast disorders: An insight with a detailed literature review. *Webmed Central Breast*, 6(1), WMC004806. doi:10.9754/journal.wmc.2015.004806

Shobeiri, F., Oshvandi, K., & Nazari, M. (2015). Clinical effectiveness of vitamin E and vitamin B_6 for improving pain severity in cyclic mastalgia. *Iranian Journal of Nursing and Midwifery Research, 20*(6), 723. doi:10.4103/1735-9066.170003

Skaane, P., Bandos, A. I., Niklason, L. T., Sebuødegård, S., Østerås, B. H., Gullien, R., . . . Hofvind, S. (2019). Digital mammography versus digital mammography plus tomosynthesis in breast cancer screening: The Oslo Tomosynthesis Screening Trial. *Radiology, 291*, 23–30. doi:10.1148/radiol.2019182394

Sushel, C., Syed, B. M., Sangrasi, A. K., Qureshi, J. N., & Talpur, A. H. (2016). Role of vitamin E in mastalgia in young women. *Journal of the Liaquat University of Medical and Health Sciences, 15*(2), 67–70.

Vedantham, S., Karellas, A., Vijayaraghavan, G. R., & Kopans, D. B. (2015). Digital breast tomosynthesis: State of the art. *Radiology, 277*(3), 663–684. doi:10.1148/radiol.2015141303

Cervicitis

Rhonda Arthur and Michelle Collins

Definition

A. Cervicitis is acute or chronic inflammation of the cervix that may be visible to the examiner, or may be identified via commentary on the Pap report.

Incidence

A. Incidence is unknown due to this condition's multiple etiologies.

Pathogenesis

A. Acute cervicitis is primarily due to infection from the following organisms:
  1. Bacteria:
     a. *C. trachomatis*
     b. *N. gonorrhoeae*
     c. *Mycoplasma*
     d. *Ureaplasma*
  2. Viruses:
     a. Herpes simplex virus type 2 (HSV-2)
     b. Human papillomavirus (HPV)
  3. *T. vaginalis*
B. Chronic cervicitis is primarily due to the following:
  1. Trauma occurring during childbirth or instrumentation
  2. Infection (see earlier)
  3. Presence of foreign bodies in the vagina (i.e., tampons, IUD strings)

Predisposing Factors

A. Vaginal birth
B. Cervical procedures: Laser, loop, or other excision procedures
C. IUDs
D. STIs

Common Complaints

A. May or may not be accompanied by vaginal discharge
B. Postcoital bleeding

Other Signs and Symptoms

A. Asymptomatic; may be found on routine gynecologic examination
B. Vaginal discharge may vary from thin to thick, white, yellow.
C. Dyspareunia
D. Vulvovaginal irritation or pruritus

Subjective Data

A. Determine onset, duration, and course of symptoms. Is there any dyspareunia, pelvic pain, fever, or urinary symptoms?
B. Determine characteristics of the vaginal discharge.
C. Review the client's history of STIs.
D. Review the client's sexual history, to include any recent change in partner, partner symptoms (if any), and use of sex toys.
E. Note the last Pap (and HPV) test results as indicated. Has the client ever had an abnormal Pap or HPV result; if so, what follow-up did she have?
F. Note first day of LMP, use and type of contraception.
G. If the client has recently been pregnant, review her records for cervical cerclage, vaginal birth with cervical laceration, or other complications.

Physical Examination

A. Check temperature, pulse, and respirations.
B. Inspect:
  1. Observe the client generally for discomfort before, during, and after the examination.
  2. Observe the external vulva for Bartholin's gland enlargement (Bartholin's gland abscess can be due to chlamydial infection), lesions, irritation, fissures, or condyloma.
  3. Note color, amount, and odor of vaginal discharge.
C. Palpate:
  1. Back: Note CVA tenderness.
  2. Abdomen: Palpate for enlarged or tender inguinal lymph nodes.
D. Pelvic examination:
  1. Speculum examination:
     a. Inspect cervix for signs of inflammation. Be aware that cervical ectropion can be noted in approximately 20% of healthy young women (especially in teens and women using combined hormonal contraception). It represents columnar epithelium that is found farther out on the ectocervix, causing the cervix to appear granular and red. Presence of cervical erosion can appear similar to normal ectropy (or ectopy, as it is also known). Ectropy is uniform, whereas inflammation may appear with edges that are more irregular and may bleed to the touch of a cotton swab. A "strawberry cervix" (petechiae) is highly suggestive of trichomoniasis.
     b. Check the cervix for friability and bleeding when the cervix is touched with a cotton-tipped swab.
     c. Assess the vagina and cervix for leukoplakia, lesions, polyps, and discharge.
     d. Assess the vaginal walls for discharge and rugae.
     e. Vesicular or ulcerated cervical lesions warrant testing for syphilis and/or chancroid.
  2. Bimanual examination:
     a. Check CMT, adnexal masses, uterine size, consistency, and tenderness.
     b. Milk Skene's glands for discharge.
     c. Palpate Bartholin's glands.

Diagnostic Tests

A. WBC count, if indicated

B. Consider testing for syphilis (rapid plasma reagin [RPR] or VDRL test).

C. Wet prep

D. Cervical cultures for gonorrhea and chlamydia

E. Pap test and/or HPV testing as indicated by guidelines

F. Urine culture and sensitivity, if indicated

G. Herpes simplex culture, if indicated

Differential Diagnoses

A. Cervicitis

B. Chlamydia

C. Gonorrhea

D. Bartholin's gland abscess

E. Cervical neoplasm

F. Cervical polyps

G. HSV-2

H. UTI

I. Cervical ulceration, or erosion, from trauma: Fingernail, cervical biopsy, recent birth, or sex toys

J. PID

Plan

A. General interventions:

1. Presumptive treatment for *C. trachomatis* and *N. gonorrhoeae* should be provided for women at increased risk (e.g., those < 25 years, those with any recent change of sex partner, those not in a mutually monogamous relationship, or those with a sex partner who has a current, or recent, STI), especially if follow-up cannot be obtained.

B. Client teaching:

1. Encourage clients to obtain routine care and Pap test evaluations per guidelines.

2. Clients should have no sexual intercourse for 1 week during treatment; they should avoid reinfection by abstaining from intercourse until sexual partners are adequately treated.

3. Avoid tampons and douches until antibiotics are completed.

▶ 4. Give the client a teaching sheet. *See Section III: Client Teaching Guides for this chapter, "Cervicitis."*

C. Pharmaceutical therapy:

1. Drug of choice for chlamydia: Azithromycin (Zithromax) 1 g orally in a single dose or doxycycline (Vibramycin) 100 mg twice daily for 7 days. Treat all partners.

2. Drug of choice for gonorrhea: Ceftriaxone (Rocephin) 250 mg by intramuscular (IM) injection plus a single dose of azithromycin (Zithromax) 1 g orally

3. Drug of choice for herpes simplex virus (HSV): Acyclovir 400 mg three times daily for 7 to 10 days for initial outbreak, acyclovir 400 mg three times a day for 5 days for recurrent outbreak or acyclovir 400 mg twice a day for suppression

4. Drug of choice for trichomoniasis: Metronidazole (Flagyl) 2 g orally in a single dose (treat all partners) or tinidazole (Tindamax) 2 g orally in a single dose. Clients should be cautioned to avoid alcohol consumption while taking and for 48 hours after the completion of oral metronidazole, and for 72 hours after completion of tinidazole due to a disulfiram-like reaction (nausea, vomiting, headache, cramps, and flushing).

5. Drug of choice for UTI: See the "Urinary Tract Infection (Acute Cystitis)" section in Chapter 12.

Follow-Up

A. Women treated for gonorrhea should be retested 3 months after treatment regardless of whether they believe their sex partners were treated.

B. Follow up with Pap and/or HPV testing as indicated by guidelines.

Consultation/Referral

A. Refer the client to an OB/GYN physician for suspected neoplasm and for cervicitis unresponsive to treatment.

B. If the cervix has a suspicious lesion, refer the client for colposcopy and/or biopsy regardless of cytology results.

Individual Considerations

A. Pregnancy:

1. Cervical inflammation is common in early pregnancy.

2. If an STI is diagnosed, follow the current CDC guidelines for the treatment of pregnant women

B. Partners:

1. A positive STI result warrants treatment of each sexual partner.

Bibliography

American Cancer Society. (2016). *What are the key statistics about cervical cancer?* Retrieved from http://www.cancer.org/cancer/cervicalcancer/detailedguide/cervical-cancer-key-statistics

American College of Obstetricians and Gynecologists. (2013). *New guidelines for cervical cancer screening.* Retrieved from http://www.acog.org/-/media/For-Patients/pfs004.pdf?dmc=1&ts=

Massad, L. S., Einstein, M. H., Huh, W. K., Katki, H. A., Kinney, W. K., Schiffman, M., & Lawson, H. W. (2013). 2012 updated consensus guidelines for the management of abnormal cervical cancer screening tests and cancer precursors. *Journal of Lower Genital Tract Disease, 17*(5 suppl 1), S1–S27. doi:10.1097/lgt.0b013e318287d329

Contraception

Rhonda Arthur and Michelle Collins

Definition

A. Contraception is the intentional prevention of pregnancy by either or both sexual partners. Contraception can be mechanical, chemical, or surgical, and is either reversible or nonreversible. Considerations in counseling regarding contraceptive choices include cost, efficacy, safety, and personal considerations such as personal belief systems and ability to use selected method.

The Centers for Disease Control and Prevention's (CDC) U.S. Medical Eligibility Criteria for Contraceptive Use is a formal adaptation of the 1996 World Health Organization's (WHO) Medical Eligibility Criteria for Contraceptive Use. This valuable document assists healthcare providers in counseling women and men and assists healthcare providers in determining safe and effective contraceptive methods individualized to client preferences and individual health issues. It is available at www.cdc.gov/reproductivehealth/unintendedpregnancy/pdf/legal_summary-chart_english_final_tag508.pdf.

Incidence

A. Women frequently visit primary care providers to request contraception and family planning education. There are 61 million women in the United States of child-bearing age. Ninety-nine percent of women aged 15 to 44 years have used at least one contraceptive method. Unfortunately, approximately 50% of all pregnancies in the United States are unintended. At greatest risk for unintended pregnancy are women at both ends of the reproductive age spectrum: teenagers and perimeno-pausal women. Consistent use of a reliable and effective contraceptive method can greatly reduce the unintended pregnancy rate. Easy access and education regarding contraceptive use is a keystone in the prevention of unintended pregnancy.

Subjective Data

A. Review the client's complete menstrual history, including age of onset, duration, frequency, regularity, and degree of discomfort with menses. Review the first day of LMP.
B. Review the client's pregnancy history.
C. Review the client's contraception and sexual history.
D. Note other medications the client is taking, including OTC medications and supplements.
E. Ask the client whether she has had a major medical disease, including hypertension, cardiovascular incident, thromboembolic disease, diabetes, migraine headaches, gallbladder disease, or liver disease.
F. Review the client's substance abuse/use history.
G. Review the client's childhood illness and immunization record.
H. Note any allergies.
I. Review any pertinent family medical history, particularly asking about family history of cardiovascular events, myocardial infarctions (MIs) prior to age 50, and thromboembolic disease.

Physical Examination

A. Check height, weight, BP, pulse, and body mass index (BMI).
B. Inspect:
   1. Note the client's overall appearance. Look at the neck (thyroid). Inspect the breast/genitalia for Tanner staging (see Appendix C: Tanner's Sexual Maturity Stages).
   2. Skin assessment: Check for central hair growth, which is responsive to androgens. Areas to inspect for coarse hair include the upper lip, chin, sideburns, neck, chest, lower abdomen, and perineum.
C. Auscultate:
   1. Auscultate the heart and lungs.
   2. If pregnancy is suspected, consider auscultating for fetal heart tones.
D. Palpate:
   1. Palpate the neck for thyroid enlargement.
   2. Palpate the abdomen for enlarged organs or uterine enlargement compatible with pregnancy.
   3. Perform a breast examination, palpating for masses. Assess for nipple discharge.
   4. Palpate the axilla for masses and lymphadenopathy.

E. Pelvic examination (note that neither a pelvic examination nor Pap testing is required for a client to receive a contraceptive prescription)
   1. Inspect the external genitalia. Note the pubic hair pattern for Tanner staging. Note any lesions, masses, or discharge.
   2. Speculum examination: Inspect the vagina and cervix. Note any vaginal discharge. Obtain a Pap and/or HPV test as well as cervical/vaginal cultures as appropriate and in accordance with guidelines for screening.
   3. Bimanual examination: Palpate the cervix and check for CMT. Palpate the size of the uterus and assess for adnexal masses.

Diagnostic Tests

A. Urine: Pregnancy test as indicated/urinalysis as indicated; not done routinely, but if indicated by symptomology
B. Serum: Complete blood count (CBC) if indicated by history and/or symptomology
C. Pap test and/or HPV test as indicated by guidelines
D. Vaginal/cervical cultures for STIs as indicated

Plan

A. General interventions:
   1. Review all methods of contraception available with the client and partner, if available.
   2. Consider all aspects of the client's history and make recommendations as appropriate.
B. Client teaching:
   1. Review anatomy and physiology of the menstrual cycle and reproduction with all clients.
   2. Review the risks, benefits, costs, use, and efficacy of contraceptive methods. Review perfect use versus typical use of method selected.
   3. Review STI prevention, and limitations of STI prevention, as related to each method.
   4. Assist the client in selecting the most appropriate method of contraception with regard to cost, efficacy, health status, ability to use correctly and consistently, and the client's personal values.
   5. Educate all clients on warning signs and information as to when to call the care provider.
   6. Educate all women of childbearing age on the availability and proper use of emergency contraceptives. *See Section III: Client Teaching Guide for this chapter, "Contraception: How to Take Birth Control Pills (for a 28-Day Cycle)."* ◄
   7. Provide all clients with information on the prevention of STIs.

Methods of Contraception

A. Abstinence: Refraining from sexual intercourse:
   1. Advantages: Easy and no cost. Perfect use offers protection against STIs and pregnancy.
   2. Disadvantages: User dependent
B. Barrier methods:
   1. Male condom:
      a. Advantages: Male condoms are easily accessible (OTC with no prescription needed) and relatively

inexpensive. Condoms do not require daily intervention and offer some protections against STIs.

b. Disadvantages: The efficacy of male condoms is technique dependent. Breakage and spillage can occur. Some condoms are made from latex, and individuals with latex allergies need to be aware and carefully check the label for latex content. Nonlatex condoms are available. Male condoms are intended for one-time use only.

c. Efficacy with perfect use of male condoms: Approximately 2 in 100 women will become pregnant each year. With typical use of male condoms, approximately 15 in 100 women will become pregnant each year.

2. Female condom:

a. Advantages: Female condoms are easily accessible (OTC with no prescription needed) and relatively inexpensive. Condoms do not require daily intervention and offer some protections against STIs.

b. Disadvantages: The efficacy of female condoms is technique dependent. Slippage and spillage can occur. The female condom is intended for one-time use only and may be inserted up to 8 hours before intercourse.

c. Efficacy with perfect use of the female condom: Approximately 5 in 100 women will become pregnant each year. With typical use of the female condom, approximately 21 in 100 women will become pregnant each year.

3. Diaphragm:

a. Advantages: Diaphragms are nonhormonal and can be used for years with proper care. They may be inserted up to 6 hours before intercourse.

b. Disadvantages: Diaphragms must be properly fitted by an experienced healthcare provider and are user controlled. Placement is crucial to contraceptive benefit, and spermicide must be used with the diaphragm. The diaphragm should be removed 6 hours after intercourse. Diaphragms carry an increased risk of toxic shock syndrome (TSS). The client must have the fit checked after childbirth and any weight gain or loss of 10 pounds or more. UTIs may be more frequent in diaphragm users, and some women may experience sensitivity or allergy to spermicide. Use during menses should be avoided due to increased risk of TSS.

c. Efficacy with perfect use of the diaphragm: Six in 100 women will become pregnant each year. With typical use of the diaphragm, 16 in 100 women will become pregnant each year.

4. Cervical cap:

a. Advantages: Cervical caps are nonhormonal and can be used for years with proper care. The cervical cap may be inserted and left in place up to 48 hours.

b. Disadvantages: Cervical caps must be properly fitted by an experienced healthcare provider and are user controlled. Placement is crucial to contraceptive benefit, and spermicide must be used; the cervical cap must be removed within 48 hours due to the risk of TSS. The FemCap is made of latex and is not appropriate for latex-allergic clients. Some women may experience sensitivity or allergy to spermicide. Use should be avoided during menses due to increased risk for TSS.

c. Efficacy with use of the cervical cap is similar to that for the diaphragm.

5. Vaginal sponge:

a. Advantages: The vaginal sponge is a nonhormonal OTC polyurethane sponge that releases the spermicide nonoxynol-9. It can be used for multiple acts of intercourse over 24 hours.

b. Disadvantages: The vaginal sponge is user-controlled. Some women may experience sensitivity or allergy to the spermicide. Use should be avoided during menses due to increased risk for TSS.

c. Efficacy with use: With perfect use of the vaginal sponge, among parous women, 20 in 100 will become pregnant each year; 9 nulliparous women will become pregnant each year. With typical use, 32 in 100 parous women and 16 in 100 nulliparous women will become pregnant each year.

C. Surgery:

1. Male sterilization:

a. Advantages: Sterilization is a very effective form of contraception. The user does not have to remember to do anything before intercourse, and it is not user dependent. Sterilization is permanent.

b. Disadvantages: Sterilization involves a surgical procedure. Though recent federal insurance changes have mandated insurance coverage for contraception, exceptions may leave coverage of the cost up to the client.

c. Risk of pregnancy after male sterilization: Approximately one in 1,000 women will become pregnant each year after their partner has had a vasectomy.

2. Female sterilization (tubal ligation) is the second most used contraceptive method in the United States.

a. Advantages: Sterilization is a very effective form of contraception. The user does not have to remember to do anything before intercourse, and it is not user dependent. Sterilization is permanent.

b. Disadvantages: Sterilization involves a surgical procedure. If pregnancy does occur after tubal ligation, there is a higher incidence of ectopic pregnancy. Though recent federal insurance program changes have mandated insurance coverage for contraception, exceptions may leave coverage of the cost up to the client.

c. After tubal ligation, five women in 1,000 will become pregnant each year.

D. IUD:

1. Hormonal (Mirena, Skyla, Kyleena, Liletta):

a. Advantages: Hormonal IUDs are very effective forms of contraception. Mirena works up to 7 years (but is currently approved for use only up to 5 years); Liletta and Kyleena are approved for use up to 5 years, and Skyla for 3 years. As far as progestin content, Mirena and Liletta have the same amount of hormone in them; Kyleena has less than that, and Skyla has the lowest amount. Having an IUD in place means that no effort is required on the woman's part (as far as ensuring contraceptive efficacy) prior to having intercourse. Women should be counseled to check that the string is present once monthly (after menses if having them). All of the hormonal IUDs may reduce menstrual flow via sustained thinning of the endometrium. Skyla, made by the same manufacturer as Mirena (Bayer), is slightly smaller than Mirena.

b. Disadvantages: Risks of progestin IUDs include uterine perforation, increased spontaneous abortion, ectopic pregnancy, ovarian cysts, and infection. Risk of infection is minimized if the IUD is placed when vaginitis is not present. IUDs do not cause ectopic pregnancies; however, if a woman conceives while she has an IUD in situ, there is greater risk that the pregnancy could be ectopic. Overall, however, because not many women will conceive while using an IUD, the overall ectopic pregnancy rate of women with an IUD in situ is still less than that of women using other forms of contraception, or no contraception at all. Any IUD must be inserted by a qualified healthcare professional who has received training in the individual insertion techniques. IUDs may be spontaneously expelled; the risk of expulsion is greatest in the first 3 months after insertion. The IUD with the smallest dose of progestin (Skyla) may result in more breakthrough spotting than those IUDs with higher progestin content.

c. With a progestin IUD in place, approximately 1.5 women per 1,000 will conceive annually

d. Effect on bleeding pattern: Progestin-containing IUDs have been associated with decreased amounts of menstrual bleeding and cramping. By the end of the first year with the IUD in situ, the majority of users will notice a significant reduction in the number of bleeding days. This makes the progestin IUDs an option for women with menorrhagia.

2. Nonhormonal (ParaGard):

a. Advantages: ParaGard is a very effective form of contraception. It may be left in place for 10 years as of current approval, though it has been proven effective for 12 years. Having an IUD in place means that no effort is required on the woman's part (as far as ensuring contraceptive efficacy) prior to having intercourse. Women should be counseled to check that the string is present once monthly (after menses if having them).

b. Disadvantages: Risks of any IUD include uterine perforation, increased spontaneous abortion, ectopic pregnancy, and infection. ParaGard must be inserted by a qualified healthcare professional trained in the insertion technique. The IUD may be spontaneously expelled; the risk of expulsion is greatest in the first 3 months after insertion. The bleeding pattern with ParaGard is different from that of the woman with a progestin-containing IUD in situ. While the user of a progestin-containing IUD may expect some irregular bleeding in the weeks and months after placement, the ParaGard user may notice increased blood volume with menses after placement. While the progestin-containing IUDs may result in menses eventually ceasing, ParaGard users tend to continue to have regular menses. This is an important difference to note, as some women want to have a monthly menses and would be very uncomfortable with not having a monthly bleed. Conversely, if a woman has a history of menorrhagia, insertion of a ParaGard may exacerbate that issue for her.

c. When using a copper IUD, approximately 1.8 women per 1,000 will conceive annually.

Women who are not appropriate candidates for an IUD include those with ongoing pelvic infections, anatomical uterine abnormalities that distort anatomy, unexplained vaginal bleeding, vaginal malignancy, and pregnancy. STI screening is not mandatory prior to IUD placement. Women who have not had STI screening in the past, or who are at increased risk for STI, should have screening done at the time of the insertion appointment. Device placement should not be delayed to wait for test results. Any positive results can be addressed with treatment without removal of the IUD. See WHO's IUD Toolkit at www.k4health.org/toolkits/iud.

E. Pharmaceutical therapy:

1. Progestin-only pills (POPs; also known as "mini-pills"):

a. Advantages: POPs are a safe hormonal alternative for women who either cannot, or prefer not to, take estrogen

b. Disadvantages: POPs cannot be taken if the client has any contraindications to progestin use. POPs must be taken daily at the same time (within a 3-hour period), requiring strict adherence to the dosing regimen.

c. Efficacy with perfect use of POPs: Three in 1,000 women per year will become pregnant. With typical use, nine in 1,000 women per year will become pregnant.

2. Injection: Long-acting depot medroxyprogesterone acetate (DMPA; Depo-Provera)

a. Advantages: Easy to use. The user only has to remember to obtain the injection every 3 months. DMPA may decrease vaginal bleeding overall, though clients may experience irregular bleeding initially. DMPA is a safe hormonal alternative for women who cannot, or prefer not to, take estrogen.

b. Disadvantages: Women cannot use DMPA if they have any contraindications to progestin use; it may cause amenorrhea or irregular vaginal bleeding in such clients. There is a risk of weight gain with DMPA use. Use of this method requires routine (3 months) visits to the provider's office for IM injections. DMPA does not provide protection against STIs. DMPA is associated with reversible decreased bone mineral density.

c. Efficacy with perfect use of DMPA: Three in 1,000 women per year will become pregnant. With typical use, 30 in 1,000 women per year will become pregnant.

d. DPMA should be administered during the first 5 days of the menstrual cycle or postpartum before resumption of intercourse (preferably, after lactation has been established). If this is not possible, or if a woman is 3 or more weeks late for return injection, administer a pregnancy test and have the client use condoms for at least 1 week after injection.

3. Contraceptive implant: Long-acting reversible etonogestrel implant (Nexplanon):

a. A single-rod subdermal radiopaque implant

b. Advantages: Progestin-containing implant is a safe hormonal alternative for women who cannot, or prefer not to, take estrogen. Nexplanon is a long-acting (3 years) reversible contraceptive.

c. Disadvantages: Women cannot use Nexplanon if they have any contraindications to progestin use. Insertion and removal complications are possible. Women may note irregular bleeding for the duration of use.

d. Only clinicians who have completed the manufacturer's training program are eligible to purchase the product. The link to request this training is www.nexplanon-usa.com/en/hcp/services-and-support/request-training/index.asp.

e. Absolute contraindications to progestin therapy:
i. Active thrombophlebitis or thromboembolic disorders
ii. Acute liver disease
iii. Known or suspected cancer of the breast
iv. Pregnancy
v. Undiagnosed, abnormal vaginal bleeding

4. Combined estrogen/progestin contraceptives: Come in three modalities—oral pills, a transdermal patch, and a vaginal ring. Advantages and disadvantages and efficacy are similar between products, but there are some differences in the delivery methods.

a. Advantages: Combined contraceptives are easy to use, convenient, rapidly reversible, and controlled by women. The transdermal patch is changed only weekly. The vaginal ring is left in place for 3 weeks, removed for 1 week, and then a new ring inserted. In addition to predictable menses, combined contraceptives decrease menstrual flow and length of menses.

b. Disadvantages: Methods are dependent on user adherence, and oral pills must be taken daily. Exposure to hormones may not be suitable for certain women based on health status and risk. See the U.S. Medical Eligibility Criteria (US MEC) for Contraceptive Use for absolute and relative contraindications. Smoking in conjunction with use of combined contraceptive increases cardiovascular risk and should be considered in prescribing. None of the delivery modalities protects against STIs. Other medications, such as anticonvulsants, may interfere with the effectiveness of combined hormonal contraceptives and should be considered in prescribing.

c. Efficacy with perfect use of combined hormonal contraceptive: Three in 1,000 women per year will become pregnant. With typical use, 80 in 1,000 women per year will become pregnant.

d. Prescribing considerations: Oral contraceptives come in combination extended cycle, combination monophasic, combination biphasic, combination triphasic, and progestin-only formulations. General considerations for pill selection include age, health history/status, family health history, and the client's preference. Alternatives for COCs should be considered in women 35 years and older who smoke, due to increased risks of thrombolytic events. For anyone who may have difficulty remembering to take a daily pill, consideration should be given to prescription of the vaginal ring, patch, or other methods. See the manufacturer's prescribing information for complete information on safety side effects and contraindications.

e. Absolute contraindications to ET:
i. Acute liver disease
ii. Cerebral vascular or coronary artery disease, MI, or stroke
iii. History of or active thrombophlebitis or thromboembolic disorders
iv. History of uterine or ovarian cancer
v. Known or suspected cancer of the breast
vi. Known or suspected estrogen-dependent neoplasm
vii. Pregnancy
viii. Undiagnosed, abnormal vaginal bleeding

f. Relative contraindications to ET:
i. Active gallbladder disease
ii. Familial hyperlipidemia

5. Spermicide (foam, film, gel, tablets, and suppositories):

a. Advantages: Spermicide is a nonhormonal OTC preparation containing nonoxynol-9. It is inexpensive and easily accessible.

b. Disadvantages: Spermicide is user-controlled and, if not used consistently, will lead to contraception failure. Some individuals may experience sensitivity or allergy to spermicide.

c. Efficacy with perfect use of spermicide: 180 in 1,000 women will become pregnant each year. With typical use of spermicide, 58 of 1,000 women will become pregnant each year.

F. Fertility Awareness Methods (FAM): Include the Standard Days Method, the TwoDay Method, and the Lactational Amenorrhea Method.

    1. Advantages: FAMs are nonhormonal and free to use

    2. Disadvantages: FAMs are user-controlled and depend on regularity of cycle and avoidance of intercourse on fertile days of cycle. They can be complex for women to use, and do not protect against STIs.

    3. Efficacy with use: With typical use of the FAM, 50 in 1,000 women will become pregnant each year.

Additional information, training, and client teaching may be found at the following websites: Association of Reproductive Health Professionals Institute for Reproductive Health (www.irh.org), Cycle Beads (cyclebeads.com), and Planned Parenthood (www.plannedparenthood.org).

G. Withdrawal:

    1. Advantages: Withdrawal is nonhormonal, inexpensive, and easily accessible.

    2. Disadvantages: Withdrawal is user-controlled. It does not protect against STIs.

    3. Efficacy with use: With typical use of the withdrawal method, 170 in 1,000 women will become pregnant each year.

Follow-Up

A. The client newly initiated on oral, ring, or patch contraceptives may be scheduled for a return visit 3 months after initiation to assess BP, use, side effects, and satisfaction. Thereafter, satisfaction with method, and desire to continue, can be addressed as annual preventive visits.

B. Clients who receive Depo-Provera injections must return every 3 months for follow-up injection. Thereafter, satisfaction with method, weight evaluation, and desire to continue can be addressed as annual preventive visits.

C. Clients with a diaphragm should return for refitting with change in weight of 10 pounds (lost or gained) or when in a postpartum state.

Consultation/Referral

A. If the contraceptive method selected is one that the practitioner is not experienced in providing (e.g., diaphragm, implant, IUD, surgical sterilization), referral to an experienced appropriate provider should be given.

Individual Considerations

A. Adults:

    1. A pelvic examination is not required and should not become a barrier to access to contraception.

    2. Discontinue combined hormonal contraceptive methods for women aged 35 years and older who smoke.

    3. Increased age and obesity increase the risk of venous thromboembolism with the use of combined hormonal contraceptive methods. These methods should be prescribed with caution and all appropriate alternative contraceptives considered.

    4. Provide anticipatory guidance regarding the need to use contraceptives until menopause is confirmed to prevent unintended pregnancy.

B. Adolescents:

    1. A pelvic examination is not required to initiate contraception and should not become a barrier to access to contraception. Long-acting reversible contraceptives (injection, implant, and IUD) and methods that require less frequent dosing (patch, ring) promote adherence and continuation and *should* be encouraged in teens.

    2. Education and counseling regarding pregnancy and STI prevention are essential.

    3. Many clients have mobile phones with reminder apps that assist in compliance with contraceptive use.

Bibliography

Bayer Pharmaceuticals. *About Skyla*. Retrieved from https://www.skyla-us.com/what-is-skyla.php

Centers for Disease Control and Prevention. (2018) *US Medical Eligibility Criteria (US MEC) for contraceptive use, 2016.* Retrieved from https://www.cdc.gov/reproductivehealth/contraception/mmwr/mec/summary.html

Cunningham, F. G., Leveno, K. J., Bloom, S. L., Spong, C. Y., Dashe, J. S., Hoffman, B. L., . . . Sheffield, J. S. (2014). *Williams obstetrics* (24th ed.). New York, NY: McGraw-Hill Education.

Cycle Beads. (2019). Retrieved from https://www.cyclebeads.com/how-family-planning-method-helps-to-plan-pregnancy-or-prevent-pregnancy

Diedrich, J. T., Desai, S., Zhao, Q., Secura, G., Madden, T., & Peipert, J. F. (2015). Association of short-term bleeding and cramping patterns with long-acting reversible contraceptive method satisfaction. *American Journal of Obstetrics and Gynecology, 212*(1), 50-.e1. doi:10.1016/j.ajog.2014.07.025

Diedrich, J. T., Zhao, Q., Madden, T., Secura, G. M., & Peipert, J. F. (2015). Three-year continuation of reversible contraception. *American Journal of Obstetrics and Gynecology, 213*(5), 662e1–662e8. doi:10.1016/j.ajog.2015.08.001

Eisenberg, D. L., Schreiber, C. A., Turok, D. K., Teal, S. B., Westhoff, C. L., Creinin, M. D., & ACCESS IUS Investigators. (2015). Three-year efficacy and safety of a new 52-mg levonorgestrel-releasing intrauterine system. *Contraception, 92*(1), 10–16. doi:10.1016/j.contraception.2015.04.006

Guttmacher Institute. (2015). *Contraceptive use in the United States.* Retrieved from http://www.guttmacher.org/fact-sheet/contraceptive-use-united-states

Hobby, J. H., Zhao, Q., & Peipert, J. F. (2018). Effect of baseline menstrual bleeding pattern on copper intrauterine device continuation. *American Journal of Obstetrics and Gynecology, 219*(5), 465.e1. doi:10.1016/j.ajog.2018.08.028

Jatlaoui, T. C., Riley, H. E., & Curtis, K. M. (2017). The safety of intrauterine devices among young women: A systematic review. *Contraception, 95*(1), 17–39. https://doi.org/10.1016/j.contraception.2016.10.006

Lange, H. L., Belury, M. A., Secic, M., Thomas, A., & Bonny, A. E. (2015). Dietary intake and weight gain among adolescents on depot medroxyprogesterone acetate. *Journal of Pediatric and Adolescent Gynecology, 28*(3), 139–143. doi:10.1016/j.jpag.2014.04.004

Liletta (levonorgestrel-releasing intrauterine system) 52 mg [Prescribing information]. Irvine, CA: Allergan and Medicines360, 2018.

ParaGard. (2014). *Prescribing information.* Retrieved from http://www.paragard.com/Pdf/ParaGard-PI.pdf

Planned Parenthood. (2019). *What are the types of hormonal IUDs?* https://www.plannedparenthood.org/learn/birth-control/iud/hormonal-iuds

Schreiber, C. A., Teal, S. B., Blumenthal, P. D., Keder, L. M., Olariu, A. I., & Creinin, M. D. (2018). Bleeding patterns for the Liletta levonorgestrel 52 mg intrauterine system. *European Journal of Contraception & Reproductive Health Care, 23*(2), 116–120. doi:10.1080/13625187.2018.1449825

Sierra, T. (2019). Helping patients select long-acting reversible contraceptives. *Journal of the American Academy of PAs, 32*(4), 23–27. doi:10.1097/01.jaa.0000554220.48629.a4

Teal, S. B., Turok, D. K., Jensen, J. T., Chen, B. A., Kimble, T. D., & Creinin, M. D. (2018). Five-year efficacy and safety of the Liletta levonorgestrel intrauterine system [13F]. *Obstetrics & Gynecology, 131*, 66S–67S. doi:10.1097/01.aog.0000533323.62976.5c

World Health Organization. (2018). *IUD Toolkit.* Retrieved from https://www.k4health.org/toolkits/iud

Zieman, M., Hatcher, R. A., Trussell, J., Nelson, A. L., Cates, W., Hatcher, R. A., & Allen, A. Z. (2015). *Managing contraception for your pocket.* Tiger, GA: Bridging the Gap Foundation.

Dysmenorrhea

Rhonda Arthur and Michelle Collins

Definition

Dysmenorrhea is painful uterine cramping felt primarily in the lower abdomen, lower back, and upper thighs.

A. Primary dysmenorrhea: Not associated with pelvic pathology; usually associated with ovulatory cycles. Occurs on the first or second day of the menstrual period, and is usually worse the first day. Affects teens and women in their 20s most often and may decrease with advancing age. Often associated with prostaglandin-induced symptoms of diarrhea, nausea, vomiting, and/or headache.

B. Secondary dysmenorrhea: Painful uterine contractions due to a pathologic etiology such as endometriosis, leiomyomata, adenomyosis, interstitial cystitis, irritable bowel syndrome (IBS), or PID. Primarily occurs in women in their 20s, 30s, and 40s.

Incidence

A. Primary dysmenorrhea is very common, affecting up to 60% of young women. Dysmenorrhea frequently leads to absenteeism from work or school and can have great impact on a woman's social life and ability to participate in physical activities. Endometriosis can be the cause, and should be considered in the differential diagnosis, particularly when the dysmenorrhea is unresponsive to treatment.

Pathogenesis

A. Primary dysmenorrhea is due to myometrial contractions that are caused by prostaglandins in the secretory endometrium. The prostaglandins cause uterine ischemia through platelet aggregation, vasoconstriction, and dysrhythmic contractions.

B. Secondary dysmenorrhea is associated with pathologic conditions such as endometriosis, cervical stenosis, tumors, adhesions, adenomyosis, myomas, polyps, infection (PID), or nongynecological causes. The pain of secondary dysmenorrhea may also be unrelated to menses.

C. In endometriosis, islands of endometrial tissue are found on peritoneal surfaces of the bladder, broad ligaments, fallopian tubes, ovaries, bowel, and cul-de-sac, as well as distant sites on the abdominal wall, vagina, lung, or other sites.

Predisposing Factors

A. Female
B. Age younger than 30 years
C. Reproductive age
D. Congenital pelvic anomaly
E. Nulliparity
F. Smoking
G. Early menarche
H. History of pelvic surgery
I. History of sexual abuse
J. BMI less than 20
K. Depression

Common Complaints

A. "I have painful periods."
B. "My menstrual cramps are terrible, particularly the first day of my cycle."
C. "My cramps are so bad I feel sick to my stomach and have diarrhea."

Other Signs and Symptoms

A. History of menstrual cramps that occur just before the onset of the menstrual period and persist through the first 24 to 48 hours
B. Pain beginning *prior to* the onset of menses, which is associated with intercourse, defecation, and urination, is often associated with endometriosis or adenomyosis. Intermenstrual bleeding is also associated with endometriosis.
C. Acute pain may be associated with infection (PID) or ectopic pregnancy.

Subjective Data

A. Obtain a complete menstrual history: Age at menarche; frequency, duration, and regularity of periods; amount of flow in number of perineal pads or tampons used.
B. Ask the client about the location of the pain; note radiation and associated symptoms such as nausea, vomiting, or diarrhea.
C. Is the pain rhythmic or spasmodic (primary) or steady (secondary)?
D. How old was the client when the pain began? Primary dysmenorrhea usually begins 2 to 3 years after menarche.
E. Inquire about the type of contraception used.
F. Obtain an obstetric history.
G. Is the pain related to the menstrual period, or does it occur before, or independent of, the menstrual period?
H. Does the client have dyspareunia?
I. Does the client have UTI symptoms?
J. What treatments have been tried, and which were effective?
K. Obtain a family history for endometriosis and dysmenorrhea.
L. Obtain a social history, particularly including use of tobacco and history of sexual abuse.
M. Obtain a gynecologic history, including any episodes of STIs, PID, prior pelvic surgery, congenital pelvic anomalies, or endometriosis.

Physical Examination

A. Check height and weight, temperature, BP, and pulse.

B. Inspect;
  1. Examine the general body habitus for female adipose fat distribution on the buttocks and thighs.
  2. Note breast development (see Tanner's Sexual Maturity Stages in Appendix C).
  3. Observe the abdomen for distention.

C. Auscultate:
  1. The heart and lungs
  2. The abdomen for bowel sounds

D. Palpate and percuss:
  1. The abdomen for masses or tenderness
  2. The lower abdomen for tenderness
  3. CVAT

E. Pelvic examination:
  1. Inspect the external genitalia for pubic hair pattern, lesions, discharge, and odor.
  2. Palpate the external genitalia for masses or areas of tenderness.

F. Speculum examination: Inspect the cervix and vagina for discharge, lesions, and cervical erosion.

G. Bimanual examination:
  1. Palpate the vagina and cul-de-sac areas for tenderness or masses.
  2. Check the cervical position, mobility, and pain with mobility (CMT).
  3. Check uterine size, mobility, shape, regularity, masses, position, contour, and tenderness.
  4. Check the adnexa for masses (cystic or solid) and tenderness.

Diagnostic Tests

Primary dysmenorrhea is often diagnosed by history, including symptoms and timing in the menstrual cycle and results of the pelvic examination. If secondary dysmenorrhea is suspected and additional information is required, the care provider may consider the following diagnostic tests:

A. Pelvic ultrasonography to rule out pelvic pathology.

B. Laboratory studies: Urinalysis, hemoglobin (Hgb), hematocrit (Hct), and WBC

C. Consider cultures for chlamydia and gonorrhea, if infection is suspected

D. Pregnancy test as indicated

E. Pap and/or HPV test as indicated per guidelines

F. Urinalysis

Differential Diagnoses

A. Dysmenorrhea: The client's history and a normal pelvic examination are used to diagnose primary dysmenorrhea.

B. Complication of pregnancy: Missed or incomplete abortion or ectopic pregnancy

C. Endometriosis or adenomyosis

D. Ruptured ovarian cyst

E. Infection: Endometritis, salpingitis, PID, or pelvic adhesions

F. Fibroid tumors

G. Adhesions

H. UTI

I. Bowel disease: Irritable bowel disease or inflammatory bowel disease (IBD)

Plan

A. General interventions:
  1. Support the client's concerns and identify the reality of discomfort. Identify primary source of pain if other diagnoses exist.

B. Client teaching:
  1. *See Section III: Client Teaching Guides for this chapter, "Dysmenorrhea (Painful Menstrual Cramps or Periods)" and "Contraception: How to Take Birth Control Pills (for a 28-Day Cycle)."* ◄
  2. Educate the client about the physiology of menstruation.
  3. Teach the client that endometriosis is one of the leading causes of infertility.
  4. Encourage activity and exercise, such as walking or swimming.
  5. Advise warm baths or heating pads.

C. Pharmaceutical therapy:
  1. NSAIDs are the drugs of choice:
    a. NSAIDs inhibit prostaglandin synthesis in the endometrium, thus decreasing uterine cramping. There is also an analgesic effect.
    b. The fenamates have been the most effective, followed by the propionic acid derivatives.
    c. Medications should be started as the menstrual period begins; may begin 24 to 48 hours prior to onset of menses for severe cases.
    d. Prostaglandin inhibitors relieve dysmenorrhea in 80% of women.
    e. Take NSAIDs with food to avoid GI upset and irritation.
  2. Medications of choice for dysmenorrhea:
    a. NSAIDs: OTC medications
      i. Arylacetic acid derivatives: Naproxen sodium (Aleve) 440 mg initially, then 220 mg every 8 to 12 hours; naproxen sodium (Anaprox) 500 mg PO initially, then 250 mg PO every 6 to 8 hours or 500 mg every 12 hours (long-acting formula); not to exceed 1,250 mg/d on the first day; subsequent doses should not exceed 1,000 mg/d. Naproxen sodium (Naprelan) 1,000 mg (taken as two 500-mg tablets) once a day. Some clients may need 1,500 mg (taken as two 750-mg or three 500-mg tablets) per day, for a limited period. However, the dose is usually not more than 1,000 mg per day.
      ii. Propionic acid derivatives: Ibuprofen (Advil, Motrin, Nuprin) 400 mg every 6 hours; ketoprofen (Orudis) immediate release: 25 to 50 mg every 6 to 8 hours as needed, with maximum dose of 300 mg/d
      iii. Anthranilic acid derivatives: Mefenamic acid (Ponstel) 500 mg initial dose, then

250 mg every 6 hours. The treatment maximum is 2 to 3 days.

    iv. Benzeneacetic acid derivatives: Diclofenac potassium (Cataflam) 50 mg three times per day. Initial dose of 100 mg may be given followed by 50 mg doses.

  b. Hormonal control:

    i. Oral contraceptive pills: Any combination pill is efficacious. Consider extended-cycle dosing to prevent having monthly periods.

    ii. Nuvaring

    iii. Depo-Provera

    iv. Mirena IUD

    v. Nexplanon

  3. Medications of choice for endometriosis:

    a. NSAIDs

    b. Oral contraceptive pills

    c. With physician consultation or referral, danazol (Danocrine). For mild cases, an initial daily dose of 200 to 400 mg given in two divided doses is recommended and may be adjusted depending on client response.

    d. With physician consultation or referral, Gn-RH agonists such as nafarelin (Synarel), leuprolide acetate (Lupron, Lupron Depot), and goserelin acetate (Zoladex) may be used.

  4. Vitamin E 400 IU daily

D. Vigorous exercise more than three times weekly has been associated with a decrease in symptomology.

E. Eating breakfast regularly has been associated with less dysmenorrhea.

F. Acupuncture has been associated with significantly lower pain from dysmenorrhea.

Follow-Up

A. The client should return in 3 months for follow-up to assess relief with medication. Encourage the client to undergo the treatment for 3 months to determine the effectiveness.

Consultation/Referral

A. If dysmenorrhea does not respond to NSAIDs or combined hormonal contraceptives, consult with an OB/GYN physician for further workup to determine the source of the pain

B. Consider consultation with OB/GYN physician for laparoscopy or hysteroscopy to rule out endometriosis or adhesions. Laser may be used to destroy endometrial implants or to lyse adhesions.

Individual Considerations

A. Pregnancy: Dysmenorrhea symptoms in the setting of pregnancy could be preterm labor.

B. Adolescents:

  1. Remember that endometriosis can occur in this age group.

C. Adults:

  1. Endometriosis can be a disabling condition interfering with work and sexual relationships. It may continue into the perimenopausal period.

Bibliography

Burbeck, R., & Willig, C. (2014). The personal experience of dysmenorrhea: An interpretative phenomenological analysis. *Journal of Health Psychology, 19*(10), 1334–1344. doi:10.1177/1359105313490313

Eittah, H. F. A. (2014). Effect of breakfast skipping on young females' menstruation. *Health Science Journal, 8*(4), 469.

Osayande, A. S., & Mehulic, S. (2014). Diagnosis and initial management of dysmenorrhea. *American Family Physician, 89*(5), 341–346.

Dyspareunia

Rhonda Arthur and Michelle Collins

Definition

A. Dyspareunia is genital or pelvic discomfort associated with sexual intercourse (upon entry or deep penetration) that interferes with sexual satisfaction. Dyspareunia may be superficial (also known as introital), relating to vulvar and vaginal pain, or it may be deep, relating to deep, pelvic pain. Vaginismus is the involuntary (often painful) contraction of the pelvic floor muscles in response to pressure or attempted penetration.

Incidence

A. Vaginismus occurs in 1% to 17% of women; dyspareunia occurs in 10% to 20% of women.

Pathogenesis

Both physical and psychosocial etiologies have been identified.

A. Physical causes:

  1. Vulvovaginal anomalies:

    a. Thick hymen

    b. Short vagina

    c. Vaginal agenesis

    d. Vaginal septum

  2. Organic dyspareunia:

    a. Episiotomy scars

    b. Bartholin's gland cyst

    c. Vulvar dystrophy

    d. Inflammation or infection, STI

    e. Vulvovaginal cancer

    f. Pelvic disease:

      i. PID

      ii. Uterine or ovarian tumors

      iii. Adenomyosis

      iv. Pelvic scarring or adhesions versus endometriosis

    g. Genital mutilation

  3. Musculoskeletal anomalies:

    a. Disk disease

    b. Myofascial pain

    c. Coccygodynia

  4. Extensive prolapse or organ displacement

  5. Urethral syndrome or other urinary tract disorders

  6. Vulvodynia

  7. GI anomalies:

    a. Constipation

    b. IBS

    c. IBD

    d. Anorexia

8. Hormonal factors:
  a. Hypoestrogenemia causing atrophic vaginitis
  b. Breastfeeding causing atrophic vaginitis
  c. Menopause causing atrophic vaginitis
B. Psychosocial causes:
  1. Childhood molestation
  2. Fear of pain, infection, or pregnancy
  3. Pelvic congestion syndrome
  4. Poor partner communication
  5. History of sexual assault, including date rape
  6. Previous trauma during intercourse
  7. Domestic violence
  8. Strict religious orthodoxy
  9. Poor sexual education; negative attitudes toward sex

Common Complaints
A. Irritation and/or burning with intercourse
B. Lack of vaginal lubrication
C. Pain and or burning upon vulvar or vaginal contact
D. Pain with deep penetration
E. Postcoital bleeding

Subjective Data
A. Review the onset, duration, and course of presenting symptoms, including the precise location and timing of pain during intercourse.
B. Review the client's medical or surgical history for physical causes (see the "Pathogenesis" section).
C. Ask: How often does pain occur (with every act of intercourse, near menses, or in certain sexual positions)? What relief measures have been tried? Is there improvement with using extra lubrication? How much relief was obtained with each measure?
D. Obtain a complete sexual history including the following:
  1. Sexual practices
  2. Sexual satisfaction; ability to achieve orgasm
  3. Perception of partner satisfaction
  4. Age at first coitus
  5. History of sexual abuse, molestation, assault
  6. Perceptions regarding sexuality
  7. Current number of sexual partners and preferences
  8. Time spent in foreplay
  9. History of recent pregnancy/birth and breastfeeding
  10. Age at onset of puberty, date of last menses, and cycle history
  11. Current method of birth control and satisfaction with method; previous methods and why they were discontinued
  12. Presence of vaginal discharge, odor, dysuria, or other physical symptoms occurring both before and after intercourse
  13. Medications, including prescription and OTC drugs
  14. Can the woman insert a tampon without pain?

Physical Examination
A. Check temperature, pulse, respirations, and BP.
B. Inspect: Observe generally for discomfort before, during, and after the examination.

Look for signs of physical or sexual abuse, cuts, bruises, and lacerations. For pain that is greatest on deep penetration, PID, ovarian cyst, endometriosis, pelvic adhesions, relaxation of pelvic support, and uterine leiomyomata are all plausible differential diagnoses.

C. Auscultate:
  1. The abdomen for bowel sounds in all quadrants; auscultation of the abdomen should precede any palpation or percussion due to the changes in intensity and frequency of sounds after manipulation.
D. Palpate:
  1. Palpate the abdomen for masses; check for suprapubic tenderness.
  2. Examine the back; assess range of motion. Observe for evidence of disk disease, myofascial pain, and coccygodynia. Palpate for CVAT.
E. Pelvic examination:
  1. Inspect: Perform a perineal examination for atrophic vaginitis. Atrophic vaginitis presents as red, shiny, smooth vaginal tissue (loss of rugae); vaginal thinning; and decreased elasticity of vaginal tissues. Vulvar inflammation may be present.
  2. Evaluate the client for vulvovaginitis. Perform a vulvar examination for Bartholin's gland enlargement, fissures, condyloma, and herpes simplex infection. Inspect for anatomical variants, including narrowed introitus, congenital vaginal malformation (septum), and pelvic relaxation (cystocele and rectocele).
  3. Q-tip test for vulvar vestibulitis. (Using a moistened cotton Q-tip, apply gentle pressure on the inner thigh, labia majora, labia minora, clitoris, and perineum.)
F. Speculum examination: Inspect for cervicitis, friability, and discharge. If the woman can insert a tampon without pain, a mechanical obstruction is unlikely.
G. Bimanual examination: Check CMT; adnexal masses; and uterine size, consistency, and position.
H. Rectovaginal examination: Palpate uterosacral ligaments for pain and nodularity and other signs of PID and endometriosis. In cases of rectal trauma, cultures may be needed to rule out STIs.

Diagnostic Tests
A. Wet prep to rule out candidiasis, trichomoniasis, and BV
B. Cervical cultures for chlamydia, gonorrhea
C. Viral cultures of lesions, if any
D. Urine culture, if applicable
E. Pelvic ultrasonography, if indicated
F. Stool culture, if applicable

Differential Diagnoses
A. Dyspareunia
B. See the Pathogenesis section.

Plan
A. General interventions:
  1. Perform a detailed physical examination after taking a thorough history.

2. Clients should be encouraged to involve their partner(s) in assessment, diagnosis, and treatment of dyspareunia.

3. A secure, trusting relationship must be established with the care provider before many clients feel comfortable discussing sexuality issues. Continuity with one provider is essential.

4. Clients with dyspareunia should be evaluated for multiple etiologies. Treat underlying pathologies such as musculoskeletal anomalies, pelvic infection, UTI, STIs, hormonal deficiencies, and GI etiologies (see specific chapters for treatment plans and drug therapy).

B. Client teaching:
  1. *See Section III: Client Teaching Guide for this chapter, "Dyspareunia (Pain With Intercourse)."*

C. Pharmaceutical therapy:
  1. Refer to specific chapters for therapies related to etiology.
  2. Vulvodynia: Consider the use of topical agents applied to the vulva or vestibule, antihistamine therapy, and/or tricyclic antidepressants.
    a. Lidocaine (Xylocaine) 2% or 5% gel applied to the vulva, vestibule, and fourchette, both nightly and prior to intercourse
    b. 2%–6% gabapentin topically
    c. Diphenhydramine (Benadryl) 25 to 50 mg orally at bedtime, or 0.1% triamcinolone acetonide cream twice daily for pruritus
    d. Botulinum toxin type A injection in the vestibular epithelium has shown reduction in pain, though the effects of long-term use have not been evaluated.
    e. Submucosal infiltration with betamethasone and lidocaine for refractory vulvodynia has shown promise.
    f. Amitriptyline 5 to 25 mg nightly; may be increased by 10 to 25 mg weekly until adequate pain control reached (maximum dose of 150 mg daily). Full relief may not be reached for 4 or more weeks.

D. Surgical therapy:
  1. Modified vestibulectomy

E. Psychological and psychosexual therapy:
  1. Cognitive behavioral therapy (CBT)
  2. Pelvic floor physical therapy
  3. Vaginal dilator therapy

F. Alternative therapies:
  1. Physical therapy combined with biofeedback and transcutaneous electronic stimulation (TENS) with intravaginal probe
  2. Acupuncture

Follow-Up
A. Refer to follow-up plans for specific etiology.

Consultation/Referral
A. Refer the client to an OB/GYN physician for removal of cysts and endometriomas. Laparoscopy is indicated if endometriosis, adhesions, or an adnexal mass is suspected.

B. Refer the client to an OB/GYN physician for vulvovaginal anomalies, including thickened hymen, shortened vagina, or vaginal agenesis.

C. Refer the client to a clinician specializing in sexual therapy for continued issues of sexual dysfunction without an identifiable physical cause.

Individual Considerations
A. Pregnancy or postpartum:
  1. Sexual intercourse may continue throughout pregnancy unless there is pain, bleeding, preterm labor, or premature rupture of the membranes. Alternative sexual positions may need to be used to facilitate client comfort, particularly in the third trimester. Sexual intercourse may resume in the postpartum period when the bleeding has decreased or stopped, and any laceration or episiotomy is healed.
  2. Breastfeeding causes hormonal changes that may result in atrophic vaginitis, as well as a vaginal environment that is similar to that of menopause. Vaginal lubrication production may also be diminished in the breastfeeding woman; counseling the client that extra lubrication may be necessary for enhanced comfort with intercourse is helpful.

B. Partners:
  1. Encourage the client to have partner(s) participate in sexual health counseling.

Bibliography
Orr, N., Wahl, K., Joannou, A., Hartmann, D., Valle, L., Yong, P., . . . Renzelli-Cain, R. I. (2019). Deep dyspareunia: Review of pathophysiology and proposed future research priorities. *Sexual Medicine Reviews, 8*(1), 3–17. doi:10.1016/j.sxmr.2018.12.007

Perez, S., & Binik, Y. M. (2016, July 29). Vaginismus: "Gone" but not forgotten. *Psychiatric Times, 33*(7), 1–3. Retrieved from https://www.psychiatrictimes.com/special-reports/vaginismus-gone-not-forgotten

Petros, P., Gold, D., & Inoue, H. (2015). Re: Vulvodynia: Integrating current knowledge into clinical practice. *Obstetrician & Gynaecologist, 17*(2), 138–139. doi:10.1111/tog.12175_4

Tharpe, N. L., Farley, C. L., & Jordan, R. G. (2016). *Clinical practice guidelines for midwifery and women's health.* Burlington, MA: Jones & Bartlett Learning.

Vieira-Baptista, P., Lima-Silva, J., Beires, J., & Donders, G. (2017). Women without vulvodynia can have a positive "Q-tip test": A cross sectional study. *Journal of Psychosomatic Obstetrics & Gynecology, 38*(4), 256–259. doi:10.1080/0167482x.2017.1327519

Emergency Contraception

Rhonda Arthur and Michelle Collins

Definition
A. Emergency contraception (EC) is a method of pregnancy prevention when either unprotected intercourse has occurred or birth control has failed (e.g., condom breakage, skipped oral contraceptive pills).

Incidence
A. Approximately 45% of the 6 million annual pregnancies in the United States are unintended. One in nine sexually active women reports using EC, with the highest use rate among women aged 20 to 24 years.

Pathogenesis
A. The hormones in oral contraceptive pills temporarily disrupt ovarian hormone production and cause

an absent or dysfunctional luteal-phase hormone pattern. This results in an out-of-phase endometrium that is unsuitable for implantation. Hormone disruption may likewise interfere with fertilization and cause disordered tubal transport. Copper in the ParaGard IUD causes an inflammatory response to occur, which renders the endometrium unsuitable for implantation and interferes with fertilization and transport.

Predisposing Factors

A. Rape
B. Failure of other means of birth control, including broken condom, dislodged diaphragm or cervical cap, expelled IUD, or lost or forgotten pill doses
C. Unprotected intercourse

Common Complaints

A. "I'm worried that I might get pregnant because the condom broke."
B. "My diaphragm slipped."
C. "I went on vacation and forgot my pills."

Other Signs and Symptoms

A. Unprotected intercourse

Subjective Data

A. Elicit a menstrual history. When was the first day of the client's LMP? Are her periods regular?
B. What form of contraception was used, if any?
C. Ask about early symptoms of pregnancy such as frequency of urination, nausea, breast tenderness, and late or missed period.
D. Has the client experienced any early signs of pregnancy? If so, discuss.
E. Ask the client about her feelings about an unplanned pregnancy.

Physical Examination

A. Check BP, pulse, and weight.
B. Inspect the abdomen for enlargement compatible with pregnancy.
C. Palpate the abdomen for uterine size; if a fundus is palpable, measure for fundal height.
D. Auscultate:
    1. Heart and lungs
    2. Abdomen. If the uterus is enlarged and is measured to be greater than 11 weeks' gestation, attempt to hear fetal heart tones with fetal Doppler.
E. Pelvic examination:
    1. Inspect the external genitalia for lesions; note the female pubic hair pattern.
    2. Speculum examination: Observe the cervix for a bluish color (Chadwick's sign). Observe for vaginal discharge; note its color and odor.
    3. Bimanual examination: Palpate the cervix for softening associated with early pregnancy. Palpate uterine size, contours, and position.

Diagnostic Tests

A. Pregnancy test: Urine HCG if the first day of the client's last menses was 4 or more weeks prior. Serum HCG can detect pregnancy sooner than urine testing can.

Differential Diagnoses

A. Pregnancy
B. Dysfunctional uterine bleeding (DUB)
C. Amenorrhea from anovulation
D. PCOS
E. Perimenopause

Plan

A. General interventions:
    1. Review the client's past medical history, contraceptive history, first date of LMP, estimated date of ovulation, date of unprotected intercourse, and number of hours since the most recent unprotected intercourses.
    2. Discuss the likely risk of pregnancy.
    3. Explore the client's feeling about continuing a pregnancy.
    4. Decide whether a physical examination and pregnancy test are needed if there is a possibility of a pregnancy from the previous month.
B. Client teaching:
    1. *See Section III: Client Teaching Guides for this chapter "Emergency Contraception—Levonorgestrel" or "Emergency Contraception—Ulipristal Acetate,"* based on the selected method.
    2. Discuss options, risks, failure rates, necessary follow-up, alteration of menstrual period, and warning signs of complications.
    3. Discuss an interim plan for contraception.
    4. Advise the client to take oral contraceptive pills as prescribed, or have an IUD inserted within 96 hours of unprotected intercourse.
    5. Treatment is most effective if taken within 72 hours for progestin–estrogen methods and within 120 hours for a progestin antagonist.
    6. Treatment is not effective in an already established pregnancy.
    7. Educate the client about the possibility of menstrual cycle disturbance with the next menses.
    8. If menstrual bleeding does not begin within 3 weeks, evaluate for possible pregnancy.
    9. EC is not associated with an increased incidence of untoward outcomes of pregnancy, should pregnancy not be averted.
    10. EC is not to be used as a primary contraceptive method.
    11. Recommendations include providing women with a prescription for EC when initiating any contraceptive method.
C. Pharmaceutical therapy:
    Choosing the best method for EC should be based on day and time of unprotected intercourse; BMI; breastfeeding; and recent (within 5 days) use of pill, patch, or ring.
    1. Copper IUD: The copper IUD is the most effective form of EC, with nearly 100% reported efficacy. It can be used up to 120 hours after unprotected intercourse.
        a. A copper IUD (ParaGard) must be inserted within 5 to 7 days after ovulation in a cycle when

unprotected intercourse has occurred. The advantage is that the IUD may be left in place for continuing contraception for 10 years.

b. Mechanism of action: The IUD leads to endometrial changes that prohibit implantation. Its main mechanism of action is to prevent fertilization through the effect of copper ions on sperm function (copper causes sperm decapitation). If fertilization has already occurred, copper ions affect the endometrium, rendering it unreceptive to implantation.

2. EC oral formulations:

a. Ella (ulipristal acetate) is a progesterone agonist/antagonist that is available only by prescription. It cannot be used in breastfeeding women, and may be less effective in women with a BMI greater than 35. However, the efficacy of ulipristal acetate may be higher in overweight and obese women than progestin-only EC products like Plan B One Step, My Way, and Next Choice. EC efficacy tends to decline as BMI increases. For women who have a BMI of 26 or greater and who use progestin-only EC, pregnancy rates are similar to women who do not use EC at all. Ella's efficacy appears to decline in women when the BMI is 35.

i. One tablet is taken orally as soon as possible after unprotected intercourse within 120 hours (5 days).

ii. Common side effects include headaches, abdominal pain, and nausea. Less common side effects include dysmenorrhea, fatigue, and dizziness.

iii. Repeated use of Ella within the same menstrual cycle is not recommended.

iv. If vomiting occurs within 3 hours of taking a dose, take another dose.

v. Because Ella and the progestin component of hormonal contraception bind to receptor sites, women wishing to use hormonal contraception after use of Ella should not do so until 5 days after Ella use, but should be counseled on alternative nonhormonal pregnancy prevention methods.

b. Levonorgestrel EC, commonly called the "morning after pill," is available under the brand names Plan B One-Step, My Way, and Next Choice; it is available in one dose (1.5 mg tablet of levonorgestrel). These progestin-only ECs are available unrestricted as OTC medicines. They are less effective for women with a BMI greater than 25 and may not be effective for women with a BMI greater than 30.

i. Levonorgestrel 1.5 mg tablet should be taken as soon as possible after unprotected sex (no later than 72 hours).

c. Using a standard packet of combined hormonal oral contraceptive pills: Two doses of a combination

TABLE 14.1   EMERGENCY CONTRACEPTION

Antiprogestin Emergency Contraception Pill			
Directions for antiprogestin pills: Take one pill within 120 hours			
Brand		**Number of Pills per Dose**	
Ella		1 white pill	
Progestin-Only Emergency Contraceptive Pill			
Directions for progestin-only pills: Take one dose within 72 hours of intercourse			
Brand	**Number of Pills per Dose**	**Ethinyl Estradiol (mcg)/Dose**	**Levonorgestrel (mg)/Dose**
Plan B One-Step	1 pill	0	1.5
My Way	1 pill	0	1.5
Next Choice One Dose	1 pill	0	1.5
COC Pills for Emergency Contraception			
Directions for COC pills: Take first dose within 72 hours and repeat dose in 12 hours			
Brand	**Number of Pills per Dose**	**Ethinyl Estradiol (mcg)/Dose**	**Levonorgestrel (mg)/Dose**
Ovral	2 white pills	100	0.50
Lo/Ovral	4 white pills	120	0.60
Nordette	4 orange pills	120	0.60
Levlen	4 orange pills	120	0.60
Triphasil	4 yellow pills	120	0.50
Tri-Levlen	4 yellow pills	120	0.50
Alesse	5 pink pills	100	0.50

COC, combined oral contraceptive.

of ethinyl estradiol and norgestrel or levonorgestrel, 12 hours apart. Table 14.1 provides the equivalent dosing that may be used as an emergency contraceptive.

   i. Method must be used within 72 hours of unprotected intercourse. Treatment is most effective if taken within 12 to 24 hours.

   ii. Side effects of nausea and vomiting with EC are common. Take each dose with food. Take the antiemetic meclizine (sold as Dramamine II or Bonine) 30 minutes before the dose of medication.

   iii. If vomiting occurs within 1 hour of taking a dose, take another dose.

   iv. Educate the client about common side effects such as breast tenderness, abdominal pain, headache, and dizziness.

Follow-Up

A. Have the client return in 4 weeks if she does not have a menstrual period. Ideally, the client should begin a reliable method of contraception the day after completing the EC dosing.

Consultation/Referral

A. Consult a provider if there is no withdrawal bleed within 4 weeks.

B. Additional information sources on EC for clients:

1. Not 2 Late is operated by the Office of Population Research at Princeton University and the Association of Reproductive Health Professionals: 888-NOT-2-LATE.

2. Websites:

   a. EC: ec.princeton.edu

   b. Planned Parenthood: www.ppfa.org

Special Considerations

A. Pregnancy: There is no increased incidence of anomalies if pregnancy does occur after the use of EC.

Bibliography

Afaxys, Inc. (2015). *Ella full prescribing information*. Retrieved from https://www.accessdata.fda.gov/drugsatfda_docs/label/2010/022474s000lbl.pdf

Batur, P., Kransdorf, L. N., & Casey, P. M. (2016, June). Emergency contraception. *Mayo Clinic Proceedings, 91*(6), 802–807.

Edelman, A., Cherala, G., Blue, S., Erikson, D., & Jensen, J. (2016). Impact of obesity on the pharmacokinetics of levonorgestrel-based emergency contraception: Single and double dosing. *Contraception, 94*(1), 52–57. doi:10.1016/j.contraception.2016.03.006

Glasier, A., Cameron, S. T., Blithe, D., Scherrer, B., Mathe, H., Levy, D., Gainer, E., & Ulmann, A. (2011). Can we identify women at risk of pregnancy despite using emergency contraception? Data from randomized trials of ulipristal acetate and levonorgestrel. *Contraception, 84*(4), 363–367. doi:10.1016/j.contraception.2011.02.009

Guttmacher Institute. (2015). *Contraceptive use in the United States*. Retrieved from http://www.guttmacher.org/fact-sheet/contraceptive-use-united-states

Moreau, C., & Trussell, J. (2012). Results from pooled Phase III studies of ulipristal acetate for emergency contraception. *Contraception, 86*(6), 673–680. doi:10.1016/j.contraception.2012.05.012

Office of Population Research at Princeton University. (2019). *The emergency contraception website*. Retrieved from https://ec.princeton.edu/questions/ecobesity.html

Planned Parenthood. (2014). *Morning-after pill (emergency contraception)*. Retrieved from http://www.plannedparenthood.org/learn/morning-after-pill-emergency-contraception

Women's Capital Corporation. (2015, August). *Plan B One-Step*. Retrieved from www.planbonestep.com

Endometriosis

Rhonda Arthur and Michelle Collins

Definition

A. Endometriosis is ectopic endometrial tissue that exhibits hormonal responsiveness, but is located outside of the uterine cavity. Bleeding from this ectopic endometrial tissue causes pelvic inflammation and scarring, resulting in chronic pelvic pain and infertility. Endometrial lesions have been found in the vagina, GI tract (especially the sigmoid colon), thoracic cavity, and limbs, and on the bladder and gallbladder. Rarely is endometrial tissue found outside of the pelvic cavity.

Incidence

A. The true incidence of endometriosis is unknown. The incidence is quoted as 10% of the general female population, and 20% of the population who present for infertility treatment. Ranges of 5% to 30% have been cited. Endometriosis is the cause of chronic pelvic pain in 25% to 38% of affected adolescents, and is rarely seen in postmenopausal women. Positive family history (mother or sister) increases the risk tenfold. A concordance among twin sisters has been observed. A higher rate of endometriosis is reported among Asian women.

Pathogenesis

A. Several theories have been proposed to explain the pathogenesis of endometriosis. Retrograde menstruation (Sampson's theory) purports that menses are suspected of "flowing backward" through the fallopian tubes, resulting in the "seeding" of endometrial tissue outside the uterus. Halban's theory suggests that endometrial cells are carried through the lymph and circulatory system and disseminated in that manner. Direct transplantation of endometrial tissue is yet another theory, as is coelomic metaplasia.

Predisposing Factors

A. Positive family history, mother and/or sister (first-degree relative)

B. Short menstrual cycles

C. Delayed childbearing

D. Uterine anomalies that lead to outflow obstruction (e.g., vaginal septum)

Common Complaints

A. Pain before period

B. Pain with intercourse

C. Pain with bowel movements; may include constipation from the fear or pain of having a bowel movement (dyschezia).

D. Vaginal spotting and/or bleeding between menses

Other Signs and Symptoms

A. Dyspareunia and/or pain that radiates to the thigh
B. Chronic, noncyclic pelvic pain
C. Abnormal vaginal bleeding: Premenstrual spotting and DUB
D. Other bowel symptoms: Diarrhea and rectal bleeding
E. Urinary symptoms: Dysuria, urgency, and hematuria

Subjective Data

A. Review the onset, duration, and course of symptoms.
B. Obtain a complete menstrual history: Menarche, interval, duration, and discomfort with menstrual cycles as well as history of dysmenorrhea.
C. Obtain the client's history of contraceptive use.
D. Assess the client's bowel habits and any recent changes or pain with defecation.
E. Interview the client regarding dyspareunia.
F. Note the client's parity and/or history of infertility.

Physical Examination

A. Check temperature, pulse, respirations, and BP.
B. Inspect:
    1. Note the general appearance of discomfort before, during, and after the examination.
    2. Perform a detailed external genitalia examination.
C. Auscultate:
    1. Abdomen for bowel sounds in all quadrants. Auscultation of the abdomen should precede any palpation or percussion due to the changes in intensity and frequency of sounds after manipulation.
D. Palpate:
    1. Palpate the abdomen for masses.
    2. Check for suprapubic tenderness.
    3. Back: Check for CVAT.
E. Pelvic examination:
    1. Speculum examination: Inspect the cervix for cervicitis; friability; and discharge color, odor, and amount. Note any cutaneous lesions of the vagina, cervix, and perineum that resemble "powder burn or chocolate spots." Laparoscopic findings frequently reveal "powder burn" lesions of endometrial implants along the uterosacral ligament, pelvic peritoneum, ovaries, sigmoid colon, and other pelvic organs.
    2. Bimanual examination: Check for CMT, adnexal masses; check uterine size, consistency, position, and mobility.

The most common indicator of endometriosis is a fixed retroverted uterus with nodularity felt along the uterosacral ligaments. Palpation of endometrial implants may result in exquisite pain for the client. Conversely, a negative pelvic exam cannot rule out the presence of endometriosis. The abdominal exam of a woman with endometriosis is commonly negative, unless ruptured endometriomas are present.

---

    3. Rectovaginal examination: The clinician may elect to perform a rectovaginal exam, though it is not required for diagnosis. A rectal examination is done because the uterus is often fixed in a retroverted position due to endometriosis. The endometrial nodules present on the posterior uterine wall, cul-de-sac, and uterosacral ligament may be distinguished better rectally. If this exam performed, the uterosacral ligaments are gently palpated for pain and nodularity. The rectum is evaluated for masses and polyps.

Diagnostic Tests

There are no specific diagnostic tests for endometriosis. Definitive diagnosis is verified by laparoscopy via tissue biopsy samples obtained and verified as endometrial tissue.

A. Serum beta-HCG to rule out ectopic pregnancy
B. WBC to rule out infection
C. Cervical cultures for chlamydia and gonorrhea, to rule out STIs and PID
D. Urine culture, if indicated
E. Transvaginal ultrasonography, to rule out cysts and masses
F. GI series or barium enema, if indicated
G. MRI may be helpful in assessing extent of disease if either bladder or bowel involvement is suspected.

Differential Diagnoses

A. Endometriosis
B. Dysmenorrhea
C. Ovarian cysts
D. PID
E. Premenstrual syndrome (PMS)
F. Mittelschmerz
G. Trauma
H. Appendicitis
I. Pregnancy: Normal, missed abortion, or ectopic
J. GI or genitourinary (GU) complaints: Diverticular disease, spastic colon, or UTI

Plan

A. General interventions:
    1. After surgical confirmation, the clinician skilled in gynecologic practice may manage the client alone, or comanage the endometriosis with a physician.
    2. Treatment plans should be individualized based on the woman's age and desire for future fertility.
B. Client teaching:
    1. Treatment goals include prevention of disease progression, alleviation of pain, and establishment or restoration of fertility. Treatment options include the following:
        a. Observation alone
        b. Medical therapy or pharmacological therapy
        c. Referral or consultation for laparoscopic therapy, including laser vaporization and removal of adhesions
    2. Continuation, or recurrence of pelvic pain, may necessitate assisting the woman to manage her chronic pelvic pain and dysmenorrhea with NSAIDs and/or other non-narcotic chronic pain therapies, such as visualization and biofeedback.
    3. Hysterectomy and bilateral salpingo-oophorectomy are the only definitive cures for women who do not wish to conserve their reproductive capacity. They

should be considered only as a last resort after failed conservative treatment.

C. Pharmaceutical therapy: Diagnosis must first be confirmed by laparoscopy:
1. First-line therapy:
a. Combined oral contraceptive (COC) pills are considered the first-line therapy and have maximum benefit when combined with NSAIDs. If the client experiences pain during the week of withdrawal bleeding, she may take active pills continuously, omitting the placebo pills of the "off week."

> COCs are being used to produce a state of pseudopregnancy that should induce regression of the disease.

b. Medroxyprogesterone acetate (MPA) 150 mg IM every 3 months
2. If symptoms persist after 3 months of COC and NSAID therapy:
a. Gn-RH agonist empiric therapy for 3 months may be initiated.
i. Leuprolide acetate (Lupron) 3.75 mg by IM injection every month
ii. Nafarelin (Synarel) nasal spray twice daily

> Use of a Gn-RH agonist, which acts to suppress ovulation, can result in side effects including hot flashes, mood changes, and other menopausal symptoms. Use is restricted to 6 months to avoid a decrease in bone density unless add-back therapy is initiated. Add-back therapy is the prescription of estrogen/progestin for a woman already on Gn-RH agonists. The expense of Gn-RH agonist therapy may preclude its use.

b. Danazol 600 to 800 mg daily for up to 6 months; less expensive than Gn-RH agonist therapy:
i. Use of danazol, which acts to produce anovulation and hypogonadotropism, can result in androgenic side effects, including acne, hirsutism, weight gain, and voice changes that may not be reversible.
ii. Other side effects, which are reversible, include decreased breast size, atrophic vaginitis, dyspareunia, hot flashes, and emotional liability.
3. Levonorgestrel IUD: There is support for reduction in menorrhagia and dysmenorrhea symptoms with use of these devices.

Follow-Up
A. Clients must return monthly while receiving Gn-RH agonist or danazol therapies to assess for symptom relief and side-effect profile.
B. Women with known endometriosis and a desire to conceive should be referred to a clinician specializing in infertility.

Consultation/Referral
A. The workup, evaluation, and medications for endometriosis are expensive. Refer the client to a gynecologist for initial management. A prudent approach is recommended with a conservative treatment option; evaluate the results before trying another option.
B. Refer the client for a surgical consultation for definitive diagnosis. Endometriosis may be suspected based on symptoms and physical examination. It cannot, however, be confirmed unless actually visualized by laparoscopy.

Individual Considerations
A. Pregnancy: Infertility may be a presenting symptom. Treatment may, therefore, be focused on endometriosis abatement and fertility support.

Resource
Endometriosis Association
8585 North 76th Place
Milwaukee, WI 53223
(414) 355-2200
www.endometriosisassn.org

Bibliography
Guttery, D. S., Blighe, K., Polymeros, K., Symonds, R. P., Macip, S., & Moss, E. L. (2018). Racial differences in endometrial cancer molecular portraits in *The Cancer Genome Atlas*. *Oncotarget*, *9*(24), 17093. doi:10.18632/oncotarget.24907

Female Sexual Dysfunction

Rhonda Arthur and Michelle Collins

Definition
A. Any persistent problem with desire, sexual response, or function, which may affect the client and her relationship. It is classified into subtypes:
1. Desire disorder: Lack of interest or desire (most common)
2. Arousal disorder: Inability to become aroused during sexual activity; absent or reduced genital sensations
3. Orgasm disorder: Delay, absence, or decreased intensity of orgasm:
a. Primary: The client has never had an orgasm.
b. Secondary: The client has achieved orgasm in the past, but is unable to achieve orgasm at the time of presentation.
4. Pain disorder: Genitopelvic pain/penetration disorder (formerly dyspareunia and vaginismus). This is described as pelvic or vulvovaginal pain during vaginal penetration, anxiety, and/or fear related to the thought of vaginal penetration, or marked tightening of pelvic floor muscles during vaginal penetration.

Incidence
A. Female sexual dysfunction affects an estimated 43% of U.S. women. This includes women who report issues with sexual desire (17%–55%), arousal difficulty (8%–28%), orgasm (25%), and pain (26%).

Pathogenesis

A. Multiple models exist to describe the phases of normal sexual function:

    1. Masters and Johnson model—consists of the stages of excitement, plateau, orgasm, and resolution

    2. Kaplan and Leif model—consists of desire, excitement, and orgasm

    3. Basson model—consists of emotional intimacy, sexual stimuli, psychological factors, and relationship satisfaction

B. Sexual dysfunction includes various biological, psychological, and social components:

    1. Biological factors: Aging; medical conditions such as diabetes and hypertension, and declining testosterone or estrogen

    2. Psychological factors: Depression or anxiety, history of sexual abuse, childhood trauma, personality disorders, body image disorders, and perceived stress

    3. Social factors: Cultural or religious values, relationship issues, career issues, financial hardship, and household responsibilities

C. Orgasm disorders can be caused by neurologic and/or vascular disease such as spinal cord injury, diabetes, or multiple sclerosis.

Predisposing Factors

A. Emotional:

    1. Depression

    2. Mood disorders

    3. Poor body image

    4. Low self-esteem

    5. Fatigue

    6. Stress

B. Poor health status:

    1. Spinal cord injury

    2. Diabetes

    3. POF

    4. Trauma

    5. Chronic illness

    6. Autoimmune disorders

    7. Cerebral vascular accident (CVA); cardiovascular disease

    8. Hyperprolactinemia

C. Partner relationship issues

D. Medications that are associated with low sexual desire in women:

    1. Antidepressants, including serotonin-specific reuptake inhibitors (SSRIs) and tricyclic antidepressants (TCA)

    2. Anxiolytics

    3. Antihistamines

    4. Anticholinergics

    5. Antihypertensives: Calcium channel blockers and angiotensin-converting enzyme (ACE) inhibitors

    6. Anti-androgenics

    7. Hormones: Combined hormonal contraception (pill, patch, ring); menopausal hormone therapy; GnRH agonists

    8. Anticonvulsants

    9. Opiates

    10. Illicit drugs

E. History of emotional, physical, or sexual abuse may contribute to low desire.

F. Advancing age:

    1. Menopausal women affected more frequently. Low sexual desire may result from decreasing hormone levels, specifically testosterone and estrogen levels. Low estrogen levels are also linked to vulvovaginal atrophy and dyspareunia, both of which may decrease sexual desire in women.

Common Complaints

A. Women:

    1. Absence of orgasm

    2. Pain during vaginal penetration

    3. Difficulty relaxing pelvic floor muscles to allow vaginal penetration

B. Both sexes:

    1. Lack of interest or desire (most common)

    2. Inability to become aroused

    3. Pain with intercourse

C. Men: Common complaints for men are specifically discussed in Chapter 11: Gastrointestinal Guidelines.

Other Signs and Symptoms

A. Vaginal discharge

B. Vulvar itching

C. Vulvar pain, described as stinging, burning, irritation

Subjective Data

A. Obtain a full medical, gynecologic, and sexual history, using open-ended questions:

    1. Assess the client for signs of depression, anxiety, and sexual concerns.

    2. Review the medication list with the client. Specifically ask about the types of medications that may contribute to low sexual desire (per the list mentioned previously).

    3. Assess for medical conditions that contribute to sexual dysfunction:

        a. Chronic diseases: Cardiovascular disease, diabetes, kidney or liver failure

        b. Neurological disorders

        c. Hormone imbalances

        d. Alcoholism

        e. Illicit drug use

        f. Evaluate for causes of pelvic pain: Vaginal dryness, vaginal discharge, or vaginal infectious causes (such as STIs, yeast infections, or PID).

    4. Evaluate for history of previous pelvic disorders or surgery (fibroids, endometriosis, malignancy, uterine/bladder prolapse, or episiotomy).

    5. Evaluate for the degree of distress that this condition may cause the client.

B. The use of self-report screening tools is recommended to identify women with low sexual desire:

    1. Decreased Sexual Desire Screener:

        a. Found at https://herhsdd.com/wp-content/themes/herhsdd/pdf/decreased-sexual-desire-screener.pdf

2. Brief Sexual Symptom Checklist for Women:
   a. Found at www.researchgate.net/figure/27761 0474_fig1_Figure-2-The-modified-Brief-Sexual -Symptom-Checklist-for-Women-BSSC-W
3. Female Sexual Function Index:
   a. Found at www.fsfiquestionnaire.com

Physical Examination

A. Check temperature, pulse, respirations, and BP.
B. Inspect:
   1. Thyroid for the presence of nodules
   2. Breasts for the presence of nipple discharge, if history warrants
   3. Skin for hirsutism, acne, alopecia, and truncal obesity; may indicate hyperandrogenism
C. Palpate:
   1. Thyroid for the presence of nodules
   2. May palpate the breasts for the presence of nipple discharge, if history warrants

Pelvic Examination

A. Inspect:
   1. Examine the external genitalia for erythema, lesions, atrophy, or unusual discharge
   2. Inspect for vulvar dermatoses, such as lichen sclerosus or lichen planus. Lichen sclerosus may look like white skin discolorations or wrinkled patches of skin. Severe cases may have bleeding or ulcerated lesions. Lichen planus may look like purple-colored lesions or bumps with flat tops. Thin white lines or blisters may appear over the lesions.
   3. Inspect for pelvic floor prolapse and pelvic floor muscle contraction
B. Palpate the external genitalia for the presence of pain.
C. Speculum examination:
   1. Assess for atrophy (common in postmenopausal women), pelvic floor muscle strength, masses, prolapse, and deep pelvic pain.
D. Bimanual examination:
   1. Check for CMT, uterine size, and position.
   2. Check the adnexa for masses or tenderness.

Diagnostic Tests

A. Laboratory tests should be performed as indicated by the history and physical examination for any medical conditions that may contribute to low desire.
B. Pap and HPV testing as indicated by guidelines, STI testing, wet prep
C. Serum testing: Thyroid function tests, prolactin level, free and total testosterone, sex hormone–binding globulin (SHBG), fasting glucose, hepatic panel, lipid panel
D. Androgen levels and testosterone levels alone are unreliable, unless the clinician suspects a hyperandrogenic condition, as evidenced by hirsutism, acne, alopecia, and truncal obesity.
E. Transvaginal ultrasound may be warranted if pelvic pain is elicited upon examination.

Differential Diagnoses

A. Arousal disorder
B. Desire disorder
C. Orgasm disorder
D. Pain disorder
E. Vulvar dermatoses, such as lichen planus or lichen sclerosis
F. Vaginal atrophy
G. Infectious issues, such as STIs, candidiasis, or BV
H. Depression, anxiety
I. Cardiovascular disease
J. Diabetes
K. Thyroid disorder
L. Neurological disorder

Plan

A. General interventions:
   1. Set realistic goals for treatment.
   2. Empower the woman to take an active role in the treatment plan. Encourage discussion about anatomy and sexual function, allowing the woman to ask questions as she is comfortable.
   3. Office-based therapy may be useful for providers who wish to include this element in their practice. The Permission, Limited Information, Specific Suggestion, Intensive Therapy (PLISSIT) Model is one office-based counseling model:
      a. Permission: Women are given permission to engage in a full discussion of the topic.
      b. Limited information: The provider gives educational information on sexual function and sexual dysfunction in the form of handouts or videos.
      c. Specific suggestion: The provider gives very specific advice tailored to each client and her presenting issues.
      d. Intensive therapy: The provider makes a referral for individual or couples therapy.
B. Client teaching:
   1. Educate about normal anatomical and sexual function.
   2. Encourage healthy lifestyle behaviors related to diet, exercise, avoiding tobacco, and minimizing stress.
   3. Educate clients about the use of vaginal lubricants to assist with vaginal dryness or dyspareunia. KY Jelly or Astroglide: Water-based glycerin-free lubricants should be first-line recommendation. Glycerin-containing lubricants can encourage the growth of bacteria. "Self-heating" lubricants may cause discomfort for women with sensitive skin in the perineal area, or for postmenopausal women (due to their thinner perineal skin).
C. Pharmaceutical therapy:
   1. Vaginal estrogen for the treatment of vaginal atrophy:
      a. Estradiol vaginal tablets (Vagifem) 10 mcg: One tablet in vagina nightly for 2 weeks, then twice a week for maintenance
      b. Estring: One ring, placed intravaginally every 3 months

c. Premarin 0.625 mg/g: Insert 0.5 g/d for 21 days on, 7 days off; may adjust dose based on client response

d. Estrace 100 mcg/g: Insert 2 to 4 g in vagina nightly for 2 weeks, then gradually taper to half the initial dose for 1 to 2 weeks, then a maintenance dose of 1 g one to three times a week for maintenance. Taper or discontinue at 3- to 6-month intervals.

2. Ospemifene (Osphena):

a. An estrogen agonist/antagonist with tissue-selective effects; used for the treatment of moderate to severe dyspareunia related to vaginal atrophy in postmenopausal females

b. Dosage: 60 mg once per day

c. If using ospemifene, prescribe opposing progestin in women with intact uterus.

d. Ospemifene is contraindicated in women with undiagnosed abnormal vaginal bleeding; those with history of venous thromboembolism, pulmonary embolism, or breast cancer; and women of childbearing age.

3. Prasterone (Intrarosa):

a. A steroid indicated for the treatment of moderate to severe dyspareunia due to menopause

b. Dosage: One vaginal insert once daily at bedtime, using the provided applicator

c. Contraindicated in clients with breast cancer, dysfunctional uterine bleeding, endometrial cancer, ovarian cancer, or vaginal bleeding, dysfunctional uterine bleeding of undetermined origin, pregnancy, and breastfeeding

Follow-Up

A. As determined by the history and physical examination findings and diagnoses made. Women placed on medications should return for follow-up 1 month after initiation to assess efficacy.

B. Postmenopausal women with vaginal bleeding should follow up immediately.

Consultation/Referral

A. Refer the client to a therapist who specializes in sexual problems:

1. Counseling may include sex therapy or CBT.

B. A pelvic floor physical therapist is an integral member of the treatment team for women with genitopelvic pain disorders.

Individual Considerations

A. Use of opposing progestin in women with an intact uterus is not necessary for all forms of vaginal estrogens. Vagifem, for example, does not have to be opposed with a progestin. Clinicians prescribing hormonal therapy should be well informed and educated on which particular formulations require opposition therapy. Additionally, estrogen should always be initiated at the lowest possible effective dose and given for the shortest duration of time. Hormone therapy should be very individualized to the woman, taking into consideration her symptoms, quality of life, and personal preference. The decision to initiate, continue, and discontinue hormone therapy is one made in partnership with the individual woman.

B. Clients with a history of breast cancer: Although risk is low, consult with the client's oncologist before initiating vaginal estrogen. Women with a history of breast cancer may be appropriate candidates for vaginal ET.

Resources

American Association of Sexuality Educators, Counselors, and Therapists
1444 I Street NW, Suite 700
Washington, DC 20005
(202) 449-1099
Email: info@aasect.org
www.AASECT.org

International Society for the Study of Women's Sexual Health
PO Box 1233
Lakeville, MN 55044
(218) 461-5115
Email: info@isswsh.org
www.ISSWSH.org

North American Menopause Society
5900 Landerbrook Drive
Suite 390
Mayfield Heights, OH 44124
(440) 442-7550
Email: info@menopause.org

Society for Sex Therapy and Research
6311 W. Gross Point Road
Niles, IL 60714
(847) 647-8832
Email: info@sstarnet.org
www.SSTARNET.org

Bibliography

American Psychiatric Association. (2013). *Diagnostic and statistical manual of mental disorders* (5th ed.). Arlington, VA: American Psychiatric Publishing.

Hilz, M. (2015). Assessment and treatment of male and female sexual dysfunction. *Journal of the Neurological Sciences, 357*(1), 498–499. doi:10.1016/j.jns.2015.09.295

Kingsberg, S. A., & Woodard, T. (2015). Female sexual dysfunction: Focus on low desire. *Obstetrics and Gynecology, 125*(2), 477–486. doi:10.1097/aog.0000000000000620

Latif, E. Z., & Diamond, M. P. (2013). Arriving at the diagnosis of female sexual dysfunction. *Fertility and Sterility, 100*(4), 898–904. doi:10.1016/j.fertnstert.2013.08.006

North American Menopause Society. (2016). *Vagina and vulvar comfort: Lubricants, moisturizers, and low-dose vaginal estrogen*. Retrieved from http://www.menopause.org/for-women/-em-sexual-health-menopause-em-online/effective-treatments-for-sexual-problems/vaginal-and-vulvar-comfort-lubricants-moisturizers-and-low-dose-vaginal-estrogen

Perez, S., & Binik, Y. M. (2016, July 29). Vaginismus: "Gone" but not forgotten. *Psychiatric Times, 33*(7), 1–3. https://www.psychiatrictimes.com/special-reports/vaginismus-gone-not-forgotten

PLISSIT Model of Sex Therapy. (n.d.). Retrieved from https://coad7404.files.wordpress.com/2014/06/plissitanonsmodel.pdf

ter Kuile, M. M., & Weijenborg, P. T. M. (2017). A woman who never could have coitus: Treatment of lifelong vaginismus. In K. M. Paarlberg & H. B. M. van de Wiel (Eds.), *Bio-psycho-social obstetrics and gynecology: A competency-oriented approach* (pp. 297–309). Cham, Switzerland: Springer.

Thomas, H. N., & Thurston, R. C. (2016). A biopsychosocial approach to women's sexual function and dysfunction at midlife: A narrative review. *Maturitas*, *87*, 49–60. doi:10.1016/j.maturitas.2016.02.009

Wright, J. J., & O'Connor, K. M. (2015). Female sexual dysfunction. *Medical Clinics of North America*, *99*(3), 607–628. doi:10.1016/j.mcna.2015.01.011

Infertility

Rhonda Arthur and Michelle Collins

Definition

A. Infertility is defined as the inability to conceive within 12 months of unprotected intercourse. For women aged 35 years and older, diagnosis is made after 6 months of unprotected intercourse.

B. A woman who has never been pregnant, and has not conceived after 12 months of unprotected intercourse, is diagnosed with "primary" infertility.

C. If a previous pregnancy has been achieved, but the woman is unable to conceive a subsequent pregnancy, the term "secondary" infertility is applicable.

Incidence

A. An estimated 12% to 18% of women are unable to conceive after 12 menstrual cycles wherein they have had unprotected sexual intercourse. Most cases of female-related infertility are related to problems with ovulation. About 10% of infertility is unexplained.

Pathogenesis

A female–male couple aged 29 to 33, without reproductive health issues, has a 20% to 25% chance of conceiving in any given month. Approximately one-third of infertility is attributed to the female partner, one-third is attributed to the male partner, and one-third is attributed to a combination of factors between both partners, with 10% of infertility unexplained. Evaluate both partners for:

A. Infrequent intercourse

B. Interpersonal problems

C. Medical causes (see Table 14.2)

Predisposing Factors

A. Predisposing factors depend on the etiology.

TABLE 14.2 PATHOGENESIS OF INFERTILITY

Male Pathogenesis	Female Pathogenesis
A. Faulty sperm production	A. Advanced maternal age
1. Azoospermia from	B. Disorder of ovulation/hypothalamic dysfunction
a. Cancer therapy	1. Anovulation
b. Adult mumps	2. Amenorrhea
c. Sertoli-cell-only syndrome	3. Polycystic ovarian syndrome
d. Hypogonadism	4. Premature ovarian failure
e. Retrograde ejaculation	a. Autoimmune
2. Oligospermia	b. Idiopathic
a. Varicocele	c. Cancer therapy
b. Small testicular size	5. Luteal-phase insufficiency
B. Reproductive tract anomaly	6. Prolactinoma
1. Blocked vas deferens	C. Ovarian factors
2. Varicocele	1. Cysts or tumor
3. Congenital obstruction of epididymis	2. Irradiation
C. Klinefelter's syndrome	D. Tubal disorders/damage/blocked
D. Exposure to physical and chemical agents	1. PID
1. Coal tar	2. *Chlamydia trachomatis*
2. Radiation	3. Postpartum infection
E. Endocrine disorders	4. Pelvic trauma (motor vehicle accident)
1. Diabetes	5. Inflammatory bowel disease
2. Low serum testosterone	6. Endometriosis
3. Pituitary tumors	7. Adhesions
4. Hyperprolactinemia	E. Uterine pathology
F. Testicular infection	1. Congenital anomalies: Duplication
G. Injury to reproductive organs/tract	2. Septate
H. Nerve damage/neurological disease: Spinal cord injury	3. Fibroids
I. Impotence/erectile difficulty: Performance anxiety	4. IUD

(continued)

TABLE 14.2 PATHOGENESIS OF INFERTILITY (*continued*)

Male Pathogenesis	Female Pathogenesis
J. Premature ejaculation	5. Asherman's syndrome
K. Early withdrawal	6. Synechiae
L. Lifestyle factors	F. Cervical factors
1. Recreational drug use	1. Anatomical abnormalities (hood)
2. Smoking	2. Previous cervical surgery (i.e., conization), which leads to mucus depletion
3. Alcohol	3. Hostile cervical mucus
4. Malnutrition	4. Presence of sperm antibodies in the cervix

M. Antispermatozoa antibodies
N. Medications
   1. Antihypertensives
   2. Antidepressants
   3. Antipsychotics
   4. Antiulcer agents/antacids
   5. Muscle relaxants
	5. Infections

	G. Lifestyle factors
	1. Recreational drug use
	2. Smoking
	H. Vaginal factors
	1. Intact hymen
	2. Septum
	3. Absent vagina
	4. Infection
	a. *Trichomonas*
	b. *Candida*
	c. Chlamydia
	d. *Mycoplasma*
	e. Bacterial vaginosis (BV)
	f. Gonorrhea
	g. *Streptococcus*
	I. Medications: Combined oral hormonal contraceptives (pill, patch, ring)
	J. Medical problems
	1. Lupus
	2. Hypothyroidism
	3. Diabetes
	4. Antiphospholipid syndrome

IUD, intrauterine device; PID, pelvic inflammatory disease.

Common Complaint

A. Inability to achieve pregnancy despite frequent acts of intercourse

Other Signs and Symptoms

A. Dependent on the pathogenesis and history

Subjective Data

A. Obtain a complete health history:
1. Age of both partners
2. General health of both partners
3. Complete pregnancy history of the female:
   a. Number of pregnancies: Term, preterm, spontaneous, and elective terminations
   b. Vaginal births or cesarean sections
   c. Recurrent miscarriages, gestational age(s)
   d. Stillbirths
   e. D&C after pregnancy loss
   f. Cerclage for incompetent cervix
4. Paternity history of the male
5. Length of infertility, including prior workup, if any
6. Coital history:
   a. Frequency
   b. Timing
   c. Use of lubricants and what kind; some lubricants have spermicidal qualities
   d. Postcoital habits: Douching or voiding
7. Adequacy of intercourse:
   a. Penetration of the vagina
   b. Ejaculation by the male

B. Obtain a complete menstrual history:
  1. Age at puberty, menarche
  2. Regularity of cycles
  3. Discomfort during menses
  4. First day of LMP
C. Obtain a complete gynecological history:
  1. Contraceptive use
  2. Medical and surgical history:
    a. D&C
    b. Laparoscopy or endometriosis
  3. Uterine anomalies
D. Take a complete nutritional and exercise history; note eating disorders:
  1. Anorexia nervosa
  2. Bulimia
E. Review female and male reproductive tract infections and treatments for past and present partners.
F. Review each individual's habits:
  1. Smoking: How much, how often, how long
  2. Recreational drugs: How much, how often, how long for each drug
  3. Alcohol: How much, how often
  4. Use of saunas or hot tubs
  5. Exercise, type, frequency, duration
G. Take a complete medication history; specifically review for:
  1. Antihypertensives
  2. Antidepressants
  3. Antipsychotics
H. Review for exposure to toxic chemicals, radiation, or known teratogens:
  1. Military war exposure
  2. Employment exposure
  3. Residential exposure:
    a. Microwaves
    b. Pesticides
I. Inquire about diethylstilbestrol (DES) exposure in utero (for either partner).
J. Review for symptoms of thyroid dysfunction:
  1. Weight gain or loss
  2. Change of bowel habits
  3. Intolerance to heat or cold
  4. Appetite changes
  5. Rapid heart rate, palpitations
  6. Changes in sleep pattern
K. Review for systemic diseases:
  1. Cardiac
  2. Collagen vascular diseases
  3. Diabetes
  4. Autoimmune disorders
L. Assess the psychosocial context of the infertility, including personal, emotional, and economic factors; family pressures to have children; expectations; timing of pregnancy; consideration of adoption; and stress from failure to conceive.

Signs and Symptoms
A. See the "Pathogenesis" section and information obtained in the "Subjective Data" section regarding past medical history.

B. History of not being able to get pregnant over the past 6 to 12 months is noted.

Physical Examination
A. Check temperature, pulse, respirations, and BP. Note height, weight, and BMI. BMI of less than 19 correlates with anovulation.
B. Inspect:
  1. Examine the breasts for the presence of nipple discharge.
  2. Note general signs and appearance of PCOS.
C. Auscultate:
  1. Abdomen for bowel sounds in all quadrants. Auscultation of the abdomen should precede any palpation or percussion due to the changes in intensity and frequency of sounds after manipulation.
D. Palpate:
  1. Neck: Examine the thyroid.
  2. Abdomen: Note tenderness and masses.
  3. Back: Check for CVAT.
E. Pelvic examination:
  1. Inspect: Perform a detailed external perineal examination looking for signs of infection, lesions, anomalies of clitoris, labia, Skene's glands, Bartholin's glands, vulva, and perineum.
  2. Speculum examination:
    a. Observe length of vagina, as well as position and characteristic of cervix, noting any anomalies.
    b. Note any vaginal discharge characteristics (thin/thick, color, consistency, and malodor).
  3. Bimanual examination: Check uterine size, consistency, contour, mobility, and CMT; check for adnexal masses.

> A fixed, immobile uterus noted on bimanual examination may indicate the presence of pelvic scarring resulting from conditions such as endometriosis or PID.

  4. Rectovaginal examination: A rectovaginal exam is not a required element of an infertility evaluation, but the clinician may sometimes feel it is warranted based on symptomology and other physical exam elements. Palpate the uterosacral ligaments for pain and nodularity; evaluate any masses and polyps of the rectum.

Diagnostic Tests
A. Male factor: Semen analysis. A semen analysis is a necessary part of the couple's infertility evaluation.
B. Female (ovarian) factor:
  1. Basal body temperature (BBT)
  2. Serum progesterone measured midway through luteal phase: Serum progesterone greater than 15 ng/mL indicates ovulation
  3. Urinary luteinizing hormone (LH) for surge
  4. FSH: A high FSH, greater than 40 m IU/mL, indicates ovarian failure
  5. TSH
  6. Serum prolactin

When nipple discharge is present, check serum prolactin and TSH to rule out hyperprolactinemia, a pituitary tumor, and thyroid dysfunction.

C. Pelvic or uterine factor:
1. Hysterosalpingogram (HSG); also done for tubal factor
2. Laparoscopy
D. Other tests:
1. Pap and HPV, as indicated by guidelines
2. Cultures for gonorrhea and chlamydia
3. Pregnancy test, if amenorrhea is present
4. CBC
5. Wet mount

Differential Diagnoses

A. Infertility
B. Sexual dysfunction
C. Hypothyroidism or hyperthyroidism
D. Hypothalamic dysfunction: Amenorrhea
E. Hyperprolactinemia, pituitary tumor
F. Menopause
G. Premature ovarian failure
H. PCOS
I. Asherman's syndrome
J. Tubal occlusion
K. Antisperm antibodies
L. Endometriosis
M. Oligo-ovulation
N. Uterine anomalies: Fibroids, synechiae
O. Pelvic adhesions

Plan

A. General interventions:
1. Semen analysis should be done early in the infertility evaluation. Typically metabolic causes are ruled out first in each partner, which would include lab work for both partners (including the semen analysis). If the first evaluation is abnormal, it should be repeated one time. Normal semen analysis includes the following:
  a. Sperm count: Greater than 20 million/mL
  b. Volume: 2.6 mL
  c. Motility: Greater than 50%
  d. Morphology: Greater than 60%
  e. Liquefaction: Within 20 to 30 minutes of ejaculation
2. The male physical examination is generally done if semen analysis is abnormal.
3. Female evaluation:
  a. BBT: Followed for several months to evaluate ovulation. Some clients' temperatures dip just before the day of ovulation and then rise. Ovulation and the development of the corpus luteum manifest as an increase in BBT by 0.6°F to 1°F above the client's baseline temperature (LH surge). The BBT provides presumptive evidence of normal oocyte production and related hormonal change, as well as guidance for the frequency and timing of intercourse. While traditionally this was tracked on paper, numerous technologies have now replaced the paper tracking (Kindara at https://www.kindara.com/the-app; Natural Cycles at https://www.naturalcycles.com; Glow at glowing.com; Ovia, Clue, and Groov available on iOS and Android).
  b. HSG (performed in radiology): Evaluates tubal patency and rules out uterine anomalies. The HSG should be scheduled for the interval between cessation of menstrual flow and ovulation to avoid retrograde flow of menstrual tissue into the tubes and the abdominal cavity.
  c. Laparoscopy: Done particularly if endometriosis is suspected as the cause. Endometrial lesions can be lasered during the procedure; thus, while it is diagnostic, it is also a treatment. Performed by a gynecologist, it is usually done in the first 2 weeks of the menstrual cycle to ensure that the client is not pregnant. Direct visualization of the pelvic organs provides data about degree of adhesion formation, presence of endometriosis or fibroids, and possibility of surgical repair of damaged tubes.
B. Client teaching:
1. Infertile couples often require extensive counseling, including grief counseling for failure to achieve pregnancy.
2. Teach the client to take BBT measurements; discuss technological aids to assist in this measurement. *See Section III: Client Teaching Guide for this chapter, "Basal Body Temperature Measurement."*
C. Pharmaceutical therapy:
1. Treatment depends on the causative factor(s).
2. Ovulation induction agents are best prescribed in collaboration with a clinician well versed in infertility treatment. Complications such as ovarian hyperstimulation can occur.

Follow-Up

A. Follow-up depends on causative factor(s).

Consultation/Referral

A. Consultation and referral are required for special testing, surgery, and assisted reproductive therapy.
B. Immediate referral to a physician skilled in infertility complications is necessary for ovarian hyperstimulation.

Individual Considerations

A. Older adults:
1. Advancing age increases the risk of age-related infertility. Women aged 35 years and older should be referred to a fertility specialist if unsuccessful in conceiving after 6 months.
2. Women aged 40 years and older should be referred as soon as possible for assisted reproductive therapy.

Bibliography

American College of Obstetricians and Gynecologists. (2015). *Gynecologic problems: Treating infertility.* Retrieved from http://www.acog.org/-/media/For-Patients/faq137.pdf?dmc=1&ts=

Centers for Disease Control and Prevention, National Center for Health Statistics. (2015). *Infertility.* Retrieved from http://www.cdc.gov/nchs/fastats/infertility.htm

Resolve: The National Infertility Association. (2019). *Fast facts*. Retrieved from https://resolve.org/infertility-101/what-is-infertility/fast-facts/

Schuiling, K. D., & Likis, F. E. (Eds.). (2013). *Women's gynecologic health* (3rd ed.). Sudbury, MA: Jones & Bartlett Learning.

Thoma, M. E., McLain, A. C., Louis, J. F., King, R. B., Trumble, A. C., Sundaram, R., & Buck Louis, G. M. (2013). Prevalence of infertility in the United States as estimated by the current duration approach and a traditional constructed approach. *Fertility and Sterility*, *99*(5), 1324–1331.e1. doi:10.1016/j.fertnstert.2012.11.037

Zhang, G., Yan, H., Chen, Q., Liu, K., Ling, X., Sun, L., . . . Tan, L. (2016). Effects of cell phone use on semen parameters: Results from the MARHCS cohort study in Chongqing, China. *Environment International*, *91*, 116–121. doi:10.1016/j.envint.2016.02.028

Menopause

Rhonda Arthur and Michelle Collins

Definition

A. Physiologic or "natural" menopause is the cessation of menses for 12 consecutive months due to the loss of ovarian follicular activity. Natural or physiologic menopause is a retrospective diagnosis recognized 12 months after the final menses. Natural menopause is generally experienced in women between 45 and 55 years of age, with the average age being 51 years.

B. Natural menopause before the age of 40 years is considered premature.

C. Premature ovarian failure is the full or intermittent loss of ovarian function before the age of 40 years. POF is thought to be caused by genetics, autoimmune disorders, surgery, or chemical interventions (such as chemotherapy or radiation).

D. Induced menopause is the abrupt cessation of menses related to chemical or surgical interventions.

E. Perimenopause describes the time "around" menopause. It is caused by fluctuations in ovarian function in the years preceding menopause. The average onset is usually in a woman's 40s (10 years prior to the age at which she will be menopausal), but may occur earlier. Due to fluctuations in ovarian function, pregnancy may still occur and unintended pregnancy should be avoided. The largest percentage of unintended pregnancies occurs at both ends of the reproductive age spectrum: teens and perimenopausal women. Perimenopausal symptoms often last several years, with the average duration being 5 years.

Incidence

A. By 2020, it is expected that more than 51 million women in the United States will be older than 51 years.

Pathogenesis

A. Physiologic menopause is due to failure of ovarian follicular development and ovarian hormone depletion. The major endocrine changes include decreasing negative feedback on the hypothalamic–pituitary system with increasing FSH and LH. When the ovaries cease to produce estrogen, they become unable to respond to FSH, resulting in the cessation of ovulation and menstruation.

Common Complaints

A. Insomnia/sleep disturbance

B. Absence of menses

C. Urogenital atrophy:
   1. Vaginal dryness
   2. Dyspareunia
   3. Dysuria/frequency

D. Vasomotor symptoms such as hot flashes/night sweats

E. Body/muscle aches

F. Intermenstrual or postcoital spotting/bleeding should be evaluated for pathologic causes.

G. Mood lability

Subjective Data

A. Determine onset, duration, and course of presenting symptoms.

B. Obtain a complete medical history, including medications; assess for risk of osteoporosis, cardiovascular disease, and breast and endometrial cancer.

C. Obtain a complete gynecological history, including menarche, interval and duration of menstrual cycles, history of dysmenorrhea, and pregnancy history. Question the client regarding sexual history and contraceptives used (condoms, combined hormonal products [pill, patch, and ring], diaphragm, IUDs), including frequency of method used.

D. What is the client's current menstrual pattern? Is there suspicion for pregnancy?

E. Review associated symptoms (hot flashes, insomnia, and GU symptoms), onset, timing, duration, and impact on daily life.

F. Assess for mood swings and dysphoria.

Physical Examination

A. Check temperature, pulse, respirations, and BP.

B. Inspect: Observe general overall appearance and obtain height, weight, and BMI.

C. Auscultate:
   1. Heart
   2. Lungs
   3. Abdomen: Auscultation of the abdomen should precede any palpation or percussion due to the changes in intensity and frequency of sounds after manipulation

D. Percuss:
   1. Abdomen for organomegaly

E. Palpate:
   1. Palpate the thyroid gland.
   2. Perform a clinical breast examination.
   3. Palpate the groin for lymphadenopathy.
   4. Palpate the abdomen for masses.

F. Pelvic examination:
   1. Inspect: Examine the vulva for Bartholin's gland enlargement, fissures, condyloma, herpes simplex, pelvic relaxation, and atrophy.
   2. Palpate: "Milk" the Skene's glands for discharge.
   3. Speculum examination: Inspect for cervicitis and friability. Evaluate vaginal discharge and bleeding for color, amount, and odor. Perform cultures and a Pap and/or HPV test as indicated by guidelines.
   4. Bimanual examination:
      a. Check CMT; evaluate the size, contour, mobility, and tenderness of the uterus. An enlarged or irregular uterus requires additional evaluation.

Over time, it is normal for the postmenopausal uterus to decrease in size.

    b. Palpate the adnexa for tenderness and masses.

Ovaries should not be palpable in postmenopausal women and require further evaluation if masses or ovaries are appreciated.

    5. Rectovaginal examination: A rectal exam to evaluate for masses, hemorrhoids, or polyps is indicated in women older than 50 years. One-time hemoccult has very low sensitivity/specificity to evaluate for blood. The woman should be sent home with the 3-day fecal occult blood test (FOBT) kit with instructions to send it back to the lab.

Diagnostic Tests

A. Consider TSH.
B. Consider urine or serum beta-HCG.
C. CBC if the client has excessive vaginal bleeding
D. Obtain a Pap and/or HPT test as indicated per guidelines.
E. Endometrial biopsy as indicated for intermenstrual spotting, or vaginal bleeding after menopause
F. Transvaginal ultrasonography for enlarged or irregular uterus
G. Additional primary care preventive screenings as indicated, such as mammogram, lipid evaluation, colorectal screening, and bone mineral density as indicated by guidelines
H. FSH greater than 40 international units (IU)/L is consistent with menopause; however, fluctuations in FSH and 17–2 estradiol (E_2) may make use of these markers unreliable, such that they are no longer recommended for determining menopausal status

Differential Diagnoses

A. Menopause
B. Perimenopause
C. Anemia
D. Cardiac abnormalities
E. Leukemia or other cancer
F. Menstrual irregularity for any cause of secondary amenorrhea
G. Pregnancy
H. Psychosomatic illness
I. Thyroid dysfunction

Plan

A. General interventions:
    1. Provide reassurance as to the cause of the absence of menses.
B. Client teaching:
    1. Discuss common symptoms of menopause.
    2. Provide education regarding healthy lifestyle changes: Regular exercise, weight control, smoking cessation, limiting use of recreational drugs and alcohol, and stress reduction.

    3. Encourage a healthy diet rich in vitamin D and calcium. Supplement the diet with calcium supplements: 1,000 mg/d for women aged 19 to 50 years; 1,200 mg/d for women aged 50 years and older. Calcium citrate is superior to calcium carbonate, as it is more absorbable and usable by the body.
        a. Vitamin D supplements: 600 IU/d until age 70 years; 800 IU/d for age 71 years and older. Consider vitamin D serum screening and, if deficient, treat accordingly. See the "Vitamin D Deficiency" section in Chapter 21.
    4. Encourage use of glycerin-free, water-soluble vaginal lubricants as needed for vaginal dryness. See the "Atrophic Vaginitis" section.
    5. Avoid overly warm environments, caffeine, alcohol, spicy food, and emotional upset; these may trigger hot flashes.
    6. Encourage good sleep hygiene practices and adequate rest.
    7. Discuss the risks and benefits of HRT. Shared decision-making between the clinician and the woman should be employed when discussing HRT initiation, continuation, and discontinuation. Care should be individualized to the woman, taking into account her preferences, menopausal symptoms, and quality of life concerns. Dosage of HRT should begin at the lowest therapeutic dose, increasing from there as needed.
    8. Assess and manage clients at increased risk for osteoporosis according to current osteoporosis guidelines.
    9. Assess and treat cardiac risk factors, including hypertension and elevated lipids, as indicated.
    10. Give the client the relevant teaching guide. *See Section III: Client Teaching Guide for this chapter, "Menopause."* ◀

C. Pharmaceutical therapy:
    1. HRT:
        a. All perimenopausal and menopausal women should be counseled regarding the risks and benefits of HRT. Benefits of HRT include the reduction of hot flashes, insomnia, night sweats, vaginal dryness, mood swings, and depression. Although HRT does reduce the risk of bone loss and fracture, due to potential risks and available effective alternative treatments for osteoporosis, HRT is not recommended specifically for the treatment of osteoporosis alone (see the "Osteoporosis/Kyphosis/Fracture" section in Chapter 21). Risks of HRT include venous thromboembolism, coronary artery disease, and cerebrovascular accident (stroke). If initiated prior to age 60, it does not appear to increase the risk of cardiovascular disease. HRT slightly elevates the risk of stroke, though the absolute risk of stroke in women younger than age 60 is very low. Estrogen-only HRT affects the risk of breast cancer only very slightly; combined estrogen–progestin formulations may increase breast cancer risk. The risk of breast cancer is higher for those clients on HRT for the longest periods,

but does decline when the HRT is discontinued. The latest evidence points to HRT potentially aiding in the prevention of chronic conditions when initiated in symptomatic women prior to the age of 60 years, or within 10 years of the onset of the menopause, considering the individual history and risks of each individual woman. Long-term unopposed ET increases the risk of endometrial cancer via the potential for endometrial hyperplasia. In considering initiation of HRT, the clinician must carefully screen and educate the woman, so that she is empowered to make an informed decision.

b. Estrogen and progesterone are recommended for treatment of moderate to severe vasomotor symptoms and moderate to severe vulvar and vaginal atrophy symptoms. For women with an intact uterus, progesterone is given with estrogen to reduce the risk of endometrial hyperplasia and, therefore, cancer. Postmenopausal women without an intact uterus generally are not prescribed progesterone products and are treated with estrogen alone.

c. Oral HRT may be given either sequentially or continuously. The sequential or "cyclical" regimen involves taking estrogen daily, with progesterone taken on the first 10 to 14 days per month. With this regimen, a withdrawal bleed will occur monthly. An alternative is a continuous regimen in which both estrogen and progesterone are taken daily. With the continuous regimen, there are no withdrawal bleeds.

2. Transdermal estrogen comes in various forms: Gels, patches, and sprays

3. Transvaginal estrogen (see Tables 14.3–14.5)

4. Absolute contraindications to use of ET also apply to use of oral and topical estrogen (i.e., breast cancer, active liver disease, and/or history of recent thromboembolic event). Vaginal estrogen creams are systemically absorbed. As with use of oral and transdermal estrogen, a progestin must be administered to women who have an intact uterus when using most of the vaginal delivery products, secondary to the risk of endometrial hyperplasia or cancer. The vaginal ring FemRing has systemic levels of estrogen and *does* require progestogen protection for the uterus. Other vaginal preparations, including the creams (if a low dose is used only twice a week), vaginal tablets, and Estring, release a very low dose of estrogen and have not shown to increase the risk of endometrial hyperplasia in the 1 year in which these products have been studied.

5. Absolute contraindications to ET:
   a. Acute liver disease
   b. Cerebral vascular or coronary artery disease, MI, or stroke

TABLE 14.3 HORMONE REPLACEMENT THERAPY*

Name	Active Ingredient	Dosage
Estrogen Sequential or Continuous Combined		
Premarin	Conjugated estrogen	0.625 mg/d
Estratab	Esterified estrogen	0.625 mg/d
Menest	Esterified estrogen	0.625 mg/d
Estrace	Micronized estradiol	1.0 mg/d
Ortho-est	Estropipate	0.625 mg/d
Progestin Only for Sequential Regimen		
Amen	Medroxyprogesterone	5–10 mg added to estrogen the first 10–14 days of the month
Cycrin	Medroxyprogesterone	5–10 mg added to estrogen the first 10–14 days of the month
Provera	Medroxyprogesterone	5–10 mg added to estrogen the first 10–14 days of the month
Prometrium	Micronized progesterone	100–200 mg added to estrogen the first 10–14 days of the month
Progestin Only for Continuous Combined Regimen		
Cycrin	Medroxyprogesterone	2.5 mg/d
Provera	Medroxyprogesterone	2.5 mg/d
Combination Packet for Continuous Combined Regimen		
Prempro	0.625 mg conjugated equine estrogen and 2.5 mg medroxyprogesterone	1 tablet orally each day
Activella	1 mg 17-beta estradiol and 0.5 mg norethindrone	1 tablet orally each day
FemHrt	5 mcg ethinyl estradiol and 1 mg norethindrone	1 tablet orally each day

*Not an exhaustive list of every HRT product; see complete prescribing reference or package insert for dosing, titration, contraindications, and side effects.

TABLE 14.4   TRANSDERMAL REPLACEMENT THERAPY*

Delivery	Name	Active Ingredient	Dosage
Transdermal patch	Climara	Estradiol	0.25–0.0375 mg/d
			0.05 mg/d
			0.06 mg/d
			0.075 mg/d
			Apply one patch weekly (lower abdomen or upper buttocks)
Transdermal patch	Combipatch	Estradiol 0.05 mg and norethindrone acetate 0.14 mg/d	Continuous combined regimen of one patch twice weekly for a 28-day cycle (lower abdomen)
		Or estradiol 0.05 mg and norethindrone acetate 0.0.25 mg/d	
Transdermal patch	Vivelle	Estradiol	0.05/d, 0.1 mg/d; one patch twice weekly to trunk
Gel-Pump	Elestrin	Estradiol	0.06% gel; one pump daily to clean dry skin of upper arm
Gel-Pump	Estrogel	Estradiol	0.75 mg/1.25 g gel; one pump daily to clean dry skin of upper arm
Spray	Evamist	Estradiol	1.53 mg/spray; one spray daily to inside of arm

*Not an exhaustive list of every HRT product; see complete prescribing reference or package insert for dosing, titration, contraindications, and side effects.

TABLE 14.5   TRANSVAGINAL REPLACEMENT THERAPY*

Delivery	Name	Active Ingredient	Dosage
Cream	Estrace	Micronized 17-beta estradiol	0.1 mg/g, one-half (2 g) to one (4 g) applicator intravaginally at bedtime every night for 1–2 weeks. When vaginal mucosa is restored, maintenance dose is one-quarter applicator (1 g) one to three times weekly in a cyclic regimen.
	Premarin	Conjugated equine estrogen	0.625 mg/g; use 0.5- to 1.0-g applicator inserted intravaginally at bedtime every night for 1–2 weeks, then every other night for 1–2 weeks, then as needed
Ring	Estring	Micronized 17-beta estradiol	7.5 mg/24 hr; insert new ring every 90 days
	FemRing	Estradiol acetate	0.05–0.1 mg/d; insert new ring every 90 days
Vaginal tablet	Vagifem	Estradiol acetate	25 mcg once daily for 2 weeks, then twice weekly
IUD	Mirena	Levonorgestrel	20 mcg daily

*Not an exhaustive list of every HRT product; see complete prescribing reference or package insert for dosing, titration, contraindications, and side effects.

c. History of or active thrombophlebitis or thromboembolic disorders

d. History of uterine or ovarian cancer

e. Known or suspected cancer of the breast*

f. Known or suspected estrogen-dependent neoplasm

g. Pregnancy

h. Undiagnosed, abnormal vaginal bleeding

6. Relative contraindications to ET:
   a. Active gallbladder disease
   b. Familial hyperlipidemia

7. Absolute contraindications to progesterone therapy:
   a. Active thrombophlebitis or thromboembolic disorders
   b. Acute liver disease
   c. Known or suspected cancer of the breast

---

*   Due to minimal central absorption of some vaginal hormonal preparations, some products **may** be appropriately prescribed for women with a history of breast cancer. Consultation with the woman's oncologist is required prior to the initiation of any HRT.

d. Pregnancy
e. Undiagnosed, abnormal vaginal bleeding

> Educate the client to notify the care provider if unusual vaginal bleeding, calf pain, chest pain, shortness of breath, hemoptysis, severe headaches, visual disturbances, breast pain, abdominal pain, or jaundice occur while being prescribed HRT.

D. Nonhormonal pharmacologic therapy for vasomotor symptoms:
1. Antidepressants: Venlafaxine (Effexor) and paroxetine (Paxil) seem to provide the best relief and reduce vasomotor symptoms by 50% to 61%. Sertraline (Zoloft) seems to be no more effective than placebo.
   a. Fluoxetine (Prozac) 20 mg/d
   b. Venlafaxine (Effexor) 37.5 to 75 mg/d
   c. Paroxetine (Paxil) 12.5 to 25 mg/d
   d. Sertraline (Zoloft) 50 mg/d
2. Anticonvulsant:
   a. Gabapentin (Neurontin) 300 mg/d and titrate to three or four times a day
3. Antihypertensive:
   a. Clonidine 0.05 to 0.1 mg twice a day
4. For nonhormonal pharmacological therapies, review prescribing literature for side effects, titrations, and discontinuation regimens
E. Nonprescription remedies/herbals:
1. Many nonprescription remedies are currently available for the treatment of menopausal symptoms: Isoflavones (soy and red clover), black cohosh, dong quai, EPO, ginseng, licorice, and vitamins E and C.
2. The provider should review with the client the lack of standardization and evidence regarding the safety and efficacy of these products. Currently, results of research are insufficient to support or refute the use of these remedies for the treatment of menopausal symptoms.
F. Acupuncture has shown mixed results.

Follow-Up
A. Follow up 3 months after initiation to assess a response to treatment, and then annually for physical examination. Perform a Pap and/or HPV test as indicated by guidelines, and a lipid panel as indicated.
B. Prior recommendations pushed for discontinuation of HRT in 5 years based on client response and risks and benefits. Current recommendations note that the decision to discontinue HRT should not be based strictly on time, but with full consideration of the woman's history, risk profile, and preferences.

Consultation/Referral
A. Consult a gynecologist if the woman experiences symptoms resistant to treatment, or vaginal bleeding from an unknown source.

Bibliography
Gambacciani, M., Cagnacci, A., & Lello, S. (2019). Hormone replacement therapy and prevention of chronic conditions. *Climacteric, 22*, 303–306. doi:10.1080/13697137.2018.1551347
Houtkooper, L., Farrell, V. A., & Mullins, V. (2017). *Calcium supplement guidelines.* https://extension.arizona.edu/pubs/calcium-supplement-guidelines
Lobo, R. A. (2017). Hormone-replacement therapy: Current thinking. *Nature Reviews Endocrinology, 13*(4), 220. doi:10.1038/nrendo.2016.164
National Institutes of Health. (2014). *Vitamin D.* Retrieved from http://ods.od.nih.gov/factsheets/VitaminD-HealthProfessional
National Institutes of Health. (2016). *Calcium.* Retrieved from http://ods.od.nih.gov/factsheets/Calcium-HealthProfessional
North American Menopause Society. (2016). *Vagina and vulvar comfort: Lubricants, moisturizers, and low-dose vaginal estrogen.* Retrieved from http://www.menopause.org/for-women/-em-sexual-health-menopause-em-online/effective-treatments-for-sexual-problems/vaginal-and-vulvar-comfort-lubricants-moisturizers-and-low-dose-vaginal-estrogen
Schuiling, K. D., & Likis, F. E. (Eds.). (2013). *Women's gynecologic health* (3rd ed.). Sudbury, MA: Jones & Bartlett Learning.
Utian, W. H., & Schiff, I. (2018). NAMS–Gallup survey on women's knowledge, information sources, and attitudes to menopause and hormone replacement therapy. *Menopause, 25*(11), 1172–1179. doi:10.1097/gme.0000000000001213

Pap Test Screening Guidelines and Interpretation

Rhonda Arthur and Michelle Collins

The Pap test is a sampling of exfoliated cells collected from the cervix for cytologic evaluation. This screening test is designed to increase detection and treatment of precancerous and early cancerous cervical lesions, and to decrease morbidity and mortality from cases of invasive cervical cancer.

In the United States, approximately 13,170 new cases of cervical cancer are diagnosed annually. Among these cases, approximately 4,250 deaths will occur. There has been a 50% reduction in cervical cancer deaths over the past 30 years due to the use of cervical cancer screening.

The following are risk factors for development of cervical cancer:
A. Early age at first intercourse: 17 or younger
B. Multiple sexual partners: More than five in a lifetime
C. Multiparity
D. Douching
E. Pessary use
F. Immunosuppression
G. Smoking
H. Male partner with a history of multiple partners or STIs (also known as "high-risk male")
I. History of STI, in particular HPV

> Sexually transmitted agents, particularly the HPV strains 16, 18, 31, 33, 39, and 42, are strongly associated with the development of cervical cancer. Virtually all cervical cancers are associated with high-risk HPV (hRHPV) infection. HPV types 16 and 18 cause 70% of all cervical cancers.

J. DES exposure in utero
K. Genetics: Although the cervical cancer in and of itself is not hereditary, some familial characteristics may leave women in the same family more vulnerable to hRHPV, or more likely to develop cervical dysplasia once exposed
L. Oral contraceptive use: Several studies have noted statistically significant positive associations between oral contraceptive use and risk of cervical cancer and

precancer. The risk appears to increase with duration of use and decreases once hormonal oral contraception is discontinued.

M. Nutritional factors: Low lutein, vitamin C, vitamin E, and lycopene levels are associated with persistent HPV.

The Pap test should include sampling from both the ectocervix and the endocervix to be considered "adequate for interpretation." The ectocervix is the cervical portion extending outward from the external cervical os. The endocervix extends upward from the external os to the internal os, where the cervical epithelium meets the uterine endometrium.

Cervical epithelium is composed of squamous and columnar cells. Squamous epithelium, appearing smooth and pink, lines the vagina and continues upward to cover variable amounts of the ectocervix. Columnar epithelium, darker red and more granular in appearance, lines the endometrium and continues downward to the cervix, lining the endocervical canal. The boundary between squamous and columnar epithelium is called the squamo-columnar junction (SCJ) and may occur anywhere on the ectocervix or endocervix.

The SCJ may regress at various times as a result of hormonal variation, particularly with menopause and during pregnancy. As new cells are formed and moved from the internal to the external cervix, those cells that formerly made up the SCJ are moved farther out to the perimeter of the os on the ectocervix. The area between the original and new SCJ is called the transformation zone. When columnar epithelium is visible on the ectocervix, appearing as a granular, red area, it is referred to as ectropion or ectopian. This condition is often seen in pregnancy and with combined oral contraceptive use.

Cervical cancer is a progressive disease with a number of histologically definable stages. Invasive cancer of the cervix, and its precursors, are detectable by cytology before they become symptomatic and before gross clinical signs appear. When symptoms are present, they usually include postcoital spotting, intermenstrual bleeding, and increased menstrual bleeding. Clients with invasive cancer may experience serosanguineous, or yellowish, vaginal discharge, which may be foul smelling and intermixed with blood.

Advanced disease may cause urinary or rectal symptoms, including bleeding. On speculum examination, advanced lesions appear as necrotic ulcers; with invasive disease, they may extend upward or protrude into the vagina.

▶ *See Section II: Procedures, "Pap Test."*

Bethesda System

The Bethesda System (a classification system developed in 2001 and used to interpret cytologic findings) was updated in 2014. When a cervical Pap sample is processed and the report issued, it includes the following information:

A. Specimen type:
1. Conventional slide method versus liquid-based preparation

B. Adequacy of the specimen:
1. Satisfactory for evaluation
2. Presence or absence of endocervical or transformational zone components
3. Quality indicators such as obscuring blood or inflammation
4. Unsatisfactory for evaluation and specific reason
C. General categorization:
1. Negative for intraepithelial lesion or malignancy
2. Other, such as endometrial cells in women older than 45 years
3. Epithelial cell abnormality: See "Interpretation/result"

If an infection is indicated as a Pap test finding, evaluate the client and treat her accordingly. Pap tests are not diagnostic for vaginal or cervical infection. Institute therapy for infections after confirmation by wet prep and/or cultures and guided by cytologic reading. For example, if Candida is identified on Pap test results, evaluate the client in the office, confirm the finding, and treat the client with appropriate antifungal therapy.

D. Interpretation/result

Negative for intraepithelial lesion or malignancy (optional to report):
1. Non-neoplastic cellular variations
2. Reactive cellular changes associated with:
   a. Inflammation
   b. Radiation
   c. IUD
3. Organisms:
   a. *T. vaginalis*
   b. Fungal organisms
   c. Shift in flora suggestive of BV
   d. Cellular changes consistent with HSV
   e. Cellular changes consistent with cytomegalovirus
4. Other: Endometrial cells (in a woman 45 years or older)
E. Epithelial cell abnormalities:
1. Squamous cell abnormalities:
   a. Atypical squamous cells of undetermined significance (ASCUS): Indicates slight cellular abnormality, without clear cause (may be due to infection or cervical trauma, for example).
   b. Atypical squamous cells, cannot exclude high grade (ASC-H): This result notes that there are abnormal cells present that have some high-grade characteristics. An ASC-H Pap result is of higher severity than an ASCUS Pap.
   c. Low-grade squamous intraepithelial lesion (LSIL): Indicates the effect of HPV, mild dysplasia, or cervical intraepithelial neoplasia (CIN) I
   d. High-grade squamous intraepithelial lesions (HSIL): Moderate and severe dysplasia, carcinoma in situ or CIN II, and CIN III
   e. Squamous cell carcinoma

2. Glandular cell:
   a. Atypical glandular cells (AGC):
      i. Endocervical cells (not otherwise specified [NOS] or specify in comments)
      ii. Endometrial (NOS or specify in comments)
      iii. Glandular (NOS or specify in comments)
   b. Atypical:
      i. Endocervical cells favor neoplastic variations
      ii. Glandular cells favor neoplastic variations
   c. Endocervical adenocarcinoma in situ
   d. Adenocarcinoma:
      i. Endocervical
      ii. Endometrial
      iii. Extrauterine
      iv. NOS
F. Other malignant neoplasms: Specify
G. Adjunctive testing
H. Computer-assisted interpretation of cervical pathology
I. Educational notes and comments appended to cytology report (optional)

Initial Management of Abnormal Pap Tests

A. ASCUS or LSIL in women aged 21 to 24 years:
   1. Repeat cytology in 12 months for the next 2 years, with colposcopy after 1 year for HSIL, ASC-H, or AGC, and colposcopy after 2 years if ASCUS or greater. This is the preferred mode of follow-up.
   2. Reflex HPV: An acceptable follow-up, with repeat cytology being the preferred modality:
      a. HPV negative: Continue routine screen with Pap test in 3 years
      b. HPV positive: Annual Pap test for 2 years with colposcopy after 1 year if HSIL, ASC-H, or AGC and after 2 years if ASCUS or greater
B. ASC-H is managed with colposcopy
C. LSIL in women aged 21 to 24 years:
   1. HPV negative: Can be managed with routine screening as follow-up
   2. LSIL with positive or no HPV test: Managed with repeat Pap at 12 months
   3. Pregnant women with LSIL in this age group can be managed the same way
D. HSIL management in women aged 21 to 24 years is colposcopy. Immediate loop electrosurgical excision procedure (LEEP) is unacceptable.
E. AGC management for all subcategories except atypical endometrial cells includes colposcopy with endocervical sampling. For women aged 35 years and older or any woman at risk of endometrial neoplasia, endometrial sampling is also indicated.
F. Unsatisfactory cytology:
   1. If HPV unknown (at any age) or HPV negative (and age 30 or greater), repeat cytology in 2 to 4 months.
   2. If HPV positive (and age 30 or greater), either repeat cytology in 2 to 4 months or perform colposcopy.
   3. If two consecutive unsatisfactory cytology tests, then colposcopy is indicated.

G. Cytology negative but absent or insufficient endocervical/transitional zone component:
   1. Aged 21 to 29 or 30 years and older with HPV negative: Conduct routine screening Pap in 3 years.
   2. Aged 30 years and older and HPV unknown: HPV testing is preferred; repeat cytology in 3 years is an acceptable route.
   3. Aged 30 years and older and HPV positive: Conduct cytology plus HPV testing in 1 year or immediate genotyping for HPV
   4. See and download American Society for Colposcopy and Cervical Pathology (ASCCP) algorithms for complete management options at www.asccp.org

---

ASCCP has a mobile device application. Look for the mobile application "ASCCP Abnormal Cervical Cancer Screening Guidelines" on iTunes.

Recommendations

According to the ACS, U.S. Preventive Services Task Force, ASCCP, and American College of Obstetricians and Gynecologists guidelines, all women should begin cervical cancer screening at age 21 years. Women younger than 21 years should not be screened regardless of the age of sexual debut. Pap alone should be performed every 3 years for women aged 21 to 29. Annual screening is not indicated for any woman. Highlights of the recommendations include:

A. Begin screening at age 21 years.
B. Women from ages 21 to 29 years should have conventional or liquid-based cytology every 3 years, and no HPV testing should be performed.
C. Women from ages 30 to 65 years should have conventional or liquid-based cytology every 3 years (acceptable route), or have conventional or liquid-based cytology plus an HPV co-test every 5 years. HPV co-testing should not be used in women younger than 30 years. Pap and HPV done together is the preferred route of cervical cancer screening in women aged 30 to 65.
D. Cervical cancer screening should cease at age 65 years in women with an adequate negative prior screening history. Women with a history of CIN II or greater should continue routine screening for at least 20 years after the diagnosis and treatment.
E. Post hysterectomy: Cervical cancer screening should cease after total hysterectomy as long as the woman does not have a history of CIN II or greater in the past 20 years, or a history of cervical cancer ever
F. HPV vaccination screen according to age-specific recommendation
G. Women who have a high-risk medical history (immunocompromised, HIV positive, DES-exposed in utero, or a history of cervical cancer) are not included in the updated routine guidelines.

The Advisory Committee on Immunization Practices recommends routine vaccination of females and males aged 11 to 12 years with three doses of nonvalent HPV vaccine and states the series can be started as young as

9 years of age. Catch-up vaccination is recommended for females aged 13 to 26 years, and males aged 13 to 21 years.

Client education regarding the prevention of cervical cancer, by avoiding exposure to HPV, should include reduction or elimination of high-risk activities. These high-risk activities include having sexual intercourse at an early age (younger than 18 years of age), having multiple sexual partners (defined as greater than five), and having partners with multiple partners. Use of condoms can reduce the risk of HPV as well as other STIs. Smoking cessation can also reduce the risk of cervical cancer. Identification and treatment of precancerous lesions can reduce the risk of invasive cervical cancer, so screening according to ASCCP guidelines should be recommended.

hRHPV Screening as Primary Screening Modality

In 2015, ASCCP issued interim guidance regarding the utilization of hRHPV testing as a primary screening modality. The following conclusions were noted in the interim guidance document: (a) Primary hrHPV testing used as primary screening has been proven to be at least as safe and effective as cytology; (b) because of the efficacy, primary hrHPV screening can be considered as an alternative to current U.S. cervical cancer screening modalities; (c) primary hrHPV screening should not be started prior to age 25; and (d) the optimal screening interval should be no sooner than every 3 years. Using the recommended algorithm, hrHPV testing is the primary screening test, and reflex testing is performed with a combination of genotyping and cytology (Pap). Women who test as hrHPV negative should follow routine screening recommendations. Women who are hrHPV positive for types 16 and/or 18 are directed to colposcopy. Women who test hrHPV positive for any of the 12 other high-risk types reflex to cytology (Pap). Women with a Pap result of ASCUS or greater are directed to colposcopy, while a negative Pap is followed up in 12 months.

Treatment Modalities

Treatment is instituted based on the severity of the lesion and the presence of pathology within the columnar epithelium of the endocervix. Treatment options include:
A. Observation and repeat cytology
B. Cryotherapy
C. Loop excision of the transformation zone
D. Laser of the transformation zone
E. Cold-knife conization

Screening Guidelines

The major healthcare organizations that establish cervical cancer screening guidelines have slightly different screening recommendations. The various recommendations are summarized in Table 14.6.

Bibliography

Centers for Disease Control and Prevention. (2015). *Human papillomavirus.* Retrieved from http://www.cdc.gov/hpv/parents/vaccine.html

Huh, W. K., Ault, K. A., Chelmow, D., Davey, D. D., Goulart, R. A., Garcia, F. A., . . . Schiffman, M. (2015). Use of primary high-risk human papillomavirus testing for cervical cancer screening: Interim clinical guidance. *Obstetrics and Gynecology, 125,* 330–337. doi:10.1097/aog.0000000000000669

Massad, L. S., Einstein, M. H., Huh, W. K., Katki, H. A., Kinney, W. K., Schiffman, M., . . . Lawson, H. W. (2013). 2012 updated consensus guidelines for the management of abnormal cervical cancer screening tests and cancer precursors. *Journal of Lower Genital Tract Disease, 17* (5 suppl 1), S1–S27. doi:10.1097/lgt.0b013e318287d329

McNamara, M., Batur, P., Walsh, J. M., & Johnson, K. M. (2016). HPV update: Vaccination, screening, and associated disease. *Journal of General Internal Medicine, 31*(11), 1360–1366. doi:10.1007/s11606-016-3725-z

Nayar, R., & Wilbur, D. C. (2015). The Pap test and Bethesda 2014: "The reports of my demise have been greatly exaggerated" (after a quotation from Mark Twain). *Acta Cytologica, 59*(2), 121–132.

Roura, E., Travier, N., Waterboer, T., de Sanjosé, S., Bosch, F. X., Pawlita, M., . . . Gram, I. T. (2016). The influence of hormonal factors on the risk of developing cervical cancer and pre-cancer: Results from the EPIC cohort. *PLoS One, 11*(1), e0147029. doi:10.1371/journal.pone.0147029

Webster, S. D. (2016). *Human papilloma virus-related cervical dysplasia.* Otterbein University, Digital Commons @ Otterbein. Retrieved from http://digitalcommons.otterbein.edu/stu_msn/145/

Pelvic Inflammatory Disease

Rhonda Arthur and Michelle Collins

Definition
A. PID is an infection of the upper genital tract. The infection can involve the uterine endometrium (endometritis), fallopian tubes (salpingitis), ovaries (oophoritis), broad ligament or uterine serosa (parametritis), and the pelvic vascular system or pelvic connective tissue.

Incidence
A. Annual incidence is difficult to obtain due to difficulty in definitive diagnosis and reporting.
B. PID is one of the leading causes of infertility in the world, as it often leads to inflammation and damage to the fallopian tubes.

Pathogenesis
A. PID is caused by organisms that ascend from the vagina and cervix into the uterus. Menses facilitates gonococcal invasion of the upper genital tract, as the luteal phase stimulates gonococcal growth and the cervical mucus barrier is removed. Infection and inflammation spread throughout the endometrium to the fallopian tubes. From there, the infectious process extends to the ovaries and peritoneal cavity.
B. The most common organisms cultured from clients with PID are *C. trachomatis, N. gonorrhoeae, M. hominis, Ureaplasma urealyticum, Bacteroides, Peptostreptococcus, Escherichia coli,* and some endogenous aerobes and anaerobes.
C. The incubation period varies with the infective organism.

Predisposing Factors
A. Age: Rates of PID are higher for women at younger ages. They are highest in the younger than 30-year-old age group (70% incidence in women younger than age 25 years). Teens are particularly susceptible because they have an immature immune system and larger zones of cervical ectopy with thinner cervical mucus.

TABLE 14.6   RECOMMENDATIONS FOR TREATING PID

	ACOG (updated last in 2009)** [ACOG endorsed ASCCP guidelines in 2013 and now recommends the same as ASCCP. Prior ACOG guidelines are provided here for context.]	ACS/ASCCP/ASCP (updated 2012)	USPTF (updated 2012)
Initial Screen	21 regardless of age at onset of sexual activity	No screening of women < 21 years of age	No screening of women < 21 years of age
Regular Screen	Every 2 years from ages 21 to 29 **At 30**: After 3 consecutive negative tests, screen every 3 years **At 30**: With negative Pap and HPV, screen every 3 years **hrHPV testing is alternative screening every 3 years for women ≥ 25 years as per SGO and ASCCP interim guidance (2016)**	**21–29:** Pap every 3 years **30–65:** "Co-testing" (Pap and HPV) every 5 years is preferred; Pap alone every 3 years is acceptable **OR** **hrHPV testing ALONE every 3 years (2015)**	**21–29:** Pap every 3 years **30–65:** Pap every 3 years, or if desired to lengthen interval, Pap plus HPV testing every 5 years **OR** **hrHPV testing ALONE every 5 years (2018)**
Special Circumstances	Screen at least yearly if high risk: Immunosuppressed, HIV, prior CA, CIN 2–3; DES exposure		
Post Hysterectomy	Screen those with prior CIN 2, 3, or CA for at least 20 years post treatment	No screening for VIN **IF** cervix removed **AND** there is no history of CIN 2, 3, or CA. Evidence of adequate negative prior screening is not required. Screening not to be resumed with a new partner.	No screening after removal of cervix **IF** there is no history of CIN 2, 3, or CA.
Dilation and Curettage (D&C)	Provider discretion based on risk and history; annual pelvic recommended; D&C for women post hysterectomy (for benign reasons)	Against screening women > 65 years who have a history of adequate screening and are not otherwise at high risk	Those with a history of adequate negative prior screening and no history of CIN 2 within the past 20 years should not be screened, even if new partner

ACOG, American College of Obstetricians and Gynecologists; ACS, American Cancer Society; ASCCP, American Society for Colposcopy and Cervical Pathology; ASCP, American Society for Clinical Pathology; CA, cancer; CIN, cervical intraepithelial neoplasia; DES, diethylstilbestrol; HPV, human papillomavirus; hrHPV, high-risk human papillomavirus; SGO, Society of Gynecologic Oncology; USPTF, United States Preventive Task Force; VIN, vulvar intraepithelial neoplasia.

B. Sexual activity: Women with multiple sexual partners are three times more likely to develop PID, when compared to women with only one partner.

C. History of PID

D. Menstruation: Supports the development and spread of PID. Women who are not currently menstruating have a decreased risk.

E. History of invasive procedures: These procedures may result in iatrogenic PID. PID is usually seen within 4 weeks of the procedure (dilation and curettage [D&C], IUD insertion, HSG, and vacuum curettage abortion).

F. There is an increased incidence of PID in African Americans and non-White women and women in lower socioeconomic groups.

G. Cigarette smoking

H. Frequent vaginal douching

Common Complaints

A. Lower abdominal pain

B. Fever or chills

C. Increased vaginal discharge, may be malodorous

D. Nausea and vomiting

E. Low back pain

Other Signs and Symptoms

A. Asymptomatic; vague and nonspecific symptoms

B. Minimal to severe pelvic pain

C. Right upper quadrant (RUQ) pain (25%)

D. Abnormal vaginal bleeding

Subjective Data

A. Determine onset, duration, and course of presenting symptoms.

B. Review the character of vaginal discharge (if any); history of recent dysmenorrhea and/or dyspareunia; any intestinal or bladder symptoms.

C. Question the client regarding sexual history: Current number of sexual partners; current or most recent sexual activity; and contraceptive used (condoms, pills, patch, ring, implant, diaphragm, IUD) and frequency of use of each method.

D. Question the client as to whether her current sexual partner has experienced any symptoms.

E. What is the client's current menstrual pattern? Is there a possibility that she is pregnant? Did the pain begin in relation to her cycle?

F. Review prior pelvic or abdominal surgeries and procedures (HSG, pregnancy termination) and when they were done.

G. Review the history and quality of pain: How long, bilateral or unilateral, what makes it better, and what makes it worse (intercourse, Valsalva maneuver with bowel movement, activity).

Physical Examination

A. Check temperature, pulse, respirations, and BP.

B. Inspect:
1. Observe the client's general overall appearance for discomfort before, during, and after the examination.

C. Auscultate:
1. The abdomen for bowel sounds in all quadrants. Auscultation of the abdomen should precede any palpation or percussion due to the changes in intensity and frequency of sounds after manipulation.

D. Percuss:
1. The abdomen for organomegaly

E. Palpate:
1. The groin for lymphadenopathy
2. The abdomen for masses
3. The levator ani muscle (left and right), the urethra, and the trigone of the bladder
4. Perform rebound, involuntary guarding, and jar tests. The jar test is performed by intentionally hitting or jarring the examination table and watching for a pain response. Pelvic discomfort is exacerbated by the Valsalva maneuver, intercourse, or movement. Abdominal or pelvic pain with PID is usually bilateral. About 25% of clients complain of RUQ pain; the pain usually occurs within 7 to 10 days of menses, is continuous, and is most severe in the lower quadrants.

F. Pelvic examination:
1. Inspect: Examine the vulva for Bartholin's gland enlargement, fissures, condyloma, herpes simplex, and pelvic relaxation.
2. Palpate: "Milk" the Skene's glands for discharge.
3. Speculum examination: Inspect for cervicitis and friability. Evaluate vaginal discharge and bleeding for color, amount, and odor. Lower abdominal, or pelvic, pain is the most common symptom of PID and typically is moderate to severe; however, many women may have subtle or mild symptoms that are not readily recognizable as PID, including abnormal bleeding, dyspareunia, or vaginal discharge.

G. Bimanual examination:
1. Check CMT; evaluate the size, contour, mobility, and tenderness of the uterus.
2. Palpate the adnexa for tenderness and masses. The classic PID presentation is lower abdominal and adnexal tenderness and CMT (chandelier sign). The pelvic area may feel hot.

H. Rectovaginal examination: Assess for adnexal thickening and masses.

Diagnostic Tests

A. CBC with differential; WBC greater than 10,500 cell/mm³

B. Quantitative beta-HCG

C. RPR, hepatitis B surface antigen, and HIV if indicated

D. Cultures for gonorrhea and chlamydia

E. Transvaginal ultrasonography

F. Laparoscopy, by referral

> Because of the similarity in symptoms between PID and ectopic pregnancy, always test the client for quantitative beta-HCG even if she claims her menses are regular and she is using reliable contraception. Vaginal cultures should also always be done as part of the STI workup. Eliciting data in the health history about hysterectomy, previous appendectomy, pregnancy terminations, and procedures, such as HSG, may provide exclusionary diagnoses.

G. Diagnostic criteria for clinical diagnosis of PID
1. Minimal criteria: Empiric treatment for PID should be initiated in sexually active women if they are experiencing pelvic or lower abdominal pain, if no cause for the illness other than PID can be identified, and if one or more of the following minimum clinical criteria are present on pelvic examination:
    a. CMT
    b. Uterine tenderness
    c. Adnexal tenderness
2. Additional routine criteria (one or more of the following support diagnosis of PID):
    a. Oral temperature greater than 101°F
    b. Abnormal cervical or vaginal discharge
    c. Elevated erythrocyte sedimentation rate
    d. Elevated C-reactive protein
    e. Laboratory documentation of cervical infection with *N. gonorrhoeae* or *C. trachomatis*

Differential Diagnoses

A. Gynecologic factors:
1. PID
2. Ectopic pregnancy
3. Pelvic endometriosis
4. Dysmenorrhea
5. Adenomyosis
6. Functional ovarian cysts
7. Endometrial polyps or fibroid
8. Pelvic relaxation
9. Anatomical abnormalities

B. GI factors:
1. Acute appendicitis
2. IBS
3. Ulcerative colitis, Crohn's disease
4. Diverticulitis
5. Hernia

C. GU factors:
1. Cystitis, urethritis interstitial cystitis
2. Ureteral obstruction
3. Carcinoma of bladder

D. Musculoskeletal factors:
1. Myofascial pain
2. Pelvic floor myalgia
3. Spinal injuries or degenerative disease
E. Neurologic factor: Nerve entrapment syndrome

Plan

A. General interventions:

1. A low threshold is needed for diagnosis of PID because of the risk of damage to reproductive health. Early treatment is imperative. Other causes of lower abdominal pain, such as IBS and endometriosis, are not likely to be impaired by empiric antibiotic therapy. The risk of ectopic pregnancy is 6 to 10 times greater for women with PID compared with uninfected women.

2. Antibiotic therapy should be instituted promptly, based on clinical diagnosis without awaiting culture results, to minimize the risk of progression of the infection and risk of transmission of the organisms to other sexual partners.

3. If a woman with an IUD in place is diagnosed with PID, the IUD does not need to be removed. The woman should receive the recommended treatment. If there is no improvement in 48 to 72 hours, the healthcare provider should consider removing the IUD.

4. Ambulatory clients should be monitored closely and reevaluated within 3 days of initiating antibiotic therapy. A decrease in pelvic tenderness should be observed within 3 to 5 days of initiation of therapy; if not, additional evaluation is warranted.

▶ B. Client teaching: *See Section III: Client Teaching Guide for this chapter, "Pelvic Inflammatory Disease."*

1. Male sexual partners (and all partners) of clients with PID must be examined, cultured when possible, and treated empirically for presumptive gonorrheal and chlamydial infection.

2. Women who do not use any contraception are at the greatest risk of PID. Transmission of STIs can be minimized with effective use of barrier contraceptives. Spermicides prevent infection with chlamydia and gonorrhea. The use of nonoxynol-9 is protective against *N. gonorrhoeae*, *Treponema palladium*, *Trichomonas*, HSV, and *Candida*.

C. Pharmaceutical therapy (see Table 14.7)

Alternative IM/Oral Regimens

Although information regarding other IM and oral regimens is limited, a few have undergone at least one clinical trial and have demonstrated broad-spectrum coverage. Azithromycin has demonstrated short-term clinical effectiveness in one randomized trial when used as monotherapy (500 mg IV daily for 1–2 doses, followed by 250 mg orally daily for 12–14 days) or in combination with metronidazole; in another study, it was effective when used as 1 g orally once a week for 2 weeks in combination with ceftriaxone 250 mg IM single dose. When considering these alternative regimens, the addition of metronidazole should be considered to provide anaerobic coverage. No data have been published regarding the use of oral cephalosporins

for the treatment of PID. Because of the emergence of quinolone-resistant *N. gonorrhoeae* (QRNG), regimens that include a quinolone agent are no longer routinely recommended for the treatment of PID. If the client has an allergy that precludes the use of cephalosporin therapy, if the community prevalence and individual risk for gonorrhea are low, and if follow-up is likely, use of fluoroquinolones for 14 days (levofloxacin 500 mg orally once daily, ofloxacin 400 mg twice daily, or moxifloxacin 400 mg orally once daily) with metronidazole for 14 days (500 mg orally twice daily) can be considered. Diagnostic tests for gonorrhea must be obtained before initiating therapy, and persons should be managed as follows:

▪ If the culture for gonorrhea is positive, treatment should be based on results of antimicrobial susceptibility testing.

▪ If the isolate is determined to be QRNG or if antimicrobial susceptibility cannot be assessed (e.g., if only nucleic acid amplification testing [NAAT] is available), consultation with an infectious-disease specialist is recommended.

Follow-Up

A. Because of the high risk of reinfection, the CDC recommends include that all women who have received a diagnosis of chlamydial or gonococcal PID should be retested 3 months after treatment, regardless of whether their sex partners were treated. If retesting at 3 months is not possible, these women should be retested whenever they next present for medical care in the 12 months following treatment. "Test of cure" is not indicated for the nonpregnant woman.

B. Hepatitis B immunization should be initiated in previously unvaccinated persons.

Consultation/Referral

Consult a gynecologist if the client diagnosis is atypical, evidence for a presumptive diagnosis is present, or hospitalization is required. General criteria for hospitalization are the following:

A. Diagnosis is uncertain.

B. Pelvic or tubo-ovarian abscess is suspected.

C. IUD in situ

D. The client is pregnant.

E. The client is an adolescent or is believed to be incapable of adhering to an outpatient regimen.

F. Outpatient therapy fails; the client is not better in 48 to 72 hours.

G. The client cannot be reevaluated in 48 to 72 hours.

H. The client is HIV positive.

I. There is generalized peritonitis or severe illness.

J. The client cannot tolerate oral medication therapies.

K. Surgical emergencies cannot be ruled out.

Individual Considerations

A. Pregnancy:

1. Fluoroquinolones are contraindicated for pregnant and nursing mothers.

2. Pregnant women with suspected PID should be hospitalized and treated with parenteral antibiotics.

TABLE 14.7 CENTERS FOR DISEASE CONTROL AND PREVENTION RECOMMENDATIONS FOR TREATING PID, FROM THE 2015 CDC STD GUIDELINES

Inpatient Therapy	Ambulatory Therapy
Cefotetan 2 g IV every 12 hours *or* cefoxitin 2 g *plus* doxycycline 100 mg IV or orally every 12 hours This regimen is continued for at least 48 hours after clinical improvement and followed by doxycycline 100 mg orally twice daily to complete a 14-day total course **OR** Clindamycin 900 mg IV every 8 hours (15–40 mg/kg/d) **Plus** Gentamicin, loading dose 2.0 mg/kg IV, followed by maintenance dose 1.5 mg/kg IV every 8 hours. Single daily dosing may be substituted. For the clindamycin/gentamicin regimen, oral therapy with clindamycin (450 mg orally four times daily) or doxycycline (100 mg twice daily) can be used to complete the 14 days of therapy. However, when tubo-ovarian abscess is present, clindamycin (450 mg orally four times daily) or metronidazole (500 mg twice daily) should be used to complete at least 14 days of therapy with doxycycline to provide more effective anaerobic coverage than doxycycline alone. ***Alternative Parenteral Regimens*** Ampicillin/sulbactam plus doxycycline has been investigated in at least one clinical trial and has broad-spectrum coverage. Ampicillin/sulbactam plus doxycycline is effective against *C. trachomatis*, *N. gonorrhoeae*, and anaerobes in women with tubo-ovarian abscess. Another trial demonstrated high short-term clinical cure rates with azithromycin, either as monotherapy for 1 week (500 mg IV daily for 1 or 2 doses followed by 250 mg orally for 5–6 days) or combined with a 12-day course of metronidazole. Limited data are available to support the use of other parenteral regimens.	IM/oral therapy can be considered for women with mild-to-moderately severe acute PID, because the clinical outcomes among women treated with these regimens are similar to those treated with IV therapy. Women who do not respond to IM/oral therapy within 72 hours should be reevaluated to confirm the diagnosis and should be administered IV therapy. *Recommended Intramuscular/Oral Regimens* Ceftriaxone 250 mg IM in a single dose **Plus** Doxycycline 100 mg orally twice a day for 14 days **With* or Without** Metronidazole 500 mg orally twice a day for 14 days **OR** Cefoxitin 2 g IM in a single dose and probenecid, 1 g orally administered concurrently in a single dose **Plus** Doxycycline 100 mg orally twice a day for 14 days **With or Without** Metronidazole 500 mg orally twice a day for 14 days **OR** Other parenteral third-generation cephalosporin (e.g., ceftizoxime or cefotaxime) **Plus** Doxycycline 100 mg orally twice a day for 14 days **With* or Without** Metronidazole 500 mg orally twice a day for 14 days These regimens provide coverage against frequent etiologic agents of PID, but the optimal choice of a cephalosporin is unclear. Cefoxitin, a second-generation cephalosporin, has better anaerobic coverage than ceftriaxone, and in combination with probenecid and doxycycline has been effective in short-term clinical response in women with PID. Ceftriaxone has better coverage against *N. gonorrhoeae*. The addition of metronidazole will also effectively treat BV, which is frequently associated with PID.

Notes: For women or their partners who cannot tolerate doxycycline or tetracycline, erythromycin 500 mg orally four times daily may be used for 10 to 14 days.

BV, bacterial vaginosis; IM, intramuscular; IV, intravenous; PID, pelvic inflammatory disease.

*The recommended third-generation cephalosporins are limited in the coverage of anaerobes. Therefore, until it is known that extended anaerobic coverage is not important for treatment of acute PID, the addition of metronidazole to treatment regimens with third-generation cephalosporins should be considered.

B. Pediatrics:
   1. Fluoroquinolones are generally contraindicated for children and adolescents younger than 18 years.
C. Partners:
   1. Sexual partners should be evaluated and treated for STIs.

Bibliography

Centers for Disease Control and Prevention. (2015a). *Sexually transmitted diseases treatment guidelines: Pelvic inflammatory disease*. Retrieved from http://www.cdc.gov/std/tg2015/pid.htm

Centers for Disease Control and Prevention. (2015b). *2015 sexually transmitted diseases treatment guidelines*. Retrieved from http://www.cdc.gov/std/tg2015/default.htm

PMS and Premenstrual Dysphoric Disorder

Rhonda Arthur and Michelle Collins

Definition

A. PMS is a psychoneuroendocrine disorder with a constellation of symptoms that occur in the luteal phase and interfere with a woman's life; this is followed by a symptom-free period. Moderate to severe forms of premenstrual distress are now classified in the American Psychiatric Association's (APA) *Diagnostic and Statistical Manual of Mental Disorders* (*DSM-5*; 2013) as premenstrual dysphoric disorder (PMDD).

Incidence

A. Virtually every menstruating woman experiences some symptoms sometimes. Twenty percent of menstruating women have symptoms serious enough to interfere with their lives, but only 2% to 5% of premenopausal women experience PMDD. Symptoms occur more commonly in women in their 30s and 40s.

Pathogenesis

A. The basis of PMS and PMDD is presumably hormonal. During the luteal phase, progesterone levels increase and estrogen levels decrease, causing a shift in the ratio of these hormones, which contributes to the symptoms experienced during PMS. These hormones are also known to interact with neurotransmitters in the brain, such as serotonin, and these interactions are thought to cause some of the symptoms experienced, such as changes in mood and pain thresholds, during PMS and PMDD.

Predisposing Factors

A. Females of reproductive age
B. First-degree female relatives affected
C. History of stressful life events
D. History of sexual and/or physical abuse

Common Complaints

A. Persistent and marked anger or irritability
B. Marked anxiety or tension
C. Markedly depressed mood and feelings of hopelessness
D. Decreased interest in usual activities
E. Easily fatigued or a marked lack of energy
F. Subjective sense of difficulty in concentrating
G. Hypersomnia or insomnia
H. A subjective sense of being overwhelmed or out of control
I. Marked change in appetite, overeating, or specific food cravings
J. Physical symptoms such as breast tenderness, headaches, edema, abdominal bloating, joint or muscle pain, and weight gain

Other Signs and Symptoms

A. The symptoms interfere with work, usual activities, or relationships.
B. The symptoms are not an exacerbation of another psychiatric disorder.
C. "I've got PMS; I'm so miserable."
D. Feelings of irritability and emotional lability

Subjective Data

A. Obtain a complete menstrual history:
   1. Age at menarche; frequency, duration, and regularity of periods
   2. Ask about premenstrual symptoms that are physical: Weight gain, edema, acne, nausea, vomiting, constipation, backache, headache, migraine, syncope, breast tenderness, breast enlargement, hot flashes, paresthesia of hands or feet, aggravation of convulsive disorder, increased appetite, food cravings (sweets, salt, or food in general), and fatigue.
   3. Ask about premenstrual symptoms that are emotional: Irritability, emotional lability, anxiety, depression, crying, palpitations, fatigue, aggression, lethargy, and sleep disturbances.
   4. Ask particularly about the timing of the symptoms. When do the symptoms begin and end in relationship to the menstrual period? Has the client kept a calendar of symptoms?
B. Ask about symptoms of dysmenorrhea. Some women confuse menstrual cramps and PMS.
C. Note the type of contraception the client uses.
D. Review the client's obstetric history.
E. Elicit the types of treatment the client has tried and the efficacy of those treatments.
F. Ask the client about the amount and type of exercise she gets.

Physical Examination

A. Check height, weight, and BP.
B. Inspect:
   1. Note overall appearance.
   2. Inspect the thyroid.
C. Auscultate:
   1. Heart
   2. Lungs
   3. Abdomen
D. Palpate:
   1. The neck, noting thyroid enlargement or nodules
   2. The abdomen, noting enlargement, masses, or tenderness
E. Pelvic examination (if indicated):
   1. Inspect the external genitalia for pubic hair pattern, lesions, or discharge.
   2. Speculum examination: Check for discharge and lesions.
   3. Bimanual examination: Check for size, mobility, shape, and tenderness of the uterus and adnexal area.
   4. No physical abnormality or changes are consistent with PMS.

Diagnostic Tests

PMS is diagnosed primarily based on the pattern of symptoms; however, the following diagnostic tests should be considered if indicated:
A. Pap and HPV testing, as indicated by guidelines
B. Screen for STIs, as indicated

C. TSH

D. Screen for psychiatric disorders, as indicated

Differential Diagnoses

A. PMS

B. Major depression

C. Dysmenorrhea

D. Substance abuse

E. Perimenopausal symptoms

F. Sexual dysfunction

G. Fibromyalgia

H. Sometimes there are underlying major medical problems like hypothyroidism, hyperthyroidism, anemia, or autoimmune disorders (such as SLE).

Plan

A. General interventions:

  1. Have the client keep a menstrual calendar or diary for at least 3 months to document occurrence of symptoms in the luteal phase.

  2. Symptomatic treatments: Treatment must be individualized.

▶ B. Client teaching: *See Section III: Client Teaching Guide for this chapter, "Premenstrual Syndrome."*

  1. Diet: Have the client eat six small meals a day to even out glucose load. Recommend avoiding caffeine to decrease irritability and facilitate sleep. Encourage the client to avoid simple sugars and eat complex carbohydrates to provide a slow, steady source of energy. She should decrease intake of salt, sugar, and fat during the most symptomatic days of her cycle.

  2. Activity: Recommend that regular exercise can mitigate symptoms. Suggest daily incorporation (walking, swimming, and stretching) of at least 30 minutes of aerobic exercise most days of the week. Encourage stress reduction activities such as imagery or yoga, CBT, support or counseling groups. Encourage smoking cessation as well as adequate sleep and rest.

C. Pharmaceutical therapy:

  1. NSAIDs for relief of muscular aches, headaches, and menstrual cramps. Follow directions for the particular NSAIDs, whether OTC or prescription.

  2. Minerals:

    a. Magnesium 300 to 500 mg/d

    b. Calcium 1,200 mg/d

    c. Chromium 200 mcg/d

    d. Zinc 30 mg/d

  3. Vitamins are used to decrease anxiety and irritability, food cravings, breast pain, depression, fatigue, and lethargy:

    a. Vitamin B$_6$ (pyridoxine) 50 to 150 mg daily (limited benefit)

    b. Vitamin E 400 to 600 mg daily (limited benefit)

  4. Herbs and botanicals:

    a. Vitex Agnus-Castus (chaste tree berry) 30 to 40 mg daily

    b. EPO 500 to 1,000 mg each day (mixed results on effectiveness)

  5. See Table 14.8 for other therapies used for PMS.

Follow-Up

A. Follow up in 3 to 4 months to assess or alter treatment and/or therapy.

Consultation/Referral

A. Consult a physician if symptoms are severe or not relieved by first-line measures.

Individual Considerations

A. Encourage the client to have her partner come to a visit. Partner education and support are helpful.

Bibliography

American College of Obstetricians and Gynecologist. (2015). *Gynecologic problems: Premenstrual syndrome (PMS)*. Retrieved from http://www .acog.org/-/media/For-Patients/faq057.pdf

American Psychiatric Association. (2013). *Diagnostic and statistical manual of mental disorders* (5th ed.). Arlington, VA: American Psychiatric Publishing.

Eittah, H. F. A. (2014). Effect of breakfast skipping on young females' menstruation. *Health Science Journal, 8*(4), 469.

Houtkooper, L., Farrell, V. A., & Mullins, V. (2017). *Calcium supplement guidelines*. https://extension.arizona.edu/pubs/calcium-supplement-guide lines

National Institutes of Health. (2016). *Calcium*. Retrieved from http://ods .od.nih.gov/factsheets/Calcium-HealthProfessional

Schuiling, K. D., & Likis, F. E. (Eds.). (2013). *Women's gynecologic health* (3rd ed.). Sudbury, MA: Jones & Bartlett Learning.

Vulvovaginal Candidiasis

Rhonda Arthur and Michelle Collins

Definition

A. Vulvovaginal candidiasis (also known as moniliasis) is a common, yeast-like fungal infection of the vulva and vagina. In 90% of the cases, the cause is *Candida albicans* infection (see Figure 14.2).

FIGURE 14.2 Vulvovaginal candidiasis. Speculum examination showing thick, curd-like plaque on vaginal wall. A slightly erythematous base is visible close to the center of the image, where some of the plaque was scraped off.

TABLE 14.8   MEDICATIONS USED WITH PMS

Drug	Dose	Purpose
Diuretics		Decreases edema peripherally and, perhaps, centrally
Oral contraceptive pills (Yaz[a])	Take on a daily basis	Evens the hormonal milieu, blocks ovulation
Spironolactone (Aldactone)	25 mg twice daily as needed	
Antidepressants		Decreases depression and anxiety and improves mood
Fluoxetine (Prozac)	10–40 mg every day or during the luteal phase (individual dose may vary); alternatively, may be taken daily	
Paroxetine (Paxil)	10–30 mg every day or during the luteal phase (individual dose may vary); alternatively, may be taken daily	
Sertraline hydrochloride (Zoloft)	25–30 mg every day or during the luteal phase (individual dose may vary); alternatively, may be taken daily	
Antianxiety Drugs		Decreases anxiety
Alprazolam (Xanax)	0.25 mg three or four times daily during luteal phase as needed	
Buspirone (BuSpar)	7.5–15 mg twice daily	
Miscellaneous Drugs		
Combined hormonal contraceptive modes (pill, patch, ring) (Yaz[a])	Take on a daily basis	Evens the hormonal milieu, blocks ovulation
Danazol (Danocrine)		Has antiestrogenic effects. *Consult with a physician. For refractory PMDD unresponsive to anything else. A treatment of last resort.*

PMDD, premenstrual dysphoric disorder; PMS, premenstrual syndrome.

[a]Has drospirenone and ethinyl estradiol.

Incidence

A. Approximately 75% of all women have at least one episode of candidiasis. It is estimated that 50% of these women have recurrences.

Pathogenesis

A. Multiple fungal species cause candidiasis, including *C. albicans* (90%), *Candida tropicalis*, *Torulopsis glabrata* (10%), *Candida parapsilosis*, and *Candida krusei*
B. *C. albicans*, *C. tropicalis*, and *T. glabrata* are part of the normal flora of the mouth, GI tract, and vagina. They may become pathogenic with changes in the vaginal pH that encourage the overgrowth of the fungus.

Predisposing Factors

A. Diabetes
B. Antibiotic use
C. Pregnancy
D. Combined hormonal contraceptive use
E. Obesity
F. Warm climate
G. Immunocompromised
H. HIV
I. Wearing tight, restrictive clothing; not changing out of damp clothing (e.g., swimsuit, exercise clothing shortly after use)
J. Corticosteroid use

Common Complaints

A. Thick, white, curd-like vaginal discharge
B. Itching, mild to intense, either on the vulva, in the vagina, or both
C. Vaginal or vulvar irritation, erythematous, and swollen
D. Discomfort during and after sexual intercourse

Other Signs and Symptoms

A. Vulvar excoriation
B. Vaginal edema or inflammation
C. Burning with urination
D. Burning with, or during, intercourse
E. Increased symptoms near menses

Subjective Data

A. Determine the onset, course, and duration of symptoms; note whether the infection is a first occurrence, recurrent, persistent, or chronic.

B. Obtain the client's medication history; include antibiotics, steroids, and birth control modality.
C. Review the client's past medical history; review systems for evidence of diabetes, HIV, or any immunocompromise.
D. Review the client's history of wearing of swimwear or tight exercise clothing.
E. Review the client's history of wearing polyester underwear, wearing underwear to bed, or wearing tight pants/jeans.
F. Review previous treatment, self-treatment measures, and compliance with previous treatments.
G. Determine whether the client is pregnant; note first day of the LMP.
H. Review sexual activity and partners. Do the partner(s) have any of the same symptoms, "jock itch," or oral candidiasis?
I. Review the use of vaginal deodorants or spray, scented toilet paper, tampons, pads, and douching.
J. Has there been any change in soaps, laundry detergent, or fabric softeners?
K. Review diet for high sugar content.

Physical Examination
A. Check temperature, pulse, and BP.
B. Inspect:
1. Inspect the vulva for inflammation, fissures, lesions, excoriation, rashes, and condyloma.
2. Examine the hairline and skin folds for inflammation, irritation, or skin breakdown.
3. Note skin changes that suggest secondary bacterial infection (erythema, drainage).

Inflammation that spares the skin folds is consistent with contact irritation. Inflammation that is within the skin folds suggests candidiasis.

C. Palpate:
1. Perform an external examination for enlarged or tender inguinal lymph nodes, vulvar masses, and lesions.
2. Back: Assess for CVAT.
D. Pelvic examination:
1. Inspect: Observe sidewalls of the vagina. Note amount, odor, and color of the discharge.

Typical discharge with *Candida* is adherent to the vaginal sidewalls and is characteristically thick, white, and curd-like (resembles cottage cheese). Sidewalls may exhibit erythema.

2. Speculum examination: Inspect the cervix for discharge and friability.
3. Bimanual examination: Check for CMT. Palpate for the size of the uterus and for adnexal masses or tenderness.

Diagnostic Tests
A. Wet prep with 10% potassium hydroxide and normal saline prep

Yeast hyphae and/or spores are determined by microscopic examination of the vaginal discharge prepared with 10% potassium hydroxide or normal saline. A positive whiff test indicates BV.

B. Test discharge with nitrazine paper

The pH in a client with candidiasis remains in the normal range of less than 4.5.

C. Consider 2-hour glucose testing if candidiasis is recurrent.
D. Consider testing for STIs as history warrants.
E. Herpes simplex culture, if lesions are present
F. Urinalysis and culture, if indicated

Differential Diagnoses
A. Vulvovaginal candidiasis
B. Vulvar dystrophy
C. Allergic vulvitis
D. BV
E. UTI
F. STI
G. HSV-2
H. Chemical vaginitis
I. Normal physiological discharge

Plan
A. General interventions:
1. Although vaginal candidiasis is treated using OTC products, encourage clients with initial presenting symptoms to have an evaluation to rule out other vaginal infections before self-treatment.
2. Consider treating partners.

Although candidiasis is not considered an STI, it can be sexually transmitted. The partner should be treated in cases of recurrent infections, even if the partner is asymptomatic.

3. For recurrent infections, consider fasting and 2-hour postprandial glucose tests to rule out diabetes mellitus.
4. Consider testing for HIV in clients with chronic candidiasis.
5. Preventive care therapies:
   a. Vinegar and water douche may be effective in mild cases: One to two tablespoons vinegar per quart warm water every 5 to 7 days or twice a day for 2 days
   b. *Acidophilus* capsules, four to six tablets daily, especially 2 to 3 days before menses
   c. Vitamin C 500 mg two to four times daily to increase vaginal acidity
   d. Daily yogurt douches or intravaginal applicator full of plain yogurt twice a day for 1 week. Have the client use *plain yogurt* with live, active cultures.

e. Boric acid crystals placed in a #0 empty capsule and inserted vaginally nightly for 14 nights

f. Grapefruit seed extract

g. Garlic: Studies have shown mixed results as to whether garlic, garlic tablets, or garlic extract is effective in treating yeast infections. Garlic has been shown to help in stopping the growth of *Candida* fungus.

h. Tea tree oil: Vaginal suppositories are available for this purpose. Research on use of tea tree oil has been mixed. It may be effective against some strains of *Candida*. As an essential oil, it must always be mixed with a carrier oil. Caution must be used when using tea tree oil, as it can irritate the skin, and the vaginal walls are particularly sensitive. Additionally, some women may be allergic, so testing on skin prior to use is recommended. Clinicians should be versed on the use of essential oils if recommending this treatment.

i. Oil of oregano: Wild oregano oil has demonstrated some ability to inhibit the growth of *C. albicans*. Capsules containing oil of oregano may be inserted into the vagina at night. As with tea tree oil, any essential oil has the potential to cause skin irritation and should be tested on a skin patch prior to use for this purpose. Clinicians should be versed on the use of essential oils if recommending this treatment.

j. Gentian violet: A purple dye that has antifungal properties. The most frequently recommended way to use it is to soak a tampon in the dye and then insert the tampon vaginally one to two times daily for 12 consecutive days. The tampon should be left for 3 to 4 hours and then removed.

k. Detoxification diet: Eliminating, or greatly reducing, consumption of coffee, alcohol, processed foods, and foods with chemical additives may contribute to reduction in recurrence.

▶ B. Client teaching: *See Section III: Client Teaching Guide for this chapter, "Vaginal Yeast Infection."*

1. Clients should be encouraged to present for evaluation whether, after appropriate therapy has been instituted, they continue to have symptoms.

2. Treatment should continue even during menstruation.

3. Recommend avoiding wearing tight clothing that will restrict airflow to the vulvar area.

4. Recommend cotton crotched underwear only, and preferably white.

5. Advise changing out of damp exercise clothing and swimwear as soon as possible after activities are finished.

6. Recommend not wearing underwear during sleep.

7. Use only mild soap (like Dove, Ivory) for washing the vulvar area.

C. Pharmaceutical therapy:

1. Vaginal antifungal creams: Mild cases may respond to 3 days of therapy; severe cases may require 10 to 14 days. Some of these preparations are available in vaginal suppository form for a 1- or 3-night regimen with proven efficacy.

a. Clotrimazole (Gyne-Lotrimin, Lotrimin, Mycelex, Mycelex-G) one applicator full at bedtime for 7 days

b. Miconazole (Monistat) one applicator full at bedtime for 7 days

c. Butoconazole nitrate (Femstat) one applicator full at bedtime for 7 days

d. Tioconazole 6.5% ointment 5 g intravaginally in a single application

e. Terconazole (Terazol) one applicator full at bedtime for 7 days

f. Terconazole vaginal antifungal cream is not available OTC.

2. Oral antifungal agents:

a. Fluconazole (Diflucan) 150 mg orally once. If treatment is not successful, the prescription may be refilled one time; if it is still unsuccessful, consider culture of the vagina, as a resistant, or uncommon, strain of *Candida* may be present (e.g., a non-*albicans* strain). Conventional pharmacological therapies are not as effective against non-*albicans* species.

Follow-Up

A. The client who presents with recurrent candidiasis (defined as four or more symptomatic episodes within 1 year) should be evaluated for HIV and/or other immunocompromised etiologies as well as diabetes mellitus.

B. If fasting and 2-hour blood glucose testing is normal, other options for recurrent candidiasis include treatment with clotrimazole, one applicator every other week, for 2 months. If the client remains symptom-free, reduce treatment to once each month, in the week before her menstrual period.

C. In case of recurrent vulvovaginal candidiasis, some recommend longer initial therapy (7–14 days of topical therapy or a 100-mg, 150-mg, or 200-mg oral dose of fluconazole every third day for a total of 3 doses [day 1, 4, and 7]) to initiate an infection-free period before initiating a maintenance regimen. Oral fluconazole (in either 100-, 150-, or 200-mg dosages) once weekly for 6 months is the first-line maintenance regimen. Topical treatments, used intermittently, are an alternative to the weekly fluconazole regimen. While suppression therapies show efficacy in reducing the number of recurrences, a significant percentage of women will have a recurrence after maintenance therapy ceases. Symptomatic women who continue to have positive cultures, despite being on maintenance therapy, should be managed in consultation with a specialist.

Consultation/Referral

A. Consult or refer the client to a clinician specializing in gynecological infections if there is no response to the previous treatments and/or recurrences continue despite maintenance therapy.

Individual Considerations

A. Pregnancy:

    1. Pregnancy may lead to an increase in vulvovaginal candidiasis episodes because of the increased glycogen content of the vagina, and the stimulatory effects of estrogen and progesterone on candidal growth. OTC antifungal creams are appropriate for use in this population if there is no rupture of membranes.

    2. Candidiasis may be transmitted from an infected mother to her newborn at birth.

B. Partners:

    1. Partners should be evaluated if the client presents with recurrences. OTC antifungal creams are appropriate for use in this population.

Bibliography

Centers for Disease Control and Prevention. (2015). *2015 sexually transmitted diseases treatment guidelines*. Retrieved from http://www.cdc.gov/std/tg2015/default.htm

15 Sexually Transmitted Infections Guidelines

Chlamydia

Jill C. Cash, Robertson Nash, and Dana Hughes

Definition
A. Chlamydia is a sexually transmitted infection (STI) (see Figure 15.1).

FIGURE 15.1 *Chlamydia trachomatis* infection. Colposcopic view of a female patient's cervix, which manifested signs of erosion and erythema because of infection.

Incidence
A. *Chlamydia trachomatis* is the most common sexually transmitted organism in the United States. In 2017, the Centers for Disease Control and Prevention (CDC) reported 1,708,569 cases of chlamydia, which is approximately 529 cases per 100,000 population, an increase of 6.9% over 2016. Health department notification is required.

Pathogenesis
A. *C. trachomatis* is an intracellular bacterium with parasitic properties. It is transmitted by sexual contact or perinatally when a vaginal delivery occurs through an infected birth canal.

Predisposing Factors
A. History of STIs
B. Multiple sexual partners
C. Early age at first coitus
D. Unprotected intercourse

Common Complaints
A. Up to 80% of those infected are asymptomatic.
B. Mucopurulent cervical, vaginal, or urethral discharge
C. Dysuria
D. Urinary frequency and urgency
E. Pelvic pain (dull or severe)

Other Signs and Symptoms
A. Cervical friability
B. Cervical motion tenderness (CMT)
C. Uterine and/or adnexal tenderness

Subjective Data
A. Elicit history of the onset of symptoms, location, frequency, and duration; aggravating and alleviating factors; and associated symptomatology.
B. Question the client about history of other STIs and sexual habits.

Physical Examination
A. Inspect:
  1. Males: Observe for anal and/or urethral discharge.
  2. Female pelvic examination: Observe for anal and/or vaginal discharge.
  3. Female speculum examination: Inspect vaginal wall and cervix for discharge and irritation.
B. Palpate:
  1. Males:
    a. Palpate inguinal lymph nodes.
    b. Palpate the groin.
  2. Females:
    a. Palpate the inguinal lymph nodes.
    b. Bimanual examination:
      i. Milk the urethra.
      ii. Palpate the periurethral and Bartholin's glands for exudate.

iii. Assess for CMT.

iv. Assess for uterine and adnexal tenderness.

Diagnostic Tests

A. Nucleic acid amplification tests (NAATs) are preferred to culture for diagnosis of *C. trachomatis*. The Food and Drug Administration (FDA) has approved NAATs for both male and female urogenital specimens collected via clean catch. It is important to obtain a thorough sexual history from the client and to screen all orifices used during sexual contact (vagina, oropharynx, rectum).

B. Other techniques for obtaining specimens include culture, antigen detections, and genetic probes.

Differential Diagnoses

A. Chlamydia

B. Gonorrhea

C. Urethritis

Plan

A. General interventions for symptomatic clients:

1. Collect samples immediately for timely treatment. Consider testing for other STIs such as gonorrhea, trichomoniasis, and human immunodeficiency syndrome (HIV).

2. Empirical treatment: People presenting with signs and symptoms of chlamydia and/or gonorrhea should be tested and treated for both infections at the time of presentation to the clinic for care. NAAT swabs should be collected from all orifices exposed to sexual contact, and urine should also be collected and tested. Absent antibiotic allergies, these clients should be treated with both ceftriaxone 250 mg intramuscular (IM) injection and azithromycin 1 g by mouth, single dose.

B. Client teaching:

▶ 1. *See Section III: Client Teaching Guide for this chapter, "Chlamydia."*

2. Inform the client of the need for partner notification and treatment. Notification is recommended for any partner with whom the client has had sexual contact within 30 days of the onset of symptoms or 60 days if asymptomatic.

3. Stress the importance of completing the treatment regimen.

4. Advise the client to avoid sexual intercourse during treatment and for 7 days following the last day of antibiotic treatment.

C. Pharmaceutical therapy:

1. In cases in which the presence of *C. trachomatis* is demonstrated and confirmed by NAAT and *Neisseria gonorrhoeae* is not present, the CDC recommends the following regimens:

a. Azithromycin 1 g by mouth in a single dose

b. Doxycycline 100 mg by mouth twice daily for 7 days

2. Alternative regimen:

a. Erythromycin base 500 mg by mouth four times daily for 7 days

b. Erythromycin ethyl succinate 800 mg by mouth four times daily for 7 days

c. Levofloxacin 500 mg orally once daily for 7 days

d. Ofloxacin 300 mg by mouth twice daily for 7 days

Follow-Up

A. The CDC now recommends that all clients follow up in 3 months for repeat culture.

Consultation/Referral

A. Consult or refer the client to a physician when treatment with the recommended dosage fails if client noncompliance and re-exposure have been ruled out.

Individual Considerations

A. Pregnancy:

1. Doxycycline, ofloxacin, and levofloxacin are contraindicated during pregnancy.

2. All pregnant women diagnosed with chlamydial infection should be retested in 3 weeks following treatment.

3. For women younger than 25 years of age, those with new partners, and/or those at a high risk for infection, repeat chlamydial testing during the third trimester.

4. All pregnant women diagnosed with chlamydial infection during the first trimester should be retested at 3 weeks following treatment, and again in 3 months after treatment.

5. The CDC recommends the following regimens for pregnant women:

a. Azithromycin 1 g orally in a single dose

b. For women intolerant to the recommended regimens:

i. Amoxicillin 500 mg by mouth three times daily for 7 days

ii. Erythromycin base 500 mg by mouth four times daily for 7 days

iii. Erythromycin base 250 mg by mouth four times daily for 14 days

iv. Erythromycin ethyl succinate 800 mg by mouth four times daily for 7 days

v. Erythromycin ethyl succinate 400 mg by mouth four times daily for 14 days

B. Pediatrics:

1. The CDC recommends the following regimens for children:

a. Weight < 45 kg: Erythromycin base or ethyl succinate 50 mg/kg/d by mouth divided into four doses daily for 14 days

b. Weight 45 kg or more but older than 8 years: Azithromycin 1 g by mouth in a single dose

c. Children 8 years and older: Azithromycin 1 g by mouth in a single dose or doxycycline 100 mg by mouth twice a day for 7 days

C. Adults: Untreated or long standing chlamydial infection in women may lead to infertility.

Bibliography

Centers for Disease Control and Prevention. (2019a). *Chlamydia*. Retrieved from www.cdc.gov/std/chlamydia/default.htm

Centers for Disease Control and Prevention. (2019b). *Reported STDs in the United States: 2017: High burden of STDs threatens millions of Americans.*

Retrieved from https://www.cdc.gov/nchhstp/newsroom/docs/fact sheets/std-trends-508.pdf

Centers for Disease Control and Prevention. (2019c). *Sexually transmitted diseases treatment guidelines, 2015*. Retrieved from https://www.cdc.gov/std/tg2015

Centers for Disease Control and Prevention. (2019d). *STDs during pregnancy*. Retrieved from https://www.cdc.gov/std/pregnancy/default.htm

Gonorrhea

Jill C. Cash, Robertson Nash, and Dana Hughes

Definition

A. Gonorrhea is a bacterial STI. Although most commonly seen in both male and female urogenital organs, *N. gonorrhoeae* can thrive in both the oropharynx and the rectum. It is important to complete a thorough sexual history of all clients presenting with concern for exposure to an STI.

Incidence

A. Gonorrhea is a CDC-reportable infection. In 2017, there were 555,608 cases reported to the CDC in the United States, which is 117 cases per 100,000 population, an increase of 18.6% since 2016. The rate of increase in infections was higher among men (19.3%) than among women (17.8%). This reflects either increased transmission or increased case ascertainment among men who have sex with men (MSM).

Pathogenesis

A. *N. gonorrhoeae,* a gram-negative diplococcus, is the causative organism. The infection begins with adherence of *N. gonorrhoeae* to the mucosal cells in the genitourinary tract or endocervix. The incubation period is typically 2 to 5 days for urethritis and 5 to 10 days for cervical infection. Rectal and pharyngeal infections are usually asymptomatic. Transmission during vaginal birth is possible and may result in conjunctivitis and blindness in neonates.

Predisposing Factors

A. History of STIs
B. Multiple sexual partners
C. Early age at first coitus

Common Complaints

A. Dysuria
B. Yellow, white, or mucoid urethral discharge in males
C. Greenish, irritating vaginal discharge in females
D. Menstrual irregularities
E. Pelvic pain
F. Fever

Other Signs and Symptoms

A. Asymptomatic
B. Uterine or adnexal tenderness
C. Mucopurulent discharge from endocervix
D. Polyarthralgias
E. Necrotic skin lesions

Subjective Data

A. Elicit history of onset, duration, and location of symptoms. Note aggravating and alleviating factors and associated symptomatology.
B. Question the client about history of other STIs and sexual habits.

Physical Examination

A. Check temperature.
B. Inspect:
    1. Inspect the skin for necrotic skin lesions.
    2. Males: Inspect for anal and/or urethral discharge; elicit the latter by milking the penis.
    3. Females:
        a. Inspect the anus and introitus for discharge; milk the urethra.
        b. Speculum examination: Inspect the vaginal walls and cervix for discharge and irritation.
C. Palpate:
    1. Examine the joints for effusion and swelling.
    2. Males: Palpate the inguinal lymph nodes.
    3. Females:
        a. Palpate the inguinal lymph nodes.
        b. Palpate the periurethral and Bartholin's glands for exudate.
        c. Bimanual examination:
            i. Assess for CMT and friability.
            ii. Assess for uterine and adnexal tenderness.

Diagnostic Tests

A. NAATs are preferred to culture for diagnosis of *N. gonorrhoeae*. The FDA has approved NAAT tests for both male and female urogenital specimens collected via clean catch. It is important to obtain a thorough sexual history from the client and to screen all orifices used during sexual contact (oropharynx, rectum).
B. During the septic joint stage, gonococci can be recovered from the joint by aspiration for culture.
C. For persons diagnosed with gonorrhea, testing should also be performed for chlamydia, syphilis, and HIV.

Differential Diagnoses

A. Gonorrhea
B. Chlamydia
C. Arthritis (rheumatoid or osteoarthritis)

Plan

A. General interventions:
    1. U.S. Preventive Services Task Force recommendations:
        a. Screening is not recommended in men and women at low risk for infection.
        b. Screening for infection is recommended for all sexually active women 24 years and younger and in older women at increased risk for infection.
        c. Current evidence is insufficient to recommend routine screening in sexually active men.
    2. Clinicians should consider their client population, clinical presentation, and local prevalence

among client population when determining screening practices.

3. Report positive test results to the health department.

4. Empirical treatment: People presenting with signs and symptoms of gonorrhea should be tested and treated for both gonorrhea and chlamydia at time of presentation to the clinic for care. NAAT swabs should be collected from all orifices exposed to sexual contact, and urine should also be collected and tested.

B. Client teaching:

1. *See Section III: Client Teaching Guide for this chapter, "Gonorrhea."*

2. Stress the importance of completing the medication regimen.

3. Inform the client of the need for partner notification and treatment. Notification is recommended for any partner with whom the client has had sexual contact within 60 days of the onset of symptoms.

C. Pharmaceutical therapy:

1. CDC recommendation: Ceftriaxone 250 mg by IM injection of a single dose *plus* azithromycin 1 g by mouth, single dose

2. If ceftriaxone is not available, the CDC recommends cefixime 400 mg by mouth in a single dose, *or*

3. For clients with severe allergy to cephalosporins, the CDC recommends azithromycin 2 g dose orally.

4. The CDC advises that quinolones no longer be used for treatment of gonorrhea due to increased bacterial resistance.

Follow-Up

A. The CDC no longer recommends a test of cure; however, clients who continue to exhibit symptoms should have culture performed.

B. All individuals should be closely monitored for treatment failure.

C. Reinforce treatment of all sexual partners within the past 60 days of diagnosis.

D. Providers are advised to report all treatment failures to the local or state public health department within 24 hours.

Consultation/Referral

A. Consult with a physician or refer the client if treatment with the recommended dosage fails and client noncompliance and re-exposure have been ruled out.

Individual Considerations

A. Pregnancy:

1. Pregnant women with *N. gonorrhoeae* infections should be treated with both ceftriaxone 250 mg IM and azithromycin 1 g by mouth, single dose.

2. If unable to tolerate penicillin, consult with an infectious disease (ID) provider.

3. Presumed or diagnosed coinfections with chlamydia should be treated with azithromycin.

B. Adults:

1. Untreated or long-standing gonorrheal infection in women can lead to infertility.

2. For clients with allergies to cephalosporins, azithromycin treatment is recommended.

C. Pediatrics:

1. Ophthalmia neonatorum prophylaxis: Perinatal exposure to the mother's infected cervix during birth can cause gonococcal conjunctivitis, which can lead to blindness if left untreated. Accordingly, the CDC recommends a single application of erythromycin (0.5%) in each eye of an infant at birth.

2. Sexual abuse should be considered. Suspect chlamydia as a cause of conjunctivitis if the infant is 30 days old or younger.

   a. Treatment:

     i. If the presence of *N. gonorrhoeae* is confirmed, treatment with a single dose of ceftriaxone 25 to 50 mg/kg IM or IV, not to exceed 125 mg, is considered the standard of care.

Bibliography

Centers for Disease Control and Prevention. (2019a). *Gonorrhea.* Retrieved from www.cdc.gov/std/gonorrhea/default.htm

Centers for Disease Control and Prevention. (2019b). *Reported STDs in the United States: 2017: High burden of STDs threatens millions of Americans.* Retrieved from https://www.cdc.gov/nchhstp/newsroom/docs/fact sheets/std-trends-508.pdf

Centers for Disease Control and Prevention. (2019c). *Sexually transmitted diseases treatment guidelines, 2015.* Retrieved from https://www.cdc.gov/std/tg2015

Centers for Disease Control and Prevention. (2019d). *STDs during pregnancy.* Retrieved from https://www.cdc.gov/std/pregnancy/default.htm

Herpes Simplex Virus Type 2

Jill C. Cash, Robertson Nash, and Dana Hughes

Definition

A. Herpes simplex is a lifelong, recurring viral disease that is transmitted by direct contact with the secretions or mucosa of an infected individual who is shedding the virus. The virus is usually characterized by painful vesicular lesions that form an ulcer, crust over, and then dry without scarring (see Figure 15.2).

FIGURE 15.2 Ulcerated lesions of genital herpes infection.

Source: Image courtesy of SOA-AIDS Amsterdam.

Incidence

A. An estimated 776,000 people in the United States are infected with the herpes virus annually. Approximately

11.9% of people from 14 to 49 years of age have genital herpes. According to the World Health Organization (WHO), more than 400 million people ages 15 to 49 worldwide have herpes simplex type 2.

Pathogenesis

A. Herpes simplex virus (HSV) is the causative organism. HSV-1 produces oral lesions, and HSV-2 produces genital lesions. Kissing, sexual contact, vaginal delivery, and autoinoculation are all possible routes of transmission. The virus remains dormant, and outbreaks can be stimulated by several factors, including stress, illness, sunlight exposure, and menstruation.

Predisposing Factors

A. Early age at first coitus
B. Multiple sexual partners
C. History of STIs

Common Complaints

A. Dysuria
B. Pruritus
C. Burning
D. Swelling sensation

Other Signs and Symptoms

A. Primary episode:
  1. Painful, itchy, vesicular, ulcerated, or crusted oral or genital lesion, singly or in clusters
  2. Flu-like syndrome: Fever, chills, headache, malaise, and myalgia
B. Recurrent episode: Less painful lesions and little or no systemic symptoms. Recurrent lesions in the same location as the previous outbreak is a significant clinical clue that the lesions are herpetic.

Subjective Data

A. Elicit history of onset of symptoms; their location, frequency, and duration; aggravating and alleviating factors; and associated symptomatology.
B. Question the client about history of other STIs and sexual habits.

Physical Examination

A. Check temperature.
B. Inspect the head, eyes, ears, nose, throat, and mucous membranes for lesions.
C. Palpate the neck and abdomen for lymphadenopathy.
D. Pelvic examination:
  1. Assess the external genitalia, perineum, and anus for lesions.
  2. Assess for inguinal lymphadenopathy.

Diagnostic Test

A. Viral culture:

> Clinical diagnosis is often reliable, but confirmation with viral culture should be attempted. Vesicles should be unroofed or crust removed to obtain the most reliable sample.

  1. The preferred method for HSV testing is either cell culture or polymerase chain reaction (PCR). NAAT is considered more sensitive.
  2. Viral isolation: Obtain vesicular fluid by swabbing the lesion with a cotton- or Dacron-tipped applicator.
  3. Place the applicator in an appropriate viral transport medium before drying.
  4. Refrigerate until ready for transport.
B. Serology: HSV-specific glycoprotein G2 (HSV-2) and glycoprotein G1 (HSV-1). **Pap smear is not a sensitive test for HSV-2.**

Differential Diagnoses

A. HSV
B. Primary syphilis
C. Chancroid
D. Lymphogranuloma venereum
E. Folliculitis
F. Candidal fissure
G. Vestibular vulvitis
H. Mucocutaneous manifestations of Crohn's disease

Plan

A. General interventions:
  1. Culture samples immediately to begin treatment.
B. Client teaching:
  1. *See Section III: Client Teaching Guide for this chapter, "Herpes Simplex Virus."* ◄
  2. Advise clients to abstain from sexual activity during prodrome or while lesions are present.
  3. Condom use should be encouraged when sexually active.
C. Pharmaceutical therapy: The CDC recommends the following treatment regimens:
  1. Primary episode:
    a. Acyclovir 400 mg by mouth three times a day for 7 to 10 days
    b. Acyclovir 200 mg by mouth five times a day for 7 to 10 days
    c. Famciclovir 250 mg by mouth three times a day for 7 to 10 days
  2. Recurrent episode: Begin during prodrome:
    a. Acyclovir 400 mg by mouth three times a day for 5 days
    b. Acyclovir 800 mg by mouth twice a day for 5 days
    c. Acyclovir 800 mg by mouth three times a day for 2 days
    d. Famciclovir 125 mg by mouth two times a day for 5 days
    e. Famciclovir 1,000 mg by mouth two times a day for 1 day
    f. Famciclovir 500 mg once, followed by 250 mg. two times a day for 2 days
    g. Valacyclovir 500 mg by mouth two times a day for 3 days
    h. Valacyclovir 1 g by mouth once daily for 5 days
  3. Daily suppressive therapy:
    a. Acyclovir 400 mg by mouth twice daily
    b. Famciclovir 250 mg by mouth twice a day

c. Valacyclovir 500 mg by mouth twice daily
d. Valacyclovir 1 g by mouth once daily
e. Discontinue after 1 year of continuous use to reassess recurrence rate.

> Clients receiving daily suppressive therapy of acyclovir 200 mg should use the lowest dose that provides relief from symptoms. Suppressive therapy has been shown to reduce the frequency of recurrences by 75% in clients with more than six recurrences per year. It does not eliminate symptomatic or asymptomatic viral shedding or the potential for transmission.

4. Topical acyclovir, famciclovir (Famvir), and valacyclovir (Valtrex) have had mixed results in clinical trials and are not currently recommended by the CDC.

Follow-Up
A. Follow-up is not recommended unless it is warranted by clinical presentation.

Consultation/Referral
A. Consult or refer the client to a physician if the client has prolonged ulceration unresponsive to therapy.

Individual Considerations
A. Adults:
1. Diagnosis is most often made via clinical presentation. Although viral testing is available, empirical treatment is recommended, versus first testing and then treating (see the "Other Signs and Symptoms" section).
2. Clients with HIV may have outbreaks of HSV lesions anywhere on their body. Do not limit the diagnosis based on the physical location of lesions.
3. Clients presenting with HSV-1/HSV-2 lesions should be tested for HIV, per the CDC recommendations.
4. Failure to isolate HSV does not mean that the client does not have HSV.
B. Pregnancy:
1. Transmission of genital herpes from an infected pregnant woman to the neonate is high, approximately 30% to 50%, when herpes is acquired during the last trimester or near delivery. The risk of transmission is much lower for pregnant women who have a history of HSV or first acquire the virus during the first half of the pregnancy.

2. All pregnant clients should be questioned and screened for HSV when they are admitted to the hospital for delivery. All women with recurrent genital herpes lesions present at the onset of labor should be delivered by cesarean section to decrease the risk of transmission of the herpes virus to the neonate.
3. Acyclovir and valacyclovir are category B drugs for pregnancy; they are considered safe to use during pregnancy. These medications can be used for treatment as well as for suppression during pregnancy. The American College of Obstetricians and Gynecologists recommends suppressive therapy beginning at approximately 36 weeks' gestation to prevent an outbreak of lesions and to increase the chance of having a vaginal delivery (see Table 15.1).
4. Culture lesions if an outbreak occurs. Lesion must be crusted for 7 days for vaginal delivery to be an option; otherwise, a cesarean delivery is recommended to avoid transmission of virus to the newborn.
5. Pregnant women without genital herpes should be advised to avoid intercourse during the third trimester with partners known or suspected of having genital herpes.
6. Acyclovir allergy: No effective alternatives to acyclovir have been identified.
C. Partners: Symptomatic partners should be evaluated and treated in the same manner as any client with genital lesions.
D. Pediatrics:
1. Transmission of HSV from mother to infant during birth is possible. The CDC recommends treatment of all infants born to mothers whose exposure to HSV was near term. Treatment is acyclovir 20 mg/kg IV every 8 hours for 14 days, unless there is disseminated disease or disease involving the central nervous system. In those cases, treatment should be extended for a total of 21 days.
E. Geriatric:
1. Genital herpes is rarely seen in the elderly. Recurrent infection of the buttocks region is not uncommon, especially in females.

Bibliography
American College of Obstetricians and Gynecologists Committee on Practice Bulletins. (2007). ACOG practice bulletin: Clinical management guidelines for obstetrician-gynecologists. No. 82 June 2007 reaffirmed in 2018. Management of herpes in pregnancy. *Obstetrics and Gynecology, 109*(6), 1489–1498. doi:10.1097/01.AOG.0000263902.31953.3e

TABLE 15.1   PHARMACOLOGICAL TREATMENT OF HERPES IN PREGNANCY

Antiviral	Acyclovir Dosage	Valacyclovir Dosage
Initial lesion outbreak	400 mg tid for 7–10 days	1 g bid for 7–10 days
Recurrent lesions	400 mg tid for 5 days	500 mg bid for 3 days
Daily suppression from 36 weeks' gestation until delivery	400 mg tid	500 mg bid

bid, twice a day; tid, three times a day.

Centers for Disease Control and Prevention. (2019a). *Genital herpes: CDC fact sheet.* Retrieved from https://www.cdc.gov/std/herpes/stdfact -herpes.htm

Centers for Disease Control and Prevention. (2019b). *Sexually transmitted diseases treatment guidelines, 2015.* Retrieved from https://www.cdc .gov/std/tg2015

Centers for Disease Control and Prevention. (2019c). *STDs during pregnancy.* Retrieved from https://www.cdc.gov/std/pregnancy/default.htm

Human Papillomavirus

Jill Cash, Robertson Nash, and Dana Hughes

Definition

A. The human papillomavirus (HPV) is an STI. Condyloma acuminata, genital warts, and venereal warts are other names for HPV.

Incidence

A. An estimated 79 million Americans are infected with HPV. Each year, there are approximately 14 million new infections in the United States and 360,000 new cases of genital warts in the United States. Certain strains of HPV are associated with cancer. Annually, in the United States, there are approximately:

12,000 women diagnosed with cervical cancer

4,000 cases of vulvar cancer

850 cases of vaginal cancer

1,200 cases of penile cancer

4,300 cases of anal cancer in women

2,200 cases of anal cancer in men

3,400 cases of oropharyngeal cancer in women

15,000 cases of oropharyngeal cancer in men

Pathogenesis

A. HPV, a slow-growing DNA virus of the papovavirus family, is the causative organism of this infection. More than 70 strains of the virus have been identified, and types 6 and 11 are most closely associated with genital warts. Types 16, 18, 31, 33, and 35 confer a high risk and are associated with cervical neoplasia. Warts may appear as early as 1 to 2 months after exposure, but most infections remain subclinical.

Predisposing Factors

A. Early first coitus
B. Multiple sexual partners
C. History of transmitted infections

Common Complaints

A. Painless genital "bumps" or warts
B. Pruritus
C. Bleeding during or after coitus
D. Malodorous vaginal discharge
E. Dysuria

Other Signs and Symptoms

A. Wart-like growths on the genital area that are elevated and rough or flat and smooth
B. Lesions occurring singly or in clusters, from <1 mm to cauliflower-like aggregates
C. Papillomas that are pale pink in color

Subjective Data

A. Elicit history of the onset of symptoms, location, frequency, and duration; aggravating and alleviating factors; and associated symptomatology.
B. Question the client about history of other STIs, sexual behaviors, recent change in sexual partner, and partner's history of STIs.

Physical Examination

A. Inspect:
 1. Inspect the external genitalia, perineum, and anus for lesions.
 2. Speculum examination in females: Inspect the vaginal walls and cervix for lesions.
 3. Application of 3% acetic acid whitens lesions (not considered diagnostic by the CDC).

Diagnostic Tests

A. Visual identification is adequate in most cases.
B. Cytology: Pap smears are useful for screening. Pap results of koilocytosis, dyskeratosis, keratinizing atypia, atypical inflammation, and parakeratosis are all suggestive of HPV.
C. Histology: Colposcopy with directed biopsy is diagnostic for subclinical lesions, dysplasia, and malignancy.
D. DNA typing: Determination of specific strains is useful in diagnosing subclinical infections (the test is costly and false negatives occur).

Differential Diagnoses

A. HPV
B. Condylomata
C. Molluscum contagiosum
D. Carcinoma

Plan

A. General interventions: Make the diagnosis promptly to begin treatment.
B. Client teaching:
 1. *See Section III: Client Teaching Guide for this chapter, "Human Papillomavirus."* ◄
 2. Explain to the client that therapy eliminates visible warts but does not eradicate the virus. No therapy has been shown to be effective in eradication of HPV. Ablation of warts may decrease viral load and transmissibility.
 3. Advise the client to abstain from genital contact while lesions are present.
C. Pharmaceutical therapy:
 1. Therapy is not recommended for subclinical infections (absence of exophytic warts).
 2. Trichloroacetic acid (TCA) 80% to 90% solution applied weekly to visible warts by the clinician until warts resolve. If unresolved after six applications, consider other therapy. *See Section II: Procedures,* ◄ *"Trichloroacetic Acid/Podophyllin Therapy."*
 3. Podophyllum resin (Podophyllin) 10% to 25% in tincture of benzoin compound applied weekly to visible warts by the clinician until warts resolve
  a. Petroleum jelly may be applied to the surrounding skin to protect unaffected areas.

b. Advise the client to wash off the resin after 4 hours. If unresolved after six applications, consider other therapy.

4. Apply TCA 80% to 90% to the warts and allow to dry; provide weekly treatment by the clinician until warts resolve.

5. Podofilox, 0.5% solution for home treatment, applied to visible warts by the client twice daily for three consecutive days, followed by 4 days without treatment. The cycle is repeated up to four times.

6. Imiquimod 5% (Aldara) cream applied to warts at bedtime, left on for 6 to 10 hours, then washed with mild soap. Use once a day, three times a week (Monday, Wednesday, and Friday), until warts resolve or up to 16 weeks.

D. Medical/surgical management: Cryotherapy, electrodesiccation, electrocautery, carbon dioxide laser, and surgical excision are options to be considered for clients with large or extensive lesions or refractory disease.

Follow-Up

A. Short-term follow-up is not recommended if the client is asymptomatic after treatment.
B. The CDC does not recommend more frequent Pap smears for women with external warts.
C. Long-term follow-up should include annual Pap smears and pelvic examinations. Encourage the client to self-examine the genitalia.

Consultation/Referral

A. Consult or refer the client to a physician when lesions persist after six consecutive treatments or when cervical or rectal warts are diagnosed.

HPV Vaccines

A. Several HPV vaccines are available for use in the United States. Gardasil protects against two to nine strains of HPV. The vaccine protecting against nine strains addresses types 6, 11, 16, 18, 31, 33, 45, 52, and 58, which are most likely to be associated with cancer, warts, and other diseases.
B. For both girls and boys, vaccination may start at as young as 9 years of age. The vaccine is recommended for girls and young women aged between 9 and 26 years. For males, the vaccine is recommended for those between 9 and 21 years of age, with an extension of administration until age 26 years for MSM and other immunocompromised males. The vaccine has been approved by the FDA for use up to age 45.
C. Administration for children 9 to 14 years of age should be two doses of IM vaccine, with the second dose given at least 5 months later. Administration for children of 15 years of age or greater consists of a three-dose series of IM injections. Dose 1 is given at month 0, with the second dose given 1 to 2 months after the first, and the third given 6 months after the first.
D. HPV vaccine is available for those younger than 19 years of age via the Vaccines for Children (VFC) program (call CDC-INFO [1-800-232-4636] for more information).
E. Uninsured clients eligible for the vaccine may be able to access client assistance programs via vaccine manufacturers.

Individual Considerations

A. Pregnancy: Podophyllum and podofilox are contraindicated during pregnancy.
B. Partners:
1. Treatment is recommended if visible lesions are present.
2. Testing sex partners for HPV is not recommended.
3. Sex partners are likely to share HPV. In most cases, the virus is likely to clear without associated health concerns. The risk of HPV warts and cancers increases greatly when the infection does not clear and becomes chronic.
4. Consistent condom usage can lower the chances of acquisition and transmission of HPV. However, the virus can infect areas not protected by condoms.
C. Adolescents: Education regarding the Gardasil vaccine is recommended for girls and boys 9 to 25 years of age to prevent the acquisition of HPV. The vaccination may help clients avoid contracting strains of HPV that increase the risk of cancers discussed earlier.
D. Geriatric:
1. Verrucous carcinoma and vulvar intraepithelial neoplasia (VIN) can be indistinguishable from condyloma. Older women are more likely to have VIN or carcinoma.
2. Diagnosis is made by biopsy; colposcopy is strongly advised.
3. Immunocompetence should be investigated in new or recurrent condyloma.

Bibliography

Centers for Disease Control and Prevention. (2019a). *Genital HPV infection: Fact sheet*. Retrieved from https://www.cdc.gov/std/hpv/stdfact-hpv.htm
Centers for Disease Control and Prevention. (2019b). *Sexually transmitted diseases treatment guidelines, 2015*. Retrieved from https://www.cdc.gov/std/tg2015
Centers for Disease Control and Prevention. (2019c). *STDs during pregnancy*. Retrieved from https://www.cdc.gov/std/pregnancy/default.htm

Syphilis

Jill Cash, Robertson Nash, and Dana Hughes

Definition

Syphilis is an STI characterized by distinct primary, secondary, and tertiary stages that occur over several years or decades. Latent or inactive periods occur between the stages. Early latent disease is less than 1 year after infection; late latent disease is more than 1 year after infection. **Health department notification of infection is required by law in all states.**

Incidence

A. In 2017, there were 101,567 new diagnoses of syphilis in the United States, with 30,644 being primary and secondary syphilis. In 2017, 79.6% of clients diagnosed were men who engaged in sexual activity with other men. There were 918 reported cases of children born with congenital syphilis in 2017.

Pathogenesis

A. *Treponema pallidum*, a spirochete bacterium, is the causative organism that infects the mucous membrane.

Predisposing Factors

A. History of STIs
B. Multiple sexual partners
C. Illicit drug use
D. Prostitution

Common Complaints

A. Genital lesion, generalized rash involving palms and soles, mucous patches, and condyloma latum are common.

Other Signs and Symptoms

A. Primary syphilis:
   1. Chancre that is painless or minimally painful (see Figure 15.3)

FIGURE 15.3 Primary syphilitic chancre of the tongue.

Source: Centers for Disease Control and Prevention/Robert E. Sumpter.

   2. Round, indurated lesion with little or no purulent exudate
   3. Regional bilateral lymphadenopathy
B. Secondary syphilis:
   1. Generalized maculopapular rash that is nonpruritic and copper colored, on palms or soles; may be erythematous or scaly
   2. Mucous patches; painless, white, mucous membrane lesions
   3. Generalized lymphadenopathy; flu-like syndrome, including fever, headache, sore throat, and malaise
   4. Patchy alopecia
C. Tertiary syphilis:
   1. Gumma: Locally destructive granulomatous tumors involving various organs or systems; commonly seen on the liver but can occur on other organs (heart, brain, skin, bone, testis)
   2. Cardiovascular: Aortic involvement, aneurysms, and valve insufficiency
   3. Neurological: Tabes dorsalis and general paresis
D. Latent syphilis: Asymptomatic

> Latent-phase syphilis manifests itself after treatment failure or no history of treatment. Spirochetes can lie dormant for years.

E. Congenital syphilis: Symptoms range from asymptomatic to fatal.

Subjective Data

A. Elicit history of onset, location, frequency, and duration of symptoms; aggravating and alleviating factors; and associated symptomatology.
B. Question the client about history of other STIs, illicit drug use, and sexual habits.

Physical Examination

A. Check temperature, pulse, respirations, and blood pressure.
B. Inspect:
   1. Inspect the skin; note lesions and rashes.
   2. Observe the head; note patchy alopecia.
   3. Examine the mouth and throat; note lesions.
   4. Inspect the genital and rectal area; note lesions and rashes.
C. Auscultate the heart and lungs.
D. Palpate the lymph nodes (neck, supraclavicular, axillary, epitrochlear, and inguinal regions).
E. Neurological examination:
   1. Assess sensory functioning.
   2. Test cranial nerves, first through twelfth.

Diagnostic Tests

Two types of tests are available for use in the diagnosis and management of syphilis—nontreponemal and treponemal—and knowledge of both is essential. Nontreponemal tests, such as the rapid plasma reagin (RPR), assess for biomarkers typically created by spirochetes. These tests are inexpensive, provide rapid results, and are easy to perform. In addition, the results are reported as titers, which facilitates monitoring the status of the infection. These are not antibody tests, however. Therefore, it is possible to have a false positive due to several conditions, including autoimmune disease, HIV, pregnancy, older age, and intravenous (IV) drug use. Accordingly, the CDC recommends a confirmatory treponemal test in all cases where the nontreponemal test is positive.

Treponemal tests, such as the *Treponema pallidum* particle agglutination (TP-PA) test, are antibody tests. Although more accurate than nontreponemal tests, treponemal tests are more expensive. A further complication of using treponemal tests as screening tools is that a treponemal test is positive for life once a person has had syphilis. When used in isolation, treponemal tests do not reveal whether an infection is active.

Interpretation of treponemal test findings is done in conjunction with review of findings from nontreponemal tests. Specifically, a fourfold drop in an initial nontreponemal titer—that is, from 1:64 to 1:4—indicates successful treatment of syphilis. In some cases, titers remain persistent over extended periods (more than 2–3 years); these individuals are referred to as sero-fast.

> Evaluate for other STIs in clients presenting with syphilis.

A. Serology: Nontreponemal tests:
1. VDRL test
2. RPR tests
3. HIV: Due to the increased likelihood of false-positive nontreponemal tests in people with HIV, all HIV-infected clients with a positive nontreponemal test should be followed with a treponemal test, as per the "Diagnostic Tests" section.

> Results are either reactive (positive) or nonreactive (negative). Titers correlate with active disease and should be quantitative. These tests are equally valid but cannot be compared because of titer differences (RPR is slightly higher than VDRL). All reactive results require confirmation with treponemal tests.

B. Serology: Treponemal tests:
1. Fluorescent treponemal antibody absorption (FTA-ABS) test
2. Microhemagglutination assay for antibody to *T. pallidum*

> Once FTA-ABS for antibody to T. pallidum, VDRL, and RPR are reactive, these tests usually remain reactive for life.

C. Cerebrospinal fluid (CSF) culture to detect neurosyphilis
D. Microscopy: *T. pallidum* cannot be seen with light microscopy; dark-field microscopic examination of the serous exudate from lesions is the definitive test for syphilis. Properly equipped labs with specially trained personnel must be available to perform this test.

Differential Diagnoses
A. Syphilis
B. HSV

Plan
A. General interventions: Staging of the disease may be difficult but guides management decisions
B. Client teaching:
1. *See Section III: Client Teaching Guide for this chapter, "Syphilis."*
2. Advise the client to abstain from sexual activity until treatment is completed.
3. Inform the client of the Jarisch–Herxheimer reaction (fever, headache, myalgia), which may occur within the first 24 hours of treatment. Antipyretics may be prescribed.
4. Discuss the importance of partner notification.
5. Stress the importance of complying with the follow-up regimen.
C. Pharmaceutical therapy: The CDC recommends the following treatment regimens:
1. Primary syphilis, secondary syphilis, and early latent syphilis:
    a. Adults: Benzathine penicillin G 2.4 million units injected IM in a single dose
    b. Pediatrics: Benzathine penicillin G 50,000 units/kg, up to the adult dose of 2.4 million units, injected IM in a single dose
2. Late latent syphilis, latent syphilis of unknown duration, and late syphilis (manage with expert consultation):
    a. Adults: Benzathine penicillin G 7.2 million units total, administered as three doses (2.4 million units each) injected IM at 1-week intervals
    b. Pediatrics: Benzathine penicillin G 50,000 units/kg, up to the adult dose of 2.4 million units, injected IM for three total doses at 1-week intervals
3. Neurosyphilis (manage with expert consultation):
    a. Adults: Aqueous crystalline penicillin G, 18 to 24 million units daily, 3 to 4 million units administered IV every 4 hours for 10 to 14 days
    b. Adults: Procaine penicillin 2 to 4 million units injected IM daily, plus probenecid 500 mg by mouth four times a day, both for 10 to 14 days
    c. Pediatrics: Penicillin desensitization, then treatment with the recommended regimen
4. Primary syphilis, secondary syphilis, latent syphilis, or late latent syphilis in (nonpregnant) clients with penicillin allergy: Doxycycline 100 mg by mouth twice daily for 2 weeks, or tetracycline 500 mg by mouth four times daily for 2 weeks
5. Latent syphilis of unknown duration or late syphilis: Treat with the aforementioned regimen for infections of less than 1 year's duration. If more than 1 year's duration, treat with the aforementioned regimen for 4 weeks.
6. For pregnant clients with penicillin allergy, penicillin treatment after desensitization is recommended for the following reasons:
    a. Penicillin is effective for preventing transmission and treating the infected fetus.
    b. Doxycycline and tetracycline are contraindicated in pregnancy.
    c. Erythromycin may not cure the infected fetus.

Follow-Up
A. Primary and secondary syphilis: Clinical and serologic examinations should be conducted at 6, 12, and 24 months. Absence of a fourfold decrease in the RPR titer within 6 to 12 months is indicative of treatment failure.
B. Latent syphilis: Clinical and serologic examinations should be conducted at 6, 12, and 24 months. Absence of a fourfold decrease in the RPR titer within 12 to 24 months is indicative of treatment failure.
C. Tertiary syphilis: Minimal evidence regarding follow-up exists. Follow-up largely depends on the nature of the lesions.
D. Neurosyphilis: CSF examination should take place every 6 months until the cell count is normal.

Consultation/Referral
A. Consult or refer the client to a physician when the recommended treatment fails and client noncompliance

and re-exposure have been ruled out, or when neurosyphilis is diagnosed.

Individual Considerations

A. Pregnancy:
1. Draw blood samples for RPR/VDRL from all prenatal clients.
2. Women in communities with high prevalence of syphilis and/or with high-risk behavior should be tested twice during the third trimester: once at 28 to 32 weeks, and again at delivery.
3. Any woman having a fetal death at more than 20 weeks' gestation should be tested for syphilis.
4. Administer the appropriate regimen of penicillin for the client's stage of syphilis. Consider a second dose of penicillin 1 week after the initial treatment.
5. Clients who are allergic to penicillin should be desensitized and treated with penicillin during pregnancy.
6. Follow-up: Perform serologic tests monthly until adequacy of treatment has been ensured.
7. The Jarisch–Herxheimer reaction may predispose women to premature labor or fetal distress if treatment occurs in the second half of the pregnancy. Advise these clients to immediately seek medical attention if they experience uterine contractions or changes in fetal movement.
8. All pregnant women diagnosed with syphilis should be offered HIV screening.

B. Pediatrics:
1. Congenital syphilis is caused by untreated infection or treatment failure in the mother.
2. Refer the client to a physician for ID consultation.
3. Medication therapy: See the "Pharmaceutical Therapy" section.

C. Partners: Identify at-risk partners who have had sexual contact with the client within these time frames:
1. Primary syphilis: 3 months plus duration of symptoms
2. Secondary syphilis: 6 months plus duration of symptoms
3. Early latent syphilis: 1 year

D. Geriatric:
1. Dementia, tremors, and pupillary changes are the result of long-term untreated syphilis.
2. The CSF should be tested using the FTA-ABS test. The VDRL is usually not adequate.
3. Syphilis is uncommon in the elderly in developed countries; however, it is very common worldwide.

Bibliography

Centers for Disease Control and Prevention. (2019a). *Reported STDs in the United States: 2017: High burden of STDs threatens millions of Americans.* Retrieved from https://www.cdc.gov/nchhstp/newsroom/docs/fact-sheets/std-trends-508.pdf

Centers for Disease Control and Prevention. (2019b). *Sexually transmitted diseases treatment guidelines, 2015.* Retrieved from https://www.cdc.gov/std/tg2015

Centers for Disease Control and Prevention. (2019c). *STDs during pregnancy.* Retrieved from https://www.cdc.gov/std/pregnancy/default.htm

Trichomoniasis

Jill Cash, Robertson Nash, and Dana Hughes

Definition

A. Trichomoniasis is an STI. Nonsexual transmission by means of fomites is possible but rare (see Figure 15.4).

FIGURE 15.4 *Trichomonas vaginalis* infection. Colposcopic view of a female patient's cervix, revealing what is referred to as a strawberry cervix.

Incidence

A. Trichomoniasis is not a CDC-reportable infection. Therefore, its exact incidence is unavailable. The CDC estimates the prevalence as 2.3 million people ages 14 to 49.

Pathogenesis

A. *Trichomonas vaginalis*, a flagellated protozoan, is the causative organism.

Predisposing Factors

A. History of STIs
B. Multiple sexual partners

Common Complaints

A. Copious, yellow-green, or watery gray vaginal discharge
B. Vaginal odor
C. Dysuria
D. Dyspareunia
E. Postcoital spotting or bleeding
F. Abdominal discomfort
G. Pruritus

Other Signs and Symptoms

A. Asymptomatic
B. Perineal irritation

Subjective Data

A. Elicit history of the onset, location, frequency, and duration of symptoms; aggravating and alleviating factors; and associated symptomatology.

B. Question the client about history of other STIs or vaginal infections, changes and characteristics of vaginal discharge, and recent change in sexual partner.

Physical Examination

A. Check temperature.

B. Inspect: Inspect the introitus for discharge and irritation.

C. Speculum examination:
   1. Inspect the vaginal walls for discharge and irritation.
   2. Inspect the cervix for discharge, erythema, punctate hemorrhages (strawberry-patch cervix), and friability.

D. Bimanual examination:
   1. Assess for CMT.
   2. Palpate for uterine and adnexal tenderness.

Diagnostic Tests

A. Wet prep: Perhaps the most common diagnostic tool, intended to visualize the presence of motile, flagellated trichomonads. An increased number of white blood cells (WBC) (>0.10 per high-power field) may be present. As per the CDC, the sensitivity of wet-mount analysis is low (51%–65%) in vaginal specimens and even lower in male urine samples.

B. NAAT methods are the current standard and are reportedly three to five times more accurate than wet-mount microscopy. New tests using vaginal, endocervical, and urine samples are becoming more widely available.

C. Pap smear: The report may include trichomonads, but sensitivity is low:
   1. If trichomonads are noted on Pap smear, the client should be reexamined and diagnosis confirmed with a wet prep.

D. Vaginal pH is usually greater than 4.5.

E. The potassium hydroxide/wet prep "whiff test" may be positive.

Differential Diagnoses

A. Trichomoniasis

B. Bacterial vaginosis

C. Vulvovaginal candidiasis

D. Chlamydia

E. Gonorrhea

F. Pelvic inflammatory disease

G. Foreign-body vaginitis

Plan

A. General interventions: Prompt diagnosis helps to initiate treatment.

B. Client teaching:
   1. *See Section III: Client Teaching Guide for this chapter, "Trichomoniasis."*
   2. Advise the client to abstain from sexual activity until treatment is complete.
   3. Advise the client to avoid alcohol consumption during and 24 hours after metronidazole treatment due to the possible Antabuse effect from the medication.

   4. Inform the client that urine may darken in color during treatment.
   5. Inform the client of a possible metallic taste in the mouth during treatment.

C. Pharmaceutical therapy:
   1. Drug of choice: Metronidazole 2 g orally in a single dose or tinidazole 2 g orally in a single dose. **Advise clients that alcohol and alcohol-containing products should be avoided at least 24 to 48 hours after the last dose of metronidazole is taken.**
   2. Alternative regimen: Metronidazole 500 mg by mouth twice daily for 7 days. The expected cure rate from either regimen is 95%.
   3. Treatment failure: The CDC recommends retreatment with metronidazole 500 mg by mouth twice daily for 7 days.
   4. If repeated failure occurs, treat with metronidazole 2 g by mouth four times daily for 3 to 5 days.
   5. Metronidazole gel is unlikely to achieve therapeutic levels in the urethra or perivaginal glands. It is a considerably less efficacious treatment than oral preparations and is *not* recommended for use.

Follow-Up

A. Immediate follow-up is not recommended if the client is initially asymptomatic or symptoms are relieved by treatment. Due to concerns about resistance, a 3-month follow-up for sexually active women is recommended.

Consultation/Referral

A. Failure to clear infection with single-dose therapy should be followed with a 7-day course of metronidazole 500 mg twice daily for 7 days for the client and sexual partner(s).

B. Should treatment with the previous regimen fail in a client felt to be adherent with medication and not subject to reinfection, consult with or refer the client to a physician for assessment of metronidazole susceptibility.

Individual Considerations

A. Pregnancy:
   1. First trimester: Metronidazole is contraindicated.
   2. Palliative treatment: Clotrimazole 1% vaginal cream one applicator full daily at bedtime for 7 days is suggested.
   3. Second and third trimesters: Metronidazole 2 g by mouth, one time
   4. Lactation: Metronidazole 2 g by mouth one time; discontinue breastfeeding during and 24 hours after treatment. Pumping and discarding milk is recommended.

B. Partners: Recommended treatment is metronidazole 2 g orally, one time.

C. Geriatrics:
   1. Uncommon pathogen in postmenopausal women
   2. Symptoms are vulvar irritation with discharge.
   3. Diagnose with wet prep.

4. Treat with metronidazole 1 g in the morning and 1 g in the evening.

D. Clients with HIV:

1. Screen all women at the first visit and annually for trichomoniasis. Treatment for trichomoniasis—multiple dose therapy: Metronidazole 500 mg twice a day for 7 days.

Bibliography

Centers for Disease Control and Prevention. (2019a). *Sexually transmitted diseases treatment guidelines, 2015*. Retrieved from https://www.cdc.gov/std/tg2015

Centers for Disease Control and Prevention. (2019b). *STDs during pregnancy*. Retrieved from https://www.cdc.gov/std/preganancy/default.htm

16 Infectious Disease Guidelines

Cat Scratch Disease

Jill C. Cash, Cheryl A. Glass, and Moya Cook

Definition

A. Cat scratch disease (CSD) is a lymphatic infection occurring 3 to 14 days after a dermal abrasion from a cat scratch. Infection causes unilateral regional adenitis; however, CSD manifestations may also include visceral organ, neurologic, and ocular involvement. There are two phases of symptoms.
1. Oroya fever: Symptoms include fever, headache, muscle aches, abdominal pain, and severe anemia
2. Verruga peruana: Symptoms include skin lesions/nodular growths that then emerge as red to purple vascular lesions. The lesions are prone to bleeding and ulceration.

Incidence

A. Incidence is less than 25,000 new cases every year; CSD is believed to be relatively common. More than 90% of cases have had a history of recent contact with cats, often kittens, which are usually healthy. Multiple cases have been observed in families, presumably resulting from contact with the same animal. There is no documentation of human-to-human transmission. Persons who are immunocompromised are more susceptible to the systemic manifestations. Dissemination to the liver, spleen, eye, or central nervous system (CNS) occurs in 5% to 14% of individuals.
B. CSD occurs worldwide.
C. Most cases (70% to 90%) of CSD occur from September through January in the United States.
D. In clients younger than 18 years, CSD is more common; 60% of those cases are in males.
E. Approximately 1% of diagnosed cases have no history of an animal scratch.

Pathogenesis

A. *Bartonella henselae* is considered to be responsible for most cases of CSD. *B. henselae* is a fastidious, slow-growing, gram-negative bacterium. Most transmission occurs from feline bites or scratches as well as cat licking to nonintact skin or mucosal surfaces like the skin and eyes. About 40% of cats carry *B. henselae* at some time in their lives. Other vectors that may be involved in the transmission of *B. henselae* to humans include dogs, monkeys, *Ixodes* ticks, and fleas from cats or kittens.
B. The incubation period for lesions to appear is 7 to 12 days after abrasion. Lymphadenopathy appears 5 to 50 days (median = 12 days) after appearance of the primary lesion.

Predisposing Factors

A. Exposure to domestic and outside cats
B. Immunocompromised state

Common Complaints

A. Swollen lymph glands (regional lymph node, groin, axillary, and cervical areas). The predominant sign is regional lymphadenopathy in an otherwise healthy person.
B. Low-grade fever
C. Body aches
D. Fatigue
E. Anorexia

Other Signs and Symptoms

A. A skin papule appears 3 to 10 days after inoculation, often found at the presumed site of inoculation. The papule progresses through erythematous, vesicular, and popular crusted stages. The papules are generally nonpruritic.
B. Headache
C. Extreme fatigue (anemia)
D. Abdominal pain in the presence of hepatosplenomegaly
E. Arthropathies of the knee, wrist, ankle, and elbows
F. Visual:
1. Unilateral eye redness/conjunctivitis is the most common ocular manifestation.
2. Loss of vision
3. Visual disturbances
4. Ocular pain (i.e., foreign-body sensation)
5. Serous discharge
G. Central nervous system:
1. Changes in level of consciousness (LOC)
2. Persistent high fever
3. Seizures within 6 weeks of lymphadenopathy

H. Cardiac:
1. Murmur
2. Dyspnea

Subjective Data

A. Review onset and duration of symptoms.
B. Elicit the history of abrasion caused by a kitten/cat or other vectors.
C. Ask the client about other symptoms such as low-grade fever and body aches.
D. Rule out other illness with review of symptoms (such as pharyngitis and mononucleosis).
E. Ask about visual loss (painless, unilateral visual loss is present with neuroretinitis).
F. Has the client had a febrile seizure?

Physical Examination

A. Check temperature, pulse, respirations, and blood pressure (BP).
B. Inspect:
1. Examine the skin for scratches, bite marks, erythema, or rash.
2. Conduct an ear, nose, and throat (ENT) examination.
3. Conduct an eye examination if indicated:
a. Visual examination: Snellen chart
b. Funduscopic examination:
i. The optic disk appears edematous.
ii. Exudates frequently surround the macula.
iii. The funduscopic examination may need to be deferred if photophobia is present.
C. Auscultate:
1. Heart
2. Lungs
D. Palpate:
1. Palpate lymph nodes: Preauricular, cervical, axillary, epitrochlear, and inguinal nodes. Unilateral tender lymph nodes (usually singular) are palpable near the scratch site. The area around the affected lymph nodes is typically tender, warm, erythematous, and indurated.
2. Abdomen to rule out organomegaly
3. Breast: Examine if indicated; mastitis is rare.

Diagnostic Tests

A. Usually none; CSD is often diagnosed by history and physical examination alone. Presenting symptoms may indicate further testing is needed:
1. Complete blood count (CBC) with differential
2. Sedimentation rate
3. *Bartonella* antibody testing
4. Disseminated polymerase chain reaction (PCR) assay
B. Warthin–Starry silver impregnation stain of lymph node, skin, or conjunctival tissue
C. Biopsy of lymph node (when malignancy is suspected)
D. Culture and sensitivity of any aspirated fluid or blood cultures. Cultures should be held for 21 days since *B. henselae* is a slow-growing bacterium. Trench fever, Carrion's disease, and endocarditis can also be diagnosed with serology.

E. Abdominal ultrasound or computed tomography (CT) scan in the presence of hepatomegaly, splenomegaly, or hepatosplenomegaly on physical examination
F. The cat-scratch skin test is no longer recommended.

Differential Diagnoses

A. CSD
B. Infectious mononucleosis
C. Kawasaki disease (KD)
D. Lyme disease
E. Malignancies that involve lymph nodes such as lymphoma and Hodgkin's disease
F. Fever of unknown origin (FUO)
G. Trench fever
H. Carrion's disease
I. Endocarditis

Plan

A. General interventions:
1. Management is usually treatment of symptoms; CSD is self-limiting, with slow resolution in 2 to 4 months.
2. Prescribe analgesics for pain.
3. Rest is advised.
4. Ice may be applied to the affected nodes.
5. About 10% of nodes will suppurate and require aspiration. However, lymph node aspiration is not recommended except to relieve severe pain. During aspiration, the needle should be moved around in several locations because microabscesses often exist in multiple septated pockets. Incision and drainage are not recommended because of the potential for chronic sinus tract formation.
B. Client teaching:
1. Lymphadenopathy usually regresses within 2 to 4 months but may persist for up to 1 year.
2. Client education on cats:
a. People should avoid playing roughly with cats.
b. Proper handwashing is recommended after handling all cats.
c. Stray cats should not be handled by children or immunocompromised people.
d. Testing cats is not recommended. Cats do not need to be removed or destroyed.
e. Always cleanse animal bites or scratches immediately with soap and water to prevent or reduce the transmission of CSD.
f. Control fleas (fleas have been found to have *B. henselae*).
3. If there are any signs of an infection after a cat bite/scratch, the client should be seen by his or her healthcare provider.
4. Disease is not contagious: There is no person-to-person transmission.
5. No vaccination is currently available.
C. Pharmaceutical therapy:
1. Acetaminophen (Tylenol) as needed
2. Nonsteroidal anti-inflammatory drugs (NSAIDs) as needed
3. Oral corticosteroids for individuals with atypical symptoms

4. Antibiotic therapy is recommended for all clients with CSD including immunocompetent clients with mild to moderate disease and lymphadenitis to prevent serious complications:

    a. Azithromycin (Zithromax) dosing for lymphadenitis:

        i. Clients weighing more than 45.5 kg: 500 mg on day 1, followed by 250 mg for 4 days

        ii. Clients weighing less than 45.5 kg: 10 mg/kg on day 1, followed by 5 mg/kg for 4 days

    b. Clarithromycin (Cipro) may be used as an alternative to azithromycin for lymphadenitis:

        i. Clients weighing more than 45.5 kg: 500 mg twice a day for a 7- to 10-day course

        ii. Clients weighing less than 45.5 kg: 15 to 20 mg/kg divided into two doses for a 7- to 10-day course

    c. Rifampin may be used as an alternative for lymphadenitis:

        i. Children: 10 mg/kg every 12 hours to a maximum dose of 600 mg/d for a 7- to 10-day course

        ii. Adults: 300 mg twice a day for a 7- to 10-day course

    d. Trimethoprim–sulfamethoxazole may be used as an alternative for lymphadenitis:

        i. Children: Trimethoprim 8 mg/kg/d, sulfamethoxazole 40 mg/kg/d in two divided doses for 7 to 10 days

        ii. Adults: One double-strength tablet twice a day

    e. For hepatosplenic disease and prolonged fever, use rifampin (as previously noted) for 10 to 14 days and add a second agent such as azithromycin or gentamicin:

        i. Azithromycin (as previously noted) for an entire 10- to 14-day course

        ii. Gentamicin loading dose 2 mg/kg, then 1.5 mg/kg over 8 hours; dose based on normal renal function and adjusted with monitoring

    f. Neurological disease/neuroretinitis: Clients diagnosed with neuroretinitis or neurological disease should be prescribed doxycycline 100 mg twice a day plus rifampin 300 mg orally twice a day (bid). Treatment should be prescribed for 4 to 6 weeks for neuroretinitis and 10 to 14 days for other neurological disease. Consult with a physician. Consult with the ophthalmologist since the client will require close monitoring.

    g. Endocarditis: The optimal antibiotic therapy and optimal duration of therapy for *Bartonella* endocarditis are unknown. Consult with a physician.

Follow-Up

A. Reevaluate the client in approximately 6 to 8 weeks if the client has mild symptoms.

B. Reevaluate in 10 days if the client is placed on antibiotics.

C. CSD is not reportable to the health department or the Centers for Disease Control and Prevention (CDC).

Consultation/Referral

A. Complications are rare; refer the client to a physician, including specialists (neurologist, cardiologist, and ophthalmologist) if infection is systemic or unresponsive to antibiotics:

1. Hearing loss
2. Neurological disability
3. Digit or limb amputations
4. Skin scarring

B. Clients diagnosed with neuroretinitis should be referred to an ophthalmologist for comanagement.

C. An infectious disease consult should be ordered for clients diagnosed with serious infections such as trench fever, Carrion's disease, and endocarditis.

Individual Considerations

A. Pediatrics:

1. If neuroretinitis is diagnosed in children younger than 8 years of age, treatment should include azithromycin or trimethoprim–sulfamethoxazole in place of doxycycline.

Bibliography

Baranowski, K., & Huang, B. (2018, November 1). Cat scratch fever. *StatPearls*. Retrieved from https://www.ncbi.nlm.nih.gov/books/NBK482139/

Spach, D., & Kaplan, S. (2018). Treatment of cat scratch disease. *UpToDate*. Retrieved from www.uptodate.com

Coronavirus Disease (COVID-19)

Cheryl A. Glass, Jill C. Cash, and Jenny Mullen

Definition

A. Coronaviruses are a large family of viruses that cause illnesses in animals or humans. Several coronaviruses are known to cause respiratory infections in humans ranging from the common cold to more severe diseases such as Middle East Respiratory Syndrome (MERS) and Severe Acute Respiratory Syndrome (SARS). The most recently discovered coronavirus causes coronavirus disease (COVID-19).

1. The first human cases of COVID-19 were identified in Wuhan City, China, in December 2019 but there is a growing pandemic of locations internationally, including the United States.

2. Currently the source of SARS-CoV-2, the coronavirus (CoV) causing COVID-19, is unknown. The SARS-CoV-2 virus most probably has its ecological reservoir in bats. The SARS-CoV, the virus which caused the SARS outbreak in 2003, jumped from an animal reservoir, civet cats, to humans and then spread between humans. It is also thought that SARS-CoV-2 jumped the species barrier and initially infected humans, but more likely through an intermediate host more likely to be handled by humans, such as a domestic or wild animal, and, as of yet, has not been identified.

3. Most estimates of the incubation period for COVID-19 range from 1–14 days, most commonly around 5 days. Not everyone needs to be tested for COVID-19. The CDC has guidance for who should be tested, but decisions about testing are at the discretion of state and local health departments and/or individual clinicians.

4. The virus that causes COVID-19 is mainly transmitted through droplets generated when an infected person coughs, sneezes, or speaks. Transmission can occur by breathing in the virus within 3 feet of a person infected with COVID-19 or by touching a contaminated surface and then touching the eyes, nose, or mouth before washing their hands.

5. The coronaviruses may persist on surfaces for a few hours or up to several days. This may vary by the type of surface, temperature, or humidity of the environment.

Incidence

A. Approximately 80% recover from COVID-19 without needing special treatment.

B. Around 1 out of every 6 people who get COVID-19 becomes seriously ill and develops difficulty breathing.

C. About 1 in every 5 people need hospital care.

Pathogenesis

A. Science indicates this genomic characterization: (1) bats and rodents are the gene sources of alphaCoVs and betaCoVs; and (2) avian species might represent the gene sources of deltaCoVs and gammaCoVs. These viruses can cause respiratory, enteric, hepatic, and neurological diseases in different animal species.

B. The first cases of the COVID-19 disease were linked to direct exposure to the Huanan Seafood Wholesale Market of Wuhan, and hypothesized to be the animal-to-human transmission as the main mechanism. However, ensuing cases were not related with this exposure process. Research then suggested that the virus could also be transmitted from human-to-human, and that symptomatic and asymptomatic people could transmit COVID-19 spread. These facts suggested that the use of isolation is the best way to contain this epidemic.

C. Research indicates that COVID-19 is capable of producing an excessive immune response in the host that in some cases has presented as a "cytokine storm." This reaction could cause extensive tissue damage. The pathogenesis of a cytokine release syndrome is an acute systemic inflammatory response that is characterized by dysfunction of multiple organs and fever.

Predisposing Factors

A. Age
1. Older adults over 60 years of age
2. Elderly over 80 years of age
3. People of any age who have serious underlying medical conditions

B. High-risk chronic conditions
1. Lung disease (COPD, asthma, pulmonary fibrosis, and cystic fibrosis)

2. Cardiac conditions (CAD, HR, and hypertension)
3. Diabetes
4. Immunocompromised or immunosuppressed (chemotherapy and other cancer treatments), autoimmune diseases (RA, lupus, MS, inflammatory bowel disease, HIV, and organ- or bone-marrow transplant patients)

C. Healthcare workers without access to appropriate personal protective equipment (PPE)

D. Living conditions
1. Residential facilities (assisted living, long-term care [LTC], and skilled nursing facilities [SNF])
2. Incarcerated populations
3. Densely populated cities
4. Homelessness

Common Complaints

A. A significant portion of individuals with coronavirus lack symptoms.

B. Symptoms may appear 2–14 days after exposure. Symptoms include:
1. Cough
2. Fever
3. Fatigue
4. Shortness of breath

Other Signs and Symptoms

A. Myalgias

B. Nasal congestion

C. Runny nose

D. Sore throat

E. Nausea/vomiting

F. Headache

G. Diarrhea

H. RED FLAGS
1. Severe shortness of breath/difficulty breathing
2. Coughing up blood
3. Chest pain or pressure
4. Skin: mottled, cold, clammy
5. Confusion
6. Cyanosis of lips or face
7. Decreased urinary output

Subjective Data

Providers and staff taking care of patients suspected of having symptoms of COVID-19 should wear personal protective equipment (PPE) for all contact with suspected patients. The sequence order of putting on PPE includes: (1) gown, (2) mask, (3) goggles/face shield, and (4) gloves.

Use caution to cover all exposed areas of the skin.

A. Determine the onset, duration, and course of symptoms.

B. Does the client currently have a fever?

C. Review the client's recent travel history including countries, plane, cruise ships, and exposure in U.S. cities considered "hot spots" within the past 14 days of appointment.

D. Are there any other family members or friends that have had close contact that had exposure and/or positive testing for COVID-19 including travel outside of the U.S. within the past 14 days of appointment?

E. Inquire about any exposure to the flu. Did the client get a flu vaccine this season?

F. Review all chronic medical conditions (see Predisposing Factors).

G. Review all prescription, OTC, and herbal medications.

H. Inquire about exacerbating factors.

I. Does the client smoke, including e-cigarettes? If so, how much, and for how long did he or she smoke?

Physical Examination

A. Check temperature, blood pressure, pulse, respirations. Always check a pulse oximetry.

1. The client may have a fairly normal examination early in the disease course.

2. The respiratory rate increases proportionally to disease severity.

B. Inspect:

1. Observe overall general appearance.

2. Note respiratory pattern.

3. Note the use of accessory muscles for breathing.

4. Inspect the eyes, ears, and throat.

5. Inspect the nose for nasal flaring.

C. Auscultate

1. Lung fields for crackles, wheezes, rhonchi, decreased breath sounds, and unequal breath sounds

2. Auscultate the heart.

D. Percuss:

1. Chest for the presence of hyperresonance and for signs of consolidation

E. Palpate

1. Liver and spleen

2. Lymph nodes

F. Mental status: Assess for decreased level of consciousness.

G. Further physical examinations are dependent on comorbidities.

Diagnostic Tests

> COVID-19 is a reportable disease to the state or local health department. Clinicians should immediately implement recommended infection prevention and control practices if a client is suspected of having COVID-19. They should also notify infection control personnel at their healthcare facility and their state or local health department if a client is classified as a Patient Under Investigation (PUI) for COVID-19.

A. Not everyone needs to be tested for COVID-19. The CDC has guidance for who should be tested, but decisions about testing are at the discretion of state and local health departments and/or individual clinicians (https://www.cdc.gov/coronavirus/2019-ncov/downloads/priority-testing-patients.pdf).

1. Priority 1: Ensure optimal care options for all hospitalized patients, lessen the risk of nosocomial infections, and maintain the integrity of the U.S. healthcare system.

   a. Hospitalized patients
   b. Symptomatic healthcare workers

2. Priority 2: Ensure those at highest risk of complication of infection are rapidly identified and appropriately triaged.

   a. Patients in long-term care facilities with symptoms
   b. Patients 65 years of age and older with symptoms
   c. Patients with underlying conditions with symptoms
   d. First responders with symptoms

3. Priority 3: As resources allow, test individuals in the surrounding community of rapidly increased hospital cases to decrease community spread and ensure health of essential workers.

   a. Critical infrastructure workers with symptoms
   b. Individuals who do not meet any of the above categories with symptoms
   c. Healthcare workers and first responders
   d. Individuals with mild symptoms in communities experiencing high COVID-19 hospitalizations

4. Non-Priority

   a. Individuals without symptoms

B. Specimens should be collected as soon as possible once a decision has been made to pursue COVID-19 testing, regardless of the time of symptom onset. Use only synthetic fiber swabs with plastic shafts. Do not use calcium alginate swabs or swabs with wooden shafts, as they may contain substances that inactivate some viruses and inhibit PCR testing.

C. Techniques:

1. Nasopharyngeal (NP) swab: Insert a swab into the nostril parallel to the palate. The swab should reach the depth equal to distance from nostrils to outer opening of the ear. Leave the swab in place for several seconds to absorb secretions. Slowly remove the swab while rotating it.

2. Oropharyngeal (OP) swab (e.g., throat swab): Swab the posterior pharynx, avoiding the tongue.

D. Interim guidelines for collecting, handling, and testing include:

1. Nasopharyngeal specimen is the preferred choice for swab-based SARS-CoV-2 testing. When collection of a NP swab is not possible, the following alternatives are considered acceptable:

   a. Allowance for healthcare worker or onsite self-collection using a flocked, tapered swab collected in the anterior nasal cavity as an acceptable specimen type if NP swab is not possible.
   b. Allowance for self- or healthcare worker–collected nasal mid-turbinate swabs as an acceptable specimen type if NP swab is not available.
   c. An OP specimen collected by a healthcare professional.
   d. Swabs should be placed in a transport tube containing viral transport medium, Amies transport medium, or sterile saline. If both NP and OP swabs are collected, they should be combined in a single tube.

2. The CDC also recommends testing lower respiratory tract specimens, if available. For patients who develop a productive cough, sputum should be collected and tested for SARS-CoV-2. The induction of sputum is not recommended.

Differential Diagnoses

A. Influenza
B. Adenovirus
C. Rhinovirus
D. Respiratory syncytial virus (RSV)
E. SARS
F. Viral or bacterial pneumonia
G. Pediatrics and adults with persistent cough: Pertussis

Plan

A. General interventions for mild symptoms are primarily supportive.
   1. Increase fluid intake.
   2. Rest.
   3. Every patient must have follow-up with the primary care provider or other team member to monitor client outcome.
B. Client teaching:
   1. Cancel or postpone travel.
   2. Comply with any local restrictions, travel advisories, avoid large gatherings to reduce the risk of catching or spreading COVID-19.
   3. Stay home if you feel unwell even with mild symptoms including low-grade fever, slightly runny nose, and headache.
   4. Seek medical attention via telemedicine or call your provider's office in advance. Calling in advance will allow healthcare providers to assess and direct you to the right health facility.
   5. Choose a room in the house that can be used to separate sick household members from others. Identify a separate bathroom for the sick person to use, if possible. Prohibit visitors who do not have essential need to be in the home.
   6. Create an emergency contact list including healthcare providers, friends, neighbors, employers, and the local public health department.
   7. Use good hygiene practices
      a. Use an alcohol-based hand sanitizer that contains at least 60% alcohol and/or practice good handwashing with soap and water. Wash your hands for at least 20 seconds.
      b. Disinfect surfaces with simple disinfectants to kill the virus and protect themselves and others.
      c. Avoid touching the eyes, mouth, or nose.
      d. Clean all foods including fruit prior to peeling.
   8. Use good respiratory hygiene practices
      a. Covering your mouth and nose with a tissue or bent elbow when coughing or sneezing. Dispose of the used tissue immediately and wash your hands.
   9. Practice social distancing
      a. The virus can spread between people interacting in close proximity. Maintain at least 6 feet distance (2 arm lengths) between yourself and anyone who is speaking, coughing, or sneezing.
      b. The CDC is additionally advising the use of simple cloth face coverings to slow the spread of the virus and help people who may have the virus and do not know it from transmitting it to others. The cloth face coverings recommended are not surgical masks or N-95 respirators.
   10. Self-isolation
      a. Guidelines for persons who are in or have recently visited areas within the past 14 days where COVID-19 is spreading should self-isolate, and monitor for symptoms.
         1. Taking your temperature 2 times a day and watch for cough or trouble breathing.
         2. Stay at home and avoid contact with others.
         3. Do not take public transportation or ride-shares.
         4. Keep 6 feet away from others.
      b. Have someone bring supplies or to go out to buy food, then wear a mask to avoid infecting other people.
      c. Have at least a 30-day supply of all medicines.
C. Pharmaceutical therapy:
   WHO does not recommend self-medication with any medicines, including antibiotics, as a prevention or cure for COVID-19. To date, there no specific antiviral medicine to prevent or treat COVID-19. However, there are several ongoing clinical trials and vaccine development.
A. Antipyretics for fever and malaise. NOTE: McNeil Consumer Healthcare, which produces the Tylenol® brand of acetaminophen, has lowered the maximum daily dose for single-ingredient Extra Strength Tylenol® (acetaminophen) products sold in the U.S. from 8 pills per day (4,000 mg) to 6 pills per day (3,000 mg). The dosing interval has also changed from 2 pills every 4–6 hours to 2 pills every 6 hours.
   1. Avoid the use of non-steroidal anti-inflammatory (NSAIDs) medications such as Motrin, ibuprofen, and Aleve. Use of NSAIDs early in the infection is thought to have a negative outcome for the patient.
B. Expectorants, such as guaifenesin with dextromethorphan (Robitussin DM, Humibid DM, Mytussin), can be used to treat minor cough from bronchial/throat irritation.
C. There are no FDA-approved vaccines available for COVID-19 or other coronaviruses. Multiple pharmaceutical companies are working to develop a COVID-19 vaccine and start clinical trials.
D. The FDA is taking the lead on a national effort to facilitate the development of, and access to, two investigational therapies derived from human blood. These are called convalescent plasma and hyperimmune globulin and are antibody-rich blood products made from blood donated by people who have recovered from the virus.

Follow-Up

A. Clients diagnosed with COVID-19 that are outpatient need to have follow-up depending on severity. Patients with mild symptoms should have phone call contact at least every 2 days up to 14 days or until symptoms have improved. If the client is symptom free on day 7, follow-up may be changed to day 10 and day 14. Clients with more acute symptoms need follow-up every 24 hours.

B. A Care Coordinator Program for COVID-19 positive patients should be instituted and a registry of the names of clients that are positive should be documented. A team protocol for physicians, nurse practitioners, nurses, and other members of the health team should be developed to follow these patients closely.

Consultation/Referral

A. Consult with a physician if the client has acute respiratory decompensation.

B. Hospitalization is recommended for clients in moderate to severe respiratory distress and RED FLAG symptoms (see Other Signs and Symptoms).

C. Mental health referrals for fear/anxiety, social isolation, and depression including the Substance Abuse and Mental Health Services Administration's (SAMHSA) Disaster Distress Helpline: 1-800-985-5990 or text TalkWithUs to 66746. (TTY 1-800-846-8517)

D. Social work referrals are indicated for assistance with financial insecurity and food insecurity.

E. Referral to home health care for continued care and support.

Individual Considerations

A. Pregnancy:

1. Dyspnea occurs in up to two thirds of clients beginning in the first or second trimester of pregnancy. Underlying pathology during pregnancy should be considered.

2. Pregnant patients who have confirmed COVID-19 or who are persons under investigation (PUI) should notify the obstetric unit prior to arrival so the facility can make appropriate infection control preparations for labor and delivery and for the neonate. It is unknown whether newborns with COVID-19 are at an increased risk for severe complications. Transmission after birth via contact with infectious respiratory secretions is a concern.

3. The American Academy of Pediatrics Initial Guidance has published guidelines on the management of infants born to mothers with suspected or confirmed COVID-19. The document was released on April 2, 2020, and is available at https://downloads.aap.org/AAP/PDF/COVID%2019%20Initial%20Newborn%20Guidance.pdf

B. Geriatrics:

1. Physical changes associated with aging increase the risk for hypoxia.

2. Elderly clients may report SOB less frequently and assume it is an expectation of aging.

C. Pediatrics:

1. Acute respiratory distress should be immediately ruled out in infants and children in an emergency department setting.

Resources

Centers for Disease Control and Prevention Information for Healthcare Professionals: https://www.cdc.gov/coronavirus/2019-nCoV/hcp/index.html

U.S. Food & Drug Administration: https://www.fda.gov/emergency-preparedness-and-response/counterterrorism-and-emerging-threats/coronavirus-disease-2019-covid-19

World Health Organization: https://www.who.int/emergencies/diseases/novel-coronavirus-2019

Bibliography

American Academy of Pediatrics Committee on Fetus and Newborn, Section on Neonatal Perinatal Medicine, and Committee on Infectious Diseases. (2020, April 2). Initial Guidance: Management of infants born to mothers with COVID-19. Retrieved from https://downloads.aap.org/AAP/PDF/COVID%2019%20Initial%20Newborn%20Guidance.pdf

Cascella, M., Rajnik, M., Cuomo, A., & Dulebohn, S. (2020, March 20). Features, evaluation and treatment Coronavirus (COVID-19), *StatPearls*. Retrieved from https://www.ncbi.nlm.nih.gov/books/NBK554776/figure/article-52171.image.f5/

Centers for Disease Control and Prevention. (2020, April 2). Coronavirus Disease 2019 (COVID-19): If you are at higher risk. Retrieved from https://www.cdc.gov/coronavirus/2019-ncov/need-extra-precautions/people-at-higher-risk

Centers for Disease Control and Prevention. (2020, February 18). Interim consideration for infection prevention and control of coronavirus disease 2019 (COVID-19) in inpatient obstetric healthcare settings. Retrieved from https://www.cdc.gov/coronavirus/2019-ncov/hcp/inpatient-obstetric-healthcare-guidance.html

Centers for Disease Control and Prevention. (2020, March 25). Interim guidelines for collecting, handling, and testing clinical specimens from persons for coronavirus disease 2019 (COVID-19). Retrieved from https://www.cdc.gov/coronavirus/2019-ncov/lab/guidelines-clinical-specimens.html

Centers for Disease Control and Prevention. (2020, February 28). Recommendations for reporting, testing, and specimen collection. Retrieved from https://www.cdc.gov/coronavirus/2019-nCoV/hcp/clinical-criteria.html

Chen, Y., Liu, Q., & Guo, D. (2020) Emerging coronaviruses: Genome structure, replication, and pathogenesis. *Journal of Medical Virology, 92*(4), 418–423. Retrieved from https://www.ncbi.nlm.nih.gov/pubmed/31967327

Farrell, S. E. (2020, January 17). *Acetaminophen toxicity*. Medscape. Retrieved from https://emedicine.medscape.com/article/820200-overview#a4

FDA U.S. Food & Drug Administration. (2020, April 3). *FDA News Release*. Coronavirus (COVID-19) update: FDA coordinates national effort to develop blood-related therapies for COVID-19. Retrieved from https://www.fda.gov/news-events/press-announcements/coronavirus-covid-19-update-fda-coordinates-national-effort-develop-blood-related-therapies-covid-19

Li, Q., Guan, X., Wu, P., Wang, X., Zhou, L., Tong, Y., Ren, R., … Feng, Z. (2020). Early transmission dynamics in Wuhan China, of novel Coronavirus-infected pneumonia. *New England Journal of Medicine, 382*(13), 1199–1207. Retrieved from https://www.ncbi.nlm.nih.gov/pubmed/31995857

McNeil Consumer Healthcare. (2016). TYLENOL® Dosage for Adults. Available at https://www.tylenol.com/safety-dosing/usage/dosage-for-adults. Accessed April 2, 2020.

World Health Organization. (2020). *Q&A on coronaviruses (COVID-19)*. Retrieved from https://www.who.int/news-room/q-a-detail/q-a-coronaviruses; Accessed April 2, 2020.

Zhou, F., Ting, Y., Du, R., Fan, G., Liu, Y. L., & Liu, Z. (2020). Clinical course and risk factors for mortality of adult inpatients with COVID-19 in Wuhan, China: A retrospective study. *The Lancet, 395*(10229), 1054–1062. Retrieved from https://www.thelancet.com/journals/lancet/article/PIIS0140-6736(20)30566-3/fulltext#seccestitle160

Cytomegalovirus

Jill C. Cash, Cheryl A. Glass, and Moya Cook

Definition

A. Cytomegalovirus (CMV) is a member of the herpesvirus family, which includes varicella-zoster virus (VZV) (chickenpox) and infectious mononucleosis (Epstein–Barr virus [EBV]). Differences in CMV genotypes may be associated with differences in virulence. CMV is responsible for a viral infection with a high rate of asymptomatic excretion. Shedding of the virus takes place intermittently. CMV can be isolated in cell culture from urine, a pharynx swab, respiratory secretions, human milk, tears, saliva, semen, cervical secretions, and body fluids such as blood and amniotic fluid. Cytomegalic cells can be found in various tissues, including the lung, liver, kidney, intestine, adrenal gland, and CNS.

B. CMV persists in latent form after a primary infection, and reactivation can occur years later, particularly under conditions of immunosuppression, transplantation, and pregnancy. It is one of the **TORCH** (toxoplasmosis, other [i.e., hepatitis and syphilis], rubella, CMV, and herpes) infections.

C. The most common illness caused by CMV is retinitis.

Incidence

A. CMV is found worldwide in people of all ages, races, and ethnic groups. Seropositivity increases with age, ranging from 40% to 100% depending on geography, cultures, child-rearing practices, and socioeconomic status. Approximately 50% of blood donors have been exposed to CMV, and 10% carry CMV in their white blood cells (WBCs). The incidence of horizontal transmission of CMV occurring in settings such as day care ranges from 10% to more than 80% from exposure to saliva and urine. Another increase in CMV incidence is noted in adolescence secondary to sexual activity.

B. In the United States, CMV is the most common congenital infection. The incidence of congenital vertical transmission of CMV ranges from 0.2% to 2.5%. Most newborns appear normal and are asymptomatic; however, 5% to 15% of congenitally infected newborns will have symptoms at delivery. Prenatal CMV infections occur from contact with maternal cervicovaginal secretions during delivery or from breast milk ingestion. Preterm infants are at greatest risk of acquiring CMV from breast milk.

C. Combination antiretroviral therapy (ART) has reduced the risk of CMV in people with human immunodeficiency virus (HIV) infection by 75%.

D. The risk of CMV is the highest in clients with HIV when their CD4 cell (T cells, T lymphocytes) counts are below 50 cells/μL. CMV is rare if the CD4 count is more than 100 cells/μL.

E. The most common illness caused by CMV is retinitis.

Pathogenesis

A. Human CMV, a DNA virus, is a member of the herpesvirus group. This virus is transmitted both horizontally (by direct person-to-person contact with virus-containing secretions) and vertically (from mother to infant before, during, or after birth). Infections have no seasonal correlation.

B. The incubation period for horizontally transmitted CMV infections in households is unknown. Primary CMV infection usually manifests itself within 4 to 7 weeks and may persist as long as 16 to 20 weeks after initial infection. CMV disease is most likely 30 to 60 days after transplant.

C. There is no treatment that will permanently eliminate CMV infection; it is a lifetime infection.

Predisposing Factors

A. Exposure to young children (especially those in daycare centers)

B. Sexual contact (cervicovaginal secretions and semen)

C. Blood transfusions: Clients with impaired immune function (e.g., bone marrow and organ transplant recipients, premature babies) are at risk for CMV infection from contaminated transfused blood

D. Hospital or occupational exposure: Universal precautions are considered adequate to prevent transmission of CMV within hospitals. Nosocomial transmission from person to person has not been documented. Isolation is not recommended.

E. Pregnancy: Pregnant healthcare workers are not restricted from caring for CMV-infected clients and should follow universal precautions.

F. Transplacental transmission

G. Ascending infection from the cervix

H. Tissue or organ transplantation

I. Household spread among family members; a young child is most frequently the index case.

J. Breast milk

Common Complaints

A. Mononucleosis-like syndrome

B. Fever

C. Overwhelming fatigue

D. Pharyngitis

E. Ulcerative lesions in the mouth

F. Loss of vision: Retinal detachment may occur in up to 50% to 60% of clients in the first year after diagnosis.

Other Signs and Symptoms

A. Mothers: Asymptomatic or mononucleosis-like syndrome

B. Fetuses:
   1. Intrauterine growth retardation (IUGR)/small for gestational age
   2. Nonimmune hydrops fetalis
   3. Microcephaly noted on ultrasound
   4. Intracerebral calcification

C. Infants after congenital exposure:
   1. Asymptomatic
   2. Skin:
      a. Jaundice at birth
      b. Petechiae and purpura of the skin
   3. Hepatosplenomegaly
   4. Anemia

5. Thrombocytopenia
6. Eyes: Chorioretinitis, retinal hemorrhage, optic atrophy
7. Seizure disorders
8. Feeding difficulties

D. Children with congenital exposure:
1. Asymptomatic
2. Development: Developmental delays, learning disability, and mental retardation
3. Ears: Progressive hearing loss (usually unilateral). Universal hearing screening programs may identify some of the otherwise asymptomatic infants.
4. Loss of vision

E. Adults:
1. Visual changes: Floaters or loss of visual fields on one side
2. Retinitis
3. Arthralgias
4. Nausea, abdominal cramping, and vomiting (includes hematemesis)
5. Prolonged fever
6. Mild hepatitis
7. Headache
8. Gastritis presents with abdominal pain; colitis presents as a diarrheal illness. CMV may infect the gastrointestinal (GI) tract from the oral cavity through the colon. The typical manifestation of disease is ulcerative lesions. In the mouth, these may be indistinguishable from ulcers caused by herpes simplex virus (HSV) or aphthous ulceration.

F. Immunocompromised persons:
1. Bacterial: Pneumonia, retinitis, myocarditis, and aseptic meningitis
2. Anemia
3. Thrombocytopenia

Subjective Data

A. Review onset of presenting signs, symptoms, and their duration.

B. Review the client's history for recent upper respiratory infection (URI) and mononucleosis-like symptoms.

C. Elicit information concerning contact with any person known to be infected with CMV.

D. Review the client's history for other family members with similar symptoms.

E. Ask the client about any occupational exposure.

F. Review the client's exposure to children in day-care centers.

G. Review recent blood transfusions and/or organ transplantation.

H. Determine the client's history for risk factors or presence of HIV:
1. If the client has known HIV, does the client know his or her last viral load CD4 count?
2. Is the client taking ART? When were the antivirals started?

I. Ask family members if the client has been confused, lethargic, or withdrawn or has exhibited personality changes (CMV encephalitis, dementia).

Physical Examination

A. Check temperature, pulse, respirations, BP, and weight; document serial weight loss.

B. Inspect:
1. Inspect the skin for jaundice and petechiae.
2. Evaluate age-appropriate developmental tasks.
3. Conduct a detailed eye examination:
   a. The CMV infection might appear as yellow-white areas with perivascular exudates and hemorrhage, having a "cottage cheese and ketchup" appearance at either the periphery or the center of the fundus.
      i. Differentiating suspected CMV retinitis and cotton wool spots is essential. Cotton wool spots appear as small, fluffy white lesions with indistinct margins and are not associated with exudates or hemorrhages.
   b. Evaluate field of vision.
4. Perform an ENT examination.

C. Auscultate:
1. Heart
2. Lungs

D. Palpate:
1. The abdomen, noting organomegaly
2. Pregnancy: Palpate fundal height and evaluate for suspected IUGR.

E. Neurological examination:
1. Assess all cranial nerves.
2. Sensation: Deficits may occur without loss of vibratory sense and proprioception).
3. Deep tendon reflexes
4. Motor skills and coordination
5. Gait
6. Conduct a hearing test.

Diagnostic Tests

A. Viral culture of a specimen from urine, cervix, vagina, nasopharynx, and saliva:
1. Viral culture is the best means of diagnosing acute CMV infections, although it does not distinguish between primary and recurrent disease. Urine contains high titers of the virus because CMV is relatively stable in urine.

B. CBC with differential: Differential WBC count reveals increased lymphocytes, many of which are atypical.

C. Total direct and indirect serum bilirubin

D. Liver function: Alanine aminotransferase (ALT) and aspartate aminotransferase (AST)

E. Serology for CMV immunoglobulin G (IgG) and immunoglobulin M (IgM): Only the recovery of the virus from a target organ provides unequivocal evidence that the disease is caused by CMV infection. However, a four-fold or greater rise in IgG-specific antibody titer is usually considered evidence of acute infection.

F. Immunocompromised clients, especially transplant recipients, may be monitored for viral surveillance weekly using surrogate markers for viremia (PCR).

G. Chest x-ray if indicated

H. CT scan if indicated to evaluate abnormalities of the brain in the presence of an abnormal neurological examination, seizures, and microcephaly

I. Sensorineural hearing evaluation

Differential Diagnoses

A. CMV

B. Other TORCH infections

C. HIV

D. Viral: Autoimmune hepatitis or hepatitis A to E

E. Enteroviruses

F. FUO

Plan

A. General interventions:
  1. Provide support for the client and family.
  2. Contact social services if long-term support will be required for these infants/families.
  3. Rest is vital.

B. Client teaching:
  1. Clients with splenomegaly should avoid activity that may increase the risk of injury to the spleen, such as contact sports and heavy lifting.
  2. Mothers infected with CMV should be discouraged from breastfeeding because CMV is secreted in breast milk. CMV-specific IgM antibodies are present in only 80% of clients with primary CMV infections and in 20% of clients with recurrent infections; therefore, a negative result does not exclude the diagnosis of CMV.
  3. Isolation is not required.
  4. Use universal precautions, especially good handwashing.
  5. Do not share eating or drinking utensils, drinks, or food with toddlers or young children.
  6. Educate about the importance of ART in treating CMV.
    a. Clients with CMV retinitis may require lifelong suppressive therapy to prevent blindness. Vision loss will not return to pre-CMV status.
    b. Report visual deterioration immediately.

C. Pharmaceutical therapy:
  1. Drug of choice: Ganciclovir (Cytovene) for CMV retinitis is the treatment both for adults and for children older than 3 months; treatment is divided into an induction and a maintenance phase:
    a. The safety of ganciclovir in pregnancy has not been established.
    b. Clients receiving ganciclovir should have blood counts monitored closely due to dose-dependent bone marrow suppression. Monitor for leukopenia, neutropenia, anemia, or thrombocytopenia. Stop ganciclovir when neutrophil counts are less than 500/mm^3. Growth factors may be necessary.
    c. The dose should be decreased in clients with impaired renal function. Monitor creatinine.
    d. Ganciclovir induction: 5 mg/kg per dose intravenously (IV) administered over 1 hour every 12 hours for 14 to 21 days, depending on the clinical and virologic response. Oral ganciclovir should not be used for induction.
    e. Ganciclovir maintenance:
      i. A single daily dose of 5 mg/kg may be administered IV every other day or 5 days a week, skipping the weekend.
      ii. Oral ganciclovir 1 g orally three times a day may be used for maintenance/prophylaxis in some clients, but poor oral availability makes it less effective than IV administration.
      iii. Ganciclovir has been associated with bone marrow suppression, such as leukopenia. This risk may be addressed by prescribing hematopoietic growth factors.
    f. Although ganciclovir has appeared to be beneficial in the treatment of some congenitally infected infants, its use is controversial and is considered mainly for high-risk clients with severe congenital CMV.
    g. Newborns: 6 mg/kg per dose administered IV over the course of 1 hour. Ganciclovir has been administered in clinical trials for infants at 6 mg/kg IV for 6 weeks.
  2. Alternative drug therapy: Foscarnet (Foscavir):
    a. Used in ganciclovir-resistant CMV retinitis and herpes simplex disease
    b. Use in children is limited, and the safe dose has not been established.
    c. The safety of foscarnet in pregnancy has not been established.
    d. Foscarnet is nephrotoxic. Meticulous attention must be paid to renal function. Small changes in creatinine require a new calculation for renal clearance. Obtain a 24-hour serum creatinine at baseline and discontinue if serum creatinine is less than 0.4 gL/min/kg.
    e. Clients must be well hydrated.
    f. Regimens:
      i. Foscarnet induction: 60 mg/kg IV every 8 hours or 90 to 120 mg/kg IV every 12 hours for 14 to 21 days for the induction of CMV retinitis
      ii. Foscarnet maintenance: 90 to 120 mg/kg IV per day as a single infusion. Infusion rate should not exceed 1 mg/kg/min.
  3. Cidofovir (Vistide):
    a. Cidofovir induction: 5 mg/kg IV once a week for 2 weeks
    b. Cidofovir maintenance: 5 mg/kg IV every 2 weeks
    c. Probenecid is given on the day of the IV infusion to reduce the renal uptake of cidofovir
  4. CMV immunoglobulin (Ig) IV: Initial dose is 150 mg/kg, followed by gradually reduced doses once every 2 weeks for 16 weeks. Currently available antiviral agents do not cure CMV disease in HIV-infected clients.

5. Ig or CMV hyperimmune globulin CytoGam may be utilized for passive immunoprophylaxis, especially in bone marrow and organ transplant recipients, to help develop antibodies and protect against CMV infection.
6. Vaccines for CMV disease are currently in clinical trials.

Follow-Up

A. Retinitis is the most common manifestation of CMV disease; clients with CNS, GI, or pulmonary disease should be assessed with a dilated retinal examination to detect subclinical retinal disease.
B. The client should be seen for reports of excessive bruising or bleeding, jaundice, or abnormal CNS functioning.
C. Monitor CBC, serum creatinine, and electrolytes (especially calcium and magnesium) every week.

Consultation/Referral

A. Consultation with an infectious disease specialist is indicated for acute infection, especially for immunocompromised clients.
B. Antivirals have many adverse effects and are best managed by a physician who has experience using these drugs.
C. Consultation with a hematologist is needed in severe cases, especially for clients with hemolytic anemia and thrombocytopenia.
D. Consultation with a neurologist is indicated for clients with meningitis, encephalitis, polyneuritis, and Guillain–Barré syndrome.
E. Consultation with an ophthalmologist is needed on an emergent basis for clients with a dilated retinal examination due to the risks of blindness. Serial dilated retinal examinations should be done after ART induction therapy and monthly thereafter.
F. Consultation with a perinatologist is indicated for pregnant clients. Evaluation may include ultrasonography, amniocentesis, and percutaneous umbilical blood sampling (PUBS).
G. Refer the client to a gastroenterologist for an endoscopic evaluation with tissue biopsies.

Individual Considerations

A. Pregnancy:
1. Routine maternal screening for CMV infection is not recommended during pregnancy. Currently available laboratory tests generally cannot conclusively determine whether a primary CMV infection has occurred during the pregnancy.
2. Between 55% and 85% of pregnant women are immune to CMV, with a higher prevalence of immunity in lower-socioeconomic-status populations.
3. Susceptible pregnant women have a 2% to 2.5% risk of acquiring primary CMV during pregnancy. Those with prior immunity have a 1% chance of reactivation of latent infection.
4. Amniocentesis for PCR to detect CMV DNA is the preferred diagnostic approach for detecting the infected fetus.

5. Recovery of CMV from the cervix or urine of women at or before the time of delivery does not warrant a cesarean section.
B. Perinatal transmission of CMV occurs by four routes:
1. In utero transplacental infections
2. Ascending infections from the cervix
3. Exposure to infected secretions from the lower genital tract during delivery
4. Ingestion of infected breast milk

Because CMV is spread by intimate contact with infectious secretions, handwashing after exposure to secretions is particularly important for pregnant healthcare workers.

C. Pediatrics:
1. Routine screening for CMV is not recommended for internationally adopted children.
2. As many as half of all neonates exposed to CMV in the lower genital tract during delivery become infected. Intrapartum or postpartum CMV acquisition does not result in adverse outcomes or sequelae except in very-low-birth-weight infants. Viral excretion from intrapartum or postpartum exposure begins at 3 to 9 weeks of life; thus, the initial viral cultures are negative.
3. The child with congenital CMV infection should not be treated differently from other children and should not be excluded from school or child-care institutions, as the virus is frequently found in many healthy children.
4. Sensorineural hearing loss is the most common sequela following congenital CMV infection. Evaluate for hearing loss at each pediatric visit.
D. Adults:
1. Occupational exposure: Risk often appears to be greatest for child-care personnel who care for children younger than 2 years.
2. Routine serologic screening for child-care staff is not currently recommended.
3. Pregnant personnel who may be in contact with CMV-infected clients should be counseled regarding the risk of acquiring CMV infection and about the need to practice good hygiene, particularly handwashing. There is no need to routinely transfer personnel to other work situations.
E. Geriatrics:
1. CMV colitis can be life-threatening for the immunocompromised older client with chronic renal disease.
2. Monitor for symptoms such as bloody diarrhea. Consider colonoscopy with biopsy for diagnosis.

Bibliography

Friel, T. J. (2019). Epidemiology, clinical manifestations, and treatment of cytomegalovirus infection in immunocompetent adults. *UpToDate*. Retrieved from www.uptodate.com/contents/epidemiology-clinical-manifestations-and-treatment-of-cytomegalovirus-infection-in-immuno competent-adults

Encephalitis

Jill C. Cash, Cheryl A. Glass, and Moya Cook

Definition

A. Encephalitis is the inflammation of cerebral tissue caused by viral agents or other toxins. The syndrome of acute encephalitis shares many clinical features with acute meningitis. Clients with either syndrome present with fever, headache, and altered states of consciousness. In most cases of encephalitis, there is some concomitant meningeal inflammation, in addition to the cephalitic component, a condition commonly referred to as meningoencephalitis.

Incidence

A. Incidence is unknown. Japanese encephalitis (JE) occurs in annual epidemics in Asia during the rainy season. The prevalence of JE (arbovirus) is related to ecological and climatic conditions that affect the natural transmission cycles during summer months (June through September). Some areas with tropical climates, such as Cambodia, Indonesia, southern Vietnam, and southern Thailand, have year-round transmission.

B. Arboviruses (Eastern or Western equine, St. Louis, and West Nile virus [WNV]) cause disease when mosquitoes are active. Walking in the woods or marshy areas with high tick populations might suggest other viral encephalitides such as Colorado tick fever or nonviral etiologies such as Lyme disease or Rocky Mountain spotted fever (RMSF).

C. Herpes encephalitis has the highest morbidity and mortality of the common viral encephalitides and may occur at any time. The mortality rate for untreated clients is 70%; fewer than 5% of survivors have normal neurological function. HSV type 1 is the most common cause of sporadic encephalitis. The most important viral etiology to rule out is HSV, because this clinical entity is usually fatal if left untreated. Survival and recovery from neurological sequelae are related to the mental status at the time of acyclovir initiation.

D. Encephalopathy is the most common CNS manifestation of HIV infection, occurring in 65% of clients with HIV/AIDS (acquired immunodeficiency syndrome).

E. Mortality depends on the etiological agent. Morbidity related to the severity of sequelae also varies according to the causative agent.

Pathogenesis

A. JE is the most common form of epidemic viral encephalitis. For the past several years, WNV has been the most common cause of proved viral encephalitis in the United States. Encephalitis may occur as a secondary infection from mumps, varicella (chickenpox), rubella, rubeola, rabies, herpes simplex types 1 and 2, EBV, HIV, and influenza. Postinfectious encephalitis, in contrast to viral encephalitis, typically occurs either as the initial infection is resolving or following subclinical illness that was not appreciated by the client.

B. The incubation period depends on the pathogen.

C. Tick-borne diseases include Russian spring–summer encephalitis and Powassan encephalitis.

Predisposing Factors

A. Military personnel and travelers

B. Age extremes are at highest risk.

C. Exposure to vectors:
1. Mosquitoes
2. Ticks
3. Bat
4. Raccoon
5. Feral dogs/cats
6. Sandflies

D. HIV-positive

E. Herpes

F. Rodent-borne arenavirus: Exposure to the secretions of mice, rats, and hamsters

G. Occupational exposure:
1. Laboratory workers
2. Healthcare workers
3. Veterinarians

H. Recreational activities (camping/hunting)

I. Recent vaccination

Common Complaints

A. Severe headache. A person with encephalitis has a severe headache throughout the entire head. Over the course of about 48 hours, the person may show a lack of energy and then lapse into a coma.

B. Stiff neck

C. Mental changes: Altered mental status, altered behavior, and personality changes

D. Decreased LOC

E. Fever

Other Signs and Symptoms

A. CNS symptoms:
1. Nuchal rigidity
2. Irritability
3. Hemiparesis: Weakness or paralysis on one side of the body
4. Flaccid paralysis: Consider WNV infection
5. Seizures
6. Exaggerated deep tendon reflexes
7. Ataxia
8. Nystagmus

B. Photosensitivity

C. Swollen or protruding eyes

D. Malaise

E. Nausea and/or vomiting

F. Dysphagia with rabies

G. Parotitis: Consider mumps encephalitis

H. Maculopapular rash

I. Tremors

Subjective Data

A. Review the onset, duration, and course of all symptoms.

B. Rule out recent history of chickenpox, rubeola, herpes, or other infections.

C. Ask the client about recent travel.

D. Question the client regarding recent mosquito or animal bites (rule out rabies).

E. Elicit a detailed sexual history.

F. Does the client have HIV?

G. Ask about recent recreational activities, including camping, spelunking, or hunting.

Physical Examination

A. Check temperature, pulse, respirations, and BP.
B. Inspect:
1. Observe general overall appearance.
2. Conduct an eye examination.
3. Examine the skin for rash, vesicles, or bites:
   a. Maculopapular rash is seen in approximately half of clients with WNV.
   b. Grouped vesicles in a dermatomal pattern suggest varicella zoster.
   c. Classic herpetic skin lesions suggest herpes encephalitis.
4. Assess dehydration status.
5. Observe for seizure activity.
6. Observe for tremors of the eyelids, tongue, lips, and extremities, which may suggest the possibility of St. Louis encephalitis or West Nile encephalitis.
C. Auscultate:
1. Lungs and monitor breathing pattern
2. Heart
D. Palpate:
1. The lymph nodes: Preauricular, posterior auricular, submental and sublingual, anterior cervical chains, and supraclavicular nodes
2. The mastoid bone
E. Neurological examination:
1. Assess LOC.
2. Assess the client for personality changes.
3. Assess for meningeal signs:
   a. Signs of meningeal irritation include nuchal rigidity.
   b. Positive Brudzinski's and Kernig's signs:
      i. Brudzinski's sign: Place the client supine and flex the head upward. Resulting flexion of hips, knees, and ankles with neck flexion indicates meningeal irritation (see Figure 16.1).

FIGURE 16.1   Demonstration of Brudzinski's sign.

      ii. Kernig's sign: Place the client supine. Keeping one leg straight, flex the other hip and knee to a bent knee to form a 90° angle. Slowly extend the lower leg. This places a stretch on the meninges, resulting in pain and spasm for the hamstring muscle. Resistance to further extension can be felt (see Figure 16.2).

FIGURE 16.2   Demonstration of Kernig's sign.

4. Check deep tendon reflexes (exaggerated and/or pathological reflexes).

Diagnostic Tests

A. CBC with differential, electrolytes, glucose, blood urea nitrogen (BUN), and creatinine
B. PCR tests for viruses
C. Serology for arboviruses
D. Lumbar puncture for the following:
1. Protein (elevated)
2. Glucose (usually normal)
3. White cell count (increased)
4. Red cell count (usually negative in a nontraumatic tap)
5. Culture (viral and bacterial): Detection of virus-specific IgM antibody in cerebrospinal fluid (CSF) is diagnostic
E. Electroencephalogram (EEG)
F. CT scan: Useful to rule out space-occupying lesions or brain abscess
G. Magnetic resonance imaging (MRI): Sensitive for detecting demyelination
H. Brain scan: Imaging studies (CT scan, MRI, brain scan) may be normal early; later, nonspecific abnormalities are seen.
I. Stool or throat cultures may be helpful if enteroviruses are suspected.
J. Skin lesions and urine may be cultured for herpes simplex and CMV).
K. Brain biopsy is the diagnostic standard.

Differential Diagnoses

A. Encephalitis
B. WNV
C. St. Louis virus
D. Chickenpox
E. Measles: Rubeola or rubella
F. Herpes
G. Rabies
H. Influenza
I. Mumps
J. Meningitis
K. Brain abscess
L. Tuberculosis

M. Syphilis
N. Intracranial hemorrhage
O. Trauma
P. Toxic ingestion
Q. Fungal meningitis
R. RMSF (tick-borne diseases)
S. Cerebral bacterial infections
T. Toxoplasmosis
U. Lyme disease
V. CSD
W. CMV
X. Nonparalytic poliomyelitis

Plan

A. General interventions:
1. If encephalitis is suspected, hospitalization is recommended for further diagnostic studies and evaluation.
B. Client teaching:
1. Prevention of vector-borne encephalitis involves mosquito and tick avoidance, use of insect repellents, and vaccination.
2. The JE vaccine is an inactivated vaccine derived from infected mouse brain and is recommended for expatriates living in Asia and for certain travelers. It is also recommended for the following clients:
a. Persons who will be residing in areas where JE virus is endemic or epidemic
b. Travelers planning prolonged stays (more than 30 days) in endemic areas during the transmission season, especially those engaging in activities such as bicycling, camping, or other unprotected outdoor activities in rural areas
3. If rabies is suspected, the domestic animal should be observed for 10 days to detect rabid behavior. If there is no indication of rabies, the animal should be immunized. Animals that show rabid behavior or wild animals should be sacrificed and their brains submitted to the local/state health department for pathology testing.
C. Pharmaceutical therapy:
1. Empirical treatment for HSV-1 should always be initiated as soon as possible if the client has encephalitis without explanation due to the high mortality and morbidity associated with this disease. Acyclovir 10 mg/kg is administered IV (given over 1 hour) every 8 hours for 14 to 21 days.
2. Antibiotics for bacterial etiology (refer to diagnosis-specific chapters)
3. Anticonvulsants for seizures
4. Other pharmaceutical therapies depend on the specific causal agent.
5. Initiate short courses of corticosteroids to control brain edema.
6. If rabies is suspected: Human rabies Ig should be given as a 20 U/kg dose.

Follow-Up

A. Follow-up varies and is specific to the causal agent.
B. Long-term management of clients with neurological sequelae includes rehabilitation services, home care, or nursing home placement for convalescent care.

Consultation/Referral

A. Refer the client to a physician and/or hospital. Consultations include a neurologist, infectious disease specialist, and neurosurgeon for managing elevated intracranial pressure.

Individual Considerations

A. Adult travelers:
1. Advise the client to take mosquito bed nets and aerosol insecticide sprays to reduce the risk of mosquito bites at night.
B. Inactivated JE vaccine series:
1. Adults 18 to 65 years: Two doses of 0.5 mL administered intramuscularly (IM) on days 0 and day 7 or day 28
2. Children 2 months to <18 years of age: Two doses of 0.5 mL administered IM on days 0 and 28
3. Children >2 months to 2 years: Two doses of 0.25 mL administered IM on days 0 and day 28

> The two-dose series should be administered at least 1 week prior to travel.

C. Geriatrics:
1. Elderly clients may be at risk for severe disease.
2. The WNV encephalitis occurs primarily in clients older than 65 years.
3. Encephalitis should be considered in all elderly clients who have progressive mental confusion
4. Herpes simplex encephalitis in the elderly may present in an atypical fashion:
a. Progressive amnestic cognitive disorder
b. Behavioral changes
c. Progressive mental confusion
d. Focal neurological deficits, which mimic stroke

Bibliography

Gluckman, S. (2017). Viral encephalitis in adults. *UpToDate*. Retrieved from www.uptodate.com/contents/viral-encephalitis-in-adults

H1N1 Influenza A (Swine Flu)

Jill C. Cash, Cheryl A. Glass, and Moya Cook

Definition

A. H1N1 influenza A, swine flu, is an influenza A virus that causes a highly contagious respiratory disease and has been reported worldwide. In 2009, the World Health Organization (WHO) designated a phase 6 global pandemic status of H1N1.
B. Persons with flu-like symptoms should promptly contact their healthcare providers. If an antiviral treatment is warranted, it should ideally be started within 48 hours from the onset of symptoms. Viral pneumonia is the primary sign of clinical deterioration.

Incidence

A. WHO declared the 2009 H1N1 pandemic to be resolved as of August 2010. However, this strain of flu still continues to circulate with other seasonal flu strains.
B. Influenza activity remained low and began increasing in late December 2015.

Pathogenesis

A. H1N1 is a new subtype of influenza A (A/H1N1) virus that is spread by human-to-human transmission. Swine flu is also transmitted from pig to person; however, persons cannot be infected with the H1N1 virus from consuming pork.

B. The primary mode of transmission is through exposure to viral strain–infected respiratory secretions from respiratory droplets (coughing or sneezing) and direct contact with contaminated surfaces. H1N1 is also spread through contaminated diarrheal stools.

C. The infectious period is 1 day before the onset of fever until 24 hours after fever ends.

Predisposing Factors

A. Age:
  1. Children younger than 5 years, especially those younger than 2 years
  2. Adults aged 25 to 64 years who have medical conditions that place them at high risk for influenza-related complications
  3. Adults aged 65 years or older

B. Pregnant women

C. Women up to 2 weeks postpartum

D. Crowded conditions

E. Institutions such as nursing homes

F. Occupational exposure: Teachers and healthcare workers

Common Complaints

A. Clinical manifestations of H1N1 influenza depend on the age and previous experience with the influenza virus. Rapid-onset respiratory illness is the most common complaint.
  1. Cough
  2. Sore throat
  3. Dyspnea/wheezing
  4. Rhinorrhea

B. Abrupt onset of fever and/or chills (temperature of 100°F [37.8°C] or greater)

C. Headache

D. Body aches

E. Altered mental status

F. Children:
  1. Apnea
  2. Tachypnea
  3. Cyanosis
  4. Dehydration
  5. Extreme irritability
  6. Febrile seizure

Other Signs and Symptoms

A. Joint pain

B. Diarrhea (common with H1N1)

C. Vomiting (common with H1N1)

Subjective Data

A. Review the onset, course, and duration of symptoms, especially fever and respiratory symptoms

B. Review symptoms of other family members or coworkers who are also ill. Did the onset of acute febrile respiratory illness occur within 7 days of close contact with a person with a confirmed case of H1N1?

C. If the client is pregnant, establish the gestational age.

D. Review the client's history for recent travel locations and travel on cruise ships/planes.

E. Evaluate living conditions for exposure risks.

F. Is the client a smoker?

G. Review all medications, including over-the-counter (OTC) and herbal products. Has the client taken any medications for the symptoms?

H. Does the client have a history of asthma or chronic obstructive pulmonary disease (COPD)?

I. Is the client immunocompromised (e.g., HIV, transplant recipient, chemotherapy)?

J. What other medical comorbidities, such as diabetes, does the client have?

Physical Examination

A. Check temperature, pulse, respirations, and BP.

B. Inspect:
  1. Observe the client's general overall appearance for pallor and for any respiratory distress.
  2. Assess hydration status, inspecting skin turgor and mucous membranes.
  3. Conduct eye and ENT examinations.
  4. Children:
     a. Observe for seizure activity.
     b. Note level of activity (playful versus lethargic).

C. Auscultate:
  1. Lung fields, observing for wheezing and crackles
  2. Heart

D. Palpate:
  1. Neck
  2. Lymph nodes: Preauricular, posterior auricular, submental and sublingual, anterior cervical chain, and supraclavicular nodes

E. Neurological examination:
  1. Assess LOC.
  2. Assess for nuchal rigidity.
  3. Assess for meningeal signs:
     a. Signs of meningeal irritation include nuchal rigidity.
     b. Positive Brudzinski's and Kernig's signs (refer to Figures 16.1 and 16.2):
        i. Brudzinski's sign: Place the client supine and flex the head upward. Resulting flexion of both hips, knees, and ankles with neck flexion indicates meningeal irritation.
        ii. Kernig's sign: Place the client supine. Keeping one leg straight, flex the other hip and knee to a bent knee to form a 90° angle. Slowly extend the lower leg. This places a stretch on the meninges, resulting in pain and spasm for the hamstring muscle. Resistance to further extension can be felt.

Diagnostic Tests

Testing is not necessary for all clients who present with influenza-type symptoms.

A. Rapid influenza antigen testing

B. Respiratory swab for H1N1 testing for detection by real-time reverse transcriptase polymerase chain reaction (rRT-PCR)

C. Viral culture
D. CBC with differential (not a required test)
E. Imaging (to rule out complications):
1. Chest x-ray
2. CT chest imaging for complications

Differential Diagnoses

A. Influenza:
1. H1N1 A (swine flu)
2. Influenza A
3. Influenza B
4. Avian flu (H5N1)
B. Pneumonia
C. Bronchitis
D. Mononucleosis
E. Respiratory syncytial virus (RSV)
F. Early HIV
G. Severe acute respiratory syndrome (SARS)
H. Meningitis

Plan

A. General interventions:
1. Management usually focuses on treatment of symptoms and is supportive:
   a. Bed rest
   b. Increased fluids
   c. Antipyretics and analgesics for fever and myalgias
   d. Encourage clients to stay home (self-isolate) if they become ill and avoid touching the eyes, nose, and mouth.
2. Community precautions:
   a. Avoid close contact with individuals who are sick.
   b. Wash hands often or use alcohol-based hand gels.
   c. Use of face masks may be advisable or required.
   d. Droplet precautions should be used and maintained for 7 days after the onset of illness or until symptoms have resolved.
B. Pharmaceutical therapy:
1. Coverage for the H1N1 swine flu is now included in the seasonal influenza vaccination; it is available in both an inactivated influenza vaccine (IIV), previously called trivalent inactivated vaccine (TIV), and a live attenuated influenza vaccine (LAIV). The influenza vaccine should be administered as prophylaxis before flu season (generally October through March). All clients older than 6 months should be encouraged to receive an annual flu vaccine.
   a. LAIV in the form of a nasal mist is targeted for use in children older than 5 years through adults up to 49 years of age. **The American Academy of Pediatrics (AAP) policy recommendations note that healthy children older than 2 years can receive either the IIV or the LAIV.**
   b. A high-dose influenza vaccine is available for adults older than 65 years.
   c. The most current information available on the flu vaccines is noted on the CDC website (www.cdc.gov).
2. Antiviral therapy:

> Antivirals started within the first 48 hours confer the greatest benefit.

   a. Neuraminidase inhibitors oseltamivir (Tamiflu) and zanamivir (Relenza) are used for both treatment and chemoprophylaxis of the H1N1 influenza A virus.
   b. In December 2012, the Food and Drug Administration (FDA) expanded the use of Tamiflu to include children as young as 2 weeks of age.
   c. Zanamivir (Relenza) is approved only for children older than 7 years.
   d. Amantadine and rimantadine antivirals are not recommended for H1N1 because of resistance to other influenza strains.
   e. WHO recommends that clients with underlying medical conditions and pregnant women should receive treatment with oseltamivir (oral) or zanamivir (inhaled) as soon as possible after symptom onset without waiting for laboratory test results.
   f. Antiviral therapy recommendations vary by type of influenza, age group, renal function, and risk factor. To prescribe the most current antiviral therapy, refer to the CDC website for the most up-to-date recommendations (www.cdc.gov) and to the current AAP *Red Book: Report of the Committee on Infectious Diseases.*
   g. Oseltamivir should not be administered with an LAIV within 2 weeks before or 48 hours after treatment.
3. Acetaminophen or ibuprofen as needed for fever and myalgia
4. Healthcare providers should refrain from recommending cough suppressants and OTC cough medicines for young children because of associated morbidity and mortality. In response to the CDC's safety concerns, manufacturers of cough and cold medications for children voluntarily changed the products' labels to state that the medications should not be used for children younger than 4 years.

Follow-Up

A. Schedule a follow-up visit within 7 to 10 days if symptoms do not improve.
B. Monitor the client for pulmonary and neurological complications.
C. The local and state health departments are the point of contact for information about current influenza activity.

Consultation/Referral

A. Refer the client to a physician or neurologist for any complications.

Individual Considerations

A. Pregnancy:

1. Pregnancy predisposes the client to an increased risk for influenzal pneumonia.

2. Flu vaccine may be given to clients in high-risk populations. Because of the risk of influenzal pneumonia, many physicians recommend that pregnant women be vaccinated when an epidemic threatens.

3. Immunization of pregnant women is considered safe at any stage of pregnancy.

4. Zanamivir is the antiviral of choice for pregnancy because of limited systemic absorption.

5. Oseltamivir is used in pregnancy for women with asthma secondary to a higher risk for complications.

6. Both oseltamivir and zanamivir are pregnancy category C drugs.

7. Breastfeeding is not contraindicated during influenza.

B. Pediatrics:

1. Influenza A/H1N1 vaccine should be offered/administered before flu season (as early as September) to children with asthma and chronic lung problems and to those who are immunosuppressed.

2. Infants who are ill with H1N1 influenza A should continue to breastfeed.

3. Aspirin or aspirin-containing products (e.g., bismuth subsalicylate [Pepto-Bismol]) should not be given to children and young adults with viral illnesses before 21 years of age due to the increased risk of Reye's syndrome.

4. Reye's syndrome has been associated primarily with influenza B, but is also associated with influenza A infections.

5. Amantadine HCl and rimantadine HCl are not effective against H1N1 infections and are not FDA approved for use in children younger than 1 year.

C. Adults:

1. Persons in high-exposure occupations, such as teachers, healthcare workers, police, and firefighters, should consider yearly immunization.

2. Vaccine should be offered/administered to persons with chronic metabolic diseases, renal dysfunction, HIV infection, and immunosuppression.

Resource

CDC: www.cdc.gov/flu/professionals

Bibliography

Dolin, R. (2019, December 3). Epidemiology of influenza. Other pandemics and antigenic shifts. *UpToDate*. Retrieved from https://www.uptodate.com/contents/epidemiology-of-influenza?search=pandemic%20H1N1&source=search_result&selectedTitle=1~95~usage_type=default&display_rank=1

Influenza (Flu)

Jill C. Cash, Cheryl A. Glass, and Moya Cook

Definition

A. Influenza is a common, acute, viral infection that is a self-limiting, febrile illness of the respiratory tract. Illness is spread person to person primarily by respiratory secretions, which can be spread from infected persons through sneezing, coughing, talking, and self-inoculation of secretions through direct contact routes. Influenza is one of the top 10 causes of death in the United States when it occurs with pneumonia.

Incidence

A. Influenza epidemics occur yearly, primarily in the winter months, in both the northern and southern hemispheres. Travelers should be reminded that the flu season differs by hemisphere and can occur on cruise ships. Attack rates may be as high as 10% to 20% of the population. Mortality is highest in the geriatric population older than 65 years, except during pandemics, when 50% of influenza deaths occur in individuals younger than 65 years. Extraordinarily high attacks have occurred in the institutionalized and semiclosed populations.

Pathogenesis

A. Influenza A and B are viruses that have the ability to undergo periodic antigenic changes of their envelope glycoproteins, the hemagglutinin and neuraminidase. Among influenza A viruses that infect humans, there are three major subtypes of hemagglutinins (H1, H2, and H3) and two subtypes of neuraminidases (N1 and N2). Influenza A outbreaks typically start abruptly, peak over 2 to 3 weeks, and last approximately 2 to 3 months. H1N1 (swine flu) is an influenza A virus.

B. Avian flu was an H5N1 and H7N7 viral infection associated with recent exposure to dead or ill poultry. Following exposure, the incubation period for human H5N1 infection is 7 days or less. Clusters of human-to-human transmission of avian flu had a typical incubation period of 3 to 5 days.

C. Influenza B outbreaks are generally less extensive and less severe. Outbreaks associated with the B virus have been reported in schools, military camps, nursing homes, and cruise ships.

D. *Haemophilus influenzae* is a gram-negative coccobacillus. *H. influenzae* infection is an invasive bacterial disease that can cause meningitis, otitis media, sinusitis, epiglottitis, septic arthritis, occult febrile bacteremia, cellulitis, pneumonia, and empyema; occasionally, this virulent organism causes neonatal meningitis.

E. The incubation period for *H. influenzae* is between 18 and 72 hours to 5 days after exposure. The exact period of communicability for *H. influenzae* is unknown, but it may be for as long as the organism is present in the upper respiratory tract.

Predisposing Factors

The primary mode of spread is via exposure to viral strain–infected respiratory secretions from respiratory droplets (coughing or sneezing) and direct contact with contaminated surfaces.

A. Adults:

1. Aged older than 65 years (dependent on the viral strain)

2. Pregnancy:

3. High-exposure jobs: Teachers, healthcare workers, police, and firefighters

4. Recent illnesses or states that lower resistance (stress, excessive fatigue, poor nutrition)

5. Immunosuppression from drugs, illness, or chronic illness (transplant recipients, lung disease, heart disease, rheumatoid arthritis)

6. Crowded living conditions, including military camps and institutions such as nursing homes

7. Travel in endemic areas

8. Avian flu: Exposure to dead or ill poultry

B. Pediatrics:

1. Chronic pulmonary disease, including broncho-pulmonary dysplasia/chronic lung disease, asthma, cystic fibrosis, or any condition that compromises respiratory function

2. Congenital heart disease or abnormalities

3. Children younger than 5 years

Common Complaints

A. Clinical manifestations of influenza depend on the client's age and previous experience with the influenza virus. Children cannot verbalize symptoms such as myalgias and headache. Respiratory symptoms may be less prominent at the onset of illness in children and adults.

B. Rapid-onset respiratory illness is the most common complaint

C. Abrupt onset of fever and/or chills (children tend to run higher fevers)

D. Joint pain

E. Headache

F. Conjunctivitis (avian flu)

Other Signs and Symptoms

A. Upper respiratory congestion (watery eyes, clear nasal drainage, headache, sore throat, and hoarseness)

B. Malaise or fatigue

C. Anorexia

D. Swollen lymph nodes

E. Nonproductive cough (persisting for weeks)

F. Muscle aches

G. GI symptoms (children tend to have more nausea, vomiting, and poor appetite)

H. Febrile seizures

I. Otitis media

Subjective Data

A. Review the onset, course, and duration of symptoms, especially myalgia and malaise.

B. Ask the client about the timing of his or her last flu vaccination.

C. Review symptoms of other family members or coworkers who are also ill.

D. Check immunization status. For children, note whether *H. influenzae* b (Hib) vaccination is up to date.

E. Review the client's history for recent travel locations and travel by cruise ships/planes.

F. Evaluate living conditions for exposure risks.

G. Is the client a smoker?

H. Review all medications, including OTC and herbal products. Has the client taken any medications for the symptoms?

I. Does the client have a history of asthma or COPD?

J. Is the client immunocompromised (e.g., HIV, transplant recipient, chemotherapy)?

K. What other medical comorbidities, such as diabetes, does the client have?

Physical Examination

A. Check temperature, pulse, respirations, and BP.

B. Inspect:

1. Observe overall appearance for pallor and for any respiratory distress.

2. Assess hydration status.

3. Conduct eye and ENT examinations.

4. Children:

a. Observe for seizure activity.

b. Note level of activity (playful versus lethargic).

C. Auscultate:

1. Lung fields, observing for wheezing and crackles

2. Heart

D. Palpate:

1. Neck

2. Lymph nodes: Preauricular, posterior auricular, submental and sublingual, anterior cervical chain, and supraclavicular nodes

E. Neurological examination:

1. Assess LOC.

2. Assess for nuchal rigidity.

3. Assess for meningeal signs:

a. Signs of meningeal irritation include nuchal rigidity.

b. Positive Brudzinski's and Kernig's signs (refer to Figures 16.1 and 16.2):

i. Brudzinski's sign: Place the client supine and flex the head upward. Resulting flexion of both hips, knees, and ankles with neck flexion indicates meningeal irritation.

ii. Kernig's sign: Place the client supine. Keeping one leg straight, flex the other hip and knee to a bent knee to form a 90° angle. Slowly extend the lower leg. This places a stretch on the meninges, resulting in pain and spasm for the hamstring muscle. Resistance to further extension can be felt.

Diagnostic Tests

Usually no diagnostic testing is required. However, if the client appears ill, consider the following:

A. CBC (WBCs)

B. Viral RNA cultures: Obtain during the first 72 hours of illness, because the quality of virus shed subsequently decreases rapidly. Some evidence indicates that a throat sampling yields an improved specimen. Nasopharyngeal secretions obtained by swab or aspirate should be placed in an appropriate transport medium for culture.

C. Rapid antigen test: Usually less sensitive in the detection of influenza A than the PCR; a negative rapid diagnostic test should be confirmed with a viral culture or other means.

D. Monospot test: Test is negative with the flu and positive with mononucleosis

E. Chest radiograph (only if pneumonia is suspected)

F. Sputum culture (complications only)

G. Lumbar puncture (complications only)

H. Rapid plasma reagin (RPR) test (for high-risk HIV factors): Negative RPR to rule out syphilis

I. PCR assay: Can differentiate between influenza subtypes; offers high sensitivity and specificity but is not readily available for clinical use

Differential Diagnoses

A. Influenza:
1. Influenza A
2. Influenza B
3. Avian flu (H5N1)
4. H1N1 (swine flu)

B. Pneumonia

C. Bronchitis

D. Mononucleosis

E. RSV

F. Early HIV

G. SARS

H. Meningitis

Plan

A. General interventions:
1. Management is usually treatment of symptoms.
2. Encourage flu vaccine for clients in susceptible populations before the flu season begins.
3. *H. influenzae*, including both type b and non-type b infection and cases in fully or partially immunized children, should be reported to the CDC through the local and state public health departments. See Chapter 1, "Health Maintenance Guidelines," for Hib immunization information.
4. Influenza-associated pediatric deaths should be reported to the CDC through the state health department.
5. Clients should expect to have a persistent cough and malaise after the initial acute phase. Healthcare providers should refrain from recommending cough suppressants and OTC cough medicines for young children because of associated morbidity and mortality. In response to the CDC's safety concerns, manufacturers of cough and cold medications for children voluntarily changed these products' labels to state that the medications should not be used for children younger than 4 years.

▶ B. Client teaching: *See Section III: Client Teaching Guide for this chapter, "Influenza (Flu)."*

C. Pharmaceutical therapy:

Influenza can alter the metabolism of certain medications, especially theophylline, possibly resulting in the development of toxicity from high serum concentrations.

---

1. Acetaminophen (Tylenol) as needed for fever
2. NSAIDs are given as needed for body aches.
3. Antivirals started within the first 48 hours confer the greatest benefit. Antiviral therapy recommendations vary by type of influenza, age group, renal function, and risk factor. To prescribe the most current antiviral therapy, refer to the CDC website for the most up-to-date recommendations (https://www.cdc.gov/flu/professionals/antivirals/summary-clinicians.htm) and to the current AAP *Red Book: Report of the Committee on Infectious Diseases.*

4. Zanamivir (Relenza) is not recommended for persons with underlying airway disease, including asthma or COPD. Zanamivir is intended for uncomplicated acute illness due to influenza A or B in adults and children 7 years and older who have been symptomatic for no more than 2 days. Zanamivir is approved only for children older than 7 years.

5. Oseltamivir (Tamiflu) is intended for adults and adolescents 13 years of age or older who have been symptomatic for no more than 2 days. Special dosing is required for children who are younger than 13 years and/or weigh less than 80 oz. In December 2012, the FDA expanded the use of oseltamivir to children as young as 2 weeks of age.

6. Vaccination:
   a. The CDC's Advisory Committee on Immunization Practice (ACIP) and the AAP recommend annual influenza vaccination for all children aged 6 months to 18 years.
   b. Flu vaccine should not be administered to persons allergic to eggs.
   c. The vaccine should be administered in the autumn before the flu season begins, at least 6 weeks before the onset of the season.
   d. Immunization is the major means of influenza prevention. Each year the vaccine is produced to address the anticipated influenza strains. The vaccine may be trivalent or quadrivalent formulations.
   e. Two types of administration of the vaccine are available:
      i. IIV, previously called TIV, is administered IM.
      ii. LAIV is administered intranasally. The AAP and the American Academy of Family Physicians approved LAIV for the 2018–2019 influenza season for individuals who are healthy, non-pregnant, and 2 to 49 years of age, and who would not otherwise receive the influenza vaccine.
      iii. Recombinant vaccine (Flublok) does not use the influenza virus in chicken eggs during the manufacturing process and is available for those clients with an egg allergy. Flublok has a shorter shelf life and expires within 9 months of the production date.
      iv. Check the CDC website's for the current *Morbidity and Mortality Weekly Report (MMWR)* giving the current recommendations on vaccines for prevention and control of influenza.
      v. A high-dose influenza vaccine is also available for adults older than 65 years.
   f. The recommended site of vaccination in adults and older children is the deltoid muscle. The

anterolateral aspect of the thigh is the preferred site for flu vaccine for small children.

g. Oseltamivir (Tamiflu) should not be administered with an LAIV within 2 weeks before or 48 hours after treatment.

Follow-Up

A. Schedule a follow-up visit within 7 to 10 days if symptoms do not improve.

B. Monitor the client for pulmonary and neurological complications.

C. Local and state health departments are the points of contact for information about current influenza.

Consultation/Referral

A. Refer the client to a physician or neurologist for any complications.

Individual Considerations

A. Pregnancy:
1. Pregnancy predisposes the client to an increased risk for influenzal pneumonia.
2. The flu vaccine may be given to clients in a high-risk population. Because of the risk of influenzal pneumonia, many physicians recommend that pregnant women be vaccinated when an epidemic threatens.
3. Immunization of pregnant women is considered safe at any stage of pregnancy. Inactivated vaccine is safe for breastfeeding mothers and their children.
4. Zanamivir is the antiviral of choice for pregnancy because of its limited systemic absorption.
5. Oseltamivir is used in pregnancy for women with asthma secondary to a higher risk for complications.

B. Pediatrics:
1. Influenza vaccine should be offered/administered before the flu season begins (as early as September) to children with asthma or chronic lung problems, or those clients who are immunosuppressed.
2. The most common pediatric complication of influenza is otitis media. However, in young infants, influenza can produce a sepsis-like picture and occasionally can cause croup or pneumonia.
3. Aspirin or aspirin-containing products (e.g., bismuth subsalicylate [Pepto-Bismol]) should not be given to children and young adults with viral illnesses before 21 years of age due to the increased risk of Reye's syndrome.
4. Reye's syndrome has been associated primarily with influenza B, but is also associated with influenza A infections.
5. Amantadine HCl and rimantadine HCl are not effective against influenza B infections and have not been approved by the FDA for use in children younger than 1 year.
6. An increased incidence of convulsions has been reported in children with epilepsy who receive amantadine.

C. Adults:
1. Persons in high-exposure occupations, such as teachers, healthcare workers, police, and firefighters, should consider yearly immunization. Vaccine should

be offered/administered to persons with chronic metabolic diseases, renal dysfunction, HIV infection, and immunosuppression.

D. Geriatrics:
1. Influenza vaccine is recommended yearly for clients older than the age of 60 years. The vaccine should be offered to nursing home residents, especially those with a history of cardiopulmonary disease. Factors that contribute to more severe infections include decreased lung compliance and decreased respiratory muscle strength.
2. Pneumococcal pneumonia and influenza are significant causes of mortality and morbidity in the elderly.

Resource

CDC: www.cdc.gov/flu/professionals

Bibliography

Centers for Disease Control and Prevention. (2019). *Influenza (flu).* Retrieved from www.cdc.gov/flu

Immunization Action Coalition. (n.d.). *Healthcare personnel vaccination recommendations.* Retrieved from www.vaccineinformation.org

NEJM Journal Watch. (2003). *FluMist: Intranasal flu vaccine.* Retrieved from www.jwatch.org/jw200308290000004/2003/08/29/flumist-intranasal-flu-vaccine

Kawasaki Disease

Jill C. Cash, Cheryl A. Glass, and Moya Cook

Definition

A. KD is an acute febrile illness associated with generalized vasculitis. It was formerly known as mucocutaneous lymph node syndrome. KD is the leading cause of acquired heart disease in American children. Death results from myocardial infarction with coronary occlusion due to thrombosis or progressive stenosis. Approximately 75% of fatalities occur within 6 weeks of the onset of symptoms, but myocardial infarction and sudden death can occur months to years after the acute episode.

B. Although a febrile seizure may occur, there is no evidence that links KD with autism or a long-term seizure disorder.

C. Long-term prognosis is unknown. Second episodes rarely occur in previously affected children. Cardiac problems are the primary cause of morbidity and mortality from pericardial effusion, myocarditis, aneurysms, ectasia (coronary artery larger than normal for the child's age), and myocardial infarction. Current American Heart Association (AHA) guidelines stratify KD by its risk of myocardial infarction:
1. Risk Level I: Normal coronary arteries on all imaging studies
2. Risk Level II: Transient coronary artery ectasia or dilation that resolves by 8 weeks after disease onset
3. Risk Level III: Small to medium coronary artery aneurysms
4. Risk Level IV: Large (greater than 6 mm) aneurysms and coronary arteries with multiple complex aneurysms without obstruction
5. Risk Level V: Coronary artery aneurysms with obstruction documented on angiography

D. For children presenting with a rash and a persistent fever (greater than 5 days) the diagnosis of KD should be held at the forefront for workup for confirmation of KD secondary to the long-term cardiovascular sequelae. Diagnosis of typical syndrome requires fever of at least 5 days duration, plus four of the following:
1. Mucous membrane changes
2. Extremity changes
3. Cervical lymphadenopathy of at least 1 cm in size is the least consistent feature of KD. When present, it tends to involve the anterior cervical nodes overlying the sternocleidomastoid muscle.
4. Rash
5. Bilateral nonexudative conjunctivitis: Present in more than 90% of clients

Incidence

A. Peak age of occurrence in the United States is between 18 and 24 months. Approximately 80% of clients are younger than 5 years. Children older than 8 years rarely have the disease. KD has been noted worldwide and affects all races. Approximately 2% of clients experience KD a second time months to years later.
B. Approximately 1 in 5 children will develop coronary artery aneurysms.
C. The risk of myocardial infarction is greatest in the first 2 years after onset of KD.

Pathogenesis

A. The etiology of KD is unknown; it may be caused by viruses or bacteria such as group A *Streptococcus* (GAS). A microbial agent is favored because of the disease's acute, self-limited course, and community-wide outbreaks.
B. The incubation period is unknown.

Predisposing Factors

A. Age: Children younger than age 5
B. Gender: Incidence is higher in boys than in girls (2:1)
C. Asian and Pacific Island ancestry
D. Siblings of children with KD (possibly genetic)
E. Epidemics generally occur during the winter and spring seasons.

Common Complaints

A. Long-term fever (1–2 weeks) that does not respond to antibiotics. The fever ranges from 101°F to greater than 104°F. Fever may rise and fall for up to 3 weeks.
B. Bilateral bulbar conjunctival injection without exudate
C. Red, tender hands and soles of feet on days 3 to 5 following fever

> The classic finding in clients with KD is swollen, indurated, erythematous, and tender palms. Desquamation of the fingers and toes occurs approximately 1 to 2 weeks after onset of the fever, and a deep groove may cross the nails (Beau's lines).

D. Cracked, red, dry lips; tongue may appear coated, slightly swollen, and look like a strawberry; mouth ulcers
E. Irritability
F. Decreased food/fluid intake
G. One or more GI symptoms (vomiting, diarrhea, or abdominal pain)
H. One or more respiratory symptoms (rhinorrhea or cough)

Other Signs and Symptoms

A. Tachycardia (disproportionate to fever), gallop rhythms, and electrocardiogram (EKG) changes, including sinus tachycardia, QRS/QT prolongation, diffuse T-wave inversions, ventricular arrhythmias, and atrioventricular (AV) conduction defects, are suggestive of myocarditis
B. Pericarditis (often subclinical): Coronary aneurysms have been detected as early as 3 days after onset of symptoms, but in most cases they appear 1 to 2 weeks later. Carditis can occur at any time during the first 3 weeks of illness and generally resolves by 6 to 8 weeks.
C. Polymorphous rash that may be maculopapular, scarlatiniform, morbilliform, erythema marginatum, or rarely vesiculopustular; frequently confluent in the perineum, where it undergoes desquamation. **Rash involves the entire body, especially in the perineal region.**
D. Swollen cervical lymph node(s): The client may have a singular enlarged lymph node, usually a cervical node, up to 1.5 cm
E. Joint pain
F. Weakness
G. Urethritis with sterile pyuria (70% of cases)
H. Mild anterior uveitis (25%–50% of cases)
I. Arthritis or arthralgia
J. Photophobia

Subjective Data

A. Review onset, course, and duration of symptoms, especially fever.
B. Elicit the initial site of the rash and the progression to other body areas.
C. Determine if the client has had any new medication and contact exposures.
D. Rule out other family members with similar symptoms.
E. Review the client's history for recent strep infection.
F. Take a thorough history of symptoms and medication or treatment type and duration.

Physical Examination

A. Check temperature, pulse, respirations, and BP.
B. Inspect:
1. Inspect the client's skin, especially the hands, feet, and nails:
a. Rash: Polymorphous; may be maculopapular, scarlatiniform, morbilliform, erythema marginatum, or rarely vesiculopustular; frequently confluent in the perineum. (Bullae and pustules are not diagnostic of KD.)

b. The rash involves the entire body; only the face is spared.

c. Fine desquamation in the groin area can occur in the acute phase.

d. Check the nail beds for detachment (periungual lifting) and transverse grooves across the finger and toenail beds (Beau's lines).

e. Observe for facial swelling.

2. Conduct a thorough eye examination:

a. Bilateral bulbar conjunctival injection without exudate

3. Conduct thorough ear and nose examinations.

4. Perform an oral examination:

a. Red fissured lips with edema

b. Tongue may appear coated and slightly swollen (generally in the first 4–5 days); strawberry tongue after the membrane is shed

c. Posterior pharynx and palate—erythematous

5. Check hydration status.

C. Auscultate:

1. Heart: A persistent resting tachycardia and the presence of an S_3 gallop are often noted.

2. Lungs

D. Palpate:

1. Palpate the lymph nodes, especially the cervical area:

a. Lymphadenopathy is primarily noted in the anterior cervical nodes overlying the sternocleidomastoid muscles.

b. Size: At least 1.5 cm

c. Lymphadenopathy is the least common clinical symptom but may be present and most prominent in an older child.

2. Check the joints for swelling and tenderness.

3. Males: Check for testicular swelling.

4. Evaluate for splenomegaly.

Diagnostic Tests

No laboratory study proves diagnosis; diagnosis rests on clinical features and exclusion of the other illnesses in the differential diagnosis.

A. CBC with differential: Neutropenia

B. Erythrocyte sedimentation rate (ESR): Elevated

C. C-reactive protein (CRP): Elevated

D. Uric acid

E. Platelet count: Elevated platelet count (1 week after onset)

F. Serum transaminase: Elevated

G. Serum albumin

H. Specialty tests: Quantitative serum IG measurements, antinuclear antibody (ANA), rheumatoid factor (RF), Venereal Disease Research Laboratory (VDRL) test, immune complexes, and complement levels

I. Urinalysis: Proteinuria and sterile pyuria

J. Echocardiogram

K. EKG

L. Angiography may be needed.

M. Chest radiograph

Differential Diagnoses

A. KD

B. Streptococcal scarlet fever

C. Rubeola

D. Cat scratch disease

E. Drug reaction

F. RMSF

G. Infectious mononucleosis

H. Toxic shock syndrome

I. Other febrile viral exanthemas

J. Syphilis

K. Lyme disease

L. Juvenile rheumatoid arthritis

M. Stevens–Johnson syndrome

N. Staphylococcal scalded skin syndrome

O. Adenovirus

Plan

A. General interventions:

1. The most severe sequela is the development of a coronary artery aneurysm; therefore, prevention and early detection are important.

2. Initial therapy should be started within 10 days of illness, which reduces the risk of coronary artery aneurysm by fivefold. Management is initially aimed at reducing inflammation.

3. Use of intravenous immunoglobulin (IVIG) therapy has drastically reduced the incidence and morbidity and mortality of cardiovascular aneurysm.

B. Client teaching:

1. Teach parents which signs and symptoms indicate when to contact the office: Arthralgias, chest pain, and palpitations

2. Disease is not communicable by means of person-to-person contact; therefore, clients do not need to be isolated from other family members.

C. Pharmaceutical therapy:

1. The AHA and the AAP recommend the following: IVIG (2 mg/kg) administered as a single infusion over 8 to 12 hours within the first 7 to 10 days of the illness shortens the duration of fever and decreases the frequency of coronary artery aneurysms and other abnormalities. **IVIG is considered the gold standard for treatment of KD.**

2. As many as 20% of clients who receive the IVIG single infusion and aspirin may have a recurrent fever and require retreatment with IVIG 2 g/kg within 24 to 48 hours of persistent fever.

3. The AHA and the AAP recommend initial use of aspirin (acetylsalicylic acid [ASA]) 80 to 100 mg/kg/d given orally four times a day until afebrile. The maximum ASA dose should not exceed 4 g/d. Then ASA 3 to 5 mg/kg should be given orally per day for 6 to 8 weeks for its antiplatelet action.

4. Aspirin is continued until laboratory markers for acute inflammation (e.g., platelet count and ESR) return to normal, unless cardiac abnormalities are detected by echocardiogram.

5. Aspirin should be rapidly discontinued upon exposure to or sign of varicella or influenza due to the increased risk of Reye's syndrome.

6. Analgesic and antipyretic medications, such as acetaminophen (Tylenol) or ibuprofen, as needed for pain and inflammation.

7. The role of glucocorticoids remains unclear for treatment of KD. A single pulsed dose of IV methylprednisolone to the single dose of IVIG (2 mg/kg) does not significantly reduce the incidence of cardiac abnormalities.

8. Scheduled routine immunizations of inactivated childhood vaccines may be given at recommended intervals except for live virus vaccines such as varicella-containing vaccines and measles for children who have received IVIG. Varicella and measles vaccination may be given for an outbreak if the child's exposure is high and as long as the vaccination is repeated in at least 11 months after administration of IVIG.

9. Ibuprofen should be avoided in children taking aspirin because it may antagonize the antiplatelet effect of the aspirin.

Follow-Up

A. The prognosis of clients following KD depends on the severity of cardiac involvement. Refer the client to a pediatric cardiologist or physician for follow-up.

Consultation/Referral

A. Consult with a physician if fever persists longer than 5 days and KD is suspected.

B. Refer all affected children to a pediatric cardiologist for coronary artery evaluation.

C. Long-term management of KD is based on the extent of coronary artery abnormalities—risk level.

Individual Considerations

A. Pediatrics:

1. Most children are hospitalized for diagnostic evaluation and supportive care. Older children with mild disease may be managed on an outpatient basis.

2. Yearly influenza vaccination is indicated in clients 6 months to 18 years of age who require long-term aspirin therapy, because children taking aspirin have an increased risk of developing Reye's syndrome.

3. Children should have limited physical activity during convalescence. Restrictions should be prescribed by the cardiologist.

Resources

AAP: www.healthychildren.org/English/health-issues/ conditions/infections/Pages/Kawasaki-Disease.aspx

AHA Scientific Statement: Diagnosis, treatment, and long-term management of KD. Available at: https://www.ahajournals.org/doi/pdf/10.1161/CIR.00000000 00000484

KD Foundation: www.kdfoundation.org

Bibliography

Kawasaki Disease Foundation. (n.d.). Retrieved from www.kdfoundation .org

Sundel, R. (2018). Kawasaki disease: Clinical features and diagnosis. *UpToDate*. Retrieved from www.uptodate.com/contents/kawasaki-disease -clinical-features-and-diagnosi

Lyme Disease

Jill C. Cash, Cheryl A. Glass, and Moya Cook

Definition

A. Lyme disease is a multisystem infection that may be acute or chronic. Lyme disease is the leading vector-borne disease in the United States.

B. Morbidity from Lyme disease usually involves neurological/cognitive dysfunction and rheumatic conditions, causing arthralgias. Approximately 15% to 55% of untreated or inadequately treated clients develop some post–Lyme disease symptoms. Posttreatment Lyme disease syndrome (PTLDS) includes cognitive disturbances, fatigue, joint/muscle pain, headaches, hearing loss, vertigo, mood disturbances, paresthesias, and difficulty sleeping.

C. Proposed criteria for PTLDS include the presence of fatigue, musculoskeletal pain, and/or cognitive difficulties within 6 months of the diagnosis and persistence of symptoms for at least 6 months after completion of accepted antibiotic therapy.

Incidence

A. There were 262,481 cases of Lyme disease confirmed in the United States between 2007 and 2016. There is a seasonal increase between the months of April and October; more than 50% of cases occur in June and July. In the United States, the incidence is highest among children aged 5 to 9 years and in adults aged 45 to 54 years.

Pathogenesis

A. *Borrelia burgdorferi*, a spirochete bacterium, is the infectious agent found in 14 species of ticks in the United States. *Ixodes scapularis* is the principal vector in the midwestern states of Wisconsin, Minnesota, and Michigan and the eastern states from Maine to Georgia. *Ixodes pacificus* is the most prevalent vector in California and Oregon. Vector transmission is usually from the deer tick to humans. Rodents and pets can also harbor deer ticks.

B. The spirochete enters the bloodstream at the time of tick feeding. The incubation period is 3 to 32 days, or about 1 to 3 weeks after the bite. Late manifestations occur several months to more than 1 year later.

Predisposing Factors

A. People of all ages are affected

B. Recreational exposure:

1. Hiking

2. Golfing

3. Hunting

4. Soccer

C. Gardening
D. Exposure to rodents such as field mice and domestic pets, which may also carry the ticks

Common Complaints
A. Flu-like symptoms
B. Fatigue
C. Headache
D. Joint pain

Other Signs and Symptoms
A. Stage 1: Acute (early localized):
  1. Rash: Erythema migrans (see Figure 16.3)

FIGURE 16.3 Erythema migrans. Distinct bull's-eye appearance denotes Stage 1 of Lyme disease.

> Approximately 80% of infected persons develop a characteristic expanding erythematous rash, called erythema migrans. It usually begins as a red macule at the site of the tick bite and spreads out to form a large annular lesion with red secondary outer rings, an intense red outer border (measuring at least 5 cm), and some clearing at the site of the bite. Appearance is a "bull's-eye" shape. The lesion is generally painless and not pruritic.

  2. Body aches
  3. Fever or chills
  4. Swollen lymph nodes
B. Stage 2: Disseminated infection (early disseminated):
  1. Malaise, debilitating fatigue
  2. Headache
  3. Photophobia
  4. Mild neck stiffness
  5. Joint or muscle pain
  6. Migratory arthralgia
  7. Rash: Diffuse erythema
  8. Itching

  9. Transient heart block:
    a. In 5% to 10% of cases, clients have cardiac involvement—a transient heart block ranging from asymptomatic, first-degree AV block to complete heart block with fainting. The cardiac phase lasts 3 to 6 weeks.
  10. Bell's palsy: A unilateral or bilateral Bell's palsy is the most common cranial nerve deficit.
  11. Mild encephalopathy
C. Stage 3: Chronic (late disease):
  1. Prolonged arthritis:
    a. Approximately 60% of complaints evolve into frank arthritis. Onset of arthritis is variable but averages 6 months from the time of initial infection. The knee is the most common site and the pattern continues to be oligoarticular.
  2. Chronic neurological deficits
  3. Distal paresthesia
  4. Radicular pain
  5. Memory loss

Subjective Data
A. Review the onset, course, and duration of symptoms.
B. Ask the client about any recent outdoor activities, such as camping, hiking, or gardening. Fewer than half of the people infected remember a tick bite. A history of a tick bite is not necessary for diagnosis.
C. Have other family members had similar symptoms?
D. Obtain a thorough history of medications.
E. Review any history of rash and course of spread.
F. Rule out late symptoms associated with Lyme disease, such as arthritis, memory loss, and distal paresthesia.
G. Has the client been previously treated for Lyme disease or RMSF?

Physical Examination
A. Check temperature, pulse, respirations, and BP.
B. Inspect:
  1. Observe general overall appearance.
  2. Observe rash pattern and type.
  3. Inspect the skin; observe for target-like pattern.
C. Auscultate:
  1. Heart
  2. Lungs
D. Palpate:
  1. Palpate the lymph nodes and mastoid bones.
  2. Examine the joints for tenderness, swelling, and range of motion.
E. Neurological examination: Evaluate for signs of meningeal irritation by means of Brudzinski's sign and Kernig's sign (refer to Figures 16.1 and 16.2).
  1. Brudzinski's sign: Place the client supine and flex the head upward. Resulting flexion of both hips, knees, and ankles with neck flexion indicates meningeal irritation.
  2. Kernig's sign: Place the client supine. Keeping one leg straight, flex the other hip and knee to a bent knee to form a 90° angle. Slowly extend the lower leg. This places a stretch on the meninges, resulting in pain and

spasm for the hamstring muscle. Resistance to further extension can be felt.

Diagnostic Tests

A. CBC with differential
B. Sedimentation rate
C. Serum antibody: Enzyme-linked immunosorbent assay (ELISA) testing for *B. burgdorferi* (not present for several weeks)
D. Western blot if ELISA is positive
E. Lyme titer or culture for spirochete (after 20 days of signs and symptoms)
F. Arthrocentesis for joint effusion
G. PCR testing
H. ALT and AST: May be mildly elevated
I. Creatine phosphokinase
J. Lumbar puncture indicated for the presence of manifestations of meningitis

Differential Diagnoses

A. Lyme disease
B. Insect or spider bite
C. RMSF
D. Cellulitis
E. Arthritis
F. Bacterial meningitis
G. Chronic fatigue syndrome (CFS)
H. Viral syndrome
I. Nummular eczema
J. Tinea corporis (ringworm)

Plan

A. General interventions:
  1. **Prophylactic therapy after a tick bite is generally not advised.** It takes 24 hours from the time of tick contact with the skin to transmit the spirochete.
  2. Start prophylactic treatment with doxycycline for tick bites that are "swollen."
  3. Wait for the development of symptoms (e.g., erythema migrans) and treat promptly if the client becomes symptomatic.
  4. There is no evidence of the existence of "chronic Lyme disease." Some symptoms (fatigue, arthralgia, headaches) may last for several months; however, long-term antibiotic treatment has not proven to be effective and can contribute to a host of other adverse problems.
B. Client teaching:
  1. Client teaching: *See Section III: Client Teaching Guide for this chapter, "Lyme Disease and Removal of a Tick."*
  2. Not all neurological signs and symptoms completely resolve (such as headache, photophobia, Bell's palsy, and third-stage symptoms).
  3. Clients with active Lyme disease should not donate blood because spirochetemia occurs in early Lyme disease. Clients who have been treated for Lyme disease in the past can be considered for blood donation.
  4. Currently there is no vaccine for Lyme disease. The Lyme disease vaccine known as LYMErix was withdrawn in early 2002. Previously vaccinated clients are not protected against Lyme disease.

  5. Nonspecific symptoms may persist for months after treatment of Lyme disease. There is no evidence that the complaints represent ongoing active infection or need repeated antibiotics.
   a. Headache
   b. Fatigue
   c. Arthralgias
C. Pharmaceutical therapy:
  1. Early localized Lyme disease:
   a. Doxycycline: 14- to 21-day antibiotic course: Warn the client about photosensitivity:
     i. Adults: 100 mg, orally, twice daily
     ii. Children older than 8 years: 2 mg/kg orally twice daily (maximum 100 mg dose)
   b. Amoxicillin: 14- to 21-day antibiotic course:
     i. Adults: 500 mg orally three times a day
     ii. Children: 50 mg/kg (maximum of 1.5 g/d) orally divided into three doses
   c. Cefuroxime (Ceftin): 14- to 21-day antibiotic course:
     i. Adults: 500 mg twice a day
     ii. Children: 30 mg/kg (maximum 1,000 mg/d), divided into two doses
  2. Lyme carditis:
   a. Ceftriaxone (Rocephin): 75 to 100 mg/kg (maximum of 2 g/d), IM or IV infusion for 14 to 28 days
   b. Penicillin: 300,000 U/kg (maximum of 20 million U/d) given by IV infusion in divided doses every 4 hours for 14 to 28 days
  3. Neurological manifestations:
   a. Facial nerve paralysis: Use oral regimen for early disease for 21 to 28 days
   b. Lyme meningitis:
     i. Ceftriaxone (Rocephin): 14- to 28-day antibiotic course:
       1) Adults: 2 g IM or IV infusion once a day
       2) Children: 50 to 75 mg/kg (maximum of 2 g/d), IM or IV infusion
     ii. Penicillin: 14- to 28-day antibiotic course:
       1) Adults: 18 to 24 million U/d IV divided into 6 daily doses
       2) Children: 200,000 to 400,000 U/kg (maximum 18–24 million U/d) IV divided into six daily doses
   c. Possible alternatives for Lyme meningitis: Doxycycline 100 mg by mouth or IV infusion for 14 to 21 days
  4. Lyme arthritis:
   a. Same oral regimen as for early localized Lyme disease for a total of 28 days
   b. Ceftriaxone (Rocephin): 75 to 100 mg/kg (maximum of 2 g/d), IM or IV infusion for 14 to 28 days
   c. Penicillin: 300,000 U/kg (maximum of 20 million U/d) given by IV infusion in divided doses every 4 hours for 14 to 28 days

5. Pregnant women:
   a. Localized early Lyme disease: Amoxicillin 500 mg three times daily for 21 days
   b. Disseminated early Lyme disease or any manifestation of late disease: Penicillin G 20 million U/d for 14 to 21 days
   c. Asymptomatic seropositivity: No treatment is necessary

6. The Jarisch–Herxheimer reaction, with increased fever, chills, and malaise, can occur transiently when antibiotic therapy is initiated. NSAIDs may be beneficial, and the antimicrobial agent should be continued.

Follow-Up

A. Follow-up depends on the stage of disease.
B. Repeat the Lyme titer in 1 to 2 months to determine the need for continuation of antibiotic therapy.

Consultation/Referral

A. Referral to a physician is indicated when the client with strong clinical evidence of Lyme disease fails to respond to prescribed antibiotics.
B. Consultation with a physician is particularly important for those clients with refractory neurological deficits or debilitating arthritis.
C. Consultation with a rheumatologist is needed for clients with persistent arthritis or fibromyalgia occurring after Lyme disease.

Individual Considerations

A. Pregnancy:
   1. Maternal–fetal transmission of infection with subsequent injury to the fetus has been reported. Antibiotic treatment should be instituted promptly in symptomatic clients.
   2. Tetracyclines are contraindicated in pregnancy. Otherwise, therapy is the same as for nonpregnant persons.
   3. There is no causal relationship between maternal Lyme disease and congenital malformations.
   4. There is no evidence that Lyme disease can be transmitted in breast milk.
B. Pediatrics:
   1. Erythema migrans is the most common manifestation of Lyme disease in children.
   2. Carditis occurs rarely in children.
   3. The AAP recommends that children not be exposed to products containing more than 30% *N,N*-diethyl-*m*-toluamide (DEET) due to potential neurotoxicity.
   4. The AAP recommends that insect repellents not be used around children younger than 2 months.
   5. DEET repellent should not be applied to children's hands.

Resources

American Lyme Disease Foundation: https://www.aldf.com

American Lyme Disease Foundation. *Lyme Disease Tick Map* [Mobile application software]. Retrieved from https://www.aldf.com/iphone-application/

Bibliography

Centers for Disease Control and Prevention. (2018). *Lyme disease*. Retrieved from www.cdc.gove/lyme/treatment/index.html

Centers for Disease Control and Prevention. (2019). *Tick removal*. Retrieved from www.cdc.gov/ticks/removing_a_tick.html

Hu, L. (2018). Clinical manifestations of Lyme disease in adults. *UpToDate*. Retrieved from https://www.uptodate.com/contents/clinical-manifestations-of-lyme-disease-in-adults?search=Clinical%20manifestations%20of%20Lyme%20disease%20in%20adults.&source=search_result&selectedTitle=1-150&usage_type=default&display_rank=1

Meyerhoff, J. O. (2019). Lyme disease. *Medscape*. Retrieved from emedicine.medscape.com/article/330178-overview

Shapiro, E. D. (2019, August 31). Lyme disease: Clinical manifestations in children. *UpToDate*. Retrieved from https://www.uptodate.com/contents/lyme-disease-clinical-manifestations-children?search=Lyme%20disease:%20Clinical%20manifestations%20in%20children.&source=search_result&selectedTitle=1-150&usage_type=default&display_rank=1

Meningitis

Jill C. Cash, Cheryl A. Glass, and Moya Cook

Definition

A. Meningitis is an acute inflammation of the meninges, or membranes lining the brain and spinal cord. A virus or noninfectious insult, such as blood in the subarachnoid space, causes aseptic meningitis. Three baseline clinical features have been independently associated with adverse outcomes—hypotension, altered mental status, and seizures.
B. Vaccines are available for three types of bacteria that cause meningitis:
   1. *Neisseria meningitidis*: Polysaccharide or conjugate vaccines are available.
   2. *Streptococcus pneumoniae*: Pneumococcus vaccine
   3. *H. influenzae* type b (Hib) vaccine
C. Bacterial meningitis is a severe infection with associated complications including brain damage, hearing loss, neurological/learning disabilities, and digit or limb amputations. Mortality rates vary in part with the organism and in part with nosocomial versus community-acquired infection.

Incidence

The attack rate of bacterial meningitis in the United States is 2.5 cases per 100,000 persons; it has a 14.3% fatality rate irrespective of appropriate treatment. Approximately 1.2 million cases of bacterial meningitis occur annually worldwide. This disease is considered one of the top 10 infectious causes of death. Meningococcal meningitis (the bacterial form) can cause severe brain damage and is fatal in 50% of cases that are not treated.

The most common organisms causing bacterial meningitis are as follows:
A. Neonates:
   1. Group B *Streptococcus* (GBS)
   2. *Escherichia coli*
   3. *Listeria monocytogenes*
B. Ages 2 to 18 years:
   1. *N. meningitidis* with portal entry in the nasopharynx
   2. *S. pneumoniae*
   3. Hib
   4. The remaining cases are caused by GBS and *L. monocytogenes*.

C. Adults up to age 60 years:
1. *S. pneumoniae*
2. *N. meningitidis*
3. *H. influenzae*
4. *L. monocytogenes*
5. GBS
D. Adults 60 years and older:
1. *S. pneumoniae*
2. *L. monocytogenes*
3. *N. meningitidis*

Acute meningitis due to infectious causes usually does not recur. However, a small number of clients with acute meningitis may develop recurrent attacks between intervals of good health. Chronic meningitis is arbitrarily defined as meningitis lasting 4 weeks or more.

Pathogenesis
A. An acute inflammation of the meninges can be caused by *S. pneumoniae*, GBS, *H. influenzae*, *L. monocytogenes*, *N. meningitidis*, gonococci (rare), *Mycobacterium tuberculosis*, *E. coli*, pol herpes, gram-positive anaerobes, and *Bacteroides*, and as a sequela of Lyme disease and varicella (chickenpox)
B. The incubation period is variable; depending on the pathogen, it is usually 1 to 10 days. Transmission occurs from person to person through droplets from the respiratory tract and requires close contact.

Predisposing Factors
A. Peak demographics:
1. Children 4 years of age or younger; peak attack rate occurs in children younger than 1 year.
2. Adolescents
3. Freshman college students living in dormitories
B. Attendance at day care, school, camps, and the military
C. Sequela of Lyme disease
D. Odontogenic infection
E. Sequela of otitis media, bacterial sinusitis, Hib infection, and varicella
F. Sickle cell disease, asplenia, Hodgkin's disease, and antibody deficiencies
G. Review history for sexually transmitted and HIV infection.
H. Penetrating wound, head trauma, spinal tap, surgery, or anatomical abnormality
I. Occupational exposure such as laboratory personnel
J. Travel exposure
K. Maternal infection and fever at the time of delivery
L. Lumbar epidural steroid injections
M. Immunosuppression

Common Complaints
A. Classic triad:
1. Nuchal rigidity
2. Fever
3. Altered mental status

Other Signs and Symptoms
A. Neonates or infants:
1. Decreased LOC
2. High-pitched cry
3. Irritability, inconsolability
4. Fever and/or temperature instability
5. Poor feeding and/or vomiting
6. Bulging fontanelles
7. Seizures
8. Respiratory distress syndrome
9. Hypotonia
B. Children or adults:
1. Sudden onset of a severe, constant headache affecting the entire head that worsens with movement; CNS symptoms (nuchal rigidity, nausea and/or vomiting, confusion, lethargy, decreased LOC)
2. Fever or chills
3. Backache
4. Photophobia
5. Difficulty swallowing
6. Facial and eye weakness and sagging eyelids
7. Seizures
8. Rash: The type of rash—macular, maculopapular, petechial, or purpuric—depends on the virus/organism
9. Anorexia
C. Chronic meningitis: Usually have subacute onset of symptoms including fever, headache, and vomiting

Subjective Data
A. Review the onset, course, and duration of symptoms, including a progressive petechial or ecchymotic rash.
B. Determine current or recent history of ear infections, URI, sinus infection, and chickenpox exposure.
C. Ask the client about any recent dental procedures, extractions, and gum procedures.
D. Review the client's recent history of tick bite and any treatments.
E. Review the client's recent history of Hib immunization.
F. Evaluate for a history of serious drug allergies.
G. Evaluate for a history of recent head trauma/fracture.
H. Obtain a full history of any ventriculoperitoneal shunt and other cranial surgery/procedures.
I. Review history for use of lumbar epidural steroid injections for pain.
J. Review all medications, including OTC and herbal products. Determine recent use of antibiotics.
K. Review for a history of illicit drug use, especially the IV route.
L. Review any recent travel locations.
M. Neonates: Review pregnancy, labor, and deliver history for treatment for GBS.

Physical Examination
A. Check temperature, pulse, respirations, and BP.
B. Inspect:
1. Observe general overall appearance.
2. Examine the skin for the presence of a petechial or ecchymotic rash.
3. Complete an ENT examination.
4. Examine mouth and teeth for dental diseases and disorders.
5. Assess the client for dehydration.
6. Observe the client for seizure activity.

7. Assess level of pain.

8. Inspect for cranial nerve palsies.

C. Auscultate:

1. Lungs; monitor breathing pattern.

2. Heart

D. Palpate:

1. Neck: Palpate the lymph nodes.

2. Head: Palpate the fontanelle in children.

3. Palpate the mastoid bones.

4. Abdominal examination: Hepatosplenomegaly

E. Neurological examination:

1. Perform a complete neurological examination.

2. Evaluate for signs of meningeal irritation by means of positive Brudzinski's and Kernig's signs (refer to Figures 16.1 and 16.2):

a. Brudzinski's sign: Place the client supine and flex the head upward. Resulting flexion of both hips, knees, and ankles with neck flexion indicates meningeal irritation.

b. Kernig's sign: Place the client supine. Keeping one leg straight, flex the other hip and knee to a bent knee to form a 90° angle. Slowly extend the lower leg. This places a stretch on the meninges, resulting in pain and spasm for the hamstring muscle. Resistance to further extension can be felt.

Diagnostic Tests

The definitive diagnosis is from bacteria isolated from CSF and the presence of elevated protein and low glucose in the CSF.

A. Lumbar puncture to obtain CSF for analysis:

1. Gram stain

2. Absolute neutrophil count

3. CSF protein

4. CSF glucose

5. Culture and sensitivity

6. WBCs (pleocytosis)

B. Laboratory tests:

1. CBC with differential

2. Metabolic panel, including electrolytes, glucose, BUN, and liver profile

3. Coagulation profile

4. Platelet count

5. Blood cultures × 2

C. Cultures of petechial or purpuric lesion scraping and synovial fluid

D. MRI or CT scan, with and without contrast: A screening CT is not necessary in the majority of the clients.

Differential Diagnoses

A. Meningitis:

1. Bacterial etiology

2. Viral etiology

3. Fungal etiology

4. Aseptic meningitis

5. Chronic meningitis

B. Neonatal sepsis or pneumonia

C. Lyme disease

D. Herpes

E. Dementia

F. Gonorrhea

G. Otitis media

H. Dental abscess

I. Chickenpox

J. Sinusitis

K. Mastoiditis

L. Intracranial abscess

M. Encephalitis

N. Subarachnoid hemorrhage

Plan

A. General interventions:

1. Treat clients aggressively because the progression of disease is often rapid. Antibiotic therapy should be initiated immediately after blood cultures are drawn and the results of the lumbar puncture are available if the clinical suspicion is high.

2. Dexamethasone should be given shortly before or at the same time as the antibiotics if clinical/laboratory evidence suggests bacterial meningitis.

3. Maintain hydration.

4. In addition to standard precautions, droplet precautions are recommended until 24 hours after initiation of effective antimicrobial therapy.

5. Chemoprophylaxis is warranted for people who have been exposed directly to a client's oral secretions through close social contact, such as sharing of toothbrushes or eating utensils as well as child care and preschool contact within 7 days before the onset of the disease in the index case. Throat and nasopharyngeal cultures are of no value in deciding who should receive chemoprophylaxis and are not recommended.

6. Airline travelers with 8 hours of contact, who are seated directly next to an infected person, should receive prophylaxis.

B. Client teaching:

1. If a child suddenly develops a severely stiff neck along with fever and irritability, he or she needs medical help immediately.

2. Advise close contacts of the client with meningococcal and *H. influenzae* meningitis that prophylactic treatment with rifampin (Rifadin) may be indicated; they should check with their healthcare providers or the local public health department.

C. Pharmaceutical therapy:

1. Dexamethasone therapy should be considered when bacterial meningitis in infants and children (older than 1 month) is diagnosed or strongly suspected on the basis of the CSF tests, Hib meningitis, and pneumococcal or meningococcal meningitis:

a. Dexamethasone should be administered 15 to 20 minutes before the first dose of antibiotics.

b. The recommended dexamethasone regimen is 0.4 mg/kg every 12 hours for a total of two doses by IV infusion for the first 2 days of antibiotic treatment. A regimen of 0.15 mg/kg every 6 hours for 4 days is also appropriate.

2. Antibiotic therapy: Broad-spectrum coverage should be initiated until culture results are available. The doses vary by the organism. All antibiotics should be administered IV for at least 7 days. Empirical therapy may require adjustment after the culture results:

  a. Cefotaxime and ceftriaxone are commonly used as empirical therapy with *S. pneumoniae*, *N. meningitidis*, and *H. influenzae*. Vancomycin may be added to cefotaxime or ceftriaxone if renal function is normal until culture and susceptibility results are available:

  b. *Listeria* has traditionally been treated with ampicillin or penicillin G; gentamicin may be added for its synergistic effect.

  c. *Pseudomonas aeruginosa* is often resistant to most commonly used antibiotics. Ceftazidime has been the most consistently effective cephalosporin therapy.

3. Chemoprophylaxis in adults includes rifampin, ceftriaxone, ciprofloxacin, and azithromycin.

4. Vaccinations: Polysaccharide (alone or conjugate) meningococcal vaccines are licensed in the United States. Two types of vaccines protect against meningococcal serogroups A, C, W, and Y: meningococcal polysaccharide vaccine (MPSV4) and meningococcal conjugate vaccine (MenACWY). Recommendations include the following:

  a. MPSV4 is administered in a single 0.5 mL dose IM. For children younger than 18 months, two doses administered 3 months apart are recommended. MPSV4 can be given concurrently with other vaccines but administered at a different site. In school-aged children and adults, MPSV4-induced protection persists for at least 3 to 5 years. MPSV4 is the only meningococcal vaccine licensed for people older than 55 years.

  b. MenACWY recommendations:

    i. Preferred vaccine for people aged 2 months to 55 years who have received this vaccine previously, or who require multiple doses

    ii. All children/teens aged 11 through 18 years: The first dose is recommended between 11 and 12 years, with a booster at 16 years of age

    iii. Children aged 2 months to 23 months with complex disorders

    iv. First-year college students younger than 22 years of age, living in a residential hall

    v. People 2 months old or older at risk during an outbreak caused by a vaccine serogroup A, C, W, or Y meningococcal disease

    vi. People 2 months of age or older traveling to a country at risk for meningitis (Mecca, Saudi Arabia)

    vii. Microbiologists who work in a laboratory are at risk of meningitis

    viii. U.S. military recruits

    ix. Anyone taking the drug eculizumab (Soliris)

    x. Anyone whose spleen has been damaged or removed

    xi. Persons diagnosed with the rare immune disorder "persistent complement component deficiency"

  c. MPSV4 and MenACWY do not prevent serogroup B meningococcal disease. New vaccines are available to protect clients from meningococcal serogroup B: Trumenba and Bexsero.

  d. Immunizations with the pneumococcus, Hib, and influenzae vaccines also protect against bacterial meningitis.

Follow-Up

A. Have the client return to the clinic in 2 to 3 days if symptoms (e.g., otitis media) are not significantly improved with antibiotic therapy.

B. Follow-up depends on the client's symptoms. Schedule a return visit after completion of antibiotics or 2 to 3 weeks after the initial examination.

C. Sequelae associated with meningococcal disease occur in 11% to 19% of clients:

  1. Hearing loss
  2. Neurological disability
  3. Digit or limb amputations
  4. Skin scarring

D. Bacterial meningitis is a disease notifiable to the local health department. All presumptive, probable, and confirmed cases should be reported.

Consultation/Referral

A. Neonate: Consult with a physician if the client is younger than 3 months. Neonates need hospitalization.

B. Child: Consult with a physician:

  1. Exceptions: Localized, nonserious infections. The child should be active, playful, drinking, and voiding.

  2. The child needs immediate consultation with a physician if lethargic and inconsolable.

Individual Considerations

A. Pregnancy:

  1. The AAP lists the following indications for selective intrapartum chemoprophylaxis in GBS-positive women:

    a. Preterm labor and delivery
    b. Preterm rupture of membranes
    c. Rupture of membranes greater than 18 hours before delivery
    d. Intrapartum fever
    e. Multiple gestation
    f. Previous offspring with invasive GBS disease

  2. Maternal: Culture introital or vaginal and anorectal samples for GBS, using a selective medium such as Todd–Hewitt broth. Vaginal colonization of GBS occurs in 5% to 40% of pregnant women, of whom 40% to 70% transmit GBS to their offspring.

  3. The most significant problem associated with pregnancy is exposure of the fetus to GBS in the maternal genital tract. In 2002, the CDC, the AAP, and the American College of Obstetricians and Gynecologists recommended universal perinatal screening for vaginal and rectal GBS colonization at 35 to 37 weeks' gestation.

4. Treat clients with positive urine culture only because recolonization occurs frequently. Antibiotics should be administered to women in labor for preterm labor, premature rupture of membranes, positive GBS cultures (past or present), and preterm premature rupture of membranes in labor.

B. Pediatrics:

1. Neonatal sepsis occurs in approximately 1% to 2% of cases. In the United States, the risk of developing Hib invasive disease during the first 5 years of life is about 1:200.

2. Neonatal GBS infections *usually* present as early onset in the first 2 days of life and as late onset in newborns up to 3 months of age.

3. Premature neonates are at the highest risk for developing symptomatic neonatal disease.

4. Neonates often appear normal at delivery, only to develop a fulminant infection with rapid deterioration. Because of the severity and fulminant course of neonatal GBS infections, the primary focus is preventing the vertical transmission of the organism.

5. Infants up to 2 years old may have meningitis without a stiff neck.

6. All infants with meningitis should undergo careful follow-up examinations, including tests for hearing loss and neurological abnormalities.

C. Adults:

1. Immunization with the pneumococcal vaccination has been shown to decrease the incidence of bacterial meningitis.

D. Geriatrics:

1. Increased mortality rate for these clients secondary to the comorbid conditions

Bibliography

Centers for Disease Control and Prevention. (2018a). *Meningococcal disease.* Retrieved from www.cdc.gov/meningococcal/about/prevention.html

Centers for Disease Control and Prevention. (2018b). *Vaccine information statement: Meningococcal ACWY vaccines (MenACWY and MPSV4) VIS.* Retrieved from www.cdc.gov/vaccines/hcp/vis/vis-statements/mening .html

Centers for Disease Control and Prevention. (2019). *Meningitis.* Retrieved from www.cdc.gov/meningitis/index.html

Domingo, P., Pomar, V., de Benito, N., & Coll, P. (2013). The spectrum of acute bacterial meningitis in elderly patients. *BMC Infectious Diseases, 13,* 108. doi:10.1186/1471-2334-13-108

Hasbun, R. (2018). Meningitis. *Medscape.* Retrieved from emedicine .medscape.com/article/232915-overview

Hersi, K., & Kondamudi, N. (2018, October 27). Meningitis. *StatPearls.* Retrieved from https://www.ncbi.nlm.nih.gov/books/NBK459360/

Immunization Action Coalition. (n.d.). *Healthcare personnel vaccination recommendations.* Retrieved from www.vaccineinformation.org

Rodrigo, H. (2019, November 21). Treatment of bacterial meningitis caused by specific pathogens in adults. *UpToDate.* Retrieved from https://www .uptodate.com/contents/treatment-of-bacterial-meningitis-caused-by -specific-pathogens-in-adults?search=Treatment%20of%20bacterial %20meningitis%20caused%20by%20specific%20pathogens%20 in%20adults.&source=search_result&selectedTitle=1~150&usage_ type=default&display_rank=1

Rodrigo, H. (2020, February 5). Clinical features and diagnosis of acute bacterial meningitis in adults. *UpToDate.* Retrieved from https:// www.uptodate.com/contents/clinical-features-and-diagnosis-of -acute-bacterial-meningitis-in-adults?search=Clinical%20features%20 and%20diagnosis%20of%20acute%20bacterial%20meningitis%20 in%20adults.&source=search_result&selectedTitle=1~150&usage_ type=default&display_rank=1

World Health Organization. (2018). *Meningococcal meningitis fact sheet.* Retrieved from www.who.int/mediacentre/factsheets/fs141/en/

Mononucleosis (Epstein–Barr)

Jill C. Cash, Cheryl A. Glass, and Moya Cook

Definition

A. Infectious mononucleosis is an acute, infectious viral disease caused by EBV. EBV is also known as human herpesvirus 4 (HHV-4). There are three classic symptoms: fever, pharyngitis, and lymphadenopathy. The spread is via intimate contact between susceptible persons and asymptomatic EBV shedders through the passage of saliva.

B. Oral shedding may occur for 6 months after the onset of symptoms but before its latency phase.

C. The fatigue related to EBV may last several months.

Incidence

A. Antibodies to EBV have been demonstrated in all population groups, with a worldwide distribution. Approximately 95% of adults are EBV seropositive. Incidence is unknown; the disease occurs primarily in adolescents and young adults. The peak incidence of infection is noted in the 15- to 24-year age range. The majority of clients with primary EBV recover uneventfully.

Pathogenesis

A. EBV, also known as HHV-4, is the primary agent of infectious mononucleosis, and persists asymptomatically for life in nearly all adults. It is associated with the development of B-cell lymphomas, T-cell lymphomas, and Hodgkin's lymphoma in certain clients.

B. The incubation period is 30 to 50 days, with an average of 11 days; it is communicable during the acute phase, which may be prolonged. Acute symptoms resolve in 1 to 2 weeks. Pharyngeal excretion may persist for up to 18 months following clinical recovery. It is estimated that once a person is infected with EBV, the virus may be intermittently shed in the oropharynx for decades.

C. EBV has been isolated both in the cervix and in male seminal fluid, suggesting the possibility of sexual transmission.

D. EBV has been noted in breast milk.

Predisposing Factors

A. Age 12 to 40 years, with peak incidence between 15 and 24 years of age

B. Exposure through oropharyngeal secretions (kiss, cough, shared food)

C. Roommates

D. Intrafamilial transmission to siblings

Common Complaints

A. Infectious mononucleosis is characterized by the following triad of symptoms:

1. Fever

2. Tonsillar pharyngitis: Exudate may have a white, gray-green, or necrotic appearance

3. Lymphadenopathy: Usually posterior cervical chains; typically symmetric

Other Signs and Symptoms

A. Fatigue: May be persistent and severe
B. Generalized aches
C. Appetite loss
D. Headache
E. Hepatosplenomegaly: Mild hepatitis is encountered in approximately 90% of individuals; splenomegaly is noted in approximately 50%. Jaundice is uncommon.
F. Otitis media (infants and children)
G. Abdominal complaints and diarrhea (infants and children)
H. Upper respiratory symptoms (more prominent in young infants)

Subjective Data

A. Review signs, symptoms, and course and duration of symptoms, specifically the triad of pharyngitis, fever, and lymphadenopathy.
B. Assess the client for recent URI and sore throat.
C. Inquire about any contact with persons known to have mononucleosis and other infections such as strep infections.
D. Review the client's history for other family members with similar symptoms.
E. Carefully review medications. A mononucleosis syndrome with atypical lymphocytosis can be induced by drugs including:
  1. Phenytoin
  2. Carbamazepine
  3. Antibiotics such as isoniazid and minocycline

Physical Examination

A. Check temperature, pulse, respirations, and BP.
B. Inspect:
  1. Conduct an ENT examination, especially focusing on the tonsils and palate:
    a. Pharynx shows lymphoid hyperplasia, erythema, and edema.
    b. Tonsillar exudates are present in about 50% of the cases.
    c. Tonsillar pillars may touch "kissing tonsils" and lead to airway compromise.
    d. Evaluate for petechiae at the junction of the hard and soft palates.
    e. Evaluate for oral hairy leukoplakia (OHL) on the lateral portions of the tongue. OHL appears as white corrugated painless plaques that cannot be scraped from the surface. (EBV-related malignancies as well as HIV may present with OHL.)
C. Auscultate:
  1. Heart
  2. Lungs
D. Percuss:
  1. Abdomen, especially the spleen area
E. Palpate:
  1. Lymph nodes, especially anterior and posterior cervical chains, axilla, and groin. Firm, tender, and

mobile lymph nodes are indicative of mononucleosis; lymphadenopathy is usually symmetric and presents in the posterior cervical chain more than the anterior chain.
  2. Abdomen, especially the spleen. Splenomegaly is noted in 50% of cases. Hepatomegaly and tenderness are noted in 10% of cases.
F. Neurological examination:
  1. Evaluate for facial nerve palsy or symptoms of meningitis. See the "Meningitis" section in this chapter.

Diagnostic Tests

A. WBC count with differential and a heterophile test

A positive heterophile antibody test is diagnostic of EBV.

B. Throat swab for rapid strep; if negative, send for culture
C. Monospot test—not recommended for general use. Results may reflect a false-positive/negative result. Results do not confirm the absence of EBV infection since the heterophile antibodies detected by this test are often not present in children.
D. Viral capsid antigen (VCA):
  1. Anti-VCA IgM: Appears early and disappears in 4 to 6 weeks
  2. Anti-VCA IgG: Appears in the acute phase of infection, peaks at 2 to 4 weeks, declines, and remains positive for a person's lifetime
  3. EBV nuclear antigen: Performed by immunofluorescent test, not sensitive early in the acute phase but appears 2–4 months after onset and remains positive for life
  4. Elevated antibody levels are not diagnostic of recent infection and can be present for years
E. Cold agglutinin titer: Markedly elevated in the setting of hemolysis (greater than 1:1,000)
F. Liver function tests: Abnormal liver function tests in a client with pharyngitis strongly suggest the diagnosis of infectious mononucleosis (80%–90% of cases have elevated liver enzymes)
G. Abdominal ultrasound if indicated for splenomegaly

Differential Diagnoses

A. Mononucleosis
B. Streptococcal pharyngitis (group A beta-hemolytic *Streptococcus* [GAS])
C. Viral syndrome
D. Hodgkin's disease
E. Hepatitis
F. CMV
G. Secondary syphilis
H. CFS
I. Acute HIV
J. Toxoplasmosis
K. Adenovirus
L. Rubella
M. Acute HIV
N. HHV type 6 (HHV-6; roseola)
O. HHV type 7 (HHV-7)

Plan

A. General interventions:

1. Make certain that the client does not have an upper airway obstruction from enlarged tonsils and lymphoid tissue.

2. Treat concurrent infections.

3. Isolation is not required; ensure good hand-washing and prevention of the spread of pharyngeal secretions.

4. Bed rest is unnecessary.

5. There is no commercially available vaccine to prevent EBV infection.

6. Splenic rupture is rare but potentially life-threatening, occurring in 1 to 2 cases per 1,000. It occurs between the 4th and 21st days of symptomatic illness, but can be the presenting symptom. The typical manifestations are abdominal pain and/or a falling hematocrit.

B. Client teaching:

1. Client teaching: *See Section III: Client Teaching Guide for this chapter, "Mononucleosis."*

2. Prolonged communicability may persist for up to 1 year.

C. Pharmaceutical therapy:

1. Acyclovir is not recommended for infectious mononucleosis.

2. Antibiotic therapy is reserved for concurrent infections such as streptococcal pharyngitis.

3. Administer analgesics, such as acetaminophen or NSAIDs, for fever, body aches, and malaise.

4. Corticosteroids may be considered in the presence of overwhelming infections including mononucleosis-related airway obstruction or other complications, such as severe hemolytic or aplastic anemia.

Follow-Up

A. Examine the client every 1 to 2 weeks.

B. The initial monospot test may be negative.

C. If splenomegaly is present, schedule an appointment to reevaluate the client before the release for contact sports. **Splenomegaly puts clients at risk for rupture secondary to blunt trauma (i.e., sports and motor vehicle accidents).**

D. Clients with the classic triad symptoms of mononucleosis should also have a diagnostic test for strep since the presenting symptoms are so similar.

Consultation/Referral

A. Consult a physician for marked tonsil enlargement and difficulty swallowing or symptoms lasting longer than 2 weeks. An emergent consultation with an otolaryngologist may be required.

Individual Considerations

A. Pregnancy:

1. Intrauterine infection with EBV is rare.

B. Pediatrics:

1. Primary EBV in young infants and children is common and frequently asymptomatic.

2. Ampicillin and penicillin may cause morbilliform rashes.

C. Geriatrics:

1. Older adults may not present with the classic triad of symptoms.

2. Lymphadenopathy is not as common in older clients.

3. Pharyngitis and myalgia are the most frequent complaints.

4. Fever may be prolonged, lasting several weeks.

Bibliography

Aronson, M. D., & Auwaeter, P. G. (2019). Infectious mononucleosis in adults and adolescents. *UpToDate*. Retrieved from www.uptodate.com/contents/infectious-mononucleosis-in-adults-and-adolescents?topicKey=ID%2F8318

Centers for Disease Control and Prevention. (2018). *About Epstein–Barr virus (EBV)*. Retrieved from www.cdc.gov/epstein-barr/about-ebv.html

Cunha, B. A. (2018). Infectious mononucleosis. *Medscape*. Retrieved from emedicine.medscape.com/article/222040-overview

Mohseni, M., & Boniface, M. (2018). Mononucleosis. *StatPearls*. Retrieved from https://www.ncbi.nlm.nih.gov/books/NBK470387/

Mumps

Jill C. Cash, Cheryl A. Glass, and Moya Cook

Definition

A. Mumps is an acute systemic viral illness. The viral illness is self-limited. Humans are the only natural host for the mumps virus. Mumps is highly contagious among clients who are not immune by vaccination or through maternal antibodies.

B. The hallmark sign of mumps is unilateral swelling of one or more salivary glands. The parotid glands are typically involved unilaterally, then bilaterally. The swelling is visible under the ears and chin (see Figure 16.4).

FIGURE 16.4 Patient diagnosed with mumps exhibiting visible swelling under the ears and chin.

C. Mumps is spread by respiratory droplets, saliva, direct contact, or fomites. Current literature indicates that clients should be isolated for approximately 5 days from the onset of symptoms.

D. CNS involvement is the most common extra-salivary complication of mumps. Meningitis and encephalitis from mumps have a good prognosis and usually resolve with complete recovery.

E. There is no specific treatment for mumps except supportive therapy; mumps is most often treated on an outpatient basis.

F. Immunization: Either the live attenuated measles–mumps–rubella (MMR) vaccine or the measles–mumps–rubella–varicella (MMRV) vaccine may be used. The CDC recommends two doses of the MMR vaccine:

1. First dose given between 12 and 15 months of age
2. Second dose given between 4 and 6 years of age
3. Persons born after 1957 who have no laboratory evidence of immunity or documentation of MMR vaccination after 12 months of age should receive at least one MMR vaccination.
4. The CDC recommends two doses of MMR for healthcare workers, students entering college, and international travelers.
5. The MMR vaccine should be given 1 month before or 1 month after any other live attenuated vaccines such as varicella.
6. Common side effects of the MMR vaccination include low-grade fever, skin rash, itching, hives, redness and swelling at the immunization site, and weakness.
7. Severe adverse side effects of the MMR vaccination include seizures; encephalopathy; thrombocytopenia; joint, muscle, and nerve pain; GI disorders; and conjunctivitis.
8. The MMR vaccine may be given with other vaccines at different injection sites and given in separate syringes.

Incidence

A. Mumps occurs worldwide. Since the implementation of the vaccine, there had been a greater than 99% decrease in the number of reported cases in the United States. Reported cases of mumps in the United States were higher in 2016 and 2017 than they had been in the previous decade.

B. The highest incidence is among African Americans.

C. Males and females are affected equally with parotitis.

D. Symptomatic meningitis is more common in males: 3:1 ratio over females

Pathogenesis

A. Mumps is caused by *Rubulavirus*, a specific RNA virus. *Rubulavirus* is in the genus *Paramyxovirus* and is a member of the Paramyxoviridae family. It shares morphologic features with the human parainfluenza; however, there is no cross-immunity between the two.

B. Mumps shares characteristics with other pediatric illnesses, including measles and rubella.

C. Mumps has an incubation of 16 to 18 days. Incubation can be as early as 7 days and as late as 23 days. Infectious period is approximately 3 days before to 9 days after the onset of symptoms. The illness lasts an average of 7 to 10 days.

Predisposing Factors

A. Lack of immunization
B. International travel
C. Immune deficiencies

D. Age groups:
  1. Primary school ages
  2. High school ages
  3. College ages
  4. Occupational exposure

E. Crowded settings such as day-care facilities and military bases

Common Complaints

A. Asymptomatic (20%–30%)

B. Prodromal symptoms may last 3 to 5 days:
  1. Low-grade fever
  2. Headache
  3. Anorexia
  4. Malaise
  5. Myalgias

C. About 48 hours after the prodromal period, the most common symptom is parotitis (30%–40%) caused by direct viral infection of the ductal epithelium:
  1. Unilateral initially, then bilateral parotitis:
    a. Tenderness/pain with pressure
    b. Edema: May last for 10 days
  2. Males:
    a. Unilateral orchitis: Uncommon in males younger than 10 years of age but occurs in 33% of postpubertal males
    b. Bilateral orchitis occurs in about 10% of cases
    c. Orchitis develops within 1 to 2 weeks of parotitis
    d. High fever
    e. Severe testicular pain accompanied by swelling and scrotal erythema
    f. Nausea, vomiting, and abdominal pain with orchitis
  3. Females: Oophoritis (7%)
  4. Aseptic meningitis: Usually presents within the first week after parotid swelling:
    a. Headache
    b. Fever
    c. Nuchal rigidity
    d. Nausea and vomiting

Other Signs and Symptoms

A. Earache on the same side as the parotitis

B. Acute pancreatitis (5% incidence):
  1. Abdominal distention
  2. Pain
  3. Fever (usually low grade)
  4. Nausea and vomiting

C. Thyroiditis

D. Mastitis

E. Encephalitis (5 cases per 1,000 mumps cases)

Potential Complications

A. Meningitis
B. Encephalitis
C. Gonadal atrophy (20%–50% in postpubertal males)
D. Sterility (rare)
E. Guillain–Barré syndrome

F. Sensorineural deafness (0.5–5 cases per 100,000 cases):
1. Up to 20% is bilateral deafness
2. Often deafness is permanent
G. Impaired renal function/glomerulonephritis
H. Miscarriage if pregnant

Subjective Data
A. Review the onset and duration of symptoms.
B. Rule out similar symptoms in other family members.
C. Review the client's immunization history.
D. Determine any new contact exposures.
E. Determine if the client is pregnant.
F. Ask the client to list all medications, including OTC and herbal products.

Physical Examination
A. Check temperature, pulse, respirations, and BP.
B. Inspect:
1. Visually inspect the face, under/behind the ears, and the chin for edema.
2. Conduct an ear, nose, throat, and mouth examination.
3. Make a visual inspection of the scrotum.
C. Auscultate:
1. Lungs (at risk for pneumonia)
2. Heart (at risk for myocarditis)
D. Palpate:
1. Palpate the parotid glands.
2. Palpate the neck and lymph glands, especially the cervical chains.
3. Palpate the abdomen.
4. Gently palpate the scrotum.
E. Neurological examination:
1. Assess hearing: May be unilateral loss
2. Evaluate for signs of meningeal irritation by means of Brudzinski's and Kernig's signs (refer to Figures 16.1 and 16.2):
   a. Brudzinski's sign: Place the client supine and flex the head upward. Resulting flexion of both hips, knees, and ankles with neck flexion indicates meningeal irritation.
   b. Kernig's sign: Place the client supine. Keeping one leg straight, flex the other hip and knee to a bent knee to form a 90° angle. Slowly extend the lower leg. This places a stretch on the meninges, resulting in pain and spasm for the hamstring muscle. Resistance to further extension can be felt.

Diagnostic Tests
A. Serum amylase level increase supports the diagnosis.
B. Serum lipase
C. Mumps IgM and IgG: Not required if the client has a classic presentation of parotitis
D. Other tests as indicated for presenting symptoms of complications

Differential Diagnosis
A. Mumps
B. CMV
C. Parainfluenza virus 1 and 3
D. Influenza A
E. HIV
F. Bacterial infection
G. Drug reaction
H. Coxsackievirus
I. EBV
J. Adenovirus
K. Bacterial infections, particularly *Staphylococcus aureus*

Plan
A. General interventions:
1. There is no medication prescribed for the mumps.
2. Symptomatic treatment is recommended for comfort.
3. Clients with complications, such as severe nausea/vomiting, may be hospitalized for IV hydration.
4. Monitor for severe complications such as meningitis or pancreatitis. Hospitalization may be required.
5. Notify the local public health department of active cases of the mumps.
B. Client teaching:
1. **The AAP and the CDC recommend that infected children not attend school/child care until 5 days after parotid swelling begins to subside.**
2. Stress universal precautions. The mumps virus can be found in the saliva, throat, and urine of the person infected.
   a. Practice good handwashing techniques.
   b. Use droplet precautions: Cover the mouth and nose with a tissue when coughing and sneezing and dispose of the tissue immediately.
   c. Do not share food or drink with the person with mumps.
3. Encourage rest.
4. Apply warm or cold packs to the parotid glands for comfort.
5. Add scrotal elevation/support and ice pack compresses.
C. Pharmaceutical therapy:
1. Antiviral agents are not indicated for mumps.
2. Ig has not been shown to be effective as a postexposure therapy.
3. Analgesics, such as acetaminophen or ibuprofen, are prescribed for headache and parotitis.
D. Dietary management:
1. There is no special diet for the mumps. However, clients should avoid acidic fluids and liquids, such as orange juice. Acid-containing foods may cause pain and difficulty swallowing with parotitis.
2. Encourage drinking of fluids.

Follow-Up
A. Follow-up is determined by the client's needs, severity of the symptoms, and the presence of complications.
B. Notify the local health department if mumps occurs in a child-care setting. Persons exempted from vaccination for medical, religious, or other reasons should be excluded for school/day care until at least 26 days after the onset of parotitis in the last person with mumps in the affected family.

Consultation/Referral

A. Consult with a physician for evaluation and need for hospital admission for complications.

Individual Considerations

A. Pregnancy:
   1. There is no evidence that the mumps causes congenital abnormalities.
   2. Vaccinated women should avoid pregnancy for 3 months after immunization.
   3. Termination of pregnancy is not indicated if the MMR vaccination is given during pregnancy.
B. Pediatrics:
   1. Infants born to mothers who have mumps a week before delivery may have clinically apparent mumps at birth or mumps may develop in the neonatal period.

Bibliography

Albrecht, M. A. (2019). Epidemiology, clinical manifestations, diagnosis and management of mumps. *UpToDate*. Retrieved from http://www.uptodate.com/contents/epidemiology-clinical-manifestations-diagnosis-and-management-of-mumps

Defendi, G. L. (2019). Mumps. *Medscape*. Retrieved from reference.medscape.com/article/966678-overview

Immunization Action Coalition. (n.d.). Healthcare personnel vaccination recommendations. Retrieved from www.vaccineinformation.org

National Vaccine Information Center. (n.d.). *Quick facts mumps*. Retrieved from www.nvic.org/vaccines-and-diseases/Mumps.aspx

Parvovirus B19 (Fifth Disease, Erythema Infectiosum)

Jill C. Cash, Cheryl A. Glass, and Moya Cook

Definition

A. Parvovirus B19, also known as "fifth disease," is considered one of the TORCH infections.
B. In children, parvovirus B19 can cause erythema infectiosum (EI), a mild febrile illness with rash. EI is also referred to as "fifth disease" since it represents one of six common childhood exanthems, each named in the order of dates they were first described. In contrast, clients with underlying hemolytic disorders can develop a transient aplastic crisis (TAC). Parvovirus B19 is an acute, communicable, viral infection that is spread by means of respiratory droplet and transplacental transmission. It can be associated with chronic hemolytic anemia and, in pregnancy, has been associated with nonimmune fetal hydrops and fetal death in 2% to 6% of cases (see Figure 16.5).

FIGURE 16.5 Infant with parvovirus B19.

C. Parvovirus B19 is the only infectious cause of TAC in more than 80% of clients with sickle cell disease.
D. The polyarthropathy associated with parvovirus B19 typically lasts 1 to 3 weeks; however, the arthritis may be prolonged, and parvovirus should be considered in the differential diagnosis of newly diagnosed rheumatoid arthritis
E. Parvovirus B19's rash may be confused with rubella.
F. There is no vaccine that can prevent parvovirus B19 infection.

Incidence

A. Parvovirus B19 occurs primarily in school-aged children between 5 and 15 years old; it rarely affects adults. Parvovirus occurs worldwide and is extremely common; however, the true incidence is unknown. Outbreaks are more usual in late winter and early spring. As many as 60% of the infections occur during the school year. Because fewer than 1% of teachers who are pregnant during EI outbreaks are expected to experience an adverse fetal outcome, exclusion of pregnant women from employment in child care or teaching is not recommended.

Pathogenesis

A. Human parvovirus B19 belongs to the *Erythrovirus* genus within the Parvoviridae family. Human parvovirus B19 is a DNA virus with preference for erythroid precursor cells. The virus replicates in the erythroid progenitor cells of the bone marrow and blood, leading to inhibition of erythropoiesis, which can result in symptoms of anemia. The parvovirus-associated rash is presumed to be at least partially immune mediated.
B. The incubation period for initial symptoms to develop is 4 to 14 days after exposure; the rash usually lasts 5 days, but can last as long as 21 days. Parvovirus B19–specific IgM antibodies are detected at days 10 to 12 and can persist for up to 5 months. Rash and joint symptoms occur 2 to 3 weeks after acquisition of infection.
C. The annual seroconversion rate among pregnant women without parvovirus B19 is 1.5%.

Predisposing Factors

A. The only known host for parvovirus B19 is humans.
B. Exposure to school-aged (through junior high) and day-care populations
C. Occupational exposure for teachers (20%), day-care workers and homemakers (9% each), and healthcare workers
D. Exposure to close contact or crowded conditions

Common Complaints

A. The clinical presentation is influenced by the infected individual's age and hematological and immunological status.
B. Approximately 25% of infected individuals are asymptomatic; 50% have nonspecific flu-like symptoms of malaise, muscle pain, and fever.
C. Classic symptoms:
   1. Red rash on the face that spreads to the rest of the body. **An erythematous, macular rash on the cheeks produces a "slap-cheek" pattern.**

2. Arthritis: Joint pain most frequently affects the hands, followed by the knees and wrists. Joint symptoms are more common in adults and may be the sole manifestation of infection. Joint pain is more common in women. The arthritis associated with acute parvovirus B19 infection does not cause joint destruction.

3. Edema

Other Signs and Symptoms

A. Adults: Chronic arthropathy
B. Child:
1. Bright-red rash on cheeks; may be confused with rubella
2. Maculopapular rash on trunk and extremities; may be pruritic
3. Circumoral pallor
4. Malaise
5. Headache
6. Sore throat and pharyngitis
7. Conjunctivitis
8. Diarrhea
C. Fetus:
1. Nonimmune hydrops fetalis
2. Stillbirth
3. Anemia

Subjective Data

A. Review the onset, duration, and course of symptoms.
B. Elicit the initial site of rash and progression to other body areas.
1. Determine if the rash is pruritic, especially on the soles of the feet.
C. Elicit job exposure for schoolteachers and day-care workers.
D. Determine if the client is pregnant.
E. Determine whether the client has had any new medication or contact exposures.
F. Rule out other family members with similar symptoms.
G. Ask about pain in the joints—usually in the hands, feet, or knees.
H. Review all medications, including OTC and herbal products.

Physical Examination

A. Check temperature, pulse, respirations, and BP.
B. Inspect:
1. Observe the rash pattern.
a. Erythematous malar "slapped-cheek sign" rash on the face is the typical facial erythema. **The facial rash is the most recognized feature.**
b. "Lacy"-patterned rash over the chest, back, buttocks, arms, and legs.
2. Conduct an ENT examination.
C. Palpate:
1. Blanch the rash area: A rash over the extremities blanches with pressure, heat or cold, and sunlight.
2. Palpate the spleen: Splenomegaly is a hallmark sign.

3. Palpate the lymph nodes: Enlarged lymph nodes, especially the posterior cervical nodes, are indicative of infection.
4. Assess the joints for tenderness, swelling, and range of motion.

Diagnostic Tests

A. CBC with differential: The hallmark laboratory finding is the dramatic decrease or absence of measurable reticulocytes.
B. Parvovirus IgG and IgM antibodies: Approximately 30% to 60% of adults have positive antibodies.
C. PCR test
D. Pregnancy test if necessary
E. Fetal assessment:
1. Ultrasonography to evaluate for fetal hydrops. Fetal ascites and pleural and pericardial effusions are evident on ultrasonogram (nonimmune hydrops fetalis).
2. PUBS to evaluate for fetal infection and anemia may be performed.

Differential Diagnoses

A. Parvovirus B19 (fifth disease)
B. Rubella
C. Aplastic crisis
D. Other viral infection
E. Contact dermatitis
F. Medication allergies
G. Chronic anemia

Plan

A. General interventions:
1. Management is usually supportive treatment of symptoms.
2. Analgesics for joint pain
3. Antipyretics for increased temperature
4. Starch bath for pruritus
5. Disease is self-limiting without treatment.
6. Immunosuppressed clients respond well to IVIG.
7. Aplastic crises may require transfusion.
B. Client teaching:
1. Educate pregnant and immunocompromised clients to avoid exposure.
2. Routine infection control practices minimize the risk of transmission, including handwashing and droplet precautions. Avoiding sharing food or drinks may partially prevent the spread of parvovirus B19.
3. The disease is most communicable before the rash appears; it is not communicable after rash outbreak.
C. Pharmaceutical therapy:
1. Acetaminophen (Tylenol) for fever
2. NSAIDs for symptomatic relief
3. Ig prophylaxis is not recommended by the CDC at this time.
4. There is no vaccine to prevent parvovirus B19.

Follow-Up

A. None is recommended, as the disease is self-limiting for low-risk population.

Consultation/Referral

A. The incidence of acute parvovirus B19 in pregnancy is 3.3% to 3.8%. Refer pregnant clients to a perinatologist for fetal evaluation for acute exposure in pregnancy.

B. Consult or refer the client to a physician immediately for exposure of immunocompromised clients, who might require a blood transfusion.

Individual Considerations

A. Pregnancy:
1. A positive IgG antibody and a negative IgM antibody indicate maternal immunity, in which case the fetus is protected from infection. A positive IgM antibody is consistent with acute parvovirus infection.
   a. If testing is negative for IgG and IgM after recent parvovirus exposure, PCR testing for maternal parvovirus B19 DNA should be performed.
2. Parvovirus B19 is not teratogenic. Fetal risks are related to the trimester of exposure. Nonimmune hydrops fetalis occurs secondary to hemolysis and inadequate production of erythrocytes. Other risks include spontaneous abortion, intrauterine growth restriction, stillbirth, and neonatal death.
3. Women who are diagnosed with acute infection beyond 20 weeks' gestation should receive periodic ultrasounds (although serial ultrasounds are commonly performed).
4. Intrauterine blood transfusion may be performed if severe anemia is confirmed.
5. Delivery and postnatal management of the hydropic infant should occur in a tertiary care center. The majority of these infants will require respiratory assistance and mechanical ventilation.

B. Pediatrics:
1. Neonates who had hydrops attributed to parvovirus B19 in utero do not require isolation if the hydrops is resolved by delivery.
2. Most children born to mothers who develop parvovirus B19 infection in pregnancy do not appear to suffer long-term sequelae; the infection does not appear to cause long-term neurological morbidity.
3. Children with abnormal red blood cells (sickle cell disease, hereditary spherocytosis, thalassemia) can develop transient aplastic anemia and may require multiple transfusions.
4. Children may attend child care or school once the rash appears since they are no longer contagious.

C. Adults:
1. Clients may have arthritis and arthralgias lasting months to years after exposure.
2. Adults may initially be asymptomatic.
3. Immunocompromised clients may develop severe, chronic anemia.
4. Working women with young children may benefit from prenatal testing and limiting exposure in pregnancy.

Bibliography

Jordan, J. A. (2019). Clinical manifestations and pathogenesis of human parvovirus B19 infection. *UpToDate*. Retrieved from www .uptodate.com/contents/clinical-manifestations-and-pathogenesis -of-human-parvovirus-b19-infection?topicKey=ID%2F8272

Kostolansky, S., & Waymack, J. (2019, January 23). Erythema infectiosum (fifth disease). *StatPearls*. Retrieved from https://www.ncbi.nlm.nih .gov/books/NBK513309/

Riley, L. E., & Fernandes, C. J. (2019, January 24). Parvovirus B19 infection during pregnancy. *UpToDate*. Retrieved from https://www .uptodate.com/contents/parvovirus-b19-infection-during-pregnancy? search=Parvovirus%20B19%20infection%20during%20pregnancy .&source=search_result&selectedTitle=1~150&usage_type=default& display_rank=1

Rheumatic Fever

Jill C. Cash, Cheryl A. Glass, and Moya Cook

Definition

A. Acute rheumatic fever (ARF) is an autoimmune inflammatory process that occurs as a sequela of a GAS tonsillopharyngitis. Rheumatic fever is a preventable disease through the detection and adequate treatment of streptococcal pharyngitis.

B. The individual who has had rheumatic fever is at very high risk of developing recurrences after subsequent GAS pharyngitis and needs continuous antimicrobial prophylaxis to prevent such recurrences (secondary prevention). The most significant complication of ARF is rheumatic heart disease, which occurs after repeated bouts of acute illness.

Incidence

A. The incidence of rheumatic fever is 19 per 100,000 worldwide, but is lower in the United States (2–14 cases per 100,000) following ineffectively treated cases of GAS URIs. ARF is most common among children 5 to 15 years. It is relatively rare in infants and uncommon in preschool-aged children. The incidence of first episodes falls steadily after adolescence and is rare after 30 years of age. The disease does not seem to have a major racial predisposition. Approximately 20% of children diagnosed with rheumatic fever have a positive history of pharyngitis; only 35% to 60% recall having any upper respiratory symptoms within the preceding 3 months.

B. Cardiac involvement is the most serious complication. Morbidity due to congestive heart failure (CHF), stroke, and endocarditis is common among individuals with rheumatic heart disease, and about 1.5% of persons with rheumatic carditis die of the disease annually. Mitral stenosis and Sydenham chorea are more common in females who have gone through puberty.

Pathogenesis

A. Rheumatic fever is caused by a preceding infection with GAS and *Streptococcus pyogenes*. Nonsuppurative inflammatory lesions of the joints, heart, subcutaneous tissue, and CNS characterize ARF. The incubation period is between 1 and 5 weeks and 6 months after GAS pharyngitis.

Predisposing Factors

A. Group A pharyngitis, untreated or inadequately treated
B. Age 5 to 15 years
C. Crowded living conditions
D. Occupational exposure: Teachers, healthcare providers, and military personnel

E. Most common in tropical countries

F. Gender: More common in females

Common Complaints

A. Sore throat (generally of sudden onset), pain on swallowing

B. Joint pain/arthralgia to frank polyarthritis is usually symmetrical and involves large joints such as the knees, ankles, elbows, and wrists. Joints feel warm, swollen, and inflamed. **Polyarthritis is the most common manifestation. Both synovitis and periarticular inflammation occur, especially in the knees and ankles. There may be erythema of the overlying skin.**

C. Fever varies from 101°F to 104°F.

Other Signs and Symptoms

A. Fatigue

B. Appetite loss

C. Sydenham chorea (more common in girls): Chorea, a CNS disorder lasting 1 to 3 months, is purposeless, involuntary, rapid movements often associated with muscle weakness, involuntary facial grimaces, speech disturbance, and emotional liability. Sydenham chorea usually resolves with permanent damage but occasionally lasts 2 to 3 years.

D. Subcutaneous nodules are firm, painless nodules that are seen or felt over the extensor surface of certain joints, particularly the elbows, knees, and wrists; in the occipital region; or over the spinous processes of the thoracic and lumbar vertebrae. The skin overlying them moves freely and is not inflamed.

E. Erythema marginatum is an evanescent, nonpruritic, pink rash with pale centers and round or wavy margins. Lesions vary greatly in size and occur mainly on the trunk and extremities; they are rarely seen on the face. Erythema is transient, migrates from place to place, and may be brought out by the application of heat.

F. Enlarged lymph nodes

G. Headache

H. Carditis: Development of new heart murmurs, cardiomegaly, and CHF

I. Pericarditis, pericardial friction rub, and/or pericardia effusion

J. Aortic regurgitation, manifested by:
1. Palpitations
2. Dyspnea on exertion
3. Angina at rest

Subjective Data

A. Review a recent history (1–3 months) of sore throat and the onset, duration, severity, and treatment of symptoms.

B. Complete a drug history. Did the client finish the prescribed antibiotics? Does the client take aspirin? **Use of aspirin can mask signs of inflammation and tends to prolong the course of the disease.**

C. Assess the client for signs and symptoms of rheumatic and scarlet fever.

D. Discuss the client's history of heart problems, chest pain, or shortness of breath.

E. Evaluate the onset and complaints of chorea: Fidgeting, clumsiness, uncoordinated erratic facial movements, including grimaces, grins, and frowns.

F. Tongue movements: Ask if the movements and other symptoms disappear with sleep.

G. Review symptoms of joint pain.

Physical Examination

A. Check temperature, pulse, respirations, and BP.

B. Inspect:
1. Inspect the joints for swelling and warmth.
2. Observe for signs of chorea (symptoms noted previously).
3. Conduct a dermal examination, especially of the trunk and proximal aspects of the extremities. Individual lesions of erythema marginatum are evanescent, moving over the skin in wavy patterns or with indented margins. The lesions may be macular and can develop and disappear in minutes, appearing to change shape while being examined.
4. Complete an ear, nose, mouth, and throat examination. Evaluate tonsillopharyngeal erythema with or without exudates. Observe for a beefy, red, swollen uvula.

C. Auscultate:
1. Auscultate the heart. Note any heart murmur, pericardial friction rub, or effusion. Characteristic murmurs of acute carditis include the high-pitched, blowing, holosystolic, apical murmur of mitral regurgitation and the high-pitched, decrescendo, diastolic murmur of aortic regurgitation heard in the aortic area. The features of CHF include tachycardia, a third heart sound, rales, and edema.
2. All lung fields. Note shortness of breath.

D. Palpate:
1. Neck lymph nodes
2. Extremities: Apical and radial pulses
3. Abdomen

E. Neuromuscular examination for chorea:
1. Have the client stick out his or her tongue for observation of a "bag of worms" when protruded.
2. Have the client grip your hand. With chorea, he or she will be unable to maintain a grip; rhythmic squeezing results.
3. Observe for the spooning sign: Flexion at the wrist with finger extension when the hand is extended
4. Observe for the pronator sign: The palms turn outward when held above the head.

Diagnostic Tests

A. No single specific laboratory test can confirm the diagnosis of ARF. The throat culture remains the key criterion for confirmation of GAS infection.
1. If a rapid antigen detection test is negative, obtain a throat culture.
2. Because of the high specificity, a positive rapid antigen test confirms a streptococcal infection.

B. ESR is usually elevated at the onset of ARF.

C. CRP is usually elevated at the onset of ARF.

D. EKG. *Note*: **Prolonged PR interval.**

E. Chest radiograph can reveal cardiomegaly and CHF.

F. Echocardiography may demonstrate valvular regurgitant lesions.

G. Tests that may rule out differential diagnoses include RF, ANA, Lyme serology, blood cultures, and evaluation for gonorrhea.

Differential Diagnoses

A. Rheumatic fever: Jones criteria (updated in 2015):
  1. Requires two major criteria or one major plus two minor criteria to support the diagnosis of ARF in a client with evidence of a preceding GAS infection
  2. Clients with a history of ARF are at risk of repeat episodes of ARF with GAS and more likely to have cardiac involvement. These clients require two major, one major plus two minor, or three minor criteria for the diagnosis of recurrent ARF. Criteria are as follows:
    a. Major criteria:
      i. Carditis: Based on clinical criteria; 50%–70% seen
      ii. Polyarthritis: 35%–66% seen
      iii. CNS involvement: Sydenham chorea—neurological disorder exhibiting abrupt, nonrhythmic, involuntary movements, muscle weakness, emotional disturbance; rare in adults, seen in 10%–30%
      iv. Erythema marginatum: Uncommon, rare in adults, less than 6% seen
      v. Subcutaneous nodules: Uncommon, rare in adults, 0%–10% seen
    b. Minor criteria:
      i. Arthralgia
      ii. Fever
      iii. Elevated ESR or CRP level
      iv. Prolonged PR interval
  3. There are three exceptions to the aforementioned criteria in which criteria do not need to be met for the diagnosis of ARF:
    a. Chorea as the only symptom
    b. Indolent carditis for clients who present months after acute GAS infection
    c. Recurrent ARF for clients with a history of ARF-associated carditis or rheumatic heart disease
  4. Criteria may also be modified for moderate- to high-risk populations.
B. Juvenile rheumatoid arthritis
C. Rheumatoid arthritis
D. Gonococcal arthritis
E. Septic arthritis
F. Sickle cell anemia
G. Infective endocarditis
H. Leukemia
I. Gout
J. Huntington's chorea
K. KD
L. Systemic lupus erythematosus
M. Lyme disease
N. Reiter's syndrome
O. Scarlet fever

Plan

A. General interventions:
  1. Bed rest is a traditional part of ARF therapy and is especially important with carditis. Bed rest is needed throughout the acute illness and should continue until the ESR has returned to normal for 2 weeks.
B. Client teaching:
  1. Reinforce the need to take the complete prescribed course of antibiotics for strep infections.
  2. Adequate treatment for streptococcal pharyngitis or skin infection is the best prevention against rheumatic fever. Strep infections are contagious, but rheumatic fever is not.
  3. Chorea is usually managed conservatively in a quiet nonstimulatory environment. Valproic acid is the preferred agent if sedation is needed. Although there is no conclusive evidence of their efficacy, IVIG, steroids, and plasmapheresis have all been used successfully in clients with refractory chorea.
  4. Diuretics are the mainstay treatment for carditis/heart failure.
C. Pharmaceutical therapy:
  1. Antibiotic treatment in clients who present with ARF is necessary regardless of the throat culture results to minimize the possible transmission of the rheumatogenic streptococcal strain. The drug of choice is penicillin, but erythromycin or sulfadiazine may be used in clients who are allergic to penicillin. Use of long-acting IM penicillin G avoids the compliance problems associated with oral regimens.
    a. Benzathine penicillin G:
      i. Adults:
        1) Primary prophylaxis for treatment of GAS pharyngitis: 1.2 million units IM in a single dose
      ii. Pediatrics:
        1) Primary prophylaxis: Children less than or equal to 27 kg: 600,000 units IM in a single dose
        2) Children less than 27 kg: 600,000 units
        3) Children more than 27 kg: 1.2 million units IM in a single dose
    b. Penicillin V: Drug of choice for GAS pharyngitis:
      i. Adults:
        1) Primary prophylaxis: 500 mg by mouth two to three times a day for 10 days
      ii. Pediatrics:
        1) Primary prophylaxis: Children less than 27 kg: 250 mg by mouth two to three times a day for 10 days
        2) Children more than 27 kg: 500 mg orally two to three times a day for 10 days
    c. Amoxicillin:
      i. Adults: Primary prophylaxis: 500 mg orally in two divided doses for 10 days
      ii. Pediatrics: 50 mg/kg/d orally in two divided doses for 10 days

d. Cephalexin:
   i. Adults: 500 mg orally twice daily for 10 days
   ii. Pediatrics: 25 to 50 mg/kg/d orally in two divided doses (maximum 1,000 mg/d) for 10 days
e. Clients with severe hypersensitivity to beta-lactam antibiotics:
   i. Azithromycin:
      1) Adults: 500 mg orally on day 1 and 250 mg once a day on days 2 to 5
      2) Children: 12 mg/kg orally on day 1, then 6 mg/kg once a day on days 2 to 5
   ii. Clarithromycin:
      1) Adults: 250 mg orally twice a day for 10 days
      2) Pediatrics: 7.5 mg/kg/d given orally every 12 hours for 10 days; do not exceed the maximum dose of 250 mg/d
   iii. Clindamycin:
      1) Adults: 300 mg orally three times a day for 10 days
      2) Pediatrics: If less than 70 kg: 7 mg/kg/dose (maximum 300 mg/dose) orally three times a day for 10 days. If greater than 70 kg: 300 mg orally three times a day for 10 days

2. Anti-inflammatory agents are the first choice of treatment for ARF-associated arthritis.

3. Naproxen is now preferred over aspirin because it has a superior side-effect profile and can be dosed twice a day. Low-dose glucocorticoids may be used if the client has an allergy or intolerance to naproxen or aspirin.
   a. Adults: Naproxen dosing is 250 to 500 mg in divided doses every 12 hours, up to a maximum of 1,250 mg per day; it should be continued until all joint symptoms have resolved
   b. Children older than 2 years of age: 10 to 20 mg/kg/d by mouth every 12 hours, up to a maximum of 1,000 mg per day
   c. Ibuprofen has been used in children younger than 2 years of age; however, no data have been published to support its use.

4. Cardiac involvement with confirmed rheumatic fever:
   a. Heart failure: Antibiotics + diuretic + angiotensin-converting enzyme inhibitors + steroid therapy
   b. Atrial fibrillation: Antibiotics + digoxin
   c. Valve leaflet or chordae tendineae rupture: Antibiotics and full assessment for an emergent valve replacement

5. Severe chorea: Antibiotics + anticonvulsants

6. Secondary antibiotic prophylaxis for procedures for chronic established changes of the heart valves

Follow-Up

A. The test of cure is a negative throat culture.
B. Clients with pharyngitis and a history of rheumatic fever and those who are symptomatic and have a household member with documented GAS infection should

receive immediate treatment without need for prior testing.

C. Since 2007, **the AHA no longer recommends prophylaxis for infective endocarditis in most clients**. The AHA prophylaxis regimen for systemic bacterial endocarditis is available at www.inesss.qc.ca/fileadmin/doc/INESSS/Outils/Guides_antibio_II/endocardite_2012_web_EN.pdf; the AHA (2017) update for high-risk clients is available at https://www.aae.org/specialty/wp-content/uploads/sites/2/2017/06/aae_antibiotic-prophylaxis-2017update.pdf.

D. The major complication is cardiac valve disease. Rheumatic fever accounts for the largest number of aortic regurgitation cases. Continuous *Streptococcus* prophylaxis in clients with prior rheumatic fever is the major means of preventing cardiac sequelae.

E. The client with carditis should be followed every 6 months and by a cardiologist with an echocardiography every 1 to 2 years.

Consultation/Referral

A. Consult and comanage the client with a physician.
B. Consult an ENT specialist if indicated for clients with intact tonsils and recurrent symptomatic strep infections for consideration of tonsillectomy.
C. Consultation with a cardiologist may be required to manage heart blocks and CHF.
D. Consultation with a neurologist or psychiatrist may be required to confirm the diagnosis of chorea and to assist in its management.

Individual Considerations

A. Pediatrics:
   1. Highest risk group; ARF is rare in children younger than 5 years.
B. Adults:
   1. ARF is rare in clients older than 40 years.
   2. Cases of arthritis following a streptococcal infection that are not supported by the Jones criteria are called poststreptococcal reactive arthritis. Many of these clients will have one major and two minor symptoms and are considered to have ARF.
C. Pregnancy:
   1. Penicillin G is a pregnancy category B drug. Fetal risk is not confirmed in humans but has been shown in some studies in animals.
   2. Erythromycin is a pregnancy category B drug.
   3. Aspirin products are pregnancy category D drugs. As fetal risk has been shown in humans, use only if the benefits outweigh the risk to the fetus.

Bibliography

American Heart Association & American College of Cardiology. (2017). *Antibiotic prophylaxis 2017 update: Endocarditis prophylaxis recommendations.* Retrieved from https://www.aae.org/specialty/wp-content/uploads/sites/2/2017/06/aae_antibiotic-prophylaxis-2017update.pdf

Pichichero, M. E. (2019, March 22). Complications of streptococcal tonsillopharyngitis. *UpToDate.* Retrieved from https://www.uptodate.com/contents/complications-of-streptococcal-tonsillopharyngitis?search=Complications%20of%20streptococcal%20tonsillopharyngitis&source=search_result&selectedTitle=1-97&usage_type=default&display_rank=1

Steer, A., & Gibofsky, A. (2018, May 18). Acute rheumatic fever: Clinical manifestations and diagnosis. *UpToDate.* Retrieved from https://www.uptodate.com/contents/acute-rheumatic-fever-clinical-manifestations-and-diagnosis?search=Acute%20rheumatic%20fever:%20Clinical%20manifestations%20and%20diagnosis&source=search_result&selectedTitle=1~150&usage_type=default&display_rank=1

Wallace, M. R. (2019, January 17). Rheumatic fever. *Medscape*. Retrieved from https://emedicine.medscape.com/article/236582-overview

Rocky Mountain Spotted Fever

Jill C. Cash, Cheryl A. Glass, and Moya Cook

Definition

A. Rocky Mountain spotted fever (RMSF) is a systemic febrile illness accompanied by a characteristic rash from the bite of an infected tick. It can involve the skin; central nervous, cardiac, and pulmonary systems; GI tract; and muscles. Ticks need 6 to 10 hours of feeding to transmit RMSF; therefore, early discovery and removal of ticks is a preventive measure.

B. In the United States, RMSF is a reportable disease and the most severe rickettsial illness.

C. Long-term sequelae are common with severe RMSF:
1. Paraparesis
2. Hearing loss
3. Peripheral neuropathy
4. Seizures
5. Bowel incontinence
6. Cerebellar and vestibular dysfunction
7. Blindness

Incidence

A. RMSF is the most common rickettsial infection in the United States. The prevalence of RMSF is highest in the southeastern and southern central states. Although RMSF is more common in rural and suburban locations, it does occur in urban areas. The incidence varies by geographic area, and cases are more common in the spring and early summer. However, RMSF has been seen in the cold-weather months in the southern United States.

B. People of all ages can be infected.

C. African Americans have a higher case-fatality rate, possibly due to the difficulty of distinguishing the rash in highly pigmented skin.

Pathogenesis

A. *Rickettsia rickettsii* is the infectious agent and is transmitted by a tick vector. *Rickettsia* also infects rodents, squirrels, and chipmunks. As many as one-third of clients with proven RMSF do not recall a recent tick bite or tick contact. RMSF is not transmitted by person-to-person contact.

B. The incubation period is usually about 1 week, but ranges from 2 to 14 days after the tick bite. It appears to be related to the size of the rickettsial inoculum.

C. Principal recognized vectors:
1. *Dermacentor variabilis* (American dog tick)
2. *Dermacentor andersoni* (Rocky Mountain wood tick)
3. *Amblyomma americanum* (Lone Star tick)
4. *Rhipicephalus sanguineus* (brown dog tick)

Predisposing Factors

A. Outdoor activities (hunting, hiking, camping)

B. Tick bite: The tick must attach and feed for 4 to 6 hours before transmitting the infection.

C. Age is not a predisposing factor, but the disease is more common in children and young adults.

D. Exposure to heavy brush areas

E. Contact with dogs and other animals with ticks

F. Transmission has occurred on rare occasion by blood transfusion.

G. Blood transmission is rare.

Common Complaints

In the early phase, most clients have nonspecific signs and symptoms that may include the following:

A. Fever

B. Sudden onset of severe headache

C. Children may present with prominent abdominal pain that may be mistaken for acute appendicitis, cholecystitis, or bowel obstruction.

D. Rash (90%) usually occurs between days 3 and 5 of illness. The typical RMSF rash begins as a pink maculopapular eruption on the ankles and wrists. The rash then spreads both centrally and to the palms of hands and soles of the feet. By the fourth day, the rash spreads centripetally and becomes petechial and papular. Hemorrhagic, ulcerated lesions may follow. In a small percentage of clients, onset of the rash is delayed (past 5 days) and/or is atypical (e.g., confined to one body region). **Urticaria and pruritus are not characteristic of RMSF, and their presence makes the diagnosis unlikely.**

E. Malaise

F. Myalgias

G. Nausea with or without vomiting

Other Signs and Symptoms

A. Deep cough

B. Edema, especially in children

C. Bleeding

D. Conjunctivitis

E. Retinal abnormalities

F. EKG abnormalities

G. Seizures

H. Dehydration

Subjective Data

A. Review the onset, course, and duration of symptoms.

B. Elicit information about a recent tick bite or removal.

C. Ask the client about any recent outdoor activities such as camping, hiking, and so on.

D. Rule out similar symptoms in other family members.

E. Review any history of rash and course of spread.

F. Elicit a history of mental or neurological changes including seizures.

G. Rule out other symptoms associated with Lyme disease, such as arthritis, memory loss, and distal paresthesia.

H. Review the client's recent history of blood transfusion.

Physical Examination

A. Check temperature, pulse, respirations, and BP.

B. Inspect:

1. Conduct an ENT examination.

2. Inspect the skin, especially on the wrist, palms, ankles, and soles of the feet.

3. Note the presence of petechiae.

4. Conduct an eye examination and evaluate periorbital edema and petechial conjunctivitis.

C. Auscultate:

1. Perform a complete heart evaluation.

2. Auscultate all lung fields.

D. Palpate:

1. All lymph nodes

2. The mastoid bones

E. Neurological examination:

1. Assess LOC.

2. Evaluate the client for signs of meningeal irritation, such as nuchal rigidity and positive Brudzinski's and Kernig's signs (see Figures 16.1 and 16.2).

Diagnostic Tests

A. Antibody titers: A fourfold rise in antibody titer is the diagnostic gold standard for RMSF. Antibodies typically appear 7 to 10 days after the onset of the illness.

B. CBC with differential

C. Platelet count: As the illness progresses, thrombocytopenia becomes more prevalent and may be severe.

D. Electrolytes

E. Liver function studies

F. Bilirubin

G. Skin biopsy: 3 mm punch biopsy

H. Lumbar puncture may be indicated.

I. Rickettsial blood cultures are highly sensitive and specific; however, only specialized laboratories perform these cultures.

Differential Diagnoses

A. RMSF is commonly mistaken for an undifferentiated viral illness during the first few days of illness.

B. Viral meningitis

C. Lyme disease

D. Mononucleosis

E. Atypical measles

F. Viral hepatitis

G. Parvovirus B19 (fifth disease)

Plan

A. General interventions:

1. **Early treatment is necessary; never delay initiation of antimicrobial treatment to confirm clinical suspicion of the disease. This is a life-threatening disease.**

2. Antibiotic therapy (see the "Pharmaceutical Therapy" section). If penicillin or a cephalosporin is administered empirically in the first few days of the illness, the subsequent rash may be incorrectly diagnosed as a drug reaction.

3. Hospitalization should be considered for most clients, especially children.

B. Client teaching:

1. Client teaching: *See Section III: Client Teaching Guide for this chapter, "Rocky Mountain Spotted Fever and Removal of a Tick," and Section II: Procedure, "Tick Removal."*

2. RMSF is not transmissible by person-to-person contact; therefore, isolation is not necessary.

3. Relapse of the illness may occur; the client should report recurrence of symptoms immediately.

4. Clients who report tick bites should be advised to inform their healthcare provider if any systemic symptoms, especially fever and headache, occur in the following 14 days.

5. All pets should be treated for ticks.

C. Pharmaceutical therapy:

> The diagnosis of RMSF can rarely be confirmed or disproved in its early phase; the cornerstone of management is empirical therapy based on clinical judgment and the epidemiological setting.

1. Drug of choice: Doxycycline 100 mg orally or IV every 12 hours for 5 to 7 days for adults or children weighing more than 45 kg. Doxycycline 2.2 mg/kg IV (maximum dose 100 mg/dose) or orally every 12 hours is the dosage for smaller children.

a. Doxycycline 200 mg initial loading dose IV may be given to critically ill clients.

b. Doxycycline is the drug of choice in all adults except for pregnant women.

c. Tetracyclines can cause dental staining when administered to children younger than 8 years. Most experts consider the risk of morbidity from rickettsial diseases greater than the minimal risk of dental staining from one short course of doxycycline.

2. Alternative drug therapy: Chloramphenicol (Chloromycetin):

a. Chloramphenicol requires frequent serum platelet counts and CBCs).

b. Not available in oral form in the United States

c. Use of chloramphenicol should be considered only in rare cases, such as in clients with severe allergy to doxycycline or in pregnancy if the mother's life is in danger.

d. Use of chloramphenicol is associated with a higher risk of fatal outcome.

3. Prophylactic therapy with doxycycline or another tetracycline is not recommended following tick exposure.

4. Severe doxycycline or tetracycline allergy in clients should be discussed with the client. Consider consulting with an allergy/immunology specialist. If the allergy is not life-threatening, administer doxycycline in a controlled setting or consult for rapid doxycycline desensitization with an allergy/immunology specialist. Anaphylactic reactions have been reported, but are rare.

5. Asymptomatic clients with seropositive results for tick-borne rickettsial disease should not be treated with antibiotics because antibodies may remain positive for several years after infection.

Follow-Up
A. See the client 24 to 48 hours after the initial visit and again at the end of antibiotic therapy (unless following lab tests for chloramphenicol therapy). RMSF progresses rapidly. Approximately 10% of clients treated as outpatients are subsequently admitted to the hospital.
B. Clients must be seen for any alteration in mental status, stiff neck, severe headaches, nausea and vomiting, severe weakness, dizziness, or high fever.
C. Hospitalization is indicated in clients who are severely ill or have complications, such as seizures, hypotension, or marked GI symptoms.
D. Several rickettsial diseases, including RMSF, are nationally notifiable diseases and should be reported to state and local health departments.

Consultation/Referral
A. Consult a physician for any suspected signs of RMSF because the client is in danger of vascular collapse and disseminated intravascular collapse.
B. Consultation with an infectious disease specialist is advised.

Individual Considerations
A. Pregnancy: Tetracyclines should not be used in pregnancy. Limited data exist for the use of doxycycline during pregnancy. Data on the risks of treatment during pregnancy are unlikely to have a substantial teratogenic risk. Prophylactic use of tetracycline is not recommended. Chloramphenicol is an alternative for RMSF; however, precautions should be taken to avoid gray baby syndrome. Short-term use of doxycycline is considered safe during lactation and, per the AAP Committee on Drugs, is "compatible with breastfeeding."

Bibliography
Cennimo, D. J. (2018). West Nile virus (WNV) infection and encephalitis (WNE). *Medscape*. Retrieved from emedicine.medscape.com/article/234009-overview
Centers for Disease Control and Prevention. (2019, September 6). *Tick bite: What to do*. Retrieved from https://www.cdc.gov/ticks/pdfs/FS_TickBite-508.pdf
Cunha, B. A. (2018). Rocky Mountain spotted fever. *Medscape*. Retrieved from emedicine.medscape.com/article/228042-overview-encephalitis

Roseola (Exanthem Subitum)

Jill C. Cash, Cheryl A. Glass, and Moya Cook

Definition
A. Roseola is a benign viral illness. It is the most common exanthem in infants and young children aged 1 to 3 years. Roseola can often be diagnosed by its classic presentation of a sudden onset of a high fever, up to 104°F, lasting 3 to 4 days. The pink-red macules and papules on the trunk and extremities occur after the client's fever defervesces. The high fever associated with roseola often triggers a febrile seizure. As many as 15% of children will experience their first febrile seizure with roseola.

Incidence
A. Incidence is unknown; 90% of cases involve children younger than 2 years. Roseola tends to be more common in females and in children with older siblings. Approximately 15% of children in the febrile phase of the illness will experience a seizure. The peak incidence of the virus occurs in the spring and autumn seasons.

Pathogenesis
A. HHV type 6 (HHV-6) has been isolated in Kaposi sarcoma (caused by HHV-8), in which roseola may contribute to tumor progression. HHV-6 may facilitate oncogenic potential in lymphoma and has been associated with CFS. HHV-6 is the causative organism; it has two variants, designated as A and B. The genomes of HHV-6A/B have been sequenced. Nearly all primary infections in children appear to be caused by HHV-6B. In the primary infection, replication of the virus occurs in the leukocytes and the salivary glands. It is present in the saliva. HHV-6 and HHV-7 are spread by respiratory droplets. The communicable period is most likely during the febrile phase.
B. The incubation period is 5 to 15 days.
C. Like other herpesviruses, HHV-6 remains latent in most clients who are immunocompetent. Following the acute primary infection, the virus remains latent in lymphocytes and monocytes and has been found in low levels in many tissues. The HHV-6 virus is a major cause of morbidity and mortality in clients who are immunosuppressed, particularly in clients with AIDS and in those who are transplant recipients.

Predisposing Factors
A. Classic age: 9 to 12 months (age range: 2 weeks to 3 years)
B. Attendance at day-care centers
C. Transplacental infection in about 1% of cases
D. Immunosuppression

Common Complaints
A. Primary infection with HHV-6 may be asymptomatic or it may cause the exanthem subitum/roseola syndrome.
B. Child with high fever (up to 105°F) for several (1–3) days: Abrupt onset of fever followed by rose-pink maculopapular rash, with rapid resolution of both, is characteristic of roseola. Rash appears after fever is resolved (see Figure 16.6).

FIGURE 16.6 Roseola rash.

C. Rosy pink rash on chest and body: Rash typically begins on the trunk or chest and spreads to the arms and neck, with mild involvement of the face and legs; rash can last several hours to 2 days and fades quickly.

D. Characteristic enanthem (Nagayama spots) consists of erythematous papules on the mucosa of the soft palate and the base of the uvula; usually present on the fourth day.

Other Signs and Symptoms

A. Drowsiness
B. Seizures (secondary to high fever)
C. Bulging anterior fontanelle (rare)
D. Encephalopathy (rare)
E. Irritability
F. Mild diarrhea
G. Otitis media
H. Respiratory distress
I. Clients who are immunocompromised may have malaise and CNS and other organ system involvement.

Subjective Data

A. Ask the parent or caregiver to describe the progression and color of the rash, onset, and duration of all symptoms.
B. Ask about the client's temperature history and the treatments administered.
C. Review other symptoms such as coryza, cough, sore throat, and watery eyes (rules out roseola).
D. Review family history of others with similar symptoms.
E. Review the client's history of febrile seizures.
F. Complete a drug history for possible allergic reaction.
G. Inquire regarding recent MMR immunization.

Physical Examination

A. Check temperature, pulse, respirations, and BP.
B. Inspect:
  1. Inspect the skin. Observe for the presence of an erythematous, pink-red, 3- to 5-mm, maculopapular rash on chest and body: Rash typically begins on the trunk or chest and spreads to the arms and neck, with mild involvement of the face and legs.
  2. Observe the client for seizure activity.
  3. Conduct an ear examination for inflamed tympanic membranes to rule out otitis media.
  4. Observe for the presence of periorbital edema, which is common in the febrile phase of infection.
  5. Conduct a nasal examination; coryza is generally not a presenting symptom of roseola.
  6. Conduct an oral/throat examination to evaluate for the presence of characteristic enanthem Nagayama spots, which appear as erythematous papules on the mucosa of the soft palate and the base of the uvula.
C. Auscultate:
  1. Heart
  2. Lungs; cough may be present.
D. Palpate:
  1. Palpate the head and the anterior fontanelle (if applicable).
  2. Palpate the neck and the cervical, suboccipital, and postauricular lymph nodes.

E. Neurological examination:
  1. Check for nuchal rigidity.

Diagnostic Tests

A. None is required unless the diagnosis is unclear.
B. Rule-out testing:
  1. CBC with differential
  2. Urinalysis and culture for urinary tract infection (UTI)
  3. Chest radiograph for pneumonia
  4. Blood cultures
  5. CSF examination if indicated
C. Skin biopsy: Rarely performed unless the diagnosis is unclear and there are other complicating medical factors.

Differential Diagnoses

A. Roseola
B. Allergic reaction
C. CMV
D. RMSF
E. Fifth disease (parvovirus B19)
F. Scarlet fever
G. Meningococcemia
H. FUO
I. Pneumococcemia
J. Herpes simplex
K. Otitis media
L. Rubella
M. Enterovirus
N. EBV
O. Measles

Plan

A. General interventions:
  1. Encourage fluids to prevent dehydration (Popsicles, Jell-O, clear fluids).
  2. Monitor for lethargy, decreased fluid intake, cough, and irritability.
B. Client teaching:
  1. Treatment is supportive.
  2. Advise parents/care provider that controlling temperature and providing supportive care is essential. Avoiding high fever, greater than 104°F, is imperative.
  3. Discomfort and body aches are often related to fever.
C. Pharmaceutical therapy:
  1. At present, there is no antiviral therapy available for HHV-6 infection.
  2. Acetaminophen (Tylenol) as needed for fever
  3. Acute or chronic antiseizure medications are not recommended for infants who have had a febrile seizure secondary to roseola.

Follow-Up

A. None is required unless other problems occur; resolution is usually rapid.
B. See the client immediately for the following:
  1. Twitching or other signs of seizure
  2. Refusal to drink liquids or signs of dehydration
  3. Loud and persistent crying; does not stop when consoled
  4. Listlessness and stiff neck

Consultation/Referral

A. Consult and/or refer the client to a physician if febrile seizures/neurological signs are present.

Individual Considerations

A. Pediatrics: Children with roseola are often playful without change in appetite, even with high fever.

Bibliography

Salvaggio, M. R. (2019, July 22). Human herpesvirus 6 infection differential diagnoses. *Medscape*. Retrieved from emedicine.medscape.com/article/219019-differential

Tremblay, C., & Brady, M. T. (2019, July 22). Roseola infantum (exanthem subitum). *UpToDate*. Retrieved from https://www.uptodate.com/contents/roseola-infantum-exanthem-subitum?search=Roseola%20infantum%20(exanthema%20subitum)&source=search_result&selectedTitle=1~150&usage_type=default&display_rank=1

White, S. W. (2018). Roseola infantum. *Medscape*. Retrieved from emedicine.medscape.com/article/1133023-overview

Rubella (German Measles)

Jill C. Cash, Cheryl A. Glass, and Moya Cook

Definition

A. Rubella, also known as German measles and 3-day measles, is primarily known as a childhood disease. Rubella is considered one of the TORCH infections and is highly contagious. The disease is preventable by immunization. Passive immunity is acquired from birth to 6 months of age from maternal antibodies.

B. The goal of immunization is to prevent congenitally acquired rubella. Routine immunization is achieved by using the MMR or MMRV vaccine. The rubella vaccine is a live attenuated virus.

C. Immunization schedule recommended by the AAP:

1. First immunization is given between 12 and 15 months of age.

2. Second immunization is given at 4 to 6 years of age when the child is entering school.

3. People who have not received the second immunization at school entry should receive their second immunization as soon as possible but optimally no later than 11 to 12 years of age.

Incidence

A. Rubella is no longer endemic in the United States as a result of an intensive vaccination campaign. The CDC declared rubella to be eliminated from the United States in 2004. Incidence is unknown. Peak season for rubella is late winter and spring.

B. The rubella vaccination is given only in about half of the world's population. Congenital rubella syndrome causes 15% of all birth defects in Russia.

C. Congenital defects arise in as many as 85% of infants if maternal rubella infection occurs during the first 12 weeks of gestation.

Pathogenesis

A. The rubella virus is an enveloped, positive-stranded RNA virus classified as *Rubivirus* in the Togaviridae family. Humans are the only source of infection. The virus is spread by nasopharyngeal, airborne respiratory droplets, and transplacental routes.

B. The incubation period for postnatally acquired rubella ranges from 14 to 23 days (usually 16–18 days). It is communicable 1 week before and 4 days after rash and illness appear. The neonate born with congenital rubella is often highly infectious and should be isolated. Neonates may continue to shed the virus for 1 year or longer.

Predisposing Factors

A. Age 5 to 9 years
B. Transplacental transmission
C. Never received rubella vaccine
D. Attendance at schools and day-care centers
E. Compromised immune system

Common Complaints

A. Low-grade fever
B. Swollen glands: Posterior auricular, suboccipital, and posterior cervical lymphadenopathy is frequently present 24 hours before rash develops.
C. Rash: Light pink to red macular rash that starts on the face and moves down the body to the trunk. The facial rash clears as the extremity rash erupts. The macular lesions rapidly become papular lesions and fade in 3 to 4 days. Exanthematous lesions remain discrete and pink, in contrast with the rash of rubeola, which is deep red and becomes confluent (Koplik's spots). Exanthem of rubella is usually preceded by 1 to 5 days of prodrome symptoms and generally last 3 days, but may persist for as long as 5 days (see Figure 16.7).

FIGURE 16.7   Rubella (German measles) rash.

Other Signs and Symptoms

A. Headache
B. Sore throat
C. Mild coryza
D. Cough
E. Malaise
F. Conjunctivitis
G. Forchheimer spots in the soft palate
H. Transient polyarthralgia and polyarthritis (older children, adolescents, and women)
I. Itching
J. Asymptomatic

Subjective Data

A. Review the onset, duration, and course of symptoms.
B. Rule out similar symptoms in other family members.

C. Review the client's immunization history, especially for recent immunization with the MMR or MMRV vaccine.
D. Determine any new medications or contact exposures.
E. Review any history of rash and the course of spread.
F. Determine if the client is pregnant.
G. If a fever is present, has the client experienced a febrile seizure?

Physical Examination
A. Check temperature, pulse, respirations, and BP.
B. Inspect:
  1. Conduct an ENT examination.
  2. Inspect the mouth for Koplik's spots. Forchheimer spots are reddish spots on the soft palate seen during the prodrome or first day of the rash.
  3. Inspect the skin.
C. Auscultate:
  1. Heart
  2. Lungs
D. Palpate:
  1. Check the lymph nodes, especially the anterior/posterior cervical chains in neck.

Diagnostic Tests
A. Blood or urine:
  1. Latex agglutination
  2. Enzyme immunoassay (ELISA)
  3. Passive hemagglutination
  4. Fluorescent immunoassay tests
B. Rubella titer: Test initially; then repeat 2 to 4 weeks after exposure)

A serologic rubella titer less than 8 indicates nonimmunity. A rubella titer greater than 1:32 indicates immunity from a past infection. A fourfold rise in the titer (about 2 weeks after exposure) indicates infection.

C. Pregnancy test if indicated
D. Tissue culture of throat

Differential Diagnoses
A. Rubella (German measles)
B. Rubeola
C. Parvovirus
D. Scarlet fever
E. Allergic reaction, contact dermatitis
F. Roseola
G. Infectious mononucleosis
H. Toxoplasmosis

Plan
A. General interventions:
  1. Primary prevention is through immunization.
  2. Vaccinating adolescents and adults in college reduces the chance of outbreaks and helps prevent congenital rubella syndrome.
  3. Generally, the course is mild; however, rest is encouraged.
  4. Treatment is supportive. Have the client increase oral fluid intake.

  5. Reinforce respiratory and nasal discharge precautions (droplet precautions); encourage good handwashing.
  6. Immunize clients preconceptually; advise them to use a method of birth control for at least 4 weeks or longer after immunization.
  7. Rubella cases should be reported to the local health department.
  8. Healthcare professionals should be immunized.
B. Client teaching:
  1. Affected clients should not return to work or school for 7 days after the onset of the rash.
  2. Pregnant clients with documented rubella infection should be counseled about the risk of fetal infection and/or compromise.
  3. Children with congenital rubella should be considered contagious until they are at least 1 year of age, unless nasopharyngeal and urine cultures are negative consecutively for rubella virus; infection control precautions should be considered in children up to 3 years who are hospitalized for congenital cataract extraction.
  4. Febrile seizures may occur in children 12 to 24 months of age
C. Pharmaceutical therapy:
  1. Acetaminophen (Tylenol) for fever and headache
  2. Antihistamines: Diphenhydramine (Benadryl) for pruritus
  3. Limited data indicate that IM Ig in a dose of 0.55 mL/kg may decrease clinically apparent shedding and the rate of viremia significantly in exposed susceptible people. The absence of clinical signs in a woman who has received IM Ig does not guarantee that infant infection is prevented. The CDC recommends limiting the use of Ig to women with known rubella exposure who decline pregnancy termination.
  4. Live-virus rubella vaccine administered within 3 days of exposure has not been demonstrated to prevent illness.
  5. Glucocorticoids, platelet transfusion, and other supportive measures are reserved for clients with complications such as thrombocytopenia or encephalopathy.

Follow-Up
A. The disease is self-limiting and has no sequelae (except congenital exposure).
B. Repeat titer 3 to 4 weeks after exposure.
C. Rubella is a disease reportable to the local or state health department.

Consultation/Referral
A. Refer the client to an obstetrician if the client is pregnant.

Individual Considerations
A. Pregnancy:
  1. Rubella infection has few consequences for an adult, but presents significant problems for a fetus. Rubella's viral teratogenic effects include cardiovascular malformation, deafness, mental retardation, cataracts, glaucoma, microcephaly, and microphthalmos.

2. If maternal infection occurs during the first trimester, 50% of the fetuses infected may abort or have complications. Approximately 30% to 50% of fetuses that acquire rubella in the first month of gestation suffer cardiac anomalies. Neural deafness is a common sequela when infection occurs in the second gestational month.

3. The rubella vaccine is a live attenuated virus; therefore, it is *not* safe to give in pregnancy. Immunization may be given postpartum; instruct the client to avoid pregnancy for the next 4 weeks or longer. The rubella vaccine may be given to a woman if she is breastfeeding.

4. Routine prenatal screening for rubella immunity should be undertaken. If a woman is found to be susceptible, the rubella vaccine should be administered during the immediate postpartum period before discharge.

5. Breastfeeding is not a contraindication to postpartum immunization of the mother.

B. Pediatrics:

1. The infected neonate must be kept in isolation in the nursery. The neonate may continue to spread the virus for 1 year or longer.

2. Cardiac and eye defects are most frequent when maternal infection occurs before 8 weeks' gestation; hearing loss and growth retardation are observed in maternal infections up to 16 weeks' gestation.

3. Other reported abnormalities include jaundice, hepatosplenomegaly, thrombocytopenia, and dermal erythropoiesis (blueberry muffin lesions).

4. The ACIP currently recommends that all children receive two doses of MMR vaccine, separated by at least 28 days, administered on or after the first birthday.

Bibliography

Edwards, M. S. (2019). Rubella. *UpToDate*. Retrieved from https://www.uptodate.com/contents/rubella

Immunization Action Coalition. (n.d.). *Healthcare personnel vaccination recommendations*. Retrieved from www.vaccineinformation.org

Rubeola (Red Measles)

Jill C. Cash, Cheryl A. Glass, and Moya Cook

Definition

A. Rubeola (red measles), also known as hard measles, is a highly communicable viral disease. The disease is preventable by immunization. Passive immunity is acquired from birth to between 4 and 6 months of age if the mother is immune before pregnancy. Immunity after measles infection is thought to be lifelong.

B. Modified measles occurs in clients who received the serum Ig following exposure to the measles virus. The incubation period may be up to 21 days. Their symptoms are generally milder.

C. Atypical measles occurs in clients who had the original killed-virus measles immunization that has incomplete immunity. Their symptoms are similar to the clinical presentation for clients who have not been vaccinated and have initial exposure.

1. The killed-virus vaccine was administered between 1963 and 1967.

2. In 1967, the live attenuated vaccine replaced the killed-virus measles vaccine.

D. In the United States, the measles vaccine is currently available in two formulations—the trivalent MMR vaccine and the MMRV vaccine.

Incidence

A. Incidence is unknown; widespread measles vaccination has led to its virtual disappearance in the United States. In 2015, WHO noted that globally there were 134,200 measles deaths (15 deaths/hour). Most of those deaths have shifted from children younger than 5 years to include older children and adolescents.

B. In temperate areas, the peak incidence of infection occurs during late winter and spring.

C. About 5% of all measles cases are due to vaccine failure.

D. There is an increased incidence in two populations: Children younger than 5 years and college students who have not been immunized.

E. Rubeola is rarely encountered in pregnancy; however, the reported mortality of congenital measles is 32%.

F. One in every 1,000 clients with measles will develop acute encephalitis. Most fatalities from measles are from respiratory tract complications or encephalitis.

G. Clients with defects in cell-mediated immunity (AIDS, lymphoma, or other malignancies) are at risk for severe, progressive measles infection.

H. A generalized immunosuppression that follows measles frequently predisposes clients to complications such as otitis media and bronchopneumonia. Laryngotracheobronchitis (croup) and diarrhea occur more commonly in young children. Two rare neurological syndromes are associated with measles:

1. Acute disseminated encephalomyelitis may occur soon after the initial clinical manifestations of measles have resolved.

2. Subacute sclerosing panencephalitis presents 7 to 10 years after the initial infection.

Pathogenesis

A. Paramyxovirus (an RNA virus) is the causative agent and is spread by respiratory droplet, direct skin contact, or transplacental passage. The incubation period lasts 7 to 14 days from exposure to onset. The disease is communicable a few days before fever to 4 days after rash appears. The measles virus replicates locally, spreads to regional lymphatic tissues, and is then thought to disseminate to other reticuloendothelial sites via the bloodstream.

B. The virus remains active and contagious in the air or on infected surfaces for up to 2 hours.

Predisposing Factors

A. Age younger than 5 years and not immunized

B. Schools: College age and not immunized with two doses. In 1989, the United States adopted a two-dose strategy; revaccination with MMR vaccine is recommended for all students and their siblings.

C. Late winter and early spring

D. Transplacental passage; presents clinically in the first 10 days of life

E. Crowded living conditions

F. Measles has been attributed to poor nutritional status and vitamin A deficiency.

Common Complaints

A. Suspected case: Febrile illness accompanied by a rash

B. Clinical case: The client is usually very ill with a fever and the three Cs: cough, coryza, and conjunctivitis. The client generally recovers rapidly after the first 3 to 4 days:

    1. Fever greater than 101°F and often exceeding 104°F

    2. Respiratory symptoms: Coryza and cough. The cough may persist for 1 to 2 weeks after the measles infection.

    3. Conjunctivitis

C. Rash: Macular rash develops on the face and neck; then lesions become maculopapular and spread to the trunk and extremities in 24 to 48 hours. The rash may appear red brown or purple red at the hairline. The rash lasts 4 to 7 days (see Figure 16.8).

FIGURE 16.8 Rubeola rash.

D. Koplik's spots on buccal mucosa. Koplik's spots are pathognomonic for measles; they appear as bluish-gray specks or "grains of sand" on a red base.

E. A probable case meets the clinical case definition but is not linked epidemiologically to a confirmed case and lacks serologic or virologic proof of disease.

F. A confirmed case meets the laboratory criteria for measles or meets the clinical case definition and is epidemiologically linked to a confirmed case.

Other Signs and Symptoms

A. Loss of appetite

B. Bronchitis

C. Photophobia

D. General lymphoid involvement

E. Myalgia

F. Pruritus

G. Diarrhea

Subjective Data

A. Review the onset and duration of symptoms such as cough, conjunctivitis, coryza, and Koplik's spots.

B. Rule out similar symptoms in other family members.

C. Review the client's immunization history.

D. Determine any new medications or contact exposures.

E. Review any history of rash and the course of spread.

F. Elicit the presence of chest pain, ear pain, and confusion (signs of complications).

G. Determine if the client is pregnant.

H. Review the client's history of tick bite (recent camping, hiking, and so forth).

Physical Examination

A. Check temperature, pulse, respirations, and BP.

B. Inspect:

    1. Conduct an eye examination: Nonpurulent conjunctivitis with lacrimation is not uncommon. Photophobia may be present.

    2. Conduct an ear examination: Otitis is a complication noted with the measles.

    3. Conduct a nasal examination: Coryza is one of the classic triad of symptoms.

    4. Conduct a throat examination: Pharyngitis encompasses all complications of the measles.

    5. Examine the mouth for Koplik's spots; they appear on buccal mucosa within 12 hours. Koplik's spots are tiny (1–3 mm) bluish-white spots on an erythematous base that cluster adjacent to the molars on the buccal mucosa. They often begin to slough when the exanthem appears.

    6. Conduct a dermal examination. The characteristic rash is maculopapular and blanches; it begins on the face and spreads centrifugally to involve the neck, upper trunk, lower trunk, and extremities. The lesions may become confluent, especially in the face, where the rash develops first. The palms and soles of the feet are rarely involved. Some petechiae may be present with the rash.

C. Auscultate:

    1. Lungs

    2. Heart

D. Palpate:

    1. Palpate the neck and lymph nodes.

    2. Generalized lymphadenopathy and splenomegaly are uncommon.

E. Neurological examination:

    1. Check for nuchal rigidity.

    2. Complete a mental status examination.

Diagnostic Tests

A. Serologic procedures are not routinely done. However, leukopenia and T-cell cytopenia often occur, and thrombocytopenia may also be seen.

B. Antibody titer at the onset of the rash; repeat antibody titer every 3 to 4 weeks.

    1. Rubeola IgG and IgM antibody levels. WHO has recommended that the diagnosis of measles be confirmed with laboratory testing.

    2. Serum IgM alone is the standard test to confirm the diagnosis of measles. At least a fourfold increase in antimeasles antibody titer is indicative of infection.

C. Chest x-ray if indicated: May show interstitial pneumonitis

Differential Diagnoses

A. Rubeola (red or 7-day measles)
B. During the prodromal period, measles may resemble a common cold, except a fever is present.
C. Rubella (German measles)
D. Roseola (exanthem subitum)
E. RMSF
F. Scarlet fever
G. Mononucleosis
H. Drug reaction
I. KD
J. Parvovirus B19
K. Toxic shock syndrome
L. *Mycoplasma pneumoniae*
M. Respiratory viruses:
   1. Rhinoviruses
   2. Parainfluenza
   3. Influenza
   4. Adenovirus
   5. RSV
N. Dengue fever should be ruled out for international travelers.

Plan

A. General interventions:
   1. Primary prevention is through immunization.
     a. For vaccination to be considered adequate for school outbreaks, two doses of measles vaccine must have been administered after the age of 12 months and separated by at least 28 days.
     b. Those who are properly vaccinated may reenter school immediately after vaccination.
     c. International travelers should receive one or two doses of the measles vaccine before travel.
   2. Encourage the client to rest.
   3. The client must be isolated 4 days from the onset of the rash, continuing up to 21 days.
   4. Encourage respiratory and nasal discharge precautions. The cough may persist for up to 2 weeks after the measles.
   5. There is no specific treatment for rubeola.
     a. Otitis media and pneumonia, both due to bacterial superinfection, should be treated with appropriate antibiotics.
     b. IV hydration may be required secondary to dehydration from diarrhea or vomiting.
   6. Monitor the client for signs of complications.
B. Client teaching:
   1. Tell the client to avoid bright lights with photophobia; may need sunglasses.
   2. Reinforce the need to comply with immunization schedules.
C. Pharmaceutical therapy:
   1. Vitamin A is recommended by WHO and the United Nations Children's Fund (UNICEF) for all children with measles in areas where vitamin A deficiency is prevalent or where the mortality from measles exceeds 1%. Vitamin A treatment can help prevent eye damage and blindness. It has been shown to reduce the number of deaths by 50%.
     a. Children younger than 6 months: 50,000 IU/d for 2 consecutive days
     b. Children 6 months to 11 months: 100,000 IU/d for 2 consecutive days
     c. Children 12 months of age and older: 200,000 IU/d for 2 consecutive days
     d. Children with ophthalmological evidence of vitamin A deficiency: A third dose of vitamin A dosage should be repeated in 2 to 4 weeks utilizing the age-specific dosing.
   2. Treatment for exposed persons:
     a. Give live measles vaccine if exposure was within 72 hours. Dose is 0.5 mL by subcutaneous injection in the outer aspect of the upper arm.
     b. Give Ig 0.25 mL/kg/dose (0.5 mL/kg for clients with HIV) by IM injection (maximum dose is 15 mL) to induce passive immunity and to prevent or modify symptoms within 6 days of exposure for the following high-risk groups:
       i. Immunocompromised individuals
       ii. Infants 6 months to 1 year of age
       iii. Infants younger than 6 months who are born to mothers without measles immunity
       iv. Pregnant women
     c. If the Ig dose exceeds 10 mL, divide the dose into several muscle sites to reduce local pain.
     d. **Do not give Ig with the live measles vaccine.**
     e. Measles is susceptible to ribavirin. Further studies are needed to determine whether this treatment should be recommended. **Ribavirin is not FDA approved for the treatment of measles.**
   3. Live measles virus vaccine should be given (except in pregnant women) approximately 3 months after Ig administration as long as client is at least 15 months of age at that time and there is no contraindication to vaccination.
   4. Children and adolescents with symptomatic HIV infection who are exposed to measles should receive Ig 0.5 mL/kg regardless of vaccination status.
   5. Exposure to measles is not a contraindication to vaccination. Available data suggest that the live measles virus vaccine, if given within 72 hours of measles exposure, provides protection in some cases. If the exposure does not result in infection, the vaccine should induce protection against subsequent measles infection.

Follow-Up

A. See the client daily for mental status examination and examination of the chest to rule out complications such as encephalitis and pneumonia.
B. Follow-up is needed 3 to 4 days after the onset of exanthem.
C. Investigate the immune status of the family and other immediate contacts; prescribe vaccine if necessary.
D. Rubeola cases should be reported to the local health department since one case is considered an outbreak.

Consultation/Referral

A. Refer the client to a physician if fever lasts for more than 4 days; this is indicative of complications. Hospitalization may be indicated for treatment of measles complications (e.g., bacterial superinfection, pneumonia, dehydration, or croup).

Individual Considerations

A. General:

1. A history of anaphylaxis after ingestion of gelatin is associated with an increased risk of anaphylaxis from the MMR or measles vaccine. This history warrants a skin test for gelatin allergy.

2. Individuals with anaphylaxis, excluding contact dermatitis, from neomycin should not receive these vaccines because they contain a small amount of this antibiotic.

3. A history of anaphylaxis after egg ingestion is *not* a contraindication to measles immunization.

B. Pregnancy:

1. Susceptible pregnant women who are exposed to rubeola should receive Ig (see the "Pharmaceutical Therapy" section) in an attempt to modify or prevent the infection.

2. Although no increase in risk of birth defects has been observed in mothers who were given live measles or MMR vaccine during pregnancy, there is a theoretical risk of such events. Measles vaccine is a live attenuated vaccine and is contraindicated in pregnancy.

3. Measles in the mother during delivery does not necessarily lead to measles in the neonate. Congenital measles (defined by the appearance of the measles rash within 10 days of birth) and postnatally acquired measles (rash appears within 14–30 days of birth) have been associated with a spectrum of illnesses ranging from mild to severe disease.

4. Measles vaccine may be administered postpartum to nonimmune mothers.

C. Pediatrics:

1. Recommendations include giving Ig 0.25 mL/kg to infants delivered from mothers with measles in the last week of pregnancy or the first postpartum week.

2. Children without evidence of measles immunity are recommended not to be admitted to school until the first dose of MMR has been administered.

3. A childhood healthcare maintenance visit between 11 and 12 years is recommended to update vaccinations.

4. Concern has been raised periodically about the possible link between receipt of MMR/MMRV and autism. A number of studies have now been performed that fail to demonstrate any such association.

5. Pediatric immunization:

a. Children older than 6 months: 1.5 mL in the outer aspect of the upper arm. Trivalent MMR vaccine should be used unless contraindicated in adults and children older than 12 months.

Bibliography

Centers for Disease Control and Prevention. (2018). *Measles (rubeola)*. Retrieved from www.cdc.gov/measles/hcp/

Chen, S. S. P. (2018a). Measles clinical presentation. *Medscape*. Retrieved from emedicine.medscape.com/article/966220-clinical

Chen, S. S. P. (2018b). Measles treatment & management. *Medscape*. Retrieved from emedicine.medscape.com/article/966220-treatment

Immunization Action Coalition. (n.d.). *Healthcare personnel vaccination recommendations*. Retrieved from www.vaccineinformation.org

Kondamudi, N., & Waymack, J. (2019, May 5). Measles. *StatPearls*. Retrieved from https://www.ncbi.nlm.nih.gov/books/NBK448068/

Scarlet Fever (Scarlatina)

Jill C. Cash, Cheryl A. Glass, and Moya Cook

Definition

A. Scarlet fever is an acute infectious disease that features a vascular response to a bacterial exotoxin usually associated with GAS pharyngitis. It may be present with pharyngitis. Scarlet fever is known as scarlatina in older literature references.

B. Scarlet fever is a nonsuppurative (inflammation without pus) complication of GAS. Development of the scarlet fever rash requires prior exposure to *S. pyogenes*.

C. There is no vaccine available for the prevention of scarlet fever.

Incidence

A. Scarlet fever is uncommon in children younger than 2 years. Recent studies indicate that GAS is responsible for as many as 30% of all pharyngitis cases in children 5 to 15 years old, and 5% to 10% of such cases in adults. The highest incidence is in children 4 to 8 years of age. By the time children are 10 years old, 80% have developed lifelong protective antibodies against streptococcal pyrogenic exotoxins.

Pathogenesis

A. GAS and some strains of *Staphylococcus* are spread by respiratory droplet means and occasionally by direct physical contact from infected wounds, skin, or burns.

B. The incubation period is 12 hours to 4 days. Scarlet fever is communicable during the incubation period and clinical illness (around 10 days), but is no longer infectious after 24 hours of antibiotic therapy.

C. Exotoxin-mediated streptococcal infections range from localized skin disorders (e.g., bullous impetigo) to the systemic rash of scarlet fever to the uncommon but highly lethal streptococcal toxic shock syndrome.

Predisposing Factors

A. Strep throat pharyngitis; family history of recurrent strep infections

B. Direct physical contact with sputum or infected skin

C. Crowded situations (e.g., schools, institutional settings) or unsanitary living conditions

D. Occurs year-round but peaks in the winter and spring

E. Age: Children 5 to 15 years of age

Common Complaints

A. Abrupt onset of fever

B. Headache

C. Sore throat

D. Bright-red rash
E. Nausea and vomiting
F. Pruritus follows with the desquamating rash.

Other Signs and Symptoms

A. Day 1: High fever (as high as 103°F–104°F), red sore throat, swollen tonsils (may have exudate), enlarged lymph nodes in neck, cough, and vomiting. Fever peaks by the second day and gradually returns to normal in 5 to 7 days. Fever abates within 12 to 24 hours after initiation of antibiotic therapy.

B. Day 2: The characteristic rash appears 12 to 48 hours after onset of fever. A bright-red rash is seen on the face, except around the mouth (see Figure 16.9). **The bright-red rash blanches on pressure, has a rough sandpaper texture, and appears first on flexor surfaces, then rapidly becomes more generalized. The rash lasts 4 to 10 days, followed by desquamation of the hands and feet that disappears by the end of 3 weeks. Rash is typically present on the face, which usually has a flushed appearance with circumoral pallor. The rash is most marked in the skin folds. The rash often exhibits a linear petechial character in the antecubital fossae and axillary folds, known as Pastia's lines.**

FIGURE 16.9 Scarlet fever.

C. Day 3:
   1. Strawberry tongue; rash on the body increases and then spreads to neck, chest, and back, and then to the entire body.
   2. Strawberry tongue appears as a thick, white coat with hypertrophied red papillae 24 to 48 hours after infection.
D. Days 4 to 5: The white coating disappears from the tongue.
E. Day 6: The rash fades and the skin begins to peel; peeling continues for 10 to 14 days; the palms of the hands and the soles of the feet are usually spared.

Subjective Data

A. Ask the client/parent about the onset and progression of the rash, its color and duration, and all other symptoms.
B. Review other symptoms related to complications, such as ear pain, chest pain, and edema.
C. Review the family history and possible contact with infected wounds or others with similar symptoms of pharyngitis.

D. Determine any new medications or contact exposures.
E. Determine if the client is allergic to penicillin.
F. Review the client's recent history of impetigo.

Physical Examination

A. Check temperature, pulse, respirations, and BP.
B. Inspect:
   1. Conduct an ear and nose examination.
   2. Inspect the mouth and throat:
      a. Exudative tonsillitis preceding scarlet fever is often accompanied by erythematous oral mucous membranes, along with petechiae, and punctuate red macules on the hard and soft palates and uvula (Forchheimer spots).
      b. Day 1 or 2: A white coating covers the dorsum of the tongue, with reddened papillae projecting through white, before becoming a strawberry red tongue.
      c. Distinctive facial finding: Circumoral pallor
   3. Inspect the skin:
      a. Note the texture of the rash: "Sandpaper" quality secondary to small 1- to 2-mm papular elevations.
      b. The red rash starts on the head, with the soles of the feet and the palms spared.
      c. The rash is most marked in the skin folds of the inguinal, axillary, antecubital, and abdominal areas and about pressure points.
      d. The rash associated with scarlet fever may have a linear petechial characteristic known as Pastia's lines in the antecubital and axillary folds.
      e. The erythematous rash blanches with pressure.
      f. The rash desquamates, with effects on the fingers and toes being most pronounced.
C. Auscultate:
   1. Heart
   2. Lungs
D. Palpate:
   1. The abdomen for organomegaly
   2. Lymph nodes in the neck: Tender and bilateral cervical nodes will be noted.

Diagnostic Tests

A. Throat culture remains the standard criterion for confirmation of GAS URI. Vigorously swab the posterior pharynx, tonsils, and any exudates with a cotton or Dacron swab under strong illumination; avoid the lips, tongue, and buccal mucosa.
B. Rapid antigen detection testing via strep throat swab
C. WBCs in scarlet fever may increase to 12,000 to 16,000 per mm^3, with a differential up to 955 polymorphonuclear lymphocytes.

Differential Diagnoses

A. Scarlet fever: Staphylococcal scarlet fever can be differentiated from streptococcal scarlet fever in the following ways:
   1. There is no circumoral pallor or strawberry tongue with staphylococcal scarlet fever.
   2. The erythematous skin is often painful or tender with staphylococcal infection.

3. Desquamation of the superficial epidermis occurs as with the streptococcal illness; if the superficial skin separates and sloughs after only a few days, the client should be classified as having scalded skin syndrome. Desquamation—one of the most distinctive features of scarlet fever—begins 7 to 10 days after the resolution of the rash and may continue up to 6 weeks.

B. KD: KD needs to be carefully differentiated from scarlet fever; KD has additional signs of conjunctivitis, cracking lips, and diarrhea.

C. Rubeola

D. Rubella

E. Toxic shock syndrome

F. Drug reaction

Plan

A. General interventions:

1. Have the client rest, with no work or school attendance. Clients should not return to work or school until they have completed a full 24 hours of antibiotics.

2. Prepare the client for skin desquamation. The desquamating rash is self-limited but may take more than 2 weeks for resolution. Skin emollients may be used.

3. Throat cultures of other household members may be necessary.

4. Acetaminophen (Tylenol) for temperature and pain relief

B. Client teaching: Reinforce the need to comply with full antibiotic treatment even if the symptoms resolve.

C. Pharmaceutical therapy:

The goal of antibiotic therapy is to prevent acute rheumatic fever, acute glomerulonephritis, and other complications.

---

1. **Tetracyclines and sulfonamides should not be used**

2. The drug of choice for streptococcal infections is penicillin by mouth or IM injection. Azithromycin and erythromycin may be substituted for clients with penicillin allergies.

   a. Adults:

   i. Penicillin V (Pen-Vee K): 250 mg orally three or four times daily for 10 days

   ii. Penicillin G benzathine (Bicillin L-A): 1.2 million units by IM injection in one dose

   iii. Erythromycin (erythromycin ethylsuccinate [EES], E-mycin, or Ery-Tab): 250 mg every 6 hours orally before meals, or 500 mg orally every 12 hours before meals for 10 days

   b. Children:

   i. Children younger than 12 years: Penicillin V (Pen-Vee K) 25 to 50 mg/kg/d orally divided into three or four doses for 10 days; do not exceed 3 g/d

   ii. Children older than 12 years: Administer penicillin V as in adults

   iii. Children less than 27 kg: Penicillin G benzathine 600,000 units IM as one dose

   iv. Children greater than 27 kg: Administer penicillin G benzathine as in adults

   v. Amoxicillin is often used in place of oral penicillin in children, since the taste of the oral suspension is more palatable. Administration of 50 mg/kg (maximum 1,000 mg) in a single dose orally for 10 days is as effective as oral penicillin V or amoxicillin given multiple times per day for 10 days. **However, strict adherence to once-daily dosing must be ensured.**

   vi. Erythromycin (E-mycin or Ery-Tab): 30 to 50 mg/kg four times a day for 10 days

   vii. Azithromycin 12 mg/kg once a day to a maximum of 500 mg/dose for 5 days (FDA approval for 5-day therapy)

3. Antihistamines may be used to control pruritus that follows the desquamating rash.

Follow-Up

A. No follow-up is needed for clients with uncomplicated illnesses. Clients should return for care if they continue to have fever and increased throat or sinus pain.

B. Consider KD if fever persists more than 4 days.

Consultation/Referral

A. Refer the client to a physician (i.e., ENT or infectious disease specialist) for complications, such as unresolved otitis media, sinusitis, bacteremia, rheumatic fever, and glomerulonephritis.

B. Consult a dermatologist if the diagnosis is unclear.

Bibliography

Pardo, S., & Perera, T. (2019, February 28). Scarlet fever. *StatPearls*. Retrieved from https://www.ncbi.nlm.nih.gov/books/NBK507889/

Toxoplasmosis

Jill C. Cash, Cheryl A. Glass, and Moya Cook

Definition

A. Toxoplasmosis is caused by an intracellular protozoan parasite, *Toxoplasma gondii*. Cats are the primary host in which *T. gondii* can complete its reproductive cycle. Humans are the intermediate host. Toxoplasmosis is acquired through contact with infected cat feces, by eating raw or undercooked meat, and by eating soil-contaminated fruit or vegetables. In less developed countries, contaminated unfiltered water is an important source of infection, as is a transfusion or organ transplantation from an infected donor (rare).

B. Emphasis should not be placed on prior exposure to cats, since clients can acquire *Toxoplasma* without direct contact with felines. Toxoplasmosis is one of the TORCH infections. It causes CNS disease in clients with AIDS and has perinatal consequences. Latent infection can persist for the life of the host.

C. There are three genotypes of *T. gondii*, designated as I, II, and III. Genotype II is generally responsible for congenital toxoplasmosis in the United States.

D. There is no vaccination available for the prevention of toxoplasmosis.

Incidence

A. Toxoplasmosis has a worldwide distribution. There is no association with cat ownership. The incidence of seropositivity in adults ranges from 10% (United States) to 80% (Africa and Europe). Rates of *Toxoplasma* encephalitis are reported to be as high as 25% to 50% in susceptible hosts. Adults most commonly acquire toxoplasmosis by environmental exposure—that is, ingestion of infectious oocysts, usually from soil contamination with feline feces.

B. Once a person is infected, the parasite lies dormant in neural and muscle tissues and will never be eliminated. Approximately 50% of all pregnant women in the United States have been previously infected and are immune, whereas those who keep cats as pets have a higher seropositivity rate. The rate of primary infection during pregnancy ranges from 1 to 8 per 1,000.

C. The global annual incidence of congenital toxoplasmosis is approximately 190,100 cases, which poses a global health burden. The severity of congenital infection depends on the gestational age at the vertical transmission. The greatest risk to the fetus is vertical transmission in the first trimester. Approximately 30% of exposed fetuses acquire the infection; however, 85% of live infants appear normal at birth.

D. Approximately 225,000 cases of toxoplasmosis are reported each year in the United States.

E. *T. gondii* is the third most common lethal foodborne disease in the United States; it is estimated to result in 5,000 hospitalizations and 750 deaths annually.

Pathogenesis

A. *T. gondii* is the causative agent and an intracellular protozoan parasite. *T. gondii* has a worldwide distribution; cats, birds, and domesticated animals serve as reservoirs. *T. gondii* is recognized as a major cause of opportunistic infection in AIDS.

B. The incubation period is estimated to be, on average, 7 days (4- to 21-day range)

C. Routine screening for toxoplasmosis in pregnancy is not currently recommended.

    1. Maternal toxoplasmosis infection is acquired orally.

    2. Fetal infection results from transmission of parasites via the placenta (vertical transmission).

    3. Neonatal infection may also occur during vaginal delivery.

Predisposing Factors

A. Food sources:

    1. Eating raw or undercooked meats, especially mutton, lamb, and pork

    2. Drinking unpasteurized goat milk

    3. Eating raw shellfish

B. Exposure to contaminated soil or garden, kitty litter, and cats

C. Immunocompromised state:

    1. HIV infection/AIDS

    2. Cancer therapy

    3. Transplant recipients

    4. Prescribed immunosuppressive drugs

D. *T. gondii* has been documented as being acquired from blood or blood product transfusion and organ (i.e., heart) or bone marrow transplant from a seropositive donor with latent infection.

E. Poor sanitary conditions

F. Consumption of contaminated unfiltered water

G. Occupational exposure:

    1. Working with meat

    2. Landscaper

H. Travel to underdeveloped country

Common Complaints

A. Approximately 80% to 90% of acute *T. gondii* infectious hosts are asymptomatic.

B. Bilateral, symmetrical, nontender cervical adenopathy

C. Approximately 30% of symptomatic clients have generalized lymphadenopathy.

Other Signs and Symptoms

A. Usually subclinical infection:

    1. Fever

    2. Arthralgia, malaise, and myalgia

    3. Headache

    4. Sore throat/pharyngitis

    5. Skin rash: Diffuse nonpruritic maculopapular rash

    6. Hepatosplenomegaly

    7. Chorioretinitis: Ocular pain and loss of visual acuity (the most-frequent permanent manifestation of toxoplasmic infection)

B. Pregnancy:

    1. IUGR or low birth weight

    2. Hydrocephaly

    3. Microcephaly

    4. Anemia

C. CNS toxoplasmosis:

    1. Headache, dull and constant, is an almost universal symptom of cerebral lesions in AIDS clients

    2. Fever

    3. Lethargy

    4. Altered mental state

    5. Seizures

    6. Weakness

    7. Hemiparesis

    8. Cranial nerve disturbances

    9. Sensory abnormalities

    10. Movement disorders

    11. Neuropsychiatric manifestations: Toxoplasmosis is a significant factor in the causation of mental retardation and blindness

Subjective Data

A. Review onset, course, and duration of symptoms.

B. Determine if the client is pregnant.

C. Review the presence of an indoor cat and contact with kitty litter.

D. Rule out other illnesses through a review of symptoms such as pharyngitis (mononucleosis).

E. Elicit the initial site of the rash and its progression to other body areas.

F. Determine any new medications and contact exposures.

G. Rule out other family members with similar symptoms.

H. Review HIV status.

I. Review ingestion of raw/rare or undercooked meats, raw shellfish, and unpasteurized goat milk.

J. Review recent travel to an underdeveloped country (untreated water).

K. Review occupational exposure.

Physical Examination

A. Check temperature, pulse, respirations, and BP.

B. Inspect:

1. Conduct an ENT examination and a careful funduscopic examination.

> A funduscopic examination may reveal yellow-white areas of retinitis with fluffy borders. Diagnosis of ocular toxoplasmosis is based on observation of characteristic retinal lesions in conjunction with toxoplasma-specific serum IgG or IgM antibodies.

2. Complete a dermal examination.

C. Auscultate:

1. Heart

2. Lungs

D. Palpate:

1. Palpate all lymph nodes, especially cervical nodes. Lymph nodes are usually smaller than 3 cm in size and nonfluctuant.

2. Abdomen

3. Joints, noting swelling, erythema, or pain with examination

E. Neurological examination: Conduct a mental status evaluation.

Diagnostic Tests

A. ELISA is the most commonly employed test due to its overall performance and cost when measuring toxoplasmosis IgG and IgM antibody titers. Maternal infections usually are confirmed by a fourfold rise in the serum IgG.

B. Serial titers: No single level of IgG antibody can be used to determine the duration of the infection. IgG-specific antibodies achieve their peak concentration 1 to 2 months after exposure and remain positive indefinitely.

C. CBC with differential

D. HIV (rule out)

E. Pregnancy test if indicated

F. Culture: Tissue smears, tissue section, and body fluids for presence of *T. gondii* may be considered in neonates. It takes 3 to 6 weeks to confirm the diagnosis.

G. CT scan or MRI: MRI is usually superior to CT scan.

Differential Diagnoses

A. Toxoplasmosis

B. EBV

C. CMV (CMV retinitis)

D. CSD

E. Tuberculosis

F. Syphilis

G. Sarcoidosis

H. Hodgkin's disease

I. Lymphoma

J. Viral syndrome

K. HIV

L. Mononucleosis

M. *Pneumocystis jirovecii* pneumonia

N. Varicella zoster

O. Fungal infection of eye

Plan

A. General interventions:

1. Treatment is rarely necessary because most clinical illnesses resolve spontaneously; the exception is during pregnancy.

B. Client teaching:

1. **Handwashing is the single most important measure to reduce transmission of *T. gondii*.**

2. Client teaching: *See Section III: Client Teaching Guide for this chapter, "Toxoplasmosis."* ◄

C. Pharmaceutical therapy:

1. Treatment is usually given for 2 to 4 weeks.

a. Nonpregnant adults: One of two regimens is typically prescribed:

i. Pyrimethamine: 100 mg loading dose, then 25 to 50 mg by mouth daily; *plus* sulfadiazine 2 to 4 g/d by mouth in divided doses; *plus* leucovorin calcium (folinic acid) 10 to 25 mg by mouth daily

ii. Pyrimethamine: 100 mg loading dose, then 25 to 50 mg by mouth daily; *plus* clindamycin 300 mg by mouth four times a day; *plus* leucovorin calcium (folinic acid) 10 to 25 mg by mouth daily

b. Pregnancy: Despite the lack of evidence of treatment efficacy, prenatal treatment is usually offered to pregnant women who are diagnosed with toxoplasmosis.

i. Spiramycin alone: 1 g orally every 8 hours without food. The drug is available in the United States for use in pregnancy from Rhone-Poulenc (Montreal, Quebec) if an Investigational New Drug number is obtained from the FDA under the "compassionate use" pathway.

ii. Three-week course of pyrimethamine 50 mg once a day orally or 25 mg twice a day; *and* sulfadiazine 3 g/d orally divided into two or three doses *alternating* with a 3-week course of spiramycin 1 g orally three times a day until delivery.

iii. Pyrimethamine 25 mg once per day by mouth *and* sulfadiazine 4 g/d orally divided into two to four doses until term

iv. Leucovorin calcium (folinic acid) 10 to 25 mg/d orally is added during pyrimethamine and sulfadiazine administration to prevent bone marrow suppression.

c. Children:

i. Trimethoprim–sulfamethoxazole 150 to 750 mg/m^2/d in two divided doses daily

ii. For children 1 month of age or older: Dapsone 2 mg/kg (maximum of 25 mg), orally every day; *plus* pyrimethamine 1 mg/kg orally every day; *plus* leucovorin 5 mg orally every 3 days

    d. Persons with compromised immune system:

      i. Trimethoprim 10 mg/kg/daily *plus* sulfamethoxazole 50 mg/kg/daily by mouth. May be considered as a non-pyrimethamine alternative for clients with AIDS who are unable to tolerate the usual adult therapy noted previously.

      ii. Administering dapsone with pyrimethamine appears to provide effective chemoprophylaxis in clients with HIV who are seropositive for *T. gondii* and who have CD4 cell counts lower than 200. However, rash, fever, and hemolytic anemia are common adverse effects, often necessitating cessation of therapy.

      iii. For clients with AIDS, after primary therapy, lifelong prophylaxis for recurrence of toxoplasmosis is required for as long as they are immunosuppressed.

Follow-Up

A. Follow up in 1 week to evaluate for secondary complications.

B. Pyrimethamine is a folic acid antagonist that can cause dose-related bone marrow suppression with resultant anemia, leukopenia, and thrombocytopenia. Sulfadiazine, another folic acid antagonist, works synergistically with pyrimethamine; it can cause bone marrow suppression and reversible acute renal failure. Clients should return for laboratory monitoring (CBC and platelet counts) weekly.

Consultation/Referral

A. Consultation is needed for all clients; comanage clients with a physician/specialist.

B. Refer the client to an obstetrician if she is pregnant.

C. The ophthalmological medication recommendation depends on the size of the eye lesion, the location, and the characteristics of the lesion (active acute versus chronic not progressing).

Individual Considerations

A. Pregnancy:

    1. Routine prenatal screening is not the standard of care secondary to costs. Many women have antibodies before pregnancy that protect the fetus.

    2. Transplacental infection increases the incidence of first-trimester spontaneous abortion, IUGR, preterm birth, neonatal anomalies, and stillbirth.

    3. Pyrimethamine is a folic acid antagonist and should not be given in the first trimester.

    4. Sulfadiazine should not be given in the third trimester secondary to the increased incidence of jaundice in the neonate.

    5. Transmission of toxoplasmosis in breast milk has not been demonstrated. Pyrimethamine is excreted in breast milk; however, WHO and the AAP classify it as compatible with breastfeeding.

B. Pediatrics:

    1. Approximately 70% to 90% of affected infants with congenital infection will be asymptomatic at birth or will present with low birth weight, enlarged liver and spleen, jaundice, and anemia.

      a. Signs of congenital toxoplasmosis at birth can include maculopapular rash, generalized lymphadenopathy, hepatomegaly, splenomegaly, jaundice, and thrombocytopenia.

      b. Cerebral calcifications may be demonstrated by radiography, ultrasound, or CT of the head.

      c. Characteristic retinal lesions (chorioretinitis) develop in as many as 85% of young adults after untreated congenital infection. Acute ocular involvement manifests as blurred vision.

      d. Ocular disease can become reactivated years after the initial infection in health and immunocompromised people.

    2. Complications including visual impairment from chorioretinitis or learning disabilities or mental retardation damage may develop several years later.

    3. Treatment consists of drug therapy for the first year of life (see the "Pharmacological Therapy" section), which appears to limit further CNS injury but does not reverse the prenatal damage already sustained by the neonate.

    4. Corticosteroids also may be administered to infants with chorioretinitis.

C. AIDS clients:

    1. Clients with AIDS who have antibodies to *T. gondii* and a CD4 count of 100 cells/mm^3 should be considered at high risk for the development of clinical disease. Reactivation of latent infection in the CNS is a common HIV- and AIDS-related complication.

    2. Clients with a CD4 count less than 100 cells/mm^3 should receive prophylaxis against toxoplasmosis. The U.S. Department of Health and Human Services provides prophylactic guidelines for treatment of opportunistic infections in adults and adolescents with HIV: https://aidsinfo.nih.gov/guidelines/html/4/adult-and-adolescent-opportunistic-infection/322/toxoplasma-gondii.

    3. Serology in HIV-infected clients is used mainly to identify those at risk for developing toxoplasmosis. Therefore, all HIV-positive clients should be tested for the presence of IgG antibodies.

Bibliography

Ayoade, F., Stevenson, A., & Chandranesan, J. (2019, January 19). Toxoplasmosis: HIV-1 associated opportunistic infections. *StatPearls*. Retrieved from https://www.ncbi.nlm.nih.gov/books/NBK441877/

Centers for Disease Control and Prevention. (2018). *Parasites: Toxoplasmosis (Toxoplasma infection)*. Retrieved from www.cdc.gov/parasites/toxoplasmosis

Gilbert, R., & Petersen, E. (2020, February 6). Toxoplasmosis and pregnancy. *UpToDate*. Retrieved from https://www.uptodate.com/contents/toxoplasmosis-and-pregnancy?search=Toxoplasmosis%20and%20pregnancy&source=search_result&selectedTitle=1~150&usage_type=default&display_rank=1

Varicella (Chickenpox)

Jill C. Cash, Cheryl A. Glass, and Moya Cook

Definition

A. Varicella, commonly called chickenpox, is a viral disease characterized by a vesicular rash that occurs in crops. It manifests as a generalized, pruritic, vesicular rash (see Figure 16.10). VZV infection causes two clinically distinct forms of disease: varicella (chickenpox) and herpes zoster (shingles).

FIGURE 16.10 Varicella rash.

1. Primary VZV results in the diffuse vesicular rash of chickenpox.
2. VZV remains dormant in the sensory nerve roots for life. Reactivation of the virus is known as shingles.
    a. With shingles, the virus migrates along sensory nerves via dermatomes. Symptoms include pain, sensory loss, and neurological complications.
    b. A diagnostic clue of shingles is sensory symptoms that do not cross the midline.
    c. Postherpetic neuralgia is a prolonged complication from shingles.
B. Varicella is considered one of the TORCH infections. Varicella infection can be fatal for an infant if the mother develops varicella from 5 days before to 2 days after delivery. A newborn is protected for several months from chickenpox if the mother had the disease before or during pregnancy. Infant immunity diminishes in 4 to 12 months.
C. Two vaccines are available for the prevention of varicella—MMRV and a monovalent varicella vaccine. The AAP notes that the quadrivalent MMRV is preferred to giving two separate injections secondary to the additional pain and the risk of the child falling behind in his or her immunization schedule.
    1. Both the monovalent and the quadrivalent immunizations carry a risk of febrile seizures. A personal or family history of seizures is considered a precaution for the administration of MMRV.
    2. The AAP also advises that with a personal or family history of seizures, the MMR and varicella vaccines should be administered as separate immunizations. The varicella vaccine may be given simultaneously with the MMR vaccine, but separate syringes and injection sites must be used. If not given simultaneously, the interval between administration of varicella vaccine and MMR should be at least 28 days apart.

Incidence

A. Infants are generally protected in the first few months through passive immunity. The peak incidence shifting from children younger than 10 years to children between 10 and 14 years of age demonstrates the highest incidence following the implementation of universal immunization in 1995. Varicella tends to be more severe in adolescents and adults. Hemorrhagic varicella is much more common among immunocompromised clients. Immunity is generally considered lifelong.
B. The rate of herpes zoster after varicella vaccination was 2.6 per 100,000 according to 1998 CDC unpublished data. The incidence of herpes zoster after natural varicella infection among healthy children younger than 20 years is 68 per 100,000; for all ages, the incidence is 215 per 100,000.
C. Varicella incidence has greatly declined since the chickenpox vaccine became available in the United States. It is predicted that varicella deaths, outbreaks, and hospitalizations will be greatly reduced through such vaccinations.
D. Seasonal incidence of VZV peaks in the months of March through May.
E. The general rate of chickenpox is 4 persons per 1,000. Approximately 1 million cases occur annually in the United States.
F. After the primary infection, the risk of shingles increases with age. The lifetime risk of herpes zoster infection is 15% to 20%.
G. The incidence of congenital varicella is 1% to 2% if the maternal infection occurs before 20 weeks' gestation.

Pathogenesis

A. Varicella (herpesvirus 3) is a member of the herpesvirus family. Humans are the only source of infection for this highly contagious virus, which may infect more than 90% of susceptible household contacts. Person-to-person transmission occurs primarily by direct contact with a client with varicella or zoster, but occasionally occurs by airborne droplet spread, from respiratory secretions spread onto the conjunctival or nasal/oral mucosal tissues, and from direct contact with vesicular zoster lesions. In utero infections also occur from transplacental passage of the virus during maternal varicella infection.
B. The incubation period is 14 to 16 days. The infection is communicable 1 to 2 days to 1 week before macular eruption and until lesions crust over (about 1 week).

Predisposing Factors

A. Exposure to someone with the varicella virus:
    1. Direct contact with skin lesions or by respiratory tract secretions
    2. Direct contact with clients with shingles can induce chickenpox in susceptible healthcare workers.
B. Compromised immune system

C. Nosocomial transmission is well documented in pediatric units, but transmission is extremely rare in newborn nurseries.
D. Late winter and early spring

Common Complaints
A. Low-grade fever
B. Mild malaise
C. Skin lesions or rash: The characteristic rash is a pruritic, vesicular exanthem occurring in crops that begin on the head and neck and progress to involve the trunk and extremities. Blisters collapse within 24 hours to 1 week and crust over to form scabs. Skin eruptions may appear almost anywhere on the body, including the scalp; penis; and inside the mouth, nose, throat, and vagina.
D. Itching
E. Myalgia 1 to 4 days before onset of rash

Other Signs and Symptoms
A. Children may have a mild prodrome to bacterial infections.
B. Adults may develop varicella pneumonitis. The risk of pneumonitis is higher in smokers than in nonsmokers.
C. Cough
D. Headache
E. Respiratory symptoms: Cough and chest discomfort. Respiratory symptoms usually develop shortly after cutaneous eruption. Respiratory failure in pregnancy can be rapid.
F. Abdominal pain lasting 1 to 2 days

Subjective Data
A. Review the onset, duration, and course of symptoms.
B. Elicit exposure information, including noting the characteristic rash, the time it started, spread of the rash or lesions, and characteristic changes.
C. Review any pulmonary or nervous system problems, such as seizures, that occur as complications.
D. Determine if the person has HIV, is immunocompromised, or is pregnant.
E. Determine the caregiver's immunity status relative to varicella.
F. Review the client's immunization history.
G. Review all medications, including OTC and herbal products.

Physical Examination
A. Check temperature, pulse, respirations, and BP.
B. Inspect:
    1. Conduct a dermal examination, especially at the hairline.
    2. Inspect the buccal mucosa.
    3. Conduct an ENT examination and a detailed eye examination.
    4. Shingles: Note locations of lesions; they usually involve only one to three dermatomes.
C. Auscultate:
    1. Heart
    2. Lungs
D. Palpate:
    1. Neck and lymph nodes

Diagnostic Tests
A. Diagnosis is usually determined by the appearance of the skin eruptions; laboratory tests are not necessary.
B. ELISA
C. Tissue culture of vesicular fluid or tissue biopsy: Requires up to a week to obtain the result
D. Varicella IgG and IgM: VZV-specific IgM is present within 5 days of onset of the rash and lasts 4 to 5 weeks. A significant increase in varicella IgG antibody by standard serologic assay can confirm a diagnosis retrospectively. These antibody tests are not as reliable in immunocompromised people.
E. Pregnancy test if indicated; if positive, order the following:
    1. Anti-VZV IgG to establish immunity
    2. Tzanck smear of suspicious lesions
    3. Culture lesion for herpes simplex
F. PCR of vesicular swabs or scrapings, scabs for crusted lesions, or tissue biopsy
G. Chest x-ray, if indicated, to rule out pneumonia
H. Genotyping of the virus is available free of charge through a specialized CDC reference lab. The CDC reference lab contact number is 404-639-0066. Merck & Company (contact number: 800-672-6372) also performs genotyping through a safety research program.

Differential Diagnoses
A. Varicella (chickenpox)
B. Herpes simplex
C. Scabies
D. Impetigo
E. Coxsackievirus
F. Insect or spider bite
G. Drug reaction
H. Secondary syphilis
I. Measles
J. Rubella
K. RMSF
L. Scabies

Plan
A. General interventions:
    1. Avoid contact with persons infected with chickenpox. Clients with varicella should avoid contact with others. Healthcare workers should be immune to varicella. Determine immunity status with varicella IgG antibody titer if this status is unknown.
    2. Strict isolation should be enforced. Varicella is contagious 1 week before the rash outbreak and until the lesions crust over (about 1 week). Isolation is a precaution until the vesicles dry.
    3. Order oatmeal baths (Aveeno) for comfort. Spray starch may also be sprayed on lesions to assist with severe itching.
B. Client teaching:
    1. Client teaching: *See Section III: Client Teaching Guide for this chapter, "Chickenpox (Varicella)."* ◄
    2. Lesions that can be covered pose little risk to a susceptible person because transmission usually occurs from direct contact with the fluid from the lesion.

Clothing or a dressing should cover lesions until they have crusted.

3. Scarring can occur from secondary infection of lesions; encourage good handwashing and no scratching.

C. Pharmaceutical therapy:

1. **Children with varicella should not receive salicylates, such as aspirin, or salicylate-containing products due to the increased risk of Reye's syndrome.** Acetaminophen (Tylenol) may be used as needed for fever.

2. Acyclovir therapy is *not* recommended routinely for treatment of uncomplicated varicella in otherwise healthy children.

3. Acyclovir is recommended if it can be initiated within the first 24 hours after the onset of rash in the following groups:

   a. Otherwise healthy, nonpregnant individuals aged 13 years or older

   b. Children older than 12 months with a chronic cutaneous or pulmonary disorder, and those receiving long-term salicylate therapy

   c. Children receiving a short, intermittent, or aerosolized course of corticosteroids (if possible, discontinue corticosteroids)

4. If therapy can be initiated within the first 24 hours of rash onset, prescribe oral acyclovir 20 mg/kg/dose in four divided doses for 5 days (maximum dose is 800 mg/dose four times daily); the usual dose for adults is 800 mg four times a day. Clients on oral acyclovir should be well hydrated during therapy.

5. Acyclovir by IV infusion is recommended for treatment of immunocompromised clients and clients with serious complications such as varicella pneumonia or encephalitis. Acyclovir IV dosage is 10 mg/kg every 8 hours for 7 days.

6. Varicella-zoster immune globulin (VZIG) is no longer available. The only manufacturer of this product has ceased its production.

7. Systemic antipruritic: Diphenhydramine HCl (Benadryl):

   a. Adults: 25 to 50 mg every 4 to 6 hours (maximum adult dosage 300 mg/d)

   b. Children:

      i. Not recommended for neonates

      ii. Children younger than 6 years: Dosage must be individualized

      iii. Children 6 to 12 years of age: 12.5 to 25 mg every 4 to 6 hours (maximum pediatric dosage 150 mg/d)

8. The varicella vaccine may be given simultaneously with the MMR vaccine, but separate syringes and injection sites must be used. If not given simultaneously, the interval between administration of the varicella vaccine and MMR should be at least 1 month.

9. Antihistamines are helpful in the symptomatic treatment of pruritus.

10. The use of corticosteroids for clients with shingles to prevent postherpetic neuralgia is controversial.

11. Treatment for postherpetic neuralgia includes gabapentin, pregabalin, tricyclic antidepressants, phenytoin, carbamazepine, cimetidine, and topical capsaicin.

Follow-Up

A. No follow-up is necessary in uncomplicated cases.

B. Have the client return to the office for any secondary skin infections, conjunctival involvement, CNS problems such as encephalitis and meningitis, or pneumonia.

Consultation/Referral

A. Refer the client to a physician if pregnant; varicella pneumonia in pregnancy is a medical emergency.

Individual Considerations

A. Pregnancy:

1. Varicella vaccine should not be administered to pregnant women.

   a. Women are advised not to get pregnant for at least 1 month following the varicella immunization.

   b. A pregnant mother or household member is not a contraindication for immunization for a child in the household.

2. When postpubertal females are immunized, pregnancy should be avoided for at least 1 month after immunization.

3. VZIG: The maternal therapy's aim is to reduce maternal morbidity; whether it protects the fetus is unknown.

4. Reporting by telephone of inadvertent immunization when the varicella-zoster–containing vaccine is given during pregnancy is encouraged: 800-986-8999 or www.merckpregnancyregistries.com/varivax.html.

5. Maternal complications of active varicella infection may include preterm labor, encephalitis, and varicella pneumonia. The mortality rate in gravid females is 10%. The profound maternal hypoxia that occurs in varicella pneumonia is associated with increased risk of spontaneous abortion and stillbirth.

6. Fetal complications of active varicella infection may include IUGR, limb reduction defects, and eye defects.

7. Acyclovir is a pregnancy category B drug. IV acyclovir is recommended for the pregnant client with serious complications of varicella. VariZIG or IVIG can be used during pregnancy for susceptible women who are exposed to VZV.

B. Pediatrics:

1. Varicella can develop between 1 and 16 days of life in infants born to mothers with active live varicella at delivery.

2. Neonates usually have no prodrome or have mild signs and symptoms with slight malaise and low-grade fever. Neonatal varicella is a serious illness associated with up to a 25% mortality rate. Complications include conjunctival involvement, secondary bacterial infection, viral pneumonia, encephalitis, aseptic meningitis, myelitis, Guillain–Barré syndrome, and Reye's syndrome.

3. Children entering day-care facilities and schools should have received varicella vaccine or have evidence of immunity.

4. Children with varicella should not receive salicylates or salicylate-containing products due to the risk for Reye's syndrome.

5. Children with varicella who have been excluded from child care may return when all lesions have dried and crusted.

C. Adults:

1. Adult clients usually have a prodrome and more severe illness than children do. Adults have a 25% increased risk of mortality.

2. Shingles (reactivated chickenpox) appears as grouped vesicular lesions distributed in one to three sensory dermatomes, sometimes accompanied by pain localized to the area. Systemic symptoms are few. The recombinant zoster vaccine (RZV) is recommended over the zoster vaccine live (ZVL) for clients aged 50 years and older.

3. A recommendation for varicella vaccination includes persons at high risk for exposure, including adolescents and adults who live in households with children.

D. Immunocompromised individuals: IV antiviral therapy is recommended for immunocompromised clients, including clients being treated with chronic corticosteroids. Therapy initiated early in the course of illness, especially within 24 hours of rash onset, maximizes efficacy. Oral acyclovir should not be used to treat immunocompromised children with varicella because of its poor bioavailability.

Bibliography

Albrecht, M. A. (2019). Vaccination for the prevention of shingles (herpes zoster). *UpToDate*. Retrieved from https://www.uptodate.com/contents/vaccination-for-the-prevention-of-shingles-herpes-zoster

Centers for Disease Control and Prevention. (2017). Shingles herpes zoster. *CDC for Health Care Professionals*. Retrieved from https://www.cdc.gov/shingles/hcp/clinical-overview.html

Immunization Action Coalition. (n.d.). *Healthcare personnel vaccination recommendations*. Retrieved from www.vaccineinformation.org

West Nile Virus

Jill C. Cash, Cheryl A. Glass, and Moya Cook

Definition

West Nile Virus (WNV) disease is a mosquito-borne viral illness caused by one of the most widely distributed arthropod-borne (arbovirus) viruses. WNV is a member of the genus *Flavivirus* group, meaning it is a single-strand RNA virus. WNV is transmitted from infected animal hosts, typically wild birds, to humans via the most common types of mosquitoes. Once a client recovers from WNV disease, he or she is thought to have a lifelong immunity to the disease. There is no immunization for WNV.

The two categories of WNV disease are nonneuroinvasive and neuroinvasive.

A. Nonneuroinvasive disease is less severe and often presents as a febrile illness.

B. Neuroinvasive disease leads to encephalitis, meningitis, and flaccid paralysis and requires much more intensive treatment.

Incidence

A. **WNV is a reportable disease, which enables the CDC to maintain significant surveillance data and statistics on this infection.** In 2018, WNV cases were reported in 49 states.

B. Approximately 20,000 new cases occur in North America each year; however, only 20% to 40% of those individuals infected with the virus develop symptoms. One in 150 clients develops severe neurological disease; 3% to 15% of those who develop severe neurological disease will die.

C. WNV was first noted in North America in 1999. It is endemic in the Middle East, Africa, and Asia.

D. Human WNV infections usually begin in midsummer and decline in September, correlating with peak mosquito activity. Mosquito bites are most likely to occur during peak feeding times during dawn and dusk. Prolonged contact or multiple mosquito bites increase the risk of developing WNV.

Pathogenesis

A. Mosquitoes become infected with WNV by feeding on an infected animal host. Wild birds are the most common source of infection, although other animals, such as horses and chickens, can also be animal hosts. The virus is delivered to the human via mosquito bite when the mosquito's saliva is deposited in the human skin cells. The virus replicates in the skin cells and migrates to the lymph nodes and various organs. Infected immune cells are able to traverse the blood–brain barrier and infect the brain parenchyma, leading to encephalitis and meningitis. The typical incubation period for WNV is 3 to 14 days.

Predisposing Factors

A. Time of year: Late summer and early fall

B. Region: Living in or traveling to a region with a higher number of reported cases

C. Work or recreational outdoor exposure

D. Homelessness

E. Age: Most likely to occur in children and young adults, with the most serious disease occurring in the elderly and infants

Common Complaints

A. Nonneuroinvasive WNV:

1. As many as 80% of persons are asymptomatic
2. Fever
3. Headache
4. Myalgia
5. Arthralgias
6. Fatigue
7. GI symptoms: Nausea, vomiting, and diarrhea
8. Maculopapular rash: Usually noted on chest, back, and arms; occurs in 20% to 50% of clients. The presence of the rash indicates a decreased risk of neuroinvasive disease.

Other Signs and Symptoms
A. Abdominal pain
B. Eye pain
C. Irregular heart rhythm

Potential Complications
A. Meningitis: Stiff neck, photophobia, focal neurological deficits, and higher fever (up to 104°F)
B. Encephalitis: Mental status changes, stupor, confusion, coma, movement disorders, focal neurological deficits, personality changes, higher fever (up to 104°F), and seizures
C. Flaccid paralysis: Cranial nerve palsy, vertigo, dysarthria, dysphagia, respiratory failure
D. Other rare complications:
   1. Cardiac dysrhythmia
   2. Myocarditis
   3. Rhabdomyolysis
   4. Optic neuritis
   5. Uveitis
   6. Chorioretinitis
   7. Orchitis
   8. Pancreatitis
   9. Hepatitis

Subjective Data
A. Review the onset, course, and duration of symptoms, especially fever, rash, headache, and myalgia.
B. Ask the client to describe any neurological symptoms, changes in mental status, stiff neck, photophobia, and seizures.
C. Review symptoms of other family members or coworkers who are also ill.
D. Ask the client to recall what activity brought about or preceded the symptoms.
E. Ask the client about steps taken to treat symptoms at home.
F. Review the client's medical history for any chronic illnesses.
G. Review all medications, including OTC and herbal products.
H. Review the client's history of mosquito bites and any preventive steps taken, such as use of insect repellent:
   1. Outdoor work activities
   2. Outdoor recreational activities
   3. Recent travel
I. Evaluate living conditions for exposure risks.

Physical Examination
Clients presenting with neurological symptoms should be quickly assessed and referred to a neurologist for immediate evaluation of symptoms.
A. Check temperature, pulse, respirations, and BP.
B. Inspect:
   1. Observe the client's general overall appearance, noting any weakness, difficulty breathing, or changes in affect, speech, or LOC.
   2. Assess hydration status.
   3. Ophthalmic examination: Assess the presence of papilledema.
   4. Inspect the face for muscle weakness or drooping.
   5. Perform a dermal inspection for the presence of a maculopapular rash, especially on the abdomen, back, and arms.
   6. Children:
      a. Observe for seizure activity.
      b. Note LOC (playful versus lethargic).
C. Auscultate:
   1. The heart for dysrhythmias
   2. All lung fields for adventitious breath sounds
D. Palpate:
   1. The skin for signs of dehydration, including poor skin turgor
   2. The neck and lymph nodes: Preauricular, posterior auricular, submental and sublingual, anterior cervical chain, and supraclavicular nodes
   3. The abdomen for tenderness and/or organomegaly
E. Mental status and neurological examination:
   1. Administer a mental status examination to look for confusion, stupor, and changes in LOC.
   2. Complete cranial nerve testing: Focus on visual fields, extraocular movement (EOM) of a transient downbeat nystagmus, facial muscle movement and strength, and gag reflex.
   3. Muscle strength testing and testing for sensation in all extremities
   4. Test reflexes:
      a. Deep tendon reflexes
      b. The Babinski reflex is performed by running the reflex hammer up the midline of the sole of the foot from the heel to the base of the toes; both feet are tested.
         i. A normal reaction is for the toes to either remain still or else to curl downward.
         ii. A positive Babinski sign is noted when the big toe points upward and the other toes fan out *except in infants.*
   5. Assess for meningeal signs:
      a. Signs of meningeal irritation include nuchal rigidity.
      b. Assess for positive Brudzinski's and Kernig's signs (refer to Figures 16.1 and 16.2).
         i. Brudzinski's sign: Place the client supine and flex the head upward. Resulting flexion of both hips, knees, and ankles with neck flexion indicates meningeal irritation.
         ii. Kernig's sign: Place the client supine; keeping one leg straight, flex the other hip and knee to a bent knee to form a 90° angle. Slowly extend the lower leg. This places a stretch on the meninges, resulting in pain and spasm for the hamstring muscle. Resistance to further extension can be felt.

Diagnostic Tests
A. **WNV IgM antibody capture enzyme-linked immunosorbent assay (MAC-ELISA) is the gold-standard diagnostic test.** A positive result would indicate WNV.
B. If there is concern that the illness could have been caused by another type of flavivirus, an additional

test—the plaque reduction neutralization test—is used to identify false-positive MAC-ELISA test results.

C. CBC with differential: Will show increased leukocytes

D. For clients with neuroinvasive disease:

1. Lumbar puncture—positive for WNV—will show pleocytosis, increased lymphocytes, increased protein, and normal glucose. The MAC-ELISA test should be performed on CSF when the lumbar puncture is completed.

2. Imaging: MRI of the brain and spinal cord is the preferred imaging test. MRI may show meningeal inflammation and bilateral lesions.

3. EEG: May show generalized slowness

Differential Diagnoses

A. Nonneuroinvasive WNV:

1. WNV

2. Other viral causes of febrile illness

B. Neuroinvasive WNV:

1. Other viral causes of encephalitis: St. Louis equine encephalitis, California encephalitis, Western and Eastern encephalitis

2. Acute poliomyelitis

3. Postpolio syndrome

4. Guillain–Barré syndrome

5. Multiple sclerosis

6. Vertebrobasilar stroke

Plan

A. General interventions:

1. Every case of WNV should be reported to the health department for surveillance purposes. Special populations may be subject to follow-up.

2. Care is primarily supportive, treating symptoms such as fever, nausea/vomiting, and diarrhea.

3. Neuroinvasive disease: Clients presenting with neurological symptoms should be quickly assessed and referred to a neurologist for immediate evaluation and treatment of acute symptoms.

B. Client teaching:

1. Educate the client about expected signs and symptoms of WNV acute febrile illness.

2. Explain signs and symptoms that would require immediate medical evaluation, such as mental status changes, stiff neck, and neurological symptoms.

3. Instruct the client to rest as needed. The client may expect fatigue to continue for up to 3 weeks.

C. Pharmaceutical therapy:

1. Utilize supportive therapy such as acetaminophen for fever, antiemetics for nausea and vomiting, and antidiarrheal medications for diarrhea.

D. Dietary management:

1. There are no specific dietary recommendations for WNV.

2. Encourage the client to drink plenty of fluids to prevent dehydration.

3. If the client is experiencing nausea and vomiting, meals should be light and nonspicy and should be taken in smaller amounts more frequently.

Follow-Up

A. Follow-up is determined by the client's needs, severity of acute symptoms, and risk of complications.

Consultation/Referral

A. Neuroinvasive disease: Refer the client to a neurologist immediately.

1. For longer-term relief from neuroinvasive disease, the client may benefit from a referral to a neuropsychologist, rehabilitation specialist, physical therapist, occupational therapist, and/or speech therapist.

B. Consider referring the client to an infectious disease specialist if there is difficulty with identifying the infectious agent.

Individual Considerations

A. Pregnancy:

1. No causal relationship has been found between WNV during pregnancy and fetal abnormalities. A small number of infants, born to women who developed WNV within 3 weeks before delivery, have been found to have symptomatic WNV disease shortly after birth.

2. If WNV is diagnosed during the last few weeks of pregnancy, a detailed examination of the newborn should be completed and steps taken to monitor for signs and symptoms of the disease in the days and weeks after the birth.

3. All cases of WNV in pregnant women should be reported to the health department so that the cases can be followed to determine the outcome of the pregnancies.

4. The virus has been found in breast milk and, in rare cases, breastfeeding has been linked to development of WNV in infants. The benefits of breastfeeding outweigh the risks of WNV disease; therefore, mothers should be encouraged to breastfeed.

5. Pregnant women can use insect repellent products containing N-diethylmetatoluamide (DEET) without adverse effects.

B. Pediatrics:

1. Infants are more likely to suffer a more serious illness with WNV. A thorough assessment and educating the parent to recognize important signs and symptoms are crucial.

2. The AAP recommends that insect repellents should not be applied to children younger than 2 months.

C. Geriatrics:

1. Older adults are more likely to suffer more serious illness and are more likely to develop neuroinvasive disease. Close attention should be given to the mental status examination and neurological examination of the elderly.

Bibliography

Centers for Disease Control and Prevention. (2018). *West Nile virus*. Retrieved from www.cdc.gov/westnile/index.html

Centers for Disease Control and Prevention. (2019). *West Nile virus neuroinvasive disease incidence by state—United States*. Retrieved from www.cdc.gov/westnile/statsmaps/preliminarymapsdata/incidencestatedate.html

Petersen, L. R. (2018). Epidemiology and pathogenesis of West Nile virus infection. *UpToDate*. Retrieved from www.uptodate.com/contents/epidemiology-and-pathogenesis-of-west-nile-virus-infection

Salinas, J. D. (2018). West Nile virus. *Medscape*. Retrieved from emedicine.medscape.com/article/312210-overview

Zika Virus Infection

Jill C. Cash and Moya Cook

Definition

A. Zika virus is an arthropod-borne virus that is transmitted by the *Aedes* species of mosquito. This virus is a member of the same family as dengue virus, yellow fever virus, and WNV. It was initially found in the rhesus monkey in 1947 and then detected in humans in 1952 in Uganda and Tanzania. The Zika virus infection has been documented in Africa, Southeast Asia, and the Pacific Islands, and has now spread to the Americas. Mosquito-borne transmission has not been reported in the United States; however, cases of infection have been reported in male and pregnant and nonpregnant female travelers who were exposed in other countries from the mosquito-borne illness.

B. Congenital microcephaly is a known pregnancy complication of Zika viral infection. Vertical transmission to the fetus occurs from the primary infected mother or can occur from an infected male to a noninfected female.

Incidence

A. The first case of congenital microcephaly in the United States was reported in January 2016 in Hawaii; the pregnant woman affected had lived in Brazil during her pregnancy. In Texas, documentation of sexually transmitted Zika virus infection occurred in February 2016. During the months of January through June 2016, reports from New York City revealed that approximately 3,605 travelers were exposed to the Zika virus in other countries, and 182 of those individuals tested positive for the Zika virus in the United States.

B. In 2017, 223 cases were reported in the United States, primarily in Florida: Of those cases, 48 were transmitted sexually, and 28 were congenital. In 2017, 452 cases were reported from travelers returning to the United States, and 7 cases of presumed mosquito-borne transmission in Florida. Currently, case counts are decreasing, with 72 cases in 2018 and no mosquito-borne transmissions; and 2 cases reported (up to June 2019) in travelers returning to the United States from affected areas.

Pathogenesis

A. The incubation period is unknown, but is thought to be within a few days to 7–12 days.

B. The Zika virus is transmitted to humans when an infected mosquito bites the person.

C. The virus is detected in urine, blood, semen, saliva, female genital secretions, breast milk, amniotic fluid, and cerebral spinal fluid.

D. The virus can be transmitted by maternal–fetal transmission, sex (vaginal, anal, and oral), blood transfusion, organ transplantation, and exposure in the laboratory from body fluids.

Predisposing Factors

A. Recent travel to Brazil or other countries at high risk for Zika virus. See the CDC website for a listing of countries: www.CDC.gov.

B. Exposure to body fluids from a person with documented infection

C. Sexual contact with a person confirmed to have Zika virus

D. Vertical transmission from an infected mother

Common Complaints

Two or more of the following symptoms appear. Symptoms may be mild and/or may not be recognized by the client.

A. Acute-onset low-grade fever

B. Maculopapular pruritic rash

C. Arthralgia of small joints (hand and feet)

D. Conjunctivitis (nonpurulent)

Other Signs and Symptoms

A. Headache

B. Malaise

C. Retro-orbital (eye) pain

D. Asthenia

E. Less common symptoms may include GI symptoms: Nausea, vomiting, diarrhea, abdominal pain, and mucous membrane ulcers

Subjective Data

A. Inquire whether the client has traveled outside of the United States in areas that are at high risk for Zika virus, such as Brazil, Sint Eustatius, and Argentina. Refer to the CDC website for an updated list of areas infected with Zika virus: www.CDC.gov.

B. Has the client had sexual contact with another person who could possibly be infected with the Zika virus? If so, were condoms used?

C. What are the client's current symptoms? When did symptoms begin, and how have they progressed?

D. Has the client had low-grade fever, joint pain, headache, eye pain, or muscle weakness?

E. Does the client have any GI symptoms, such as nausea, vomiting, and abdominal pain?

F. Has the client noted any skin rash or irritation?

G. What has the client used for symptoms that have presented? Did the treatment(s) improve symptoms? Has the client taken any medications before the appointment to help with fever or pain?

Physical Examination

A. Check temperature, pulse, respirations, and BP.

B. Inspect:
   1. The skin for rash. Note if a maculopapular, pruritic rash is present.
   2. The eyes for erythema and drainage. Perform an ophthalmic examination. Note eye pain.

C. Auscultate:
   1. Heart
   2. Lungs

D. Palpate:
   1. The abdomen for tenderness, rebound tenderness, and masses

2. The back for costovertebral angle (CVA) tenderness
3. A joint examination should be performed in the hands, feet, and other joints in which the client is complaining of joint pain
E. Neurological examination:
1. Perform a neurological examination if Guillain–Barré syndrome is suspected. See Chapter 19, Neurological Guidelines, "Guillain-Barré Syndrome," for assessment guidelines.

Diagnostic Tests
A. CBC: Usually normal
B. The FDA has issued two diagnostic tests for Zika virus: Zika MAC-ELISA and Trioplex rRT-PCR assay. Only certain laboratory centers are qualified to run these complex tests.
C. Clinicians are encouraged to contact the state or local public health department for testing instructions. The FDA website may be used for further instructions.
D. **The Zika virus is a nationally notifiable condition.** All state, local, and territorial health departments must notify the CDC of positive results.

Differential Diagnoses
A. Zika virus
B. Other viruses: Dengue fever, parvovirus, rubella, enterovirus, adenovirus
C. GAS
D. Measles
E. Malaria
F. Leptospirosis
G. Guillain–Barré syndrome

Plan
A. General interventions:
1. There is no vaccine or treatment available for Zika virus.
2. Treatment is recommended for presenting symptoms such as low-grade fever, joint pain, and conjunctivitis, along with comfort measures.
3. Mosquito bite prevention is highly recommended to avoid this virus.
4. Confirmation of the diagnosis is essential for proper care and management.
5. Pregnant women should avoid traveling to areas at high risk for Zika virus.
6. Sexual contact should be avoided with clients diagnosed with Zika virus.
B. Client teaching:
1. Client teaching: *See Section III: Client Teaching Guide for this chapter, "Zika Virus Infection."*
2. Advise travelers to avoid going to areas that have a high risk for Zika virus, such as Brazil. Refer to the CDC website for a list of countries at risk for the Zika virus: www.CDC.gov.
3. The *Aedes* mosquito is most active during daytime hours, but precautions must also be used at dusk and at night.
4. Educate the client regarding preventive measures for the Zika virus.
   a. Advise clients to wear loose, long-sleeved, light-colored clothing (shirts and pants) to avoid mosquito bites. Treat clothing with insecticide, such as permethrin.
   b. Apply insect repellent that contains *N*-diethylmetatoluamide (DEET) when outside.
   c. Apply insect repellent after sunscreen.
   d. If traveling in exposed areas, use mosquito bed nets while sleeping, if areas are not screened in or screens are not used in windows. Treat bed nets with insecticide.
   e. Avoid mosquito insect breeding areas, such as standing water (e.g., pools, water-filled buckets). Empty out containers with standing water.
   f. **Advise women to avoid becoming pregnant while traveling to high-risk areas as well as to avoid pregnancy up to 8 weeks after such travel.**
5. Practice safe sex, using condoms, or abstain from sexual activity with clients diagnosed with Zika virus.
6. **Pregnant women with confirmed Zika virus should use condoms or abstain from sex for the duration of the pregnancy.**
7. **Men with confirmed Zika virus should use condoms or abstain from sex for at least 6 months after the onset of the virus.**
8. **Couples in which the man has traveled to a high-risk area but did not develop symptoms should use condoms or abstain from sex for at least 8 weeks to prevent potentially spreading the virus.**
C. Pharmaceutical therapy:
1. No medication is currently available for prevention or treatment of Zika virus infection.
2. The CDC recommends using analgesics such as acetaminophen (Tylenol) for the treatment of arthralgia and fever.
3. NSAIDs and aspirin should be avoided due to the risk of dengue infection and risk of hemorrhage.

Follow-Up
A. Depending on symptoms, the client should be reevaluated in 24 to 48 hours either by office visit or by phone.
B. If the client has myalgia, joint pain, and fever, or if symptoms worsen or new symptoms present, advise the client to return for a follow-up evaluation.
C. If the client begins having muscle weakness and/or symptoms of Guillain–Barré syndrome, the client should make a follow-up appointment immediately with the provider or go to the ED for evaluation. See Chapter 19, Neurological Guidelines, "Guillain–Barré Syndrome," for assessment and client education guidelines.
D. Blood work that is sent to the laboratory for screening for the Zika virus may take up to 3 weeks for final interpretation of results. Advise the client that precautions should be taken while waiting on results.
E. **All positive results are reportable to the CDC.**

Consultation/Referral
A. Consult with the collaborating physician if a client presents with complaints relating to Zika virus.
B. Consider referral to an infectious disease specialist for evaluation and management.

Individual Considerations

A. Pediatric:

1. Presenting symptoms in children may be the same as in adults. Other symptoms may include poor feeding, irritability, difficulty walking or bearing weight, and joint pain with active/passive movement of joints.

2. Neurological complications (brain ischemia, myelitis, meningoencephalitis) have been documented in children who were exposed to the virus in utero.

B. Pregnancy:

1. Congenital microcephaly and fetal loss have been reported in newborns exposed to the Zika virus in utero.

C. Adults:

1. Guillain–Barré syndrome has been documented as a complication of Zika virus. Further evaluation is necessary if Guillain–Barré syndrome is suspected.

Bibliography

Centers for Disease Control and Prevention. (2019a). *2019 case counts in the U.S.* Retrieved from https://www.cdc.gov/zika/reporting/2019-case-counts.html

Centers for Disease Control and Prevention. (2019b). *Zika virus.* Retrieved from www.cdc.gov/zika

LaBeaud, A. (2019). Zika virus infection: An overview. *UpToDate.* Retrieved from www.uptodate.com/contents/zika-virus-infection-an-overview

17 Systemic Disorders Guidelines

Chronic Fatigue Syndrome (CFS; Systemic Exertion Intolerance Syndrome)

Julie Adkins and Jenny Mullen

Definition

A. Fatigue is one of the most common symptoms confronting the practitioner in an office practice. A client with chronic fatigue is characterized as having fatigue with multiple associated symptoms for longer than 6 months in which these symptoms have a profound impact on daily activities and are moderate to severe symptoms that occur over half the time. The fatigue is not relieved by rest.

Incidence

A. Fatigue accounts for 1% to 3% of visits to generalists as an isolated symptom or diagnosis. Psychiatric disorders are involved in <50% of cases. The Centers for Disease Control and Prevention (CDC) estimates that up to 2.5 million people meet criteria for chronic fatigue syndrome (CFS), and approximately 84% to 91% are undiagnosed. The CDC indicates that the CFS disorder results in a significant economic impact of a $17 to $24 billion annual productivity loss (not including U.S. citizens' medical/disability costs).

B. The average onset is in the third decade of life. Fatigue is seen predominantly four times more in women than in men, and the highest prevalence is in people aged 40 to 60 years, but it can affect people of all ages, including teens and children.

Pathogenesis

A. Fatigue is a sensitive but nonspecific indicator of underlying medical and/or psychological pathology. It is reportedly more often due to unknown cause or to psychiatric illness than to physical illness, injury, medications, drugs, or alcohol.

B. The Institute of Medicine (IOM) indicated chronic fatigue is caused by changes in the immune system's response to stress/infection. Possible systemic dysfunctions include chronic production of cytokines, low-functioning natural killer cells, differences in markers of T-cell activation, and disruptions within hypothalamic–pituitary–adrenal axis. The long-term effects of CFS can lead to a serious illness affecting multiple body systems, which the IOM reports as myalgic encephalomyelitis chronic fatigue syndrome (ME/CFS). Clients suffering from ME/CFS experience three primary symptoms: a sizable drop in activity level for ≥ 6 months; postexertional malaise that includes decrease in mental acuity; and relentless sleep difficulties. An overview of the CDC and IOM's management education can be found at https://www.cdc.gov/me-cfs/index.html.

Predisposing Factors

A. Hyperthyroidism
B. Hypothyroidism
C. Cardiac disease: congestive heart failure (CHF)
D. Neurally mediated hypotension
E. Infections: endocarditis, hepatitis
F. Respiratory disorders: chronic obstructive pulmonary disease (COPD) and sleep apnea
G. Anemia
H. Arthritides and related disorders
I. Cancer
J. Alcoholism
K. Side effects from drugs such as sedatives and beta-blockers
L. Psychological conditions such as insomnia, depression, anxiety, and somatization disorder
M. Female gender
N. Viruses such as Epstein–Barr virus and herpes virus

Common Complaints

A. Sudden onset of profound fatigue with other symptoms
B. Unrefreshing sleep
C. Extreme exhaustion lasting more than 24 hours after physical or mental exercises
D. Loss of memory and concentration
E. Joint pain that moves around without swelling or redness
F. Muscle fatigue
G. Swollen lymph nodes in neck/armpits

Other Signs and Symptoms

A. Headache with new pattern and intensity
B. Overexertion
C. Poor physical conditioning
D. Stress
E. Undernutrition and poor appetite
F. Emotional problems: depression, anxiety, and somatization disorder

Subjective Data

A. Review history for onset, duration, and course description of the fatigue.
B. Ask the client about significant losses, low self-esteem, and occurrence of crying spells and suicidal thoughts. High prevalence of depression and suicide is present in this client population.
C. Ask the client about a history of any abuse of hypnotic drugs, alcohol, or tranquilizers.
D. Review medications, both over-the-counter (OTC) and prescription drugs.
E. Review the client's medical history for cardiac, thyroid, and other medical conditions.
F. Review sleep and insomnia history.
G. Review history for family illness, new baby, or postpartum period.
H. Establish last menses to rule out pregnancy.
I. Review exercise patterns.
J. Review diet with 24-hour recall.
K. Elicit history of fever, night sweats, weight loss, and enlarged lymph node(s).
L. Inquire about recent major life changes, such as moving or a change in job.
M. Establish usual weight, and review recent weight gain or loss, over what period.
N. Review any recent infections, flu, or mononucleosis.
O. Review high-risk sexual practices and intravenous drug use to rule out HIV exposure.
P. Review recent history for transfusion of blood products to rule out hepatitis or HIV exposure.
Q. Obtain history of the client's daily living and working habits.

Physical Examination

A. Check temperature, pulse, respirations, blood pressure, and weight; check for postural hypotension.
B. Inspect:
  1. Observe general overall appearance. Skin: conduct dermal examination for changes in pigmentation, purpura, dryness, rashes, jaundice, pallor, splinter hemorrhages, or petechiae.
  2. Eyes: Conduct a funduscopic examination to rule out Roth's spots and tuberculoma.
  3. Check sclerae for icterus.
  4. Throat: Inspect pharynx for petechiae at the junction of the hard and soft palates to rule out mononucleosis.
  5. Extremities: Inspect the joints for inflammation.
C. Auscultate:
  1. Heart
  2. Lungs

D. Percuss:
  1. Abdomen for organomegaly, masses, ascites, and hepatic tenderness.
E. Palpate:
  1. Palpate the neck, to rule out goiter.
  2. Palpate all lymph nodes (neck, axilla, and groin) for size, degree of tenderness, and distribution.
  3. Complete clinical breast examination for masses.
  4. Palpate the abdomen for organomegaly, masses, and ascites.
  5. Palpate the joints for tenderness.
  6. Assess the genitalia for masses and tenderness to rule out infection.
F. Neurologic examination:
  1. Complete mental status assessment.
G. Rectal examination:
  1. Assess for masses, prostatic pathology, and occult blood.

Diagnostic Tests

A. Complete blood count (CBC) with differential and peripheral smear
B. Erythrocyte sedimentation rate (ESR)
C. Calcium, albumin, blood urea nitrogen (BUN), and creatinine
D. Glucose
E. Transaminase (aminotransferase): Viral hepatitis is associated with elevation in transaminase.
F. HIV serum test
G. Thyrotropin-stimulating hormone (TSH) to rule out hyperthyroidism or hypothyroidism
H. Heterophile test to rule out acute mononucleosis
I. Monospot
J. Epstein–Barr virus
K. Sleep study

Differential Diagnoses

A. Hypercalcemia
B. Mild renal failure
C. Early diabetes mellitus
D. Hypothyroid or hyperthyroidism
E. Cardiac disease
F. Anemia
G. Anicteric hepatitis
H. Connective tissue disease
I. Immune hyperactivity
J. Disturbed sleep
K. Occult neoplasm
L. Infection: history of fever, sweats, weight loss, and diffuse adenopathy. These symptoms also suggest HIV, especially with high-risk behaviors (see "Human Immunodeficiency Virus" section).

Plan

A. General interventions:
  1. Find out the client's view of his or her illness before proceeding with client education.
  2. Manage underlying disease (refer to specific chapters).
  3. Managing CFS can be as complex as the illness itself. There is no cure and symptoms vary over time.

Treating the most disruptive symptoms first is paramount, and then monitoring medications and supplements, managing activities and exercise, and improving health and quality-of-life issues are the primary goals.

4. Cognitive behavioral therapy and exercise therapy have been shown to be beneficial to the CFS client.

5. Evaluate the client for the possibility that he or she is confusing focal neuromuscular disease with generalized lassitude.

B. Client teaching:

1. Discuss and review the evidence for the diagnosis and offer a careful explanation of symptoms. Many clients think they have a medical problem producing fatigue symptoms.

2. Review the diagnostic criteria for depression (see Chapter 22, "Psychiatric Guidelines") and describe the neurochemical mechanisms by which depression leads to fatigue. Refer the client for individual counseling or group therapy.

3. Review the idiopathic nature of CFS and its nonprogressive nature. Inform the client that CFS has a gradually improving clinical course and has the chance of full recovery. Symptoms are self-limited, usually clearing within 12 to 18 months. People with chronic fatigue 2 years or less are more likely to improve than the person for whom it has taken more time to diagnose.

4. Encourage the client to begin a gentle exercise program and to engage in life's activities.

5. Provide nutritional education.

C. Pharmaceutical therapy:

1. For postural hypotension:

a. Increase dietary sodium.

b. Antihypotensive agent: fludrocortisone 0.1 mg daily

2. Low-dose antidepressant therapy for disordered sleep:

a. Amitriptyline HCl 25 mg every bedtime

b. Imipramine HCl 25 to 50 mg at bedtime; may increase dosage up to 300 mg daily

c. Doxepin HCl 10 to 20 mg daily at bedtime

d. Short-term hypnotic: zolpidem (Ambien) 5 to 10 mg at bedtime

3. Nonsteroidal anti-inflammatory drugs (NSAIDs) for symptomatic relief of myalgia, arthralgia, or headache

4. Correct anemia with iron supplements, if applicable.

Follow-Up

A. Follow up in 2 weeks to reevaluate status, and then monthly depending on signs and symptoms.

B. Follow up closely whether the client is depressed.

Consultation/Referral

A. Consult a physician if no improvement is seen with therapies. Emphasize the legitimacy of the client's symptoms and summarize the workup, its rationale, and its findings.

B. Refer the client to a mental health professional as indicated by depression and/or suicidality.

Individual Considerations

A. Pediatrics:

1. Between 0.2% and 2.3% of children and adolescents suffer from CFS. It is more prevalent in adolescents than in younger children and is more likely to develop after an acute flu-like illness or mononucleosis. Gradual onset may also occur.

B. Adults:

1. Fatigue is most often explained by common factors such as overexertion, poor physical conditioning, inadequate quantity or quality of sleep, obesity, undernutrition, stress, and emotional problems.

C. Geriatrics:

1. Chronic fatigue commonly presents in the elderly population. Assess and evaluate the following possible causes: multiple medication side effects, grief from loss (loved ones or socioeconomic status changes), end of life issues that could be causing stress and sleep disruptions, poor nutritional intake, or drinking excess alcohol.

Resource

Fact sheets may be obtained with information about child, adolescent, and adult CFS at the CDC at www .cdc.gov.

Chronic Fatigue Immune Dysfunction Syndrome (CFIDS) Association
PO Box 220398
Charlotte, NC 28222-0398
704-365-2343
Available 24 hours a day, 7 days a week

Bibliography

Centers for Disease Control and Prevention. (2019e, May 8). *Myalgic encephalomyelitis/ chronic fatigue syndrome*. National Center for Emerging and Zoonotic Infectious Diseases. Retrieved from https:// www.cdc.gov/me-cfs/index.html

Institute of Medicine. (2015). *Beyond myalgic encephalomyelitis/chronic fatigue syndrome: Redefining an illness*. Washington, DC: National Academies Press.

National Institute on Aging. (2016, July 2). *Fatigue in older adults*. NIH Health Information. Retrieved from https://www.nia.nih.gov/health/ fatigue-older-adults

Roberts, J., & Bronze, M. (2018). *Chronic fatigue syndrome (CFS)*. MedScape. Retrieved from https://emedicine.medscape.com/article/ 235980-overview#a5

Fevers of Unknown Origin

Julie Adkins and Jenny Mullen

Definition

A. The criteria for fevers of unknown origin (FUO) are an illness of at least 3-week duration, fever >101.0°F (38.3°C) on several occasions, and remaining undiagnosed after 1 week of study in the hospital. Because of cost factors, the criterion requiring 1 week of hospitalization is often bypassed.

Incidence

A. In adults, infections account for 30% to 40% of the cases. Cancer accounts for 20% to 30% of the cases of FUO. In children, infections are the most common cause of FUO, accounting for 30% to 50% of the cases; cancer is a rare cause of FUO in children. Autoimmune disorders occur with equal frequency in adults and children. Infection, cancer, and autoimmune disorders combined account for 20% to 25% of FUO in clients who have been febrile for 6 months or longer. Various miscellaneous diseases account for another 25%. Approximately 50% of FUO remain undiagnosed but have a benign course, with symptoms eventually resolving. Between 5% and 15% of FUO cases defy diagnosis even after exhaustive studies.

Pathogenesis

There are five categories of causes of FUO.

A. Infection: Most common systemic infections are tuberculosis (TB), cat-scratch disease (CSD), Epstein-Barr virus, cytomegalovirus (CMV), and HIV. Least common are organ-based infections such as endocarditis, tooth abscess, chronic mastoiditis, chronic prostatitis, vascular graft infections, and cholecystitis. Geographic and travel-related infections must be considered, which would include tick-borne infections and regional infections.

B. Neoplasms: Most common are lymphoma, renal cell carcinoma, and leukemia. Least common are multiple myeloma; cancers of breast, liver, pancreas or colon; and metastases to brain or liver.

C. Noninfectious inflammatory autoimmune disorders: Most common are Still's disease, systemic lupus erythematosus (SLE), giant cell arteritis, and polyarteritis nodosa. Least common would include gout, sarcoidosis, and antiphospholipid syndrome.

D. Miscellaneous causes: These include hyperthyroidism, thyroiditis, sarcoidosis, Whipple's disease, familial Mediterranean fever, recurrent pulmonary emboli, alcoholic hepatitis, drug fever, factitious fever, and others.

E. Undiagnosed FUO

Predisposing Factors

A. Upper respiratory infection
B. Urinary tract infection
C. Viral illnesses
D. Drug allergy, especially to antibiotics
E. Connective tissue disease
F. TB
G. HIV
H. Parasite infection

Common Complaints

A. The client feels "sick all over," with malaise and fatigue.
B. The client has chills all over the body with high fever.

Other Signs and Symptoms

A. Tachycardia
B. Sensation of warmth or flushing
C. Piloerection
D. Myalgias
E. Mild inability to concentrate, confusion, delirium, or even stupor
F. Labial herpes simplex outbreak or fever blisters
G. Children: seizures
H. Rigors or shaking most likely indicates infectious origin.

Subjective Data

A. Review the onset, course, and duration of symptoms.
B. Review family, occupational, and social history.
C. Review sexual practices, including monogamy and oral, rectal, and vaginal sexual habits; recreational habits; and any new changes.
D. Elicit information regarding use of intravenous drugs.
E. Review if the client has had this illness before. How was it treated?
F. Review travel during the last month.
G. Review any new hobbies, changes at home or work, or other new events.
H. Review the client's history for contact with any friends or family members who have been sick and do not seem to be getting any better.
I. Review the client's history for eating any uncooked meat and dietary changes during the past month.
J. Review the child's history specifically for febrile seizures.
K. Review for risk factors for thrombophlebitis (see Chapter 10, "Cardiovascular Guidelines").

Physical Examination

A. Check temperature, pulse, respirations, blood pressure, weight, and height.
B. Inspect:
    1. Conduct funduscopic examination to rule out retinopathy, Roth's spots, and choroidal tubercles.
    2. Examine the ears, nose, and throat. Inspect the mouth.
    3. Observe the skin and mucous membranes.
    4. Perform transillumination of sinus cavities for evidence of sinusitis.
    5. Inspect body for skin rashes or wounds.
C. Auscultate:
    1. Heart for murmurs and rubs
    2. Lungs for rales, consolidation, and effusion
D. Percuss:
    1. Sinuses for tenderness
    2. Chest for consolidation
    3. Abdomen
E. Palpate:
    1. Neck, axilla, and groin for lymphadenopathy
    2. Thyroid gland
    3. Abdomen for organomegaly, masses, tenderness, guarding, rebound, suprapubic tenderness, and costovertebral angle tenderness (CVAT)
    4. Musculoskeletal system for bone or joint swelling, tenderness, increased warmth; check lower extremities for evidence of phlebitis, asymmetrical swelling, calf tenderness, and palpable cord

5. Elderly: palpate scalp for tender arteries.

6. Infants: palpate fontanelles.

F. Neurologic examination:

1. Assess for signs of meningeal irritation (Brudzinski's and Kernig's signs) and presence of focal deficits.

2. Conduct mental status examination.

G. Genitorectal examination, if applicable:

1. Female: conduct pelvic examination for cervical discharge, adnexal masses, lesions, and pelvic inflammatory disease (PID) symptoms.

2. Male: conduct prostate and testicular examination for tenderness and masses; check penis for discharge, rash, and lesions.

3. Both: conduct rectal examination for discharge, tenderness, and masses; check stool for occult blood specimen.

Diagnostic Tests

A. CBC with differential

B. Sedimentation rate

C. Urinalysis and urine culture

D. Blood glucose

E. Liver function test

F. Blood cultures

G. Consider serology for suspected infections or pathology (refer to Chapter 16, "Infectious Disease Guidelines"). Suspected infections include Epstein-Barr virus, Q fever, Lyme disease or other tick-borne diseases, hepatitis, syphilis, and CMV.

H. Suspected collagen disease: antinuclear antibodies (ANAs) and rheumatoid factor

I. Suspected TB: tuberculin skin test, sputum, and urine cultures

J. Immunologic studies: enzyme-linked immunosorbent assay (ELISA), Western blot test, and antistreptolysin O (ASLO) titer

K. Suspected mononucleosis: heterophile antibody test

L. Suspected *Salmonella*: Widal's test

M. Suspected thyroiditis: thyroid profile

N. Suspected malaria or relapsing fever: direct examination of blood smears

O. Imaging: depends on suspected infection:

1. Chest, sinus radiographic films

2. Gastrointestinal (GI) studies: proctosigmoidoscopy; evaluate gallbladder function

3. CT scan of abdomen and pelvis, abdominal ultrasonography

4. MRI is better than CT scan for detecting lesions of the nervous system.

P. Suspected embolism: ventilation–perfusion (V/Q) scan

Q. Suspected endocarditis or atrial myxoma: echocardiography

R. Radionuclide studies: Gallium scan and radium-labeled immunoglobulin are useful in detecting infection and neoplasm.

S. Laparotomy in the deteriorating client if the diagnosis is elusive despite an extensive evaluation. Any abnormal finding should be aggressively evaluated. Headache necessitates a lumbar puncture to rule out meningitis; biopsy any skin from an area of rash to look for cutaneous manifestations of collagen vascular disease or infection; enlarged lymph nodes should be aspirated or biopsied and examined for cytologic features to rule out neoplasm and send for culture.

Differential Diagnoses

A. Systemic and localized infections

B. Neoplasms

C. Autoimmune disorders

D. Thrombophlebitis

E. Miscellaneous causes (see "Definition" section)

Plan

A. General interventions:

1. Observe the client taking his or her own temperature to document the presence of a fever to make sure the temperature is not self-induced.

2. Treatment should be directed toward the underlying cause once a diagnosis is made.

B. Client teaching:

1. Instruct the client to keep a record of temperatures, preferably rectal, taken each evening, when elevations are most likely to occur.

2. Reassure the client that there is nothing abnormal about temperatures in the range of 97.0°F to 99.3°F.

3. Instruct the client on use of physical cooling aids, such as exposure of skin to cool ambient temperature, bedside fan, and sponging with cool water or alcohol.

4. Explain to the client that immersion in an ice water bath may be indicated for hyperthermic emergencies.

C. Pharmaceutical therapy:

1. Start therapeutic trials if a diagnosis is strongly suspected:

   a. Antituberculous drugs for TB

   b. Tetracycline for brucellosis

   c. If the client shows no clinical response in 2 weeks, stop therapy and reevaluate.

2. Symptomatic antipyretic therapy: salicylates or acetaminophen every 4 hours

Follow-Up

A. Follow up in 24 to 48 hours.

B. Indications for admission to the hospital: fever remains elevated beyond 101°F for weeks and ambulatory diagnostic efforts have been unsuccessful.

Consultation/Referral

A. Consult with a physician for diagnosis and comanagement if indicated.

B. Refer the client to a specialist (infectious disease) if unable to differentiate definitive diagnosis.

Individual Considerations

A. Pregnancy:

1. Refer the client for perinatal consultation.

2. High fevers early in the first trimester have been associated with an increase in neural tube defects.

3. Maternal fevers may cause fetal tachycardia.

B. Pediatrics:

1. Toxic-appearing infants and children should be hospitalized and given parenteral antibiotic therapy following prompt diagnostic testing that includes white blood cell (WBC); urinalysis; and cultures of blood, urine, and cerebrospinal fluid. Consult a physician.

2. Infants under 28 days, regardless of appearance, are generally hospitalized and given parenteral antibiotic therapy following prompt diagnostic testing with WBC, urinalysis, and cultures.

3. Aspirin products should not be given to children due to the risk of Reye's syndrome.

4. Consider inflammatory bowel disease in older children and adolescents.

C. Geriatrics:

1. Generally 25% to 35% of FUO cases in populations older than 65 years are commonly a result of TB, Hodgkin's lymphoma, and temporal arteritis; whereas, 12% to 23% account for malignancies.

2. Elderly clients often present with nonspecific symptoms.

Bibliography

Chan-Trak, K. (2015). *Fever of unknown origin*. Medscape. Retrieved from http://emedicine.medscape.com/article/217675

Gompf, S., & Bronze, M. (2018, March 1). *Fever of unknown origin (FUO)*. MedScape. Retrieved from https://emedicine.medscape.com/article/217675-overview#a5

Ternak, G. (2014). Fever of unknown origin in the elderly: Clinical approach. *Journal of Gerontology & Geriatric Research*, *3*(4), e1. doi:10.4172/2167-7182.S1.004. Retrieved from https://www.omicsonline.org/proceedings/fever-of-unknown-origin-in-the-elderly-clinical-approach-18188.html

Human Immunodeficiency Virus (HIV)

Beverly R. Byram and Dana Hughes

Definition

A. Acquired immunodeficiency syndrome (AIDS) is a chronic, life-threatening condition caused by the HIV, which is a retrovirus that targets helper T (CD4) cells. This retrovirus contains a viral enzyme called reverse transcriptase that allows the virus to convert its RNA to DNA, and then integrates to take over the cell's own genetic material. Once taken over, the new cell begins to produce new HIV retrovirus. This process kills the CD4 cells that are the body's main defense against illness and interferes with the body's ability to fight off infection—bacteria, viruses, and fungi—that causes the disease. The term AIDS is used to define a severely compromised immune system.

Incidence

A. According to the CDC, by the end of 2016, there were approximately 1.1 million persons over the age of 13 living with HIV in the United States. Approximately 14% of those were unaware of their HIV status. In 2017 an estimated 43% of those living with HIV were African American, 26% White, and 26% Hispanic. Asians/Pacific Islanders represent 2.5% and American Indians/Alaskan Natives represent <1%.

B. The largest population living with HIV comprises men having sex with men (MSM), followed by persons infected by high-risk heterosexual contact, those infected by intravenous drug users (IVDUs), and those exposed through both MSM and IVDU.

C. The widespread use of antiretroviral therapy (ART) has altered the course of HIV disease. In 2012, HIV was reclassified as a chronic illness. More than 50% of deaths in HIV-positive persons on highly active antiretroviral therapy (HAART) are related to conditions other than AIDS.

The U.S. Preventive Services Task Force (USPSTF) recommends HIV screening for all people between the ages of 15 and 65 years as well as younger and older people at high risk of HIV infection. Older adults have unrecognized risks and tend to present symptoms late in the course of infection. Clinical recommendation for early detection is to devise a routine risk-based screening to identify HIV regardless of age. This screening could prompt immediate ART, which is critical for successful outcomes.

D. Due to the rapidity of changing technology and knowledge, refer to the website at https://www.cdc.gov/hiv/default.html for the newest statistics.

Pathogenesis

A. HIV belongs to a subgroup of retroviruses called lentiviruses or "slow" viruses. The course of infection of the virus is characterized by a long interval between infection and the onset of serious symptoms. CD4 cells are the primary target of the HIV.

B. Primary HIV infection is followed by a burst of viremia during which the virus is easily detected in peripheral blood per HIV polymerase chain reaction (PCR) viral load (VL). During the "window period," the first 2 to 4 weeks following the infection, persons may test negative for the HIV antibody with fourth-generation antigen and antibody screening tests. During this time, the person can be highly infectious to sexual partners. In this time of early infection with high VL, the CD4 cells can decrease by 20% to 40%. Within 2 to 4 weeks after the exposure to the virus, up to 70% of infected clients experience a flu-like illness related to acute infection. The immune system fights back to reduce the HIV levels with killer T cells (CD8) that attack and kill the infected cells. The client's CD4 cell count may rebound by 80% to 90%. A client can remain symptom-free for a long time, often years. During this time there is low-level replication of HIV but an ongoing deterioration of the immune system. Enough of the immune system remains intact to prevent most infections. The client is infectious during this time.

C. The final phase of HIV occurs when a sufficient number of CD4 cells are destroyed and when production of new CD4 cells cannot match destruction. Clients exhibit fatigue, fever, and weight loss. This failure of the immune system leads to AIDS.

D. An HIV-infected person can live an average of 8 to 10 years before developing clinical symptoms. The signs and symptoms of HIV are not uniformly expressed in

all people. A small portion of clients develop AIDS and die within months of the infection. Approximately 5% of infected clients, known as "long-term nonprogressors," have no signs of disease after 12 or more years.
E. Most AIDS-defining conditions are marked by a CD4 count of <200 cells or the appearance of one or more of the opportunistic infections (OIs). Bacteria, viruses, or fungi that would not cause illness in a healthy immune system cause OIs. These infections are often severe and sometimes fatal.

Predisposing Factors

A. Gay or bisexual men or prostitutes
B. Needle sharing by IVDU
C. Perinatal infection: mother-to-child transmission
D. Open wound and mucous membrane exposure to body fluids of infected person
E. Recipients of transfusion of contaminated blood or blood products (rare since 1985)

Common Complaints

A. Fatigue: often severe
B. Fever: longer than 1 month
C. Night sweats: drenching
D. Loss of appetite
E. Weight loss
F. Rash

Other Signs and Symptoms

A. Lymphadenopathy: enlarged lymph nodes often involving at least two noncontiguous sites
B. Anemia
C. Neutropenia
D. Thrombocytopenia
E. Cough
F. Dyspnea
G. Asymptomatic whitish patches on sides of tongue: hairy leukoplakia
H. Thrush: oral candidiasis
I. Odynophagia: esophageal candidiasis, CMV esophagitis
J. Chronic vaginal candidiasis
K. Skin changes: rashes, dry skin, and seborrheic dermatitis
L. Purplish, nonblanching nodules found on the skin, mucous membranes, and viscera: Kaposi's sarcoma
M. Muscle wasting
N. Chronic diarrhea: longer than 1 month
O. Hepatosplenomegaly
P. Cardiomyopathy
Q. Chronic bacterial infections, including community-acquired pneumonias
R. TB
S. Sexually transmitted infections (STIs)
T. Peripheral neuropathy
U. Dementia
V. Children: failure to thrive

Subjective Data

A. Review symptoms: onset, course, and duration.
B. Ask about previous HIV testing including dates and reasons for testing.

C. Past medical history: hospitalizations, comorbidities, immunizations, normal weight, pain, chronic lymph node disorders, and any changes of skin overlying lymph nodes
D. Past surgical history
E. Sexual history: number of partners in the past year, number of lifetime partners, any previous partner known to be HIV positive or have STIs, and any previous partner known to have been incarcerated:
   1. Women: history of abnormal Paps, contraception, and condom use with partner
   2. Men: MSM, heterosexual, bisexual, receptive anal intercourse, and condom use
F. Past mental health history: past and current mental health diagnosis and treatment
G. Substance use: tobacco, alcohol, and drugs
H. History of IVDU: needle sharing and when last used drugs
I. Transfusion or blood product history before 1985
J. Lived or traveled outside of the United States: when and for how long
K. Assess the presence of persistent fever with no localizing symptoms.
L. Assess the client's support system. Who knows the diagnosis?

Physical Examination

A. Height, weight, blood pressure, pulse, respiratory rate, and temperature
B. Inspect:
   1. General observation: general appearance, including fat distribution signs of wasting
   2. Skin: evaluate for rashes, seborrhea, folliculitis, moles, Kaposi's sarcoma, warts, herpes, dry skin, skin cancer, fungal infections, molluscum contagiosum, jaundice, and needle marks.
   3. Head and neck: head, eyes, ears, nose, and throat (HEENT):
      a. Assess visual acuity.
      b. Retina examination for abnormal findings: cotton wool spots, broken blood vessels, CMV retinitis (inflammation, bleeding and vision loss), red fleshy mass on conjunctiva (Kaposi's sarcoma)
      c. Evaluate sclera for icterus.
      d. Oral examination for thrush, hairy leukoplakia, mucosal Kaposi's sarcoma, gingivitis, aphthous ulcers, and dental health
C. Auscultate:
   1. Pulmonary auscultation for air movement and abnormal breath sounds
   2. Cardiac evaluation for normal and abnormal heart sounds
D. Palpate:
   1. Thyroid
   2. Lymphatic evaluation of regional versus generalized swelling: specific location, size, and texture of nodes
   3. Abdomen to evaluate the presence of hepatosplenomegaly, masses, tenderness, pain, or rebound tenderness
   4. Breast examination (female)

E. Rectal/vaginal examination:
1. Both genders: inspect for the presence of ulcers and warts in the vagina, perineum, and rectum.
2. Females: perform bimanual examination, collect Pap smear, obtain specimens for STI testing, and perform a digital rectal examination. Consider anal cytology if abnormal Pap smear.
3. Males: testicular examination, digital rectal examination, anal cytology if MSM
F. Neurologic examination:
1. Assess mental status.
2. Assess cranial nerves, including gait, strength, deep tendon reflexes, evaluation of proprioception, vibration, pinprick, temperature, and sensation in distal extremities.
G. Psychiatric examination: screen for depression.

Diagnostic Tests

A. Repeat HIV testing if the client does not have a confirmed lab copy of diagnosis.
B. CBC, with differential, including platelets
C. Complete chemistry profile
D. Fasting lipid profile
E. VDRL test and rapid plasma reagin (RPR) test
F. Serologies for toxoplasmosis
G. CD4/CD8 cells and CD4/CD8 ratio
H. HIV RNA VL
I. HIV-resistance genotype and integrase strand transfer inhibitors (INSTI) genotype if under previous exposure
J. HLA-B 5701 (risk of abacavir hypersensitivity reaction syndrome)
K. Hepatitis serologies: hepatitis A virus (HAV) serology (antibody), hepatitis B virus (HBV) complete serology profile, and hepatitis C virus (HCV) serology (antibody)
L. Cultures for *gonorrheal/chlamydia* (GC)/*chlamydia*—anal, vaginal, and oral
M. Urinalysis
N. Pap smear
O. Anal cytology with MSM; recommended for women with abnormal Pap smear
P. TB screening: T-spot, QuantiFERON, or purified protein derivative (PPD). Chest x-ray yearly in case of a history of TB treatment. Refer to a TB clinic if screening is positive.

Differential Diagnoses

A. Other diseases that lead to immune suppression or are related to symptoms
B. Cancer
C. Chronic infections
D. TORCH infections: toxoplasmosis, other (syphilis, varicella-zoster, parovirus B19), rubella, CMV, and herpes
E. Syphilis
F. TB
G. Endocarditis
H. Infectious enterocolitis
I. Bowel disorders: antibiotic-associated colitis, inflammatory bowel disease, or malabsorptive symptoms
J. Endocrine diseases

K. Neuropathy
L. Alcoholism
M. Liver disease
N. Renal disease
O. Thyroid disease
P. Vitamin deficiency
Q. Chronic meningitis

Plan—Clinical Guidelines per National Institutes of Health: AIDSinfo.NIH.gov

A. General interventions:
1. Refer and comanage the client with HIV/AIDS clinician.
2. Identify and treat substance abuse.
3. Explain to the client that at each visit you will review history, conduct a physical examination, and run laboratory studies to assess health status.
4. Discuss health habits: smoking, nutrition, and exercise.
5. Discuss treatment plan:
   a. HAART
   b. Therapy for OIs and malignancies
   c. Prophylaxis for OIs: *Pneumocystis carinii* pneumonia (PCP) and *Mycobacterium avium* complex (MAC) according to CD4 count and treatment strategy
   d. Managing side effects of medications and comorbidities
   e. Immunizations
B. Client teaching:
1. Discuss living with HIV disease.
2. Discuss transmission prevention strategies: safer sex practices and condom use.
3. Provide contact information for AIDS service organizations (ASOs).
4. Discuss the client's concerns, including notification of sexual partner(s) and needle-sharing partner(s).
5. Discuss birth control and family-planning issues. Offer preconception counseling.
6. *See Section III: Client Teaching Guide for this chapter, "Reference Resources for Clients With HIV/AIDS."* ◄
C. Pharmaceutical therapy:
1. Treatment with HAART: always consult with an infectious disease HIV/AIDS specialist for treatment options.
   a. HAART: There are approximately 30 individual medications from seven classes of drugs as well as numerous pills that are combinations of two to four of these medications. Recommendations for new HIV diagnoses are a minimum of three drugs from a minimum of two classes. Classes:
      i. Nucleoside/nucleotide reverse transcriptase inhibitors (NRTIs)
      ii. Nonnucleoside reverse transcriptase inhibitors (NNRTIs)
      iii. Protease inhibitors (PIs)
      iv. Integrase inhibitors (INIs)
      v. Fusion inhibitors (FIs)

vi. Entry inhibitors (EIs)

vii. Pharmacokinetic enhancer

viii. Combination antiretrovirals

ix. Chemokine receptor antagonist

x. Post-attachment inhibitors

2. Prophylaxis and treatment for OIs: may discontinue prophylaxis if sustained an immune reconstitution on HAART:

a. PCP. Prophylaxis if CD4 count <200 or client has oral candidiasis.

i. First line: Bactrim DS (TMP-SMZ), 1 tablet three times weekly or 1 tablet daily (if toxoplasmosis positive)

ii. Alternatives: dapsone, atovaquone, and aerosolized pentamidine

b. MAC prophylaxis if CD4 count is <50:

i. First line: Zithromax 1,200 mg weekly

ii. Alternative: clarithromycin

3. Managing side effects of HAART and complications of HIV therapy: multiple complications of long-term HIV infection and treatment with HAART:

a. Lipodystrophy syndrome, bone marrow suppression, cardiovascular disease, CNS side effects, GI intolerance, hepatic failure, hepatoxicity, hyperlipidemia, insulin resistance, diabetes, lactic acidosis/hepatic steotosis, nephrotoxicity, osteonecrosis, osteopenia, peripheral neuropathy, nephrolithiasis, urolithiasis, crystalluria, hypogonadism, and psychiatric complications

4. Immunizations:

a. Hepatitis A and B series: if not immune, recommended dosing as per renal failure

b. Tetanus: Tdap

c. Pneumococcal conjugate vaccine (PVC): PVC13 followed by PVC23 per recommendations

d. Yearly influenza vaccines

e. HPV vaccine series for women and men up to age 45 years

Follow-Up

A. Schedule return visit within 4 weeks after initial visit to discuss staging HIV/AIDS, living with HIV/AIDS, and to start HAART regimen.

B. PPD yearly unless there is a history of positive PPD, then yearly chest x-ray.

C. Pap smear:

1. Initially, if normal, repeat in 6 to 12 months, then yearly if remains normal. For women over 30 if negative cytology and negative HPV, repeat Pap smear and HPV testing in three years.

2. If abnormal, follow the guidelines by the American Society of Colposcopy and Cervical Pathology (ASCCP).

D. Some clinicians advocate for anal Pap smears for men, but there are no set guidelines at present.

Consultation/Referral

A. Refer the client to a specialist in HIV for management of continued care and pharmacological therapy.

B. Refer the client to a nutritionist for baseline evaluation and diet counseling.

C. Refer pregnant women to a perinatologist.

D. Ophthalmology examination yearly for CMV screening and vision changes

E. Dental referral

F. Hepatology referral if chronic, active hepatitis B and/or hepatitis C

Individual Considerations

A. Adults:

1. Preconception counseling: Clinical Guidelines per National Institutes of Health—AIDSinfo.NIH.gov. The goal is to avoid transmission of HIV to partner and fetus. Use ovulation kits (basal body charts) to determine the most fertile time for pregnancy.

a. Discordant couples:

i. HIV-positive female and HIV-negative male:

1) Self-insemination (methods: syringe, turkey baster, cervical cap)

2) Use of preexposure prophylaxis (PrEP) for HIV-negative partner

3) Advice regarding Undetectable = Untransmittable (U = U)

ii. HIV-positive male and HIV-negative female:

1) Sperm washing/IVF: very expensive; often cost-prohibitive

2) HIV-positive male partner on HAART and HIV VL as close to undetectable as possible

3) Unprotected sex during ovulation times only and no other

4) Use of PrEP for uninfected partner

iii. HIV-positive male and HIV-positive female: avoid superinfection:

1) Both partners on HAART and VL as close to undetectable as possible

2) Unprotected sex during ovulation times only and no other

B. Pregnancy:

Clinical Guidelines per National Institutes of Health—AIDSinfo.NIH.gov

1. Antepartum:

a. HAART starting as soon as possible and maintaining treatment if already on pregnancy-approved HAART

b. Goal of therapy is undetectable HIV VL.

c. Sustiva should not be used in pregnancy during first trimester.

d. Vaginal delivery can be offered if HIV VL is <1,000.

2. Intrapartum:

a. Continue oral HAART.

b. Zidovudine intravenously (IV) 2 mg/kg in the first hour and then 1 mg/kg throughout delivery if VL is not detectable

c. C-section if HIV VL >1,000

3. Postpartum:

a. HAART for mother is continued.

b. Infant receives zidovudine 2 mg/kg every 12 hours for the first 4 weeks of life if mother has undetectable HIV VL. If mother's VL is unknown or the aforementioned is undetectable, the baby should receive combination therapy.

c. Breastfeeding is not recommended.

C. Pediatrics:

Clinical Guidelines per National Institutes of Health—AIDSinfo.NIH.gov

1. Perinatal transmission in the United States has been reduced to <2% due to HAART.

2. Infants born to HIV-infected mothers test positive for HIV antibody ELISA test. Transplacentally acquired antibody may persist in the child for up to 18 months.

3. Clinical and laboratory evaluation of the child must be done postpartum. Initial HIV RNA VL testing should be done at birth, 14 to 21 days, 1 to 2 months, and 4 to 6 months postpartum.

4. Children who are HIV positive from vertical transmission should be followed by pediatric infectious disease clinicians.

5. All routine immunizations are recommended for HIV-infected children except for severely immunocompromised HIV-infected children who should not receive live-virus vaccines.

D. Prophylaxis:

1. PrEP is a prevention method for HIV-negative partners.

a. Truvada is FDA approved for use as PrEP for heterosexual and MSM–HIV-negative partners.

i. One tablet is taken daily to reduce the risk of infection.

ii. Those taking PrEP should be monitored for potential side effects.

2. Postexposure prophylaxis (PEP): Clinical Guidelines per National Institutes of Health—AIDSinfo.NIH.gov:

a. Depending upon exposure type and severity, postexposure ART should be started as quickly as possible and be taken for 4 weeks postexposure.

b. Expert consultation should be obtained as quickly as possible (National HIV/AIDS Clinician's Consultation Center PEPline: 1-888-448-8765).

c. Follow with occupational health for regular clinical assessment and labs

d. Perform HIV testing: baseline, 6 weeks, 3 months, 6 months, and 1 year

e. HIV testing with HIV RNA VL if an illness compatible with seroconversion illness occurs (fever, lymphadenopathy, pharyngitis, rash)

f. Advise transmission precautions during first 3 to 6 months postexposure (use condoms, refrain from donating blood, discontinue breastfeeding).

Resource

National HIV/AIDS Clinician's Consultation Center: Warmline

800-933-3413

PEPline 888-448-4911

Perinatal HIV Hotline 888-448-8765

Resources for patients living with HIV (paying for care and medications, housing, jobs, legal issues, stigma and more): https://www.cdc.gov/hiv/basics/livingwithhiv/resources.html

Bibliography

AIDSInfo. (2018a). *Guidelines for the use of antiretroviral agents in adults and adolescents living with HIV.* Department of Health and Human Services. Retrieved from https://aidsinfo.nih.gov/contentfiles/lvguidelines/adultandadolescentgl.pdf

AIDsInfo. (2018b). *Recommendations for the use of antiretroviral drugs in pregnant women with HIV infection and interventions to reduce perinatal HIV transmission in the United States.* Department of Health and Human Services. Retrieved from https://aidsinfo.nih.gov/contentfiles/lvguidelines/PerinatalGL.pdf

AIDSInfo. (2019). *Guidelines for the prevention and treatment of opportunistic infections in HIV-infected adults and adolescents.* Department of Health and Human Services. Retrieved from https://aidsinfo.nih.gov/guidelines/html/4/adult-and-adolescent-opportunistic-infection/326/mac

The AIDS Infonet. (2019). *Reliable, up-to-date treatment information.* Retrieved from www.aidsinfonet.org

AIDSmeds. (2019, April 25). *Currently approved drugs for HIV: A comparative chart.* Retrieved from http://www.aidsmeds.com/articles/DrugChart_10632.shtml

American Academy of HIV Medicine. (2019). *Fundamentals of HIV medicine for the HIV specialist.* Washington, DC: Author. Retrieved from http://www.AAHIVM.org

The Body. (n.d). *Physical health issues: The latest. Side effects of HIV/AIDS and HIV medications. The body: HIV/AIDS resource.* Retrieved from http://www.thebody.com/index/treat/side_effects.html#general

The Body. (2019). *The complete HIV/AIDS resource.* Retrieved from http://www.thebody.com

Centers for Disease Control and Prevention. (2018a, July 23). *Opportunistic infections.* Retrieved from www.cdc.gov/hiv/basics/livingwithhiv/opportunisticinfections.html

Centers for Disease Control and Prevention. (2018b, May 23). *Updated guidelines for antiretroviral postexposure prophylaxis after sexual, injection drug use, or other nonoccupational exposure to HIV—United States, 2016.* Retrieved from stacks.cdc.gov/view/cdc/38856

Centers for Disease Control and Prevention. (2019a, February 9). *Recommendations for HIV prevention with adults and adolescents with HIV.* Retrieved from https://www.cdc.gov/hiv/guidelines/personswithhiv.html

Centers for Disease Control and Prevention. (2019b, March 19). *HIV among African American gay and bisexual men.* Retrieved from https://www.cdc.gov/hiv/risk/racialethnic/bmsm/facts/index.html

Centers for Disease Control and Prevention. (2019c, April). *HIV in the United States: At a glance.* Retrieved from https://www.cdc.gov/hiv/basics/statistics.html

Centers for Disease Control and Prevention. (2019d, April 25). *HIV surveillance report: Diagnoses of HIV infection in the United States and dependent areas, 2017.* Retrieved from https://www.cdc.gov/hiv/pdf/library/reports/surveillance/cdc-hiv-surveillance-report-2017-vol-29.pdf

Centers for Disease Control and Prevention. (2019e, May 14). *HIV testing.* Retrieved from https://www.cdc.gov/hiv/testing/index.html

Centers for Disease Control and Prevention. (2019f, June). *Monitoring selected national HIV prevention and care objectives by using HIV surveillance data–United States and 6 U.S. dependent areas-2010. HIV surveillance supplemental report.* Retrieved from https://www.cdc.gov/hiv/topics/surveillance/reports

Clinician Consultation Center, University of California, San Francisco (2020). Retrieved from http://nccc.ucsf.edu/

Eisinger, R. W., Dieffenbach, C. W., & Fauci, A. S. (2019). HIV viral load and transmissibility of HIV infection: Undetectable equals untransmittable. *Journal of American Medical Association, 321*(5), 451–452. doi:10.1001/jama.2018.21167

Günthard, H. F., Saag, M. S., Benson, C. A., del Rio, C., Eron, J. J., Gallant, J. E., . . . Volberding, P. A. (2016). Antiretroviral drugs for treatment and prevention of HIV infection in adults: 2016 recommendations of the international antiviral society-USA panel. *Journal of the American Medical Association, 316*(2), 191–210. doi:10.1001/jama.2016.8900. Retrieved from https://www.iasusa.org/content/antiretroviral-drugs-treatment-andprevention-hiv-infection-adults-2016-recommendations

Panel on Antiretroviral Guidelines for Adults and Adolescents. (2018, October 25). *Guidelines for the use of antiretroviral agents in HIV-1-infected adults and adolescents.* Washington, DC: Department of Health and Human Services. Retrieved from https://aidsinfo.nih.gov/guidelines/html/1/adult-and-adolescent-arv/0

Panel on Antiretroviral Therapy and Medical Management of HIV-Infected Children. (2019, April 16). *Guidelines for the use of antiretroviral agents in pediatric HIV infection.* Washington, DC: Department of Health and Human Services. Retrieved from https://aidsinfo.nih.gov/guidelines/html/2/pediatric-arv/0

Panel on Opportunistic Infections in HIV-Infected Adults and Adolescents. (2019, March 28). *Guidelines for the prevention and treatment of opportunistic infections in hiv-infected adults and adolescents.* Washington, DC: Department of Health and Human Services. Retrieved from https://aidsinfo.nih.gov/contentfiles/lvguidelines/adult_oi.pdf

Panel on Treatment of HIV-Infected Pregnant Women and Prevention of Perinatal Transmission. (2018, December 7). *Recommendations for use of antiretroviral drugs in pregnant HIV-1-infected women for maternal health and interventions to reduce perinatal HIV transmission in the United States.* Washington, DC: Department of Health and Human Services. Retrieved from https://aidsinfo.nih.gov/guidelines/html/3/perinatal/0

Rathbun, R. C., & Bartlett, J. (2019, April). Antiretroviral therapy for HIV infection. *Drugs and Diseases: Medscape, 2019,* e1–e40. Retrieved from https://emedicine.medscape.com/article/1533218-overview#a1

Saag, M. S., Benson, C. A., Gandhi, R. T., Hoy, J. F., Landovitz, R. J., Mugavero, M. J., . . . Volberding, P. A. (2018). Antiretroviral drugs for treatment and prevention of HIV infection in adults: 2018 recommendations of the international antiviral society-USA panel. *Journal of the American Medical Association, 320*(4), 379–396. doi:10.1001/jama.2018.8431. Retrieved from https://www.iasusa.org/2018/07/24/antiretroviral-drugs-treatment-prevention-hiv-infection-adults-2018-recommendations-of-the-international-antiviral-society-usa-panel/

U.S. Food and Drug Administration. (2018, May 14). *Antiretroviral drugs used in the treatment of HIV infection.* Retrieved from http://www.fda.gov/ForClients/Illness/HIVAIDS/Treatment/ucm118915.htm

U.S. Preventive Services Task Force Recommendation Statement. (2018, November). *Recommendations in progress: Screening for HIV. USPSTF.* Retrieved from https://www.uspreventiveservicestaskforce.org/Page/Document/UpdateSummaryFinal/human-immunodeficiency-virus-hiv-infection-screening

U.S. Public Health Service. (2018, March). *Preexposure prophylaxis for the prevention of HIV infection in the United States–2017 update. CDC US public health service.* Retrieved from https://www.cdc.gov/hiv/pdf/risk/prep/cdc-hiv-prep-guidelines-2017.pdf

Idiopathic (Autoimmune) Thrombocytopenic Purpura

Julie Adkins and Jenny Mullen

Definition

A. Idiopathic thrombocytopenic purpura (ITP) is an autoimmune disorder in which an immunoglobulin G (IgG) autoantibody is formed that binds to platelets. Blood is able to clot through the ability of platelets clumping together to plug small holes in damaged blood vessels. The platelet count is <150,000 mm^3.

Incidence

A. Acute ITP occurs commonly in childhood, frequently precipitated by a viral infection. It is seen in children of 1 to 6 years of age and middle-aged adults of 30 to 40 years of age. There is a 2:1 female-to-male predominance. The adult form is usually a chronic disease (>6 months) and seldom follows a viral infection. Clients ≥ 60 years old have a predicted 5-year mortality rate (47.8%) compared to younger adults (2.2%). Spontaneous remission has occurred in >80% cases with children; however, it is rare for adults.

B. In the United States, the incidence of ITP has up to 66 cases per million citizens per year. Intracranial hemorrhage is the most significant complication, and the hemorrhage mortality rate is 5% for adults and 1% for children.

Pathogenesis

A. ITP results from production of antiplatelet antibodies that leads to peripheral destruction and sequestration of platelets. It is not clear which antigen on the platelet surface is involved. Relative bone marrow failure may be causative for reduction in platelet production. Platelets are not destroyed by direct lysis. Destruction takes place in the spleen, where splenic macrophages with Fc receptors bind to antibody-coated platelets. The primary cause of long-term morbidity and mortality is hemorrhage, whether spontaneous or accident-induced trauma.

Predisposing Factors

A. Infections
B. Chronic alcoholism
C. Sepsis
D. AIDS
E. Immune disorders, such as SLE
F. Drug use
G. Chronic lymphocytic leukemia (CLL)
H. Pregnancy

Common Complaints

A. Purple spots and bruises on skin
B. Nosebleeds
C. Mouth and gum bleeding

Other Signs and Symptoms

A. Purpura, petechiae, and hemorrhagic bullae in the mouth
B. Tendency to bleed easily—easy bruising
C. Menorrhagia—abnormal heavy menstruation
D. No systemic illness: The client feels well and is not febrile.

Subjective Data

A. Determine when the client or caregiver first noticed symptoms; note whether the symptoms have changed or progressed.
B. Rule out pregnancy as a cause of nosebleeds.
C. Ask whether the client is feeling well except for the bleeding or bruising.

D. Determine whether the client has a fever.

E. Obtain medication history for OTC and prescribed medications.

F. Determine the client's history of immune disorders, recent infections, alcoholism, and pregnancy.

G. Establish usual weight and any recent weight loss.

Physical Examination

A. Check temperature, pulse, respirations, blood pressure, and weight.

B. Inspect:
1. Observe general appearance.
2. Conduct dermal examination for purpura and petechiae.
3. Conduct eye examination; check sclera for hemorrhages.
4. Examine the mouth for dental caries and poor hygiene, mouth petechiae, and hemorrhagic bullae.

> Normally, the spleen should not be palpable.

C. Auscultate:
1. Heart
2. Lungs
3. Abdomen for bowel sounds and bruits

D. Percuss:
1. Abdomen
2. Liver
3. Spleen

E. Palpate:
1. Abdomen
2. Liver
3. Spleen
4. Lymph nodes (cervical, axillary, and groin); assess for adenopathy

Diagnostic Tests

A. Platelet count

> The major concern during the initial phase is risk of cerebral hemorrhage when platelet count is less than 5,000 platelets/µL.

B. IgG

> Increased levels of IgG appear on the platelet count in the presence of thrombocytopenia.

C. CBC with differential and peripheral smear

> Peripheral smear shows normal white blood cells (WBCs) and red blood cells (RBCs), platelets low in count with large size.

D. Bleeding time is prolonged.

E. Coagulation tests: prothrombin time (PT), partial thromboplastin time (PTT), and fibrinogen—usually normal. Platelet-associated antibodies may be detected.

> Coagulation studies are normal.

F. Bone marrow aspiration, per specialist

> Bone marrow may appear normal or have increased megakaryocytes (early form of platelets) with thrombocytopenia.

Differential Diagnoses

Thrombocytopenia may be produced in two ways: by abnormal bone marrow function or by peripheral destruction of platelets.

A. Abnormal bone marrow function:
1. Aplastic anemia
2. Hematologic malignancies
3. Myelodysplasia: This can be ruled out only by examining the bone marrow.
4. Megaloblastic anemia
5. Chronic alcoholism

B. Non–bone marrow disorders:
1. Immune disorders:
   a. ITP
   b. Drug induced from medications being taken
   c. Secondary to CLL and SLE
   d. Posttransfusion purpura
2. Hypersplenism resulting from liver disease
3. Disseminated intravascular coagulation (DIC)
4. Thrombotic thrombocytopenic purpura
5. Sepsis
6. Hemangiomas
7. Viral infection
8. AIDS
9. Pregnancy
10. Hypothyroidism

Plan

A. General interventions:
1. Comanage the client with a physician for medication therapy.

B. Client teaching:
1. Instruct the client to avoid trauma; advise that the client cannot participate in *contact sports*.
2. Instruct the client to avoid salicylates; they impair platelet function.
3. Prednisone therapy benefits:
   a. Prednisone increases platelet count by increasing platelet production.
   b. Long-term therapy may decrease antibody production.
   c. Bleeding often diminishes 1 day after beginning prednisone.

d. Platelet count usually begins to rise within a week; responses are almost always seen within 3 weeks.

e. About 80% of clients respond to treatment and the platelet count usually returns to normal.

C. Pharmaceutical therapy:

1. Initial treatment:

a. Prednisone 1 to 2 mg/kg/d:

i. High-dose therapy should be continued until the platelet count is normal, and the dose should then be gradually tapered.

ii. In most clients, thrombocytopenia recurs if prednisone is completely withdrawn.

iii. High-dose therapy should not be continued indefinitely in an attempt to avoid surgery.

2. Alternative drug therapy:

a. High-dose intravenous immunoglobulin (IVIg) 400 mg/kg/d for 3 to 5 days is highly effective in rapidly raising the platelet count.

i. This treatment is expensive, costing approximately $5,000 or more.

ii. The beneficial effect lasts only 1 to 2 weeks.

iii. This therapy should be reserved for emergency situations such as preparing a severely thrombocytopenic client for surgery.

b. Thrombopoietin receptor agonists: Drugs that boost platelet production, such as romiplostim (Nplate) and eltrombopag (Promacta), stimulate the bone marrow to produce more platelets. Side effects include headache, dizziness, nausea, and vomiting. There is also an increased risk of blood clots.

3. Platelet transfusions are an option rarely used. Transfusions may be necessary in emergency situations along with intravenous methylprednisolone and intravenous immune globulin.

4. Avoid aspirin, NSAIDs, or warfarin, which interfere with platelet function and blood clotting.

D. Surgical management:

1. Splenectomy is the most definitive treatment. Most adults ultimately undergo splenectomy.

2. Splenectomy is indicated if clients do not respond to prednisone initially or require unacceptably high doses to maintain an adequate platelet count.

Exogenous platelets survive no better than the client's own platelets. In many cases, platelets survive less than a few hours. This therapy is reserved for cases of life-threatening bleeding in which enhanced hemostasis for even an hour may be of benefit.

Follow-Up

A. The client must be monitored very closely by a physician. Perform daily to weekly platelet counts; frequency depends on the severity and course.

B. Prognosis for acute ITP: 80% respond and fully recover within 2 months; 15% to 20% progress to chronic ITP.

C. Prognosis for chronic ITP: 10% to 20% recover fully; remainder continue to have low platelet counts and may see a remission or relapse over time.

D. The principal cause of death from ITP is intracranial hemorrhage.

Consultation/Referral

A. After diagnosis, refer the client to a hematologist.

Individual Considerations

A. Pregnancy:

1. Rule out hemolysis, elevated liver enzymes, low platelets (HELLP) syndrome, infection, and DIC as causes of thrombocytopenia.

2. There is an increased incidence of spontaneous abortions and hemorrhage at the time of delivery from genital tract injury.

3. Antepartum management: conduct fetal blood sampling and testing when the mother has a known history of ITP.

4. Intrapartum management:

a. Avoid fetal hypoxia, which can decrease the fetal platelet count.

b. Avoid prolonged labor.

c. Conduct continuous fetal monitoring.

d. Epidural anesthesia may be used if the platelet count is at least 100,000 cells/mm^3.

5. Postpartum management: Breastfeeding is not recommended because of the possible transmission of antiplatelet antibodies through breast milk.

B. Pediatrics:

1. Viral infections frequently precipitate ITP.

2. It usually has an acute course that is self-limited.

C. Geriatrics:

1. There is usually another cause for low platelets in geriatrics, and ITP is uncommon in this population.

2. Persons older than 60 years must be evaluated for other causes such as myelodysplastic syndromes, acute leukemia, or bone marrow infiltration.

3. Persons with ITP aged 70 years or older are at risk of spontaneous bleeding and adverse events of treatment. First-line treatments for the elderly are steroids and IVIg, yet steroids are not recommended for the geriatric population, and IVIg could cause renal failure.

Bibliography

Kessler, C. (2015). *Immune thrombocytopenic purpura (ITP)*. Medscape. Retrieved from emedicine.medscape.com

Lambert, M. L., & Gernsheimer, T. B. (2017). Clinical updates in adult immune thrombocytopenia. *Blood. 129*, 2829–2835. doi:10.1182/blood-2017-03-754119

Mahévas, M., Michel, M., & Godeau, B. (2016). How we manage immune thrombocytopenia in the elderly. *British Journal of Haematology, 173*(6), 844–856. doi:10.1111/bjh.14067

Mayo Clinic. (2016). *Idiopathic thrombocytopenia purpura (ITP). Mayo Clinic disease and conditions*. Retrieved from https://www.mayoclinic.org/diseases-conditions/idiopathic-thrombocytopenic-purpura/symptoms-causes/syc-20352325

Silverman, M., & Shlamovitz, G. (2017). *Idiopathic thrombocytopenia purpura (ITP) in emergency medicine*. MedScape. Retrieved from https://emedicine.medscape.com/article/779545-overview#a6

Iron-Deficiency Anemia (Microcytic, Hypochromic)

Julie Adkins and Jenny Mullen

Definition

A. Microcytic anemia is characterized by small, pale red blood cells (RBCs) and depletion of iron (Fe) stores. The hematocrit (Hct) is <41% in males, with a hemoglobin (Hgb) <13.5 g/dL. In females, the Hct is <37% with an Hgb <12 g/dL.

Incidence

A. Iron deficiency is the most common cause of anemia worldwide; it is particularly prevalent in women of child-bearing age. Approximately 4% to 8% of premenopausal young women in the United States are iron deficient. It is estimated to occur in 20% of adult women, 50% of pregnant women, and 3% of adult males in the United States, yet does not commonly transpire in the absence of bleeding.

Pathogenesis

A. Anemia is acquired; it develops slowly and in stages. Iron loss exceeds intake so that stored iron is progressively depleted. As stored iron is depleted, a compensatory increase in absorption of dietary iron and in the concentration of transferrin occurs. Iron storage can no longer meet the needs of the erythroid marrow; the plasma-transferring level increases and the serum iron concentration declines, resulting in a decrease in iron available for RBC formation.

Predisposing Factors

A. Female with heavy menses
B. Chronic blood loss, GI blood loss
C. Family history or personal history of anemia
D. Poor diet, including strict vegetarian diets. Vegetarian diets do not include iron-rich foods.
E. Excessive cow's milk intake (children who drink >16 to 24 oz a day). Excessive cow's milk intake interferes with iron absorption and irritates the intestinal lining.
F. Closely spaced pregnancies
G. Lactation
H. Pica
I. Chronic hemoglobinuria due to an abnormally functioning cardiac valve
J. Chronic aspirin use or NSAID use
K. Repeated blood donation
L. Decreased iron absorption due to gastric surgery
M. Taking too many antacids that contain calcium
N. Postgastric bypass surgery
O. GI diseases such as celiac disease, irritable bowel syndrome (IBS), ulcerative colitis, Crohn's disease, and peptic ulcer disease
P. Chronic kidney disease

Common Complaints

A. Fatigued all of the time
B. Heart feels like it is racing, beating hard
C. Out of breath on exertion
D. Loss of appetite
E. Nausea and vomiting
F. Headaches throughout day
G. Weak and dizzy

Other Signs and Symptoms

> Clinical presentation depends on severity, client's age, and the ability of the cardiovascular and pulmonary systems to compensate for the decreasing oxygen-carrying capacity of the blood.

A. Initial: Exercise-induced dyspnea and mild fatigue symptoms may be minimal until the client has significant anemia.
B. As Hct falls, dyspnea and fatigue increase.
   1. Malaise
   2. Drowsiness
   3. Sore tongue and mouth
   4. Skin pallor
   5. Pale mucous membranes and conjunctiva
   6. Pale nail beds
   7. Tachycardia
   8. Palpitations
   9. Tinnitus
   10. Pica symptoms (craving ice or clay)
   11. Brittle nails
   12. Hair loss
C. Severe anemia:
   1. Atrophic glossitis, cheilitis (lesions at the corner of the mouth)
   2. Koilonychia (thin concave fingernails with raised edges)

Subjective Data

A. Inquire about onset, course, and duration of symptoms.
B. Ask the client about past history of GI bleeding.
C. Take careful history of GI complaints that might suggest gastritis, peptic ulcer disease, or other conditions that might produce GI bleeding.
D. Ask if there has been a change in stool color or bleeding from hemorrhoids.
E. In menstruating women, ask about blood loss during menses.
F. Ask about dietary intake of iron-rich foods.
G. Inquire about pica habits, intake of nonfood items such as clay, dirt, detergent, and the like.
H. Obtain medication history, especially use of aspirin and other NSAIDs.
I. Rule out history of anemia, blood-clotting problems, sickle cell disease, glucose-6-phosphate dehydrogenase (G6PD) deficiency, or other hereditary hemolytic disease.
J. Review occupation and activities with exposure to lead or lead paint.
K. Has the client experienced palpitations, chest pain, dizziness, or shortness of breath?

Physical Examination

A. Check temperature, pulse, respirations, blood pressure, and weight. Check for postural hypotension. Children: plot weight, height, and head growth parameters on growth chart (see Table 17.1).

TABLE 17.1 NORMAL HEMOGLOBIN AND HEMATOCRIT VALUES FOR CHILDREN

Age (Years)	Hgb (%)	Hct (%)
1–2	>11.0	>33.0
2–5	>11.2	>34.0
5–8	>11.4	>34.5
8–12	>11.6	>35.5
12–18	>12.0	>36.0

Hct, hematocrit; Hgb, hemoglobin.

B. Inspect:
1. Inspect general appearance; the client may be pale, lethargic, or without overt signs if anemia is mild.
2. Conduct eye examination; check conjunctivae for paleness.
3. Examine oral mucosa, corners of the mouth (for cheilitis); note appearance of the tongue (atrophy of the papillae; smooth, shiny, beefy red appearance), angular stomatitis, or pale gums.
4. Examine the skin for dryness and perfusion.
5. Examine nails for brittleness, flattening, ridges, and concave or spoon shape.
C. Auscultate:
1. Heart for systolic flow murmurs
D. Percuss:
1. Abdomen
E. Palpate:
1. Abdomen for tenderness and enlargement of the liver and spleen
F. Rectal examination:
1. Assess for masses and obtain stool for occult blood.

Diagnostic Tests

A. Initial:
1. CBC with differential and peripheral smear
2. Serum ferritin level, serum iron, total iron-binding capacity (TIBC), reticulocyte count, RBC indices
3. Serum iron concentration: absent iron storage equals ferritin value <30 ng/mL
4. Urinalysis
5. Stool for occult blood
B. Follow-up:
1. TIBC: serum TIBC and serum ferritin rise
2. Hct 3 to 4 weeks after treatment. Treatment should continue for at least 4 to 6 months after the Hct returns to normal.
3. GI series, if indicated
4. Endoscope, if indicated
5. Ultrasonography, if indicated

Differential Diagnoses

A. Inadequate intake of iron
B. Any condition that causes acute or chronic blood loss
C. Hemolytic diseases such as sickle cell and G6PD deficiency
D. Anemia of chronic disease (thalassemia, sideroblastic anemias)
E. Lead poisoning
F. Neoplasm

Plan

A. General interventions:
1. Identify source of anemia.
2. Discuss dietary sources of iron-rich foods.
3. Infants should ingest formula enriched with iron and iron-enriched cereals.
B. Client teaching:
1. Stress the importance of dietary intake of foods high in iron. Iron in food is absorbed better than most vitamins. Vitamin C increases absorption of iron. Suggest taking iron with a glass of orange juice or vitamin C supplement.
2. Tea and milk reduce iron absorption; avoid large consumptions.
3. Provide iron supplements as indicated.
4. Encourage the client to stop smoking if applicable.
C. Pharmaceutical therapy:
1. Oral iron replacement:
   a. Adult:
      i. Begin 6-month trial of ferrous sulfate tablets 300 to 325 mg three times daily before meals or with orange juice or vitamin C 250 mg 1 hour before meals. Food decreases iron delivery by 50%.
      ii. Iron supplement (Slow Fe) one time-release capsule daily or Niferex-150 Forte daily
      iii. If the client has been prescribed an antacid, oral iron supplements should be taken 2 hours before or 4 hours after taking the antacid to avoid absorption interaction.
   b. Children:
      i. Liquid iron 3 mg/kg/d in a single dose
      ii. Chewable vitamin with an iron supplement one tablet every day for mild cases
2. Alternative drug therapy: Parenteral iron is indicated if the client cannot tolerate or absorb oral iron or if iron loss exceeds oral replacement.
   a. Iron dextran injection (Imferon)
   b. Iron sorbitex injection (Jectofer):
      i. Parenteral iron therapy is expensive.
      ii. It is associated with significant side effects: anaphylaxis, phlebitis, regional adenopathy, serum sickness-type reaction, and staining of intramuscular injection sites.
      iii. Dose is based on the client's weight.
      iv. Do not administer parenteral iron along with oral iron.

Follow-Up

A. Follow-up of adults is variable, depending on the source of blood loss. Manage signs of anemia

B. It is advisable to see the client after 3 to 4 weeks, both to monitor the hematologic response and to answer questions about the medication, which may result in improved compliance.

C. If the client's Hgb level has increased by 1.0 g/dL in 3 to 4 weeks, continue iron supplementation for an additional 3 to 6 months. The Hct should return to normal after 2 months of iron therapy. However, client should keep taking iron supplements for another 6 to 12 months to replace the body's iron storage in the bone marrow.

D. Determine the effectiveness of iron replacement therapy during the first 2 weeks of therapy by checking the reticulocyte count.

Consultation/Referral

A. Refer the client to a physician for the following:
  1. Hgb is not increased by 1.0 g/dL after 1 month of treatment.
  2. The therapeutic trial should not be continued beyond 1 month because the Hgb concentration has not increased and client compliance with recommended regimen is not a factor.
  3. There is a steady downward trend in Hct despite treatment.
  4. There is a significant drop in Hct over previous readings (rule out lab error first).
  5. Laboratory findings show Hgb <9.0 g/dL or Hct <27%. Suspect underlying inflammatory, infectious, or malignant disease

B. Refer the client for nutrition consultation, if indicated.

Individual Considerations

A. Pregnancy:
  1. Check Hct at initial prenatal visit, 28 weeks, and 4 weeks after initiating therapy.
  2. Laboratory findings of Hgb >13 g/dL and Hct >40% may indicate hypovolemia. Be alert for signs of dehydration and preeclampsia.
  3. Currently, there are no universal evidence-based thresholds for transfusing packed RBC for iron-deficient anemia. However, for pregnant women with Hgb ≤ 6 g/dL there is a potential for abnormal fetal oxygenation and other system compromises to the fetus. Refer these clients to the high-risk OB/GYN specialist for further evaluation and treatment.
  4. Counsel the client on proper diet and refer to a dietitian.
  5. Recommend one to two iron tablets a day in addition to prenatal vitamins containing iron.
  6. If unable to tolerate vitamins, recommend children's chewable Flintstones vitamins with iron, two orally daily.

B. Pediatrics:
  1. Place medication in back of mouth to reduce staining of teeth.
  2. All infants must be on iron-fortified formula or breast milk.
  3. Inform caregiver not to give cow's milk to infants younger than 12 months old.
  4. Educate parents about iron-rich foods that are age-appropriate: cereals, bran, dried fruit, red meat, and beans.
  5. Obtain height and weight of infants and children, plot on growth chart, and compare with previous parameters.

C. Adults:
  1. Bleeding is the usual cause of anemia in adults. In adult men and postmenopausal women, bleeding is usually from the GI tract.
  2. In premenopausal women, menstrual loss may be the underlying cause of anemia.
  3. Smokers may have higher Hgb levels; therefore, anemia may be masked if standard Hgb levels are used.

Bibliography

American Society of Hematology. (2016). *Iron deficiency anemia*. Retrieved from www.hematology.org

Chaudhry, H., & Kasarla, M. (2019, March 2). *Microcytic hypochromic anemia*. StatPearls. Retrieved from https://www.ncbi.nlm.nih.gov/books/NBK470252/

Harper, J., & Besa, E. (2018). *Iron deficiency anemia*. MedScape. Retrieved from https://emedicine.medscape.com/article/202333-overview#a2

Weinstein, R. (2016, November). *Red blood cell transfusion: A pocket guide for the clinician*. American Society of Hematology. Retrieved from https://www.hematology.org/Clinicians/Guidelines-Quality/Quick-Ref/6976.aspx

Lymphadenopathy

Julie Adkins and Jenny Mullen

Definition

A. Lymphadenopathy is enlargement of a lymph node, manifested in benign, self-limiting diseases and in those that are incurable and fatal. Only small lymph nodes in the neck, axilla, and groin are palpable in normal individuals. Palpable nodes in other regions, or any node exceeding 0.5 cm in size, are potentially abnormal. Localized lymphadenopathy must alert further workup for etiologies related to the region associated with the lymphatic drainage pattern. When two or more regions are involved, it is referred to as generalized lymphadenopathy, which could indicate an underlying systemic disease. The body has approximately 600 lymph nodes.

B. There are different categories of lymphadenopathy:
  1. Localized adenopathy
  2. Hilar adenopathy
  3. Generalized lymphadenopathy
  4. Other lymphatic abnormalities that present in other ways, such as lymphangitis, lymphadenitis, and lymphedema

Incidence

A. Lymphadenopathy is a very common presenting symptom. Age is an important diagnostic factor: palpable adenopathy in childhood generally occurs from 38% to 45%; in clients younger than 30 years, the cause proves to be benign in 80% of cases; and with clients older than age 50, the rate of benign disease falls to 40%.

B. In primary care clients with unexplained lymphadenopathy, approximately three-fourths of clients will present with localized lymphadenopathy and one-fourth with generalized lymphadenopathy. Lymphadenopathy in children is commonly caused by benign self-limiting diseases, such as viral disease.

C. In the United States, mortality causes for lymphadenopathy are primarily from malignancies (e.g., leukemia, lymphomas), and morbidity is associated with autoimmune disorders (e.g., juvenile rheumatoid arthritis, SLE).

Pathogenesis

A. Lymphatic fluid channels progress throughout the body and regionally converge to form lymph nodes. The primary function of lymph nodes is to originate, process, and monitor the immune response to antigen-presenting cells. Anatomically, the lobules contain compartments of T-cells, B-cells, and macrophages. Lymph nodes integrate blood vessels between intravascular and extravascular spaces, which results in antigenic preparedness for the immune response to initiate prompt action against cellular threats.

B. Inflammation and infiltration are responsible for pathologic enlargement. Localized lymphadenopathy may represent the spread of disease from an area of drainage. The left supraclavicular node is referred to as the "sentinel" node, which is in contact with the thoracic duct and drains much of the abdominal cavity. The right supraclavicular node drains the mediastinum, lungs, and esophagus. Generalized lymphadenopathy often results from infection, malignancy, hypersensitivity, and metabolic disease.

Predisposing Factors

A. High risk of exposure to HIV
B. Occupational exposure
C. History of pharyngitis, upper body infections (head and neck), or intraoral infection
D. Exposure to animals: Cats, sheep, cattle, rodents, deer ticks
E. Travel to the Southwest United States
F. Exposure to bird droppings
G. Lacerations sustained from gardening
H. Exposure to TB
I. History of sexual exposure resulting in STIs
J. History of tobacco abuse
K. Cancer
L. Medications:
   1. Anticonvulsant drugs that cause skin rash, fever, hepatosplenomegaly, and eosinophilia (e.g., phenytoin [Dilantin])
   2. Hydralazine
   3. Para-aminosalicylic acid
   4. Allopurinol

Common Complaints

A. Sore throat
B. Fever
C. Fatigue and malaise
D. Loss of appetite

E. Loss of weight
F. Swollen, painless lumps in neck, axilla, supraclavicular, iliac, and inguinal areas

Other Signs and Symptoms

A. May feel "good" except for finding enlarged lymph node
B. Node location(s): For inguinal enlargement, rule out conditions that may resemble inguinal or femoral lymphadenopathy—hernias; ectopic testicular, endometrial, or splenic tissue; lipomas; varices; and aneurysms. If inguinal area is painful and tender, it is most frequently caused by STIs.
C. Skin rash
D. Bruising or petechiae
E. Pruritus
F. Erythema of skin or scalp
G. Skin eruption
H. Night sweats
I. Abdominal pain, enlarged and tender abdomen
J. Joint pain

Subjective Data

A. A comprehensive and detailed history is necessary for diagnosis (see "Predisposing Factors" section).
B. Review the onset, course, and duration of symptoms.
C. What does the client note with respect to location, tenderness or painfulness, softness or hardness, and mobility of lymph nodes? Has the client noticed more than one enlarged lymph node?
D. Review the client's history of intravenous drug use. Review risk factors for HIV.
E. Review history for hobbies, specifically gardening and camping, and occupation (see "Lyme Disease" and "Toxoplasmosis" in Chapter 16, "Infectious Disease Guidelines").
F. Review medications: prescription, OTC, and herbal remedies.
G. Determine whether the client has a fever or a known valvular heart disease.
H. Review any other associated symptoms or signs.
I. Review any recent exposure to family and friends with infections. Has the client had recent immunizations?
J. Review recent dental problems or abscessed teeth.
K. Note whether the client is a smoker. If so, how much, for how long, and when did the client quit smoking?
L. Review the client's history for recent cat scratches (see "Cat Scratch Disease" in Chapter 16, "Infectious Disease Guidelines").
M. Review the client's history for recent travel.
N. Review the client's history for new sexual partners, to rule out STIs.
O. Review usual weight and any recent weight loss, noting how much and over what period of time.
P. Elicit information about similar symptoms in the past, when they occurred, how they were treated (antibiotics, biopsy), and the success of the treatment.
Q. Elicit information about alcohol intake, noting how much, how long, and whether the client has quit and how long ago.

Physical Examination

A. Check temperature, pulse, respirations, blood pressure, and weight.

B. Inspect:
1. Conduct a funduscopic examination.
2. Examine the eyes, ears, nose, and throat.
3. Conduct a dermal examination and check mucous membranes for a primary inoculation site, which may be a clue to a diagnosis of CSD.

C. Auscultate:
1. Heart
2. Lungs

D. Percuss:
1. Sinuses for tenderness, and transilluminate for evidence of sinusitis.

E. Palpate:
1. Abdomen
2. Conduct a clinical breast examination. Palpate mass to determine if it is a lymph node, if applicable.
3. All nodal areas for localized and generalized lymphadenopathy
   a. Hard, fixed nodes suggest metastasis, and a biopsy should be taken promptly. Size alone is not itself diagnostic; any node larger than 3 cm suggests neoplastic disease.
4. Scalp in the elderly for the tender arteries of cranial arteritis
5. Neck for thyroid gland tenderness or masses
6. Musculoskeletal system examination:
   a. Assess and palpate for bone or joint swelling, tenderness, and increased warmth.
   b. Examine lower extremities for evidence of phlebitis: asymmetric swelling, calf tenderness, and palpable cord.

F. Genitorectal examination:
1. Conduct careful external evaluation for herpetic lesions, masses, discharge, erythema, chancroid, scabies, and pediculosis.
2. "Milk" urethra for discharge
3. Note any folliculitis if the client regularly shaves the genital area.
4. Female pelvic examination: look for cervical discharge, cervical motion tenderness, adnexal tenderness, and mass or "heat" in the pelvis.
5. Males: examine the prostate and testicles for tenderness and masses, and the penis for discharge and rash.
6. Examine the rectum for discharge, tenderness, masses, and fistulas.

Diagnostic Tests

A. CBC with differential

B. Peripheral blood smear: The most useful laboratory test, it may be helpful in the diagnosis of chronic leukemia, infectious mononucleosis, and other viral illnesses.

C. Blood chemistries

D. Liver function tests, especially alkaline phosphatase

E. Angiotensin-converting enzyme (ACE)

F. ANA and rheumatoid factor

G. RPR and microhemagglutination assay for antibody to *Treponema pallidum* (MHA-TP), to rule out syphilis

H. Heterophile test, to rule out mononucleosis

I. ELISA and Western blot, to rule out HIV

J. Uric acid: Elevations may reflect lymphoma or other hematologic malignancies.

K. Blood cultures

L. Urethral or cervical cultures and smears

M. Throat culture

N. Chest x-ray

O. Mammogram with ultrasonography of suspicious breast area, if indicated

P. After consultation:
1. Abdominal ultrasonography or CT scan, if indicated
2. Biopsy or fine-needle aspiration: Fine-needle aspiration is used to obtain a cytologic diagnosis of a suspected cancer. False-negative results may occasionally occur.
3. Lymph node biopsy: Lymph node biopsy is the definitive test to confirm or rule out a suspected neoplastic process.
4. Mediastinoscopy

Q. Tuberculin skin testing of PPD and the ACE determination can facilitate assessment.
1. If the client tests *negative for ACE and PPD* and is Caucasian, then bronchoscopy and mediastinoscopy may be necessary to rule out lymphoma. If the client tests *positive for ACE but negative for PPD,* then the probability is very high that sarcoidosis is the cause.
2. If the client tests *negative for ACE but positive for PPD,* then primary TB is likely.

Differential Diagnoses

A. Four categories for lymphadenopathy:
1. Infections:
   a. Mononucleosis
   b. AIDS or AIDS-related complex (ARC): Generalized adenopathy in an asymptomatic HIV-infected client indicates a high risk of progression to AIDS. The lymphadenopathy represents follicular hyperplasia in response to HIV infection.
   c. Toxoplasmosis
   d. Secondary syphilis
2. Hypersensitivity reactions:
   a. Serum sickness
   b. Phenytoin and other drugs
3. Metabolic diseases:
   a. Hyperthyroidism
   b. Lipidoses
4. Neoplasia:
   a. Leukemia
   b. Hodgkin's disease, advanced stages
   c. Non-Hodgkin's lymphoma

B. Causes can be isolated by site of the enlarged nodes (see Table 17.2).

TABLE 17.2 CAUSES OF LYMPHADENOPATHY BY SITE OF ENLARGED NODES

Anterior Auricular Viral conjunctivitis Trachoma	**Axillary** Breast malignancy Breast infection Upper extremity infection
Posterior Auricular Rubella Scalp infection	**Epitrochlear** Syphilis (bilateral) Hand infection (unilateral)
Submandibular or Cervical (Unilateral) Buccal cavity infection Pharyngitis (can be bilateral) Nasopharyngeal tumor Thyroid malignancy	**Inguinal** Syphilis Genital herpes Lymphogranuloma venereum chancroid Lower extremity or local infection
Cervical (Bilateral) Mononucleosis sarcoidosis Toxoplasmosis pharyngitis	**Any Region** Cat scratch fever Hodgkin's disease Leukemia Metastatic cancer Sarcoidosis Granulomatous infections
Supraclavicular (Right) Pulmonary malignancy Mediastinal malignancy Esophageal malignancy	**Hilar Adenopathy**
Supraclavicular (Left) Intra-abdominal malignancy Renal malignancy Testicular or ovarian malignancy	Sarcoidosis (unilateral or bilateral) Fungal infection (histoplasmosis, coccidioidomycosis) Lymphoma (unilateral or bilateral) Bronchogenic carcinoma (unilateral or bilateral) Tuberculosis (unilateral or bilateral)

Plan

A. General interventions:

1. Pay careful attention to nodal history and characteristics on physical examination.

2. Make a careful assessment to establish the palpable mass is a lymph node. Chronicity alone is not always serious.

B. Client teaching:

1. As indicated by the particular disease process causing the lymphadenopathy. See the relevant guidelines.

C. Pharmaceutical therapy:

1. Dependent on the underlying etiology

Follow-Up

A. Follow the client closely to evaluate resolution of lymphadenopathy and disease process.

B. Follow-up depends on the diagnosis.

Consultation/Referral

A. Consultation with a physician may be useful if a period of observation is needed.

B. Refer the client to a specialist after initial workup, if indicated.

C. Refer the client to an oncologist or oncologic surgeon if the client is suspected of having a malignancy, to consider the need for biopsy or best approach to obtaining a tissue diagnosis.

Individual Considerations

A. Pediatrics:

1. Palpable nodes in the anterior cervical triangle of the neck are common in children and usually suggest infection as a cause.

2. Kawasaki disease is seen among children and young adults; it is also known as mucocutaneous lymph node syndrome (see Chapter 16, "Infectious Disease Guidelines").

B. Adults:

1. Hodgkin's lymphoma is one of the most common cancers of young adults.

C. Geriatrics:

1. Regional lymphadenopathy occurs often in the elderly when carcinomas metastasize to lymph nodes.

Bibliography

Freeman, A., & Matto, P. (2019, May 10). *Adenopathy*. StatPearls. Retrieved from https://www.ncbi.nlm.nih.gov/books/NBK513250/

Kanwar, V. (2016). *Lymphadenopathy*. Medscape. Retrieved from www.emedicine.medscape.com

Pernicious Anemia (Megaloblastic Anemia)

Julie Adkins and Jenny Mullen

Definition

A. Pernicious anemia is a megaloblastic, macrocytic, normochromic anemia caused by a deficiency of intrinsic factor in the gastric juices produced by the stomach, which results in malabsorption of vitamin B12 necessary for DNA synthesis and maturation of RBCs. There is a production of abnormally large and oval red cells with a mean corpuscular volume (MCV) in excess of 100 fL (femto-liters). The anemia can be severe, with hematocrit (Hct) as low as 10% to 15%.

Incidence

A. Estimates of pernicious anemia in the United States are approximately 151 per 100,000 people. Its prevalence is 0.1% and increases up to 2% in clients ≥ 60 years old. The prevalence in European, Scandinavian, and African decent increases in older adults up to 4.3%. Both sexes are equally affected. It is rarely seen in persons younger than 35 years, but it can occur in individuals in their 20s. There is an increased incidence in those with other immunologic disease.

Pathogenesis

A. Pernicious anemia is possibly due to an autoimmune reaction involving the gastric parietal cell that results in nonproduction of intrinsic factor and atrophy of gastric mucosa. Vitamin B12 deficiency can result from inadequate intake, impaired absorption, increased requirements as in pregnancy, or faulty utilization. Poor intake is rare, occurring most often in strict vegetarians. People get this vitamin from eating foods such as beef, liver, poultry, shellfish, tuna, eggs, fortified breakfast cereals, and dairy products.

Predisposing Factors

A. People of northern European, Scandinavian, and African descent
B. Ages >60 years
C. Immunologic disease
D. Loss of parietal cells following gastrectomy
E. Overgrowth of intestinal organisms
F. Crohn's disease
G. Ileal resection or abnormalities
H. Fish tapeworm
I. Congenital enzyme deficiencies
J. Diet: strict vegetarian diets
K. Medications: aminosalicylate sodium, proton pump inhibitors, phenobarbital, methotrexate, acyclovir, and 5-fluorouracil
L. Alcoholism
M. Hashimoto's thyroiditis
N. Addison's disease, Graves' disease, myasthenia gravis, or type 1 diabetes
O. Increased erythropoiesis: response to hemorrhage, hemolytic anemia
P. Pancreatic insufficiency
Q. *H. pylori* gastritis

Common Complaints

> Classic presentation involves sore tongue and numbness and tingling in the extremities, hands, or feet.

A. Weakness and dizziness
B. Sore, red, and shiny tongue
C. Numbness, burning, tingling sensation of arms or legs
D. Feel heart "jumping out of skin"
E. Edema of lower extremities
F. Anorexia
G. Diarrhea

Other Signs and Symptoms

A. Dyspnea on exertion
B. Pallor
C. Fatigue
D. Tachycardia
E. Exercise intolerance
F. Angina
G. Glossitis
H. Mucositis
I. Peripheral paresthesia
J. Palpitations
K. Abdominal tenderness, organomegaly
L. Neurological changes: dementia and spinal cord degeneration occur with advanced stages of pernicious anemia

Subjective Data

A. Inquire about onset, duration, and course of presenting symptoms.
B. Ask the client to describe usual bowel habits. Has there been any blood in stools?
C. If GI complaints are present, inquire about the presence of red, burning tongue; abdominal complaints; and/or presence of diarrhea or constipation.
D. If neurologic complaints are present, inquire about the presence of pins-and-needles paresthesia and weakness, unsteadiness due to proprioceptive difficulties, lethargy, and fatigue.
E. Inquire about dietary intake, using a 24-hour recall.
F. Ask about alcohol consumption: How much? How long?
G. Obtain medication history: OTC and prescription drugs
H. Obtain past medical history, specifically if the client has a history of gastrectomy, resection of ileum, or other GI disorders.
I. Review usual weight and recent loss.

Physical Examination

A. Check temperature, pulse, respirations, blood pressure, weight, and height for children; plot on graph.
B. Inspect:
    1. Observe general, overall appearance; observe walking.
    2. Conduct oral examination for characteristic red, shiny tongue.
    3. Conduct dermal and eye examinations for color: Affected clients are slightly icteric.
    4. Evaluate the look of the person related to age: Affected clients show premature aging or graying.
C. Auscultate:
    1. Heart sounds
    2. Lungs
    3. Abdomen for bowel sounds
D. Percuss:
    1. Abdomen for tenderness and organomegaly
E. Palpate:
    1. Abdomen for masses
    2. Evaluate pedal edema.

F. Neurologic examination:
1. Assess deep tendon reflexes (DTRs) and mental status.
2. Assess for paresthesia involving hands and feet.
3. Observe for gait disturbances.
4. Ask the client to perform finger-to-nose test. Poor finger–nose coordination may be seen.
5. Observe Romberg's test. Elicit Babinski's sign. Positive Romberg's and Babinski's signs may be present.
6. Assess for memory loss. Differentiate among mild forgetfulness, dementia, or altered thought processes.

Diagnostic Tests

A. CBC with differential and peripheral smear: Macroovalocytes and hypersegmented neutrophils may be present on peripheral blood smear. (They are absent in the setting of concurrent iron deficiency.)
B. Serum vitamin B12 level: <100 pg/mL
C. Serum folic acid levels, serum iron, serum ferritin, and TIBC
D. Serum intrinsic factor antibody
E. Lactate dehydrogenase (LDH)
F. Urinalysis
G. Stool for occult blood
H. Oral Schilling test with and without intrinsic factor
I. GI radiographic studies
J. Gastric analysis: Achlorhydria is found on stimulation testing.
K. Bone marrow aspiration
L. A woman with low B12 levels may have a false-positive Pap smear due to vitamin B12 effects on the epithelial cells.

Differential Diagnoses

Differential diagnosis of anemia by red cell morphology can be undertaken (MCV, mean corpuscular hemoglobin concentration [MCHC]). Common causes of each type of anemia are as follows:
A. Normochromic, normocytic: normal MCV = 80 to 100, MCHC = 32% to 36%:
1. Aplastic anemia
2. Chronic disease
3. Early iron deficiency
4. Hemolysis
5. Hemorrhage
B. Microcytic: MCV = 50 to 82, MCHC = 24 to 32:
1. Chronic disease
2. Iron deficiency
3. Thalassemia
C. Macrocytic: MCV >100, MCHC >36:
1. Antimetabolites
2. Folic acid deficiencies
3. Vitamin B12 deficiencies
4. Chronic alcoholism

Plan

A. General interventions:
1. Most common method of determining vitamin B12 deficiency is by serum vitamin B12 assay.

2. Most common method of demonstrating folate deficiency is by measurement of serum folic acid levels.
3. Red cell indices and peripheral smear should be done to determine classification of anemia to facilitate workup.
4. Red cell distribution width (RDW) determination can assist in detecting red cell heterogeneity previously available only by examination of the peripheral smear. The RDW determination overcomes the problems of detecting coexisting microcytic and macrocytic anemias.
B. Client teaching:
1. *See Section III: Client Teaching Guide for this chapter, "Pernicious Anemia."* ◄
2. Neurologic symptoms usually improve with treatment; however, some neurologic deficits may not be reversible.
C. Pharmaceutical therapy:
1. Vitamin B_{12} (cyanocobalamin or hydroxocobalamin) 100 mg intramuscularly or subcutaneous administration daily for 1 week
a. Decrease the frequency and administer a total of 2,000 mg during the first 6 weeks of therapy (weekly for 1 month)
b. Maintenance treatment requires lifelong administration of 100 mg intramuscular injection monthly depending on B_{12} levels. Some people may require lifelong administration at different intervals such as every 2 weeks.
c. Nascobal (intranasal cyanocobalamin) one spray in one nostril one time per week
2. Recommended daily allowance for vitamin B_{12}:
a. Neonates and infants up to 6 months: 0.3 mcg/d
b. Children older than 6 months to 1 year: 0.5 mcg/d
c. Children 1 to 3 years: 0.7 mcg/d
d. Children 4 to 6 years: 1.0 mcg/d
e. Children 7 to 10 years: 1.4 mcg/d
f. Adults and children older than 11 years: 2.0 mcg/d
g. Pregnant women: 2.2 mcg/d
h. Breastfeeding women: 2.6 mcg/d
3. Concomitant iron supplementation during first month of therapy. Rapid blood cell regeneration increases iron requirements and can lead to iron deficiency.

Follow-Up

A. The client must be seen in 2 weeks to determine response to treatment: increased reticulocyte count and increased Hct; diminution in neurologic signs and symptoms.
B. Evaluate the client monthly when giving vitamin B_{12} injections.
C. Endoscopy every 5 years is used to rule out gastric carcinoma. People with pernicious anemia may have gastric polyps and are more likely to develop gastric cancer and gastric carcinoid tumors.

D. Check the client every 6 months for Hct and check his or her stool for occult blood.

E. Hct value rises 4% to 5% per week in uncomplicated cases.

Consultation/Referral

A. Refer the client to a dietitian.

B. Rapid reticulocytosis should be seen following treatment; it peaks in 7 to 10 days.

C. Consult a physician if no change is seen.

Individual Considerations

A. Pregnancy:

    1. Lactovegetarians and ovolactovegetarians do well in pregnancy.

    2. Vegetarian women who eat neither eggs nor milk products should take vitamin B12 supplements during pregnancy and lactation.

B. Pediatrics:

    1. Congenital disorder usually is seen before 3 years of age.

C. Adults:

    1. Disorder rarely is seen in clients younger than age 35 years.

D. Geriatrics:

    1. Disorder most commonly is seen in the geriatric population.

    2. Follow up elderly clients with assessment of cardiovascular symptoms 48 hours after initiating therapy.

    3. Rapid blood cell regeneration increases iron requirements and can lead to iron deficiency.

Bibliography

Rodriguez, N., & Shackelford, K. (2019, April 10). *Pernicious anemia.* StatPearls. Retrieved from https://www.ncbi.nlm.nih.gov/books/NBK540989/

18 Musculoskeletal Guidelines

Neck and Upper Back Disorders

Julie Adkins and Jenny Mullen

Definition
A. Nonspecific disorders: Self-limited, usually benign disorders with unclear etiology, such as regional upper back and neck pain and shoulder pain adjacent to the neck. Pain can occur as a result of injury or through strain or poor posture over time.

B. Degenerative disorders: Consequences of aging or repetitive use, or a combination thereof, such as degenerative disk disease and osteoarthritis (OA).

C. Potentially serious neck or upper back disorders: Fractures, dislocation, infection, tumor, progressive neurological deficit, or cord compression. Examples include muscle strains, overuse injuries, sports injuries, and auto accidents; all can result in muscular irritation of the shoulder girdle, causing upper back pain.

D. Three general types of neck pain:
   1. Acute—lasts less than 4 weeks
   2. Subacute—lasts 4 to 12 weeks
   3. Chronic—lasts 3 months or longer

E. Seven vertebrae of the cervical spine surround the spinal cord and canal. The neck includes skin, neck muscles, arteries, lymph nodes, thyroid gland, parathyroid gland, esophagus, larynx, and trachea. Any condition affecting these tissues of the neck can cause neck pain.

Incidence
A. Exact numbers are unknown. Neck pain is common among adults but can occur at any age. Neck pain is estimated to be one of the top five disorders in the United States, with as many as 20% of people reporting incidents of neck pain. For children through geriatrics, a variety of ergonomic factors and posture have increased the risk of neck pain, which has been augmented from the use of technology devices (e.g., smartphones, computers).

B. OA is primarily present in up 50% of all neck pain cases in individuals older than age 50. Men have a higher percentage of cervical disk problems (40%) than women (28%) in individuals aged 55 to 64. In children and adolescents, increased stresses regarding flawed flexion of the neck associated with neck pain have led to cervical degeneration and are correlated with other developmental, psychosocial, medical, and social complications.

C. The pain may go away in a few days or weeks. Pain may also radiate to other body parts. Neck pain and upper back disorders can cause headaches or occipital neuralgia.

Pathogenesis
Cervical strain is irritation and spasm of the upper back and cervical muscles. The upper portion of the trapezius and the levator scapulae muscles, rhomboid major and minor muscles, and the long cervical muscles are most often affected. Neck pain can be identified by location:

A. C1 and C2: At the top of the cervical spine, these control the head; irritation may cause headaches.

B. C3 and C4: Regulate the diaphragm that is instrumental in breathing. C4 can radiate pain to the lower neck and shoulder.

C. C5: If impinged or irritated, shoulder pain and weakness can affect the top of the upper arms.

D. C6: If impinged or irritated, weakness can affect the biceps and the wrists. Pain, tingling, and numbness can radiate through the arm to the thumb.

E. C7: Compression causes weakness of the back of the upper arm or pain can radiate down the back of the arm and into the middle finger.

F. C8: Compression causes weakness with the handgrip as well as numbness and tingling down the arm to the little finger.

Predisposing Factors
A. Whiplash-like injuries
B. Cervical strain
C. Cervical arthritis
D. Holding the head in a forward posture or odd position
E. Sleeping on a pillow too high or too flat
F. Stress/tension

Common Complaints
A. Aching neck
B. Tightness and tenderness in neck area
C. Stiffness and tightness in shoulders
D. Stiff neck and a headache on awakening

Other Signs and Symptoms

A. Limited range of motion (ROM)

B. Back pain: Guarding with cervical motion

C. Numbness in upper extremities

D. Muscle weakness

Subjective Data

A. What are presenting symptoms? Note pain, numbness, weakness, or stiffness.

B. Was there any type of injury, either recently or in the past?

C. Is the pain located primarily in the neck, upper back, or shoulder? Is there any radiation noted?

D. How do these symptoms limit the client's activity?

E. How long can the client sit, stand, walk, or do overhead work?

F. Is the client able to lift? If so, how much weight is bearable? Compare with normal weight.

G. How long has the client had these symptoms?

H. How have the symptoms evolved, from the beginning of discomfort until now?

I. If the client has a previous history of a similar or the same pain, what therapy was used in the past and what were the results?

J. Does the client have any medical problems?

Physical Examination

Infection may include severe cervical spasms (nuchal rigidity), elevated temperature, chills, hypotension, and tachycardia.

A. Check temperature, blood pressure, and pulse.

B. Inspect:

1. Observe stance and gait.

2. Note the client's coordination and use of extremities.

C. Auscultate:

1. Heart

2. Lungs

D. Palpate:

1. Palpate trigger points in the upper back, paracervical, and rhomboid muscles.

2. Palpate for any bony tenderness in the neck, shoulders, and upper back.

3. Perform ROM tests.

4. Assess the client for reduced ipsilateral and contralateral bending of the neck.

5. Check for fracture, or inability to move the neck due to pain, and severe cervical midline vertebral pain. Note tenderness and the client holding head for stability; look for possible neurological deficits.

6. Reflexes:

a. Assess deep tendon reflexes (DTRs) bilaterally.

b. Biceps reflex tests the fifth and sixth cervical nerve roots.

c. Brachioradialis reflex tests the fifth and sixth cervical nerve roots.

d. Triceps reflex tests the seventh and eighth cervical nerve roots.

7. Strength:

a. Shoulders: Test muscle strength in the shoulders. Ask the client to shrug the shoulders against resistance.

b. Extremities:

i. Elbows: Abduction, elbow flexion, or supination tests the fourth and fifth cervical disks. Check for weakness of elbow extension and ulnar wrist flexion, indicating seventh cervical nerve impairment.

ii. Wrists/hands: Check for weakness of radial wrist extension, indicating fifth and sixth cervical disk problems. Check for weak finger abduction and adduction, indicating seventh and eighth cervical nerve impairment.

iii. Measure circumference at the forearm and the upper arm for muscle atrophy. The dominant arm will be at least 1/4 inch greater than the nondominant arm.

8. Sensory:

a. Test light touch, pinprick, and pressure sensations in the forearm and hand. Possible cervical spinal cord compromise is indicated by paresthesia of the upper extremities, weakness of the upper or lower extremities, and difficulty walking.

E. Percuss:

1. Back, spine, and neck areas. Tumor is indicated by tenderness to vertebral percussion and cachexia.

Diagnostic Tests

A. Perform radiographic studies for clients with nontraumatic neck pain and the following criteria:

1. Serious pathology is suspected.

2. Unsatisfactory response to conservative care

3. Unexplained progression of symptoms

4. Possible change in treatment

5. Concern of infection

6. Unexplained symptoms, such as weight loss, fever, or chills

7. Neurological symptoms that continue to progress

8. Concern or history of malignancy

B. Radiography of the cervical spine may include:

1. X-ray: Recommended for nontraumatic pain in all clients as recommended previously

2. Magnetic resonance imaging (MRI): Symptoms worsening or signs of neurological disease, symptoms longer than 6 weeks, or concern over malignancy or infection

3. CT of spine

4. Myelogram

5. Electromyography (EMG): Useful for more pain experienced in the extremities than in the neck

6. Nerve conduction studies: Evaluates nerve damage

7. Bone scan: Assessment for malignancy

Differential Diagnoses

A. Regional neck pain

B. Cervical strain

C. Cervical arthritis
D. Cervical nerve root compression with radiculopathy
E. Rotator cuff tendinitis
F. Rotator cuff tendon tear
G. Post-laminectomy syndrome
H. Spinal stenosis
I. Torticollis, which may be present at birth or caused by injury or disease

Plan

A. General interventions:
 1. Correct posture and lifestyle modifications (e.g., exercise, strengthening) are imperative for the client to remain free of pain. Client education and therapy depend on individual diagnosis.
B. Client teaching:
 1. Teach the client to use local applications of cold packs during the first 3 days of acute complaints and hot pack applications thereafter.
 2. Encourage the following changes in lifestyle:
  a. Sitting straight with shoulders held high
  b. Sleeping with the head and neck aligned with the body and a small pillow under the neck
  c. Driving with shoulders slightly shrugged, using arm rests
  d. Avoiding carrying objects with a strap over the shoulders
 3. Encourage daily stretching exercises, including shoulder roll, scapular pinch, and neck stretches
 4. Have the client perform ROM exercises daily.
 5. Advise the client to avoid extremes of ROM, prolonged periods in one position, and any other aggravating activity.
 6. Explain relaxation techniques and stress reduction.
 7. Massage may be useful to help relax muscles in the back and neck.
 ▶ 8. Provide the client with a teaching sheet. *See Section III: Client Teaching Guide for this chapter, "RICE Therapy and Exercise Therapy," if applicable.*
C. Pharmaceutical therapy:
 1. Nonprescription medications: Acetaminophen or nonsteroidal anti-inflammatory drugs (NSAIDs), topical pain relief patches, muscle rubs
 2. Prescription medications: NSAIDs and/or muscle relaxants for nighttime use
  a. Motrin (ibuprofen) 400 to 800 mg orally three times a day as needed. Use prescribing precautions found in the prescribing literature.
  b. Aleve (naproxen) 200 to 500 mg twice a day as needed. See the Monthly Prescribing Reference (2016) for guidance on prescribing.
  c. Flexeril (cyclobenzaprine) 5 to 10 mg orally three times a day as needed. Use of Flexeril for periods longer than 2 to 3 weeks is not recommended. Dosing adjustments should be considered for clients with liver impairment and/or elderly clients. Advise clients that driving and the use of machinery is not recommended while taking this medication. See the Monthly Prescribing Reference (2016) for guidance on prescribing.
  d. Soma (carisoprodol) 250 to 350 mg orally three times a day as needed. Precautions should be given for no driving or use of machinery while taking this medication. Use caution in clients with compromised liver and/or kidney function. Soma should not be used for long-term use greater than 2 to 3 weeks. See the Monthly Prescribing Reference for guidance on prescribing.
 3. Trigger injections of cortisone and anesthetics may be used as necessary.
D. Nonpharmacological interventions:
 1. Active craniocervical flexion exercise with upper cervical passive mobilization
 2. Manual pressure release (MPR) and muscle energy technique (MET) may be used and adjunct physiotherapeutic interventions for neck pain reduction.

Follow-Up

A. Evaluate the client after 2 weeks of conservative treatment if pain continues after 2 to 3 weeks despite adequate therapy, ordered radiography, and physical therapy. Treatment options include ultrasonography, massage, and gentle cervical traction beginning at 5 pounds for 5 to 10 minutes once a day. A soft cervical collar may be worn while doing physical work.

Consultation/Referral

A. Consult or refer the client to a physician if there is still no improvement after adequate time for healing and no relief is noted with physical therapy and medications.

Individual Considerations

A. Adults:
 1. Neck and upper back problems are more commonly seen in adults.
 2. Insomnia appears to be associated with musculoskeletal pain (primarily neck pain) rather than subjective sleepiness.
B. Pediatrics:
 1. Sports are the primary cause for head and neck/spinal injuries in children. Football, cheerleading, hockey, and gymnastics are the sports most commonly associated with athlete head/spinal injuries.
C. Geriatrics:
 1. Use precautions when treating older adults with NSAIDs. Consider using lower-dose medications for older clients.
 2. Long-term medications should also be taken into consideration when assessing for interactions between medications.
 3. Beers criteria should be considered when prescribing muscle relaxants and pain medication for elderly clients.

Bibliography

Amrit, K., Komal, M., & Mahesh, M. (2018). To compare the immediate effects of active cranio cervical flexion exercise versus passive mobilization of upper cervical spine on pain, range of motion and cranio cervical flexion test in patients with chronic neck pain. *Indian*

Journal of Physiotherapy and Occupational Therapy, 12(3), 22–27. doi:10.5958/0973-5674.2018.00050.3

Baselice, S. (2018). Neck pain statistics. *The Original TENS Units*. Retrieved from https://www.tensunits.com/blog/2018/07/15/neck-pain-statistics/

Fares, J., Fares, M., & Fares, Y. (2017). Musculoskeletal neck pain in children and adolescents: Risk factors and complications. *Surgical Neurology International*, 8(72), e1–e9. doi:10.4103/sni.sni_445_16

Genebra, C. V., Maciel, N., Bento, T., Simeão, S. & Vitta, A. (2017). Prevalence and factors associated with neck pain: A population-based study. *Brazilian Journal of Physical Therapy*, 21(4), 274–280. doi:10.1016/j.bjpt.2017.05.005

Gross, A. R., Paquin, J. P., Dupont, G., Blanchette, S., Lalonde, P., Cristie, T., . . . Bronfort, G.; Cervical Overview Group. (2016). Exercises for mechanical neck disorders: A Cochrane review update. *Manual Therapy*, 24, 25–45.

Kashyap, R., Iqbal, A., & Alghadir, A. (2018). Controlled intervention to compare the efficacies of manual pressure release and the muscle energy technique for treating mechanical neck pain due to upper trapezius trigger points. *Journal of Pain Research*, 11(12), 3151–3160. doi:10.2147/JPR.S172711

Katsifaraki, M., Nilson, K., Wærsted, M., Knardahl, S., Lie, J. A., Bjørn, B., Härmä, M, & Matre, D. (2018). The association of sleepiness, insomnia, sleep disturbance and pain: A study amongst shift-working nurses. *Sleep and Biological Rhythms*, 16(1), 133–140. doi:10.1007/s41105-017-0135-5

Lin, I. (2019). What does high value care for musculoskeletal pain look like? Eleven consistent recommendations from high-quality clinical practice guidelines. *BIM*, 3, e1–e5. Retrieved from https://bodyinmind.org/best-practice-care-musculoskeletal-pain/

Lin, I., Wiles, L., Waller, R., Goucke, R., Nagree, Y., Gibberd, M., Straker, L., & Sullivan, P. (2019). What does best practice care for musculoskeletal pain look like? Eleven consistent recommendations from high-quality clinical practice guidelines: Systematic review. [Abstract]. *British Journal of Sports Medicine*, 53(5). doi:10.1136/bjsports-2018-099878

Lin-Fen, H., Ying-Chen, K., Chia-Cheng, L., Ya-Fang, L., Yu-Chia, L., & Vincent, H. (2018). Comparison between corticosteroid and lidocaine injection in the treatment of tennis elbow: A randomized, double-blinded, controlled trial. *American Journal of Physical Medicine & Rehabilitation*, 97(2), 83–89. doi:10.1097/PHM.0000000000000814

Shim, J. (2016). *Causes of upper back pain*. Retrieved from www.spine-health.com

Video

Jasper, D. (2015) *How to find trigger points for neck pain (MPR)* [Video]. Available from https://www.youtube.com/watch?v=WDsdNz2xzZ8

Video

Nutting, P. (2016). *Muscle energy techniques* [Video]. Available from https://www.youtube.com/watch?v=qWps4buNITc

Plantar Fasciitis

Julie Adkins and Jenny Mullen

Definition

A. Plantar fasciitis is an inflammatory condition in the plantar fascia (foot) that causes pain in the arch of the foot and radiates to the heel. The plantar fascia connective tissue runs across the bottom of the foot and connects the bottom of the tuberosity of the calcaneus to the heads of the metatarsal bones.

Incidence

A. Plantar fasciitis is the most common cause of heel pain in the United States. The prevalence of plantar fasciitis is lowest in those aged 18 to 44, and highest in those aged 45 to 64. Females are 2.5 times more likely to report plantar fasciitis than males. Greater than 61% report having pain every day, and approximately 54% report that their pain (moderate to severe) interferes with normal work activities.

B. Body mass index (BMI) is strongly associated with plantar fasciitis: Those with a BMI ≥ 30 are five times more likely to have plantar fasciitis than those with a BMI ≤ 25.

C. Current National Institutes of Health (NIH) research indicates that one-quarter of respondents with plantar fasciitis use opioids (28%) to treat pain. The most common OTC products used to treat plantar fasciitis are NSAIDs (49%) and acetaminophen (27%); a small percentage of clients use herbal products or other nonvitamin, nonmineral dietary supplements.

Pathogenesis

A. Repetitive small tears in the plantar fascia cause collagen breakdown at the medial tubercle of the calcaneus.

Predisposing Factors

A. Athletes: Overuse injury from running

B. Tight or weak muscles/tendons: Achilles tendon, heel cord, gastrocnemius, soleus muscle

C. Poor arch support/improper footwear: Poor support in shoes

D. Anatomical abnormalities: Low arch support, flat foot, high arch, tibial torsion, overpronated foot, leg length discrepancy, forefoot varus, thinning of fat pad

E. Overweight/obesity

Common Complaints

A. Severe, stabbing foot pain in the bottom of the foot, especially first thing in the morning

B. Burning pain when walking

C. Stiffness in the foot/heel

D. May be worse in the morning, improve during the day, and then get painful at the end of the day

E. Increased foot pain with walking after long periods of standing or sitting

Other Signs and Symptoms

A. Both heels may be affected.

B. Pain is located at the medial tubercle of the calcaneus, medial of the longitudinal arch.

C. Heel spurs may or may not be present.

D. Pain worsens with standing for long periods of time.

Subjective Data

A. Ask the client when pain began, when it occurs, and how long it lasts.

B. Does pain occur with walking, running, and standing?

C. Is the pain constant or stabbing? Rate pain on a pain scale of 1 to 10.

D. Locate the pain site. Does pain radiate into toes or leg?

Physical Examination

A. Check pulse and blood pressure.

B. Inspect:
   1. Examine feet bilaterally.
   2. Note swelling, discoloration, or rash.

C. Auscultate:
  1. Heart
  2. Lungs
D. Palpate:
  1. Palpate both feet, noting tenderness and any point tenderness. Point tenderness will be noted over the insertion on the medial heel (calcaneus medial tubercle).
  2. Perform passive dorsiflexion of the toes and ankle. Have the client stand on tips of toes to see if this elicits pain.

Diagnostic Tests

A. An x-ray may be performed but is often normal and not needed. Perform an x-ray if tumor, spur, or fracture is suspected.
B. MRI should be ordered if thickening of proximal plantar fascia is noted or rupture of proximal fascia is suspected

Differential Diagnoses

A. Plantar fasciitis
B. Heel pain
C. Heel spur

Plan

A. General interventions:
  1. Conservative treatment includes no long periods of standing for the next 6 to 8 weeks.
  2. Proper foot care and support are recommended.
B. Client teaching:
  1. Shoe arch supports are imperative for relief. New shoes may provide this support or additional arch supports may be needed to insert into the shoe to provide adequate support.
  2. Suggest getting proper shoe fitting for running if the client is an athlete.
  3. The client should avoid walking on hard surfaces and never go barefoot, even indoors. Avoid wearing sandals and flip-flops.
  4. Ice therapy may help with pain control and swelling.
  5. For severe cases, a corticosteroid lidocaine injection 1 to 1.5 mL injected directly into the most tender area on the sole of the foot may be helpful.
  6. Exercises:
     a. Roll the foot arch with a tennis ball or a frozen bottle of water for 20 to 30 minutes each evening to help stretch the plantar fascia.
     b. Perform calf stretches against a wall: Leaning forward against the wall while extending one leg behind you and one leg in front of you, stretch the leg; then reverse.
C. Pharmaceutical therapy:
  1. NSAIDs such as ibuprofen (Motrin) 800 mg three times daily or naproxen (Naprosyn) 500 mg by mouth twice a day for comfort.
D. Nonpharmacological therapy:
  1. Orthotic footwear as prescribed by podiatry
  2. The Low-Dye taping technique can be used to improve pain while waiting on the arrival of orthotic

footwear. This technique is also recommended as an alternative footwear for clients who are unable to tolerate orthoses or accommodating insoles. Suggested demonstration of the technique: https://www.youtube.com/watch?v=OvhPCNhodmI
  3. The concept of Mulligan's physical intervention is to mobilize movement in the extremities while sustaining natural apophyseal glides of the spine. The design is intended to reduce pain and increase the client's ROM.
  4. Consider referring the client to a physical therapist for this advanced technique, and for stretching exercises unique to the plantar fasciitis client.

Follow-Up

A. Recommend follow-up in 4 weeks following treatment. Pain should slowly improve with aggressive treatment management. The client must be compliant with instructions given for improvement. It may take 6 to 12 months for complete resolution.
B. Complications of foot, knee, hip, or back problems may occur if a change of gait occurs in an effort to minimize pain with walking.
C. If pain worsens, consider a diagnostic workup (x-ray or MRI).

Consultation/Referral

A. Refer the client to a podiatrist if conservative treatment therapy fails after 6 weeks.

Individual Considerations

A. Plantar fasciitis has become common with school-age children who are becoming more involved with recent popular trends of marathons, dancers, and sports that involve running/jumping. In most cases stretching exercises, rest, and OTC meds alleviate the pain and injury resolves after 4 to 6 weeks.

Bibliography

American Orthopedic Foot and Ankle Society. (2016). *Plantar fasciitis*. Retrieved from www.aofas.org/footcaremd/conditions/ailments-of-the-heel/pages/plantar-fascitis.aspx

Karls, S. L., Snyder, K. R., & Neibert, P. J. (2016). Effectiveness of corticosteroid injections in the treatment of plantar fasciitis. *Journal of Sport Rehabilitation*, 25(2), 202–207. doi:10-1123/jsr.2014-0234

Munir, S., Babur, M., Sultana, B., Kafeel, S., & Aslam, H. (2018). Effectiveness of Mulligan's mobilization techniques in the treatment of plantar fasciitis. *International Journal of Rehabilitation Sciences*, 7(2), 7–9. Retrieved from http://ijrs.org/ojs/index.php/IJRS/article/view/237

National Institutes of Health, National Center for Complementary and Integrative Health. (2019). *Analysis data on the prevalence and pharmacologic treatment of plantar fasciitis pain*. Retrieved from https://nccih.nih.gov/research/results/spotlight/Plantar-Fasciitis-Pain

Shah, S. A. (2019). Plantar fasciitis. *KidsHealth*, e1–e3. Retrieved from http://fugazi.kidshealth.org/en/teens/plantar-fasciitis.html

Verbruggen, L., Thompson, M., & Durall, C. (2018). The effectiveness of Low-Dye taping in reducing pain associated with plantar fasciitis. *Journal of Sport Rehabilitation*, 27(10), 94–98. doi:10.1123/jsr.2016-0030

Video

SLO Motion Shoes. (2015). *Low Dye-taping: Supportive taping technique* [Video]. Available from https://www.youtube.com/watch?v=OvhPCNhodmI

Sciatica

Julie Adkins and Jenny Mullen

Definition

A. Sciatica is a sharp or burning pain, usually associated with numbness, that radiates down the posterior or lateral leg and that can result in neurosensory and/or motor deficits. Sciatica indicates abnormal function of the lumbosacral nerve roots or one of the nerves in the lumbosacral plexus.

Incidence

A. The prevalence of sciatica in the general population is 40%, though only 5% or fewer of all clients have any neurosensory or motor deficits. Peak incidence occurs approximately in the fourth decade of life; the condition rarely manifests before age 20. Occupational predispositions are as follows: machine operators, truck drivers, poor ergonomics with computers and technology devices over long periods of time, and employment that require physically awkward positions. The most common cause of sciatica is herniated disks, 95% of which occur at the L4 to L5 or L5 to S2 level.

Pathogenesis

A. Pressure on the nerve from a herniated disk, from bony osteophytes, a compression fracture, or any other extrinsic pressure (e.g., pelvic mass or epidural process, "wallet sciatica") causes progressive sensory, sensorimotor, or sensorimotor visceral loss. Typically, sciatica affects only one side of the body. The nerve may be "pinched" on the inside or outside of the spinal canal as it passes into the leg.

Predisposing Factors

A. Inflexibility
B. Obesity
C. Trauma
D. Bony osteophytes
E. Herniated or slipped disk
F. Piriformis syndrome
G. Spinal stenosis
H. Spondylolisthesis
I. Smoking

Common Complaints

A. Pain around the buttocks area may occur suddenly or develop gradually
B. Pain often associated with numbness traveling down the lateral or posterior leg
C. Numbness
D. Paresthesia

Other Signs and Symptoms

A. Difficulty walking with affected leg
B. Positive straight leg raises
C. Decreased sensation

Subjective Data

A. Elicit information about the onset of symptoms, duration, and what makes pain better or worse.
B. Inquire about previous episodes of pain or trauma.

C. Have the client point to the area of pain, numbness, or tingling.
D. Are symptoms unilateral or bilateral?
E. Question the client about loss of bowel or bladder control or other deficits and/or changes.
F. Does the client notice leg weakness or difficulty walking?

Physical Examination

A. Check pulse and blood pressure.
B. Inspect:
   1. Gait and movement of the back and extremities
   2. Spine: Examine flexion and extension of the spine.
C. Palpate:
   1. Spinous processes for tenderness
   2. Examine neurological function of the back and lower extremity.
      a. Straight leg raising sign is positive. A positive sign is pain reproduced at greater than 70 degrees and less than 30 degrees of hip joint flexion. If pain is reproduced between 30 and 70 degrees, then consider further evaluation for lumbar disk herniation.
      b. Dorsiflexion of ankle is positive.
      c. Check for loss of sensation in a radicular pattern. Light-touch pinprick and two-point discrimination are not present.
      d. Look for decrease or loss of DTRs.
      e. Check muscle strength of the lower extremities.
      f. Check for motor weakness.
      g. Check for cauda equina syndrome, indicated by urinary retention, radicular symptoms, and saddle anesthesia.

> Cauda equina syndrome is a surgical emergency, characterized by bowel and bladder dysfunction; saddle anesthesia at the anus, perineum, or genitals; and widespread or progressive loss of strength in the legs or gait disturbances.

Diagnostic Tests

A. Radiography, when red flags for fracture, cancer, or infection are present
B. CT scan or MRI, when cauda equina, tumor, infection, or fracture is suspected. MRI is the test of choice for clients with prior back surgery.

Differential Diagnoses

A. Sciatica of unknown etiology
B. Lumbosacral strain
C. Herniated disk
D. Bony osteophytes, spinal stenosis
E. Compression fracture
F. Neoplasm of spine
G. Pelvic mass
H. Epidural process causing progressive sensory, sensorimotor, or sensorimotor visceral loss
I. Meralgia paresthetica

Plan

A. General interventions:
   1. Care for these clients should evolve over a three-step process. See the following.

B. Client teaching:
1. Step 1 (2–4 days):
   a. Bed rest for severe radiculopathy only
   b. Limit walking and standing to 30 to 40 minutes each day.
   c. Recommend application of heat or cold packs to the site as needed.
2. Step 2 (7–14 days):
   a. Reevaluate the neurological and back examination; tell the client, "Let pain be your guide," when resuming normal daily activities.
   b. Have the client perform gentle stretching exercises.
   c. Encourage walking on flat surfaces.
   d. Educate the client regarding proper care of the back, with regard to exercises, posture, and so forth.
   e. Provide handouts on back exercises/stretches for the client.
   f. Physical therapy may be implemented at this time if no significant improvement is noted.
3. Step 3 (2–3 weeks):
   a. Reevaluate the client, noting the degree of improvement with examination.
   b. Continue muscle toning and reconditioning exercises.
   c. If improvement is noted, gradually increase physical activities.
   d. Reinforce healthy care of the back.
   e. Continue physical therapy until the client can perform exercises without assistance or until released by the physical therapist.
C. Pharmaceutical therapy:
1. NSAIDs as needed: Naproxen (Naprosyn) 500 mg initially, followed by 250 mg every 6 to 8 hours
2. Acetaminophen may also be used as needed, especially if the client is not able to tolerate ibuprofen.
3. For more severe pain not relieved by NSAIDs, consider acetaminophen (Tylenol) with codeine for a short duration. Narcotics should not be used for more than 2 weeks.
4. Muscle relaxants: Muscle relaxants should not be used for more than 2 weeks.
   a. Cyclobenzaprine (Flexeril) 10 mg one to three times daily
   b. Muscle relaxants place clients at risk for drowsiness. Warn the client not to mix medications with alcohol because it may potentiate the medication.

Follow-Up
A. Initial follow-up is needed in 1 to 2 weeks. See the "Plan" section for the recommended stepwise approach.

Consultation/Referral
A. If cauda equina syndrome is suspected, prompt referral to a physician is necessary.
B. If pain is severe enough that narcotics are needed, consult with a physician.
C. If bilateral sciatica is associated with vertebral collapse, osteoporosis, neoplasia, and/or vascular disease, consult with a physician.

Individual Considerations
A. Pregnancy:
1. Sciatica pain is common due to physiological changes of the pelvis as pregnancy progresses to term.
2. Avoid use of NSAIDs.
3. Physical therapy may be used as indicated.
B. Adults:
1. For adults older than 50 years presenting with no prior history of backache, consider a differential diagnosis of neoplasm. The most common metastasis is secondary to a primary site in the breast or prostate, or to multiple myeloma. Pain is most prominent in the recumbent position and rarely radiates into the buttock or leg.
C. Geriatrics:
1. Bilateral sciatica is associated with vertebral collapse, osteoporosis, neoplasia, and/or vascular disease. Refer the client to a physician immediately.
2. Use caution when prescribing medications for pain to the elderly due to the risk for drowsiness and potential falls.
3. Consider the Beers criteria when prescribing medications for pain.

Bibliography

Cherian, R., & Li, Y. (2018). Clinical electrodiagnostic features of non-traumatic sciatic neuropathy. *Muscle & Nerve*, *59*(3), 309–314. doi:10.1002/mus.26380

Davis, D., & Vasudevan, A. (2019). *Sciatica*. National Library of Medicine, National Institutes of Health. Retrieved from https://www.ncbi.nlm.nih.gov/books/NBK507908/

Dengler, J., Kools, D., Pflugmacher, R., Gasbarrini, A., Prestamburgo, D., Gaetani, P., . . . Sturesson, B. (2019). Randomized trial of sacroiliac joint arthrodesis compared with conservative management for chronic low back pain attributed to sacroiliac joint. *Journal of Bone & Joint Surgery, American Volume*, *101*(5), 400–411. doi:10.2106/JBJS.18.00022

Euro, U., Knekt, P., Rissanen, H., Aromaa, A., Karppinen, J., & Heliövaara, M. (2018). Risk factors for sciatica leading to hospitalization. *European Spine Journal*, *27*(7), 1501–1508. doi:10.1007/s00586-017- 5182-8

Mayo Clinic. (2019). Sciatica. *Patient Care & Health Information*, e1–e7. Retrieved from https://www.mayoclinic.org/diseases-conditions/sciatica/symptoms-causes/syc-20377435

Poquet, N., & Lin, C. W. (2016). Management strategies for sciatica (PEDro synthesis). *British Journal of Sports Medicine*, *50*(4), 253–254. doi:10.1136/bjsports-2015-095268

Steffens, D., Hancock, M. J., Pereira, L. S., Kent, P. M., Latimer, J., & Maher, C. G. (2016). Do MRI findings identify patients with low back pain or sciatica who respond better to particular interventions? A systematic review. *European Spine Journal*, *25*(4), 1170–1187. doi:10.1007/s00586-015-4195-4

Sprains: Ankle and Knee

Julie Adkins and Jenny Mullen

Definition
Sprains are ligament stretching or partial tears from forceful stress on the joint. Sprains are categorized as follows:
A. Grade 1: Microscopic tears without ligament tearing or joint instability
B. Grade 2: Partial tearing of involved ligaments and laxity of the joint with moderate function loss
C. Grade 3: Ligament tearing with severe function loss and joint instability

Incidence

A. *Ankle* sprains are among the most common injuries seen in primary care. It is estimated that more than 23,000 ankle sprains occur each day in the United States. Female athletes have a 25% more occurrence than male athletes, with female basketball players at a higher risk for first-time injury than those participating in different sports.

B. *Knee* injuries are among the 10 most common causes of occupational injury and worker compensation claims. Approximately 74,000 knee sprain injuries occur annually in the United States. Such injuries are most common in high school athletes. Recent research indicates that the average amount of time lost per knee sprain injury is 23 to 24 days.

C. Current statistics for knee/ankle injury causes: Falls, 80.2%; collision with object, 11%; and hit by moving object, 8.8%

D. Rehabilitation process trajectory for returning to play/work:

1. Grade 1: Approximately 10 days
2. Grade 2: Approximately 20 days
3. Grade 3: Approximately ≥60 days

Pathogenesis

A. Sudden stress to a supporting ligament causes ligament stretching or tearing. Sprains are usually the result of jumping, falling, or rotating a joint.

B. Ankle sprains are most often inversion sprains, with symptoms occurring on the lateral side of the joint

C. Eversion injuries affect the medial side.

D. Knee sprains most often involve the patellofemoral joint.

Predisposing Factors

A. Previous injury to ankle or knee
B. Athletic activities
C. Patellofemoral instability
D. Use of a standing electric scooter

Common Complaints

A. "I twisted my ankle or knee."
B. "I stepped off of a step and came down on the side of my foot."
C. Swelling, pain, weakness of ankle or knee from a previous injury

Other Signs and Symptoms

A. First degree: Minimal pain; mild to moderate pain with stress, little swelling; minimal tenderness with palpation; little functional loss; unimpaired weight bearing or walking; internal microdamage with full continuity

B. Second degree: Moderate pain with ROM; swelling; marked tenderness on palpation; moderate loss of function; difficulty with weight bearing or walking; mechanical dissociation with partial loss of continuity

C. Third degree: Severe pain, especially with passive inversion; severe swelling, marked tenderness; marked decrease in ROM; intolerant of weight bearing or walking; joint instability; discoloration of skin; complete rupture of a ligament

Subjective Data

A. Inquire about history of trauma.

B. Have the client describe the injury: Time, place, activity, predisposing factors, and time the symptoms developed.

C. Determine if the symptoms are acute or chronic.

D. Inquire about the type and location of the pain.

E. Have the client describe the pain and what conditions aggravate or relieve the pain.

F. Ask if there are symptoms of popping, clicking, locking, recurrent swelling, or giving way of the joint.

G. Ask if there is pain or other symptoms elsewhere, such as the low back, hip, or leg.

H. Explore the client's history of any previous ankle or knee injury.

I. Determine if the current injury was evaluated and treated previously.

J. Have the client describe the ability to bear weight on the extremity and to tolerate ROM.

K. Review the client's medical history for arthritis, gout, cancer, autoimmune disorders, or metabolic disease.

Physical Examination

A. Check temperature, pulse, respirations, and blood pressure.

B. Inspect:

1. Observe ambulation. Note overall appearance and facial grimaces during the examination.
2. Inspect the injured area for swelling, discoloration, and deformity. Compare the injured side to the uninjured side.

C. Palpate:

1. Palpate the injured site for tenderness.
2. Palpate the joints above and below the injured site.
3. Perform ROM (active and passive) and resisted ROM to evaluate strength.
4. Check for catching or locking of the knee on extension.
5. Assess neurovascular status of the knee or ankle and distal extremity.
6. *Ankle*: Palpate for a tender sulcus in the anterolateral aspect on inversion of the ankle. Assess for pain aggravated by forced ankle inversion. Perform an isometric test of plantar flexion and eversion. Perform the anterior drawer test and talar tilt test.
7. *Knee:* Palpate for tenderness on the medial and lateral joint line. Perform McMurray's test to detect a torn meniscus (*see the Section II: Procedure, "Evaluation of Sprains"*). Symptoms of sprained knees include:

   a. Meniscus tear: Locking of knee with flexion and giving way of knee

   b. Collateral ligament tear or strain: Pain at lateral or medial sides

   c. Anterior cruciate tear: Popping sound at the injury site and immediate swelling

   d. Posterior cruciate tear or strain: Pain in the interior knee

e. Patellofemoral syndrome: Popping or snapping, pain under the patella with motion, and pain on stairs or hills

f. Tendinitis: Pain over the patellar tendon

g. Prepatellar bursitis: Swelling over the patella with inability to kneel due to swelling

h. Nonspecific effusion: Effusion that becomes worse with exercise

8. *See Section II: Procedure, "Evaluation of Sprains."*

Diagnostic Tests

A. Radiography of extremity, if fracture is suspected

B. MRI, if mechanical symptoms and effusion persist

C. Bone scans or MRI are usually reserved for clients who have failed to respond after 6 to 12 weeks of therapy.

Differential Diagnoses

A. Ankle sprain:
   1. Fracture
   2. Acute dislocation
   3. Infection
   4. Ligament strain
   5. Tendinitis or tenosynovitis
   6. Nonspecific foot or ankle pain

B. Knee sprain:
   1. Fracture
   2. Dislocation
   3. Septic arthritis
   4. Infected prepatellar bursitis
   5. Inflammation
   6. Tumor
   7. Meniscus tear
   8. Collateral ligament tear
   9. Anterior cruciate tear
   10. Posterior cruciate tear
   11. Collateral ligament strain
   12. Cruciate ligament strain
   13. Patellofemoral syndrome, or chondromalacia
   14. Effusion, nonspecific
   15. Patellar tendinitis
   16. Prepatellar bursitis
   17. Nonspecific knee pain

Plan

A. General interventions:
   1. Reinforce the degree of injury and the need to take care of the extremity to prevent further damage.
   2. Prescribe an exercise program to prevent stiffness, restore function, improve ROM, and restore normal flexibility and strength.
   3. A mild ankle sprain may require 3 to 6 weeks of rehabilitation, a moderate sprain may require 2 to 3 months of rehabilitation, and a severe sprain may require 8 to 12 months of therapy to return to full activity.
   4. Wrapping the ankle with a three-way ankle joint mobilization improves dynamic postural control, balance, and weight-bearing dorsiflexion ROM.

B. Client teaching:
   1. Educate clients on the risks and benefits protective knee and ankle gear and bike helmets when riding electric standing scooters.
   2. *See Section III: Client Teaching Guide for this chapter, "RICE Therapy and Exercise Therapy"; "Ankle Exercises" or "Knee Exercises."*

C. Pharmaceutical therapy:
   1. Drug of choice:
      a. NSAIDs to reduce pain and inflammation
      b. Consider one of the following: Aspirin, ibuprofen, indomethacin, or piroxicam. Do not use these medications in the long term.
      c. If there is increased risk for bleeding, acetaminophen with codeine may be used for pain.
   2. Injectable medication:
      a. Methylprednisolone acetate (Depo-Medrol) may be used if symptoms continue to be present 6 to 8 weeks after injury.
      b. Repeat injection in 4 to 6 weeks if symptoms have not been reduced by 50%.

Follow-Up

A. Schedule the initial follow-up in 2 weeks to evaluate current therapy or sooner if problems arise

B. Follow-up appointments should be scheduled according to treatment/therapy.

Consultation/Referral

A. Refer the client to a physician if fracture is suspected.

B. Refer the client to physical therapy as needed.

C. Refer the client to a physician or orthopedic surgeon if therapy is unproductive and symptoms have not begun to regress within 6 weeks.

Individual Considerations

A. Pediatrics:
   1. In prepubertal or peripubertal clients, knee ligaments usually do not tear. Instead, the growth plate may open up on one side. This age group needs stress radiography to check for fracture of the growth plate.

B. Adults:
   1. Clients with a history of mild-to-moderate knee OA who practice walking as a regular exercise report benefits of strengthened mobility and quality of life.

C. Eleven best-practice recommendations across musculoskeletal pain conditions:
   1. Client-centered care: Implement interventions unique to client preferences, with effective communication that includes shared decision-making.
   2. Identify clients with high risk for serious pathology or demonstrating unusual (red flag) signs/symptoms.
   3. Evaluate psychosocial dynamics.
   4. Radiological imaging is not recommended unless:
      a. Suspected pathology
      b. Conservative care is ineffective
      c. Unexplained progression of signs/symptoms
      d. Unresolved condition mandates treatment changes

5. Exam must include screening for neurological ability, mobility, and muscle strength.

6. Evaluate client progress with standard outcome measures.

7. Provide client education regarding the condition and care plan management

8. Address parameters of physical activity and exercise during and post treatment.

9. Manual therapy must serve as an adjunct to other evidence-based treatments.

10. Offer evidence-based nonsurgical care prior to surgery.

11. Design a maintenance program and resumption of work with the client.

D. RICE and MEAT:

   1. RICE = Rest, Ice, Compression, Elevation. This method is generally recommended immediately following a musculoskeletal injury. However, ice and rest over an extended period of time might impede the healing process. This treatment might be all that is needed for minor injuries. If swelling continues after a few hours and pain is not diminishing, the client must consider further assessment from a medical clinician.

   2. MEAT = Movement, Exercise, Analgesics, Treatment. This method is best implemented when the client collaborates with the medical clinician and/or physical therapist. Maintaining ROM would increase blood flow to the injured area and promote healing. A progressive exercise plan (guided by the healthcare provider) would be created to increase strength, improve balance, and facilitate a healing timeline that avoids reinjury. Medication, advanced neuromuscular modalities, and therapeutic exercises would help restore, retrain, and expedite recovery.

Bibliography

American Academy of Family Physicians. (2019). *Musculoskeletal (MSK) clinical recommendations & guidelines*. Retrieved from https://www.aafp.org/patient-care/browse/topics.tag-musculoskeletal.html

Brisson, N., Gatti, A., & Maly, M. (2019). Pain is not associated with steps per day in persons with mild-to-moderate symptomatic knee osteoarthritis: A mixed models analysis of multiple measurements over 3 years. *Arthritis Care & Research, 71*(3), 331–447. doi:10.1002/acr.23842

Duffy, S. (Ed.). (2019). *Monthly prescribing guide* (Vol. 1–4). London, UK: Prescribing Reference, Inc.

Fraser, J., Koldenhoven, R., Jaffri, A., Park, J., Saliba, S., Hart, J., & Hertel, J. (2018). Foot impairments contribute to functional limitation in individuals with ankle sprain and chronic ankle instability. *Knee Surgery, Sports Traumatology, Arthroscopy, 26*(7), e1–e11. doi:10.1007/s00167-018-5028-x

Herman, D., Weppner, J., & Raiser, S. (2016). Medial and lateral collateral ligament injuries. *American Academy of Physical Medicine and Rehabilitation*, e1–e6. Retrieved from https://now.aapmr.org/medial-and-lateral-collateral-ligament-injuries/

Janssen, K. W., van der Zwaard, B. C., Finch, C. F., van Mechelen, W., & Verhagen, E. A. (2016). Interventions preventing ankle sprains; previous injury and high-risk sport participation as predictors of compliance. *Journal of Science and Medicine in Sport/Sports Medicine Australia, 19*(6), 465–469. doi:10.1016/j.jsams.2015.06.005

Kosk, K., & Gribble, P. (2018). The effect of joint mobilization on dynamic postural control in patients with chronic ankle instability: A critically appraised topic. *Journal of Sport Rehabilitation, 27*(1), 103–108. doi:10.1123/jsr.2016-0074

Mana, S. (2018). Treating an acute injury: Go for M.E.A.T. and R.I.C.E. physiotherapy. *Lifemark*. Retrieved from https://www.lifemark.ca/blog-post/treating-acute-injury-go-meat-over-rice

Mitchell, H., Rothenberg, M. D., & Graf, B. (2016). Evaluation of acute knee injuries. *Postgraduate Medicine, 93*(3), 75–86.

Ortho Bullets. (2019). Trauma high-yield topics. *General Trauma*. Retrieved from https://www.orthobullets.com/topic/dashboard?id=1&specialty=1&expandLeftMenu=true

Runde, M. & Van Vooren, J. (2019). Do the benefits of NSAIDs outweigh the risks when treating ankle sprains? *Evidence-Based Practice, 22*(2), 24. doi:10.1097/EBP.0000000000000160

Trivedi, T., Lui, C., Antonio, A. L., Wheaton, N., Kreger, V., Yap, A., Schriger, D., & Elmore, J. (2019). Standing electric scooter riders underestimate risks. *JAMA Network Open Emergency Medicine, 2*(1), e1–e9. doi:10.1001/jamanetworkopen.2018.7381

Weerasekara, I., Osmotherly, P., Snodgrass, S., Marquez, J., Zoete, R., & Rivett, D. (2018). Clinical benefits of joint mobilization on ankle sprains: A systemic review and meta-analysis. *Physical Medicine and Rehabilitation, 99*(7), 1395–1412. doi:10.1016/j.apmr.2017.07.019

Wirfs, M. J. (2018). *The APRN's complete guide to prescribing drug therapy*. New York, NY: Springer Publishing Company.

Young, C., Sherwin, S., Andary, M., Bernhardt, D., Bessman, E., Bozzelle, J., ... Windsor, R. (2019). What is the prevalence of ankle sprains? *Medscape Sports Medicine*, e1–e32. Retrieved from https://www.medscape.com/answers/1907229-95137/what-is-the-prevalence-of-ankle-sprains

Video

Rusin, J. (2017). *3-way ankle joint mobilization* [Video]. Available from https://www.youtube.com/watch?v=oVnR0LPo3ag

19 Neurological Guidelines

Alzheimer's Disease

Julie Adkins, Jill C. Cash, and Kimberly Waltrip

Definition
A. Alzheimer's disease and related dementias (ADRD) involve memory loss that eventually affects an individual's level of independence. Alzheimer's disease (AD) is a brain disorder that is irreversible and progressive. The disease slowly destroys memory and cognition, then eventually impairs task performance. Cognitive deterioration is permanent and progressive. Impairments, such as memory disturbance, severely interfere with activities of daily living (ADLs), but do not affect level of consciousness (LOC). Insidious disease onset and gradual, progressive cognitive decline without other specific causes of dementia are also present.

Incidence
A. AD, the most common type of dementia, is the sixth leading cause of death in the U.S. population, and the fifth leading cause of adult deaths at ages 65 years and older. In 2014, ADRD affected an estimated 5.0 million adults aged 65 years and older, or 1.6% of the population. These diseases have significant impact on clients, families, communities, and healthcare systems.
B. Approximately 6.1 million people were diagnosed with AD or mild cognitive impairments in 2017. Based on this estimate, 15.0 million cases are anticipated by 2060. Another projection doubles ADRD disease burden in the United States to 3.3% by 2060, with an estimated 13.9 million cases.
C. Age is the primary risk factor for ADRD. Race and ethnicity are also important risk factors to consider upon noting the disparities in ADRD prevalence. The prevalence of ADRD is highest in African Americans—specifically, 64% higher compared to the prevalence in Caucasians. Hispanics are 1.5 times more likely than non-Hispanic whites to have ADRD.

Pathogenesis
A. The degenerative disease process involves cell loss within the basal forebrain, cerebral cortex, and other areas where plaques and tangles accumulate and block essential cellular processes, which in turn destroys neurons. Neuronal death causes memory loss, changes in personality, and other signs and symptoms of AD.
B. Obesity has been identified as a major risk factor for developing AD due to the increased adipokine dysregulation, which leads to subsequent release of pro-inflammatory adipokines that decrease anti-inflammatory adipokines

Predisposing Factors
A. Age older than 50 years
B. Severe head trauma
C. Genetic defects, such as Down syndrome
D. Family history of AD
E. Obesity
F. African American or Hispanic race

Common Complaint
A. Significant memory loss

Other Signs and Symptoms
Ten warning signs of AD
A. Memory loss that interrupts ADLs
B. Loss of all intellectual capacities, such as executing or following plans, solving problems
C. Difficulty completing routine tasks at home or work
D. Confusion with time or place
E. Problems understanding visual images or spatial relationships
F. Difficulty speaking or writing words
G. Losing things without the ability to retrace steps and locate what is missing
H. Poor judgment in daily routine
I. Withdrawal from work or social activities
J. Changes in mood or personality (www.alz.org/national/documents/checklist_10signs.pdf)

Subjective Data

> Family members can be reliable resources for obtaining an accurate client history.

A. Determine onset, course, and duration of symptoms.
B. Note loss of immediate, recent, or remote memory, such as trouble remembering appointments, difficulty recalling recent events, and inability to find personal belongings.
C. Determine the client's ability to make reasonable judgments, such as answering the phone when it rings, or exiting a burning building.
D. Assess the client's ability to perform ADLs, including bathing, cooking meals, and housekeeping.
E. Discuss the client's sleep–wake cycle.
F. Assess for associated signs and symptoms of depression, such as decreased appetite, lack of pleasure in usual activities, melancholy mood, and other related findings.
G. Note language difficulties and problems expressing oneself.
H. Note any recent physical illness.
I. Review the medication history.
J. Discuss alcohol intake and abuse factors.
K. Review any past medical history of head trauma, hypertension (HTN), cerebrovascular accident (CVA), cancer, metabolic problems, neurological disorders, infections, gastric surgery (vitamin B_{12} deficiency), and emotional or psychiatric problems.

Physical Examination

A. Check temperature, blood pressure, pulse, respirations, and weight.
B. Inspect:
  1. Inspect the client's general appearance for hygiene and nutritional deficits.
C. Auscultate:
  1. Heart
  2. Lungs
D. Neurological examination:
  1. Perform a complete neurological examination.
  2. Perform the standardized Mini-Mental State Examination (MMSE), available at https://pdfs. semanticscholar.org/4370/72f1421146674eaf98e11c c9079311f23fcb.pdf.
  3. The clock-draw test (CDT) may also be administered and used as a screening tool. The CDT is available at www.sralab.org/rehabilitation-measures/clock -drawing-test. See Section II: Procedure, "Clock-Draw Test."

> Rule out other specific causes of dementia, including cardiovascular disease (CVD).

Diagnostic Tests

A. Complete blood count (CBC)
B. Comprehensive metabolic profile (CMP)
C. Thyroid function studies
D. Folate and vitamin B_{12} levels
E. Homocysteine
F. Methylmalonic acid
G. Vitamin D level
H. Rapid plasma reagin (RPR) to screen for neurosyphilis
I. CT scan of the head

Differential Diagnoses

A. AD
B. Drug interactions
C. Delirium
D. Depression
E. Cerebrovascular disease
F. Vascular dementia (secondary to small-vessel disease)

Plan

A. General interventions:
  1. Identify the stage of impairment:
    a. **Stage 1:** No impairment: No evidence of symptoms
    b. **Stage 2:** Very mild decline: No symptoms of dementia, memory lapses
    c. **Stage 3:** Mild decline: Difficulties with memory and concentration
    d. **Stage 4:** Moderate decline: Cognitive impairment with complex tasks, difficulty solving math problems, forgetting one's personal history
    e. **Stage 5:** Moderately severe decline: Unable to remember phone number or address, confusion about day of the week, difficulty dressing self according to season or weather conditions
    f. **Stage 6:** Severe decline: Difficulties recalling personal history, identifying family members, dressing appropriately; behavioral changes and client wandering secondary to inability to recognize the environment and becoming lost
    g. **Stage 7:** Extremely severe decline: Unable to communicate appropriately with others, assistance required with ADLs, pathological and/or certain primitive reflexes, difficulty swallowing
  2. Provide supportive measures. Explain exam findings and possible treatment options to the client and family.
  3. Treatment may address coexisting diseases, thyroid disease, and vitamin B_{12} deficiency.
  4. Discuss options such as cognitive stimulation therapy (CST), where musical, occupational, and other mind-stimulating activities are used to improve cognition and quality of life (QoL).
  5. Ensure a safe environment for the client at all times (e.g., locks and alarms on doors, relinquishing driving privileges).
  6. Emphasize the importance of exercise: Daily exercise improves cerebral perfusion, memory, attention, executive function, and processing speed.
B. Client teaching:
  1. Educate clients, family, and the community about interventions and strategies that lower the risk for AD. Obesity is a significant, modifiable risk factor. Lifestyle changes, such as adherence to healthy diet

and/or calorie restriction, exercise, cognitive stimulation, and social participation, are recommended to decrease AD risk.

2. Support groups are encouraged for the client and/or family. Therapy sessions may be beneficial to both.

3. Provide the client with support group information for the Alzheimer's Association online at www.alz.org, and via phone at 1-800-272-3900 (24/7 Helpline).

4. Encourage families who require legal and financial advice to contact the Alzheimer's Disease Family Relief Program at 1-800-437-2423 soon after AD diagnosis, before any crises occur.

C. Pharmaceutical therapy:

1. Cholinesterase inhibitors:

   a. Rivastigmine (Exelon; for mild-to-moderate disease), 1.5 to 6 mg twice daily or via transdermal patch starting at 4.6 mg/d, then titrate up to 9.5 mg/d or increase to the maximum effective dose at 13.3 mg/d, as indicated

   b. Donepezil (Aricept; for all stages of disease):

      i. 5 mg at bedtime, then to 10 mg/d after a month

      ii. 23 mg extended-release tablets are available for clients with moderate-to-severe disease, who have taken 10 mg at bedtime for at least 3 months

   c. Galantamine (Razadyne; for mild-to-moderate disease):

      i. 4 mg twice daily with meals for 4 weeks, then may increase to maximum dose at 12 mg twice daily. For missed doses, the client or family will need to retitrate doses.

      ii. Extended-release version, 8 mg/d; after 4 weeks, may increase dose to 16 mg/d, or increase to the maximum dose at 24 mg/d

2. N-methyl-D-aspartate (NMDA) receptor antagonist:

   a. Memantine (Namenda) 5 mg/d, increase dose an additional 5 mg each week; can also adjust dose to 5 mg twice daily, and increase to the maximum dose at 20 mg twice daily:

      i. Use the titration pack for the first 4 weeks.

      ii. Do NOT prescribe more than 5 mg twice daily to clients with severe renal impairment.

   b. Namzaric (donepezil and memantine) is also available to clients with moderate-to-severe disease who are taking donepezil, 10 mg/d.

3. Assess the client for secondary behaviors of dementia. Psychosis, delusions, hallucinations, anxiety, depression, and insomnia may occur and should be treated accordingly. Cognitive and behavioral interventions should be initiated for additional client assistance with behavioral modification. The benefits and risks must be weighed, and pharmacological treatment may be necessary for clients exhibiting extreme, aggressive behaviors with irritability and/or insomnia. Treatment with antipsychotics is very controversial due to the potential side effects and extreme complications associated with these medications.

4. Antidepressants:

   a. Nortriptyline (Pamelor), 30 to 50 mg/d

   b. Sertraline (Zoloft), 50 mg/d; can increase dose 50 mg each week, up to the maximum dose at 200 mg/d

   c. Paroxetine (Paxil), 10 mg/d for older adults; can increase dose 10 mg each week to 40 mg/d

   d. Escitalopram (Lexapro), 10 mg/d; can increase dose to 20 mg/d after 1 week

   e. Monitor selective serotonin reuptake inhibitor (SSRI) use for weight loss, decreased seizure threshold, and/or tremors.

   f. Do NOT use with monoamine oxidase inhibitors (MAOI).

   g. Monitor coumadin and lithium levels closely.

Follow-Up

A. Follow-up will vary, depending on the client's status and the needs of the client and family. Follow-up is recommended every 3 months to follow disease progression. Monitor clients monthly when new medications are introduced.

Consultation/Referral

A. Consider referrals for a home health nurse and/or nurse assistant, social worker, occupational therapy (OT), and/or physical therapy (PT).

B. Consult a physician regarding medications for secondary behavioral symptoms.

Individual Considerations

A. Adults:

1. AD should be considered in adults at early ages to avoid risk factors.

2. Lifestyle and dietary changes should be encouraged to lower the risk of AD. Exercise, a healthy diet, and maintaining a healthy weight (body mass index [BMI]) can decrease AD-associated risk factors.

3. Assess for common AD medication side effects: Nausea, vomiting, decreased appetite, increasingly frequent bowel movements, constipation, headache, confusion, and dizziness.

B. Geriatrics:

1. AD is most prevalent in older adults.

2. Long-term prognosis: Average life expectancy varies from 7 to 10 years after onset of early symptoms, but clients with dementia can live 20 years or more.

3. The use of probiotics in the elderly has been shown to improve the anti-inflammatory properties of the gut. However, any behavioral changes should be monitored closely.

Bibliography

Alzheimer's Association Diagnostic Evaluation Clinical Practice Guideline Workgroup (AADx-CPG Workgroup). (2018). First practice guidelines for clinical evaluation of Alzheimer's disease and other dementias for primary and specialty care. In A. Atri (Ed.), *Alzheimer's Association international conference (AAIC) 2018* (pp. 1–8). Chicago, IL: Alzheimer's Association. Retrieved from https://www.alz.org/aaic/downloads2018/Sun-clinical-practice-guidelines.pdf

Mendiola-Precoma, J., Berumen, L. C., Padilla, K., & Garcia-Alcocer, G. (2016). Therapies for prevention and treatment of Alzheimer's disease. *BioMed Research International, 2016.* doi:10.1155/2016/2589276

Scheltens, N. M., Galindo-Garre, F., Pijnenburg, Y. A., van der Vlies, E. A., Smits, L. L., Koene, T., . . . van der Flier, W. M. (2016). The identification of cognitive subtypes in Alzheimer's disease dementia using latent class analysis. *Journal of Neurology, Neurosurgery, and Psychiatry, 87*(3), 235–243. doi:10.1136/jnnp-2014-309582

Bell's Palsy

Julie Adkins, Jill C. Cash, and Kimberly Waltrip

Definition

A. Bell's palsy and idiopathic peripheral facial palsy are acute clinical syndromes characterized by rapid onset of unilateral facial paralysis. Bell's palsy typically occurs from herpes simplex virus (HSV-1) activation. Signs and symptoms of Bell's palsy are rapid and progressive. Symptoms present within 24 hours to a week, usually reaching peak severity at 72 hours. Partial to complete weakness/paralysis in half of the face affects motor control of the eyebrows, eyelids, forehead, and corners of the mouth. Clients may be unable to close the eyelid or mouth on the affected side. If forehead muscles are unaffected, central nervous system (CNS) pathology must be considered. Other reported symptoms include changes in eye tearing, taste (anterior two-thirds of the tongue), salivation, and sound sensitivity. Bell's palsy can affect both sides, but only in rare cases.

Incidence

A. The incidence of Bell's palsy ranges from 15 to 20 cases per 100,000, with 40,000 newly diagnosed cases each year (1:60 lifetime risk). Recurrence varies between 8% and 12%. Approximately 70% of Bell's palsy cases will completely resolve without treatment.
B. Age, gender, and race are not risk factors, but a higher number of cases are diagnosed in middle-aged and older adults. Onset is at a median age of 40 years. Nearly 70% of facial paralysis cases are attributed to Bell's palsy.

Pathogenesis

A. The pathogenesis of Bell's palsy is often considered idiopathic, but potential etiologies may be genetic, metabolic, autoimmune, or vascular. An event or stressor triggers activation of a latent virus, usually HSV, within the geniculate ganglion of the facial nerve. Viral activation results in re-expression of dormant viral particles and neural inflammation, leading to facial nerve entrapment, ischemia, and degeneration.

Predisposing Factors

A. Diabetes
B. Pregnancy
C. Recent infection or immunization
D. Family history of Bell's palsy
E. HTN
F. Hypothyroidism
G. Obesity
H. Preeclampsia

Common Complaints

A. Acute onset of unilateral facial weakness with an inability to close one eye
B. Sagging of one eyelid
C. Absence of nasolabial fold
D. Mouth drawn to affected side

Other Signs and Symptoms

A. Ipsilateral retroauricular pain preceding, or occurring with paralysis
B. Hyperacusis or sensitivity to sound
C. Dysgeusia or altered taste in the anterior two-thirds of the tongue
D. Facial paresthesia
E. Drooling
F. Decreased tearing; increased while eating

Subjective Data

A. Elicit onset, duration, and course of symptoms.
B. Obtain the client's description of all neurological symptoms present.
C. Note associated symptoms, such as altered taste and visual or hearing disturbances.
D. Ask about any predisposing factors, such as trauma, infection, or pregnancy.
E. Review the client's family history for other cases of Bell's palsy.
F. Review the client's past medical history, especially for any cerebrovascular or cardiac risk factors. Any contraindications to steroid use must be examined further before treatment.

Physical Examination

A. Check temperature, pulse, respirations, and blood pressure.
B. Inspect:
    1. Symmetry of facial appearance and expression
    2. Observe symmetry of the eyes, and for a weak or absent corneal reflex on the affected side.
    3. Assess the skin for a maculopapular rash or herpetic/zoster lesions, especially in and behind the affected ear.
    4. Perform a complete ear examination to rule out infection.
    5. Examine the mouth and nose for lesions; examine the oral cavity for food pocketing secondary to xerostomia and injury on the affected side from chewing.
C. Auscultate:
    1. Heart
    2. Lungs
D. Neurological examination:
    1. Perform a complete neurological examination, testing all 12 pairs of cranial nerves (CNs).
    2. **Assess ALL muscles innervated by the facial nerve, specifically for motor control versus paralysis of muscles in the forehead, eyelid, and cheek/around the mouth. Partial or complete paralysis may be present.**

> Subjective, decreased sensation may be present in the trigeminal nerve distribution.

Diagnostic Tests

A. Lyme disease antibodies (2-step test): Positive or equivocal enzyme immunoassay (EIA) followed with a positive immunoblot (Western blot) in clients with secondary facial weakness from Lyme disease

B. Skull radiography, computed tomography (CT) scan, or magnetic resonance imaging (MRI): No pathology specific to Bell's palsy, but may show evidence of fracture line, stroke (CVA), mass (tumor), or bony erosion secondary to infection

C. Electromyographic (EMG) and nerve conduction velocity (NCV) studies: EMG/NCV testing will evaluate the severity and extent of any peripheral nerve damage, and may provide additional information regarding a client's prognosis

D. Lumbar puncture (LP): Indicated only when other conditions are suspected. Cerebrospinal fluid (CSF) should be sent for cytology.

Differential Diagnoses

A. Bell's palsy

B. Guillain–Barré syndrome (GBS)

C. Stroke

D. Lyme disease

E. Sarcoidosis

F. Ramsey–Hunt syndrome (varicella zoster virus/VZV), herpes zoster oticus

G. Cerebellopontine angle (CPA) masses, such as vestibular schwannoma (acoustic neuroma) or hemangioma

H. Middle ear disease, such as purulent otitis media or neoplasms

I. Parotid gland mass

Plan

A. General interventions:

1. Symptoms usually resolve within 1 to 3 weeks and may be managed with short-term steroids and acetaminophen as needed for discomfort.

2. PT may be beneficial for facial muscle weakness or contractures.

3. Reinforce the client's need for reassurance and emotional support to family members and significant others.

> Recovery may require 3 to 6 months or longer; complete resolution of symptoms occurs in approximately 80% of Bell's palsy cases.

B. Client teaching:

1. See *Section III: Client Teaching Guide for this chapter, "Bell's Palsy."*

2. Provide eye protection using the following:

    a. Instill methylcellulose drops (artificial tears) as needed and use an ocular lubricant like Refresh or Systane Ultra at bedtime.

    b. Tape the eye closed, especially at night.

    c. Wear dark glasses when outdoors to minimize exposure.

3. Application of moist heat packs may be useful for pain as needed.

C. Pharmaceutical therapy:

1. Prednisone: Adults take 80 mg daily with breakfast for the first 3 days, then 40 mg daily for 3 days, followed by 20 mg daily for 3 days, and then steroids are discontinued.

> Recent studies suggest that a brief course of prednisone offers modest benefits with minimal risks.

2. Acyclovir, 400 mg five times daily for 10 days. Consider acyclovir for clients without renal insufficiency and no other contraindications to therapy.

3. Analgesics, such as acetaminophen, when necessary (prn) for ear pain.

Follow-Up

A. For clients with severe symptoms, schedule follow-up in 3 to 4 days, then again in 2 weeks.

B. If symptoms worsen or do not resolve within 4 weeks, have the client return for additional follow-up and possible referral.

Consultation/Referral

A. Consult a neurologist for the following:

1. Signs and symptoms fail to resolve significantly after 4 to 6 weeks. Only 5% to 8% of clients report distressing residual signs and symptoms, such as contracture of facial muscles at rest and synergistic mass innervation from defective nerve regeneration, as evidenced by "crocodile tears" secondary to abnormal secretory fibers that were intended for salivary glands versus ipsilateral eyelid shutting.

2. Other CN involvement or other aberrant neurological exam findings are present.

3. Between 5% and 7% of clients experience recurrence of symptoms. Known causes of recurrent palsy include sarcoidosis, diabetes, leukemia, and infectious mononucleosis.

4. Bilateral facial palsies

B. Consult an ophthalmologist for persistent ocular pain or development of corneal abrasions or ulcerations.

C. Consult a neurosurgeon and/or an otolaryngologist if neural decompression is considered.

Individual Considerations

A. Pregnancy:

1. The incidence of Bell's palsy increases throughout pregnancy, with the highest incidence during the third trimester or immediately postpartum. Prednisone can be prescribed during pregnancy.

Bibliography

National Institute of Neurological Disorders and Stroke. (2016). *Bell's palsy fact sheet*. Retrieved from http://www.ninds.nih.gov/Disorders/Client-Caregiver-Education/Fact-Sheets/Bells-Palsy-Fact-Sheet

Carpal Tunnel Syndrome

Julie Adkins, Jill C. Cash, and Kimberly Waltrip

Definition

A. Carpal tunnel syndrome (CTS) is a nerve entrapment condition of the median nerve of the wrist. The median nerve extends down the forearm, then passes through the carpal tunnel space before entering the hand. Such compression can alter sensation in the thumb, first and second fingers, and possibly third finger. Median nerve compression from injury, inflammation, or edema within the carpal tunnel can also cause numbness, tingling, arm and/or hand pain, and functional impairment.

Incidence

A. Estimated overall lifetime prevalence of CTS ranges between 8% and 10%, regardless of employment or occupation. CTS typically affects individuals between ages 30 and 60 years, occurring nearly twice as often in females, and more frequently with increasing age.

Pathogenesis

A. The carpal bones and the transverse carpal ligament form the carpal tunnel, a rigid, hollow structure surrounding the median nerve that enters the hand. The median nerve contains spinal nerve roots C6, C7, C8, and T1 that innervate the forearm, wrist, and hand. Median nerve compression occurs when the flexor tenosynovium swells, increases pressure within the carpal tunnel space, and blocks nerve conduction. Subsequent numbness and discomfort in the hands and fingers result from repetitive wrist flexion and extension that causes this increased pressure.

B. Potential causes of CTS include inflamed, thickened, or fibrotic flexor tendons around the median nerve; inadequate space within the carpal tunnel; lesions, cysts, or masses that compress the median nerve; chronic disease processes that cause edema or inflammation, such as rheumatoid arthritis (RA), diabetes mellitus (DM), and thyroid or endocrine disease; blunt trauma or structural changes; mechanical overuse; and infectious diseases, such as tuberculosis (TB) and leprosy. Consider multifactorial causes of CTS. Genetic factors are important, for example, when individuals and family members have small carpal tunnel spaces or other anatomical anomalies that alter nerve structure or function.

Predisposing Factors

A. Female gender
B. Hobbies or occupations that require repetitive wrist or hand movement, or the use of vibrating tools
C. Pregnancy
D. Genetic predisposition
E. Aging

Common Complaints

A. Pain
B. Tingling, numbness, and/or burning (paresthesia) reported in the thumb and first, second, and third fingers; altered sensation that radiates upward from the wrists, hands, and fingers into the forearm
C. Dropping objects because of weak handgrip or grasp, numbness, or lost proprioception
D. Symptoms with increased severity at night

Other Signs and Symptoms

A. Paresthesia in wrists, hands, and fingers
B. Localized pain in radial three fingers
C. Weakened grasp and/or handgrip
D. Decreased manual dexterity
E. Nocturnal wrist pain
F. Referred pain to the elbow and/or shoulder
G. Irreversible neural damage from long-term compression can occur, in addition to ischemic changes, and possible axonal death, muscle atrophy, and/or pain

Subjective Data

A. Assess the onset, duration, and timing of presenting symptoms.
B. Note the progression of symptoms since the initial occurrence.
C. Determine whether symptoms increase with hand or wrist use, and decrease when at rest.
D. Identify factors that precipitate, aggravate, and alleviate symptoms.
E. Inquire whether numbness and tingling awaken the client at night.
F. Ask the client to describe the pain, whether it radiates up the upper extremity, and if symptoms are bilateral.
G. Document the client's occupation, hobbies, and daily activities that require hand or wrist use.
H. Ask the client what treatment and/or relief measures have been used, and the effectiveness of each.

Physical Examination

A. Check temperature, blood pressure, and pulse.
B. Inspect:
   1. Hands for atrophy, noting any palmar deformities or wasting in the hand muscles
   2. Bone deformities in the hand, such as ulnar deviation and/or swan neck deformity associated with RA, and for wrist deformities that suggest osteoarthritis (OA)
   3. Assess for any edema, abrasions, or ecchymoses that may indicate trauma or injury.
C. Palpate:
   1. Perform a sensorimotor exam of the hand and arm.
   2. Perform a two-point discrimination test on the hand, forearm, and upper arm: Assess the client's ability to discern between two sharp stimuli applied at different points; more than a 5-mm difference between applied stimuli is considered an aberrant finding.
   3. Perform Tinel's test: Percuss or lightly tap the ventral wrist over the transverse carpal ligament; Tinel's sign is present if the client reports tingling or "pins and needles" sensations in the fingers.

4. Perform Phalen's test:
   a. Maintain the client's shoulders in neutral position, extend the elbows on a flat surface, and hold the forearms in vertical position. Passively flex the client's wrists without overpressure and hold in forced flexion for 60 seconds or until symptoms occur.
      i. Positive test findings: Palmar numbness, tingling, and/or pain reported in the first, second, third, and radial half of the fourth fingers within 60 seconds of forced flexion.
   b. Document the time client symptoms were reported.
5. Perform a manual carpal compression test:
   a. Apply pressure over the transverse carpal ligament. Paresthesia reported within 30 seconds is a positive test finding.
   b. Document the time client symptoms were reported.

Diagnostic Tests
A. EMG and NCV studies are only ordered to rule out other pathology.
B. MRI is rarely ordered to rule out soft-tissue masses and lesions.
C. If an underlying systemic illness or condition exists, consider the following:
   1. Erythrocyte sedimentation rate (ESR)
   2. Blood glucose
   3. Thyroid profile
   4. Inflammatory disease studies

Differential Diagnoses
A. CTS
B. Peripheral neuropathy (PN)
C. Cervical radiculopathy secondary to spondylosis or cervical disk herniation
D. Brachial plexus lesion
E. Trauma
F. Thenar atrophy and neuropathy
G. OA
H. Neurological disorders: Polyneuritis, multiple sclerosis (MS)
I. Connective tissue diseases
J. Aromatase inhibitor use
K. Tendonitis

Plan
A. General interventions:
   1. Help the client identify causative agents, eliminate overuse activity if possible, decrease repetitive use, or use alternative methods to perform the same manual task(s).
   2. Recommend frequent breaks to rest the arms and wrists as much as possible.
   3. Encourage daily stretching exercises.
   4. Give instructions on applying wrist splints at bedtime during sleep:
      a. Wear wrist splints every night for at least 6 to 8 weeks.

      b. If symptoms are present after a month, continue splint use for another 1 to 2 months and treat with corticosteroids (oral or injection).
B. Client teaching:
   1. Instruct the client on wrist splint application:
      a. Splint the wrist in neutral position and 0° extension at night and as needed during the day.
   2. Demonstrate stretching exercises.
   3. Stress the importance of rest and elimination of the causative activity.
   4. Reinforce that improvement or recovery may require up to 6 months.
   5. Encourage the use of ergonomic adaptive aids appropriate for specific manual tasks.
   6. Alternate between manual tasks or jobs and other activities.
C. Pharmaceutical therapy:
   1. Nonsteroidal anti-inflammatory drugs (NSAIDs) as needed: Ibuprofen (Motrin), 600 to 800 mg three times daily, or naproxen (Naprosyn), 500 mg twice daily
   2. Vitamin B_6 100 mg/d
   3. Consider corticosteroid injections to decrease inflammation within the carpal tunnel space (methylprednisolone, 40 mg/mL with 1% lidocaine/1 mL):
      a. Contraindicated with hand muscle weakness and/or hand muscle atrophy, or advanced sensory loss
      b. Do NOT administer multiple injections; limit to one injection every 6 months per wrist.
      c. Risks with corticosteroid injections include increased median nerve compression, wrong-site injection into the median or ulnar nerve, and a ruptured digital flexor tendon.
   4. For clients who decline injection, oral corticosteroids provide short-term relief:
      a. Prednisone, 20 mg/d for 10 to 14 days; do not use for more than 4 weeks to avoid side effects.
   5. Consider other nonsurgical treatments or surgical referral for recurrent symptoms after two corticosteroid injections.

Follow-Up
A. Depending on treatment, the practitioner may schedule follow-up in 1 month to evaluate the client's status.

Consultation/Referral
A. Refer to an orthopedic or neurosurgeon for severe symptoms that may require carpal tunnel release.
B. Consider PT and/or OT consults:
   1. Custom-fitted wrist splints from OT are recommended for CTS. Refer to OT for evaluation and treatment.
   2. Median nerve movement may be restored with nerve and tendon gliding exercises.
   3. Carpal bone mobilization can be performed by PT to move the bones and joints in the wrist. Refer to PT for evaluation and treatment.

Individual Considerations

A. Pregnancy:

1. CTS is the most frequent complaint during pregnancy. Approximately 15% of pregnancy-related CTS cases will progress and continue several months postpartum.

Bibliography

Erickson, M., Lawrence, M., Jansen, C. W. S., Coker, D., Amadio, P., & Cleary, C. (2019). Hand pain and sensory deficits: Carpal tunnel syndrome. *Journal of Orthopaedic & Sports Physical Therapy, 49*(5), CPG1–CPG85. doi:10.2519/jospt.2019.0301

Faust, K., & Jennings, C. (2016). *Carpal tunnel syndrome.* Retrieved from www.orthoinfo.aaos.org/topic.cfm?topic=A00005

Sears, E. D., Meerwijk, E. L., Schmidt, E. M., Kerr, E. A., Chung, K. C., Kamal, R. N., & Harris, A. H. S. (2019). Variation in nonsurgical services for carpal tunnel syndrome across a large integrated healthcare system. *Journal of Hand Surgery, 44*(2), 85–92. doi:10.1016/j.jhsa.2018.11.002

Guillain–Barré Syndrome

Julie Adkins, Jill C. Cash, and Kimberly Waltrip

Definition

A. GBS is an acute, immune-mediated polyneuropathy of the peripheral nervous system (PNS) that often follows an infection.

B. GBS is the most common cause of acute neuromuscular, flaccid paralysis in the United States.

C. GBS is not contagious or curable.

D. GBS usually presents with ascending, progressive, multifocal, symmetric muscle weakness and paresthesia. The first symptom of GBS includes weakness and/or tingling sensations in the lower extremities. The stage of greatest weakness usually occurs within the first 2 to 4 weeks after symptom onset. By the third or fourth week, most clients reach nadir during GBS progression.

E. GBS is considered monophasic and remits spontaneously, with recurrence in 3% of clients. Most clients recover, and up to 85% ambulate independently. However, morbidity occurs in 20% of clients. Approximately 20% to 20% will have persistent disability as defined by measures such as the Overall Disability Sum Score (ODSS; see Table 19.1). An electronic version of the ODSS is available online at farmacologiaclinica.info/scales/overall-disability-sum-score. This application grades the upper extremities (0–5 scale) and the lower extremities (0–7 scale) to provide an overall score. A total score of 0 equals no disability, while a total score of 12 equals maximum disability.

F. Several variants of GBS are described as follows:

1. Miller Fisher syndrome (MFS) often follows an infection, especially *Campylobacter jejuni* gastroenteritis. Ophthalmoplegia, areflexia, and ataxia occur, but previous reports indicate other CNs have been affected as well.

2. Acute inflammatory demyelinating polyradiculoneuropathy (AIDP): Approximately two-thirds of GBS cases occur after infections from *C. jejuni,* cytomegalovirus (CMV), *Mycoplasma pneumoniae*, or influenza virus.

3. Acute motor axonal neuropathy (AMAN; pure motor involvement) is more commonly diagnosed in Asia.

4. Acute sensorimotor axonal neuropathy (AMSAN)

5. Acute panautonomic neuropathy (rare)

6. Bickerstaff's brainstem encephalitis (BBE) affects the CNS.

a. Pharyngeal–cervical–brachial (regional variant); pharyngeal, neck, and upper-extremity muscles are mostly affected.

Incidence

A. The global incidence of GBS varies between 0.4 and 2 per 100,000, and is slightly higher in males. An estimated 100,000 clients contract GBS annually.

B. GBS affects all age groups, but is more common in older adults, starting at age 50 and up.

C. The incidence of GBS in children is between 0.6 and 2.4 cases per 100,000.

D. Approximately 80% to 90% of clients become non-ambulatory over the course of GBS.

E. Relapses are not uncommon in adults who have been treated with intravenous immunoglobulin (IVIG) and plasmapheresis.

F. Approximately 30% have residual weakness after 3 years.

G. GBS severe enough to require mechanical ventilation is associated with partial recovery and up to 20% mortality.

H. Approximately 5% of clients with GBS die from medical complications such as sepsis, pulmonary emboli, and cardiac arrest related to dysautonomia.

Pathogenesis

A. GBS is believed to be an immune-mediated response linked to an infection that precedes a patchy demyelination of multiple peripheral motor nerves. The sensory disturbance is quickly followed by a rapid progressive limb weakness and sometimes paralysis. Similarities between peripheral nerve membranes and antiganglioside antibodies formed after infection have contributed to the understanding of GBS pathology, especially the axonal variant. Up to 70% of clients with GBS report an illness or infection 1–6 weeks before the onset of GBS signs and symptoms. However, antiganglioside antibodies are not present in all clients, and the specific role of these antibodies in GBS is still unknown.

B. The AIDP variant of GBS is the most commonly diagnosed in the United States, although less is known about the related pathophysiology. Numerous types of infections are associated with GBS, especially those involving the gastrointestinal (GI) and respiratory systems. For example, multiple GBS cases were reported during an outbreak of the Zika virus. Other case reports cite other potential causes associated with GBS, including various medications and surgeries.

TABLE 19.1   OVERALL DISABILITY SUM SCORE (ODSS) FOR GUILLAIN–BARRÉ SYNDROME (GBS)

Area of Body	Activities	Functional Ability Scale for Each Activity	Disability Scale Grade
Arm disability	A. Dressing the upper body (excludes buttons/zippers) B. Washing and brushing hair C. Turning a key in a lock D. Using a knife and fork (use of spoon applies if a fork/knife have never been used) E. Using buttons and zippers	Not affected Affected, but does not prevent activity Prevents activity	0 = Adequate function for all activities 1 = Minor signs/symptoms (S/Sx) in one or both arms, but does not affect activity 2 = Moderate S/Sx in one or both arms affecting, but not preventing, any activity 3 = Severe S/Sx in one or both arms preventing at least one, but not all, activities 4 = Severe S/Sx in both arms preventing all functions; purposeful movements are still possible 5 = Severe S/Sx in both arms preventing all purposeful movements

Leg disability	A. Do you have any problems walking?
	B. Do you walk with a walking aid?
	C. How do you get around for 25 feet (10 m)?
	  1. Without aid
	  2. With one stick or crutch or holding someone's arm
	  3. With two sticks or crutches or one stick and a crutch and holding someone's arm
	  4. With a wheelchair
	D. If you use a wheelchair, can you stand and walk a few steps with help?
	E. If you are restricted to bed most of the time, are you able to make some purposeful movements?
		No
		Yes
		Does not apply
			0 = Walking is not affected
			1 = Walking is affected, but does not appear to be upon assessment
			2 = Walks independently, but gait is visibly affected
			3 = Usually uses unilateral support (stick, crutch, one arm) to walk 25 feet or 10 m
			4 = Usually uses bilateral support (stick, crutch, two arms) to walk 25 feet or 10 m
			5 = Usually uses a wheelchair to travel 25 feet or 10 m
			6 = Restricted to wheelchair, unable to stand and walk a few steps with assistance, but makes some purposeful leg movements
			7 = Restricted to wheelchair or bed most of the day, no purposeful leg movements (e.g., unable to reposition legs in bed)

Source: Adapted from Merkies, I. S., Schmitz, P. L., van der Meche, F. G., Samihn, J. P., van Doorn, P. A., & INCAT Group. (2016). *Overall disability sum score: Overall disability scale online calculator*. Retrieved from http://farmacologiaclinica.info/scales/overall-disability-sum-score/

Predisposing Factors

A. Illness:

1. Up to two-thirds of GBS clients have contracted a viral upper respiratory infection (URI) or gastroenteritis 10 to 14 days before symptom onset.

2. *C. jejuni* gastroenteritis

3. CMV is reported as the second most common infection preceding GBS.

4. Epstein–Barr virus (EBV)

5. *M. pneumoniae*

6. HIV

7. *Haemophilus influenzae*

8. Enteroviruses

9. Hepatitis A and B

10. HSV

11. *Chlamydophila* (formerly *Chlamydia*) pneumonia

12. Zika virus

B. Trauma

C. Surgery

D. Parturition

E. Immunization:

1. In 1976, a small increase in GBS cases occurred after administration of influenza A/H1N1 vaccine. Today, the chance of developing GBS is up to seven times more likely after a flu infection versus after immunization against the flu.

F. No genetic factor is associated with GBS.

Common Complaints

A. Classic clinical features:

1. Ascending, progressive, fairly symmetric muscle weakness:

 a. Difficulty walking

 b. Nearly complete paralysis of the following:

   i. All extremities, starting in the proximal legs (most common presentation)

   ii. Facial muscle weakness from facial nerve involvement, oropharyngeal weakness from glossopharyngeal, vagus, and/or hypoglossal CN involvement

    iii. Respiratory and neck muscles: Respiratory failure occurs in up to 30% of GBS cases.

    iv. Bulbar (ocular) muscles

  2. Deep tendon reflexes (DTRs) are absent or hyporeflexia is present.

B. Acute weakness in hands, dropping things, difficulty picking up small objects or buttoning buttons, inability to feel different textures

C. Acute onset of persistent tingling or pins and needles; "crawling-skin" sensation in feet, possibly in hands; and an inability to feel pain

D. Prominent low back pain (LBP)

E. Approximately 85% of clients with GBS complain of moderate to severe pain. Joint, muscle, lumbar, and radicular pain are several types of pain reported in GBS.

Other Signs and Symptoms

A. Sinus tachycardia or other arrhythmias

B. Bilateral, generally symmetric, muscle weakness that does not improve with rest

C. Urinary retention

D. Ileus–gastric motility disorders

E. Severe residual fatigue (may persist for years)

F. Inability to sweat

G. Facial or pharyngeal weakness versus plegia

Subjective Data

A. Ask about any dyspnea. If shortness of breath (SOB) is reported, determine whether the client requires immediate transport via ambulance to the nearest hospital.

B. Elicit information regarding the onset and duration of symptoms.

C. Ask questions regarding any change or progression of symptoms.

D. Document any recent URIs, flu, gastroenteritis, other infections, recent trauma, or surgery: Determine whether an associated fever occurred.

E. Ask about paresthesias that precede motor weakness by approximately 24 to 48 hours.

F. Ask about any recent exposures to environmental hazards, such as lead, pesticides, volatile solvents, or ticks.

G. Investigate any complaints of pain (onset, location, characteristics, timing, aggravating and alleviating factors, and duration), including whether pain preceded or followed motor weakness. More than 50% of clients with GBS report severe pain.

Physical Examination

A. Check temperature, pulse, respiration, and blood pressure (e.g., persistent hypotension, HTN alternating with hypotension, or orthostatic hypotension). HTN is present in about one-third of clients with GBS and can be labile or precede hypotension.

B. Inspect:

  1. Observe overall appearance.

  2. Assess for gait disturbance.

  3. Assess for any difficulty breathing or respiratory distress.

C. Auscultate:

  1. Heart rate and rhythm: Tachycardia is common, but bradycardia and other arrhythmias may be present.

  2. Auscultate all lung fields.

  3. Auscultate all abdominal quadrants for bowel sounds or dysfunction. GI motility disorders occur in 15% of severe GBS cases.

D. Palpate:

  1. Palpate the extremities.

  2. Note muscle tone and size.

  3. Assess DTRs for areflexia (absent reflexes) or hyporeflexia (diminished); test motor strength in all extremities.

  4. Assess for symmetric motor weakness (incidence of ankle and knee weakness is higher than biceps and triceps weakness).

  5. Palpate the abdomen and assess for urinary retention.

E. Neurological examination:

  1. Perform a complete neurological examination. Generally, no sensory deficits to touch or pinprick are noted, but decreased proprioception or vibration may be present. GBS may progress rapidly in approximately 50% of clients, sometimes within hours, to severe respiratory muscle weakness and respiratory failure. The patellar reflex is usually lost.

Diagnostic Tests

Prompt treatment mandates a diagnosis of GBS based solely on client history and physical exam findings. Additional testing can be useful for atypical cases or rare subtypes of disease. These labs and diagnostic tests include the following:

A. LP:

  1. CSF analysis is primarily ordered to rule out other infectious diseases.

  2. Two weeks after symptom onset, approximately 80% of clients with GBS have elevated CSF protein levels and white blood cell (WBC) counts that are within range.

B. Needle EMG and NCV studies are used to confirm the presence, type, pattern, and severity of neuropathy.

C. Negative inspiratory force (NIF) testing is ordered when GBS is suspected. Clients at high risk for respiratory complications require serial NIFs. Clients who cannot perform a NIF of −20 to −30 cm H_2O should be considered very high risk.

D. Ganglioside antibody testing includes anti-GM1, anti-GD1A, anti-GT1A, and anti-GQ1B. These tests range in sensitivity up to 60% (anti-GM1 antibodies in AMAN) and to greater than 90% (anti-GQ1B antibodies in MFS). However, the turnaround time for lab results precludes their usefulness during initial clinical decision-making.

E. Serum blood testing: Electrolytes, liver function tests (LFTs), creatine phosphokinase (CPK), and ESR

F. MRI can be used to rule out other causes of quadriparesis or facial diplegia, such as transverse myelitis (TM) or intracranial pathology.

Differential Diagnoses

A. GBS
B. Myasthenia gravis (MG)
C. Poliomyelitis
D. Acute intermittent porphyria
E. West Nile encephalomyelitis
F. Tick paralysis (Lyme neuroborreliosis)
G. Diphtheria
H. HIV
I. Cervical myelopathy
J. Sarcoidosis
K. Poisoning:
   1. Heavy metal toxicity (arsenic, lead, mercury, thallium)
   2. Hexacarbon abuse (glue-sniffing neuropathy)
   3. Organophosphate poisoning
   4. Botulism
L. Zika virus

Plan

A. General interventions:
   1. Early diagnosis is crucial to appropriate management. Potential diagnosis of GBS requires *immediate* admission to a progressive care unit or ICU with an experienced neurologist to manage GBS. The most critical treatments maintain the body's function during recovery.
B. Client teaching:
   1. Educate the client and family on "GBS."
   2. Inform the client and family that GBS has no cure, but various treatments may lessen the severity of GBS symptoms and shorten recovery time.
   3. Recovery may require several weeks or months. Reinforce the critical aspects of GBS that warrant ICU admission and treatment for paralysis and severe complications.
   4. Along with physical impairments and weakness, the client may experience emotional problems after sudden onset of GBS, including a new dependence on family and friends for physical and emotional support.
   5. Offer professional resources for the client and family:
      a. National Library of Medicine: https://medlineplus.gov/guillainbarresyndrome.html
      b. National Institute of Neurological Disorders and Stroke: "Guillain–Barré Syndrome Fact Sheet," June 2018; NIH Publication No. 18-NS-2902
      c. National Institutes of Health's Brain Research through Advancing Innovative Neurotechnologies (BRAIN) Initiative: https://braininitiative.nih.gov
      d. GBS/CIDP Foundation International: https://www.gbs-cidp.org

C. Pharmaceutical therapy:
   1. Pain therapy:
      a. Gabapentin (Neurontin), 1,800–5,400 mg daily in three divided doses, adjust for renal clients with creatinine clearance (CrCl) below 60 mL/min; add one 300 mg tablet every 3 to 5 days as tolerated, until client reports adequate relief
      b. Carbamazepine (Tegretol), 100–1,200 mg daily in two divided doses, starting with one 100 mg tablet at bedtime, then increasing to 100 mg twice daily after 1 week; add one 100 mg tablet each week as tolerated, until client reports adequate relief:
         i. Check CBCs and LFTs once a month for 3 months, then once every 3 months during carbamazepine administration.
         ii. Female clients must utilize barrier methods of birth control.
      c. Refer to the client to a neurologist if opioids are necessary.
      d. Tricyclic antidepressants (TCAs), such as amitriptyline (Elavil), imipramine (Tofranil), nortriptyline (Pamelor), and desipramine (Norpramin), have achieved effectiveness at doses of 25 to 75 mg daily (amitriptyline, imipramine) and 50 to 150 mg daily (nortriptyline, desipramine).
         i. Amitriptyline, imipramine, or nortriptyline: Start with 10 mg daily, then increase by 10 mg every 3 to 7 days as tolerated, and up to 75 mg daily (amitriptyline, nortriptyline) or 150 mg daily (imipramine), if necessary.
         ii. Desipramine: Start with 25 mg daily, then increase by 25 mg every 3 to 7 days as tolerated, and up to 150 mg daily, if necessary.
         iii. Avoid or use TCAs with great caution in clients with angle-closure glaucoma, urinary retention, orthostatic hypotension, cardiac dysrhythmias, or heart failure (HF), and in older adults.
         iv. Blurred vision, dry mouth, and sedation are side effects that may preclude continued use of TCAs.
   2. Immunizations:
      a. Immunizations are not recommended during the acute phase of GBS, and for up to 1 year after onset of signs and symptoms.
      b. Influenza, tetanus, and typhoid immunizations are most commonly associated with GBS relapse.
D. Hospital medical management:
   1. Plasmapheresis (plasma exchange), five treatments
   2. IVIG administration, 0.4 mg/kg daily for 5 days
   3. Steroids demonstrate NO benefit in the treatment of GBS.
   4. HTN should be treated with short-acting IV medications due to dysautonomia.

5. The presence of at least four of the following six factors indicates the need for respiratory support or mechanical ventilation:
    a. Onset of symptoms less than 7 days
    b. Inability to cough
    c. Inability to stand
    d. Inability to lift the elbows
    e. Inability to lift the head
    f. Elevated liver enzymes
6. The American Society of Hematology (ASH) has made the following conditional recommendation for venous thromboembolism (VTE) prophylaxis: Low-molecular-weight heparin (LMWH) (low certainty based on current evidence) or fondaparinux (very low certainty based on current evidence), instead of low-dose unfractionated heparin (LDUH).
7. The ASH suggests using intermittent pneumatic compression devices (ICDs) or graduated compression stockings for clients who are not receiving anti-coagulants (conditional recommendation, very low certainty based on the evidence of effectiveness).

Follow-Up

A. Clients usually follow up with neurology after discharge from the hospital or inpatient rehabilitation settings.
B. Full recovery can take up to 3 years in severe cases, with 30% of clients reporting residual weakness, and 3% of clients experiencing recurrence. Severe fatigue after GBS occurs in two-thirds of adults.
C. The most critical treatment maintains body functions during neurological recovery. Rehabilitation with an interdisciplinary team includes physical, occupational, speech, and respiratory therapists, as needed. Treatment focuses on proper limb positioning, posture, orthotics, exercise, strengthening swallowing muscles, airway protection, and improving pulmonary function.
    1. Foot and wrist drop are not uncommon and may require orthotics per PT/OT recommendations.
    2. Joint contracture requires active and passive range of motion (ROM) exercises (aROM and pROM).
D. Psychological treatment and/or mental health visits for counseling may be required to facilitate acceptance and adjustment.
E. The Centers for Disease Control and Prevention (CDC) developed the Vaccine Adverse Event Reporting System (VAERS) to monitor vaccine safety. The CDC and the U.S. Food and Drug Administration (FDA) co-manage and utilize the VAERS as an early-warning system for possible side effects after immunization.

Consultation/Referral

A. Consult with a physician if GBS is suspected.
B. Refer to neurology based on client history and clinical exam findings.
C. Refer to PT, OT, and speech therapy (ST) for evaluation and treatment of gross and/or fine motor deficits, impaired speech and/or swallow, and splinting and/or adaptive equipment.

Individual Considerations

A. Pediatrics:
    1. GBS is the most common cause of acute flaccid paralysis in healthy infants and children.
    2. No current evidence supports an increased risk of GBS from the H1N1 flu vaccine.
    3. The Pediatric Evaluation of Disability Inventory Computer Adaptive Test (PEDI-CAT) is designed to assess children from birth to age 20 years for physical and behavioral conditions in daily activities, mobility, and social/cognitive domains.
B. Geriatrics:
    1. Age older than 55 years is a poor prognostic factor.

Resources

CDC Vaccine Adverse Event Reporting System (VAERS) website: vaers.hhs.gov
GBS/CIDP Foundation International: www.gbs-cidp.org

Bibliography

Centers for Disease Control and Prevention. (2015, October 16). *Guillain–Barré syndrome and flu vaccine*. Retrieved from https://www.cdc.gov/flu/protect/vaccine/guillainbarre.htm

Ding, X., Jiang, H., Hu, X., Ren, H., & Cai, H. (2018). Guillain–Barré syndrome and low back pain: Two cases and literature review. *Open Medicine, 13*(1), 503–508. doi:10.1515/med-2018-0074

Merkies, I. S., Schmitz, P. L., van der Meche, F. G., Samihn, J. P., van Doorn, P. A., & INCAT Group. (2016). *Overall disability sum score: Overall disability scale online calculator*. Retrieved from http://farmacologiaclinica.info/scales/overall-disability-sum-score/

National Institutes of Health. (2016). *Guillain–Barré syndrome fact sheet*. Retrieved from www.ninds.nih.gov/Disorders/Client-Caregiver-Education/Fact-Sheets/Guillain-Barre-Syndrome-Fact-Sheet

Schünemann, H. J., Cushman, M., Burnett, A. E., Kahn, S. R., Beyer-Westendorf, J., Spencer, F. A., . . . Wiercioch, W. (2018). American Society of Hematology 2018 guidelines for management of venous thromboembolism: Prophylaxis for hospitalized and nonhospitalized medical patients. *Blood Advances, 2*(22), 3198–3225. doi:10.1182/bloodadvances.2018022954

Headache

Julie Adkins, Jill C. Cash, and Kimberly Waltrip

Definition

A. Headache refers to pain or discomfort in the head, face, or neck from inflammation and/or spasms of associated cranial vessels, nerves, and/or muscles. Primary headaches are significant causes of missed days of school and work, decreased productivity at work (presenteeism), and disability in children and adults. These disorders typically occur early in individuals, while the incidence of new primary headache decreases after ages 40 to 50.
B. Various types of primary headaches include tension-type headache (TTH), trigeminal autonomic cephalalgias, such as cluster headaches, and new daily-persistent headaches (NDPH; see Table 19.2):
    1. Migraines are discussed separately in this chapter under the section "Migraine Headache."
    2. Posttraumatic headaches typically occur within 7 days after head trauma.

TABLE 19.2   INTERNATIONAL HEADACHE SOCIETY CLASSIFICATION OF HEADACHES (ICHD-3)

NDPH[a]	TTH[b]	Cluster Headache	MOH[c]
NDPH is persistent, daily headache from the time of onset that is clearly remembered. Headache pain has no characteristic symptoms and may be similar to migraine, TTH, or have elements of each.	**Infrequent episodic** headaches are typically bilateral, pressing or tightening in quality, and of mild to moderate intensity, lasting minutes to days. Headache pain does not worsen with routine physical activity, no associated nausea is noted, but photophobia or phonophobia may occur. **Frequent episodic** headaches are typically bilateral, pressing or tightening in quality, and of mild to moderate intensity, lasting minutes to days. Headache pain does not worsen with routine physical activity, no associated nausea is noted, but photophobia or phonophobia may occur. **Chronic TTH** evolves from **frequent episodic TTH**, as daily or very frequent headache episodes that are typically bilateral, pressing or tightening in quality, and of mild to moderate intensity, lasting hours to days, or unremitting. Headache pain does not worsen with routine physical activity, but may be associated with mild nausea, photophobia, or phonophobia.	Headache attacks occur with severe, unilateral pain that is orbital, supraorbital, temporal, or a combination of these, lasting 15 to 180 minutes, from once every other day to eight times daily. This type of pain is associated with ipsilateral, injected conjunctiva, lacrimation, nasal congestion, rhinorrhea, forehead and facial diaphoresis, miosis, ptosis and/or eyelid edema, and/or restlessness or agitation. Alcohol, histamine, or nitroglycerin can provoke attacks.	Headache occurs on 15 or more days per month with a preexisting primary headache, and develops from regular overuse of acute or symptomatic headache medication (on 10 or more versus 15 or more days per month, depending on the medication) for more than 3 months. MOH usually resolves in the majority of clients after discontinued overuse.
Diagnostic Criteria			

A. Persistent headache fulfills criteria B and C	A. Episode
	  1. **Infrequent:** At least 10 headache episodes occur on average less than 1 day/month, or less than 12 days/year, that fulfill B–D criteria.
	  2. **Frequent:** At least 10 headache episodes occur on average 1 to 14 days for more than 3 months (12 or more and less than 180 days a year), that fulfill B–D criteria.
	  3. **Chronic:** Headaches occur on average 15 days or more per month for longer than 3 months (180 days or more a year), that fulfill criteria B–D
		A. At least five headache episodes occur that fulfill B–D criteria.	A. Headaches occurring 15 days or more per month, with a preexisting headache disorder that fulfill B criteria.

B. The distinct onset of headache pain is clearly remembered and evolves into continuous and unremitting pain within 24 hours.	B. Duration
	  1. **Infrequent** and **frequent** headaches last from 30 minutes to 7 days.
	  2. **Chronic** headaches last hours to days, or are unremitting
		B. Severe to very severe unilateral, orbital, supraorbital, and/or temporal pain lasts between 15 and 180 minutes, if untreated.	B. Regular overuse greater than 3 months of one or more medications for acute and/or symptomatic treatment of headache, with medication overuse defined as:
			  1. 10 or more days per month of ergot derivatives, triptans, opioids, combination

(continued)

TABLE 19.2   INTERNATIONAL HEADACHE SOCIETY CLASSIFICATION OF HEADACHES (ICHD-3) (*continued*)

NDPH[a]	TTH[b]	Cluster Headache	MOH[c]
			analgesics, and a combination of medications from different drug classes that are not individually overused 2. 15 or more days per month of nonopioid analgesics, acetaminophen, and NSAIDs, including ASA
C. Headache pain is present longer than 3 months. **NDPH** may present similar to migraine or TTH. Even when criteria for chronic migraine and/or TTH may be fulfilled, NDPH is the default diagnosis whenever the headache meets criteria for this disorder.	C. At least two of the following pain characteristics are present: 1. Bilateral location 2. Pressure/tightening, nonpulsating quality 3. Mild to moderate intensity 4. Headache does not worsen with routine physical activity, such as walking or climbing stairs	C. Either or both of the following occur with headache: 1. At least one of the following signs or symptoms ipsilateral to the headache a. Ipsilateral, conjunctival infection and/or lacrimation b. Ipsilateral nasal congestion and/or rhinorrhea c. Ipsilateral eyelid edema d. Ipsilateral, diaphoretic forehead and face e. Ipsilateral miosis and/or ptosis 2. Restlessness or agitation typically evidenced by pacing back and forth, and the inability to lie down	None
None	D. Other signs/symptoms 1. Both of the following occur with **infrequent** and **frequent TTH**: a. No nausea or vomiting b. Either photophobia or phonophobia 2. Both of the following occur with **chronic TTH**: a. Either photophobia, phonophobia, or mild nausea b. Neither moderate or severe nausea, nor vomiting	D. Frequency of headache varies from one attack every other day to eight attacks daily.	None
E. Not better attributed to other ICHD-3 diagnoses	E. Not better attributed to other ICHD-3 diagnoses	E. Not better attributed to other ICHD-3 diagnoses	None

[a]The client must clearly recall and unambiguously describe the daily headache as unremitting at the moment of onset that escalates to continuous/unremitting pain.

[b]Previously known as common, muscle contraction, stress, ordinary, or psychogenic headache.

[c]Previously known as rebound, drug-induced, or medication misuse headache.

ASA, acetylsalicylic acid; ICHD-3, *The International Classification of Headache Disorders*, third edition; MOH, medication-overuse headache; NDPH, new daily-persistent headache; NSAID, nonsteroidal anti-inflammatory drug; TTH, tension-type headache.

Source: Adapted from Vincent, M., & Wang, S. (2018). Headache Classification Committee of the International Headache Society (IHS). *The International Classification of Headache Disorders*, 3rd edition. *Cephalalgia, 38*(1), 1–211. doi:10.1177/0333102417738202

3. TTHs are the most frequent type and can also occur with postconcussive syndrome.

C. NDPHs have many similarities to TTHs and migraines. The most significant symptom associated with TTH is increased pericranial tenderness upon palpation. Diagnosis of TTH versus mild migraine without aura can be challenging when both disorders commonly occur in clients. Other types of headaches should be ruled out, such as posttraumatic headache, low CSF volume (pressure) headache, high CSF pressure headache, and headaches attributed to infection. NDPH has unique daily, unremitting symptoms from or near the moment of onset, and typically occurs in individuals with no headache history. Two subtypes of NDPH are identified:

1. Self-limiting: Typically resolves without treatment within several months
2. Refractory: Resistant to aggressive treatment

Incidence

Primary headaches account for more than 90% of all headaches, and the incidence depends on age, gender, and type.

A. TTHs are the most common primary headaches, affecting 30% to 78% of the population. The onset of TTH generally occurs around ages 25 to 30, with a peak prevalence at 30 to 39 years. Up to 15% of children and adolescents have experienced TTHs, while 4% have experienced migraines.

B. Headaches occur in 90% of school-aged children.

C. Cluster headaches typically occur in adults between 20 and 40 years old, but have been reported in children as young as age 3. The prevalence of cluster headaches occurs in less than 1% of the population, affecting males three times more than females.

D. In many countries, more than 50% of individuals with headaches on 15 or more days per month have medication-overuse headache (MOH). The majority of MOHs improve after discontinuing the overused medication; therefore, preventive treatment is more effective in such clients.

E. MOHs are reported by 20% to 36% of adolescents with daily headaches:

1. Medication overuse is defined when the following are used **15** or more days in 1 month: Acetaminophen, nonopioid analgesics, NSAIDs (including aspirin or acetylsalicylic acid [ASA])
2. Medication overuse is also defined when the following are used **10** or more days in 1 month: Ergot derivatives, triptans, combination analgesics, opioids, and combinations of medications from different drug classes that are not overused individually

Pathogenesis

A. Different types of headaches have different origins. Many individuals experience combinations of different types of headaches. Headache etiology ranges from systemic illness, such as infection; medical disorders, such as tumors or hemorrhage; medications, drug use, and/or stress. TTHs arise from contracted scalp and neck muscles. Cluster headaches have an uncertain etiology, but seem to originate from extracerebral vasodilation.

B. Review environmental and seasonal factors. Headaches may be cyclic when allergic rhinitis occurs in the spring and summer, and in the fall and winter when carbon monoxide poisoning occurs from gas heater use.

C. Medications commonly associated with headaches:

1. Nitroglycerin (Nitrostat, Rectiv)
2. Nifedipine (Procardia, Adalat)
3. Dipyridamole (Persantine)
4. SSRIs

Predisposing Factors

A. Tension, stress
B. Cervical or lumbar spine disorders
C. Medications
D. Bruxism
E. Sleep disorders (e.g., snoring, insomnia)
F. Foods, caffeine, and/or alcohol
G. Hormonal changes
H. Family history of headache
I. Sexual activity
J. Cough
K. Physical exertion/exercise
L. Viral/infectious etiologies
M. Poorly fitted dentures
N. Faulty/inefficient gas heat
O. Trigeminal neuralgia (TGN)
P. Valsalva maneuvers
Q. Trauma to the head and/or neck

Common Complaints

A. Depending on the type of headache, other symptoms may coexist, such as lacrimation, nasal congestion, restlessness, and visual changes.
B. Pain and location depend on the type of headache.
C. Headache characteristics vary by type of headache.

Other Signs and Symptoms

A. Crying
B. Behavioral problems

Subjective Data

A. Use the following acronym for subjective information: **PQRST**

P: Provocation or worsening of triggering factors that stimulate headaches
Q: Quality and severity of pain
R: Region or location of headache
S: Strength or intensity of pain based on a pain scale of 0 to 10, with 10 describing the worst pain ever experienced
T: Time, including the onset, frequency, and duration of headaches

B. Assess whether the client has frequent migraine headaches. Ask if the current headache is the first or worst headache the client has ever experienced.

C. If recurrent headaches are reported, note the frequency and patterns of similar headaches.

D. Ask whether the client has identified potential triggers of recurring headaches such as foods, beverages, stressors, and smells or odors (e.g., perfumes, cigarette smoke).

E. Identify the location of pain and whether the pain radiates from that location.

F. Describe the type of pain (e.g., throbbing, aching, dull, sharp, constant, or burning).

G. Assess the presence of associated signs and symptoms, such as nausea or vomiting, photophobia, noise sensitivity, or seeing halos around lights.

H. Determine whether the client experiences any neurological and/or prodromal symptoms that precede a headache.

I. Review previous interventions the client used to alleviate and/or prevent headaches, including the effectiveness of each.

J. Inquire about past diagnostic evaluations of headaches.

K. Note any family history of headaches.

L. List current medications, including any over-the-counter (OTC) medications and herbal supplements.

M. Review the client's past medical history for head trauma, allergies, ventriculoperitoneal (VP) shunt insertion or removal, and/or other neurological diagnoses.

N. Determine whether a pregnant client is in the second or third trimester.

O. Assess whether the client is febrile or has a recent history of infection.

P. Rule out gas exposure that can cause carbon monoxide poisoning.

Physical Examination

Physical exam findings may be within range, unless the client presents with a headache.

A. Check temperature, blood pressure, pulse, and respirations; if febrile, assess for meningeal signs.

B. Inspect:
1. Observe overall appearance for signs of discomfort, photosensitivity (sunglasses worn indoors), and LOC.
2. Examine the eyes with an ophthalmoscope; perform a dilated fundoscopic examination to rule out papilledema, retinal tear, and posterior vitreous detachment:
    a. Assess the optic disk, optic cup, retinal vessels, and fovea:
        i. Observe optic vessels for pulsations.
        ii. Asscss for a blurred optic disk margin and color changes in the optic disk that vary from the typical yellow-orange.
    b. Signs and symptoms of papilledema include optic disk swelling, hemorrhage, and yellow, hard exudates. Visual acuity is usually preserved:
        i. Fundoscopic exam changes with increased intracranial pressure (ICP): Initially, pulsations in retinal vessels are lost; then blurring of the optic disk margin occurs. Retinal hemorrhage is possible.
        ii. Assess for the presence of a pale, white optic disk with distinct margins. Optic atrophy is a late finding with increased ICP.

    c. Assess CN II function with visual field testing:
        i. Face the client at eye level, 12 inches away. Ask the client to cover his/her right eye with the right hand and look at your eyes. Instruct the client to maintain eye contact and say "now" when he/she sees your fingers enter his/her peripheral vision from the upper, lateral, and lower directions. Repeat with the client's left eye covered by the left hand.
    d. Aberrant pupil exam findings are associated with migraine and cluster headache.
    e. Headache with a dilated, fixed pupil is considered a medical emergency in cases of subarachnoid hemorrhage (SAH) from ruptured aneurysms or arteriovenous malformations (AVMs).
3. Inspect the ears, nose, and throat.

C. Auscultate:
1. Listen for bruits over the neck, eyes, and head that may indicate arteriovenous fistula (AVF) or AVM, intracranial hemangioma, or carotid artery dissection/disease.

D. Palpate:
1. Palpate the head, eyes, ears, temporomandibular joint (TMJ), sinuses, and temporal and neck arteries.
2. Palpate the cervical vertebrae, surrounding muscles, and shoulder regions. Identify any potential trigger areas. Occipital nerves extend halfway between the middle of the posterior neck and laterally from that location. Pain may be reproduced upon palpation of this particular trigger area.
3. Examine the spinal and neck muscles.
4. Assess cervical ROM.

E. Neurological examination:
1. Extraocular movements (EOM)
2. Pupil size, responses to light (direct and consensual) and accommodation
3. Ask the client to stand from a seated position without assistance or support.
4. Ask the client to walk on tiptoes and heels.
5. Tandem gait
6. Romberg test
7. Assess for symmetry during motor and sensory exams, DTRs, and coordination tests.
8. Assess for nuchal rigidity during neck flexion.

Diagnostic Tests

Tests are selected based on client history and physical examination findings.

A. Sinus x-rays (XRs) can rule out sinusitis or lesions.

B. Sleep studies will detect obstructive sleep apnea (OSA).

C. Head CT or MRI is only indicated when significant physical examination findings are present, such as the following:
1. Papilledema or optic nerve swelling
2. Pathological reflexes
3. Hemifacial weakness or hemiparesis
4. Gait and/or balance disturbances
5. Diplopia
6. Vision loss

7. Pupil changes
8. Confusion

D. Neuroimaging is appropriate for individuals, especially children, with any signs and symptoms of intracranial pathology.

E. Lab tests are rarely indicated for headache, unless infectious etiology is suspected.

Differential Diagnoses

A. Headache:
1. Tension (TTH)
2. Cluster
3. MOH
4. Migraine
5. Combination headache
6. NDPH

B. Sinusitis

C. Meningitis: Acute headache occurs with fever, lethargy, nausea and/or vomiting, irritability, photophobia, and systemic bacterial or viral infection

D. Space-occupying mass or lesion: Subacute, progressive pain develops over time; new onset of symptoms occurs in adults older than age 40

E. Temporal arteritis: New onset of throbbing, continuous headache occurs on either or both sides of the forehead in adults older than age 50. Presenting symptoms include temporal artery swelling and constriction; weak or absent pulses; scalp and/or temporal tenderness; jaw pain that may worsen upon chewing; musculoskeletal pain in the extremities, hips, gluteals, and/or lumbar area; vision loss or changes; systemic symptoms (fever, anorexia, malaise); and an ESR of 50 mm/hr or higher.

F. Carotid dissection: Sudden headache occurs with neck pain radiating to the scalp, face, ear, or eye; onset is often related to extreme neck flexion/extension or trauma. Symptoms may include partial Horner's syndrome, pulsatile tinnitus, ipsilateral tongue weakness, dysphagia, hemiparesis or numbness on one side of the body, cervical artery bruit or tenderness, diplopia, and syncope.

G. TMJ disorders: Pain or tenderness occurs in one or both TMJs. Symptoms may include earache, facial pain, pain or difficulty with chewing, difficulty opening or closing the mouth with a locked TMJ, and clicking and/or grating sensation when opening the mouth or chewing.

H. Carbon monoxide poisoning

I. TGN

J. Pregnancy-induced hypertension (PIH)

K. Medication-induced headache occurs as a side effect of current medications (individual and/or combinations of medications used). Review the client's medication list for potential causes of headache.

Plan

A. General interventions:
1. Encourage the client to identify and avoid associated triggers such as food, alcohol, and odors.
2. Encourage hydration, adequate nutrition and sleep, and daily exercise to reduce tension.
3. Educate the client on stress management techniques, including biofeedback, yoga, meditation, and massage.
4. Instruct the client to take medications as prescribed, and to maintain a headache diary.
5. Advise that alcohol consumption can exacerbate cluster headaches.
6. Recommend ice/heat for musculoskeletal tension.
7. Individual and/or family psychotherapy may be considered for signs/symptoms of catastrophization, somatization, generalized anxiety disorder (GAD), and/or depression.
8. Complementary and alternative medicine (CAM) and therapies:
   a. Nutraceuticals:
      i. Magnesium, 400 to 600 mg daily
      ii. Riboflavin or vitamin B_2, 400 mg daily
      iii. Coenzyme Q10, 100–150 mg daily
   b. Acupuncture
   c. Oxygen/hyperbaric oxygen therapy
   d. Transcutaneous electrical nerve stimulation (TENS) unit
   e. Chiropractic manipulation of the spine (inconclusive evidence of effectiveness)
   f. PT
   g. Continuous positive airway pressure (CPAP)
   h. Biofeedback
   i. Relaxation training

B. Client teaching:
1. Encourage the client to maintain a headache diary that includes any associated factors to identify headache triggers.
2. Advise clients with menstrual headaches to avoid triggers, such as alcohol, tyramine- or phenylethylamine-containing foods, missing meals, and sleeping late.
3. Discuss sleep hygiene guidelines (see Chapter 22, Psychiatric Guidelines, "Sleep Disorders" section).
4. Biofeedback, breathing exercises, and visualization techniques are helpful for muscle-related, nonmenstrual headaches. Prevention must be stressed, in addition to lifestyle changes and daily exercise.
5. When clients overuse various analgesics for headaches, paroxysmal migraines can convert into chronic daily headaches. Caution clients about the consequences of medication overuse and this particular effect.
6. The highest incidence of MOHs occurs with opioids, butalbital-containing combination medications, and ASA/acetaminophen/caffeine combination medications, as well as triptans. The preferred treatment for MOH is discontinuation of the overused medication(s).

C. Pharmaceutical therapy: **Treatment should begin at the lowest effective dose, then increase as tolerated to achieve the desired outcome while avoiding overuse. Limit use of acute headache medications to no more** than 2 days a week or 10 days a month, to prevent MOH. Client education on dose adjustment, expectations of treatment, side effects, and adverse medication-related events may improve adherence.

1. NSAIDs:

    a. ASA, 650 to 1,000 mg; maximum dose: 4,000 mg/d

    b. Ibuprofen (Advil), 400 to 800 mg every 8 hours; maximum dose: 2,400 mg/d

2. Combination medications:

    a. Acetaminophen, butalbital, and caffeine (Fioricet) with or without codeine, 1 to 2 tablets every 4 hours as needed; maximum dose: 6 tablets/d

    b. ASA, butalbital, and caffeine (Fiorinal), 1 to 2 tablets every 4 hours as needed; maximum dose: 6 tablets/d

    c. Isometheptene mucate, dichloralphenazone, and acetaminophen (Epidrin or Migratine), one to two capsules every 4 hours as needed; maximum dose: 8 capsules/d for adults with TTH

    d. Acetaminophen, ASA, and caffeine (Excedrin), 2 tablets every 6 hours as needed; maximum dose: 4,000 mg of ASA or acetaminophen

3. Cluster or vascular headaches:

    a. Verapamil is the agent of choice for prevention therapy with cluster headaches

    b. Propranolol (Inderal) or carbamazepine (Tegretol), 80 mg daily in divided doses; maximum dose: Between 160 and 240 mg daily

    c. Oxygen therapy at 100% nonrebreather mask (NRB) has reported effectiveness for cluster headaches.

4. Menstrual headaches:

    a. Estrogen supplements or continuous cycling are used to decrease headaches. Instruct the client to begin estrogen 2 days before an anticipated migraine and continue for 7 days.

    b. Naproxen, 275 to 550 mg every 2 to 6 hours (maximum dose: 1,500 mg/d); instruct the client to begin 7 days before menses and take as needed.

    c. Ibuprofen (Advil), 600 mg every 8 hours daily

    d. Fluoxetine (Prozac), 10 to 20 mg daily, for individuals with premenstrual syndrome (PMS) and luteal phase defect

5. Medications that may be used for preventive treatment include ergot derivatives, anticonvulsants, antidepressants, TCAs, muscle relaxants, and antihistamines.

6. Medications for chronic daily and NDPH are combinations of those prescribed for TTH and migraine.

7. Continually inform the client on the hazards of medication dependency and associated patterns.

Follow-Up

A. Examine the client in 2 weeks to evaluate effectiveness of treatment.

B. Review the client's headache diary to facilitate identification of any headache triggers.

Consultation/Referral

A. Consult neurology or another physician for headaches caused by acute problems other than migraine and/or TTH.

B. Severe headache episodes require a neurology or physician consult for treatment with opioid agonists and antagonists, narcotics, and neuroleptics.

C. Consult neurology if headaches are not relieved by the prescribed treatment regimen.

Individual Considerations

A. Pregnancy:

    1. PIH often presents with a headache.

B. Pediatrics:

    1. Antihistamines, biofeedback, and relaxation techniques are useful preventive interventions.

    2. Avoid ASA-containing medications to reduce the risk of Reye's syndrome in children. Accurate diagnosis of headache is essential.

    3. Prescribed medications for children are age dependent.

C. Adults:

    1. Premenopausal women may see improvement with continuous, instead of cyclic, estrogen therapy.

D. Geriatrics:

    1. Headaches decrease with age, while serious causes of headache increase. Examples of such causes include the following:

        a. Temporal arteritis

        b. TGN

        c. OSA

        d. Postherpetic neuralgia

        e. Cervical spondylosis

        f. SAH

        g. Intracranial hemorrhage (ICH)

        h. Intracranial neoplasm

        i. Postconcussive syndrome

    2. Hypnic headache occurs only in older individuals.

    3. Consider neuroimaging for older individuals with unusual headache presentations.

    4. Rule out chronic subdural hematoma (SDH) in individuals with headache and a history of falls; order a head CT or MRI for evaluation.

    5. Older individuals with headache may not exhibit any other signs or symptoms.

    6. Prescribe medication at the lowest effective dose and increase as tolerated in older individuals:

        a. Naproxen and hydroxyzine are common rescue medications for older individuals with migraine or TTH.

        b. Caffeine and lithium are preventive medications for hypnic headaches.

        c. Evaluate renal function before prescribing NSAIDs.

    7. All contraindications for medication use must be considered before treatment; for example, CVD is common in older individuals, therefore ergot derivatives are contraindicated.

Bibliography

American Academy of Family Physicians. (2016). Headache. *American Family Physician*. Retrieved from http://www.aafp.org/afp/topicModules/viewTopicModule.htm?topicModuleId=10

Cruccu, G., Finnerup, N. B., Jensen, T. S., Scholz, J., Sindou, M., Svensson, P., . . . Nurmikko, T. (2016). Trigeminal neuralgia: New classification and diagnostic grading for practice and research. *Neurology, 87*(2), 220–228. doi:10.1212/WNL.0000000000002840

Vincent, M., & Wang, S. (2018). Headache Classification Committee of the International Headache Society (IHS). *The International Classification of Headache Disorders*, 3rd edition. *Cephalalgia, 38*(1), 1–211. doi:10.1177/0333102417738202

Zakrzewska, J. M., & Linskey, M. E. (2016). Trigeminal neuralgia. *American Family Physician, 94*(2), 133–135. Retrieved from https://www.aafp.org/afp/2016/0715/p133.html

Migraine Headache

Julie Adkins, Jill C. Cash, and Kimberly Waltrip

Definition

A. Migraine headaches are a common medical complaint responsible for significant disability and decreased quality of life. The economic impact involves lost days of work and school, decreased social interaction, and lost productivity while at work (presenteeism). Three types of migraines are described by the International Headache Society IHS by type, with diagnostic criteria (see Table 19.3).

B. Migraine headaches have been associated with an increased risk of cerebral ischemia and cardiac ischemia.

Incidence

Headaches are one of the most common medical complaints. The exact incidence of migraines is unknown, especially when clients self-treat, are underdiagnosed, and are misdiagnosed (a common occurrence). Approximately 39 million people suffer from migraine headaches in the United States alone; however, several subsets of migraineurs are noted in the literature. An estimated 6% of men and 18% of women in the United States have migraines, but fewer than 50% see a healthcare provider for treatment. Migraines are heterogenous in frequency, duration, and disability.

A. 3% incidence in preschoolers

B. Up to 10% incidence in school-aged children:

1. Boys with migraines outnumber girls with migraines before age 7 years.

2. Boys and girls are equally likely to have migraines between ages 7 and 11 years.

3. After puberty, girls have more migraines than do boys.

C. 23% incidence in adolescents

D. Approximately 1 billion people suffer from migraines worldwide. Typical onset of migraine occurs during the teenage years or early 20s. Migraine headaches are most common from age 30 through the 40s, then improvement occurs and continues after age 50.

E. An estimated 38% of clients with migraines require preventive treatment and care, but current use has been reported in only 3% to 13% of this headache subpopulation. Treatment and intervention improve migraine headache in 60% of clients.

Pathogenesis

A. Migraine headaches were previously viewed as mostly vascular events. Sensitization of pain pathways and a possible origin of headache within the CNS have received more attention over the years. Current pathophysiological concepts of migraine aura include a possible dysfunction of neuromodulatory structures in the brainstem and cortical spreading depression (CSD). The mechanisms of action in highly receptor-specific medications, such as (serotonin 5-HT) 5-HT1B/D receptor agonists (triptans), 5-HT1F receptor agonists, and calcitonin gene-related peptide (CGRP) receptor antagonists have provided additional insight into migraine pathophysiology. These

---

TABLE 19.3   INTERNATIONAL HEADACHE SOCIETY CLASSIFICATION OF MIGRAINES (ICHD-3)

Migraine Without Aura	Migraine With Aura (Six Subtypes)	Chronic Migraine
This clinical syndrome is characterized by headache with specific features and associated symptoms, and is also most likely to worsen with frequent use of symptomatic medication. The recurrent headache attacks last 4 to 72 hours and meet the diagnostic criteria.	The recurrent headache manifests with transient focal neurological symptoms that usually precede or occur with headache pain. These symptoms develop gradually over 5 to 20 minutes and last for less than 60 minutes. A typical aura consists of visual and/or sensory and/or speech symptoms. Some clients also experience a prodromal phase, occurring hours or days before the headache, and/or a postdromal phase following headache resolution. Prodromal and postdromal symptoms include hyperactivity versus hypoactivity, depression, specific food cravings, repetitive yawning, fatigue, and neck stiffness and/or pain.	Chronic migraine meets the criteria for migraine without aura that occurs with a frequency of at least 15 headache days per month, for longer than 3 months' duration. On at least eight days of the month, the features of migraine headache must be present.

(*continued*)

TABLE 19.3   INTERNATIONAL HEADACHE SOCIETY CLASSIFICATION OF MIGRAINES (ICHD-3) (*continued*)

Diagnostic Criteria	Diagnostic Criteria	Diagnostic Criteria

A. At least five attacks fulfill criteria B–D
B. Headache attacks last 4 to 72 hours (untreated or unsuccessfully treated)
C. Headache has at least two of the following four characteristics:
  1. Unilateral location
  2. Pulsating quality
  3. Moderate or severe pain intensity
  4. Aggravation by or causing avoidance of routine physical activity (e.g., walking or climbing stairs)
D. During headache, at least one of the following occur:
  1. Nausea and/or vomiting
  2. Photophobia and phonophobia
E. Not better attributed to another ICHD-3 diagnosis
	A. At least two attacks fulfill criteria B–C
	B. One or more of the following fully reversible aura symptoms:
	  1. Visual (most common)
	  2. Sensory
	  3. Speech and/or language
	  4. Motor
	  5. Brainstem
	  6. Retinal
	C. At least three of the following six characteristics:
	  1. At least one aura symptom spreads gradually over ≥5 minutes
	  2. Two or more aura symptoms occur in succession
	  3. Each individual aura symptom lasts 5 to 60 minutes
	  4. At least one aura symptom is unilateral
	  5. At least one aura symptom is positive
	  6. Aura is accompanied, or followed within 60 minutes, by headache
	D. Not better attributed to another ICHD-3 diagnosis
		A. Chronic migraine subsumes headache attacks of all types, subtypes, or subforms, This headache (migraine-like or tension-type-like) occurs in the absence of MOH, on 15 days or more per month for at least 3 months. Criteria B and C must be fulfilled.
		B. These particular headaches occur in a client who has had at least five attacks fulfilling criteria B–D for migraine without aura, and/or criteria B and C for migraine with aura
		C. On 8 or more days per month for longer than 3 months, headaches must fulfill any of the following:
		  1. Criteria C and D for migraine without aura
		  2. Criteria B and C for migraine with aura
		  3. Client believes the headache was a migraine at onset that was also relieved by a triptan or ergot derivative
		D. No medication overuse and not better attributed to another ICHD-3 diagnosis

ICHD-3, *The International Classification of Headache Disorders*, third edition; MOH, medication-overuse headache.

Source: Adapted from Vincent, M., & Wang, S. (2018). Headache Classification Committee of the International Headache Society (IHS). *The International Classification of Headache Disorders*, 3rd edition. *Cephalalgia, 38*(1), 1–211. doi:10.1177/0333102417738202

medications have demonstrated efficacy for acute treatment of migraines. Regarding a migraine with aura, the aura consists of neurological symptoms that usually precede headache, but may occur upon onset or continue as the headache progresses.

Predisposing Factors

A. Family history of migraines
B. Chronic use of OTC analgesics (rebound headache)
C. Posttraumatic brain injury
D. Exposure to triggers, such as food, odors, light, sound, sleep, weather changes, hormonal changes, and/or stress
E. Menstruation
F. Obesity
G. Daily habitual snoring is a modest risk factor
H. Estrogen use

Common Complaints

A. Unilateral headache (usually bilateral in children)
B. Frontotemporal area (rarely occipital in children)
C. Photophobia, or sensitivity to light (young children may cover their eyes)
D. Phonophobia, or sensitivity to sound (young children may cover their ears)
E. Osmophobia, or hypersensitivity/aversion to smells/odors
F. Nausea with/without vomiting
G. Prodromal phase, no aura present: Fatigue, reduced concentration, agitation, craving, irritability, depression, frequent yawning, or hyperexcitability, within hours or 1 to 2 days before onset of headache
H. Postdromal phase, no aura present: Fatigue, reduced concentration, and neck stiffness may occur after the headache resolves and continue for up to 48 hours.

Other Signs and Symptoms

A. Muscle tension and neck pain
B. Cutaneous allodynia (pain from stimulus to skin or scalp)
C. Sinus congestion
D. Abdominal pain (with or without nausea, vomiting, and/or headache in children)

Subjective Data

A. Use the following acronym for subjective information: **PQRST**
  P: Provocation or worsening of factors stimulating headaches
  Q: Quality of pain, severity of pain
  R: Region of headache
  S: Strength of pain; evaluate pain on a scale of 1 to 10
  T: Time, including onset, frequency, and duration of headaches
B. Assess whether the client frequently has migraine headaches. Ask the client: Is this particular headache the first or worst ever experienced?
C. If recurrent headaches exist, note frequency and patterns of similar headaches.

D. Document whether the client has ever identified potential triggers of recurring headaches such as dietary factors, stressors, and odors (e.g., perfumes, cigarette smoke).

E. Identify the location of the pain, along with radiation if present.

F. Describe the type of pain: Throbbing, constant, or burning

G. Assess the presence of associated symptoms: Nausea or vomiting, photophobia, and noise sensitivity.

H. Determine whether the client experiences any neurological, prodromal, and/or postdromal symptoms associated with the headache.

I. Review the methods used in the past to abort and/or prevent headaches and subsequent effectiveness.

J. Inquire about past diagnostic evaluations for headaches.

K. Document a family history of headaches.

L. List current medications, including OTC and herbal products.

M. Review the client's medical history for head trauma, infection, allergies, VP shunt insertion, or other neurological diagnoses.

Physical Examination

No aberrant physical examination findings may be present unless the client presents with a headache.

A. Check temperature, blood pressure, pulse, and respirations (especially if meningeal signs are present).

B. Inspect:
1. Observe overall appearance for signs and symptoms of discomfort, photosensitivity (use of sunglasses indoors), and LOC.
2. Examine the eyes; perform a dilated funduscopic examination.
3. Assess the ears, nose, and throat.

C. Auscultate:
1. Listen for bruits at the neck, over the eyes, and in the head for clinical signs of AVM.

D. Palpate:
1. Palpate the head, eyes, ears, TMJ, sinus cavities, temporal, and neck arteries.
2. Palpate cervical vertebrae, cervical muscles, and shoulder areas. Identify potential anatomical triggers: Occipital nerves extend halfway between the middle of the posterior neck and lateral to this area. Pain may be reproduced upon palpation.
3. Examine the spine and neck muscles.
4. Assess cervical ROM.

E. Neurological examination:
1. EOM
2. Pupil response
3. Rising from a seated position without any assistance
4. Walking on tiptoes and heels
5. Tandem gait
6. Romberg test
7. Assess for symmetry upon testing motor, sensory, DTRs, and coordination

Diagnostic Tests

A. Neuroimaging, CT, and MRI are based on the history and physical examination:
1. No neuroimaging is warranted for adults and children with stable headaches, examinations with no aberrant findings, and no evidence of seizures.
2. Neuroimaging should be considered for children with headaches with aberrant neurological exam findings and/or seizures.
3. Neuroimaging should be considered for children with severe headaches, changes in headaches, or associated neurological dysfunction.
4. An emergent head CT without contrast should be obtained when a client complains of "the worst headache ever," and whenever focal neurological findings, nuchal rigidity, or altered mental status are present.
5. The presence of personality changes, depression, and a migraine may suggest a temporal lobe mass.
6. The presence of orbital bruit requires neuroimaging.
7. Neuroimaging is recommended for adults with onset of headache at ages older than 40 years.
8. Neuroimaging should be considered for onset of headache with exertion, cough, or sexual activity.

B. An LP may be indicated in children with altered mental state or focal exam findings.

C. Sinus films can rule out sinusitis, a mass, or lesion.

D. Laboratory tests are not required for most clients with typical symptoms and a negative physical examination:
1. A urine drug screen may be indicated to rule out opioid and illicit substance use.
2. Complete metabolic panel (CMP)
3. CBC
4. Thyroid-stimulating hormone (TSH)
5. ESR

Differential Diagnoses

A. Migraine:
1. Migraine with aura
2. Migraine without aura

B. Other types of headaches:
1. MOHs
2. Common headache
3. Cluster headache
4. Combination headache
5. Chronic daily headache
6. TTH
7. Hypnic headaches (typically occur after age 50, but younger adults may be affected as well)

C. Sinusitis

D. Mass or space-occupying lesion: Subacute and progressive pain, new onset for adults older than age 40

E. Temporal arteritis: New onset of progressive headache in adults older than age 50

F. Carotid dissection can present with a sudden headache, partial Horner's syndrome, and neck pain radiating to the scalp, face, ear, or eye.

G. TMJ syndrome

H. Meningitis

I. Brain abscess
J. Encephalitis
K. Idiopathic intracranial HTN

Plan

A. General interventions: Four main approaches to migraine therapy:
   1. Nonpharmacological interventions:
      a. Adjust habits to maintain a routine pattern of sleeping at all times, even on weekends and vacations.
      b. Do not skip breakfast. Eat regularly scheduled meals with one or two snacks.
      c. Avoid food triggers identified in the migraine diary.
      d. Drink no more than two caffeinated beverages per day.
      e. Maintain adequate hydration.
      f. Exercise at least 30 minutes on 3 to 7 days a week.
      g. Apply cold compresses to affected area(s).
   2. Behavioral interventions:
      a. Relaxation techniques such as yoga, deep breathing, meditation, and guided imagery
      b. Biofeedback, as an adjunct to relaxation training
      c. Cognitive behavioral therapy (CBT)
      d. Psychiatric therapy
   3. Complementary and alternative interventions:
      a. Acupuncture
      b. Nutraceuticals, such as magnesium, coenzyme Q10, and butternut root extract
      c. Vitamins: Riboflavin (vitamin B_2)
      d. Herbal products (not regulated by the FDA), including butternut root extract
      e. PT
      f. Hypnosis
      g. TENS, chiropractic manipulation, and occlusal adjustment should be considered with caution.
      h. Onabotulinumotoxin A has been tested extensively and has been approved by the FDA to treat chronic migraine headaches.
   4. Pharmacological interventions:
      a. Clients must understand why medications must be taken as prescribed. When various analgesics for headaches are overused, paroxysmal migraines can convert into chronic daily headaches.
B. Client teaching:
   1. Encourage the client to maintain an accurate, current headache diary at all times; an example of a migraine diary is available at www.webmd.com/migraines-headaches/guide/headache-diary. The diary may help the client identify triggers for the migraine headaches.
      a. Examples of food triggers: Aspartame, saccharin, red wine, alcohol, chocolate, aged cheese, oranges, tomatoes, avocado, nuts, onions, tyramine, phenylethylamine, monosodium glutamate (MSG), and the nitrates and nitrites found in hot dogs, luncheon meat, and sausage
      b. Examples of odor triggers: Tobacco smoke, perfumes, and strong smells

   c. Examples of visual triggers: Strobe lights, bright lights/sunlight, fluorescent lights, and glare
   d. Other triggers: Medications, barometric pressure changes, too much or too little sleep, and high altitude
   2. The 2014 American Heart Association (AHA)/American Stroke Association (ASA) guidelines for the prevention of strokes in women suggest strong recommendations for smoking cessation, based on the increased stroke risk in female smokers who have migraine headaches with aura.
C. Pharmaceutical therapy: **Selected drug prophylaxis depends on preexisting comorbidities such as cardiac, respiratory, psychiatric, sleep, and GI disorders** (see Table 19.4).
   1. A number of common medications prescribed for migraines are not FDA approved for migraine therapy, such as amitriptyline (Elavil), nortriptyline (Pamelor), and SSRIs.
   2. Antiepileptic medications, including valproic acid (Depakote) and topiramate (Topamax), are FDA approved for migraine prophylaxis. Topiramate should be prescribed with caution in clients with a history of renal calculi, and the importance of adequate hydration must be emphasized.
   3. Beta-blockers are approved for migraine prophylaxis, but must be prescribed with caution when clients have comorbidities such as asthma, depression, diabetes, and thyroid disease.
   4. Several triptans and one triptan/NSAID combination are available to treat migraines. Triptans are widely used for menstrual migraines. Triptans should be used cautiously in clients with cardiovascular comorbidities. Several triptans are not approved for use in children. Triptans should not be administered within 24 hours of an ergot.
   5. Dihydroergotamine mesylate (Migranal) nasal spray is contraindicated during pregnancy or in clients with a history of CVD, angina (chest pain), uncontrolled HTN, myocardial infarction (MI), CVA, or severe hepatic or renal disease. Use ergot derivatives selectively, not long term or more than three times per week. The vasoconstriction from these medications is associated with a greater risk of CVA.
   6. Ergots and triptans should not be given within 14 days of an MAOI.
   7. Antiemetics are prescribed as needed for nausea/vomiting associated with migraines.
   8. Multiple drugs are used off-label for migraines.
   9. Three new drugs have been FDA approved for prophylactic treatment: erenumab (Aimovig), fremanezumab (Ajovy), and galcanezumab (Emgality). These subcutaneous (SC) injections have a lower side-effect profile and have not been reported to cause adverse reactions of HTN or exacerbate depression.
   10. The American Migraine Foundation reported that onabotulinumotoxin A (Botox) is FDA approved for chronic migraines and that one treatment usually lasts approximately 10–12 weeks.

TABLE 19.4   MEDICATIONS FOR MIGRAINES

Medication	Class	Instructions for Adult Dosing	Acute vs. Prophylaxis
Sumatriptan (Imitrex)	Triptan	Initially 25 to 100 mg; may repeat in 2-hour intervals without exceeding the maximum dose of 200 mg/24 hr. Subcutaneous and intranasal formulations are also available.	Acute treatment
Sumatriptan (Alsuma)	Triptan	Initially 6 mg subcutaneous; may repeat in 1 hour without exceeding the maximum dose of 12 mg/24 hr.	Acute treatment; also indicated for cluster headaches
Sumatriptan iontophoretic system (Zecuity)	Triptan	This TDS uses a low electrical current for drug delivery. A patch delivers 6.5 mg of sumatriptan through the skin for more than 4 hours. No more than two patches should be applied in a 24-hour period. A second patch should not be applied within 2 hours of applying the first patch.	Acute treatment of migraine with and without aura
Rizatriptan (Maxalt)	Triptan	Initially 5 to 10 mg; may repeat in 2-hour intervals without exceeding the maximum dose of 30 mg/24 hr. Oral or disintegrating tablets are also available.	Acute treatment
Zolmitriptan (Zomig)	Triptan	Initially 2.5 to 5 mg; may repeat in 2 hours without exceeding the maximum dose of 10 mg/24 hr. Oral or disintegrating tablets are also available.	Acute treatment
Naratriptan (Amerge)	Triptan	Initially 1 to 2.5 mg; may repeat in 4 hours without exceeding the maximum dose of 5 mg/24 hr.	Acute treatment
Almotriptan (Axert)	Triptan	Initially 6.25 to12.5 mg; may repeat in 2 hours without exceeding the maximum dose of 25 mg/24 hr.	Acute treatment
Eletriptan (Relpax)	Triptan	Initially 40 mg; may repeat in 2 hours without exceeding the maximum dose of 80 mg/24 hr.	Acute treatment
Frovatriptan (Frova)	Triptan	Initially 2.5 mg; may repeat in 2 hours without exceeding the maximum dose of 7.5 mg/24 hr.	Acute treatment
Sumatriptan with naproxen sodium (Treximet)	Triptan + NSAID	1 tablet contains 85 mg of sumatriptan and 500 mg of naproxen sodium. Initially administer 1 tablet; may repeat in 2 hours without exceeding the maximum dose of 2 tabs/24 hr.	Acute treatment
Dihydroergotamine mesylate (Migranal)	Ergot derivative	Intranasal spray only; start with 1 spray in each nare; may repeat in 15 minutes without exceeding the maximum dose of 6 sprays/24 hr and no more than 8 sprays/wk.	Acute treatment
Ergotamine tartrate + caffeine	Ergot derivative	Initially 2 tablets at onset; may repeat 1 tablet every 30 minutes without exceeding the maximum dose of 6 tablets/24 hr and no more than 10 tablets/wk. Suppositories are also available.	Acute treatment; also indicated for cluster headaches
Propranolol (Inderal)	Beta-blocker	Initially 80 mg daily; may titrate up to 240 mg/24 hr.	Migraine prophylaxis
Timolol	Beta-blocker	Initially 10 to 15 mg twice daily; may titrate up to 30 mg/24 hr.	Migraine prophylaxis
Topiramate (Topamax)	Antiepileptic (AED)	Requires weekly titration Week 1: 25 mg at bedtime every night Week 2: 25 mg every morning and 25 mg at bedtime every night Week 3: 25 mg every morning. and 50 mg at bedtime every night Week 4: 50 mg every morning and 50 mg at bedtime every night without exceeding the maximum dose of 100 mg/24 hr.	Migraine prophylaxis
Valproic acid (Depakote)	Antiepileptic (AED)	500 mg daily for 1 week, then increase dose up to 1,000 mg/24 hr.	
Amitriptyline	Antidepressant	Initially 75 mg daily in divided doses *or* 50 to 100 mg at bedtime without exceeding the maximum dose of 150 mg/24 hr.	Migraine prophylaxis

TABLE 19.4   MEDICATIONS FOR MIGRAINES (continued)

Medication	Class	Instructions for Adult Dosing	Acute vs. Prophylaxis
Nortriptyline (Pamelor)	Antidepressant	Initially 25 mg, three to four times daily without exceeding the maximum dose of 150 mg/24 hr.	Migraine prophylaxis
Fluoxetine (Prozac)	SSRI	Initially 20 mg every morning, then increase as needed after several weeks. Doses higher than 20 mg/d should be administered in divided doses at morning and again at 12 p.m. without exceeding the maximum dose of 80 mg/24 hr.	Migraine prophylaxis
Erenumab (Aimovig)	CGRP inhibitors	70 mg subcutaneously once monthly	Migraine prevention
Galcanezumab-gnlm (Emgality)	CGRP inhibitors	240 mg (two consecutive injections of 120 mg each) once as a loading dose, followed by monthly doses of 120 mg injected subcutaneously	Migraine prevention
Fremanezumab-vfrm (Ajovy)	CGRP inhibitors	225 mg subcutaneously every month, OR 675 mg subcutaneously every 3 months (quarterly) administered as three consecutive subcutaneous injections of 225 mg each	Migraine prevention
Onabotulinumotoxin A (Botox)	Acetylcholine release inhibitor and a neuromuscular blocking agent	Total dose 155 units, as 0.1 mL (5 units) intramuscular injections per each site divided across 7 head/neck muscles every 3 months (quarterly)	Prophylaxis for chronic migraines

AED, antiepileptic drug; CGRP, calcitonin gene-related peptide; NSAID, nonsteroidal anti-inflammatory drug; SSRI, selective serotonin reuptake inhibitor; TDS, transdermal system.

Follow-Up

A. Schedule follow-up with the client in 2 weeks to evaluate treatment effectiveness.

B. Review the client's headache diary and discuss identifying headache triggers or patterns, such as premenstrual signs and symptoms. Refer to content from the headache diary when considering whether additional tests and consultations are necessary.

C. Monitor LFTs and CBC at least every 3 months with antiepileptic drug (AED) prophylaxis.

Consultation/Referral

A. Consult a physician if headaches are caused by acute problems other than migraine and/or TTHs.

B. If medications do not improve headache, refer the client to neurology.

C. Send the client to the ED for any neurological, life-threatening signs and symptoms.

Individual Considerations

A. Pregnancy:

1. Many medications are contraindicated in pregnancy.

B. Pediatrics:

1. Avoid using aspirin-containing products to avoid the risk of Reye's syndrome.

2. The cause of headache must be accurately identified in this client population.

3. Adolescents may see improvement when estrogen levels are constant, instead of cyclic.

4. Options for medication management are selected based on age. Antiepileptic drugs (AEDs), antidepressants, antihistamines, calcium-channel blockers, and NSAIDs are prescribed to children with headaches.

C. Geriatrics:

1. Headaches decrease after the age of 50 years. A new headache after age 50 years is often associated with epilepsy, essential tremor, ischemic stroke, mood disorders, asthma, or a patent foramen ovale.

2. Consider neuroimaging for older adults who present with unusual headaches.

3. Consider chronic SDH in clients who fall frequently or whose falls were not witnessed by others. Order a head CT or MRI for evaluation. Older adults may not exhibit any signs or symptoms other than a headache.

4. Consider all contraindications before prescribing medications. For example, many older adult clients may have CVD that contraindicates the use of ergot derivatives.

Bibliography

Allergan. (2019, June). *Botox (onabotulinum toxin A): Highlights of prescribing information.* Retrieved from https://www.allergan.com/assets/pdf/botox_pi.pdf

American Headache Society. (2019). The American Headache Society's position statement on integrating new migraine treatments into clinical practice. *Headache, 59*(4), 1–18. doi:10.1111/head.13456

American Migraine Foundation. (2017). *Botox for migraine.* Retrieved from https://americanmigrainefoundation.org/resource-library/botox-for-migraine/

Vincent, M., & Wang, S. (2018). Headache Classification Committee of the International Headache Society (IHS). *The International Classification of Headache Disorders,* 3rd edition. *Cephalalgia, 38*(1), 1–211. doi:10.1177/0333102417738202

Mild Traumatic Brain Injury

Kimberly D. Waltrip

Definition

Head injury includes any structural damage or functional impairment of the scalp, skull, meninges, blood vessels, and/or brain, secondary to traumatic force(s) against the head or body. Signs and symptoms can occur immediately after head injury, such as (a) loss of consciousness or decreased LOC; (b) no recall of recent events pre- or post-injury; (c) disorientation; and (d) deficits in motor strength, balance, vision, sensation, and speech. Severity of head injury is determined by the subsequent, disrupted brain function occurring within 24 hours post-injury. Other associated signs and symptoms include nausea/vomiting, headache, sensitivity to light and/or sound, changes in personality or mood, disrupted sleep, and inattention. Deficits after mild traumatic brain injury (mTBI) may not be detected without overt signs and symptoms. Radiographic testing after mTBI is negative for anatomical pathology, such as cerebral edema or hemorrhage. *Concussion* describes immediate and transient signs and symptoms of mTBI. Concussion can cause confusion, a transient loss of consciousness, and/or decreased level of consciousness. However, loss of consciousness is reported in less than 10% of concussive injuries. Serious complications of mTBI include asymptomatic extradural hematoma, fatal thrombosis of the basilar artery, and hemorrhage from preexisting conditions, such as fibrous dysplasia or essential thrombocytopenia.

Incidence

A. An estimated 3.8 million traumatic brain injuries (TBIs) occur in the United States each year. The majority of TBIs are classified as mTBIs and concussions. Many individuals with mTBI do not seek medical attention. The underreported and untreated cases of mTBI are factors to consider during assessment and diagnosis. Most individuals with TBI recover fully within several days to weeks. However, approximately 10% to 15% of individuals with mTBI have persistent symptoms a year after injury.

Pathogenesis

A. Head injury can produce two types of injury: Primary and secondary:

    1. Primary injury occurs upon initial impact or traumatic force against the head or body. Upon impact, the rapidly shifting position of the head or body sets the brain in motion within the cranial vault. The brain is confined without extra space and has no buffer or cushion to absorb an impact. Injury occurs upon the brain's contact with the skull, and with shearing or sliding. These mechanical injuries are described as focal or diffuse. Localized contusions, lacerations, and skull fractures are *focal* injuries, while concussion and diffuse axonal injury (DAI) are considered widespread or *diffuse*. Primary injuries do not require surgical intervention.

    2. Secondary injury is caused by a flow–metabolism mismatch that occurs after the primary brain injury. Secondary injury includes ischemic and hypoxic changes in the brain, cerebral edema, ICH, and any effects of prolonged, ICP, hydrocephalus, and infection. Secondary injury presents with delayed onset of signs and symptoms, occurring within seconds to minutes, hours, or days.

Predisposing Factors

A. Motor vehicle accident (MVA)
B. Assault or abuse
C. Sports- and recreation-related trauma
D. Ages of increased incidence:
    1. 0 to 4 years
    2. 15 to 19 years
    3. 65 years and older
E. Military occupation (combat-related, exposure to blasts)
F. Falls

Common Complaints

A. Headaches that are often constant, generalized in nature; clients may report frontal headache pain; symptoms may persist for days or weeks.
B. Brief amnestic epoch surrounding the initial injury
C. Faintness
D. Nausea and/or vomiting
E. Changes in vision (slight blurring is commonly reported)
F. Drowsiness
G. Confusion

Other Signs and Symptoms

Other presenting signs, symptoms, and complaints are identified within the following four categories: physical, emotional, cognitive, and sleep disturbance.
A. Physical:
    1. Reported or observed injury to the head or body
    2. Dizziness
    3. Fatigue
    4. Impaired balance
    5. Photophobia
    6. Sensitivity to noise
    7. Numbness/tingling
    8. Seizures, delayed onset after initial injury
B. Emotional:
    1. Irritability
    2. Anxiety
    3. Depression
    4. Labile mood
C. Cognitive:
    1. Difficulty concentrating
    2. Impaired memory:
        a. Short-term memory loss
        b. Repetition
    3. Confusion
    4. Slow responses or difficulty processing information
    5. Changes in reaction time
    6. Changes in speech

7. Disorientation
8. Fatigue
D. Sleep disturbance:
1. Feeling "drowsy"
2. Difficulty falling asleep
3. Sleeping more or less than usual

Subjective Data

A. Obtain a description of injury from the client or witness of the traumatic event, if possible. Identify the cause of the head injury, how it occurred (direct or indirect impact), and what type of force was exerted.

B. Confirm the client's LOC at the time of injury and afterward. Inquire about retrograde and anterograde amnesia, which may predict increased severity of injury. Ask about the precipitating event, its duration, and whether anyone witnessed the client's injury.

C. Review initial and current symptoms per the "Common Complaints" and "Other Signs and Symptoms" sections. Include the description, location, severity, and onset of symptoms. Document everything reported or observed since the initial injury. (Clients often report symptoms that recur or worsen on exertion.)

D. Obtain the client's medical history, especially any details of previous head injuries. Learning disabilities, such as attention deficit hyperactivity disorder (ADHD), developmental disorders, depression, anxiety, sleep disorders, and mood disorders should be documented because of the potential effects on client recovery.

E. Review current medications; certain medications like warfarin (Coumadin) can be predisposing factors for complications.

F. Document any recreational drug and/or alcohol history.

G. Ask family members and significant others if they have noticed any related signs or symptoms, behavioral changes, or evidence of seizure activity.

Physical Examination

A. Check temperature, pulse, respirations, and blood pressure.

B. Inspect:
1. Observe overall appearance. Note LOC.
2. Inspect the skin and head for obvious injury. Periorbital ecchymosis ("raccoon's eyes"), postauricular/mastoid ecchymosis (Battle's sign), or evidence of a CSF leak (otorrhea, rhinorrhea) can indicate basilar skull fracture.
3. Examine the eyes for the presence of papilledema, such as optic disk swelling caused by increased ICP, proptosis, and periorbital edema.
4. Examine the ears for hemotympanum or possible laceration to the external canal, nose, and throat.
5. Examine for any facial fractures.
6. Examine for any cervical spine trauma (e.g., vertebral malalignment, abnormal curvature, reports of pain or tenderness); if necessary, immobilize the client's head and neck (C-spine precautions) and refer to orthopedics or neurosurgery for further evaluation.

C. Auscultate:
1. Over the globes of the eyes if warranted (bruit may indicate traumatic carotid–cavernous fistula)
2. Carotid arteries bilaterally if warranted (bruit may indicate carotid dissection)
3. Heart and lungs, if cardiovascular etiology is suspected
4. Abdomen, if other incidental injuries are suspected (e.g., from a contact sport or MVA)

D. Palpate:
1. Palpate for instability of the facial bones, including the zygomatic arch; may detect a palpable step-off with orbital rim fractures
2. If appropriate, palpate the abdomen and the entire posterior spine to rule out any other incidental injuries.

E. Neurological examination:
1. Assess mental status and memory. Determine whether the client is awake, alert, cooperative, and oriented to *person*, *place*, *time*, and *situation*. Transient impaired memory is one of the most common deficits after a head injury.
2. Assess CN function:
   a. Ophthalmoscopic/visual examination (CN II)
   b. Pupillary size and response (CN III)
   c. EOMs (CNs III, IV, and VI)
   d. Facial sensation and muscles of mastication (CN V)
   e. Facial expression and taste (CN VII)
3. Perform a motor examination on all four extremities.
4. Perform a sensory examination on all four extremities.

Diagnostic Tests

A. A plain film of the skull is no longer recommended for any minor traumatic injury. If the client has a suspected skull fracture or clinical indications for imaging, a CT scan is preferred. This type of imaging will usually reveal any linear or basilar skull fractures.

B. Order and perform CT scan within 1 hour for the following:
1. Decreasing LOC during or after the injury
2. Focal neurological deficits
3. Potential, penetrating, or depressed skull fractures
4. Increasing or persistent, severe headache with nausea and/or vomiting
5. Seizures, post-injury
6. Alcohol, drug, or substance intoxication
7. Posttraumatic amnesia (PTA) over 5 minutes' duration, or when other signs and symptoms are present
8. Unreliable or questionable accuracy regarding the history of client injury
9. Use clinical judgment regarding certain comorbidities and conditions:
   a. Coagulopathy
   b. Persistent alcohol, drug, or substance intoxication
   c. Multitrauma or multisystem injuries

d. Concurrent medical problems

e. Clients older than age 65

C. Consider anteroposterior (AP) and lateral spine films for suspected soft-tissue injury or vertebral fracture, especially if the client has experienced an amnestic episode or cannot recall the initial injury.

D. Drug screen

E. Blood alcohol level

Differential Diagnoses

A. Concussion or mTBI

B. Contusion

C. ICH

D. Shearing injury

E. Skull fracture

F. SAH, traumatic

G. SDH

H. Epidural hematoma (EDH)

I. Vascular occlusion or dissection

J. DAI

Plan

A. General interventions:

1. Initial observation until client's neurological exam returns to baseline, then discharge to home if the following are noted after mTBI:

a. Awake, alert, oriented (AAO) × 4, demonstrating improvement after concussion

b. No risk factors that warrant a head CT, or negative head CT results when risk factors are present

c. No signs, symptoms, or conditions indicating the need for prolonged hospital observation or admission

2. Direct admission to the hospital for decreased LOC, seizure activity, focal deficits, penetrating or depressed skull fracture, vomiting, serious facial injuries, and positive head CT findings

3. Hospitalization may be required if the client has an injured middle meningeal artery, or if venous sinus or posterior skull fractures are suspected. Posterior fossa hematomas can present suddenly; assess blood pressure readings for a wide pulse pressure.

4. Consider possible secondary injuries including cerebral edema, infarction, hemorrhage, hydrocephalus, and infection.

5. The client should not be impaired by alcohol or other drugs when leaving the healthcare setting, to ensure neurological function and detect any evolving deficits.

6. Hospital admission should be considered for certain clients without home observation or supervision.

7. Discuss suspected abuse with a client in a private setting.

B. Client teaching:

1. *See Client teaching: Section III: Client Teaching Guide for this chapter, "Head Injury: Mild."*

2. Provide instruction regarding safety and accident prevention on the following:

a. Wear safety helmets as indicated for occupational role.

b. Use safety belts.

c. Never drive or operate machinery under the influence of alcohol or other substances.

d. Use age-appropriate car seats and booster seats for children.

e. Remove scatter rugs and other objects that would increase the risk for falls.

f. Place nonslip mats in the shower and bathtub.

g. Install grab bars in the shower and bathtub.

h. Install safety gates at the bottom and top of the stairs in homes with small children.

i. Always keep stairs, floors, and hallways clean and uncluttered.

j. Install handrails in stairways.

k. Wear adequate, correct protective gear specific to athletic games and work.

l. Wear helmets for biking, city scooters, and other sports.

m. **Exercise caution upon returning to work, school, or sports:**

i. **Return-to-work (RTW) and return-to-play (RTP) recommendations vary per client,** depending on age, history of previous injuries, severity of injury, resolution of symptoms, job requirements, or specific sport, including the position played.

ii. Typical instructions include client rest until symptoms resolve, avoiding overexertion and strenuous exercise until cleared by healthcare provider, and return to full-time work or contact sports only as directed by occupational or sport-specific guidelines.

C. Pharmaceutical therapy:

1. Analgesics: Acetaminophen, 650 mg every 6 to 8 hours as needed for headache (do not exceed 3,000 mg daily)

2. TCAs or triptans may be used for posttraumatic migraines.

Follow-Up

A. Clients with injuries mild enough to be discharged may be observed. Clients with nonfocal examinations in the outpatient setting do not require routine follow-up, unless otherwise indicated.

B. Postconcussive symptoms may continue for some period of time, usually resolving around 3 months, but possibly after years. The use of the Rivermead Post-Concussion Symptoms Questionnaire (RPQ) may be helpful for serial evaluation; it is available at www.tbi-impact.org/cde/mod_templates/12_F_06_Rivermead.pdf.

Consultation/Referral

A. Refer all clients to the emergency department for the following signs and symptoms:

1. Focal neurological deficit(s)

2. Decreasing LOC

3. Persistent headaches, nausea, and/or vomiting

4. Seizures and any evidence of skull fractures

5. Neuropsychological dysfunction

B. Refer to a neurologist for evaluation of postconcussive symptoms with continued complaints—specifically irritability, fatigue, headaches, difficulty concentrating, dizziness, and/or memory problems. Further evaluation, including MRI and electroencephalogram (EEG) testing, may be needed.

C. Refer to a psychologist specifically trained to perform neuropsychological testing, as indicated for clients with mild head injury. The assessment will evaluate brain function in the areas of attention/concentration, initiation/planning, motor/sensory skills, visual perception, learning and memory, language, speed of processing information/reaction time, and complex problem-solving.

D. Refer to a psychiatrist for evaluation and treatment of any associated disorders emerging within a month or more after mTBI, and with increased signs and symptoms of anxiety, depression, or posttraumatic stress disorder (PTSD) secondary to assault or combat.

E. Consult OT for driving assessments of older adults with mTBI after MVA.

Individual Considerations

A. Pediatrics:
  1. Children are at risk for TBI caused by falls and sports injuries.
  2. Teens are at increased risk for TBI caused by sports, MVAs, and at-risk behaviors.
B. Geriatrics:
  1. Falls are the primary risk factor for head injury in older adults.
  2. MVAs are the second most common risk factor for adults older than age 65 years, due to vision problems, slower reaction times and reflexes, and alcohol and medication use.
  3. Medications, such as aspirin and anticoagulants, increase the complications of head injury.

Resources

Brain Injury Resource Center: www.headinjury.com
CDC Injury Prevention & Control: Traumatic Brain Injury: www.cdc.gov/headsup/parents/index.html
Concussion Fact Sheet for Parents: www.cdc.gov/headsup/pdfs/schools/tbi_factsheets_parents-508-a.pdf
Injury Association of America: www.biausa.org
National Collegiate Athletic Association (NCAA) has concussion fact sheets for student athletes and for coaches: www.ncaa.org/sport-science-institute/concussion-educational-resources
National Institutes of Health (NIH): www.nichd.nih.gov/health/topics/tbi/rcsources/patients-consumers

Bibliography

Barker-Collo, S., Theadom, A., Starkey, N. J., Kahan, M., Jones, K., & Feigin, V. (2019). Long-term factor structure of the Rivermead Post-Concussion Symptom Questionnaire in mild traumatic brain injury and normative sample. *Brain Injury, 33*(5), 618–622. doi:10.1080/02699052.2019.1570339

Centers for Disease Control and Prevention & National Center for Injury Prevention and Control. (2019). *Heads Up*. Retrieved from https://www.cdc.gov/headsup/index.html

Croke, L. (2019). Mild TBI in children: Guidance from the CDC for diagnosis and treatment. *American Family Physician, 99*(7), 462–464. Retrieved from https://www.aafp.org/afp/2019/0401/p462.html

Ellenbogen, R. G., Batjer, H., Cardenas, J., Berger, M., Bailes, J., Pieroth, E., . . . Sills, A. (2018). National Football League Head, Neck and Spine Committee's concussion diagnosis and management protocol: 2017–18 season. *British Journal of Sports Medicine, 52*(14), 894–902. doi:10.1136/bjsports-2018-099203

Ferry, B., & DeCastro, A. (2019). *Concussion: StatPearls* [Internet]. Treasure Island, FL: StatPearls Publishing. Retrieved from https://www.ncbi.nlm.nih.gov/books/NBK537017/

Fremont, P. (2019). Managing a patient with a sport-related concussion. *Canadian Family Physician, 65*(3), 198–199. Retrieved from www.cfp.ca

Giza, C., Greco, T., & Prins, M. L. (2018). Concussion: Pathophysiology and clinical translation. *Handbook of Clinical Neurology, 158,* 51–61. doi:10.1016/B978-0-444-63954-7.00006-9

Scorza, K. A., & Cole, W. (2019). Current concepts in concussion: Initial evaluation and management. *American Family Physician, 99*(7), 426–434. Retrieved from https://www.aafp.org/afp/2019/0401/p426.html#.XLyd6gVrzTM.mendeley

Wells, E. M., Goodkin, H. P., & Griesbach, G. S. (2016). Challenges in determining the role of rest and exercise in the management of mild traumatic brain injury. *Journal of Child Neurology, 31*(1), 86–92. doi:10.1177/0883073815570152

Multiple Sclerosis

Kimberly D. Waltrip

Definition

MS is an autoimmune, degenerative disease that damages neuronal axons and breaks down myelin. The process of inflammatory demyelination varies in progression, with recurrent relapse and remission of symptoms over time. The most common symptoms include visual disturbances, spastic paraparesis, and bladder dysfunction. The course of MS is typically intermittent, with periodic exacerbations occurring in various areas of the CNS. MS can also present more acutely regarding the severity, progression, and variety of symptoms. Early diagnosis is difficult, but crucial to treatment. An attack or exacerbation of MS lasts at least 24 hours, without associated fever or any infectious process. Complete recovery after the first attack is common, often presenting as a *clinically isolated syndrome (CIS)*, but typically converting to MS within 5 years. Subsequent progression with exacerbations leads to diminished function over time.

The loss of myelin leads to neurological deficits involving vision, speech, gait, writing, memory, and/or the swallowing or cough reflexes. Clients typically use the emergency department when they experience relapse; 80% present with exacerbations of previous MS-related deficits. Diagnosis is supported when at least one reported exacerbation correlates with MS-related findings obtained from the neurological examination, MRI, or visual evoked potential (VEP) studies when any visual disturbances have been noted.

MS is classified as relapsing–remitting (RR) or progressive, and further described as *active* versus *not active, with* or *without progression*. Progressive MS is further differentiated with the following two subtypes:

A. *RR* affects approximately 85% of clients with MS. Exacerbations of symptoms and periodic remission occur.

B. *Primary progressive (PP)* is a less common form of MS, accounting for around 10% of MS cases.; PPMS progresses slowly without periods of relapse or remission.

C. *Secondary progressive (SP)*: It is not unusual for clients with RRMS to progress to secondary progressive MS (SPMS) over time. Progression of the disease process continues with or without periods of remission. Symptoms do not necessarily decrease or stabilize in terms of severity.

Incidence

A. An estimated 2.5 million individuals are living with MS worldwide. In the United States, approximately 913,625 are diagnosed with MS, with prevalence estimates up to 363 per 100,000. Symptoms can present between 10 and 80 years of age, but onset usually occurs between ages 20 and 50, with an average age of 32 years. MS is one of the leading causes of disability in young adults and is difficult to accurately diagnose. There is no specific test for diagnosing MS, and signs/symptoms may not be easily recognized. Therefore, the true prevalence and incidence of MS are unknown, especially given that U.S. physicians are not required to report newly diagnosed cases. In 2014, the MS Prevalence Initiative was launched to determine the best method for estimating the number of MS cases in the United States. An algorithm was developed for use with various administrative databases of client information to estimate prevalence and the relationships between geography and triggering factors for MS.

Pathogenesis

A. The cause of MS is unknown. A suspected combination of genetic predisposition and a trigger (e.g., viral infections, environmental factors, metabolic issues) may create an autoimmune disorder that facilitates the degenerative disease process. Autoimmune attacks on the myelin sheaths of nerves initiate an inflammatory response, which is followed by eventual plaque formation and scarring, the hallmark characteristics of MS. There is a loss of saltatory conduction. Axonal death occurs during this acute inflammatory response, which explains any permanent disability. The associated inflammation and edema around an MS lesion, along with myelin and axonal loss, contribute to the associated neurological deficit. A limited amount of remyelination and the eventual resolution of inflammation will allow a certain amount of recovery with remission. Over time, multiple plaques will continue to develop in diffuse areas of the CNS. With each attack, there is a lesser degree of recovery with subsequent decrease in function.

Predisposing Factors

A. Family history of MS
B. Female gender (women are two times more likely than men to develop MS)
C. Ages 20 to 50 years (onset can vary from age 10 years to 59 years)
D. Caucasian race (northern European ancestry)
E. Environment (living in temperate zones, e.g., Canada, northern United States, Europe):
    1. A northern latitude is associated with prevalence, but no direct link has been established at this time. Distance from the equator—specifically, the lack of direct sunlight as a cause of vitamin D

deficiency—may be a contributing factor in the development of MS.
F. Previous viral infections, such as EBV or varicella zoster, may increase susceptibility.
G. Smoking

Common Complaints

A. Sensory loss (e.g., paresthesia) is often reported early in the course of the disease.
B. Visual disturbances: Diplopia on lateral gaze occurs in 33% of clients; blurred vision, loss of vision, eye pain
C. Urinary incontinence, frequency, hesitancy, or urgency; more than 90% of clients with MS report bladder dysfunction.
D. Fatigue affects up to 90% of clients with MS.
E. Weakness in one or more extremities
F. Gait disturbance; 50% of clients with MS will require assistance with ambulation within 15 years of disease onset.

Other Signs and Symptoms

A. Babinski response
B. Spasticity, usually in the lower extremities
C. Depression; occurs in nearly 50% of MS clients; also affects memory, attention, and concentration
D. Hyperreflexia
E. Loss of proprioception
F. Impotence (males)
G. Impaired cognition:
    1. Subjective difficulties with attention span, concentration, short-term memory, planning, and judgment
    2. Dementia is reported in 3% of clients with late-stage MS.
H. Dysarthria
I. Reduced libido (males and females)
J. Constipation
K. Pain
L. TGN (rare)
M. Dysphagia; may also have recurrent respiratory infections secondary to aspiration

Subjective Data

A. Establish location and onset of symptoms. Is this the first time the client has experienced the symptom in question? Was the onset acute or insidious?
B. Ask the client to describe the quality and severity of the symptom, and how it has evolved over time, including duration. Is there an RR pattern? Is there progression regarding severity of the symptom?
C. Ask the client if any factors aggravate or alleviate the symptom. Does hot weather/environment (e.g., hot tubs, saunas, and overexertion) aggravate the condition? Does rest help? Did the symptom resolve on its own?
D. Establish if there have been any known viral or bacterial infections before any reported symptoms
E. Evaluate visual complaints, including the presence of scotoma, decreased color perception, diplopia, decreased acuity, or painful EOMs. Is visual deterioration induced by exercise, a hot meal, or a hot bath (i.e., Uhthoff phenomenon)?

Physical Examination

A. Check temperature, blood pressure, pulse, and respirations.

B. Inspect:

1. Conduct a complete eye examination (Snellen eye chart, test CNs II, III, IV, and VI):

a. Fifty percent of clients with MS present with retrobulbar involvement, yet funduscopy results are negative for any related pathology.

b. Anterior involvement causes papillitis; look for the presence of macular star.

c. Assess pupillary response bilaterally; look for pendular nystagmus or sinusoidal involuntary oscillations of one or both eyes, and/or loss of smooth eye pursuit.

2. Mental status (orientation to person, place, time, and situation); also test short-term memory and ability to plan (impaired planning is another cognitive issue secondary to MS)

3. Assess for discomfort or pain: Location, onset, duration, timing/setting, aggravating factors, alleviating factors, and any other associated data

4. Observe overall appearance for signs of depression, especially with progression of MS-related symptoms.

C. Neurological and musculoskeletal examination:

1. Sensory: Test for perception of sharp versus dull stimulus, heat versus cold stimulus, local pain perception, proprioception; use the tuning fork to evaluate sense of vibration

2. Motor strength: Test all extremities and assess for any increased tone (spasticity), clonus, and/or tremors

3. Heel-to-toe tandem gait testing (assess for ataxia, any cerebellar involvement); Romberg test

4. Finger-to-nose testing, heel-to-shin testing (rule out dystaxia)

5. Test DTRs; assess for Babinski response, hyperreflexia.

Diagnostic Tests

A. Diagnosis of MS is problematic because of the heterogeneous clinical and radiological findings that vary between clients and within clients over time. MS lesions can also be confused with nonspecific MRI and other disease-specific findings in the general population. Diagnosis is therefore based on a combination of clinical, radiological, and laboratory findings that meet the following criteria:

1. MRI confirmation of CNS damage in two or more locations, such as the brain, optic nerves, or spinal cord

2. MRI confirmation of CNS damage that occurred at different times

3. All differential diagnoses have been ruled out.

B. MRI is the designated radiological test to support clinical diagnosis of MS. An MRI of the head will reveal any associated plaques of MS.

1. MRI cannot determine whether the identified lesions are specific to MS when other diseases may have similar findings.

2. TM lesions identified with MRI may convert to MS over time.

C. CSF analysis: Characteristics specific to MS include the presence of oligoclonal bands (in 85%–90% of clients with MS), elevated immunoglobulin G (IgG; >12%), and elevated WBCs (>5%). These findings are not present in the remaining 5% to 10% of clients with MS.

D. Evoked response tests (ERT) or evoked potential (EP) studies: Several different types of tests/studies evaluate brain function and the PNS using EEG with NCV:

1. Brain auditory evoked response (BAER) studies can detect subtle changes in brainstem function.

2. VEP studies focus on visual interpretation and perception, evaluating optical responses to strobe light and/or frequent pattern reversal (typically checkerboard patterns).

3. Somatosensory evoked potential (SSEP) studies evaluate nerve conduction from the extremities via the spinal cord to the brain.

E. CBC with differential

F. Serum glucose levels will rule out hypoglycemia and chronic hyperglycemia as potential causes of neurological findings.

Differential Diagnoses

A. MS

B. CNS lymphoma

C. CNS infection

D. Acute disseminated encephalomyelitis (ADEM)

E. Tumor: Brainstem, cerebellar, or spinal cord

F. Amyotrophic lateral sclerosis (ALS)

G. Systemic lupus erythematosus (SLE)

H. Syringomyelia

I. Progressive multifocal leukoencephalopathy (PML)

J. Sarcoidosis

K. Sjögren's syndrome

L. Acute TM

M. MG

N. GBS

O. CVA

P. Diabetes mellitus

Q. Spinal cord compression (stenosis, ruptured disk)

R. Behcet's disease

S. Neuromyelitis optica (NMO)

Plan

A. General interventions:

1. Energy effectiveness strategies: Aerobic exercise, equipment modifications, specific cooling techniques specific to client's lifestyle

2. Environmental and transportation modifications: Home, workplace, recreational, ADLs, and executive function areas

3. Collaborate with OT/PT to evaluate and implement gait training, exercises for deconditioning, assistive devices, mobility equipment (manual/motorized).

4. Supportive footwear, fall prevention program, textured surfaces, sensory precautions, larger grips

B. Client teaching:

1. Educate on heat sensitivity and how it can aggravate symptoms: Individuals with MS must avoid hot tubs, saunas, and prolonged exposure to hot/humid conditions, and choose appropriate clothing for the season:

a. Approximately 60% of individuals with MS experience heat sensitivity, facilitating a *pseudoexacerbation* in which symptoms may worsen, but do not necessarily indicate additional axon/myelin degeneration.

2. For visual disturbances, advice on resting the eyes at various times during the day may be helpful; for double vision, an eyepatch may be used temporarily.

3. Stress the importance of exercise and its effect on MS-related fatigue and spasticity; overactivity/overwork is another issue to address at this time. Rest periods are needed during exacerbations of MS.

4. Teach Kegel exercises and timed voiding (habit training) to improve bladder function; also advise individuals with MS to avoid alcohol and caffeinated beverages.

5. Advise on increasing daily water intake, dietary fiber intake, and physical activity for increased bowel motility.

6. Educate on signs and symptoms of infection, especially urinary tract infections (UTIs), and how infection can trigger exacerbations.

7. Teach self-intermittent catheterization (SIC) when necessary for urinary retention.

8. Discuss the purpose and availability of local MS support groups.

9. Discuss counseling for adaptive coping techniques, improving family dynamics/relationships with significant others, adjusting to physical disability, and addressing anticipatory grief issues.

10. Educate on all medications, including side effects and any follow-up for pertinent laboratory tests or other testing.

11. Suggest pertinent strategies for short-term memory and planning ability: Individuals with MS can benefit from writing things down, making lists, drawing pictures, and allocating more time for planning.

C. Pharmaceutical therapy: **Medications are prescribed specifically for the type of MS for the specific symptoms experienced and may include any combination of the following medications:**

1. Disease-modifying therapies (DMTs) suppress the immune system to slow progression of MS, decreasing the frequency and severity of exacerbations, and reducing MS-related plaques):

a. Injectable medications (recommended for first-line therapy):

i. Interferons beta-1a and beta-1b: Avonex, Betaseron (extavia), Rebif

ii. Glatiramer acetate: Copaxone (glatopa; 20 mg and 40 mg)

iii. Peginterferon beta-1a: Plegridy

b. Oral medications:

i. Aubagio (teriflunomide): Recommended for first-line therapy

ii. Gilenya (fingolimod): Recommended for second-line therapy

iii. Tecfidera (dimethyl fumarate): Recommended for first-line therapy

iv. Mayzent (siponimod): Recommended for second-line therapy

v. Mavenclad (cladribine): Recommended for first- or second-line therapy

c. Intravenous infusions:

i. Lemtrada (alemtuzumab): Recommended for second- or third-line therapy

ii. Novantrone (mitoxantrone): Recommended for third-line therapy

iii. Rituxan (rituximab): Off-label use for RRMS when second-line medications have been ineffective

iv. Ocrevus (ocrelizumab): Recommended for first- or second-line therapy (progressive types, RRMS)

v. Tysabri (natalizumab): Recommended for second-line therapy

2. Short-term steroid use (e.g., methylprednisolone or prednisone for 3–5 days) may shorten a period of exacerbation. Long-term use is not recommended. IV steroids may be prescribed initially, then converted to oral steroids (prednisone, dexamethasone), and tapered off over time.

a. H.P. Acthar Gel (ACTH) is an option when individuals cannot tolerate the side effects of high-dose corticosteroids, do not respond to corticosteroid therapy, have no available IV infusion services, or when individuals have difficult/inadequate peripheral IV access.

3. Ampyra (dalfampridine) is an FDA-approved drug that has been shown to improve ambulation and possibly decrease fatigue in the MS population. Dalfampridine is a potassium-channel blocker that targets channels located on the outside of nerve fibers, subsequently improving nerve conduction when myelin sheaths are damaged.

4. Antivert (meclizine) may be prescribed for dizziness or vertigo.

5. Various medications (antiepileptics, antidepressants) may be considered for treatment of neuropathic or spasticity-related pain:

a. Dilantin (phenytoin)

b. Elavil (amitriptyline)

c. Klonopin (clonazepam)

d. Neurontin (gabapentin)

e. Pamelor, Aventyl (nortriptyline)

f. Tegretol (carbamazepine)

6. MS-related spasticity may be treated with the following drugs:

a. Botox (onabotulinumotoxin A) injections

b. Klonopin (clonazepam; watch for sedation, dependence increases after 4 weeks)

c. Lioresal (baclofen)

d. Valium (diazepam; watch for sedation, dependence increases after 4 weeks)

e. Zanaflex (tizanidine)

f. Dantrium (dantrolene; use only when other drugs are ineffective, as it can cause liver damage).

g. Intrathecal (IT) pump placement is another option for continuous IT administration of baclofen or clonidine for spasticity.

7. Stool softeners (Colace, Dulcolax, Pericolace), bulk-forming agents (Metamucil), and/or laxatives (Milk of Magnesia, MiraLAX) may be prescribed for complaints of constipation, depending on the severity of symptoms.

8. Flomax (tamulosin) or Hytrin (terazosin) can be used to improve urinary flow.

9. Ditropan (oxybutynin), Tofranil (imipramine), and Detrol (tolterodine) are several examples of medications commonly used to treat bladder spasms.

10. Options for treatment of depression include the following:

a. Selective serotonin–norepinephrine reuptake inhibitors (SSNRIs): Cymbalta (duloxetine hydrochloride), Effexor (venlafaxine)

b. SSRIs: Prozac (fluoxetine), Zoloft (sertraline), Paxil (paroxetine)

c. **Individuals with protracted, painful, and/ or progressive medical conditions are at risk for suicide.**

11. Provigil (modafinil), Symmetrel (amantadine), or Prozac (fluoxetine) can be used to treat fatigue symptoms.

12. Laniazid, Nydrazid (isoniazid), and Klonopin (clonazepam) can be prescribed for tremors.

13. Nuedexta (dextromethorphan and quinidine) for pseudobulbar affect

14. Stem cell transplantation for RRMS: Recent clinical trial results indicate that stem cell therapy may be more effective than DMTs, which could cause reversal of MS symptoms while offering a way to "reset" the immune system.

Follow-Up

A. A neurologist who specializes in MS management should coordinate and prescribe therapies for this client population. Collaboration with a primary care nurse practitioner or physician for follow-up depends on the individual's clinical presentation, diagnosis, and treatment.

Consultation/Referral

A. Neurology referral and consultation for management of MS

B. Ophthalmology for visual disturbances, optic neuritis

C. Urology for genitourinary (GU) disturbances (impotence in males, UTIs, and other urinary symptoms of hesitancy, frequency, incontinence, and urgency)

D. OT will address any barriers or problems with performing ADLs, deficits in fine motor skills (coordination, strength in the upper extremities), and prescribe any necessary adaptive equipment

E. ST will address any issues with language, cognition, or swallowing (including any evaluations necessary for feeding tube placement and for specific dietary recommendations).

F. PT will address gait disturbances, motor weakness, spasticity, and ROM, and prescribe any necessary adaptive equipment for impaired physical mobility.

G. Psychiatry referral and consultation for pharmacological management of depression and/or dementia may be necessary in specific cases; also consider referrals to psychology or licensed professional counselors (LPCs) for any behavioral therapy or counseling needs.

H. Social work (SW) referrals may be necessary for assistance with insurance issues, locating community resources, applying for disability, arranging home healthcare, obtaining placement in a skilled nursing facility, and counseling (individual and family).

Individual Considerations

A. Pregnancy:

1. Symptoms of MS may stabilize or remit during pregnancy, but 20% to 40% of clients with MS experience a relapse within 3 months postpartum.

2. No evidence suggests that pregnancy affects the long-term course of MS. There is no acceleration in the rate of disability or disease progression over time.

3. Neither epidural anesthesia nor breastfeeding has an adverse effect on the rate of relapse or progression of disability with MS.

4. There are no accepted guidelines for recommending for or against pregnancy in females with MS. MS history and current neurological deficits should be considered independently per client.

5. Pregnancy may affect the treatment regimen; some of the medications used to treat MS are known teratogens. For instance, glucocorticoids may cause neonatal adrenal suppression and maternal glucose intolerance.

a. IVIG is an alternative to consider during pregnancy or while breastfeeding, after weighing the risks and benefits carefully before administration. The adverse effects are few, but may present complications that can be severe (e.g., aseptic meningitis, thromboembolism).

B. Pediatrics:

1. MS is rarely diagnosed in children younger than 16 years.

2. Children with MS generally have a similar clinical presentation to adults. Most diagnoses of pediatric MS are classified as RRMS.

C. Geriatrics:

1. The occurrence of MS is rare in individuals older than 60 years of age.

2. Spinal infarcts are seen more often in older individuals when evaluating specific inflammatory lesions.

Resources

Multiple Sclerosis Association of America: mymsaa.org

Multiple Sclerosis Foundation: msfocus.org

National Multiple Sclerosis Society: www.nationalmssociety .org

Bibliography

Burt, R. K., Balabanov, R., Burman, J., Sharrack, B., Snowden, J. A., Oliveira, M. C., . . . Helenowski, I. B. (2019). Effect of nonmyeloablative hematopoietic stem cell transplantation vs continued disease-modifying therapy on disease progression in patients with relapsing–remitting multiple sclerosis: A randomized clinical trial. *Journal of American Medical Association*, *321*(2), 165–174. doi:10.1001/jama.2018.18743

Gullo, H. L., Hatton, A. L., Bennett, S., Fleming, J., & Shum, D. H. K. (2016). Habitual and low-intensity physical activity in people with multiple sclerosis. *Brain Impairment*, *17*(1), 77–86. doi:10.1017/BrImp.2016.9

McCarthy, C., & Thorpe, J. (2016). Some recent advances in multiple sclerosis. *Journal of Neurology*, *263*(9), 1880–1886. doi:10.1007/s00415-016-8124-1

National Multiple Sclerosis Society. (n.d.). *Assessment and interventions*. Retrieved from https://www.nationalmssociety.org/For-Professionals/Clinical-Care/Managing-MS/Rehabilitation/Rehabilitation-Paradigm/Assessment-and-Intervention

Rae-Grant, A., Day, G. S., Marrie, R. A., Rabinstein, A., Cree, B. A. C., Gronseth, G. S., . . . Pringsheim, T. (2018). Comprehensive systematic review summary: Disease-modifying therapies for adults with multiple sclerosis. *Neurology*, *90*(17), 789–800. doi:10.1212/WNL.0000000000005345

Roy, S., Benedict, R. H., Drake, A. S., & Weinstock-Guttman, B. (2016). Impact of pharmacotherapy on cognitive dysfunction in clients with multiple sclerosis. *CNS Drugs*, *30*(3), 209–225. doi:10.1007/s40263-016-0319-6

Wallin, M. T., Culpepper, W. J., Campbell, J. D., Nelson, L. M., Langer-Gould, A., Marrie, R. A., . . . LaRocca, N. G. (2019). The prevalence of MS in the United States. *Neurology*, *92*(10), e1029 LP–e1040. doi:10.1212/WNL.0000000000007035

Myasthenia Gravis

Julie Adkins, Jill C. Cash, Cheryl A. Glass, and Kimberly Waltrip

Definition

A. MG is a chronic autoimmune neuromuscular disorder that affects the neuromuscular junction and is characterized by fatigability and weakness of voluntary muscles. The hallmark of MG is muscle weakness that increases during periods of activity and improves after periods of rest.

B. There are two clinical forms of MG: ocular and generalized. In ocular MG, the weakness is limited to the eyelids and extraocular muscles. In generalized MG, the weakness commonly affects ocular muscles and a variable combination of bulbar, limb, and respiratory muscles.

Incidence

A. MG prevalence is 70 to 320 per 1 million people. There are two peaks in MG incidence that are age and gender related: One is women in their 20s and 30s, and the other is men in their 60s and 70s. Nevertheless, MG can occur at any age. Cases of neonatal MG are temporary and usually disappear within 2 to 3 months after birth. MG in juveniles is uncommon.

Pathogenesis

A. MG is believed to be an antibody-mediated autoimmune attack that destroys variable numbers of acetylcholine receptors (AChR) at the postsynaptic junction. The decrease in AChRs results in weakness with repeated activities and recovery after rest. MG is often associated with thymic hyperplasia or tumors; the thymus plays an unclear role in the autoimmune process of MG. The thymus is large in infants, grows until puberty, and then gets smaller with age. In MG, the thymus gland remains large and abnormal.

Predisposing Factors

A. Inherited by autosomal recessive mutations

B. Children may have congenital myasthenic syndromes.

C. Factors that trigger or worsen exacerbations:
1. Tapering of immunosuppressive medications
2. Pregnancy and postpartum period
3. Medications including antibiotics, bisphosphonates, diazepam, lithium, phenytoin, beta-blockers, calcium-channel blockers, procainamide, quinidine, high-dose prednisone, magnesium, anesthetic agents

Common Complaints

A. Classic triad: Ptosis, diplopia, and dysphagia:
1. Fluctuating symptoms such as droopy eyelid(s)
2. Blurry or double vision
3. Sense of choking

B. Prolonged chewing/fatigable chewing

C. Slurring of speech

D. Easy fatigability manifested by worsening muscle contraction (not a sensation of tiredness)

E. Symptoms are more pronounced with fatigue or in the evening.

Other Signs and Symptoms

A. Selected voluntary muscles that fatigue with activity

B. Motor function that improves with rest, but then decreases with use

C. Signs of impending MG crisis:
1. Sudden onset of inspiratory distress
2. Difficulty swallowing
3. Visual difficulty
4. Tachycardia
5. Rapid onset of weakness

Subjective Data

A. Establish onset of symptoms and possible progression.

B. Ask the client what makes the symptoms better or worse: Does rest help?

C. Ask if the client feels better in the morning, or in the afternoon, or in the evening.

D. Look for difficulties with chewing or swallowing.

E. Review medications, nutraceuticals, and herbal products the client is currently taking or has recently taken as noted earlier.

Physical Examination

Both the presentation and course of MG are highly variable; therefore MG can be very difficult to diagnose.

A. Check temperature (if infection is suspected), pulse, respiration, and blood pressure.

B. Inspect:
    1. Observe overall appearance.
    2. Perform a complete eye examination. Subtleties of eye movement dysfunction are often key in differentiating MG from other disorders.
    3. Observe for respiratory insufficiency: May require mechanical ventilation
C. Palpate:
    1. Assess DTRs; note normal to increased reflexes.
D. Neurological examination:
    1. Perform a complete neurological examination with particular focus on muscular strength and ocular exam:
        a. Muscle strength:
            i. Weakness is increased with repetition or sustained activity; arm raise cannot be sustained.
            ii. Neonatal hypotonia and/or reduced movements
            iii. Facial weakness
        b. Eyes:
            i. Upward or lateral gaze cannot be maintained for longer than 30 seconds. Ptosis may be increased by holding up the opposite eyelid with the examiner's finger (curtain sign).
            ii. Ptosis occurs with repetitive lid closure.
            iii. Ice pack test: Fill a plastic bag or glove with ice and place over the closed eyelid for 2 minutes. Remove the ice and evaluate the degree of ptosis. This test is very sensitive with prominent ptosis.
        c. Facial expression:
            i. Clients may appear expressionless.
            ii. Have the client attempt to smile to evaluate the "myasthenic sneer" (mid-lip rises but the outer corners of the mouth fail to move).
        d. Voice: Voice quality (sounds nasal) or speech changes (low intensity) when counting out loud to 100.

> Normal coordination, normal sensory perception, and normal pupillary response are noted in MG.

Diagnostic Tests

A. Antibody titer for anti-acetylcholine receptor antibody (anti-AChR-ab) is positive in 90% to 100% of clients with generalized MG but in only 50% to 70% of those who have ocular MG. May also perform MuSK antibody titer. Both antibody titers will be negative in approximately 6% to 12% of clients.
B. Cholinesterase-inhibiting drug test: Improvement in strength following injection of edrophonium (Tensilon)
C. Rheumatoid factor and antinuclear antibodies to rule out autoimmune disorders
D. Thyroid function studies to rule out Graves's disease or hyperthyroidism (essential with ocular MG)

E. Repetitive muscle stimulation test: Decremental response
F. Chest x-ray may identify a thymoma.
G. Single-fiber EMG and/or repetitive nerve stimulation (RNS) studies are diagnostic studies performed for diagnosis.

> Initial diagnostic tests may be equivocal with some negative test results, but this does not absolutely rule out MG.

Differential Diagnoses

A. MG: The most common disorder of neuromuscular transmission. **It is important to maintain a high index of suspicion and include MG in the differential diagnosis for any client presenting with variable muscle weakness even without eye signs.**
B. Incomplete extraocular nerve palsy
C. Polymyositis
D. Brainstem transient ischemic attack (TIA)
E. ALS
F. Brainstem vascular accident: "Dizziness" is a symptom rarely seen with MG but often associated with brainstem ischemia
G. GBS
H. Brainstem tumor
I. Hyperthyroidism or hypothyroidism
J. **Cholinergic crisis: Although it is useful to distinguish myasthenic crisis (weakness from MG exacerbation) from cholinergic crisis (weakness from too much medication), both can rapidly lead to respiratory failure. Transportation to an emergency department for evaluation should not be delayed by attempts to differentiate the two.**
K. Eaton–Lambert myasthenic syndrome: Often associated with bronchogenic carcinoma but may precede detection of the carcinoma by as many as 2 years
L. SLE
M. RA

Plan

A. General interventions:
    1. MG is primarily managed by a neurologist, given the difficulty in diagnosing it, the variable course of the disease, and the highly individualized medication regimen required.
    2. The course of MG fluctuates most during the first 3 to 5 years after diagnosis.
    3. Autoimmune disorders, such as thyroid disease, RA, and SLE, should also be screened for in clients diagnosed with MG.
B. Client teaching:
    1. *See Section III: Client Teaching Guide for this chapter, "Myasthenia Gravis."* ◀
    2. Clients should have a Medic Alert tag and always carry a list of their medications and dosing schedules in case of an emergency.

C. Pharmaceutical therapy:

1. **Many medications can cause worsening of myasthenic symptoms, so changes and additions of any medication require consultation with the client's neurologist. Cholinesterase-inhibiting medications:**

a. Pyridostigmine (Mestinon) 60 and 180 mg sustained release (SR); titrate as needed, with usual dose up to 600 mg/d. Pyridostigmine is able available in syrup 60 mg/5 mL for clients who require fractions of 60 mg doses.

b. Neostigmine methylsulfate (Prostigmin) 0.25 to 0.5 and 1.0 mg/mL concentrations, titrated with starting dose 0.5 mg SC or intramuscular (IM) every 3 to 4 hours

2. Prednisone may be used when the client is an inpatient and then tapered on an outpatient basis.

3. Long-term immunosuppression with steroid-sparing agents: Azathioprine, mycophenolate mofetil, cyclosporin, tacrolimus, methotrexate, Rituximab, and cyclophosphamide

4. IVIG

5. Effectiveness of medication regimen is gauged by changes in ptosis, diplopia, dysphagia, chewing ability, and muscle fatigue.

6. Care should be used with medications that may worsen symptoms of weakness.

D. Medical and surgical management:

1. Thymectomy is an early consideration; an MRI of the chest is obtained once the diagnosis is made to assess for thymic enlargement.

Thymectomy lessens the severity of MG, but rarely results in complete elimination of the need for medication.

---

2. Plasmapheresis, or plasma exchange to remove antibodies, is used emergently for the management of myasthenic crisis. Opinion is mixed regarding its use in the long-term management of MG.

3. A myasthenic crisis occurs when the muscles that control breathing are weakened to the point of requiring ventilation. This usually is triggered by an infection, fever, or adverse reaction to a medication.

Follow-Up

A. Clients with MG require lifelong management by a neurologist, given the variable course of both the disease and the client's response to treatment.

B. The client is initially followed every 1 to 2 months, then every 3 to 4 months.

Consultation/Referral

A. If MG is suspected, consult with a physician and consider neurological referral.

Individual Considerations

A. Pregnancy:

1. MG is considered high risk for both the woman and the fetus.

a. Pregnancy requires management by the client's neurologist and a perinatologist.

2. MG frequently manifests for the first time during pregnancy and/or postpartum period. Refer the client to a perinatologist.

B. Pediatrics:

1. There are three forms of MG in children:

a. Transient neonatal myasthenia: Results from transplacental transfer of maternal AChR-Abs

b. Congenital myasthenic syndromes

c. Juvenile myasthenia gravis (JMG): Mainly affects extraocular muscles

2. Children should be followed by a multidisciplinary team that includes a pediatric neurologist and pediatric ophthalmologist.

3. Thymoma is rare in children but should be imaged after JMG has been diagnosed. Thymectomy is not recommended in prepuberal children.

C. Adults:

1. Oral contraceptives, levonorgestrel, and estrogen have been reported to worsen myasthenic symptoms.

Resources

Myasthenia Gravis Foundation of America: https://myasthenia.org/

Bibliography

Bird, S. J. (2018, August 1). Clinical manifestations of myasthenia gravis. *UpToDate*. Retrieved from https://www.uptodate.com/contents/clinical-manifestations-of-myasthenia-gravis

Finnis, M. F., & Jayawant, S. (2011). Review article, juvenile myasthenia gravis: A paediatric perspective. *Autoimmune Diseases*, *2011*(404101), 1–7. doi:10.4061/2011/404101

Jordan, A., & Freimer, M. (2018). Recent advances in understanding and managing myasthenia gravis. *F1000Research*, *7*(F1000 Faculty Rev), 1727–1732. doi:10.12688/f1000research.15973.1

Jowkar, A. (2018, August 2). Myasthenia gravis. *Medscape*. Retrieved from https://emedicine.medscape.com/article/1171206-overview

Myasthenia Gravis Foundation of America. (2019a). *MG crisis, MG exacerbations & crisis*. Retrieved from https://myasthenia.org/What-is-MG/MG-Management/MG-Crisis

Myasthenia Gravis Foundation of America. (2019b). *Treatment and strategies & goals*. Retrieved from https://myasthenia.org/What-is-MG/Treatment-Strategies-Goals

Myasthenia Gravis Foundation of America & Howard, J. F. Jr. (2015). *Clinical overview of MG*. Retrieved from https://myasthenia.org/For-Professionals/Clinical-Overview-of-MG

Peragallo, J. H. (2017). Pediatric myasthenia gravis. *Seminars in Pediatric Neurology*, *24*(2), 116–121. doi:10.1016/j.spen.2017.04.003

University of Arkansas for Medical Sciences. (2018). *Drugs that may worsen myasthenia gravis*. Retrieved from https://neurology.uams.edu/wp-content/uploads/sites/49/2018/03/Drugs-that-may-worsen-Myasthenia-Gravis.pdf

Neurocognitive Disorders (Dementia)

Julie Adkins, Jill C. Cash, Cheryl A. Glass, and Kimberly Waltrip

Definition

A. Neurocognitive disorders are characterized by deficits in cognitive function, with a significant decline from a previous level of function. Decline may be evident in one or more areas of function, including attention, language, memory, visuospatial skills, or executive function (complex tasks such as organizing, sequencing, judgment, and reasoning).

B. Neurocognitive disorders include AD, vascular dementia, Lewy body dementia, and other dementias (frontotemporal dementia, Parkinson's dementia, HIV dementia, neurosyphilis, and Korsakoff's dementia).

C. Clinical features that differentiate these disorders:
   1. AD:
      a. Gradual onset and a course of progressive decline
      b. Memory, language, and visuospatial deficits
      c. Depressive symptoms, which may precede diagnosis
      d. Delusions, hallucinations, agitation, and apathy
   2. Vascular dementia:
      a. Symptoms are similar to AD. However, it is not related to AD pathology, but rather is due to chronic blood flow reduction to the brain causing dementia.
      b. Subtle worsening of cognitive function in a stepwise course of progression: Slower speed of thought, difficulty concentrating and learning, language less fluent, trouble with word-finding, mild visuospatial deficits, and mood changes (apathy, depression, or anxiety).
   3. Lewy body dementia:
      a. Visual hallucinations and delusions
      b. Extrapyramidal symptoms (muscle rigidity, parkinsonism)
      c. Fluctuating mental status
      d. Increased sensitivity to antipsychotic medications
   4. Frontotemporal dementia:
      a. Change in personality
      b. Hyperorality
      c. Impairment in executive function, with relatively well-retained visuospatial skills
      d. Loss of social awareness
      e. Aphasia

D. The diagnosis of dementia must be differentiated from delirium, a disturbance in cognition that develops over a short period and is characterized by an alteration in attention that fluctuates in severity during the course of the day. Delirium may be the consequence of an acute medication condition, hospitalization, or medication/substance induced. Delirium typically may last weeks to months, with gradual improvement in cognition.

Incidence

A. Worldwide, an estimated 47.5 million people have dementia; this number is expected to increase to 75.6 million by the year 2030. Dementia is present in 5% to 20% of persons older than 65 years, and in up to 30% of those 85 years and older. It accounts for more than 50% of nursing home admissions and is the condition most feared by aging adults. One in three senior adults will die with a diagnosis of AD or another form of dementia. The incidence is higher in women, with almost two-thirds of persons with AD being female.

Pathogenesis

The following includes the pathogenesis of each type of dementia.

A. AD:
   1. Cortical atrophy is most prominent in the temporal and hippocampal regions of the brain.
   2. There is extracellular deposition of beta-amyloid protein.
   3. Intracellular neurofibrillary tangles contribute to neuronal loss; tau proteins are a major component.
   4. Decreased levels of acetylcholine
   5. The Apo E epsilon 4 allele of chromosome 19 has been associated with familial and late-onset AD.

B. Vascular dementia:
   1. Microvascular changes of the brain
   2. Cortical and subcortical infarctions

C. Lewy body dementia:
   1. Extensive cortical neuritic plaques
   2. Presence of Lewy bodies (intraplasmic spherical neuronal inclusion bodies) in the brainstem, cortex, and neocortex.

D. Frontotemporal dementia:
   1. Atrophy of the frontal and temporal regions of the brain

E. A number of diseases alter cerebral metabolism and result in dementia, such as Huntington's chorea and Parkinson's disease (PD). Some other diseases can produce or mimic dementia, but may be arrested or reversed. These conditions are classified as pseudodementia, such as hypothyroidism or depression.

Predisposing Factors

A. Definite risks:
   1. Advanced age
   2. Atrial fibrillation (Afib)
   3. Depression
   4. Family history
   5. Down syndrome

B. Possible risks:
   1. Delirium
   2. Head trauma
   3. Heavy smoking

Common Complaints

Interview the client, family members, and/or friends/caretakers who spend quality time with the client to assess for social, neurological, and cognitive changes experienced by the client.

A. Memory impairment

B. Change in behavior and inability to perform normal activities of self-care

Other Signs and Symptoms

A. Disoriented to date and/or place

B. Naming difficulties (anomia)

C. Impaired recent recall

D. Decreased insight

E. Impaired judgment

F. Social withdrawal

G. Problems managing finances; inability to pay bills and to balance checkbook; spending money in unusual ways

H. Getting lost in familiar environments

I. Lack of safety awareness; leaving the stove on, taking medications incorrectly, increased vulnerability to strangers

> Impairment of remote memory carries a graver prognosis than the loss of recent memory alone.

Subjective Data

A. Elicit onset and duration of symptoms; commonly, this information comes from family members.

B. Question the family members and/or caregivers regarding personality changes in the client, or any changes in personal hygiene.

C. Review the client's history for sexually transmitted infections.

D. Is there a loss of interest in things the client used to find important?

E. Review medications, specifically those medications with anticholinergic side effects, including OTC products such as diphenhydramine.

F. Evaluate the client's history for any recent major life events, such as the death of a spouse, a move to a new living environment, or loss of purpose following retirement.

Physical Examination

A. Check temperature (if infection is suspected), blood pressure, pulse, respiration, and weight.

B. Inspect:
1. Observe general appearance; note grooming, interest in conversation, and apathy.
2. Note the presence of slurred speech and slowed body movements.
3. Inspect the nail beds and mucous membranes for anemia.

C. Auscultate:
1. Heart
2. Lungs
3. Abdomen

D. Palpate:
1. Thyroid

E. Neurological examination:
1. Perform a complete neurological examination, including CNs, gait, motor function, and cerebellar function.
2. Note facial asymmetry, distal weakness, and any focal neurological findings
3. Complete a mental state examination with the instrument of choice. See the "Diagnostic Tests" section.
4. Assess functional status; may use a functional assessment tool such as Physical Self-Maintenance Scale, available at https://aging.ufl.edu/files/2012/05/ADLTable.pdf; Instrumental Activities of Daily Living Scale; or Reisberg Functional Assessment Staging (FAST) Scale, available at https://www.crisisprevention.com/CPI/media/Media/Specialties/dcs/How-to-Assess-Cognitive-Functioning.pdf.

5. Complete depression screening with the instrument of choice:
   a. Geriatric Depression Scale (GDS): https://consultgeri.org/try-this/general-assessment/issue-4.pdf
   b. Client Heath Questionnaire (PHQ)-9: https://www.phqscreeners.com
   c. Beck Depression Inventory: https://www.ismanet.org/doctoryourspirit/pdfs/Beck-Depression-Inventory-BDI.pdf

Diagnostic Tests

A. MMSE: https://www.bgs.org.uk/sites/default/files/content/attachment/2018-07-05/mini-mental_state_exam.pdf

B. Pfeiffer's short, portable, mental status questionnaire (or other mental examination of choice): geriatrics.stanford.edu/culturemed/overview/assessment/assessment_toolkit/spmsq.html

C. The CDT may also be administered and used as a screening tool: https://www.sralab.org/rehabilitation-measures/clock-drawing-test (see Section II: Procedures)

D. Rule out possible reversible causes of dementia; not all are required, so use discretion:
1. Thyroid function tests, to rule out either hypothyroidism or hyperthyroidism
2. CBC
3. Vitamin B_{12} level: Anemia or B_{12} deficiency
4. Serum chemistry profile: Hyponatremia
5. Toxicology screen or serum drug screen: Toxicity or intoxication
6. VDRL, fluorescent treponemal antibody absorption (FTA-ABS), or microhemagglutination assay for antibody to *Treponema pallidum* (MHA-TP; CSF) to confirm syphilis
7. HIV-1 antibody titer: AIDS–dementia complex
8. LFTs: Liver disease
9. CT scan or MRI: Vascular dementia, tumor, chronic SDH, normal pressure hydrocephalus, and AIDS–dementia complex
10. EKG: Creutzfeldt–Jakob disease
11. Neuropsychological evaluation

> The history is the key to the diagnosis of dementia. The physical examination may be normal. Dementia is not a normal part of aging; normal aging intelligence scores decrease by only about 10% by age 80 years. A thorough search for a potentially reversible cause is required.

Differential Diagnoses

A. Dementia

B. Depression and adverse reactions to medications are the most common reversible causes of dementia.

C. Use the **DEMENTIA** mnemonic:
   D: Drugs or depression
   E: Emotional upset
   M: Metabolic—for example, vitamin B_{12} deficiency or hypothyroidism

E: Ear or eye impairment or sensory impairment

N: Normal-pressure hydrocephalus

T: Tumors or masses—for example, SDH

I: Infection or sepsis

A: Anemia

D. AD

E. Dementia with Lewy bodies

F. PD with dementia

G. Vascular dementia

H. Frontotemporal dementia

Plan

A. General interventions:

    1. The goal is to treat identifiable abnormalities

    2. Caring for clients with dementia can be overwhelming. Caregivers need support when caring for these clients as well.

    3. Encourage healthy behaviors including regular exercise, healthy diet, and stress management.

    4. Maintain brain function through involvement in stimulating social activities.

    5. Consider driving evaluation for safety if the client is still driving.

    6. Recommend the use of a safe-return bracelet.

    7. Evaluate the home for safety features.

    8. Arrange for supportive care for the family and the client.

    9. Information regarding support groups for caregivers and family is helpful.

B. Client/family teaching:

    1. *See Section III: Client Teaching Guide for this chapter, "Dementia."*

    2. Educate the family and the client regarding the diagnosis, disease process, and progression.

    3. Discuss advance directives and planning for future care needs.

    4. Encourage the client and family caregivers to become involved in dementia support groups.

    5. Avoid medications such as anticholinergic medications, including diphenhydramine, hydroxyzine, TCAs, and oxybutynin.

    6. Recommended handbook for the family: *The 36-Hour Day: A Family Guide to Caring for People Who Have Alzheimer's Disease, Related Dementias and Memory Loss* (Mace & Rabins, 2012), can be ordered through online retailers.

C. Pharmaceutical therapy:

    1. No medications have been found to decrease the rate of decline in cognitive behavior. However, studies have shown that clients can be treated with medications for agitation, hallucinations, and depression and to improve mental alertness. Studies indicate that clients with a diagnosis of mild to moderate AD, vascular dementia, Lewy body dementia, and Parkinson's dementia may trial and benefit from a cholinesterase inhibitor:

        a. Donepezil (Aricept): Start 5 mg daily at bedtime for 4 weeks, then 10 mg/day at bedtime

            i. Donepezil 23 mg extended-release tablets are available for clients with moderate-to-severe

disease, who have taken 10 mg at bedtime for at least 3 months

        b. Rivastigmine (Exelon): 1.5 to 6 mg twice daily or via transdermal patch starting at 4.6 mg/d, then titrate up to 9.5 mg/d or increase to the maximum effective dose at 13.3 mg/d, as indicated

        c. Galantamine (Razadyne): 4 mg twice daily with meals for 4 weeks; then may increase to maximum dose at 12 mg twice daily. For missed doses, the client or family will need to retitrate doses.

            i. Razadyne ER: 8 mg/d; after 4 weeks, may increase dose to 16 mg/d, or increase to the maximum dose at 24 mg/d

    2. Clients with moderate-to-severe AD: *N*-methyl-D-aspartate (NMDA) receptor antagonist:

        a. Memantine (Namenda): 5 mg/d, increase dose an additional 5 mg each week; can also adjust dose to 5 mg twice daily, and increase to the maximum dose at 20 mg twice daily. Use the titration pack for the first 4 weeks.

            i. Do NOT prescribe more than 5 mg twice daily to clients with severe renal impairment.

            ii. Namzaric (donepezil and memantine) is also available to clients with moderate-to-severe disease who are taking donepezil 10 mg/d.

        b. Namenda XR: 7 mg daily, titrate by 7 mg/wk increments to recommended maintenance dose of 28 mg daily

Follow-Up

A. Routine follow-up in 1 month to evaluate the client's status, response to medication, and side effects

B. Clients and families have an ongoing need for education and support in learning to deal with the diagnosis.

C. Subsequent follow-up visits can be scheduled every 3 to 6 months.

Consultation/Referral

A. Refer the client to a neurocognitive specialist if the diagnosis is unclear.

B. Refer clients and families to support groups in the community.

C. Geriatric psychiatry may be appropriate for management and treatment of behavioral and psychological symptoms of dementia.

D. Refer to social services or geriatric case management for assistance with respite care and placement options.

Individual Considerations

A. Pediatrics:

    1. A client who presents at a young age with dementia requires a thorough workup to evaluate the cause of the symptoms.

B. Geriatrics:

    1. Irreversible dementia or AD begins in the fourth to fifth decade of life and is characterized by loss of recent memory, inability to learn new information, language problems, mood swings, and personality changes.

Resources

Alzheimer's Association: https://www.alz.org

Family Caregiver Alliance: https://www.caregiver.org/vascular-dementia

Lewy Body Dementia Association: https://www.lbda.org

National Institute on Aging, Alzheimer's Disease Education and Referral Center: https://www.nia.nih.gov/alzheimers

Bibliography

Alzheimer's Association. (2016). What is dementia? Retrieved from https://www.alz.org

Alzheimer's Association & Centers for Disease Control and Prevention. (2018). *Healthy Brain Initiative, state and local public health partnerships to address dementia: The 2018–2023 road map* (3rd ed.). Chicago, IL: Alzheimer's Association. Retrieved from https://www.cdc.gov/aging/pdf/2018-2023-Road-Map-508.pdf

Annear, M. J., Eccleston, C. E., McInerney, F. J., Elliott, K. E., Toye, C. M., Tranter, B. K., & Robinson, A. L. (2016). A new standard in dementia knowledge measurement: Comparative validation of the Dementia Knowledge Assessment Scale and the Alzheimer's Disease Knowledge Scale. *Journal of the American Geriatrics Society, 64*(6), 1329–1334. doi:10.1111/jgs.14142

Delgado-Alvarado, M., Gago, B., Navalpotro-Gomez, I., Jiménez-Urbieta, H., & Rodriguez-Oroz, M. C. (2016). Biomarkers for dementia and mild cognitive impairment in Parkinson's disease. *Movement Disorders, 31*, 861–881. doi:10.1002/mds.26662

Kim, K., Han, J. W., So, Y., Seo, J., Kim, Y. J., Park, J. H., . . . Kim, K. W. (2017). Cognitive stimulation as a therapeutic modality for dementia: A meta-analysis. *Psychiatry Investigation, 14*(5), 626–639. doi:10.4306/pi.2017.14.5.626

Parkinson's Disease

Julie Adkins, Jill C. Cash, Cheryl A. Glass, and Kimberly Waltrip

Definition

A. PD is an idiopathic, progressive, chronic neurological syndrome characterized by a combination of akinesia or bradykinesia, or reduction of spontaneous activity and movement; rigidity, or increase in spontaneous muscle tone and involuntary movements; tremor; and postural instability.

Incidence

A. PD affects nearly 1 million people in the United States and more than 6 million people worldwide. One percent of the population older than 50 years has PD. The mean age of onset is 55 to 60 years; however, the mean age at diagnosis is 70.5 years.

Pathogenesis

A. For reasons that are unclear, degenerative changes occur in the basal ganglia and deplete the dopaminergic neurons in the substantia nigra, resulting in dopamine reduction in the striatum. This interrupts neuronal circuits and produces akinesia and rigidity. The pathophysiology of tremor is less clear, but thalamic involvement is implicated. Symptoms are caused by loss of neurons that produce dopamine. Certain nerve cells (neurons) in the brain break down or die.

Predisposing Factors

A. Advancing age

B. Antecedent encephalitis

C. Arteriosclerosis

D. Trauma

E. Toxins

F. Drugs, particularly phenothiazines

G. Familial neurodegenerative diseases in which parkinsonism is a prominent feature

H. Presence of Lewy bodies

Common Complaints

Cardinal symptoms:

A. Tremor at rest: May be intermittent, but progresses over time

B. Rigidity: Joints are more rigid; increased resistance to passive movement; appears unilaterally and then progresses to the opposite side; usually asymmetrical; appears as decreased movement in arm swing when ambulating, stooped posture, and cogwheel rigidity—resistance with tremor

C. Bradykinesia, or slow voluntary movement, especially with daily activities such as cutting food, dressing self, and so forth. When walking, shorter steps are taken, shuffle-step, feeling of unsteadiness with walking; postural instability.

D. Impaired balance and coordination with increase in fall risks

Other Signs and Symptoms

A. Micrographia (handwriting that decreases in size when writing out name)

B. Voice changes: Fading, softness, hoarseness, and mumbling

C. Decreased frequency of swallowing/saliva escaping mouth

D. Dysphagia

E. Neuropsychiatric changes: Cognitive impairment/dementia/memory loss, sleep disturbance, fatigue, anxiety, depression, pain, and sensory changes

F. Oily, greasy skin

G. Excessive perspiration

H. Constipation

I. Urinary hesitancy or frequency

J. Visual loss: Impaired vision, reflex, upward gaze, convergence, and decreased blinking

K. Decreased ability to smell

L. Restless legs

Subjective Data

A. Elicit information regarding onset of symptoms. Note changes in progression of symptoms.

B. Talk with the client and the family to establish if there have been behavioral changes, problems with activities such as eating or getting out of chairs, or personality changes.

C. Determine if other family members have had similar symptoms.

D. Ascertain the client's medical history, including current medications, both prescription and OTC.

E. Particularly in clients younger than 55 years, investigate substance abuse and exposure to herbicides or pesticides.

Physical Examination

A. Check temperature (if indicated), pulse, respiration, blood pressure, and weight; note orthostatic hypotension.

B. Inspect:

1. Observe overall appearance.

2. Note asymmetric tremor at rest.

3. Note subtle facial masking, decreased frequency, and amplitude of eye blinks.

4. Note posture and gait disturbances: Festination, or shuffling, increasingly tiny steps; usually walking with arms down to side; difficulty turning; freezing, or inability to continue to move.

C. Palpate:

1. Palpate extremities, noting increased tone in resting muscles.

D. Neurological examination:

1. Perform a complete neurological examination. Assess all CNs. Assess DTRs.

2. Assess rapid alternating movements. Note difficulty with rapid alternating movements such as tapping fingers or turning palm alternately up and down.

3. Check cogwheel phenomenon, which is stepwise rigidity of movement with PROM, rather than anticipated smooth movement through ROM. Best tested in wrists.

4. Perform mental state examination.

5. Assess the progression of the disease state with the scale of choice. The International Parkinson and Movement Disorder Society site hosts a list of rating scales and questionnaires at www.movementdisorders.org.

6. Scales commonly used include:

a. Unified Parkinson's Disease Rating Scale evaluates ADLs, motor function, behavior and mood, and complications of therapy. Points are assigned for every item based on responses, observations, and physical examination. https://img.medscape.com/fullsize/701/816/58977_UPDRS.pdf

b. Modified Hoehn and Yahr Scale measures the progression and disability of Parkinson's symptoms over time from no signs of disease (Stage 0) to being wheelchair bound or bedridden (Stage 5). https://emedicine.medscape.com/article/2172546-overview

c. Unified Dyskinesia Rating Scale (UDysRS) is used for evaluation of involuntary movements. http://www.movementdisorders.org/MDS-Files1/PDFs/UDysRS_English_FINAL.pdf

Diagnostic Tests

A. There is no definitive diagnostic test for PD. Diagnosis is based on a person's medical history and neurological examination.

B. Consider serum blood tests or other testing to rule out other conditions causing symptoms.

C. Urinalysis to rule out UTI with any urinary symptoms

D. Brain CT scan or MRI to exclude mass lesion, multiple infarcts, or normal-pressure hydrocephalus

E. MRI of cervical spine if there is increased gait disturbance after a fall

Differential Diagnoses

A. PD

B. Essential tremor

C. Multi-infarct dementia

D. AD

E. Brain tumor

F. Progressive supranuclear palsy

G. Normal-pressure hydrocephalus

H. Shy–Drager syndrome

I. Hypothyroidism

J. Hereditary disease such as Huntington's chorea or Wilson's disease

K. Chorea: Not generally seen in PD; its development in a client with PD is generally a medication side effect and should be discussed with the client's neurologist.

Plan

A. General interventions:

1. Encourage regular exercise to maintain or improve flexibility.

2. The client should follow a diet that is high in fiber and calcium, with adequate fluid intake, to limit complications caused by constipation and osteoporosis. In some clients, protein intake may need to be timed to limit interactions with medications such as levodopa.

3. Emphasize the importance of the nonmotor symptoms being addressed and adequately treated. Encourage the family to notify the provider if these symptoms are not being controlled. Anxiety, depression, fatigue, mood changes, and behavioral issues need to be addressed and controlled to ensure adequate quality of life for the client and the family.

4. Home safety evaluations are recommended because the symptoms of PD place clients at high risk of falls and accidental injury.

5. Surgery, such as pallidotomy or thalamotomy, is an option for severe PD in which tremor is poorly controlled with medications.

6. Deep brain stimulation (DBS) is an option for clients who do not respond well to medications.

B. Client teaching:

1. *See Section III: Client Teaching Guide for this chapter, "Managing Your Parkinson's Disease."* ◀

C. Pharmaceutical therapy:

1. No single DMT can stop or slow the progression of PD. Polypharmacy is the hallmark rather than the exception with PD. Always comanage clients with a neurologist.

2. Lower doses of several medications, rather than high doses of a single agent, aid in maximizing function while minimizing side effects.

3. Drug dosages are always tapered, not stopped abruptly.

4. First-line drug: Levodopa, combined with carbidopa, a decarboxylase inhibitor, is the mainstay of treatment. Sinemet is the levodopa/carbidopa combination drug most often used:

a. The dose and dosing frequency are very individualized.

b. Clients are often on a combination of SR and short-acting preparations.

c. See the literature for individual dosing. Titrate the dose up every 3 days for adjustments.

d. Long-term use is often associated with adverse effects requiring careful medication dosage.

5. Second-line therapy: Dopamine agonists. Generally given in conjunction with levodopa, these allow use of lower doses of levodopa that can delay or reduce levodopa-associated problems. Examples include pramipexole (Mirapex) and ropinirole (Requip).

6. Ergot derivatives

a. Bromocriptine and pergolide are the two dopamine agonists most often used:

i. Bromocriptine mesylate (Parlodel) is initiated at 1.25 mg daily or twice a day and increased slowly to 10 to 25 mg daily.

ii. Pergolide mesylate (Permax) is initiated at 0.05 mg daily and increased slowly to 2 to 3 mg in divided doses three times a day.

b. Non-ergot drugs are preferred because of fewer side effects:

i. Pramipexole (Mirapex) 0.125 mg three times daily up to 4.5 mg/d maximum is useful for tremors

ii. Ropinirole (Requip) 0.25 mg three times daily, maximum 24-hour period

7. Neuroprotective agents:

a. Selegiline (Eldepryl), MAO-B inhibitor 5 mg at breakfast and at lunch, may have neuroprotective effects and slow progression of symptoms

i. Often an initial treatment, a drug is usually continued throughout the course of the disease.

ii. Maximum dose is 10 mg/d.

b. Amantadine (Symmetrel) is used as short-term monotherapy in clients younger than 60 years with mild to moderate PD in which akinesia and rigidity are more prominent than tremor:

i. Its effects tend to wane, and it should be tapered once other antiparkinsonian drugs are started.

ii. The usual dose is 100 to 300 mg twice daily. Adjust the dose gradually.

c. Caution should be used with neuroprotective agents because of the interactions with other medications and foods that can precipitate high blood pressure to dangerous levels. Advise clients to avoid foods high in tyramine, such as some cheeses, tofu, yeast extracts, and so forth.

8. Anticholinergics: These are useful for treating resting tremor, but not akinesia or impaired postural reflexes:

a. The centrally acting drug trihexyphenidyl HCl (Artane) is the most common anticholinergic used:

i. Usually started at 0.5 to 1.0 mg twice daily with food, with dose slowly increased to 2 to 3 mg three times daily

ii. Dosage should always be tapered, never stopped abruptly.

iii. Use is not recommended in clients older than 60 years or with dementia.

b. Benztropine mesylate (Cogentin) 0.5 to 1 mg at bedtime may also be used in PD. Maximum is 6 mg/d. Increase every 6 to 7 days.

9. Sleep disorders are common in PD and respond well to TCAs, benzodiazepines, diphenhydramine, or low-dose chloral hydrate.

10. Excessive daytime sleepiness should first be evaluated as a symptom of depression before it is attributed to medications or effects of PD.

As PD progresses, clients often develop clear "on" and "off" times of medication effectiveness and functional ability; therefore, medication schedules are very carefully customized to maximize "on" times.

Follow-Up

A. PD requires lifelong management by a neurologist.

B. The frequency of appointments depends on the severity of disease and the client's response to medication. Depression and neuropsychiatric side effects of medications are often seen in clients with PD; therefore, any office visit should involve screening for these effects. Inquire particularly about memory loss, vivid dreams or nightmares, hallucinations, symptoms of depression or anxiety, and occurrence of panic attacks. Discuss findings with the client's neurologist, as medication adjustments could be required.

Consultation/Referral

A. Managing PD requires referral to a neurologist to initiate and adjust medications.

B. If a client with PD requires the addition of medication for other conditions, consult the client's neurologist to evaluate for possible serious adverse effects.

C. Prescribe PT for walking and balance and evaluation of assistive devices.

D. Prescribe an ST evaluation of dysarthria and dysphagia to assess aspiration risk.

E. A multidisciplinary team is required for the evaluation and treatment with DBS.

F. Involvement with a support group can be helpful for the client and family. Information about PD and local support groups can be obtained from:

1. American Parkinson's Disease Association: https://www.apdaparkinson.org/

2. National Parkinson Foundation: https://www.parkinson.org

3. International Parkinson and Movement Disorder Society: https://www.movementdisorders.org

4. Michael J. Fox Foundation for Parkinson's Research: https://www.michaeljfox.org/

a. Parkinson's 360° Real Talk for Clients and Families: https://www.michaeljfox.org/sites/default/files/media/document/PD360_MJFF_WEB_BOOK.pdf

Individual Considerations

A. Pediatrics:
1. PD is uncommon in people younger than 40 years of age. When PD is seen in the pediatric age group, it is usually because of secondary factors.
B. Geriatrics:
1. PD is most commonly seen in this population.

Bibliography

American Association of Neurological Surgeons. (2019). *Parkinson's disease*. Retrieved from https://www.aans.org/en/Patients/Neurosurgical-Conditions-and-Treatments/Parkinsons-Disease

Besser, L. M., Litvan, I., Monsell, S. E., Mock, C., Weintraub, S., Zhou, X. H., & Kukull, W. (2016). Mild cognitive impairment in Parkinson's disease versus Alzheimer's disease. *Parkinsonism & Related Disorders, 27*, 54–60. doi:10.1016/j.parkreldis.2016.04.007

Chou, K. L. (2019, April 17). Clinical manifestations of Parkinson disease. *UpToDate*. Retrieved from https://www.uptodate.com/contents/clinical-manifestations-of-parkinson-disease

Christensen, B. (2014, November 26). Modified Hoehn and Yahr Scale. *Medscape*. Retrieved from https://emedicine.medscape.com/article/2172546-overview

Delgado-Alvarado, M., Gago, B., Navalpotro-Gomez, I., Jimeńez-Urbieta, H., & Rodriguez-Oroz, M. C. (2016). Biomarkers for dementia and mild cognitive impairment in Parkinson's disease. *Movement Disorders, 31*, 861–881. doi:10.1002/mds.26662

Kang, M. Y., & Ellis-Hill, C. (2015). How do people live life successfully with Parkinson's disease? *Journal of Clinical Nursing, 24*(15–16), 2314–2322. doi:10.1111/jocn.12819

Mayo Clinic. (2019). *Parkinson's disease*. Retrieved from https://www.mayoclinic.org/diseases-conditions/parkinsons-disease/symptoms-causes/syc-20376055

Michael J. Fox Foundation. (2016). *Parkinson's 360° guide to Parkinson's medications*. Retrieved from https://www.michaeljfox.org/sites/default/files/media/document/PD360_MJFF_WEB_BOOK.pdf

U.S. Department of Health & Human Services, NIH National Institute on Aging. (2017, May 16). *Parkinson's disease*. Retrieved from https://www.nia.nih.gov/health/parkinsons-disease

Restless Legs Syndrome

Julie Adkins, Cheryl A. Glass, and Kimberly Waltrip

Definition

A. Restless legs syndrome (RLS), also known as Willis–Ekbom disease (WED), is a neurological disorder usually involving throbbing, pulling, creeping, or other unpleasant sensations of the legs with sometimes an overwhelming urge to move them. Symptoms occur usually at night when in a relaxing, resting position, but can increase in severity throughout the night. Moving the legs usually relieves the discomfort, causing disorders of sleep. Left untreated, RLS can cause exhaustion and fatigue, which is often associated with daytime problems with concentration and memory, and can cause depression.
B. Recently, RLS has been identified as a risk factor for cardiovascular disease including stroke.

Incidence

A. As many as 5% to 15% of adults may have RLS. Moderate to severe symptoms affect 2% to 3% of adults. An additional 5% have the milder form.
B. Prevalence varies by gender, region, and ethnicity:
1. RLS occurs in both men and women, but the incidence is about twice as high in women.
2. Northern European countries have the highest prevalence of RLS.

C. RLS may begin at any age. Symptoms seem to become more frequent and last longer with age.
D. Children can also have RLS; almost 1 million school-age children are affected and one-third have moderate to severe symptoms.

Pathogenesis

A. RLS is classified as a movement disorder, as people are required to move their legs to get any relief. More than 80% of people with RLS also may experience periodic limb movement of sleep (PLMS), a condition that involves leg twitching or jerking movements during sleep occurring every 15 to 40 seconds. Although many clients with RLS develop PLMS, most people with PLMS do not have RLS or any other cause of PLMS. Periodic limb movement disorder (PLMD) may be a variant of RLS and responds to similar treatments.
B. The cause of RLS is unknown; however, it may have a genetic component. Nearly half of all people with RLS also have a family member with the condition.
C. Evidence indicates that low levels of iron in the brain may be responsible for RLS.
D. Considerable evidence suggests that RLS is a dysfunction in the brain's basal ganglia that uses the neurotransmitter dopamine. Disruption of this pathway frequently results in involuntary movements.
E. Alcohol and sleep deprivation may aggravate or trigger RLS symptoms.

Predisposing Factors

A. Alcohol use
B. Sleep deprivation
C. Chronic diseases such as uremia secondary to renal failure, diabetes, anemia, and PN
D. Certain medications such as antiemetics, antipsychotic drugs, antidepressants, and some cold and allergy medications
E. Pregnancy, especially during the third trimester
F. Family history of RLS
G. Parkinson disease
H. MS
I. Varicose veins

Common Complaints

A. **A classic feature of RLS is that the symptoms are worse at night, with a distinct symptom-free period in the early morning**
B. Uncomfortable sensations in the legs with an irresistible urge to move the limb. Sensations may occur on only one side of the body, but most often affect both sides.
C. Need to keep legs in motion, such as by pacing the floor, moving legs while sitting, and tossing and turning in bed

Other Signs and Symptoms

A. May vary from day to day, in severity and frequency, and from person to person
B. Triggering factors may include long car trips; sitting for long periods of time, such as at a movie theater or on long-distance flights; immobilization of a cast; or relaxation exercises.

C. Worsening of symptoms occurs with sleep deprivation.
D. In severe cases, interruption and impairment of daytime function occur.

Subjective Data

A. Ask the client to describe the sensations (urge to move legs) that he or she is complaining of. Do sensations occur in one leg or both legs?
B. What makes symptoms worse? What makes symptoms better?
C. What does the client do to make the sensations better?
D. Do symptoms occur during rest or activity? Is there a particular activity that usually makes the symptoms worse or better? Do they improve with movement?
E. How often are symptoms present? Do the symptoms occur during the daytime or nighttime? Daily, nightly, several times a day, once a week, and so forth?
F. Does the client have other medical or behavioral conditions that can be attributed to the symptoms that occur?
G. Are symptoms triggered by rest, relaxation, or sleep?
H. Determine sleep patterns and disturbances.
I. Review current medications being taken and discuss chronic conditions.
J. Inquire regarding the amount of alcohol ingested each day.
K. Inquire regarding the use of tobacco.
L. If the client is pregnant, are symptoms new during the pregnancy or has she always had the symptoms?

Physical Examination

A. Check blood pressure, pulse, respirations, and weight.
B. Inspect:
    1. Overall appearance and hygiene.
C. Auscultate:
    1. Heart
    2. Lungs
D. Neurological examination:
    1. Perform a full neurological examination.

Diagnostic Tests

A. Diagnosis of RLS is made by history alone; it does not require additional testing except for a serum ferritin level.
B. Polysomnogram is not required for the diagnosis of RLS. A sleep study is reserved for clients in whom the diagnosis is in question.

Differential Diagnoses

A. **RLS: There is no specific test for RLS. The basic criteria for diagnosing the disorder are:**
    1. Symptoms are worse at night and are absent or negligible in the morning.
    2. A strong and often overwhelming need or urge to move the affected limb(s), often associated with paresthesias or dysesthesias
    3. Sensory symptoms that are triggered by rest, relaxation, or sleep
    4. Sensory symptoms that are relieved with movement, in which the relief persists as long as the movement continues
    5. None of the previously noted symptoms is caused by another medical condition.

B. Sleep apnea
C. Alcoholism
D. Specific vitamin deficiencies
E. Pregnancy (third trimester)
F. PD
G. MS

Plan

A. General interventions:
    1. Activities that worsen symptoms should be discontinued.
    2. Medications can be prescribed and are effective for many clients.
    3. Some chronic conditions may contribute to RLS, such as diabetes, PN, or vitamin deficiency, and should be evaluated.
B. Client teaching:
    1. Advise the client to discontinue activities that worsen symptoms.
    2. Lifestyle changes may be suggested, such as discontinuing use of alcohol, tobacco, and caffeine.
    3. Bedtime rituals should be encouraged. Regular sleep patterns should be encouraged. Avoid exercise at least 1 to 2 hours before bedtime. Encourage relaxation techniques before going to bed.
    4. The use of relieving techniques, such as massage, warm bath, or warm/cold compresses, is encouraged.
C. Pharmaceutical therapy:
    1. Dopaminergic agents (increase dopamine) are recommended first-line treatment for frequent or nightly symptoms. However, caution should be used. Long-term use can lead to worsening symptoms as early as a few months after initiation of these drugs. This is reversible with withdrawal of the medication. Medications are best initiated at low doses and taken 1 to 2 hours before bedtime to allow for sufficient absorption.
        a. U.S. FDA-approved non-ergotamine dopamine agonists for moderate-to-severe RLS include:
            i. Ropinirole (Requip): 0.25 mg orally at bedtime; may titrate the dose every three nights, for a maximum dose of four tablets at bedtime, until symptoms are resolved.
            ii. Pramipexole (Mirapex): Initial dose: 0.125 mg, one tablet at bedtime; may increase dose every three nights, for a maximum dose of four tablets at bedtime, until symptoms are resolved; requires dosage adjustment in renal impairment
            iii. Rotigotine (Neupro) transdermal patch: 1 mg/24 hr patch; apply new patch nightly at alternating sites; may increase patch weekly to a maximum dose of 3 mg/24 hr
        b. Levodopa formulation:
            i. Levodopa/carbidopa or levodopa/benserazid: 50/12.5 mg starting dose; may increase to maximum dose of 200/50 mg.
    2. Pregabalin 2 mg starting dose; may increase to a maximum dose of 300 mg until symptoms improved

3. Gabapentin enacarbil (Horizant) is also FDA approved for RLS treatment:

    a. Recommended dose: 600 mg once daily taken with food about 5 p.m.

    b. Should not be cut, crushed, or chewed

    c. **Not recommended for client with a CrCl < 30 mL/min or on hemodialysis**

4. Analgesics, such as acetaminophen (Tylenol), NSAIDs, and opioids, may be used as needed for pain.

5. Benzodiazepines, such as clonazepam 0.5 to 2.0 mg at bedtime, may be used as needed. Benzodiazepines should be avoided in the elderly.

6. Iron supplemental to restore iron

7. Vitamin deficiencies should be treated with appropriate vitamins as diagnosed.

Follow-Up

A. Follow up in 1 to 2 weeks to evaluate effect(s) of medications.

B. Evaluate severity or minimization of symptoms.

C. Reassure clients that a diagnosis of RLS does not indicate the onset of another neurological disorder such as PD.

Consultation/Referral

A. Consider referral to a neurologist if symptoms are not improving with treatment.

Individual Considerations

A. Pregnancy:

    1. Symptoms are usually worse in the third trimester.

B. Pediatrics:

    1. Diagnosing RLS can be difficult in children because of the child's difficulty describing symptoms, such as where it hurts, when and how often it occurs, and how long symptoms last.

    2. Pediatric RLS can sometimes be misdiagnosed as "growing pains" or attention deficit disorder.

    3. Families need advice on recommended hours of sleep and naps for age.

    4. Iron supplementation should be co-administered with vitamin C:

        a. Adolescents 12 years and older: Ferrous sulfate 65 mg of elemental iron per tablet, 1 to 2 tablets/d

        b. Children younger than 12: Ferrous sulfate 3 mg/kg/d of elemental iron to a maximum of 130 mg elemental iron daily

    5. Nonpharmacological interventions should be tried before moving to medications:

        a. Gabapentin is the first-line medication for children 6 years or older

        b. Benzodiazepines, clonidine, and dopamine agonists are medications used for RLS in children 6 to 18 years of age

C. Geriatrics:

    1. Symptoms progress with age. Other chronic diseases are also usually present; it can be difficult to pinpoint the diagnosis of RLS because of other chronic problems.

    2. Be alert to side effects of medications used for treatment for RLS (dizziness, somnolence, and dyskinesia). Perform a fall risk assessment when prescribing medications for RLS.

Resources

Restless Legs Syndrome Foundation: www.rls.org

National Sleep Foundation: https://www.sleepfoundation.org/

Bibliography

Heim, B., Djamshidian, A., Heidbreder, A., Stefani, A., Zamarian, L., Pertl, M. T., . . . Högl, B. (2016). Augmentation and impulsive behaviours in restless legs syndrome: Coexistence or association? *Neurology, 87* (1), 36–40. doi:10.1212/WNL.0000000000002803

Klingelhoefer, L., Bhattacharya, K., & Reichmann, H. (2016). Restless legs syndrome. *Clinical Medicine, 16* (4), 379–382. doi:10.7861/clinmedicine.16-4-379

Lee, C. S., Kim, T., Lee, S., Jeon, H. J., Bang, Y. R., & Yoon, I. Y. (2016). Symptom severity of restless legs syndrome predicts its clinical course. *American Journal of Medicine, 129*(4), 438–445. doi:10.1016/j.amjmed.2015.12.020

Ondo, W. G. (2019, May 20). Clinical features and diagnosis of restless legs syndrome and periodic limb movement disorders in adults. *UpToDate.* Retrieved from https://www.uptodate.com/contents/clinical-features-and-diagnosis-of-restless-legs-syndrome-and-periodic-limb-movement-disorder-in-adults

Picchietti, D. L. (2018, March 7). Restless legs syndrome and periodic limb movement disorder in children. *UpToDate.* Retrieved from https://www.uptodate.com/contents/restless-legs-syndrome-and-periodic-limb-movement-disorder-in-children

Suzuki, K., Miyamoto, M., Miyamoto, T., & Hirata, K. (2015). Restless legs syndrome and leg motor restlessness in Parkinson's disease. *Parkinson's Disease, 2015*, 490938. doi:10.1155/2015/490938

Seizures

Julie Adkins, Cheryl A. Glass, and Kimberly Waltrip

Definition

A. Epilepsy is a disease of the brain that is defined by any of the three following conditions, as identified by the International League Against Epilepsy (ILAE):

    1. At least two unprovoked (or reflex) seizures occurring more than 24 hours apart

    2. One unprovoked (or reflex) seizure and a probability of further seizures similar to the general recurrence risk (at least 60%) after two unprovoked seizures, occurring over the next 10 years

    3. Diagnosis of epilepsy syndrome

B. The ILAE's clinical definitions also state that epilepsy is considered to be resolved for individuals who had an age-dependent epilepsy syndrome but are now past the applicable age or those who have remained seizure-free for the past 10 years, with no seizure medications for the past 5 years.

C. The 2017 ILAE classification of epilepsies defines three seizure types:

    1. Focal onset:

        a. Focal awareness seizure (FWS)

        b. Focal impaired awareness seizure (FIAS)

        c. Focal motor seizure (FMS)

        d. Focal nonmotor seizure (FNMS)

        e. Focal to bilateral tonic–clonic seizure (FBTCS)

2. Generalized onset:
   a. Generalized tonic–clonic seizure (GTCS)
   b. Generalized absence seizure (GAS)
   c. Generalized motor seizure (GMS)
   d. Generalized epileptic spasm (GES)
3. Unknown onset (motor and nonmotor):
   a. Unknown-onset tonic–clonic seizure (UTCS)

D. Accurate classification of seizures is dependent on observations of witnessed seizures, full medical history including comorbidities, and clinical findings. The 2017 basic classification is based on where the seizure begins in the brain, level of awareness, and other features of seizures.

1. Focal-onset seizures—generally only in one area of the brain:
   a. Motor symptoms: Jerking (clonic), tense or rigid muscles (tonic), muscular limpness or weak (atonic), brief muscle twitching (myoclonus), or epileptic spams; may also have automatisms or repeated automatic movements such as clapping or rubbing hands, lip smacking or chewing, or running
   b. Nonmotor symptoms do not affect movement: Changes in sensation, emotions, cognition change, lack of movement (behavior arrest), or autonomic function changes (GI sensations, waves of heat or cold, goosebumps, racing heart rate)
2. Generalized motor seizures involve networks on both side of the brain at the onset:
   a. Motor seizures, generalized tonic–clonic: Seizure with stiffening and jerking; this loosely corresponds to "grand mal"
   b. Nonmotor seizures: Primarily absence seizures and correspond to the old term "petit mal"; involve brief changes in awareness, staring, and sometimes automatic or repeated movements like lip-smacking
3. Unknown-onset seizures may initially fall into the unknown onset category and later the seizure type becomes clear:
   a. Motor seizures are described as tonic–clonic or epileptic spasms.
   b. Nonmotor seizures include a behavior arrest: The movement stops, and the person may stare and not make any other movements.
4. Focal to bilateral seizure starts on one side or part of the brain and spreads to both sides.

E. Awareness: Whether a person is aware during a seizure is one of the main factors affecting a person's safety. Awareness is used instead of consciousness, because it is simpler to evaluate.

1. Focal aware: The person's awareness remains intact, even if they are unable to talk or respond during a seizure (previous term: simple partial).
2. Focal impaired awareness: Impaired or affected awareness at any time of the seizure, even if a person has a vague idea of what happened (previous term: complex partial seizure)

3. Awareness unknown: Unable to determine if a person is aware or not, such as an unwitnessed seizure
4. Generalized seizures: All presumed to affect a person's awareness or consciousness in some way. There are no special terms to describe awareness in generalized seizures.

F. Lennox–Gastaut syndrome (LGS) is a rare form of epilepsy consisting of multiple seizure types. It includes cognitive impairment and drop seizures. Clients with LGS may require antiseizure medications, steroids or immune globulin, vagus nerve stimulation (VNS), surgical resection, and ketogenic diet.

G. Eclampsia may occur anytime in pregnancy from the second trimester to the puerperium. It is notable for the occurrence of one or more generalized convulsions and/or coma in women with preeclampsia (in the absence of other neurological conditions):

1. Eclampsia is self-limited; delivery is the treatment.
2. The tonic–clonic seizure generally lasts 60 to 75 seconds.
3. Fetal bradycardia lasts 3 to 5 minutes, but does not necessitate an emergent cesarean section delivery. Compensatory fetal tachycardia and transient fetal heart rate decelerations occur. Delivery should be considered for the lack of improvement in 10 to 15 minutes after maternal/fetal resuscitative interventions.
4. Seizures caused by eclampsia generally resolve within a few hours to days postpartum. Hemolysis, elevated liver enzymes, low platelets (HELLP) syndrome develops in approximately 10% to 20% of women with preeclampsia/eclampsia.

H. Idiopathic seizures, gelastic seizures, dacystic seizures, posttrauma, and nonepileptic seizures are other types noted in the literature.

Incidence

A. Epilepsy is the fourth most common neurological disease and affects people of all ages. An estimated 3.4 million Americans are affected by epilepsy. There are 150,000 new cases of epilepsy every year. One in 26 people in the United States will develop epilepsy at some point in their lives.
B. Stroke is the leading cause of new-onset epilepsy in adults after age 65 years.
C. Eclampsia:
   1. Mild preeclampsia: 0.5%
   2. Severe preeclampsia: From 2% to 3%
   3. Forty-eight hours postpartum: Up to 33%
D. Photosensitivity seizures are more common in children and adolescents.

Pathogenesis

A. Epilepsy is a functional disorder of the brain in which neurons signal abnormally. The exact causes of epilepsy and eclampsia are unknown.

Predisposing Factors

A. Tumors
B. Alcohol/drugs

C. Cerebral infarction/stroke
D. Hypoglycemia
E. AD
F. Posttrauma (head injury)
G. Surgery
H. Pregnancy (eclampsia)
I. Febrile illness
J. Photosensitivity
K. Risk factors for recurrent seizures:
  1. Identifiable brain disease
  2. Mental retardation
  3. Abnormal neurological examination/EEG
  4. Seizures: Onset after age 10 years
  5. Multiple types of seizures
  6. Family history/genetics
  7. Poor response to AEDs/combination therapy at time of withdrawal
  8. Chronic alcoholism
L. Eclampsia risk factors:
  1. Nulliparous
  2. PIH
  3. Teens to lower 20s and again older than 35 years
  4. Other conditions to be ruled out:
    a. Stroke
    b. Hypertensive disease
    c. Space-occupying lesion
    d. Metabolic disorders (hypoglycemia, uremia, water intoxication)
    e. Meningitis or encephalitis
    f. Drug use (methamphetamine, cocaine)
    g. Idiopathic epilepsy
    h. Thrombotic thrombocytopenia purpura (TTP)
M. Breath holding in children

Common Complaints

A. Aura: Epigastric discomfort, fear, or unpleasant smells
B. Automatisms (swallowing, chewing, fumbling, picking clothes, or lip smacking)
C. Stiffening, then jerking of limbs
D. Staring with/without repetitive motor behaviors
E. Eclampsia:
  1. Headache: Severe or persistent frontal or occipital
  2. Blurred vision
  3. Photophobia
  4. Right upper quadrant pain/epigastric pain
  5. Altered mental status
  6. Nausea and vomiting
  7. Hyperreflexia

Other Signs and Symptoms

A. Lack of memory of seizure
B. Impaired consciousness
C. Postictal:
  1. Confusion
  2. Amnesia
  3. Fatigue
  4. Headaches
  5. Loss of urine or bowel control

> Seizures longer than 5 to 10 minutes require emergent care. If the client has a persistent headache after a rest period, unconsciousness with failure to respond, unequal pupil size or excessively dilated pupils, or weakness of the limbs, immediate medical attention is essential.

Subjective Data

A. Obtain a history from the client or a person who witnesses the seizure:
  1. Have the witness describe the duration, part of the body affected, and qualities of the seizure.
  2. Does the client have a recollection of the seizure?
  3. How long did it take to feel better after the seizure?
B. Evaluate if the client has ever had seizures, and ask whether this was an isolated event:
  1. Were there any warning symptoms before the seizure?
  2. What kind of warning was noted?
C. Did the client have a fever or an active/recent infection?
D. Do a thorough review of the client's medical history, including head injury, pregnancy, diabetes, and cancer.
E. Ask if there is a family history of seizures.
F. Take a full medication history, including OTC and herbal products:
  1. Is the client on an AED?
  2. Has the client missed any doses?
  3. When was the last blood level checked to evaluate therapeutic dosing?
G. Review alcohol intake. Alcohol interferes with the efficacy of AEDs.

Physical Examination

A. Check temperature (if indicated to rule out infection), blood pressure, and pulse.
B. Inspect:
  1. Assess LOC, orientation
  2. Perform a general overall examination for secondary injuries from fall or striking objects.
C. Auscultate:
  1. Lungs for possible aspiration
D. Palpate (if applicable for any injuries):
  1. Elevate neck for nuchal rigidity.
E. Neurological examination:
  1. CNs testing
    a. Wrinkle forehead, raise eyebrows.
    b. Smile and show teeth.
    c. Stick out the tongue/lateral tongue movement
    d. Ocular movements
    e. Visual field
    f. Finger-to-nose test
  2. Motor strength:
    a. Shrug shoulders
    b. Test muscle strength: Grasp hands and squeeze.
    c. Check reflexes of biceps, triceps, patellar, brachioradial, and Achilles tendon.
  3. Sensory testing: Pinprick
  4. Gait and posture

Diagnostic Tests

A. Diagnosis is confirmed by the client's history, witness accounts, neurological examination, blood work, and clinical testing such as EEG.

B. EEG is essential in all cases of undiagnosed transient loss of consciousness, especially in the elderly to rule out cardiac arrhythmias as the sudden loss of consciousness.

C. MRI is the gold standard for neuroimaging.

D. Blood glucose

E. Drug/alcohol screen

F. Serum level of anticonvulsant

G. LP if indicated for signs of infection/meningitis

Differential Diagnoses

A. Seizures

B. Brain tumor

C. CNS infection

D. Drug/alcohol use

E. Stroke/TIA

F. Hypoglycemia

G. Trauma

H. Migraine

I. Ménière's disease

J. Syncope:
   1. Long QT and cardiac syncope
   2. Reflex anoxic
   3. Orthostatic intolerance
   4. Hyperventilation
   5. Compulsive Valsalva maneuver
   6. Vasovagal

K. Psychogenic:
   1. Daydreaming/inattention
   2. Panic attacks
   3. Dissociative states
   4. Hallucination in psychiatric disorder
   5. Fabricated/factitious illness

L. Breath holding (children)

M. Sleep-related conditions:
   1. Sleep-related rhythmic movement disorders
   2. Hypnogogical jerks
   3. Parasomnias

Plan

A. General interventions:
   1. Emergency transport may be required. Seizures longer than 5 to 10 minutes require emergent care. If the client has a persistent headache after a rest period, unconsciousness with failure to respond, unequal pupil size or excessively dilated pupils, or weakness of the limbs, immediate medical attention is essential.
   2. Obtain a consultation with a neurologist for a thorough evaluation.
   3. States vary on the driving requirements/restrictions for clients with epilepsy. Individual state driving requirements are noted on the Epilepsy Foundation website: www.epilepsy.com/search/site/Seizure%20Severity%20 Questionnaire?f[0]=bundle%3Adriving_laws.
      a. A person with epilepsy has the risk of MVA while driving. It is considered similar or slightly higher than in clients with other medical conditions (diabetes, cardiovascular disease) and compares with the risk of MVA with persons with sleep apnea, alcoholism, dementia, and cellular phone use.
      b. Regulatory agencies, as a measure of driving risk, require having a seizure-free interval of 3 to 12 months (state dependent). In studies, the seizure-free interval was the strongest predictor of MVA.
      c. Clinicians must warn clients about possible driving risks after reduction of medications or missing AED doses and must consider the clients' neurological deficits other than seizures (e.g., cognition and visual field deficits) when making recommendations about driving. The risk factors for an MVA for persons with epilepsy are as follows:
         i. Medication noncompliance:
            1) Forgetting when to take the medication
            2) Drug schedule is too complicated
            3) Affordability
            4) Unable to get medications on time due to insurance restriction or mail-order delays
            5) Stopping medications against medical advice:
         ii. Recent history of alcohol or drug abuse
         iii. Uncorrectable brain function or metabolic disorder
         iv. Structural brain disease
         v. Frequent seizure recurrence after seizure-free intervals
         vi. Prior crashes caused by seizures

B. Client teaching:
   1. Keeping a seizure diary is extremely helpful in identifying seizure trends, maintaining drug compliance, monitoring side effects, and evaluating the need for changing the course of therapy. The frequency or time of day that seizures occur is used in the adjustment of AED dosage and timing of administration. The Epilepsy Foundation's self-management tool *My Seizure Diary* focuses on self-monitoring, tracking, and development of a response plan. The *My Seizure Diary* platform includes a fully responsive web application on diary.epilepsy.com as well as native mobile operating system and Android companion apps. The mobile operating system and Android companion apps are available from the online media library and online digital distribution service.
   2. Seizure triggers:
      a. Most common cause is missed AED dose and/or sudden discontinuation of medications
      b. Sleep deprivation

c. Alcohol/drug intake

d. Stress

e. Hormone fluctuations

f. Pregnancy

g. Photosensitivity/strobe or flashing light/intense lights

h. TV and video games (flicker frequency)

i. Contrasting visual patterns (grids, checkerboard, and stripes)

j. Computer monitors

k. Visual fire alarms

l. Sunlight shimmering off water/through trees/through window blinds

m. OSA

3. Review the importance of medication adherence:

a. Give oral and written dosing instructions.

b. Refill the prescription before running out.

c. Take the medication on a schedule (set a watch alarm, use a pill container, mark off the calendar). Taking an extra pill when a seizure aura occurs will not stop the seizure, as the medication is not absorbed fast enough.

d. New-prescription interaction profiles should be evaluated before starting new drugs.

e. Clients should not use supplements, herbals, or OTC medications without checking with their healthcare provider.

4. Excessive alcohol use (more than 3 drinks a day) increases the likelihood of seizures. Clients should have no more than 1 to 2 drinks a day.

5. Encourage the client to use a Medic Alert identification such as a bracelet or charm: https://www.medicalert.org/product/catalog/medical-ids/bracelets.

6. First aid for grand mal seizure:

a. Stay calm.

b. Time the seizure. Call 911 if the seizure lasts longer than 5 to 10 minutes.

c. Clear the area to prevent harm from surrounding objects.

d. Turn the person to the side and do not put anything in his or her mouth.

e. Do not hold the person down.

f. Place a soft object under the head to prevent head injury.

g. CPR is not necessary unless the person stops breathing after the seizure.

h. Stay with the person and reassure him or her.

i. Help get the person home; call family or friends.

j. Immediate transport to the emergency department is necessary for known conditions such as:

i. Diabetes/hypoglycemia

ii. Heat exhaustion

iii. Pregnancy

iv. Infection/high fever

v. Poisoning

vi. Head injury

7. First aid for generalized nonmotor seizures:

a. Stay calm.

b. Guide the client away from any dangers.

c. Block access to hazards.

d. Do not restrain the person.

e. Stay with the person until full awareness returns.

C. Pharmaceutical therapy:

1. There is controversy concerning whether to start AED therapy for the first seizure. AEDs are generally started after a second seizure.

2. The prescription of AEDs should be individually weighed with a risk-versus-benefit decision that includes factors such as age; gender; family planning/desire for pregnancy; current driver; type/recurrence of seizure; abnormal EEG; concurrent medications used for other comorbid conditions; history of depression, anxiety, suicidal ideation, and hepatic and renal disease; cost; client preference and lifestyle issues; and side-effect profile of medications (see Table 19.5).

3. A neurological consultation should be obtained for full evaluation and prescription of AED, with a neurologist or primary healthcare provider managing subsequent follow-up.

4. A single-agent AED is started and titrated slowly to the lowest dose that is the most effective in seizure control with the least number of side effects:

a. Ideally, the client should be maintained on one AED; however, combination therapy may be required or the first agent discontinued.

b. When a second AED is required, the second medication is started by titration, a therapeutic level is achieved, and the first AED is subsequently tapered off. During this period of time, there is an increase in side effects.

c. Switching to a generic formulation has been noted to increase seizure activity.

d. Rectal diazepam gel (Diastat) may be prescribed for use at home for clients with a history of prolonged seizures.

5. Cannabidiol (CBD) is used as an adjunctive therapy in the treatment of epilepsy, particularly in Dravet syndrome and LGS, and has been found to be superior to placebo in clinical trials. There are limited data available regarding the risk of rebound seizures following abrupt or rapid discontinuance of CBD treatment.

6. Stevens–Johnson syndrome (SJS) and toxic epidermal necrolysis (TEN) can occur up to 4 months after the institution of AEDs, including carbamazepine (Tegretol), oxcarbazepine (Trileptal), phenytoin (Dilantin), and lamotrigine (Lamictal).

7. Women should be routinely prescribed folate supplements of 0.4 to 0.8 mg/d. The folic acid recommendation is 4 mg/d for 1 to 3 months before conception when the client is on valproate or carbamazepine (Tegretol).

TABLE 19.5   ANTIEPILEPTIC MEDICATIONS

Generic (Brand Name)	Seizure Type	First-Line Treatment
ethosuximide (Zarontin)	Absence seizures	Adjunctive treatment
lacosamide (Vimpat)	Partial seizures	Adjunctive treatment
zonisamide (Zonegran)	Partial seizures	Adjunctive treatment
rufinamide (Banzel)	LGS	Adjunctive treatment
divalproex sodium (Depakote)	Absence seizures	First-line treatment
	Complex partial seizure	
phenytoin (Dilantin)	Tonic–clonic seizures	First-line treatment
	Psychomotor and neurosurgical-induced seizures	
felbamate (Felbatol)	Partial seizures LGS	Not first line in partial seizures and used as an adjunctive for LGS
tiagabine (Gabitril)	Partial seizures	Adjunctive treatment
levetiracetam (Keppra)	Partial onset seizures	Adjunctive treatment for all types of seizures
	Myoclonic seizures	
	Generalized tonic–clonic seizures	
clonazepam (Klonopin)	Absence seizures LGS	First-line treatment
	Myoclonic seizures	
lamotrigine (Lamictal)	Partial seizures LGS	First-line treatment for LGS
pregabalin (Lyrica)	Partial onset seizure	Adjunctive treatment
primidone (Mysoline)	Focal and psychomotor seizures; tonic–clonic seizures	Not first-line treatment
gabapentin (Neurontin)	Partial seizures	Adjunctive treatment
carbamazepine (Tegretol)	Partial or mixed seizures	First-line treatment
	Generalized tonic–clonic seizures	
topiramate (Topamax)	Partial onset seizures	First-line treatment and adjunctive for LGS
	Generalized tonic–clonic seizures LGS	
oxcarbazepine (Trileptal)	Partial seizures	Monotherapy or adjunct treatment
valproate	LGS	First-line treatment in LGS
magnesium sulfate (MgSO$_4$)	Eclamptic tonic–clonic seizure	First-line treatment

LGS, Lennox–Gastaut syndrome.

8. Other treatment includes neuromodulator devices utilized when AEDs do not control seizures. The neuromodulation device sends electrical stimulation to the brain's nerve cells:
   a. VNS therapy
   b. Responsiveness neurostimulation (RNS) therapy
   c. External trigeminal nerve stimulation (eTNS)

Follow-Up

A. Follow-up by primary healthcare providers depends on the frequency of seizures, toxicity profile of AED, and other comorbid conditions.

B. Subsequent visits include the following evaluations:
   1. Drug compliance
   2. Seizure log/diary:
      a. Epilepsy.com makes the Seizure Severity Questionnaire available for download for individual use by clients to describe their most common type of seizure: https://www.epilepsy.com/sites/core/files/atoms/files/ssq_0.pdf

   3. Drug concentrations, blood counts, and hepatic and renal function
   4. Premenstrual serum levels when there is an increase in seizure activity the week before menstruation
   5. Yearly drug levels are required for clients on a stable dose with no seizures.

C. There is an increased risk of suicide associated with several AEDs. Evaluation of the client 1 week after institution of therapy is prudent. Instructions should be given to notify the office concerning depression:
   1. Perform serial depression/suicide screening.
   2. Treat psychiatric comorbid conditions promptly.

D. Osteopenia and osteoporosis are noted with long-term therapy with AEDs; therefore, a dual-energy x-ray absorptiometry (DEXA) scan is warranted:
   1. Vitamin D and calcium may be prescribed with AEDs.
   2. Encourage weight-bearing exercises.

E. Clients taking AEDs need regular dental/oral care.

F. Each state has the legal prerogative to grant driving privileges. Clinicians cannot grant or suspend driving privileges:

1. Six states require clinicians to report their clients with seizures (California, Delaware, Nevada, New Jersey, Oregon, and Pennsylvania).

2. Some states require a letter sent to the Motor Vehicle Department stating, "My patient has seizures and has been advised not to drive."

3. All states require drivers with epilepsy or seizures to report their condition.

4. Commercial driving restrictions are stricter. Restrictions for commercial vehicles involved in intrastate commerce vary among individual states. The U.S. Department of Transportation (DOT) allows people with a history of epilepsy who have been seizure-free and off medication for 10 years to obtain a commercial driver's license (CDL).

G. Consider a sleep study to evaluate for OSA.

Consultation/Referral

A. A neurology consultation is necessary for the evaluation and medication initiation and the use of a ketogenic diet.

B. A neurosurgical consultation is necessary to evaluate a VNS or surgical options.

1. VNS has been approved for intractable epilepsy refractory to medications.

C. Refer to an obstetrician.

Individual Considerations

A. Pregnancy:

1. Preconception counseling and a planned pregnancy are imperative:

a. Discuss the teratogenicity of AEDs:

i. Attempt to decrease to monotherapy.

ii. Taper doses of AEDs to the lowest possible dose.

iii. If there is an absence of seizures for 2 to 5 years, consider a complete withdrawal of AEDs.

iv. First-trimester use of one AED has been associated with a two- to five-fold increase in major fetal anomalies such as neural tube defects, cleft lip and palate, and cardiac anomalies.

b. Increase folic acid to 4 mg/d to help prevent neural tube defects.

c. Stress the need for regular prenatal care.

d. Offer maternal alpha-fetoprotein screening test.

e. A fetal echocardiogram may be considered to diagnose cardiac defects.

f. All care providers, including nurses, pediatricians, and anesthesiologists, should be aware that the client has epilepsy on admission.

2. Oral contraceptives are less effective in clients on AEDs. The failure rate is 0.7 to 3.1 per 100 women. Women taking enzyme-inducing AEDs should use a backup method or alternative birth control. Enzyme-inducting AEDs include:

a. Dilantin (phenytoin)

b. Phenobarbital

c. Tegretol (carbamazepine)

d. Zarontin (ethosuximide)

e. Felbatol (felbamate)

f. Topamax (topiramate)

g. Trileptal (oxcarbazepine)

3. Estrogen and progesterone act on the temporal lobe, where partial seizures often begin. Seizure patterns may change during menopause.

B. Pediatrics:

1. A ketogenic diet may be prescribed under a physician's care.

C. Geriatrics:

1. Seizures are likely to begin from 60 to 80 years of age.

2. Management may be more difficult dependent on comorbidities and the use of other medications.

3. Older clients have an increased rate of falls and loss of independence.

4. After stroke and dementia, epilepsy is the most common serious neurological disorder in the elderly.

5. Focus on cardiovascular and neurological systems in the clinical physical evaluation in the elderly.

6. BEERS criteria include cautions about commonly prescribed AEDs in the elderly:

a. Phenytoin:

i. Most commonly prescribed AED in the elderly

ii. Use caution, as phenytoin interacts with digoxin and warfarin.

iii. Causes sedation

b. Sodium valproate:

i. Ataxia and tremor are not uncommon.

ii. Can cause reversible extrapyramidal symptoms

c. Carbamazepine:

i. Hyponatremia can occur, especially with coadministration of a diuretic.

ii. Increases warfarin metabolism

d. Lamotrigine:

i. Requires a slow titration in the elderly

e. Levetiracetam:

i. Mood and behavioral problems may occur.

f. Ginkgo biloba is the most commonly used herbal for seizures in the elderly.

Bibliography

Aleyadeh, W., Hutt-Centeno, E., Ahmed, H. M., & Shah, N. P. (2019). Hypertension guidelines: Treat patients, not numbers. *Cleveland Clinic Journal of Medicine, 86*(1), 47–46. doi:10.3949/ccjm.86a.18027

Epilepsy Foundation. (2019). *State driving laws.* Retrieved from https://www.epilepsy.com/search/site/driving?f[0]=bundle%3Adriving_laws

Epilepsy Foundation. (n.d.-a). *Diagnosis.* Retrieved from http://www.epilepsy.com/learn/diagnosing-epilepsy

Epilepsy Foundation. (n.d.-b). *Febrile convulsions (3 months to 5 years).* Retrieved from http://www.epilepsy.com/information/professionals/about-epilepsy-seizures/idiopathic-epileptic-seizures-and-syndromes-1

Epilepsy Foundation. (n.d.-c). *First aid for seizures.* Retrieved from http://www.epilepsy.com/learn/treating-seizures-and-epilepsy/first-aid/first-aid-resources

Epilepsy Foundation. (n.d.-d). *Injuries from seizures.* Retrieved from http://www.epilepsy.com/get-help/staying-safe/types-injuries

Epilepsy Foundation. (n.d.-e). *Photosensitivity and epilepsy.* Retrieved from http://www.epilepsy.com/learn/triggers-seizures/photosensitivity-and-seizures

Epilepsy Foundation. (n.d.-f). *Seizure provoking triggers.* Retrieved from http://www.epilepsy.com/learn/triggers-seizures

Epilepsy Foundation. (n.d.-g). *Seizures.* Retrieved from http://www.epilepsy.com/learn/types-seizures

Epilepsy Foundation. (n.d.-h). *Suicide risk.* Retrieved from http://www.epilepsy.com/article/2014/3/antiepileptic-drugs-and-suicidality

Epilepsy Foundation. (n.d.-i). *Treatment.* Retrieved from http://www.epilepsy.com/learn/treating-seizures-and-epilepsy

Seizure, Febrile (Child)

Julie Adkins, Cheryl A. Glass, and Kimberly Waltrip

Definition

Febrile seizures are the most common seizure of early childhood. The average age of onset is 3 months to 5 years of age. Febrile seizures are of short duration, usually less than 5 minutes, and are generalized tonic–clonic convulsions; 4% to 16% have focal features. The seizures are associated with fever in the absence of CNS infection, acute electrolyte imbalance, or any other defined cause for a seizure. Seizures lasting longer than 15 minutes require immediate medical attention. The majority of children with febrile seizures do not develop epilepsy.

There are two types of febrile seizures:

A. Simple febrile seizures are brief (less than 15 minutes) and generalized, and do not recur within a 24-hour period. More than 90% of febrile seizures are simple.

B. Complex febrile seizures have at least one of the following features: Duration lasting longer than 15 minutes, multiple seizures in 24 hours, and focal features:

    1. Complex febrile seizures may indicate meningitis, abscess, or encephalitis.

    2. A severe type of complete febrile seizure, febrile status epilepticus, is defined as a single seizure or series of seizures without interim recovery, lasting at least 30 minutes.

    3. The majority of seizures occur in children between the ages of 12 and 18 months, but can occur at any age.

Incidence

A. Two to five percent of the population of children up to the age of 5 years develop seizures with a febrile illness:

    1. The incidence in the world varies from 0.35% to 10%.

    2. Febrile seizures occur in all races. Approximately 35% of children have recurrent febrile seizures during subsequent illnesses. An estimated 24% of children have a family history of febrile seizures, and 4% have a family history of epilepsy.

B. Viral illnesses (e.g., roseola, gastroenteritis, influenza) are the predominant cause of febrile seizures.

C. The risk of febrile seizures has been noted to increase slightly after administration of the measles, mumps, rubella, varicella (MMRV) vaccine at age 12 to 15 months. The risk is increased approximately 5 to 12 days after the first MMRV vaccine is given. The risk is not higher in older children receiving a second dose of MMRV vaccine.

D. Although the risk is small, DTaP (diphtheria, tetanus, acellular pertussis)/IPV (polio)/Hib (*Haemophilus influenzae* type b) vaccination has been associated with an increased risk of febrile seizures on the days of the first and second vaccinations.

E. Risk of febrile seizure has been noted to increase the first 24 hours after receiving the trivalent inactivated influenza vaccine (IIV3) at the same time as the pneumococcal 13-valent conjugate (PCV13) vaccine or the DTaP vaccine. It was not shown to occur when vaccines are given separately on different days. There has been an increased risk of seizure when giving the PCV13 alone.

Pathogenesis

A. Fever is characterized by a cytokine-mediated rise in core temperature as well as immunological, neurological, endocrinological, and physiological changes. A febrile seizure is an abnormal electrical discharge of neurons in the cerebral cortex causing tonic–clonic muscular contractions, induced by fever in children.

B. Febrile seizures have been identified from a combination of genetic and environmental factors. They are linked to an autosomal dominant inheritance, and a few other genes and chromosomal loci have been identified.

Predisposing Factors

A. Fever:

    1. Temperature at least greater than 100.4°F (38.0°C). Most seizures occur with fever greater than 102.2°F (39°C).

    2. More likely to occur with the maximal rate of temperature rise

    3. May occur early or late in the course of the febrile illness

    4. May occur before fever is apparent

B. Family history of febrile seizures

C. Family history of seizures

D. Age:

    1. Occurs between 3 months and 5 years

    2. Median age of onset is 18 months.

E. Recent childhood immunizations

F. Other neurological abnormalities

G. Viral infections

H. Bacterial infections

I. Day care

Common Complaints

A. Fever

B. Generalized tonic–clonic seizure lasting less than 5 minutes

C. Staring and loss of muscle tone

D. Staring and muscle stiffness/rigidity

Other Signs and Symptoms

A. An altered state of consciousness after the seizure

B. Vomiting

C. Decreased feeding

Subjective Data

A. Ascertain whether the child had a fever at the time of the seizure.

B. Ask the caregiver to describe how the child appeared before the seizure: Lethargic, normal, or irritable.

C. Review what happened during the seizure: Jerky movements of one extremity, blinking, and general convulsions with loss of consciousness.

D. After the seizure, determine whether the child was very sleepy, confused, or normal.

E. Review what other symptoms, such as vomiting or diarrhea, the child has and what treatments have been given before presentation.

F. Note if this has ever happened before. If so, was it the same?

G. Assess the client's medical history and developmental course.

H. Review all prescription medications, OTC products, and recent immunizations. Specifically evaluate recent antibiotic use; partially treated meningitis must be considered.

I. Elicit information about any family history of any type of seizures.

J. Is anyone else in the family/day care ill?

Physical Examination

A. Check temperature, pulse, respirations, blood pressure, and pulse oximetry.

B. Inspect:

1. Observe overall appearance. Observe for seizure activity and LOC: Unable to arouse? If able to arouse, is the client having trouble staying awake?

2. Presence of difficulty breathing, grunting, and retractions

3. Presence and quality of crying: Weak, high-pitched, or continuous crying

4. Inspect the head for the presence of a bulging fontanelle (if applicable)

5. Evaluate the eyes for the presence of petechiae: Are they sunken?

6. Ears: Evaluate the tympanic membrane

7. Nasal examination for signs of sinusitis and nasal flaring

8. Oral examination for dry mucous membranes, erythema, and enlarged tonsils

9. Dermal examination: Evaluate for the presence of cyanosis and pallor; check skin tone and turgor; evaluate for the presence of a rash.

10. Nails: Check for prolonged capillary refill. A capillary refill of 3 seconds or greater is an intermediate risk for serious illness such as meningococcal disease.

11. Check for nuchal rigidity/stiffness.

C. Auscultate:

1. Heart

2. All lung fields for crackles and decreased breath sounds

3. All quadrants of the abdomen

D. Palpate:

1. Fontanelle (if applicable for age)

2. Evaluate lymphadenopathy.

3. Palpate the abdomen for masses, tenderness, and rebound.

E. Neurological examination:

1. Perform a complete neurological examination, assessing all CNs.

2. Be alert for signs and symptoms of CNS infection: Stiff neck, lethargy, and confusion are highly indicative of CNS infection. The neurological examination should be normal. Any abnormal neurological findings are inconsistent with febrile seizures.

Diagnostic Tests

A. Pulse oximetry

B. CBC

C. Blood chemistries are not indicated with febrile seizures unless electrolyte imbalance or other specific indications exist. Seizures that continue for more than 5 minutes should have electrolytes and glucose evaluated.

D. Urinalysis

E. EEG is not indicated for febrile seizures; however, if neurological signs are present or seizures are recurrent, an EEG and neurological workup should be done.

F. LP is indicated if there are positive neurological signs, especially in children 12 to 18 months and infants younger than 12 months who present after their first febrile seizure.

G. Consider chest x-ray for respiratory problems.

H. Consider stool cultures if indicated for diarrhea.

I. CT and MRI are not required for children with first simple febrile seizures. A CT scan should be considered with complex febrile seizures.

Differential Diagnoses

A. Febrile seizure

B. Shaking chills from fever

C. Metabolic imbalances: Hypoglycemia, hyponatremia, and hypomagnesemia

D. Syncope

E. CNS infection: Encephalitis, meningitis, and abscess

F. Epilepsy

G. Brain tumor

H. Trauma/EDH

I. Chemical ingestion

Plan

A. General interventions:

1. Tepid sponge baths have not been shown to be effective in preventing febrile seizures and are not recommended for treating fever.

2. Children with fevers should not be undressed or overwrapped.

3. Support the client with positioning to prevent aspiration; maintain the airway, and administer oxygen.

4. Do not try to pry the jaws open to place an object between the teeth.

B. Client teaching:

1. *See Section III: Client Teaching Guide for this chapter, "Febrile Seizures (Child)."* ◄

2. Advise the family that neurological sequelae, intellectual impairment, and behavioral disorders are rare following febrile seizures.

3. Advise parents that, if a child has a seizure, to lay the child on his or her side and do not try to restrict the child's movements or convulsions. Nothing should be placed in the mouth.

4. Recommend timing the seizure to see how long the seizure lasts. Seizures that last 5 minutes or longer need immediate attention, and the child should be taken to the emergency department by calling 911.

5. Never leave a child alone during a seizure.

C. Pharmaceutical therapy:

1. Antipyretic agents do not prevent febrile seizures and are not used for prophylaxis. Ibuprofen (Motrin) or acetaminophen (Tylenol), using age/weight-appropriate doses every 4 hours, may be given for temperature elevation of 104°F (37.9°C).

2. Antibiotics are not indicated for a fever without an apparent source.

3. The American Academy of Pediatrics' Committee on Quality Improvement and Management, Subcommittee on Febrile Seizures, concluded that on the basis of the risks and benefits of effective therapies, neither continuous nor intermittent anticonvulsant therapy is recommended for children with one or more simple febrile seizures.

Follow-Up

A. See the client for repeat seizures and as needed.

B. Seizures lasting longer than 15 minutes require immediate medical attention.

Consultation/Referral

A. Consult a neurologist for uncontrolled or repeated seizures. When no fever is present, it may signal the onset of epilepsy and the client should be referred. Children who have experienced prolonged febrile seizures are more likely to develop a particular type of epilepsy known as temporal lobe epilepsy (TLE).

B. When meningitis cannot be eliminated by history and physical examination, the child should be admitted to the hospital.

C. If seizures are continuous, this is a medical emergency. The client should be sent to the hospital immediately by ambulance, and a neurologist should be consulted.

Individual Considerations

A. Pediatrics:

1. Approximately 30% to 35% of children who have had one febrile seizure are at risk of having another seizure.

Bibliography

Duffy, J., Weintraub, E., Hambidge, S. J., Jackson, L. A., Kharbanda, E. O., Klein, N. P., . . . DeStefano, F. (2016). Febrile seizure risk after vaccination in children 6 to 23 months. *Pediatrics*, *138*(1), 1–12. doi:10.1542/peds.2016-0320

Jeong, J. H., Lee, J. H., Kim, K., Jo, Y. H., Rhee, J. E., Kwak, Y. H., . . . Noh, H. (2014). Rate of and risk factors for early recurrence in clients with febrile seizures. *Pediatric Emergency Care*, *30*(8), 540–545. doi:10.1097/PEC.0000000000000191

Leung, A. K., Hon, K. L., & Leung, T.N. (2018). Febrile seizures: An overview. *Drugs in Context*, *7*, 212536. doi:10.7573/dic.212536

National Institute of Neurological Disorders and Stroke. (2019, May 12). *Febrile seizures fact sheet*. Retrieved from https://www.ninds .nih.gov/Disorders/Patient-Caregiver-Education/Fact-Sheets/Febrile -Seizures-Fact-Sheet#3111_4

Smith, D. K., Sadler, K. P., & Benedum, M. (2019). Febrile seizures: Risks, evaluation, and prognosis. *American Family Physician*, *99*(7), 445–450. Retrieved from https://www.aafp.org/afp/2019/0401/p445.html

Tejani, N. R. (2018, December 18). Febrile seizures. *Medscape*. Retrieved from https://emedicine.medscape.com/article/801500-overview

Stroke

Jill C. Cash, Cheryl A. Glass, and Kimberly Waltrip

Definition

Strokes are a medical emergency. Treatment for HTN is effective in reducing incidence of stroke across all ages and populations and is a major component of primary and secondary stroke prevention.

A. Because of the aging population, it is estimated that by 2030 approximately 4% of the U.S. population will have had a stroke. The risk of having a stroke increases with age 65 and older and is especially prominent in the population age 80 years or older.

B. Strokes are the fifth leading cause of death for men, but the third leading cause of death in women

C. Strokes are the leading cause of disability in the United States:

1. Nearly half of stroke survivors have residual deficits, including weakness or cognitive dysfunction 6 months after stroke.

D. Stroke mortality varies by geographic location. The United States has a "Stroke Belt" in the southeastern states, including Georgia, North Carolina, and South Carolina. Within this Stroke Belt, the "buckle" region has an approximate 40% increased rate of strokes. The Pacific Northwest states also have high stroke mortality rates.

E. Types of stroke:

1. TIAs (see the "Transient Ischemic Attacks" section in this chapter)

2. Ischemic stroke: 87% of all cases:

    a. Cerebral thrombosis

    b. Cerebral embolism

3. Hemorrhagic stroke: 13% of stroke cases; intracerebral hemorrhage or SAH:

    a. Aneurysm

    b. AVM

Incidence

A. Incidence of stroke differs by gender, race, and ethnicity: Ischemic stroke is greater in Hispanics/Latinos and Blacks:

1. Hispanic women and men have the highest rates of diabetes, HTN, and obesity. Stroke is the third leading cause of death in Hispanic women. The average age for stroke among non-Hispanic Whites is 80 years of age; among Hispanics, it is 67 years of age.

2. African American men and women are more likely to have a stroke than any other population the United States. They are more likely to have strokes at a younger age and have more-severe strokes related to HTN, sodium intake, sickle cell anemia, smoking, obesity, and diabetes.

3. Stroke is the fifth leading cause of death in men, killing almost the same number of men each year as prostate cancer and AD combined in white males.

4. One in five women in the United States will have a stroke in her lifetime.

B. Nearly 60% of stroke deaths are in women; stroke kills twice as many women as breast cancer does.

1. Pregnancy-related HTN is the leading cause of both hemorrhagic and ischemic stroke in pregnant and postpartum women.

2. Presence of migraine with aura, contraceptive use, and smoking leads to a sevenfold higher odds of stroke in women.

C. One out of four people with stroke will have another stroke within 5 years.

D. History of stroke and/or TIA: Averages 10% yearly risk for a stroke.

E. The risk of a stroke within 90 days of a TIA may be as high as 17%, with the greatest risk during the first 7 days.

F. The rate of ischemic stroke in clients with Afib is 5% per year.

G. Hemorrhagic strokes account for 13% of strokes.

H. Brain AVMs occur in less than 1% of the general population and affect about one in 2,000 to 5,000 people. AVMs are more common in males than in females.

Pathogenesis

A. Ischemic strokes are a complication related to atherosclerotic deposits. Plaque builds up and occludes blood flow. The lack of blood flow to the brain causes ischemic changes. The symptoms exhibited depend on the location and severity of the ischemia. Ischemic strokes are also a complication of a cerebral embolism.

B. Hemorrhagic strokes are related to an aneurysm/rupture of a blood vessel or an AVM.

Predisposing Factors

A. Cardiac causes:
1. Afib: Increases risk for stroke fivefold
2. Mitral and aortic valve disease
3. Rheumatic heart disease
4. Atrial and ventricular septal defects
5. Carotid artery stenosis
6. Thrombosis
7. Embolism

B. Modifiable risk factors:
1. HTN
2. Smoking/exposure to smoke
3. Diabetes
4. Dyslipidemia
5. Obesity is an independent risk factor for stroke
6. Physical inactivity
7. Sickle cell disease

C. Nonmodifiable risk factors:
1. Age: The age of stroke onset is older for women, with the majority of events occurring after age 70.
2. Gender: Several factors increase the stroke risk for women:

    a. Pregnancy
    b. Preeclampsia/eclampsia: Twice the risk for stroke
    c. Hormone therapy (HT)
    d. Contraceptive use
    e. Migraine with aura

3. Race/ethnicity: Stroke risk is increased in Blacks and Hispanic/Latinos.

4. Family history/genetic predisposition: Inherited coagulopathies

D. TIA

E. Migraine with aura

F. Iatrogenic anticoagulation

G. Illicit drug use (i.e., cocaine or methamphetamines)

H. Postsurgical complications

I. Cerebral amyloidosis

Common Complaints

A. **Signs and symptoms depend on the affected vessel and surrounding brain tissue.**

B. Acute onset of focal neurological deficit:
1. Partial or total loss of consciousness
2. Headache: Often described as the worst headache ever)
3. Limb weakness or numbness
4. Contralateral hemiparesis
5. Facial weakness/drooping
6. Speech difficulty: Ranges from a total loss of speech to the inability to express and comprehend
7. Dysphagia: Ranges from an inability to chew and swallow to swallowing liquids that may lead to aspiration
8. Visual changes: Loss of vision, blurring, double vision
9. Ataxia

Other Signs and Symptoms

A. Cognitive changes
B. Behavioral changes
C. Nausea and vomiting
D. Fatigue
E. Seizures

Potential Complications

A. Long-term sequelae are dependent on the location and severity of the ischemia or hemorrhage.
B. Death

Subjective Data

A. Ask detailed questions about symptoms before, during, and after the incident:
1. Review the exact timing of onset of symptoms.
2. How intense were the symptoms?
3. What were the duration and the presence of any fluctuation of symptoms?
4. Has there been a pattern that is becoming more frequent or escalating in symptoms?

B. Interview the client, family members, witnesses, and emergency personnel for their description of behavior, speech, gait, memory, and movement.

C. Review the client's medical history:
1. Previous TIA or stroke
2. Previous/recent surgeries, specifically carotid or cardiac surgeries and any procedures such as coronary artery bypass graft (CABG) or stents
3. Afib
4. HTN
5. Pregnancy or recent delivery history
6. Migraine headaches
7. Seizures
8. CNS infection
9. Illicit drug use
10. Presence of any metabolic disorders
11. Recent trauma: Blunt or torsion injury to the neck
D. Focus on precipitating factors and state of consciousness after the acute event.
E. Review all medications, including anticoagulants, oral contraceptives, HT, OTC, and especially substances not prescribed, as well as illicit drugs such as cocaine.
F. Herbals that alter bleeding time and interact with warfarin:
1. Feverfew
2. Garlic
3. Ginkgo biloba
4. Ginger
5. Ginseng

Physical Examination

> Clients presenting with acute symptoms should be quickly assessed for the need to call emergency services (911) for immediate transport to the hospital. Time is of the essence for treatment with tissue plasminogen activator (tPA).

A. Check blood pressure, pulse, respirations, and pulse oximetry. Obtain weight and height so as to calculate BMI.
B. Inspect:
1. Observe overall appearance, LOC, ability to interact, language, difficulty swallowing, tremors, and spasticity, as well as memory skills.
2. Observe the client walking (cerebellar system).
3. Dermal exam:
    a. Overall hydration status
    b. Look for post-carotid endarterectomy scars, presence of a pacemaker, implantable cardioverter-defibrillator, or other cardiac surgical scars.
4. Check pupil size and reactivity to light.
5. Perform a funduscopic exam to evaluate optic disk margins, retinal plaques, and pigmentation. A "cherry red spot" may be evident in the macula in clients with central retinal artery occlusion.
C. Auscultate:
1. Heart for rate, rhythm, murmurs, or rubs
2. Lungs, noting respiratory rate and pattern
3. Carotid arteries for the presence of bruit
4. Abdomen for abdominal bruits for artery stenosis or aortic aneurysm
D. Palpate:
1. Palpate extremities for pulses and peripheral edema.

E. Neurological exam:
1. CN testing:
    a. Wrinkle forehead, raise eyebrows.
    b. Smile and show teeth.
    c. Stick out the tongue/lateral tongue movement.
    d. Ocular movements
    e. Visual field
2. Motor strength:
    a. Shrug shoulders.
    b. Test muscle strength: Grasp hands and squeeze.
    c. Check reflexes of biceps, triceps, patellar, brachioradial, and Achilles tendon.
3. Sensory testing: Pinprick
4. Gait and posture (cerebellar system evaluation):
    a. Ocular movements
    b. Gait
    c. Finger-to-nose test
    d. Heel-to-knee test

Diagnostic Tests

There is no "gold standard" for the diagnosis of CNS infarction.

A. CT scan
B. MRI
C. Other imaging:
1. Computed tomographic angiography (CTA) to look for abnormalities including aneurysm
2. Magnetic resonance angiography (MRA) to locate a large-vessel occlusion
3. Cerebral angiography/cerebral arteriography to locate size and location of blockages
4. Duplex Doppler studies
D. Laboratory tests:
1. Emergent labs:
    a. Glucose
    b. Serum chemistry profile
    c. Coagulation and hypercoagulability testing
    d. CBC
2. Urgent labs:
    a. ESR
    b. Cardiac enzymes
    c. Lipid profile
3. Other laboratory tests based on history:
    a. Urine drug screen
    b. Blood alcohol level
    c. Antiphospholipid antibodies
E. EKG to identify cardiac dysrhythmia

Differential Diagnoses

A. Cardiovascular accident:
    a. Ischemic stroke
    b. Hemorrhagic stroke
B. TIA
C. AVM
D. Aortic dissection
E. Thrombosis
F. CNS infection
G. Trauma
H. Brain tumor

I. Demyelination
J. Intoxication

Plan

A. General interventions:

1. Primary general care: Respiratory and cardiac care, fluid and electrolytes management, control blood glucose, stabilize blood pressure control, implement treatment for hyperthermia, and prevent systemic or bleeding complications.

2. Some clients will need sent to the emergency department immediately. Intravenous tissue plasminogen activator (tPA) must be given within 3 to 4.5 hours (specific to the client's comorbidities and history) of the time when symptoms first began.

B. Client teaching:

1. Therapeutic lifestyle changes (TLCs), including physical activity, diet, weight management, and smoking cessation, are recommended for all clients.

2. Physical activity:

a. All adults should avoid inactivity. Some physical activity is better than none, and adults who participate in any amount of physical activity gain some health benefits.

b. American College of Cardiology (ACC)/AHA guidelines on lifestyle management and physical activity recommendations advise adults to engage in 40 minutes of aerobic physical activity three to four times a week. The aerobic exercise should involve moderate-to-vigorous intensity to reduce blood pressure, low-density lipoprotein-cholesterol (LDL-C), and non-high-density lipoprotein-cholesterol (HDL-C).

c. Therapy or cardiac rehabilitation, at least on initiation of an exercise regimen, may be considered for individuals with disability after ischemic stroke.

C. Pharmaceutical therapy:

1. **Reperfusion therapy with the intravenous thrombolytic drug Alteplase IV recombinant tPA (r-tPA), utilized in the hospital setting, is considered the gold-standard treatment for ischemic stroke. Use of r-tPA to reduce the effects of stroke is time dependent. Treatment should be initiated as quickly as possible (within 3 hours of symptom onset). Delayed hospital arrival is the single most important reason for the failure to administer tPA within the window of 3 or 4.5 hours.**

a. The AHA/ASA 2018 Guidelines for the Early Management of Clients With Acute Ischemic Stroke recommend:

i. r-tPA to be initiated within 3 hours of symptom onset for medically eligible clients with an acute ischemic stroke; administration of r-tPA within 3 hours is equally recommended for clients <80 and >80 years of age.

ii. r-tPA can be initiated for medically eligible clients within 3 to 4.5 hours of acute symptom onset.

iii. In clients with acute ischemic stroke who have an unclear time and/or unwitnessed symptom onset and in whom treatment cannot be initiated within 4.5 hours of symptom onset, **the guidelines recommend against r-tPA therapy.**

iv. Prior to initiation of r-tPA, a noncontrast head CT and glucose are the only required tests. Centers should attempt to obtain a noncontrast head CT within 20 minutes of the client's arrival to the emergency department.

1) If the CT reveals an acute ICH, r-tPA should not be administered.

2) Clients with initial blood glucose levels < 50 mg/dL or > 400 mg/dL that are subsequently normalized may be treated with r-tPA if otherwise medically eligible.

2. Antiplatelet therapy is used for both the management of acute ischemic stroke and the prevention of stroke:

a. Aspirin (ASA) is the most commonly used antiplatelet therapy. Administration of aspirin is recommended in clients with acute stroke within 24 to 48 hours after stroke onset. For clients treated with IV tPA, aspirin administration is generally delayed for 24 hours:

i. High-dose aspirin: 150 mg to 325 mg/day

ii. Lower-dose aspirin: 75 to 100 mg daily

iii. Lower doses of aspirin are associated with milder GI symptoms and less GI hemorrhage

b. Clopidogrel (Plavix) 75 mg once daily as monotherapy

c. For clients with recently symptomatic atherosclerotic intracranial large-artery stenosis, dual platelet therapy with aspirin plus clopidogrel for 90 days, followed by antiplatelet monotherapy, is recommended:

i. Clopidogrel 300 mg loading dose, then 75 mg daily for 90 days, plus aspirin 75 mg daily for the first 21 days

ii. Dual antiplatelet therapy with aspirin and clopidogrel is not recommended for *stroke prevention.*

d. Dipyridamole as monotherapy or as dual therapy for secondary stroke prevention:

i. Immediate-release: 50 to 100 mg three times a day is not routinely recommended for secondary prevention of ischemic stroke.

ii. Aspirin plus extended-release dipyridamole 25 mg/200 mg twice a day is used as an alternative for clients intolerant to aspirin.

e. Ticlopidine 500 mg daily for secondary stroke prevention is not considered as a first-line antiplatelet therapy for stroke prevention because of cost and side effects. The most serious side effect/complication with ticlopidine is severe neutropenia, requiring biweekly to weekly CBCs for the first 3 months of therapy.

f. Cilostazol 100 mg twice a day. This phosphodiesterase 3 inhibitor is used mainly for intermittent claudication in clients with peripheral artery disease, but has also been found effective for preventing cerebral infarction in Asian ethnic groups. High-quality data are lacking regarding the use of cilostazol for secondary stroke prevention in non-Asian ethnic groups.

g. Long-term anticoagulant therapy is required for the secondary prevention of Afib (see Chapter 10, "Cardiovascular Guidelines," for an in-depth review of Afib). Note: The CHA_2DS_2-VASc score evaluates the risk of ischemic stroke in clients with Afib. To calculate a CHA_2DS_2-VASc score, go to http://clincalc.com/cardiology/stroke/chadsvasc .aspx In general, the lower the score, the stronger the consideration for oral anticoagulation is. The lone exception is when the client has a score of 1 due to gender alone.

3. Statin therapy with intensive lipid-lowering effects is recommended to reduce the risk of stroke and cardiovascular events among clients with ischemic stroke or TIA presumed to be of atherosclerotic origin and a LDL-C level ≥ 100 mg/dL with or without evidence for other clinical ASCVD (see Chapter 10, "Cardiovascular Guidelines," in the section "Atherosclerosis and Hyperlipidemia").

4. AHA/ACC initiate or resume blood pressure therapy for prevention and reoccurrence of TIA or ischemic stroke to achieve a systolic pressure less than 140 mmHg and a diastolic pressure less than 90 mmHg. The ideal target is not known, but a goal of less than 130/80 mmHg may be reasonable. (see Chapter 10, "Cardiovascular Guidelines," in the "Hypertension" section).

5. Further adjuvant therapy must be managed under the direction of a neurologist after a full evaluation.

D. Dietary management:

1. Advise the client that diet modification is the first line of therapy for hyperlipidemia.

2. Explain the cholesterol-lowering diet. Give the client dietary recommendation sheets. See Appendix B for low-fat/low-cholesterol and DASH dietary approaches to stop HTN.

3. Weight reduction:

a. Explain that weight reduction in clients who weigh more than 20% over their ideal body weight can lower LDL-C and triglyceride levels.

b. Start by setting small, realistic, attainable goals such as losing 5–10 pounds, which encourages successful attempts.

4. Other key dietary recommendations:

a. Counsel clients with a history of stroke or TIA to follow a Mediterranean-type diet instead of a low-fat diet. The Mediterranean-type diet emphasizes vegetables, fruits, and whole grains and includes low-fat dairy products, poultry, fish, legumes, olive oil, and nuts. It also limits intake of sweets and red meat.

b. Clients with ischemic stroke, TIA, or hemorrhagic stroke who are heavy drinkers should eliminate or reduce their consumption of alcohol. Limit intake of alcohol to light to moderate amounts. One drink per day for women and up to two drinks per day for men may be reasonable. Nondrinkers should be counseled not to start drinking.

c. Lower sodium intake. Consume no more than 2,400 mg/d of sodium. Further reductions to 1,500 mg/d of sodium are associated with greater reduction in BP. Even a modest reduction in salt intake for more than or equal to 4 weeks leads to a reduction in BP.

5. Healthcare providers should strongly advise every client with stroke or TIA who has smoked in the past year to quit. It is reasonable to advise clients after a TIA or ischemic stroke to avoid passive tobacco smoke. *See Section III: Client Teaching Guide "Nicotine Dependence."*

E. Surgery:

1. Mechanical thrombectomy

2. Carotid endarterectomy (CAE)

3. Carotid angioplasty and stenting (CAS)

4. Extracranial–intracranial (EC/IC) bypass

5. Endovascular stenting

6. Open surgical procedures, including vertebral artery endarterectomy and vertebral artery transposition

Follow-Up

A. Follow-up is determined by the client's needs, the severity of the stroke, and whether complications are present.

B. Cardiac rhythm studies for more than 24 hours should be considered for nonvalvular Afib (NVAF).

C. Sleep apnea is present in approximately half to three-fourths of clients with stroke or TIA. Consider a sleep study and treatment with continuous positive airway pressure (CPAP).

D. AHA/ASA recommend that clients with sickle cell disease and prior strokes/TIA have chronic blood transfusions to reduce hemoglobin S to less than 30% of total hemoglobin.

E. Evaluate for depression at each office visit.

F. Stroke rehabilitation may include:

1. ST

2. OT

3. PT

G. Rehabilitation sites include:

1. Rehabilitation facility

2. Skilled nursing facility (SNF)

3. Assisted living facility

4. Home

H. Identify area support groups for the client and/or caregivers.

I. Fitness for driving varies by state.

Consultation/Referral

A. Neurology

B. Cardiology, if applicable

C. Hematologist

D. Maternal–fetal medicine for high-risk pregnancy

Individual Considerations

A. Pregnancy:

1. Pre-pregnancy HTN increases the risk for PIH and stroke during pregnancy

2. The highest risk for stroke occurs in the third trimester of pregnancy and postpartum due to venous stasis, edema, and hypercoagulable state

B. Pediatrics:

1. Strokes may occur in neonates, infants, children, and young adults:

a. Infants and children: Incidence of stroke is 1.6 to 7.9 per 100,000 annually.

b. Incidence in young adults: 3.4 to 11.3 per 100,000 annually:

i. Higher incidence in boys than girls, and primarily in young Black adults

ii. Increased prevalence of risk factors for arterial ischemic stroke:

1) Genetic conditions

2) Congenital heart problems

3) Vasculopathies

4) Hematological conditions

5) Infections

6) Head and neck trauma

7) Smoking in younger adults

8) Increased use of illicit drugs

C. Women:

1. Women older than 85 years of age have one of the highest risks of ischemic stroke. The increased risk may be accounted for by women living longer than men.

2. Women have a higher rate of SAH as well as a higher risk of rupture.

3. Major risk factors for stroke in women are oral contraceptives, pregnancy, and HT.

4. Postmenopausal status:

a. Research indicates that natural menopause is not associated with a risk of stroke.

b. Women with hysterectomy with bilateral oophorectomy have a slightly elevated risk of total stroke compared with women with hysterectomy with ovarian conservation.

c. The 2014 AHA/ASA guidelines for prevention of stroke make the following HT recommendations for women:

i. HT, in the form of conjugated equine estrogen (CEE) with or without medroxyprogesterone, should not be used for primary or secondary prevention of stroke in postmenopausal women.

ii. Selective estrogen receptor modulators, such as raloxifene, tamoxifen, or tibolone, should not be used for primary prevention of stroke.

5. Women with asymptomatic carotid stenosis should be screened for other treatable risk factors for stroke; appropriate lifestyle changes and medical therapies should be instituted.

D. Men:

1. More men are diagnosed with diabetes than women, which increases men's risk for stroke.

2. Men commonly drink more alcohol than women, which increases their risk for stoke.

3. Only one in four men engages in daily exercise; not getting enough physical activity increases their risk for stroke.

4. Three of four American men are overweight or obese, which increases risk for stroke.

E. Geriatrics:

1. Worldwide, the elderly population is quickly growing. In the United States, geriatric clients 85 years of age or older constitute 2% of population; this proportion is predicted to double by 2060. Incidence of strokes doubles in octogenarians. making preventive measures a prominent focus for clinicians regarding the "very elderly."

2. Ten percent of intracerebral hemorrhages from cerebral amyloidosis occur in the elderly.

Resources

American Heart Association: https://www.heart.org/HEARTORG/GettingHealthy/GettingHealthy_UCM_001078_SubHomePage.jsp

American Stroke Association (formerly National Stroke Association): https://www.stroke.org/

Bibliography

Aleyadeh, W., Hutt-Centeno, E., Ahmed, H. M., & Shah, N. P. (2019). Hypertension guidelines: Treat patients, not numbers. *Cleveland Clinic Journal of Medicine, 86*(1), 47–46. doi:10.3949/ccjm.86a.18027

Bushnell, C., McCullough, L. D., Awad, I. A., Chireau, M. V., Fedder, W. N., Furie, K. L. . . . Walters, M. R. (2014). Guidelines for the prevention of stroke in women: A statement for healthcare professionals from the American Heart Association/American Stroke Association. *Stroke, 45*(5), 1545–1588. doi:10.1161/01.str.0000442009.06663.48

Centers for Disease Control and Prevention & National Center for Injury Prevention and Control. (n.d.). *Men and stroke.* Retrieved from https://www.cdc.gov/stroke/docs/Men_Stroke_Factsheet.pdf

Fox, C. (2019, July 9a). Ischemic stroke in children: Clinical presentation, evaluation, and diagnosis. *UpToDate.* Retrieved from https://www.uptodate.com/contents/ischemic-stroke-in-children-clinical-presentation-evaluation-and-diagnosis

Fox, C. (2019, July 9b). Ischemic stroke in children: Management and prognosis. *UpToDate.* Retrieved from https://www.uptodate.com/contents/ischemic-stroke-in-children-management-and-prognosis

George, A. (2018, May 2). Acute stroke in sickle cell disease. *UpToDate.* Retrieved from https://www.uptodate.com/contents/acute-stroke-in-sickle-cell-disease

Jauch, E. C. (2017, September). Acute management of stroke. *Medscape.* Retrieved from http://emedicine.medscape.com/article/1159752-overview#a8

Medic Alert Foundation. (2019). *Medical ID bracelets.* Retrieved from https://www.medicalert.org/product/catalog/medical-ids/bracelets

Powers, W. J., Rabinstein, A. A., Ackerson, T., Adeoye, O. M., Bambakidis, N. C., Becker, K. . . . Tirschwell, D. L. (2018). 2018 guidelines for the early management of patients with acute ischemic stroke, a guideline for healthcare professionals from the American Heart Association/American Stroke Association. *Stroke, 49*, e46–e99. doi:10.1161/STR.0000000000000158

Silver, B. (2019, May 3). Stroke prevention. *Medscape.* Retrieved from https://emedicine.medscape.com/article/323662-overview

Strouse, J. J., Lanzkron, S., & Urrutia, V. (2011). The epidemiology, evaluation and treatment of stroke in adults with sickle cell disease. *Expert Review in Hematology, 4*(6), 597–606. doi:10.1586/ehm.11.61

U.S. Burden of Disease Collaborators. (2018). The state of U.S. health, 1990–2016: Burden of diseases, injuries, and risk factors among U.S. states. *Journal of the American Medical Association, 319*(14), 1444–1472. doi:10.1001/jama.2018.0158

Transient Ischemic Attack

Julie Adkins, Cheryl A. Glass, and Kimberly Waltrip

Definition

A. TIAs are brief focal brain deficits, spinal cord issues, or retinal ischemia (without acute infarction) caused by vascular occlusion. **TIAs are a medical emergency.**
B. Symptoms generally last less than an hour; however, they may have permanent sequelae. TIAs are a risk factor for recurrent risk of stroke. Approximately 15% of diagnosed strokes are preceded by TIAs. TIAs can be difficult to diagnose, as symptoms are transient. Assume that all stroke-like symptoms signal an emergency.
C. **Presence of neurological deficit suggests a stroke rather than a TIA.**

Incidence

A. The prevalence of TIAs in the United States is between 200,000 and 500,000 per year. The population prevalence is about 2.3%, or approximately 5 million Americans.
B. The early risk of stroke is approximately 5% at 2 days after a TIA, and as high as 11% at day 7 after a TIA.
C. The risk of a stroke within 3 months of a TIA is 10% to 15%.
D. The risk of death from coronary artery disease and stroke is as high as 6% to 10%, depending on other risk factors. More than one-third of those who have a TIA will have a major stroke within a year if risk factors are not addressed.
E. More men (101/100,000) than women (70/100,000) are affected. An increased number of Black adults are affected by TIAs (98/100,000) compared to White adults (81/100,000).

Pathogenesis

A. The pathogenesis is a neurological event secondary to a temporary reduction of blood flow to the brain from a partially occluded vessel or related to an acute thromboembolic event.

Predisposing Factors

A. HTN:
    1. Systolic blood pressure greater than 140 mmHg
    2. Diastolic blood pressure greater than 90 mmHg
B. Atherosclerosis
C. African American
D. Age older than 40 years
E. Hypotensive episodes
F. Oral contraceptives/HT
G. Afib
H. Smoking
I. Familial hyperlipidemia
J. Diabetes mellitus
K. Valvular heart disease
L. Infective endocarditis
M. Migraine with aura
N. Common nutraceuticals that alter bleeding time and interact with warfarin:
    1. Feverfew
    2. Garlic
    3. Ginkgo biloba
    4. Ginger
    5. Ginseng
O. Drugs that interact with warfarin can be found at https://www.drugs.com/drug-interactions/warfarin.html.

Common Complaints

Signs and symptoms depend on the affected vessel and surrounding brain tissue.
A. Acute onset of focal neurological deficit:
    1. Limb weakness or numbness
    2. Facial weakness
    3. Speech difficulty, ranging from mild to aphasia
    4. Visual loss/blurring
    5. Ataxia
B. Acute change in LOC or confusion
C. Posterior circulation TIAs: Headache may be one of the prodromal symptoms that precedes a stroke by days or weeks.
D. Basilar artery occlusion TIAs: Vertigo, nausea, and headaches may occur as early as 2 weeks or more before the onset of stroke.

Other Signs and Symptoms

A. Dysarthria
B. Dysphagia
C. Near syncope
D. Hemiparesis
E. Temporary monocular blindness
F. Behavior changes
G. Difficulty with balance and vertigo
H. Dizziness
I. Diplopia

Subjective Data

If a TIA is suspected, call 911; symptoms of a TIA and a major stroke are not always distinguishable.
A. Ask detailed questions about symptoms before, during, and after the spell:
    1. Review the exact timing of onset of symptoms.
    2. How intense were the symptoms?
    3. What was the duration and the presence of any fluctuation of symptoms?
    4. Has there been a pattern that is becoming more frequent or escalating in symptoms?
B. Interview the client, family members, witnesses, and emergency personnel for their description of behavior, speech, gait, memory, and movement.
C. Focus on precipitating factors and state of consciousness after the acute event.
D. Question the client about risk factors such as HTN, smoking, cardiac disease, and heredity.
E. Review all medications, including anticoagulants, OTC, herbals, and illicit drug use such as cocaine.

F. Review the medical history:
1. Recent surgeries, specifically carotid or cardiac surgeries
2. Seizures
3. CNS infection
4. Illicit drug use
5. Presence of any metabolic disorders
6. Recent trauma (blunt or torsion injury to the neck)
7. Afib
8. Migraine headaches

Physical Examination

A. Check temperature (if an infectious process is suspected), pulse, respiration, and blood pressure, including orthostatic blood pressure and pulse, and pulse oximetry.
B. Inspect:
1. Observe overall appearance, LOC, ability to interact, language, difficulty swallowing, tremors, spasticity, and memory skills.
2. Observe the client walking (cerebellar system).
3. Dermal examination:
   a. Overall hydration status
   b. Look for post–carotid endarterectomy scars, presence of a pacemaker, implantable cardioverter-defibrillator, or other cardiac surgical scars.
4. Check pupil size and reactivity to light.
5. Perform a funduscopic examination to evaluate optic disk margins, retinal plaques, and pigmentation.
C. Auscultate:
1. Heart for rate, rhythm, murmurs, or rubs
2. Lungs, noting respiratory rate and pattern
3. Carotid arteries for the presence of bruit
4. Abdomen for abdominal bruits signaling artery stenosis or aortic aneurysm
D. Palpate:
1. Extremities for pulses and peripheral edema
E. Neurological examination:
1. CN testing:
   a. Wrinkle forehead, raise eyebrows.
   b. Smile and show teeth.
   c. Stick out the tongue, lateral tongue movement.
   d. Ocular movements
   e. Visual field
2. Motor strength:
   a. Shrug shoulders.
   b. Test muscle strength: Grasp hands and squeeze.
   c. Check reflexes of biceps, triceps, patellar, brachioradial, and Achilles tendon.
3. Sensory testing: Pinprick
4. Gait and posture (cerebellar system evaluation):
   a. Ocular movements
   b. Gait
   c. Finger-to-nose test
   d. Heel-to-knee test

Diagnostic Tests

A. Pulse oximetry
B. Laboratory tests:
1. Emergent labs:
   a. Glucose
   b. Serum chemistry profile, including creatinine
   c. Coagulation and hypercoagulability testing
   d. CBC
2. Urgent labs:
   a. ESR
   b. Cardiac enzymes
   c. Lipid profile
3. Other laboratory tests based on history:
   a. Urine drug screen
   b. Blood alcohol level
   c. Antiphospholipid antibodies
   d. RPR for syphilis
C. MRI or CT scan within 24 hours of symptom onset
D. Carotid Doppler ultrasonography identifies clients with urgent surgical needs.
E. Cardiac imaging to evaluate cardioembolic sources
F. EKG to evaluate dysrhythmias (such as Afib)
G. LP to rule out infection, demyelinating disease, and SAH
H. EEG as indicated for seizure activity
I. Consider cardiac Holter monitor for suspected intermittent Afib

Differential Diagnoses

A. TIA
B. Ischemic stroke
C. SAH/SDH
D. Migraine
E. Hypoglycemia/hyperglycemia
F. Epilepsy—postictal period
G. Malignant HTN
H. Brain tumor
I. Bell's palsy
J. MS
K. Syncope
L. Drug induced
M. Concussion
N. Vertigo

Plan

A. General interventions:
1. Carefully assess the client to diagnose TIA on a timely basis.
2. Perform a full workup to determine the underlying disease process.
3. Prevent stroke through modification of risk factors.
B. Client teaching:
1. *See Section III: Client Teaching Guide for this chapter, "Transient Ischemic Attack."* ◀
C. Pharmaceutical therapy: **The mainstay of treatment for TIA is pharmacological management with antithrombotic agents:**
1. Antiplatelet therapy:
   a. Aspirin 50 to 325 mg/d: **Aspirin should not be administered concomitantly with coumarin anticoagulants.**
   b. Dipyridamole (Persantine) 200 mg/d; may be given as an adjunct with warfarin therapy.

c. Aspirin + dipyridamole extended release (Aggrenox) 25/200 mg twice a day

d. Clopidogrel (Plavix) 75 mg/d:

i. Aspirin is not routinely recommended with clopidogrel because of the risk of hemorrhage.

ii. No dosage adjustment is necessary with clopidogrel for elderly clients or clients with renal disease.

e. Ticlopidine (Ticlid) 250 mg twice a day is a second-line antiplatelet therapy for clients who cannot tolerate or do not respond to aspirin therapy. In some circumstances, it can be an alternative to clopidogrel.

f. Warfarin (Coumadin) 5 to 15 mg; titrate for a goal international normalized ratio (INR) of 2.0 to 3.0.

2. Antihypertensive therapy as indicated to maintain blood pressure below 140/90 mmHg with an angiotensin-converting enzyme (ACE) inhibitor or an angiotensin receptor blocker alone or in combination with a diuretic.

3. Initiate a daily statin to achieve a goal of LDL-C less than 100 mg/dL.

D. Medical and surgical management:

1. Treat TIAs with antiplatelet drugs as soon as intracranial bleeding is ruled out.

2. Consider carotid endarterectomy.

3. Lipid control

4. Glucose control

5. Smoking cessation

6. Eliminate or reduce alcohol consumption.

7. Start an exercise plan for losing weight. Recommend starting with about 30 minutes of exercise three times per week as tolerated.

Follow-Up

A. Rapid transfer is essential for a client with positive symptoms for risk stratification.

B. Clients with a suspected TIA who are not admitted to the hospital should have rapid access (within 12 hours) for an urgent assessment and evaluation with CT or MRI brain scan, EKG, and carotid Doppler testing.

C. Clients managed in the outpatient setting should be fully educated about the need to return to the clinic or emergency department immediately if symptoms recur.

D. Specific follow-up depends on etiology, severity, frequency, and duration of TIAs.

E. Follow-up laboratory testing as indicated (e.g., CBC, cholesterol, prothrombin time, and INR. [PT/INR])

F. Monitor the client for occult bleeding if started on antiplatelet, antithrombic medications.

Consultation/Referral

A. TIA should be viewed as a medical emergency because these clients have salvageable neurological function; consult with a physician.

B. Cardiology and neurology consultations should be obtained when cardioembolic TIAs are treated with anticoagulation therapy.

C. Ophthalmological consultation is indicated to assess the nature of transient visual symptoms.

D. Vascular surgeon consultation is necessary for clients with significant stenosis or occlusion. Clients with symptomatic carotid artery stenosis should have a surgical evaluation immediately.

Individual Considerations

A. Pediatrics: TIA etiologies in children include:

1. Congenital heart disease with cerebral thromboembolism

2. Drug abuse (e.g., cocaine)

3. Clotting disorders

4. CNS infection

5. Marfan disease

6. Tumor

B. Adults:

1. TIAs that occur in the younger adult population should be evaluated for embolism.

2. Anticoagulation is not recommended for women younger than 65 years of age with Afib who are otherwise at low risk for stroke. Antiplatelet therapy is recommended for this population.

C. Geriatrics:

1. TIAs are most commonly seen in this population.

2. Screen for Afib in women, especially those older than 75 years of age.

3. Assess swallowing function of geriatric clients following a TIA event, especially in clients with cognitive impairment. Implement preventive measure for aspiration pneumonia and choking when eating/drinking.

Resources

The ABCD2 Score for TIA estimates the risk of a stroke after a TIA: https://www.mdcalc.com/abcd2-score-tia

The National Institutes of Health Stroke Scale (NIHSS) is a stroke scale that evaluates the effect of an acute cerebral infarct. The 15-item stroke scale requires less than 10 minutes to complete.

- Online training certification course for NIHSS: https://www.stroke.org/nih-stroke-scale/

- Online NIHSS: https://www.mdcalc.com/nih-stroke-scale-score-nihss

Bibliography

Aleyadeh, W., Hutt-Centeno, E., Ahmed, H. M., & Shah, N. P. (2019). Hypertension guidelines: Treat patients, not numbers. *Cleveland Clinic Journal of Medicine, 86*(1), 47–46. doi:10.3949/ccjm.86a.18027

Fox, C. (2019, July 9a). Ischemic stroke in children: Clinical presentation, evaluation, and diagnosis. *UpToDate*. Retrieved from https://www.uptodate.com/contents/ischemic-stroke-in-children-clinical-presentation-evaluation-and-diagnosis

Fox, C. (2019, July 9b). Ischemic stroke in children: Management and prognosis. *UpToDate*. Retrieved from https://www.uptodate.com/contents/ischemic-stroke-in-children-management-and-prognosis

Jauch, E. C. (2017, September). Acute management of stroke. *Medscape*. Retrieved from http://emedicine.medscape.com/article/1159752-overview#a8

Nanda, A. (2016). Transient ischemic attack. *Medscape*. Retrieved from http://emedicine.medscape.comarticle/1910519-overview

Schünemann, H. J., Cushman, M., Burnett, A. E., Kahn, S. R., Beyer-Westendorf, J., Spencer, F. A., . . . Wiercioch, W. (2018). American Society of Hematology 2018 guidelines for management of venous thromboembolism: Prophylaxis for hospitalized and nonhospitalized medical patients. *Blood Advances*, 2(22), 3198–3225. doi:10.1182/bloodadvances.2018022954

Vertigo

Julie Adkins, Jill C. Cash, Cheryl A. Glass, and Kimberly Waltrip

Definition

A. Vertigo is the illusion of self or environmental movement, typically rotating, spinning, tilting, even a sensation that one is going to fall down. Older clients have an increased risk of falls and depression secondary to vertigo.

B. Vertigo is often classified as either central or peripheral in origin.

Incidence

A. Approximately 5% to 10% of the general population experience dizziness, vertigo, and imbalance. Incidence reaches up to 40% in clients older than 40 years.

B. Approximately 0.5% of the population consults a primary healthcare provider each year regarding vertigo.

C. Both sexes, as well as all age groups, are affected.

D. Benign paroxysmal positional vertigo (BPPV) is the most common cause of vertigo, excluding CNS lesions:

1. The prevalence of BPPV is 2.4%.

2. BPPV rarely occurs in people younger than 35 years unless there is a history of head trauma.

3. BPPV recurs in approximately one-third of clients after 1 year and in about 50% in all clients treated after 5 years.

E. About 20% of clients with migraines experience vertigo, motion sickness, and mild hearing loss.

Pathogenesis

A. Distinguishing between peripheral and central vertigo is critical because the evaluation, treatment, and progress vary significantly. Central vertigo suggests brainstem dysfunction affecting the vestibular nuclei or their connections. This may be secondary to a structural lesion such as a neoplasm or ischemia.

B. Vertigo due to vascular insufficiency is rarely isolated; instead, other symptoms of brainstem involvement are usually also seen, such as diplopia, dysphagia, motor weakness, or disruption in sensation. Neoplasms are usually slow growing, and the vestibular dysfunction is often insidious.

C. Central vertigo secondary to brainstem or cerebellar ischemia usually lasts for 20 minutes to 24 hours. The client may be unable to ambulate during acute attacks of vertigo. Other considerations for causes of central vertigo include MS, seizures, and migraines.

D. Vertigo of peripheral origin is more common and may be caused by dysfunction of the inner ear or vestibular nerve. The most commonly diagnosed peripheral vestibular disorder is BPPV, yet its cause is unknown. The most common explanation is free otoconia within the semicircular canals that are dislodged by trauma, infection, or degeneration. The debris relocates when the head is repositioned and provokes vertigo. Causes of labyrinthine dysfunction include infection, trauma, ischemia, or toxins such as drugs or alcohol.

E. Ménière's disease causes vertigo, hearing loss, and ringing of the ears. The exact cause is unknown, but a hypothesis is a buildup of fluid in the inner ear.

F. Viral infections may lead up to vestibular neuritis (labyrinthitis). The vertigo experienced with vestibular neuritis is sudden and severe and may last days.

G. Other possible causes of vertigo are psychogenic, cardiovascular, metabolic, head trauma, and migraines.

H. Medications that cause dizziness:

1. Anticonvulsants
2. Antidepressants
3. Antipsychotics
4. Anxiolytics/sedatives
5. Antihypertensives
6. Nitrates
7. Diuretics
8. Insulin/oral hypoglycemic agents

Predisposing Factors

A. Head or body movement:

1. Rolling over in bed
2. Getting out of bed
3. Bending down from the waist
4. Looking up

B. Fear or anxiety

C. Stress

D. Recent infection, usually upper respiratory in cases of vestibular neuronitis

E. Family history, especially in cases of vertiginous migraine

F. Head trauma

G. Migraines

H. Idiopathic with no cause identified

I. Hypoglycemia

J. Alcohol intoxication

K. Medication side effects

L. Cerebellar or brainstem stroke

M. Tumors

N. MS

O. Dehydration

Common Complaints

A. Dizziness with or without change in body positioning

B. Nausea/vomiting

C. Tinnitus

D. Aural fullness

E. Hearing loss

Other Signs and Symptoms

A. Central origin, including vascular insufficiencies, strokes, neoplasms, migraine, MS, seizures:

1. Double vision
2. Dysarthria
3. Dysphagia
4. Paresthesias
5. Changes in motor or sensory examination
6. Mild to moderate vertigo

7. Multiple episodes of vertigo lasting seconds to minutes in duration with vascular insufficiency and seizures

8. Constant complaints of vertigo with neoplasms or strokes

9. Multiple episodes of vertigo lasting hours with migraines

10. Single episodes of vertigo with MS

11. Dix–Hallpike test: Habituation is common with delayed nystagmus

B. Peripheral origin, including BPPV, Ménière's disease, labyrinthitis, vestibular dysfunction, vestibular neuritis, and acoustic neuroma:

1. No associated signs of brainstem dysfunction

2. Vertigo, usually described as severe

3. Multiple episodes of vertigo lasting hours with Ménière's disease

4. Single or multiple episodes of vertigo with labyrinthitis

5. Vestibular dysfunction, described as constant vertigo

6. Severe nausea or vomiting

7. Hearing loss or tinnitus; aural fullness may be present, as well as a roaring sound.

8. Triad of vertigo, tinnitus, and hearing loss is suggestive of Ménière's disease.

9. Dix–Hallpike test: No habituation; nystagmus occurs immediately.

Subjective Data

A. Elicit onset, frequency, duration, and course of presenting symptoms:

1. Is this recurrent or new?

a. Acute vertigo is seen with trauma, stroke, meningitis, otitis media, mastoiditis, drug use, vestibular neuronitis, MS, and labyrinthitis.

b. Recurrent vertigo is seen in migraines, BPPV, motion sickness, seizures, and Ménière's disease.

B. Elicit from the client a verbal description of the sensation(s) experienced. Ask the client to describe the symptoms by using words other than "dizzy." The word "dizzy" is nonspecific; alternative descriptions may include light-headedness, unsteadiness, motion imbalance, spinning, floating, or a tilting sensation.

C. Note triggering and alleviating factors.

D. Query the client regarding associated symptoms such as hearing loss, tinnitus, nausea, difficulty with gait, aural fullness, or other neurological manifestations such as nystagmus.

E. Ask the client if he or she has ever fallen down as a result of the dizziness when symptoms are present.

F. Review the client's past medical history, including recent infections; trauma; risk factors for cardiovascular disease such as smoking, diabetes, and hyperlipidemia.

G. Review OTC medications, herbal products, and medication use: Aminoglycosides, antibiotics, diuretics, antihypertensives, and antidepressants.

H. Has the client had any previous treatments for vertigo, such as an Epley procedure?

I. Has the client had any previous testing?

1. Audiometric testing

2. Electronystagmogram (ENG)/videonystagmography (VNG) to evaluate balance

3. Rotational/balance platform test

4. CT or MRI

5. Computerized dynamic posturography (CDP) to evaluate postural stability/motor control

Physical Examination

A. Check temperature (if infection is suspected), pulse, respirations, and blood pressure; note orthostatic hypotension.

B. Inspect:

1. Observe overall appearance.

Generalized muscle weakness may be observed.

---

2. Note gait: Difficulty with tandem gait. Note global weakness.

3. Inspect the eyes: Assess for nystagmus; a few beats of nystagmus on extreme lateral gaze may be normal.

4. Ear examination: Rule out otitis media.

5. Evaluate for aphasia, which may indicate a stroke.

C. Auscultate:

1. Auscultate the heart, neck, and carotid arteries: **Physical examination may reveal cardiovascular abnormalities such as a carotid bruit.**

2. Auscultate the lungs: Deep inspirations may cause dizziness.

3. Auscultate the abdomen.

D. Palpate:

1. Extremities; note pulses and edema.

E. Neurological examination:

1. Perform a complete neurological examination.

2. Perform Rinne and Weber's test.

3. Assess CNs: **Brainstem involvement is frequently seen with a detailed neurological examination. Signs of cerebellar dysfunction include difficulty with finger-to-nose testing, rapid alternating supination or pronation of hands, and gait disturbance.**

4. Perform Romberg test: The client stands with feet together and closes his or her eyes. A positive result is when the client sways. This may be seen with vestibular disease and acoustic neuroma.

5. The Dix–Hallpike test (also called the Nylen–Bárány maneuver test) is a provocative positional test. Perform the Dix–Hallpike test: While the client is seated on the middle third of the examination table, turn the client's head 45° toward the affected side (problem ear). While holding the head in that position, assist the client to the reclining position past the supine position. There is a distinctive nystagmus with BPPV, in which involuntary eye movement (predominantly in a rotating fashion) begins slowly, progresses

to a fast phase, and then enters a resetting phase. The nystagmus generally lasts less than 20 seconds and reverses itself upon the client sitting upright.

   a. Use caution when performing the Dix–Hallpike test with clients who have cervical stenosis, severe kyphoscoliosis, spinal cord injuries, and significant vascular disease such as vertebral artery stenosis.

6. Test for nuchal rigidity if fever is present.

> The Dix–Hallpike maneuver is considered the gold standard for diagnosing BPPV. However, a negative test does not rule out BPPV if the client is asymptomatic on the date of the test. If a positive response is observed on the initial side, no further testing is required.

Diagnostic Tests

A. Laboratory testing:
   1. Thyroid function studies: To rule out hypothyroidism
   2. VDRL: To rule out secondary or early tertiary syphilis, which can have symptoms similar to Ménière's disease
   3. CBC: To rule out infection or severe anemia
   4. Electrolytes: To rule out hyponatremia, hypokalemia, and dehydration
   5. Urine drug screen (if indicated)
   6. Cardiac panel (if indicated)
   7. Urinalysis to rule out a UTI in the elderly
B. CT scan for head trauma
C. MRI with and without contrast to assess for mass, especially if a central origin is suspected
D. Bithermal caloric test: The definitive procedure for identifying vestibular pathology. Cold irrigation is an inhibitory stimulus; warm irrigation is an excitatory stimulus. The three most important findings from the caloric tests are unilateral weakness, bilateral weakness (peripheral vestibular disease), and failure of fixation suppression (FFS) of caloric-induced nystagmus (central cerebellar disease).
E. Electronystagmography: Most useful in chronic peripheral disorders to determine the degree and progression of vestibular deficit
F. Audiogram: Test for possible hearing loss.
G. Rotating chair test: Interprets the slow component velocity of the nystagmus response with bilateral canals stimulated
H. LP if meningitis is suspected

Differential Diagnoses

A. Vertigo
B. Vascular insufficiencies
C. Stroke
D. Neoplasms
E. Migraine
F. MS
G. Seizures
H. BPPV
I. Ménière's disease
J. Labyrinthitis
K. Vestibular dysfunction
L. Vestibular neuritis
M. Acoustic neuroma
N. Syncope
O. Multiple sensory defects
P. PD
Q. Adverse reaction to medications

Plan

A. General interventions: Treatment of vertigo depends on the underlying pathology and duration of the symptoms:
   1. Acute vertigo: Maintain the client on bed rest, with the reassurance that most clients with acute vertigo recover spontaneously over a period of several weeks to months.
   2. Chronic vertigo: Refer the client for PT with emphasis on vestibular rehabilitation:
      a. The Cawthorne Cooksey physical exercise regimen encourages eye, head, and body movements to facilitate recalibration of the vestibulo-ocular and vestibulospinal reflexes.
      b. Encourage ambulation when tolerated to induce the central compensatory mechanism.
   3. Ménière's disease: The client needs bed rest in the acute phase and nutritional therapy, with restrictions of sodium, caffeine, alcohol, and tobacco.
   4. BPPV:
      a. The client needs bed rest for acute symptoms.
      b. Canalith repositioning procedures (CRP) provide immediate resolution of vertigo in 85% to 95% of clients. Epley procedure: The CRP is safe, simple, inexpensive, quick, and easy to perform. It is likely to be unsuccessful in clients with bilateral positional nystagmus, and it is not recommended for clients with acute vertigo, many of whom may have vestibular neuronitis. See Section II: Procedure, "Canalith Repositioning (Epley) Procedure for Vertigo." Contraindications to performing the Epley procedure are:
         i. Recent neck fracture or neck instability
         ii. A history of unstable carotid disease
         iii. Recent retinal detachment
         iv. Any physical condition that prevents the client from lying down quickly or rolling over as required for the procedure
      c. As an alternative, meclizine may be used for 1 to 2 weeks, and then the client is reassessed. Stop meclizine on the day the client returns; it may suppress the positional nystagmus.
      d. For clients with severe positional vertigo during the Dix–Hallpike maneuver, premedicate with a prochlorperazine (Compazine) 25 mg suppository 1 hour before performance of the CRP.
      e. If the Dix–Hallpike test is positive on the left, use a left-sided CRP. Conversely, if it is positive on the right, use a right-sided CRP. If the client has bilateral disease, refer the client to an otolaryngologist or treat the more symptomatic side first.

f. After the Epley procedures, different types of recommendations are made to prevent the otoconia from returning to their posterior semicircular canal:

    i. Wear a cervical collar for two nights after the maneuver.

    ii. Stay upright for 24 hours after the procedure or have the head elevated 30° for one to two nights after the procedure.

    iii. Avoid sleeping with the affected ear down.

    iv. Counsel the client to avoid abrupt head changes for 1 week after the procedure.

    v. Avoid exercise, such as yoga and sit-ups, that would make similar motions.

    vi. Avoid looking up, such as looking at items on the top shelves at the grocery.

    vii. Symptoms may reoccur after tilting backward in dental chairs.

    viii. Symptoms may reoccur after turning in the hairdresser's chair and/or tilting backward for a shampoo.

B. Client teaching:

  1. Encourage compliance with bed rest and exercises.

C. Pharmaceutical therapy: **The American Academy of Otolaryngology—Head and Neck Surgery does not recommend the use of vestibular suppressant medications to control BPPV. The American Academy of Neurology also reports that there is no evidence to support the routine use of vestibular suppressant therapy as treatment for BPPV.**

  1. Antihistamines prevent the histamine response in sensory nerve endings and blood vessels that are affected when treating vertigo:

    a. Meclizine (Antivert)

    b. Dimenhydrinate (Dramamine)

  2. Benzodiazepines: Diazepam (Valium, Diastat)

  3. Phenothiazine derivative to treat emesis:

    a. Promethazine (Phenergan, Promethegan)

    b. Prochlorperazine (Compro)

  4. Beta-adrenergic agonists: Ephedrine

  5. Anticholinergic agents:

    a. Glycopyrrolate (Robinul, Cuposa)

    b. Scopolamine (transdermal)

  6. Ménière's disease:

    a. Diuretics such as hydrochlorothiazide and triamterene (Dyazide) together will help with vertigo, but may not reduce hearing loss.

    b. TCAs may be used in resistant cases.

  7. Antivirals are not useful for treatment of vestibular neuritis.

  8. Steroids have been used in the treatment of vestibular neuritis.

  9. Vestibular migraines respond to antimigraine medications.

D. Surgery:

  1. Pneumatic equalization tubes

  2. BPPV surgery: Canal partitioning or canal plugging

  3. Vestibular nerve section (vestibular neurectomy) is a treatment for intractable violent episodes of BPPV.

  4. Labyrinthectomy to remove the semicircular canals, utricle, and saccule—the balance organs. This procedure is considered only when a client has already lost all hearing function in the affected ear.

  5. Chemical labyrinthectomy: Gentamicin infusion destroys the vestibular hair cells.

Follow-Up

A. The American Academy of Otolaryngology—Head and Neck Surgery Foundation recommends managing clients with BPPV as follows:

  1. CRP/Epley procedure should be offered unless there is a risk for impaired mobility or balance or the client is at increased risk of falls.

  2. Clients should be reevaluated in 1 month after an Epley procedure/CRP to confirm that the procedure resolved the symptoms of vertigo.

  3. The recurrence rate after an Epley procedure is 30% to 50%.

B. Follow up as needed according to the origin of the diagnosis and the client's needs.

C. If indicated, transfer to the emergency department/call 911 for cardiovascular and cerebrovascular symptoms for treatment of stroke or cardiac events.

Consultation/Referral

A. Refer the client to a physician if the client does not experience improvement in 2 to 4 weeks. If symptoms worsen, consider referring the client to an ear, nose, and throat specialist.

B. Refer the client to an otolaryngologist for testing:

  1. Audiometric testing

  2. ENG to evaluate balance

  3. Rotational/balance platform test

C. Occupational and physical therapists are helpful in addressing home safety and providing a structured balance-rehabilitation program.

Individual Considerations

A. Pediatrics:

  1. The most common causes of dizziness in children are otitis media, migraine headaches, and BPPV.

  2. Concussion: Nausea, vertigo, and nystagmus are classic symptoms of a concussion.

  3. Drug overdoses and other poisons cause vertigo and nystagmus.

B. Geriatrics:

  1. Normal aging affects degeneration of neural structures that manage balance performance and equilibrium. Disequilibrium is one of the most frequent complaints from geriatric clients to their healthcare providers; vestibular disorders account for 48% of dizziness reported.

  2. Possible etiologies for vertigo in the elderly:

    a. CNS: Vestibular neuritis, late-onset Meniere's disease, TIA/stroke, vestibular migraine

b. Cardiovascular: Arrhythmia, CHF, heart valve disease, postural hypotension, occluded anterior vestibular artery

c. Age-related disorders: Presbystasis, labyrinthitis, breast/prostate neoplasia, musculoskeletal disorders, somatosensory, and proprioception losses

3. Vestibular abnormalities may mimic stroke/TIA symptoms and must be further explored to determine the appropriate treatment. Vertigo and balance dysfunctions have improved with pharmacological treatments and PT.

4. Evaluate need for an assistive device.

5. **Many of the medications used for vestibular suppression, individually and especially in combination, are on the American Geriatrics Society's Beers Criteria list of potentially inappropriate medications for older adults:**

a. Medications include antihypertensives, benzodiazepines, antiepileptics, and hypnotics/anxiolytics.

b. Review all medications for side-effect profiles and consider deprescribing.

Resources

American Speech–Language–Hearing Association (ASHA): https://www.asha.org/

Vestibular Disorders Association: https://www.vestibular.org

Bibliography

American Academy of Neurology Professional Association Model Policy. (n.d.). *Canalith repositioning procedure (CRP)*. Retrieved from https://www.aan.com/uploadedFiles/Website_Library_Assets/Documents/3.Practice_Management/1.Reimbursement/1.Billing_and_Coding/5.Coverage_Policies/Coverage%20Policies%20-%20Canalith.pdf

American Academy of Otolaryngology—Head and Neck Surgery. (2018, August). *Ménière's disease*. Retrieved from https://www.enthealth.org/conditions/menieres-disease/

Vestibular Disorder Association. (n.d.[a]). *Benign paroxysmal positional vertigo (BPPV)*. Retrieved from http://vestibular.org/understanding-vestibular-disorders/types-vestibular-disorders/benign-paroxysmal-positional-vertigo

Vestibular Disorder Association. (n.d.[b]). *Ménière's disease*. Retrieved from http://vestibular.org/menieres-disease

Vestibular Disorder Association. (n.d.[c]). *Surgical procedures for vestibular dysfunction*. Retrieved from http://vestibular.org/understanding-vestibular-disorders/treatment/vestibular-surgery

Vestibular Disorder Association. (n.d.[d]). *Vestibular neuritis and labyrinthitis*. Retrieved from http://vestibular.org/labyrinthitis-and-vestibular-neuritis

20 Endocrine Guidelines

Addison's Disease

Jill C. Cash and Mellisa A. Hall

Definition
A. Primary adrenal insufficiency resulting in glucocorticoid and mineralocorticoid insufficiency

Incidence
A. Approximately 40 to 60 cases per million people; idiopathic autoimmune disease is more common in women and children. There is no racial predilection.

Pathogenesis
A. Autoimmune dysfunction of the adrenals accounts for up to 80% of cases; 10% to 20% of cases are attributed to tuberculosis. At least 90% of the adrenal gland is destroyed, resulting in chronic cortisol deficiency, reduced aldosterone, and decreased adrenal androgens. As a result, volume and sodium depletions occur with potassium excess. The risk of death in clients with Addison's disease is twofold that of the general population due to higher rates of cardiovascular disease (CVD), cancer, and infectious disease.

Predisposing Factors
A. Other autoimmune disorders:
   1. Insulin-dependent diabetes mellitus (IDDM)
   2. Pernicious anemia
   3. Thyroid disorders
B. Disseminated tuberculosis
C. Gonadal failure
D. Hypoparathyroidism
E. Vitiligo
F. Alopecia areata
G. Chronic active hepatitis
H. Metastatic disease (especially lung and breast cancer)
I. AIDS
J. Certain medications (e.g., ketoconazole, anticoagulant)
K. Fungal disease
L. Bleeding diathesis (e.g., disseminated intravascular coagulation [DIC])

M. Sepsis
N. Metabolic stress
O. Trauma
P. Bilateral nephrectomy
Q. Pituitary tumors

Common Complaints[a]
A. Weakness
B. Fatigue
C. Anorexia
D. Nausea
E. Diarrhea
F. Abdominal pain
G. Weight loss
H. Hyperpigmentation
I. Hypoglycemia (more often in children)
J. Low libido
K. Salt craving

Other Signs and Symptoms
A. Proximal muscle weakness
B. Failure to gain weight (children)
C. Muscle and joint pain
D. Reduced axillary/pubic hair in women
E. Amenorrhea
F. Hypotension
G. Anemia with:
   1. Lymphocytosis
   2. Eosinophilia
   3. Neutropenia
   4. Hyponatremia
   5. Hyperkalemia
   6. Hypoglycemia
   7. Hypercalcemia
H. Positive antiadrenal antibodies
I. Low plasma cortisol or failure to rise after corticotropin (adrenocorticotropic hormone [ACTH]) administration
J. EKG changes: decreased voltage, prolonged PR and QT intervals, and general slowed rhythm

---

a   Usually presenting as insidious and nonspecific.

> Missed or delayed diagnosis can lead to acute adrenal crisis, a medical emergency evidenced by sudden low back, abdominal, or leg pain; severe vomiting or diarrhea; hypotension; and loss of consciousness.

> Plasma ACTH level differentiates among primary (adrenal) and secondary (pituitary) or tertiary (hypothalamus) etiologies (high plasma ACTH with primary insufficiency whereas normal or low with secondary insufficiency). The clinician can use ACTH–corticotropin-releasing hormone (CRH) to distinguish between pituitary and hypothalamic etiologies.

Subjective Data

A. Determine the extent of fatigue.
B. Elicit degree and location of weakness.
C. Question the client regarding appetite, nausea, or diarrhea.
D. Evaluate food intake.
E. Determine the amount of weight loss or weight gain (children).
F. Discuss hypopigmentation or hyperpigmentation and whether it occurs on unexposed areas as well as exposed areas of the skin.
G. Note the presence of abdominal, muscle, and joint pain.
H. Assess for light-headedness and/or fainting and when it occurs.
I. Inquire about the client's history of cancer or fungal infections.
J. Note last date of tuberculosis evaluation (purified protein derivative [PPD]) and results.
K. Determine HIV status or risk.
L. For women, discuss pubic and axillary hair distributions and note menstrual patterns.
M. Inquire about libido.
N. Inquire regarding cold intolerance.
O. Ask about recent illness and treatments.
P. Determine client's occupation to assess safety risk if weakness or dizziness present.

Physical Examination

A. Check pulse, respirations, and blood pressure (BP); pulse and BP while seated and standing; and weight.
B. Inspect:
   1. Observe overall appearance.
   2. Note hair distribution and skin pigmentation, especially sun-exposed surfaces.
C. Auscultate:
   1. The heart, lungs, and abdomen
D. Palpate:
   1. The abdomen
E. Musculoskeletal: perform complete musculoskeletal examination

Diagnostic Tests

A. Serum chemistry, electrolytes, blood urea nitrogen (BUN), creatinine, glomerular filtration rate (GFR)
B. Complete blood count (CBC)
C. PPD
D. Rapid ACTH test: Rapid ACTH stimulation test excludes or establishes adrenal insufficiency but does not differentiate between primary and secondary adrenal insufficiencies. With abnormal results (plasma cortisol <18–20 mcg/dL) proceed to plasma ACTH levels.
E. Plasma ACTH level
F. Serum creatinine kinase (CK) levels

G. Antiadrenal antibodies: A negative adrenal antibody test is observed in only 30% to 50% of persons with idiopathic Addison's disease and does not rule out adrenal insufficiency of autoimmune etiology.
H. CT scan of adrenals

Differential Diagnoses

A. Secondary adrenal insufficiency (usually after exogenous glucocorticoid therapy)
B. Hypothalamic/pituitary lesions
C. Diabetic coma
D. Salt-losing nephritis
E. Acute infections
F. Occult cancer
G. Anorexia nervosa
H. Hemochromatosis
I. Acute poisoning
J. Myasthenia gravis
K. Pigmentation due to racial/ethnic variations
L. Premature primary ovarian failure
M. Testicular failure
N. Pernicious anemia
O. Cancer
P. Iatrogenic Cushing's syndrome

Plan

A. General interventions:
   1. If primary adrenal insufficiency is established, and the cause is not apparent, order adrenal CT scan to look for metastatic disease, sarcoidosis, and tuberculosis.
B. Client teaching:
   1. *See Section III: Client Teaching Guide for this chapter, "Addison's Disease."* ◀
   2. Teach the client regarding adrenal crisis and encourage treatment before symptoms begin.
   3. Encourage the client to avoid contacts that predispose him or her to infections.
C. Pharmaceutical therapy:
   1. Hydrocortisone (drug of choice) or prednisone in three doses (every 8 hours), or two-thirds in the morning and the remainder in the afternoon or early evening; 12 to 15 mg cortisol/m^2 body surface area. Most adults need a total of 20 to 30 mg/d.
   2. Increase hydrocortisone dose or add prednisone if ill. If accompanied by diarrhea, excessive sweating, or fever, the client should double the routine dose.
   3. Simultaneously decrease fludrocortisone about 50% to avoid salt retention and elevated BP.
      a. Total daily stress dose is about 100 to 400 mg hydrocortisone.

4. If serum aldosterone is undetectable, mineralo-corticoid replacement is likely necessary in addition to glucocorticoid.

5. Abrupt discontinuation of exogenous glucocorticoid administration after a course as short as 3 weeks may induce temporary secondary adrenal insufficiency, leading to decreased cortisol but normal or near-normal aldosterone production. This insufficiency may occur up to 12 months after discontinuation of glucocorticoid therapy.

6. Pediatrics:

   a. Treat adrenal enzyme defects with hydrocortisone 10 to 20 mg/m²/d in three divided doses: 25% in morning and afternoon and 50% at night

   b. Fludrocortisone acetate typically 0.05 to 0.2 mg/d every day or two divided doses

Follow-Up

A. Plasma renin activity: When less than 10 ng/mL, this is a probable indication of adequate fludrocortisone dose.
B. Serum and urinary cortisol and serum ACTH to monitor hydrocortisone dose. Urinary-free cortisol greater than 70 mcg/24 hr indicates excessive hydrocortisone dose, whereas values less than 20 mcg/24 hr indicate inadequate hydrocortisone dose.
C. Monitor BP and serum electrolytes to determine fludrocortisone dose.
D. Do annual adrenal function studies.

Consultation/Referral

A. If Addison's disease is suspected, consult with a physician.
B. Consider Addison's disease in any client with unexplainable hypotension and hyperkalemia.

Individual Considerations

A. Pregnancy:
   1. Due to changes in plasma cortisol, diagnosis is based on lack of rise in plasma cortisol concentration after ACTH administration.
   2. If nausea and vomiting are problems, intramuscular glucocorticoid may be necessary.
   3. Delivery requires increased glucocorticoid dose similar to surgery.
B. Pediatrics:
   1. Leading causes of Addison's disease are hereditary enzymatic defects resulting in congenital adrenal hyperplasia (CAH), as well as idiopathic causes.
   2. Although rare in pediatrics, common presentations include malaise, nausea, vomiting, and weight loss. Poor vascular tone, hyperpigmentation, hyponatremia, hyperkalemia, and ketonemia are classic findings.
   3. Medications should be adjusted with the child's growth.
C. Geriatrics:
   1. Urinary excretion rate of cortisol decreases by about 25%; serum level and response to ACTH stimulation are unchanged.

Safety consideration: Clients receiving long-term replacement should carry a medication card as well as wear a medical alert bracelet or necklace. Parenteral therapy is required if clients are unable to take required replacement medication orally.

Bibliography

Donohoue, P. A. (2017, November). Treatment of adrenal insufficiency in children. *UpToDate*. Retrieved from http://www.uptodate.com

Lee, A. (Ed.). *NPPR: Nurse practitioners' prescribing reference.* (2019). New York, NY: Haymarket Media. Retrieved from https://www.empr.com/

Nieman, L. K. (2017, May). Diagnosis of adrenal insufficiency in adults. *UpToDate*. Retrieved from http://www.uptodate.com

Nieman, L. K. (2018, October). Treatment of adrenal insufficiency in adults. *UpToDate*. Retrieved from http://www.uptodate.com

Prescriber's Letter. (2019, March). Consider the new Beer's criteria when prescribing meds for older adults. Retrieved from https://prescriber.therapeuticresearch.com/Content/Articles/PRL/2019/Mar/Consider-the-New-Beers-Criteria-When-Prescribing-Meds-for-Older-Adults

Cushing's Syndrome

Jill C. Cash and Mellisa A. Hall

Definition

A. Cushing's syndrome is a cluster of symptoms, signs, and biochemical abnormalities arising from glucocorticoid overproduction. It is depicted by an increase of ACTH from the anterior pituitary, which stimulates the adrenal glands to release an overproduction of cortisol. Iatrogenically induced Cushing's syndrome is the most common cause (e.g., inadvertently induced from medications, treatments, or diagnostic tests).

Incidence

A. Two to four new endogenous cases per 1,000,000 are diagnosed annually; it is five times more frequent in women. Cushing's syndrome is usually diagnosed 3 to 6 years after its onset, and occurs more often in women between 50 and 60 years old.

Pathogenesis

The cause is exogenous (chronic glucocorticoid or ACTH administration) or endogenous (increased ACTH secretion). The endogenous type is due to either excessive pituitary or ectopic ACTH secretion (ACTH dependent), resulting in signs of androgen excess or autonomous cortisol overproduction (ACTH independent [of ACTH regulation]), as well as depressed ACTH production and absent signs of androgen excess. The etiology of spontaneous Cushing's (adults) comprises:
A. 70% to 80% pituitary ACTH hypersecretion (90% pituitary adenoma, 10% pituitary hyperplasia)
B. 10% to 15% autonomous adrenal tumor (adenoma or carcinoma)
C. 5% to 15% ectopic ACTH secretion (nonpituitary neoplasm, usually lung)
D. Less than 1% bilateral nodular hyperplasia without ACTH.

Among children younger than 12 years, the cause is usually iatrogenic. Cortisol excess precipitates generalized protein catabolism, reduced intestinal calcium reabsorption, elevated hepatic gluconeogenesis and glycogenosis, impaired collagen production leading to atrophy of connective and fatty tissues, impaired immune and inflammatory responses, and accelerated atherosclerosis.

Predisposing Factors

A. Exogenous glucocorticoid administration (oral, inhaled, injected, topical)
B. Megestrol acetate use
C. Excessive alcohol intake
D. Pituitary adenoma
E. Thoracic tumors
F. Adrenal neoplasms
G. Tumors of the pancreas
H. Thyroid and thymus disease
I. Pheochromocytoma

Common Complaints

A. Excessive coarse hair on face, chest, and back
B. Rapid weight gain
C. Easy bruising
D. Muscle weakness
E. Oligo- or amenorrhea
F. Impotence or decreased libido
G. Depression
H. Poorly controlled diabetes
I. Irregular menses
J. Resistant hypertension in young adults
K. Osteoporosis in young adults

Other Signs and Symptoms

A. Cervicodorsal "buffalo hump" and supraclavicular fat pad
B. Hirsutism in women
C. Acne and/or folliculitis
D. Increased intraocular pressure
E. Purple striae
F. Increased BP
G. Polydipsia/polyuria, increased serum glucose, and glycosuria
H. Osteopenia/osteoporosis
I. Mood lability/changes
J. Growth deceleration (children)
K. Delayed skeletal maturation (children)
L. Spontaneous hypokalemia
M. Erythrocytosis
N. Round face
O. Bruising

Subjective Data

A. Ask whether the client has taken exogenous glucocorticoids.
B. Determine whether the onset of complaints was acute or subacute.
C. Assess for bruising and determine whether bruising was precipitated by trauma.
D. Assess for muscle weakness and, if present, whether it is proximal weakness.
E. Review the client's menstrual history, including characteristics of menstrual periods.
F. Identify the client's family history of similar problems.
G. Question the client regarding any vision impairment.
H. Rule out the presence of abdominal pain.
I. Review the client's history of neoplasms and location.
J. Identify the current pattern of sexual function.
K. Question the client regarding mood swings or recent treatment for psychiatric disorder.
L. Identify the pattern of weight gain and effectiveness of weight-loss interventions, if implemented.
M. Assess for the presence of leg or arm pain.
N. Review the client's history of fractures, especially if postmenopausal.
O. Determine the amount of alcohol consumed.
P. Ask about the history of high BP readings.

Physical Examination

A. Check BP, pulse, height, and weight. Compare serial BP readings.
B. Inspect:
    1. Inspect the skin, noting hair distribution, lesions, bruising, and striae.
    2. Observe the face and note shape.
    3. Observe the neck.

Note that a "moon-shaped" face and fat pads in posterior neck ("buffalo hump") are characteristics of clients with Cushing's syndrome.

---

    4. Complete a funduscopic examination. Be alert for cataracts, glaucoma, and/or signs of benign intracranial hypertension.
C. Auscultate:
    1. Auscultate the heart and lungs.
    2. Hypercoagulable state should be considered with risk for pulmonary embolism.
D. Musculoskeletal:
    1. Complete musculoskeletal examination. Be alert for septic necrosis of femoral and/or humeral head.
    2. Assess for kyphosis or back pain associated with osteoporosis and long-term cortisol excess.
E. Peripheral vascular:
    1. Assess for deep vein thrombosis due to the hypercoagulable state.

Initial Diagnostic Tests

A. Serum electrolytes
B. CBC and glucose
C. 24-hour urine-free cortisol (at least two measurements)
D. Late-night salivary cortisol (at least two measurements)
E. Late-night serum cortisol (typically inpatient study)
F. Overnight dexamethasone suppression test, 1 mg
G. Bone density studies

The overnight dexamethasone suppression test has a false positive rate of 20% to 30%; false positives can occur with obesity, stress, depression, alcoholism, pregnancy, or medications that increase the hepatic metabolism of cortisol and dexamethasone (e.g., antiseizure drugs, estrogen, and rifampin). The false negative rate is less than 3%. Use the low-dose dexamethasone test as an alternative.

The 24-hour urinary-free cortisol is the most sensitive and specific test and is the best choice for screening.

If any of the earlier initial lab screenings are positive, the client should be referred to endocrinology for additional evaluation.

Differential Diagnoses
A. Depression
B. Severe obesity
C. Chronic stress
D. Familial cortisol resistance
E. Medication induced (e.g., phenytoin, phenobarbital, primidone)
F. Pituitary adenoma
G. Adrenal and other neoplasms
H. Alcoholism
I. Nephrolithiasis
J. Psychosis

Plan
A. General interventions:
  1. Taper glucocorticoid dose as appropriate for the underlying disease.
  2. Begin alcohol detoxification if applicable.
  3. Consider hormone replacement therapy for post-menopausal women.
B. Client teaching:
  1. *See Section III: Client Teaching Guide for this chapter, "Cushing's Syndrome."*
C. Pharmaceutical therapy:
  1. Calcium 1,000 mg/d and vitamin D 400 IU/d
  2. Mitotane (Lysodren) for control of adrenocortical carcinoma progression
  3. Metyrapone inhibits adrenal steroid biosynthesis.
  4. Ketoconazole (most useful for blocking adrenal steroidogenesis) and suramin inhibit adrenal steroid biosynthesis. Ketoconazole is associated with hepatic failure and drug-to-drug interactions, resulting in fatal ventricular arrhythmias. An endocrinologist should be consulted before the use of oral ketoconazole.
    a. Ketoconazole should be started at a dose of 200 mg two or three times daily and increased rapidly to 400 mg three times daily; higher doses are seldom more effective. Increase every 4 to 7 days. Avoid use in pregnancy.
  5. Hydrocortisone may be given in physiologic doses to avoid adrenal insufficiency.
  6. Mifepristone (restricted use in United States) is given for ectopic ACTH production or adrenal carcinoma. Mifepristone is an abortifacient.

Most persons on a daily steroid program for more than 2 to 4 weeks have some degree of hypothalamic–pituitary–adrenal axis suppression.

D. Medical/surgical management:
  1. If noniatrogenic etiology, surgery is the treatment of choice followed by irradiation and/or chemotherapy.

Follow-Up
A. At the provider's discretion, 1 to 2 weeks after tests are complete follow up to discuss results and possible therapy.

Consultation/Referral
A. If Cushing's syndrome is suspected, consult with an endocrinologist regarding treatment and therapy.

Individual Considerations
A. Pregnancy:
  1. Urinary-free cortisol increases in the third trimester, but women still have normal 17-hydroxycorticosteroids and normal diurnal variability of serum cortisol. Dexamethasone testing is not recommended in the initial screening for Cushing's syndrome during pregnancy.
B. Pediatrics:
  1. It is possible to differentiate between exogenous obesity and Cushing's syndrome by the child's growth rate. Exogenous obesity is characterized by normal or slightly increased growth rate.

Resource
National Adrenal Diseases Foundation: www.nadf.us/links-resources/international-adrenal-disease-groups-resources

Bibliography
Centers for Disease Control and Prevention, NCHS National Center for Health Statistics. (n.d.). *Clinical growth charts.* Retrieved from https://www.cdc.gov/growthcharts
Kairys, N., & Schwell, A. (2019, May 5). Cushing disease. *StatPearls.* Retrieved from https://www.ncbi.nlm.nih.gov/books/NBK448184/
Lee, A. (Ed). *NPPR: Nurse practitioners' prescribing reference.* (2019). New York, NY: Haymarket Media. Retrieved from https://www.empr.com/
Nieman, L. K. (2017, September). Establishing the diagnosis of Cushing's. *UpToDate.* Retrieved from http://www.uptodate.com
Nieman, L. K. (2019, February). Causes and pathophysiology of Cushing's syndrome. *UpToDate.* Retrieved from http://www.uptodate.com
Nieman, L. K. (2019, February). Epidemiology and clinical manifestations of Cushing's syndrome. *UpToDate.* Retrieved from http://www.uptodate.com
Skelton, J. A. (2018, October). Management of childhood obesity in the primary care setting. *UpToDate.* Retrieved from http://www.uptodate.com

Diabetes Mellitus (DM)

Jill C. Cash and Mellisa A. Hall

Definition
Diabetes is a group of diseases characterized by high levels of blood glucose with a defect in insulin secretion or action caused by a chronic disorder of carbohydrate, fat, and protein metabolism. There are four categories of

diabetes: type 1, type 2, gestational, and diabetes from secondary causes.

A. Type 1 diabetes, formerly referred to as IDDM or juvenile-onset diabetes, is an endocrine condition in which there is complete destruction of pancreatic beta cells or a complete absence of insulin.

B. Type 2 diabetes, formerly referred to as noninsulin-dependent diabetes mellitus (NIDDM) or adult-onset diabetes, describes a condition in which individuals have an impairment in insulin production and/or insulin resistance.

C. Gestational diabetes is diagnosed during pregnancy. It usually resolves when the pregnancy is completed. It will increase the woman's risk of developing type 2 diabetes later in life.

D. Diabetes resulting from secondary causes is due to genetic defects and/or diseases of the pancreas, such as cystic fibrosis or pancreatic cancer. Other causes of this type of diabetes can be drug-/chemical-induced diabetes from medications or therapies used when treating HIV/AIDS and in clients who receive treatments after organ transplantation.

Incidence

A. It is estimated that more than 29.1 million Americans have diabetes, 9.3% of the population. Diagnosed cases account for 21 million, with an estimated 8.1 million who have not been diagnosed. Type 1 diabetes accounts for less than 10% of diagnosed cases. There are 1.9 million new cases reported a year, not counting people 19 years old or younger. The incidence of type 2 diabetes has been rising in the children and adolescent populations and is correlated with the increasing incidence of childhood obesity.

B. People with diabetes are more prone to have unhealthy low-density lipoprotein cholesterol (LDL-C) and therefore are at increased risk for atherosclerotic cardiovascular disease (ASCVD). The incidence of CVD is four times higher in adults with diabetes. The risk of stroke is two to four times higher because 60% to 65% of the clients have hypertension.

Pathogenesis

A. Type 1 diabetes is an inherited defect causing an alteration in immunologic integrity, placing the beta cell at risk for inflammatory damage. The mechanism of damage is autoimmune. Environmental factors that may influence the etiology of diabetes include viral illnesses: mumps, coxsackievirus, cytomegalovirus, and hepatitis. Other factors that may influence the disease include diets high in dairy products, emotional and physical stress, and/or environmental toxins.

B. Type 2 diabetes involves impaired insulin secretion, insulin resistance, and/or an abnormally elevated glucose production by the liver. Genetics and obesity are major risk factors.

C. The severity of carbohydrate intolerance in gestational diabetes is unknown. Women identified at risk have screening done during the 24th and 28th weeks of gestation.

D. Genetic defects and medications/chemicals are thought to affect the beta-cell function and alter insulin function. Hemoglobin A1C (HgbA1C) levels may not be interpreted correctly in clients with blood disorders such as anemia/hemoglobinopathies. See www.ngsp.org/interf.asp for a complete list of laboratory methods recommended to be used to measure HgbA1C values for clients with hemoglobin variants (sickle cell trait, HbC, HbS, HbE, HbD trait, or elevated HbF).

Predisposing Factors

A. Body mass index (BMI) greater than or equal to 27 kg/m²

B. Physical inactivity

C. First-degree relative with type 1 or type 2 diabetes

D. HgbA1C greater than or equal to 5.7%, impaired glucose tolerance (IGT) or impaired fasting glucose (IFG) on previous testing

E. Native American, Hispanic, Asian, African American, and Pacific Islander heritage

F. Hypertension with systolic pressure greater than 140 mmHg and diastolic pressure greater than 90 mmHg

G. High-density lipoprotein (HDL) level of 35 mg/dL or less and/or triglyceride level of greater than or equal to 250 mg/dL

H. Female gender and a history of giving birth to babies larger than 9 pounds or history of gestational diabetes

I. History of IGT or fasting glucose

J. Acanthosis nigricans or severe obesity

K. Polycystic ovary syndrome (PCOS)

L. History of CVD

M. The U.S. Preventive Services Task Force (USPSTF) recommends screening for abnormal blood glucose as part of cardiovascular risk assessment in adults aged 40 to 70 years who are overweight or obese.

Common Complaints

A. Classic triad of symptoms:
   1. Polyuria
   2. Polydipsia
   3. Polyphagia

B. Weight loss

C. Lack of energy

D. Recurrent infections (urinary tract, vaginal, skin breakdown that is slow to heal)

E. Asymptomatic

Other Signs and Symptoms

A. Weakness

B. Fatigue

C. Nausea and vomiting

D. Abdominal pain

E. Anorexia

F. Sexual dysfunction, including impotence or dyspareunia

G. Itching

H. Visual disturbances

I. Signs and symptoms related to nephropathy, neuropathy, and/or retinopathy

Subjective Data

A. Obtain a detailed history regarding the onset, duration, and course of presenting symptoms.
B. Question the client regarding all characteristic signs and symptoms of diabetes.
C. Determine the client's nutritional status, 24-hour recall, weight history, and eating patterns.
D. Review the family history of diabetes or other endocrine disorders.
E. Note predisposing factors to diabetes.
F. Review the client's social history, including smoking, alcohol, and exercise.

Physical Examination

A. Check pulse, respirations, BP, and weight, with serial weight reviews, waist circumference.
B. Inspect:
   1. Observe overall appearance.
   2. Perform oral examination. Diabetic clients are prone to thrush, gingivitis, plaque, and infections. A dental examination should be done every 6 months.
   3. Complete funduscopic examination. Proliferative diabetic retinopathy is the leading cause of new blindness in adults in the United States. Clients with diabetes are 25 times more at risk for blindness and have four to six times the increased risk for cataracts and twice the increased risk for glaucoma.
   4. Inspect the skin, including feet with monofilament testing, hands, fingers, and skin folds for erythema and insulin injection sites.
C. Auscultate:
   1. The heart
   2. The lungs
   3. The carotid arteries
D. Percuss:
   1. The chest
   2. The abdomen
   3. Assess deep tendon reflexes (DTRs)
E. Palpate:
   1. The neck (thyroid)
   2. The abdomen
   3. The extremities for edema and assess peripheral pulses
F. (other)

Diagnostic Tests

A. Serum glycosylated HgbA1C of 6.5% or higher
B. Fasting plasma glucose: greater than or equal to 126 mg/dL. All clients should have a baseline fasting blood sugar (fasting for at least 8 hours) performed at 45 years of age, then repeated every 3 years. The baseline should be performed earlier if any predisposing factors exist.
C. Random plasma glucose: greater than or equal to 200 mg/dL with symptoms of diabetes
D. Oral glucose tolerance test (OGTT): after a 75-g glucose load, a 2-hour plasma glucose greater than or equal to 200 mg/dL. IGT is a fasting plasma glucose of greater than or equal to 126 mg/dL.

> According to the Diabetes Control and Complications Trial, an HgbA1C of 7.2% or below decreases the risk of retinopathy, neuropathy, and nephropathy by 50% to 70%.

Differential Diagnoses

A. Benign pancreatic insufficiency
B. Pheochromocytoma
C. Cushing's syndrome
D. History of corticosteroid use
E. Stress hyperglycemia
F. Acromegaly
G. Hemochromatosis
H. Somogyi phenomenon: early-morning hyperglycemia due to very early morning (2:00–3:00 a.m.) hypoglycemia

Plan

A. General interventions:
   1. Establish, review, and evaluate individual goals with the client on a routine basis
   2. Center goals around normal metabolic control and the prevention and delay of complications while maintaining a flexible, normal, high-quality life.
   3. After a new diagnosis is made and treatment has begun, be alert for an initial remission or a honeymoon phase with decreased insulin needs and better control that may last 3 to 6 months.
   4. Include the following in the treatment plan:
      a. Exercise:
         i. Develop a consistent, individualized exercise plan with the client to improve insulin sensitivity, blood sugars, weight reduction, and reduction of cardiovascular complications
         ii. Evaluation by a healthcare provider, including a complete physical examination and EKG. EKG must precede any exercise program.
         iii. Generally, the goals for physical activity are to reduce LDL-C and non-HDL-C and to lower the BP. The exercise should be of moderate to vigorous intensity.
         iv. Exercise should not be done if the fasting blood sugar is greater than 250 mg/dL and ketones are present in the urine or if the glucose level is greater than 300 mg/dL at any time regardless of the presence of ketones.
         v. Because exercise can lower the blood sugar concentration, special precautions such as medication adjustment and meal planning should be done before and after exercise if the client is taking insulin or a glucose-lowering medication.
      b. Self-monitoring blood glucose (SMBG): The process of monitoring the client's blood gives valuable information to the client on a daily basis and assists the provider in identifying trends.
         i. Several different meters are available with a variety of options. A certified diabetes educator can show examples of different types

before the client purchases one. Insurance formularies should be considered when recommending a glucometer.

ii. Frequency of testing depends on the type of medication the client is taking and the client's compliance and use of sliding scale prior to meals and at bedtime.

iii. Additional testing should be done at times of changes in medication, meal plans, and/or exercise and during illness or stress.

iv. Continuous blood glucose (CBG) monitoring is recommended for clients with hypoglycemia unawareness or frequent nocturnal hypoglycemia. Additional fingerstick glucose checks are required with CBG monitoring if hypoglycemia occurs.

c. Psychosocial support: It is important from the beginning of treatment to give the client a sense of control.

i. Consistent involvement of family members will influence compliance.

ii. Assess and discuss psychosocial issues at each visit, including depression.

B. Client teaching:

1. *See Section III: Client Teaching Guide for this chapter, "Diabetes."*

2. Topics in the educational plan include the pathophysiology of diabetes, procedures for SMBG and medication therapies, recognition and treatment of hypoglycemia, and instructions for special situations such as illness and traveling.

3. Include preventive care, instructions for family members, and the importance of a MedicAlert tag (available at www.medicalert.org/product/catalog/medical-ids).

4. Smoking cessation and avoidance of all tobacco products should be advised to all clients. Counseling regarding smoking/tobacco cessation methods and classes should be offered.

C. Pharmaceutical therapy:

1. Type 1 diabetes depends on exogenous insulin for treatment.

2. Type 2 diabetes is dependent on the severity of disease at the diagnosis. If HgbA1C is less than 7.5%, pharmaceutical treatment should be initiated along with an exercise program and nutrition plan. If HgbA1C is less than 7.5%, lifestyle modifications alone may be considered for 3 to 6 months, with a reassessment of HgbA1C to determine the need for pharmaceutical therapy.

a. Monotherapy for type 2 diabetes: Metformin is the preferred oral medication for type 2 diabetes. If using monotherapy at the maximum dose and goal is not achieved after 3 months, a second oral medication should be added. Insulin may eventually be required for clients who are not controlled on oral agents.

i. Insulin should be considered initially for clients presenting with glucose levels 300 mg/dL and higher or an HgbA1C of 10% or greater.

b. Add a second and third medication when glucose control is not achieved with metformin alone. Oral combination therapies:

i. Two-drug combination options:
1) Metformin + sulfonylurea (SU)
2) Metformin + thiazolidinedione (TZD)
3) Metformin + dipeptidyl peptidase-4 (DPP-4) inhibitor
4) Metformin + glucagon-like peptide-1 (GLP-1) receptor agonist (RA)
5) Metformin + insulin (basal) alone or with prandial (rapid acting before meals)
6) Metformin + sodium-glucose cotransporter 2 inhibitor (SGLT2 Inh)

ii. Three-drug combination options:
1) Metformin + SU + TZD, DPP-4 inhibitor, GLP-1 RA, or insulin
2) Metformin + TZD + SU, DPP-4-I, GLP-1-RA, or insulin
3) Metformin + DPP-4 inhibitor + SU, TZD, or insulin
4) Metformin + GLP-1 RA + SU, TZD, or insulin
5) Metformin + insulin (basal) + TZD, DPP-4-I, or GLP-1-RA
6) Metormin + DPP-4 inhibitor + SGLT2 Inh, or insulin

iii. Complicated, uncontrolled clients on previously mentioned therapy require insulin.

c. Criteria for initiation of insulin therapy:
i. Glucose level at diagnosis of type 2 diabetes is greater than 300 mg/dL
ii. HgbA1C greater than or equal to 10%
iii. Ketonuria

> Although clients with type 2 diabetes do not depend on exogenous insulin, many will require supplemental insulin during times of stress, illness, injury, pregnancy, or routinely along with oral medication (see Tables 20.1 and 20.2).

d. Additional medications that may need to be considered:

i. Angiotensin-converting enzyme (ACE) inhibitors are the antihypertensive drugs of choice to retard renal dysfunction associated with diabetes.

ii. ACE inhibitors or angiotensin II receptor blockers (ARBs) are recommended for clients with an elevated urinary albumin excretion (30–299 mg/24 hr).

iii. Calcium channel blockers may reduce microalbuminuria and proteinuria.

iv. Aspirin therapy (75–162 mg/d) is recommended for primary prevention in clients with type 1 or type 2 diabetes with an increased risk of CVD (age 50 years or older) with one or more risk factors, such as hypertension, smoking, obesity, dyslipidemia, albuminuria, or a family history of CVD. For clients who

TABLE 20.1 ACTION TIMES OF INSULIN

Insulin	Onset	Peaks	Duration
Lispro/aspart/glulisine	10 minutes	1.5 hours	3 hours
Regular	20 minutes	3–4 hours	8 hours
NPH	1.5 hours	4–12 hours	22 hours
Lente	2.5 hours	7–15 hours	24 hours
Ultralente	4 hours	10–24 hours	36 hours
75 NPH/25 Rapid Acting	<15 minutes	1–6 hours	13–22 hours
70 NPH/30 Reg	0–1 hour	Dual	12–20 hours
50 NPH/50 Rapid Acting	0–1 hour	Dual	12–20 hours
Detemir	1 hour	None	>24 hours
Glargine	1 hour	None	>24 hours
Degludec	1 hour	None	≥42 hours
Afrezza (inhalation)	10 minutes	20 minutes	2.5–3 hours

NPH, neutral protamine Hagedorn.

TABLE 20.2 DIABETES MEDICATION/CLASS

Drug	Brand Name	Drug Class
Acarbose	Precose	Alpha-glucosidase inhibitor
Ertuglifloxin	Steglatro	SGLT2 Inh
Ertuglifloxin + metformin	Segluromet	SGLT2 Inh + biguanide
Ertuglifloxin + sitagliptin	Steglujan	SGLT2 Inh + DDP-4 Inh
Pioglitazone + metformin	ActoPlus Met	Thiazolidinedione plus biguanide
Glimepiride	Amaryl	Sulfonylurea
Insulin glulisine	Apidra	Rapid-acting insulin
Rosiglitazone + metformin	Avandamet	Thiazolidinedione plus biguanide
Rosiglitazone + glimepiride	Avandaryl	Thiazolidinedione plus sulfonylurea
Exenatide	Byetta	Incretin mimetic
Exenatide extended release	Bydureon	GLP-1 receptor agonist
Glyburide	DiaBeta	Sulfonylurea (second generation)
Pioglitazone + glimepiride	Duetact	Thiazolidinedione plus sulfonylurea
Glucagon	N/A	Antihypoglycemic
Metformin extended release	Glucophage	Biguanide
Glipizide extended release	Glucotrol	Sulfonylurea (second generation)
Glyburide + metformin	Glucovance	Sulfonylurea plus biguanide
Glyburide micronized	Glynase PresTab	Sulfonylurea (second generation)
Miglitol	Glyset	Alpha-glucosidase inhibitor
Insulin lispro	Humalog	Rapid-acting insulin
NPH/regular insulin	Humulin 70/30 Humulin 50/50	Short- and intermediate-acting insulin Short- and intermediate-acting insulin
Regular insulin	Humulin R	Rapid-acting insulin
NPH insulin	Humulin N	Intermediate-acting insulin
Sitagliptin + metformin	Janumet	Dipeptidyl peptidase-4 inhibitor plus biguanide
Sitagliptin	Januvia	Dipeptidyl peptidase-4 inhibitor
Insulin glargine	Lantus	Long-acting insulin

(*continued*)

TABLE 20.2   DIABETES MEDICATION/CLASS (*continued*)

Drug	Brand Name	Drug Class
Insulin detemir	Levemir	Long-acting insulin
Linagliptin	Tradjenta	Dipeptidyl peptidase-4 inhibitor
Liraglutide	Victoza	GLP-1 receptor agonist
Metformin + glipizide	Metaglip	Biguanide plus sulfonylurea
Glyburide	Micronase	Sulfonylurea (second generation)
Nateglinide	Starlix	Glinide
Insulin isophane + regular insulin	Novolin 70/30	Short- and intermediate-acting insulin
Insulin aspart	NovoLog	Rapid-acting insulin
Insulin aspart protamine/insulin aspart	NovoLog Mix 70/30	Short- and intermediate-acting insulin
Insulin lispro protamine/insulin lispro	Humalog Mix 75/25 Humalog Mix 50/50	Rapid and intermediate-acting insulin Rapid and intermediate-acting insulin
Nateglinide	Starlix	Insulin secretagogue
Insulin isophane suspension NPH	Novolin	Intermediate-acting insulin
Saxagliptin	Onglyza	DPP-4 Inh
Pioglitazone	Actos	Thiazolidinedione
Pioglitazone + glimeperide	Duetact	Thiazolidinedione + sulfonylurea
Repaglinide + metformin	Prandimet	Meglitinide analog plus biguanide
Pramlintide	Symlin	Amylin analog/amylinomimetic
Repaglinide	Prandin	Meglitinide analog
Rosiglitazone	Avandia	Thiazolidinedione
Rosiglitazone + glimeperide	Avandaryl	Thiazolidinedione + sulfonylurea
Dapagliflozin	Farxiga	SGLT2 Inh SGLT2 Inh with DPP-4 Inh
Dapagliflozin + metformin ext release	Xigduo XR	SGLT2 Inh + biguanide
Dapagliflozin + saxagliptin	Qtern	SGLT2 Inh + DDP-4 Inh
Empagliflozin + linagliptin	Glyxambi	SGLT2 Inh + DDP-4 Inh
Canagliflozin + metformin	Invokamet	SGLT2 Inh + biguanide
Canagliflozin	Invokana	SGLT2 Inh
Empagliflozin	Jardiance	SGLT2 Inh
Empagliflozin + metformin	Synjardy	SGLT2 Inh + biguanide
Alogliptin + metformin	Kazano	DPP-4 Inh + biguanide
Alogliptin + pioglitazone	Oseni	DPP-4 Inh + thiazolidinedione
Saxagliptin + metformin	Kombiglyze XR	DPP-4 inh + biguanide
Empagliflozin + linagliptin	Synjardy	SGCT2 Inh + biguanide
Albiglutide	Tanzeum	GLP-1 receptor agonist
Lixisenatide	Adlyxin	GLP-1 receptor agonist
Semaglutide	Ozempic	GLP-1 receptor agonist
Insulin glargine	Toujeo	Long-acting (basal) insulin
Insulin degludec	Tresiba	Long-acting (basal) insulin
Dulaglutide	Trulicity	GLP-1
Dapagliflozin	Xigduo XR Afrezza	SGLT2 Inh + biguanide Insulin for oral inhalation
Colesevelam	Welchol	Bile acid sequestrant
Chlorpropamide	Diabinese	Sulfonylurea (first generation)

DPP-4 Inh, dipeptidyl peptidase-4 inhibitor; GLP-1, glucagon-like peptide-1; NPH, neutral protamine Hagedorn; SGLT2 Inh, sodium-glucose co-transporter 2 inhibitor.

have a history of CVD with an allergy to aspirin, clopidogrel 75 mg/d should be used.
e. Some medications adversely affect diabetes:
i. Nicotinic acids affect glycemic control by increasing the insulin resistance.
ii. Beta-blockers may mask symptoms of hypoglycemia.
iii. Thiazide diuretics increase insulin resistance.
3. The American College of Cardiology (ACC)/ American Heart Association (AHA) published guidelines on the primary prevention and treatment of cholesterol in people with DM and LDL-C of 70 to 189 mg/dL. These include:
a. Moderate-intensity statin therapy initiated or continued for adults with DM 40 to 75 years of age
b. High-intensity statin therapy is reasonable for adults with DM 40 to 75 years of age with a greater than or equal to 7.5% estimated 10-year ASCVD risk unless contraindicated. (Use the lifetime risk calculator to define percentage of risk.)
c. In adults with DM who are younger than 40 years or older than 75 years of age, it is reasonable to evaluate the potential for ASCVD benefits and for adverse effects for drug–drug interactions and to consider client preferences when deciding to initiate, continue, or intensify statin therapy.
D. Dietary/physical activity management:
1. Nutritional plan: The client should meet with a dietitian who has experience with diabetes nutritional therapy.
2. Eating patterns and ideal percentage of calories from protein, carbohydrates, and fat should be individualized for each client and determined along with a dietitian.
3. Involve the family to improve compliance with the individualized meal plan
4. Overweight/obese clients are encouraged to set a goal of healthy eating strategies to enhance weight loss. Along with dietary management, exercise programs should be encouraged as soon as the primary care provider has approved that the client is safe to perform physical exercise on a routine basis. It is recommended to perform at least 150 min/wk of moderate intensity physical exercise for at least 3 days a week, with not more than 2 consecutive days of rest. Resistance training is recommended for all clients with type 2 diabetes at least 2 days a week after authorized by the primary care provider.

Follow-Up

A. Determine follow-up appointments by the type of diabetes, age, client compliance, any treatment changes, and presence of any complications related to diabetes or other health problems
B. A glycosylated hemoglobin determination every 3 months can assist the provider in measuring the control. There are several computer software packages that print

the glucometer readings for assessing the compliance; this can be done by the provider or the client.
C. The American Diabetes Association management goals:
1. Preprandial glucose 80 to 120 mg/dL
2. A glucose level of less than 180 mg/dL 1 to 2 hours after meals
3. A bedtime glucose level of 100 to 140 mg/dL
4. HgbA1C target less than 8% is for the elderly, those with limited life expectancy, a history of significant hypoglycemic episodes, or the presence of extensive microvascular/macrovascular complications.
5. The American Diabetes Association and the ACC/AHA recommend diabetics with hypertension, clients with cardiovascular risks, and clients more than or equal to 18 years old with chronic kidney disease be treated to a systolic blood pressure (SBP) goal of less than 130 mmHg and to a diastolic blood pressure (DBP) of less than 80 mmHg.
6. Other goals are cholesterol less than 200 mg/dL, triglycerides less than 150 mg/dL, HDLs greater than 35 mg/dL, and LDLs less than 100 mg/dL and less than 70 mg/dL if heart disease is present.
D. Tests or examinations and recommendations should include a dilated funduscopic examination by an ophthalmologist to screen for retinopathy every 2 years, monofilament foot examination at each follow-up, an annual flu vaccination and other adult vaccines as recommended, serum creatinine, BUN, GFR, lipid panel, urinalysis, and urine for albuminuria. Additional tests may be needed if complications develop.

Consultation/Referral

A. Refer to the physician if the client experiences the following:
1. Diabetic ketoacidosis
2. Pediatric clients with hyperglycemia/new onset diabetes (type 1 or type 2)
3. Severe or frequent hypoglycemia that is unresponsive to conventional pharmaceutical therapy
4. Hyperosmolar hyperglycemic nonketotic syndrome
5. Pregnancy
6. Symptoms from an acute complication related to retinopathy
7. Nephropathy is often present at the time of diagnosis of type 2 diabetes mellitus (T2DM). Diabetic nephropathy is the leading cause of end-stage renal failure requiring dialysis.
8. Neuropathy: 60% to 70% of clients experience impaired sensation or pain in feet/hands, carpal tunnel syndrome; over half of all amputations of lower extremities are related to diabetes. All clients should be screened for neuropathy at the diagnosis of type 2 diabetes and at 5 years after the diagnosis of type 1 diabetes, and then annually. Early diagnosis is imperative to prevent nerve damage from occurring. Tight control of the blood glucose levels can slow down the progression of nerve damage but cannot reverse

neuronal loss. The pain experienced with neuropathy can be treated with oral medications. Pregabalin and duloxetine are both Food and Drug Administration (FDA) approved for neuropathic pain. Other medications that may be used include opioids such as tramadol and morphine, along with venlafaxine, amitriptyline, gabapentin, or valproate.

9. Persistent uncontrolled diabetes

Individual Considerations

A. Pregnancy/preconceptual:

1. Women considering pregnancy should be switched to insulin or an oral agent with safe pregnancy rating before conception and during pregnancy.

    a. Fetal anomalies increase proportionally to uncontrolled diabetes.

    b. HgbA1C goal before conception is less than 7%.

    c. Gestational diabetes screening may be completed by performing the "one-step" 2-hour 75-g OGTT or a "two-step" approach with 1-hour 50-g nonfasting Glucola followed by a 3-hour 100-g OGTT for clients who test positive for the 1-hour screening.

2. Hypertensive medications may need to be changed if considering pregnancy because ACE inhibitors, angiotensin receptor blockers, direct renin inhibitors, and diuretics are contraindicated during pregnancy.

3. Increased monitoring of blood glucose is necessary during pregnancy.

B. Pediatrics:

Screening should begin at 10 years of age or the onset of puberty if younger than 10 years. Screening is recommended every 3 years. Criteria for screening for diabetes include the following:

1. Overweight (BMI >85th percentile for age and sex, or weight for height, or weight >120% for height)

2. Risk factors that include:

    a. Family history of T2DM in a first- or second-degree relative

    b. Race/ethnicity (Native American, African American, Latino, Asian American, Pacific Islander)

    c. Insulin-resistance conditions (hypertension, dyslipidemia, PCOS, acanthosis nigricans, birth weight small for gestational age)

    d. Maternal history of diabetes or gestational diabetes

3. Children are encouraged to perform at least 60 minutes of physical activity on a daily basis.

4. Children diagnosed with type 1 diabetes should also be screened for celiac disease by ordering laboratory studies that include immunoglobulin A (IgA) antitissue transglutaminase or antiendomysial antibodies. If positive, the child should be referred to a gastroenterologist and rheumatologist.

5. Children with Type 1 diabetes should also be screened for thyroid disease by ordering a thyroid-stimulating hormone (TSH) level test. If normal, screen every 1 to 2 years.

C. Elderly:

1. Risk for hypoglycemia should be reviewed in clients using insulin or oral agents that can cause hypoglycemia. Medical alert bracelets and emergency care for hypoglycemic episodes should be reviewed during each follow-up.

2. Treatment goals for older diabetic clients should be individualized and based on life expectancy. The risk of hypoglycemia due to medication use or knowledge of previous hypoglycemic episodes requires a relaxed HgbA1C goal of 8%.

Bibliography

American Diabetes Association. (2019). Standards of medical care in diabetes—2019. *Diabetes Care, 37*(1), 11–34. Retrieved from http://clinical.diabetesjournals.org/content/37/1/11

Atkinson, M. A. (2016). Type 1 diabetes mellitus. In S. Melmed, K. S. Polonsky, P. R. Larsen, & H. M. Kronenberg (Eds.), *Williams textbook of endocrinology* (13th ed., pp. 1451–1483). Philadelphia, PA: Elsevier.

BMI Calculator. (n.d.-a). *BMI calculator*. Retrieved from http://www.bmi-calculator.net

BMI Calculator. (n.d.-b). *Waist to hip ratio calculator*. Retrieved from http://www.bmi-calculator.net/waist-to-hip-ratio-calculator

Centers for Disease Control and Prevention. (2018, March). *Diabetes Home.* Retrieved from https://www.cdc.gov/diabetes/statistics/prevalence_national.htm

Centers for Disease Control and Prevention. (n.d.-a). *Adult BMI calculator: English version*. Retrieved from https://www.cdc.gov/healthyweight/assessing/bmi/adult_bmi/english_bmi_calculator/bmi_calculator.html

Centers for Disease Control and Prevention. (n.d.-b). *BMI percentile calculator for child and teen: English version*. Retrieved from https://nccd.cdc.gov/dnpabmi/calculator.aspx

Centers for Disease Control and Prevention, NCHS National Center for Health Statistics. (n.d.). *Clinical growth charts*. Retrieved from https://www.cdc.gov/growthcharts

Durnwald, C. (2019, February) Diabetes mellitus in pregnancy: Screening and diagnosis. *UpToDate.* Retrieved from http://www.uptodate.com

Grundy, S. M., Stone, N. J., Beam, C., Bailey, A. L., Beam, C., Birtcher, K. K., . . . Yeboah, J. (2018). 2018 Guideline on the management of blood cholesterol. A report of the American College of Cardiology/American Heart Association Task Force on Clinical Practice Guidelines. *Journal of the American College of Cardiology, 139*(25), e1082–e1143. doi:10.1161/CIR.0000000000000625

Laffel, L., & Svoren, B. (2018, March). Epidemiology, presentation, and diagnosis of type 2 diabetes mellitus in children and adolescents. *UpToDate.* Retrieved from http://www.uptodate.com

Lee, A. (Ed.). *NPPR: Nurse practitioners' prescribing reference*. (2019). New York, NY: Haymarket Media. Retrieved from https://www.empr.com/

Levitsky, L. L., & Misra, M. (2019, January). Epidemiology, presentation, and diagnosis of type 1 diabetes mellitus in children and adolescents. *UpToDate.* Retrieved from http://www.uptodate.com

McCulloch, D. K., & Robertson, R. P. (2018, November). Pathogenesis of type 2 diabetes mellitus. *UpToDate.* Retrieved from http://www.uptodate.com

Munshi, M. (2019, March). Treatment of type 2 diabetes mellitus in the older patient. *UpToDate.* Retrieved from http://www.uptodate.com

National Institutes of Health. (2015). *Third report of the National Cholesterol Education Program (NCEP) expert panel on detection, evaluation, and treatment of high blood cholesterol in adults (ATP III): final report.* Bethesda, MD: Author. Retrieved from https://www.nhlbi.nih.gov/files/docs/guidelines/atp3xsum.pdf

National Lipid Association. (2018, November). *2018 AHA/ACC/AACVPR/AAPA/ABC/ACPM/ADA/AGS/APhA/ASPC/NLA/PCNA guideline on the management of blood cholesterol: Executive summary.* A report of the American College of Cardiology/American Heart Association Task Force on Clinical Practice Guidelines. Retrieved from http://www.onlinejacc.org/content/accj/early/2018/11/02/j.jacc.2018.11.002.full.pdf

Rees, A., Levy, M., & Lansdown, A. (2017). *Clinical endocrinology and diabetes at a glance.* Chichester, West Sussex, England: John Wiley & Sons.

Skelton, J. A. (2018, October). Management of childhood obesity in the primary care setting. *UpToDate*. Retrieved from http://www.uptodate.com

U.S. Department of Health and Human Services. (2015, October). *Screening for abnormal blood glucose and type 2 diabetes mellitus: U.S. Preventive Services Task Force recommendation statement*. Retrieved from https://www.uspreventiveservicestaskforce.org/Page/Document/RecommendationStatementFinal/screening-for-abnormal-blood-glucose-and-type-2-diabetes

U.S. Department of Health and Human Services. (2018, November). *National Diabetes Statistics report*. Centers for Disease Control and Prevention. Retrieved from https://www.cdc.gov/diabetes/data/statistics/statistics-report.html

U.S. Department of Health and Human Services. (2019, February). *Physical activity guidelines for Americans*. Retrieved from https://www.hhs.gov/fitness/be-active/physical-activity-guidelines-for-americans/index.html

Weinstock, R. D. K. (2019, April) Self-monitoring of blood glucose in management of adults of non-pregnant adults with diabetes mellitus. *UpToDate*. Retrieved from https://www.uptodate.com/contents/self-monitoring-of-glucose-in-management-of-nonpregnant-adults-with-diabetes-mellitus

Galactorrhea

Jill C. Cash and Mellisa A. Hall

Definition

A. The production of a milky discharge excreted from the nipple occurring beyond the 6-month period of pregnancy and/or breastfeeding cessation.

Incidence

A. It is estimated that 50% to 80% of women during their reproductive years will experience galactorrhea at some time in their life.

Pathogenesis

A. The pathogenesis depends on the etiology. Physiologic galactorrhea is caused by pregnancy. The anterior pituitary gland secretes prolactin, which stimulates milk production. Milk production is normal for 6 months after pregnancy and/or after breastfeeding has ceased. The majority of cases are from a benign etiology. Malignancy is responsible for 5% to 15% of cases. Malignancy evidenced by nipple discharge is more common after age 60.

Predisposing Factors

A. Reproductive women (15–50 years old)
B. Medications: oral contraceptives, first- and second-generation antipsychotics, tricyclic antidepressants, selective serotonin reuptake inhibitor (SSRI) antidepressants, antiemetics, opioid analgesics, and antihypertensives (verapamil and methyldopa)
C. Stress (surgery, trauma)

Common Complaint

A. Milky discharge from the nipple

Subjective Data

A. Note the onset, duration, and course of presenting symptoms.
B. Ask whether the client has been pregnant and/or breastfed within the past 6 months. If so, how long did she nurse?
C. Review her menstrual history and pattern.
D. Ask her to describe the discharge, noting color, consistency, and/or presence of blood.
E. Determine the mechanism of production of discharge: spontaneous or with manual expression.
F. Assess for any palpable mass in the breast.
G. Review current medications, including use of oral contraceptives.
H. Note any previous experience with galactorrhea. Discuss testing performed and treatment, if any.
I. Identify any family history of breast cancer or other tumors.

Physical Examination

A. Check pulse, respirations, and BP.
B. Inspect:
  1. Inspect the breast and nipples for symmetry.
  2. Assess the discharge.
  3. Inspect the skin; note dimpling, retraction, and irregularities.
  4. Eyes: complete funduscopic examination.
  5. Perform visual field testing.
C. Palpate:
  1. Palpate the breasts for masses and fibrocystic changes.
  2. Squeeze the nipple to induce discharge.
  3. Palpate the axillary lymph nodes.
  4. Palpate the neck, thyroid, and lymph nodes.

Diagnostic Tests

A. Prolactin level: normal level is 1 to 20 ng/mL.
B. TSH

> Many cases of galactorrhea are considered idiopathic. Usually endocrine studies will be normal.

C. Beta human chorionic gonadotropin (beta hCG)
D. Hemoccult of breast discharge
E. Breast discharge for pathology
F. Periareolar ultrasound (all ages)
G. CT or MRI of sella turcica if pituitary mass is suspected
H. Mammogram in women older than 30 years if tumor is suspected
I. Breast sonography
J. Ductography/ductoscopy
K. Breast MRI
L. Skin-punch biopsy for abnormal skin presentations

Differential Diagnoses

A. Fibrocystic disease
B. Mastitis
C. Breast tumor
D. Medication induction
E. Breast cancer: bloody nipple discharge, painless, firm fixed mass
F. Pituitary adenoma: can produce permanent visual field loss and headaches
G. Hypothalamic disorders

H. Chiari-Frommel: galactorrhea occurring after 6 months postpartum
I. Pregnancy

Plan

A. General interventions:
  1. Treat underlying cause of nipple discharge.
  2. If induced by medications, consider stopping medications if the side effect outweighs benefits.
  3. If benign cause, no treatment is necessary with medication. Monitor symptoms. If symptoms progress, re-evaluate.
B. Client teaching:
  1. Teach self-examination of the breast.
C. Pharmaceutical therapy:
  1. No pharmaceuticals are advised with the exception of tapering or discontinuing medications that are causing the discharge. This course is recommended only after cautious consideration of why the medication is being used (antipsychotics).

Follow-Up

A. Monitor prolactin level every 6 to 12 months.
B. Recommend yearly vision evaluation.
C. Order MRI of brain at 1 year, then every 2 to 5 years if symptoms persist.

Consultation/Referral

A. Consult a physician regardless of normal imaging results if breast tumor is suspected with bloody discharge or palpable mass noted.

Individual Considerations

A. Pregnancy:
  1. Galactorrhea during pregnancy is an expected physiologic response.
  2. If galactorrhea persists after pregnancy/lactation has ceased for 6 months, a full workup evaluation is required.
B. Adult men: Galactorrhea is rare in men; however, it can occur with prolactinoma.

Bibliography

Golshan, M. (2018, February). Nipple discharge. *UpToDate*. Retrieved from http://www.uptodate.com
Lee, A. (Ed.). *NPPR: Nurse practitioners' prescribing reference*. (2019). New York, NY: Haymarket Media. Retrieved from https://www.empr.com/

Gynecomastia

Jill C. Cash and Mellisa A. Hall

Definition

A. Gynecomastia is an enlargement of the breast tissue in males.

Incidence

A. Common in newborns; approximately 40% to 69% of adolescent boys will experience breast enlargement. It is also seen in men (between the ages of 50 and 80 years) with excessive weight gain.

Pathogenesis

A. Male breast duct proliferation occurs due to a hormonal imbalance of estrogen. Pathologic conditions such as pituitary tumors, systemic disorders, kidney disease, thyroid disorders, and liver disease can cause symptoms to occur. Medications can also induce symptoms. These medications include antiandrogens, antidepressants, cimetidine, ranitidine, omeprazole, chemotherapeutic agents, amiodarone, diltiazem, nifedipine, digoxin, methyldopa, reserpine, hormones, and sedatives.

Predisposing Factors

A. Newborn
B. Puberty
C. Age (men older than 65 years)
D. Family history
E. Klinefelter's syndrome
F. Malnutrition with severe weight loss
G. Peutz-Jeghers syndrome
H. Obesity in males
I. Medications associated with androgen and estrogen effects

Common Complaint

A. Enlargement of breast tissue with or without discomfort

Other Signs and Symptoms

A. Asymptomatic
B. Type I: Nodule present under areolar tissue area
C. Type II: Nodule palpable under and beyond areolar area
D. Type III: Breast enlargement without contour separation of tissue

Subjective Data

A. Identify when breast development first appeared.
B. Determine whether enlargement is unilateral or bilateral.
C. Review the progression of enlargement.
D. Note any pain, discharge, or masses that are palpable.
E. List current medications, drugs, and alcohol and substance abuse.
F. Review the client's medical history.
G. Note the client's family history of gynecomastia or breast malignancy.
H. Explore nutritional intake.
I. Discuss the client's level of physical activity (sports, hobbies, etc.).
J. Note use of herbal products or anabolic steroids.

Objective Data

A. Inspect breasts bilaterally and surrounding nodes for enlargement or skin changes.
B. Palpate breast tissue systematically and surrounding nodes. Gynecomastia can usually be appreciated once the glandular tissue reaches 0.5 cm or larger.
C. Palpate testes for masses or atrophic changes.

D. Check BMI.

E. Assess BP.

Diagnostic Tests

A. Prolactin level

B. TSH

C. hCG

D. Serum luteinizing hormone (LH)

E. Testosterone level

F. Estradiol level

G. Mammography with ultrasound as needed for suspicious breast masses in adult males

Differential Diagnoses

A. Obesity: fatty breast enlargement without glandular involvement

B. Breast cancer: fixed, firm nodule in tissue with dimpling and/or breast discharge

C. Neurofibroma

D. Lipoma

Plan

A. General interventions:

1. Identify any pathologic condition. If none is identified, reassure the client that normal resolution will occur over time.

B. Client teaching:

1. Reinforce weight reduction if weight gain is a factor in the condition.

C. Pharmaceutical therapy:

1. Antiestrogens (tamoxifen)

2. Androgens (testosterone replacement)

3. Aromatase inhibitors (anastrozole)

Follow-Up

A. Follow-up is dependent on etiology and/or client needs.

B. Follow up pubertal boys every 4 to 6 months for evaluation of development or regression.

Consultation/Referral

Consult a physician or refer to an endocrinologist if the male client:

A. Is noted to have breast enlargement for longer than 2 years

B. Is a pubertal boy without genital development

Individual Consideration

A. Newborns: commonly seen in newborns due to maternal estrogen. This breast enlargement spontaneously regresses over time.

Bibliography

BMI Calculator. (n.d.). *BMI calculator*. Retrieved from http://www.bmi-calculator.net

Braunstein, G. D. & Anawalt, B. D. (2019a, February). Causes, evaluation, and management of gynecomastia. *UpToDate*. Retrieved from http://www.uptodate.com

Braunstein, G. D. & Anawalt, B. D. (2019b, February). Epidemiology, pathophysiology, and causes of gynecomastia. *UpToDate*. Retrieved from http://www.uptodate.com

Centers for Disease Control and Prevention. (n.d.-a). *Adult BMI calculator: English version*. Retrieved from https://www.cdc.gov/healthyweight/assessing/bmi/adult_bmi/english_bmi_calculator/bmi_calculator.html

Centers for Disease Control and Prevention. (n.d.-b). *BMI percentile calculator for child and teen: English version*. Retrieved from https://nccd.cdc.gov/dnpabmi/calculator.aspx

Lee, A. (Ed). *NPPR: Nurse practitioners' prescribing reference*. (2019). New York, NY: Haymarket Media. Retrieved from https://www.empr.com/

Hirsutism

Jill C. Cash and Mellisa A. Hall

Definition

A. An excessive production of an androgenic hormone causes the development of male features in females, particularly hair distribution.

Incidence

A. Approximately 8% to 10% of women develop hirsutism after puberty.

Pathogenesis

A. The pathogenesis depends on the etiology: excessive amounts of androgenic hormones from the ovary, adrenal gland, and/or a hormonal imbalance. The two major adrenal gland conditions responsible for hirsutism or virilism are CAH and Cushing's syndrome.

Predisposing Factors

A. Females who have a family history of endocrine disorders

B. Usually occurs in the second to third decade of life

C. Southern European ancestry

D. PCOS

E. CAH

F. Ovarian tumors

G. Adrenal tumors

H. Cushing's syndrome

I. Hyperthecosis

J. Severe insulin-resistance syndrome

K. Medications

L. Obesity

M. Medications containing androgens, including oral contraceptives

Common Complaint

A. An excessive amount of hair production on the upper lip, chin, and/or chest

Other Signs and Symptoms

A. Irregular periods

B. Infertility

C. Acne

D. Virilization (temporal hair recession, large muscle mass, deep voice)

Subjective Data

A. Note the age of onset, duration, and distribution pattern of the excessive hair growth.

B. Review any previous experiences with similar symptoms. What were the diagnosis, treatment, and results?

C. Note the client's menstrual history. Note amenorrhea and galactorrhea. Has the client ever had a history of infertility?

Physical Examination

A. Check pulse, respirations, and BP, BMI (>30 kg/m²), central obesity pattern.

B. Inspect:

1. Look for excessive hair growth on face, breasts, abdomen, back, and shoulders.

2. Assess for signs of virilization.

3. Confirm expected development of secondary sexual characteristics.

4. Assess for acne.

5. Assess for striae acanthosis nigricans and skin tags.

C. Palpate: perform a pelvic examination to assess for enlarged ovaries or masses.

Diagnostic Tests

A. Total testosterone (>200 ng/dL needs further workup)

B. Free serum testosterone

C. TSH, follicle-stimulating hormone (FSH), LH, and prolactin levels

D. Dehydroepiandrosterone sulfate (DHEA-S). A lab value greater than 700 ng/dL needs further workup.

E. 24-hour urine: 17-ketosteroid assay

F. Pelvic ultrasound

G. CT of ovaries/adrenal glands if abnormally elevated blood tests

Differential Diagnoses

A. Hypothyroidism: elevated TSH

B. Ovarian tumor: testosterone level greater than 200 ng/dL

C. Adrenal tumor: DHEA greater than 800 mcg/dL

D. Excessive steroid use: the client medicates self with excessive steroids.

E. Cushing's syndrome: centripetal obesity and muscle wasting

Plan

A. General interventions:

1. Medications are not recommended for mild cases. Hair removal by other mechanisms is recommended as the client desires (plucking, waxing, bleaching, etc.).

2. Moderate to severe cases require treatment with medications. Drug therapy may stop excessive hair growth. Current hair growth will not spontaneously resolve. Hair removal may also be desired until the drug shows an effect.

3. If acne is severe, institute appropriate therapy (see "Acne Vulgaris" in Chapter 4, "Dermatology Guidelines").

B. Client teaching:

1. If obese, reinforce weight loss management. Consider nutritional consult.

2. Educate the client that it may take 3 to 6 months on medication to see results.

C. Pharmaceutical therapy:

1. Use combined oral contraceptives daily if no contraindication; any brand is effective.

2. Use high-estrogen pills to increase steroid-binding globulins if no contraindication.

3. Use high-progesterone pills to influence the clearance of testosterone.

4. Antiandrogens:

a. Spironolactone

b. Cyproterone acetate

c. Finasteride

d. Flutamide

5. Gonadotropin-releasing hormone (GnRH) agonists

6. Topical therapy (Vaniqua): cream to be applied twice daily to reduce growth of unwanted facial hair. Results should be noted after 4 to 6 weeks of use.

Ovarian and/or adrenal tumor must be ruled out before medication therapy is instituted.

Follow-Up

A. Follow-up depends on the treatment. If medication is used, follow up in 3 months to evaluate effectiveness.

Consultation/Referral

A. Consult a physician if abnormally elevated laboratory results exist or if Cushing's syndrome is suspected.

B. Refer to a physician if there is no improvement after 3 months of medication treatment.

C. Refer clients who have virilization and elevated testosterone levels to an endocrinologist.

Individual Considerations

A. Pregnancy:

1. If conception occurs, discontinue medications, which may be teratogenic to the fetus.

2. If anovulation is diagnosed, fertility measures are needed if pregnancy is desired.

B. Geriatrics:

1. Hirsutism may be seen in women after menopause.

2. Hirsutism that occurs in the middle to late years in life should be closely monitored for adrenal hyperplasia and adrenal and/or ovarian tumors.

Bibliography

Barbieri, R. L. (2018, June). Treatment of hirsutism. *UpToDate*. Retrieved from http://www.uptodate.com

Barbieri, R. L., & Ehrmann, D. A. (2017, June). Pathogenesis and causes of hirsutism. *UpToDate*. Retrieved from http://www.uptodate.com

Barbieri, R. L., & Ehrmann, D. A. (2018, May). Evaluation of premenopausal women with hirsutism. *UpToDate*. Retrieved from http://www.uptodate.com

BMI Calculator. (n.d.). *BMI calculator*. Retrieved from http://www.bmi-calculator.net

Centers for Disease Control and Prevention. (n.d.-a). *Adult BMI calculator: English version*. Retrieved from https://www.cdc.gov/healthyweight/assessing/bmi/adult_bmi/english_bmi_calculator/bmi_calculator.html

Centers for Disease Control and Prevention. (n.d.-b). *BMI percentile calculator for child and teen: English version*. Retrieved from https://nccd.cdc.gov/dnpabmi/calculator.aspx

Lee, A. (Ed.). *NPPR: Nurse practitioners' prescribing reference*. (2019). New York, NY: Haymarket Media. Retrieved from https://www.empr.com/

Hypogonadism

Jill C. Cash and Mellisa A. Hall

Definition

A. Hypogonadism in men is the failure of the testes to produce physiological levels of testosterone and a normal number of spermatozoa.

B. Generally, hypogonadism is defined as the reduction or absence of hormone secretion or other physiological activity of the gonads, which are the testes or ovaries.

Incidence

A. An estimated 40% of men older than 45 years of age have below-normal values of serum testosterone. Studies indicate that testosterone levels decrease approximately 100 ng/dL every 10 years.

Pathogenesis

A. Hypogonadism in men can be the result of testicular dysfunction or nondevelopment (primary hypogonadism) or dysfunction of the pituitary or hypothalamus (secondary hypogonadism). The two clinical manifestations of impaired spermatogenesis are infertility and decreased testicular size. There are several possible clinical manifestations of testosterone deficiency, which are determined by its time of onset during reproductive development.

1. In utero first or second trimesters: incomplete virilization of external genitalia, incomplete development of Wolffian ducts to form male internal genitalia

2. Third trimester in utero: micropenis

3. Prepuberty: incomplete pubertal maturation, eunuchoid body habitus, poor muscle development, and reduced peak bone mass

4. Postpuberty: decreased energy, mood, and libido; decrease in sexual hair, hematocrit, muscle mass and strength, and bone mineral density

Predisposing Factors

A. Hypogonadism associated with Klinefelter's syndrome

B. Chemotherapy

C. Radiation therapy

D. Excessive alcohol consumption

E. Painful testicular swelling

F. Anosmia associated with Kallmann's syndrome

G. Use of medications that cause hypogonadism: ketoconazole or extended-release opiates

Common Complaints

A. Decreased vigor and libido

B. Depression

C. Adolescent and young adult males—failure to begin or complete puberty

Other Signs and Symptoms

A. Fatigue

B. Difficulty concentrating

C. Hot flashes

D. No change in deepening of the voice

Subjective Data

A. To client or parent: history of known chromosomal abnormalities in family or client

B. History of cryptorchidism

C. History of muscular weakness

D. History of varicocele unresolved within 6 months of birth

E. Known infections affecting the scrotum and testes

F. Therapeutic radiation to area

G. History of chemotherapy

H. History of long-term ketoconazole, glucocorticoid, or long-acting opiate use

I. Known testicular trauma

J. Known torsion

K. History of autoimmune disorder

L. Alcohol consumption (amount, duration, and frequency)

M. Chronic illnesses including cirrhosis, chronic renal failure

N. HIV

O. Decreased spontaneous erections

Physical Examination

A. Inspect:

1. Testes for appropriate size

2. Upper and lower body musculatures

3. Full/dense male-pattern beard

4. Expected Tanner development for age

5. Testes should be bilaterally descended.

6. Rule out eunuchoid appearance.

7. Gynecomastia

8. Clinical findings of hypogonadism develop gradually and become obvious after puberty.

9. Inspect penis for hypospadias.

10. Long-term alcohol abuse: Palmar erythema, rhinophyma, telangiestasia, hand tremor

B. Palpate:

1. The scrotum and testes for masses

2. The breasts for masses

Diagnostic Tests

A. Serum testosterone (morning total); repeat to confirm.

B. Measurement of free testosterone if total testosterone is not near the lower limit

C. Avoid lab tests during acute illness.

Differential Diagnoses

A. Moderate obesity

B. Nephrotic syndrome

C. Hypothyroidism

D. Use of glucocorticoids, progestins, and androgenic steroids

E. Acromegaly

F. DM

G. Hepatic cirrhosis

H. Hypopituitarism

I. Malnutrition

J. Klinefelter's syndrome

K. Depression

L. Psychological sexual dysfunction

Plan

A. General interventions:

1. Testosterone replacement's effect on reducing adverse health outcomes in the general population is unknown.

2. Testosterone levels vary significantly with circadian rhythms, illness, and medications.

3. Measurement of bone mineral density is recommended to assess fracture risk.

4. LH and FSH concentrations can help distinguish between primary and secondary hypogonadism.

5. Differentials for secondary hypogonadism should evaluate for pituitary neoplasia, hyperprolactinemia, hemochromatosis, obstructive sleep apnea (OSA), and genetic disorders.

6. Testosterone replacement should be initiated only after a baseline prostate-specific antigen (PSA) and digital prostate examination. PSA levels should be followed again in 3 months once replacement therapy started, and then annually.

7. Hematocrit should be measured prior to replacement therapy, at 2 months, and then annually. Erythrocytosis leading to hypercoagulable states is a risk with testosterone replacement. Erythrocytosis is an indication to cease or reduce replacement therapy.

B. Client teaching:

1. Both men and women with hypogonadism can lead normal lives with hormone replacement therapy.

2. Hormone replacement should continue throughout life.

3. Potential side effects of testosterone replacement therapy should be discussed before therapy, including gynecomastia, worsening benign prostatic hyperplasia (BPH), sleep apnea, peripheral edema, potential increased risk for myocardial infarction (MI), and cerebrovascular accident (CVA).

4. Reduced sperm production and fertility is a potential side effect of testosterone replacement.

5. Clients using topically absorbed testosterone gel or creams can transfer testosterone to female partners or children by direct skin-to-skin contact.

C. Pharmaceutical therapy:

1. Injectable testosterone: 50 up to 400 mg intramuscular (IM) every 2 weeks

2. 1% testosterone gel

3. Transdermal testosterone patch

4. Buccal testosterone

5. Implanted subcutaneous testosterone pellets

Follow-Up

A. Clients receiving hormone replacement should be reevaluated every 6 months or more frequently, including screening for prostate cancer as recommended.

B. Testosterone replacement is contraindicated in metastatic prostate cancer and breast cancer. Routine screening should be performed.

Consultation/Referral

A. Physician consultation before initiating testosterone therapy is advised.

B. Endocrinology referral is recommended for males not responsive to the replacement therapy.

C. Clients with primary hypogonadism should be referred to an endocrinologist for initial workup and management.

Individual Considerations

A. Geriatrics: Current recommendations are *not* in favor of testosterone therapy for all older males. Providers should cautiously consider the benefits compared to the risks for older males. The benefits of testosterone replacement are unproven, and the long-term risks are unknown.

B. HIV clients: Short-term testosterone replacement should be considered for HIV men with low testosterone, weight loss, and muscular wasting.

Bibliography

Lee, A. (Ed.). *NPPR: Nurse practitioners' prescribing reference*. (2019). New York, NY: Haymarket Media. Retrieved from https://www.empr.com/

Prescriber's Letter. (2019, March). *Consider the new Beer's criteria when prescribing meds for older adults*. Retrieved from https://prescriber .therapeuticresearch.com/Content/Articles/PRL/2019/Mar/Consider -the-New-Beers-Criteria-When-Prescribing-Meds-for-Older-Adults

Resnick, B. (Ed.). (2017). *GNRS Geriatric nursing review syllabus: A core curriculum in advanced practice geriatric nursing* (5th ed.). New York, NY: American Geriatrics Society.

Sizar, O., & Schwartz, J. (2019, April 2). Hypogonadism. *StatPearls*. Retrieved from https://www.ncbi.nlm.nih.gov/books/NBK532933/

Snyder, P. J. (2018, April). Clinical features and diagnosis of male hypogonadism. *UpToDate*. Retrieved from http://www.uptodate.com

Metabolic Syndrome/Insulin Resistance Syndrome

Jill C. Cash and Mellisa A. Hall

Definition

A. Metabolic syndrome is an association of several complex disorders: obesity, insulin-resistant type 2 diabetes, hypertension, and hyperlipidemia. This coexistence of conditions leads to ASCVD. Metabolic syndrome is considered a proinflammatory and prothrombotic state. Elevated triglycerides and low high-density lipoprotein cholesterol (HDL-C) are strong predictors of vascular events. Triglycerides and the waist circumference are considered the strongest predictors for the development of metabolic syndrome.

B. The inclusion of type 2 diabetes in the definition of metabolic syndrome is debated. Currently, there is no consensus on definition for metabolic syndrome in children. The Adult Treatment Panel (ATP) III defines metabolic syndrome in adults as the coexistence of any three of five conditions (see Table 20.3).

C. Complications associated with metabolic syndrome include T2DM, fatty liver disease, cirrhosis, chronic kidney disease, PCOS, OSA, and gout.

D. Metabolic syndrome is noted in the literature under other names, including insulin resistance syndrome and obesity dyslipidemia syndrome. Previously, the term "syndrome X" was used; however, syndrome X is noted to have normal coronary arteries and the occurrence of angina.

Incidence

A. Increase in incidence is age-dependent; overall incidence is estimated at 24% in Americans over 20 years old. Although there is not yet a diagnostic criterion for insulin resistance in the pediatric population, studies have

TABLE 20.3   ADULT TREATMENT PANEL III CRITERIA FOR METABOLIC SYNDROME

Metabolic Syndrome Traits	Definition
Central/abdominal obesity	Adult waist circumference: Men >40 inches (102 cm) Women >35 inches (88 cm)
	Obesity in children 6 years to <10 years: waist circumference ≥90th percentile
	Obesity ages 10 to <16 years: ≥ 90th percentile ≥16 years use adult criteria
Serum triglycerides	Adults: ≥150 mg/dL *or* drug treatment for elevated triglycerides
	Children: >100 mg/dL
Serum HDL cholesterol	Adults: <40 mg/dL in men; <50 mg/dL in women; *or* drug treatment for low HDL cholesterol
	Children: ≥35 mg/dL
BP	Adults: ≥130/85 *or* drug treatment for hypertension
	Children: ≥90th percentile for age, sex, and height
FPG	Adults: ≥100 mg/dL *or* drug treatment for elevated blood glucose
	Children: ≥110 mg/dL

BP, blood pressure; FPG, fasting plasma glucose; HDL, high-density lipoprotein.

Source: Adapted from National Institutes of Health. (2015). *Third report of the National Cholesterol Education Program (NCEP) expert panel on detection, evaluation, and treatment of high blood cholesterol in adults (ATP III): Final report*. Bethesda, MD: Author. Retrieved from https://www.nhlbi.nih.gov/files/docs/guidelines/atp3xsum.pdf.

indicated a significant rise in childhood obesity, which has caused metabolic syndrome to be diagnosed in children. The incidence in children is 4.2% to 8.4% (dependent on ethnicity).
B. Asians living in the United States and Mexican Americans have the highest age-adjusted prevalence. Among African Americans and Mexican Americans, the prevalence is higher in women than in men.
C. Ethnic background:
  1. Native Americans are at the greatest risk (60% females and 45% males).
  2. Mexican Americans have the highest prevalence (31.9%).
  3. Black and Hispanic females are 1.5 times more likely than non-Hispanic White females to have the syndrome.

Pathogenesis
A. The exact etiology is unknown; however, abdominal obesity has been associated with insulin resistance. Vascular endothelial dysfunction occurs secondary to insulin resistance, hyperglycemia, hyperinsulinemia, and adipokines. Along with high BP and abnormal lipids, vascular inflammation places the individual at high risk of a cardiovascular insult.

Predisposing Factors
A. Genetic predisposition
B. Weight gain, especially central/abdominal obesity
C. Female, especially postmenopausal
D. Childhood obesity
E. Smoking
F. High-carbohydrate diet, especially soft drink consumption

G. Lack of exercise:
  1. Sedentary lifestyle
  2. Television or other electronic device use more than 2 hours per day
H. Insulin resistance

Common Complaints
A. Complaints are all related to the individual coexisting comorbid symptoms.

Other Signs and Symptoms
A. All are related to the individual coexisting comorbid symptoms.

Subjective Data
A. Review the client's medical history related to comorbid conditions, including obesity, hypertension, and any abnormal laboratory testing (fasting lipids, triglycerides, insulin, and glucose levels).
B. Review the client's family history including T2DM.
C. Review all prescription medications, over-the-counter (OTC) drugs, and herbals.
D. Review the client's current level of exercise.
E. Review the client's usual diet (24-hour recall) noting high fat and high glucose consumption, including fast-food and processed food consumption.
F. Review the client's reproductive history.

Physical Examination
A. Check height, weight, waist circumference, BP, pulse, and respirations.
B. Calculate the BMI and waist-to-hip measurement. Several Internet sites have BMI, body fat, and waist-to-hip ratio calculators. Document on a growth chart BMI results for visual teaching support for client and parent.

C. Make general observations for acanthosis nigricans and skin tags (insulin resistance).

D. A full physical examination is guided by the client's medical history and presenting signs and symptoms.

Diagnostic Tests

A. Fasting plasma glucose

B. Fasting lipid panel

C. Triglycerides

D. Consider thyroid function

E. Consider C-reactive protein (CRP; optional)

Differential Diagnoses

A. Cushing's syndrome

Plan

A. General interventions:

1. Aggressive lifestyle modification focusing on increased physical activity and weight reduction is a cornerstone for treatment.

B. Client teaching:

1. Dietary recommendations include a low-fat, low-cholesterol, and/or dietary approaches to stop hypertension (DASH) diet. Decrease simple sugar consumption, as well as saturated and trans fats and cholesterol (see Appendix B).

2. Exercise recommendations include a minimum of 30 minutes a day of walking at a brisk pace or other activity at a moderate intensity. Start by using a pedometer, walking at breaks, or performing household work.

3. Weight loss of 5% to 10% or more should be encouraged (gradual weight loss of 1–2 kg/mo). Even small losses are associated with health benefits.

4. BP control strategies include a low-sodium diet (DASH), smoking cessation, and alcohol in moderation.

5. Counsel on smoking cessation.

6. Abdominoplasties do not lower the risk for coronary artery disease (CAD) or insulin sensitivity.

C. Pharmaceutical therapy:

1. Currently, the treatment for metabolic syndrome is to treat each individual component/diagnosis for the individual.

2. Insulin-resistant clients with impaired glucose testing may benefit from metformin.

3. Statins for elevated lipids

4. Low-dose aspirin may be prescribed related to the client's risk of CVD, with an increased risk of the client having a prothrombotic state.

5. Oral hypoglycemic agents used to treat type 2 diabetes are not currently recommended for the prevention of metabolic syndrome, unless the client has an impaired fasting glucose or abnormal glucose tolerance testing.

6. Hypertension should be controlled with appropriate antihypertensives.

D. Bariatric surgery may be considered in adults with elevated BMIs and numerous comorbidities.

Follow-Up

A. Follow-up involves assessing clients for metabolic syndrome at a minimum of 3-year intervals for anyone with one or more risk traits. Follow-up testing includes the following:

1. BMI calculation

2. Waist-to-hip calculation

3. Fasting lipid profile

4. Fasting glucose or other diabetic screening methods (HgbA1C, fasting insulin levels, gamma-glutamyl transferase [GGT])

5. BP

Consultation/Referral

A. Refer to an obstetrician/gynecologist for consultation and management for infertility/pregnancy.

B. Refer to a specialist for any comorbid condition as needed.

Individual Considerations

A. Individual considerations for pregnancy, pediatrics, and geriatrics are specific to their comorbid condition.

Bibliography

BMI Calculator. (n.d.-a). *BMI calculator*. Retrieved from http://www.bmi-calculator.net

BMI Calculator. (n.d.-b). *Waist to hip ratio calculator*. Retrieved from http://www.bmi-calculator.net/waist-to-hip-ratio-calculator

Bray, G. A. (2018, October). Obesity in adults: Overview and management. *UpToDate*. Retrieved from http://www.uptodate.com

Centers for Disease Control and Prevention. (2018, March). *Diabetes Home*. Retrieved from https://www.cdc.gov/diabetes/statistics/prevalence_national.htm

Centers for Disease Control and Prevention. (n.d.-a). *Adult BMI calculator: English version*. Retrieved from https://www.cdc.gov/healthyweight/assessing/bmi/adult_bmi/english_bmi_calculator/bmi_calculator.html

Centers for Disease Control and Prevention. (n.d.-b). *BMI percentile calculator for child and teen: English version*. Retrieved from https://nccd.cdc.gov/dnpabmi/calculator.aspx

Freeman, A., & Pennings, N. (2019, March 8). Insulin resistance. *StatPearls*. Retrieved from https://www.ncbi.nlm.nih.gov/books/NBK507839/

Grundy, S. M., Bailey, A. L., Beam, C., Birtcher, K. K., Blumenthal, R. S., Braun, L. T., … Yeboah, J. (2018). 2018 Guideline on the management of blood cholesterol, A report of the American College of Cardiology/American Heart Association task force on clinical practice guidelines. *Journal of the American College of Cardiology*. doi:10.1016/j.jacc.2018.11.003

Klish, W. J. (2018a, October). Clinical evaluation of the obese child and adolescent. *UpToDate*. Retrieved from http://www.uptodate.com

Klish, W. J. (2018b, December). Comorbidities and complications of obesity in children and adolescents. *UpToDate*. Retrieved from http://www.uptodate.com

Klish, W. J. (2018c, December). Definition; epidemiology; and etiology of obesity in children and adolescents. *UpToDate*. Retrieved from http://www.uptodate.com

Lee, A. (Ed.). *NPPR: Nurse practitioners' prescribing reference*. (2019). New York, NY: Haymarket Media. Retrieved from https://www.empr.com/

Lim, R. B. (2018, June). Patient information: Weight loss surgery and procedures: Beyond the basics. *UpToDate Online*. Retrieved from http://www.uptodate.com

Mantzoros, C. (2018, May). Insulin resistance: Definition and clinical spectrum. *UpToDate*. Retrieved from http://www.uptodate.com

Meigs, J. B. (2019, January). The metabolic syndrome (insulin resistance syndrome or syndrome X). *UpToDate*. Retrieved from http://www.uptodate.com

Moore, J. X., Chaudhary N., & Akinyemiju T. (2017). Metabolic syndrome prevalence by race/ethnicity and sex in the United States, National

Health and Nutrition Examination Survey, 1988–2012. *Preventing Chronic Disease 14*, (160287). doi:10.5888/pcd14.160287

National Institutes of Health. (2015). *Third report of the National Cholesterol Education Program (NCEP) expert panel on detection, evaluation, and treatment of high blood cholesterol in adults (ATP III): final report.* Bethesda, MD: Author. Retrieved from https://www.nhlbi.nih.gov/files/docs/guidelines/atp3xsum.pdf

National Lipid Association. (2018, November). *2018 AHA/ACC/AACVPR/AAPA/ABC/ACPM/ADA/AGS/APhA/ASPC/NLA/PCNA guideline on the management of blood cholesterol: Executive summary.* A Report of the American College of Cardiology/American Heart Association Task Force on Clinical Practice Guidelines. Retrieved from http://www.onlinejacc.org/content/accj/early/2018/11/02/j.jacc.2018.11.002.full.pdf

Perreault, L. (2018a, October). Obesity in adults: Health consequences. *UpToDate.* Retrieved from http://www.uptodate.com

Perreault, L. (2018b, June). Patient information: Losing weight: beyond the basics. *UpToDate Online.* Retrieved from http://www.uptodate.com

Perreault, L. (2019a, February). Obesity in adults: Drug therapy. *UpToDate.* Retrieved from http://www.uptodate.com

Perreault, L. (2019b, June). Obesity in adults: Prevalence, screening, and evaluation. *UpToDate Online.* Retrieved from http://www.uptodate.com

Prescriber's Letter. (2019, March). *Consider the new Beer's criteria when prescribing meds for older adults.* Retrieved from https://prescriber.therapeuticresearch.com/Content/Articles/PRL/2019/Mar/Consider-the-New-Beers-Criteria-When-Prescribing-Meds-for-Older-Adults

Skelton, J. A. (2018, October). Management of childhood obesity in the primary care setting. *UpToDate.* Retrieved from http://www.uptodate.com

U.S. Department of Health and Human Services. (2019, February). *Physical activity guidelines for Americans.* Retrieved from https://www.hhs.gov/fitness/be-active/physical-activity-guidelines-for-americans/index.html

Polycystic Ovary Syndrome (PCOS)

Jill C. Cash and Mellisa A. Hall

Definition

PCOS is characterized by ovulatory dysfunction and hyperandrogenism. PCOS was previously called Stein–Leventhal syndrome. PCOS is a risk factor for metabolic syndrome, infertility, glucose intolerance, and T2DM. PCOS itself is not considered a disease; instead, it is a syndrome of coexisting conditions (see Table 20.4).

The Androgen Excess Society diagnostic criteria for PCOS:

A. Hyperandrogenism
B. Ovarian dysfunction
C. Exclusion of other androgen excess or related disorders
   Although obesity is one of the hallmarks of PCOS, lean women may also have insulin resistance/PCOS. The

diagnosis of PCOS is based on medical history, physical examination, and laboratory tests. Aggressive lifestyle modification is the mainstay of all adolescents and women with PCOS.

Incidence

A. The incidence of PCOS is up to 15% in the literature. It is the most common cause of infertility. It is also the most common worldwide endocrinopathy in women, with 5 to 7 million women in the United States experiencing its effects.

Pathogenesis

A. The exact etiology is unknown; however, PCOS is noted to have insulin resistance and abnormal pituitary function, as well as abnormal steroidogenesis.

Predisposing Factors

A. Obesity
B. Genetic predisposition, including Mexican American women
C. Metabolic syndrome
D. Women with oligo-ovulatory infertility
E. Type 1, type 2, or gestational diabetes
F. History of premature adrenarche
G. First-degree relatives with PCOS
H. Antiepileptic medications

Common Complaints

A. Hirsutism
B. Menstrual problems
C. Obesity
D. Infertility

Other Signs and Symptoms

A. Acne
B. Alopecia (male pattern)
C. Hyperhidrosis
D. Acanthosis nigricans
E. Seborrhea

Subjective Data

A. Review the client's menstruation history:
   1. Premature puberty (younger than 8 years)
   2. Primary amenorrhea: lack of menses by age 15 years
   3. Oligomenorrhea: missing four periods per year

TABLE 20.4   PCOS-ASSOCIATED SYMPTOMS

Signs	
Hirsutism	Excessive hair growth on face, shoulders, upper back
Menstrual irregularity	Severe acne
Obesity	Alopecia
Polycystic ovaries	Oligomenorrhea
	Amenorrhea
	Dysfunctional uterine bleeding
	>34.5 inches (88 cm) waist circumference for women and adolescents ≥16 years
	≥90th percentile for ages 10 to <16 years
	Noted on pelvic ultrasound

PCOS, polycystic ovarian syndrome.

4. Dysfunctional uterine bleeding (DUB): bleeding at irregular intervals, heavy cycles, periods longer than 7 days

B. Review the client's history of weight gain, increased waist circumference, and obesity.

C. Review the client's history of any skin/hair changes.

D. Review the family history for the presence of diabetes, metabolic syndrome, and infertility.

Physical Examination

A. Check height, weight, waist circumference, BP, pulse, and respirations.

B. Calculate the BMI and waist-to-hip measurement. Several Internet sites have BMI, body fat, and waist-to-hip ratio calculators.

C. Inspect:
1. Skin
   a. Evaluate hirsutism (upper lip, chin, nape of the neck, periareolar, abdomen—linea alba).
   b. Pigmentation patterns for acanthosis nigricans (neck, axilla)
2. Observe fat distribution.

D. Perform pelvic examination to evaluate enlarged ovaries and pelvic masses.

Diagnostic Tests

A. Fasting glucose

B. OGTT if fasting glucose is elevated between 100 mg/dL and 125 mg/dL

C. Thyroid function tests (TSH, free thyroxine [T4])

D. Random serum cortisol to rule out Cushing's syndrome

E. Serum LH and prolactin to rule out hypothalamic and pituitary diseases

F. Ultrasound to rule out ovarian pathology (as indicated: not required for definitive diagnosis)

G. Insulin-like growth factor (IGF-I)

H. DHEA-S to rule out adrenal hyperandrogenism

I. Free and total testosterone

J. Lipid profile

K. Endometrial biopsy if indicated for women without menses for 1 year

L. Pregnancy test before start of pharmaceutical therapy and history of anovulation

Differential Diagnoses

A. PCOS

B. Adrenal disorders:
1. CAH
2. Cushing's syndrome
3. Cortisol resistance

C. Hyperprolactinemia

D. Acromegaly

E. Insulin resistance (types 1 and 2 diabetes)

F. Thyroid dysfunction

G. Virilizing tumors

H. Drug induced:
1. Anabolic steroids
2. Valproic acid

Plan

A. General interventions:
1. Aggressive lifestyle modification focusing on increased physical activity and weight reduction is a cornerstone for treatment.

B. Client education:
1. Exercise recommendations include a minimum of 30 minutes a day of walking at a brisk pace or other activity at a moderate intensity. Start by using a pedometer, walking at breaks, or performing household work.
2. Weight loss of 5% to 10% or more. Gradual weight loss of 1 to 2 kg/mo is recommended. Even small amounts of weight loss are associated with health benefits.
3. Weight loss may cause a resumption of ovulation and the ability to get pregnant.
4. High-fiber, low-fat diet and reduction of refined sugar
5. Hair removal can be achieved with shaving, waxing, or use of depilatories. Electrolysis and laser treatment are more expensive therapies for hirsutism.

C. Pharmaceutical therapy:
1. Oral contraceptive pills (OCPs) are the most commonly used treatment for endometrial hypertrophy prevention and hirsutism.
   a. Due to sodium and water retention, weight reduction while on OCPs is more difficult.
   b. Oral contraceptives that contain 30 to 35 mcg of ethinyl estradiol and progestins, such as norethindrone (Ortho Micronor), norgestimate (Ortho-Tri-Cyclen), desogestrel (Desogen and Ortho-Cept), or drospirenone (Yasmin), are prescribed for PCOS.
2. Metformin (Glucophage) is used to manage oligomenorrhea, cause weight loss, lower insulin levels, and induce ovulation for women with PCOS.
   a. Start metformin 500 mg at the evening meal. The dosage can be increased by 500 mg/wk in divided doses up to the maximum of 2,000 mg/d.
   b. Titrate slowly because of the gastrointestinal side effects (diarrhea)
   c. Check a metabolic panel before and every 3 to 6 months to evaluate for lactic acidosis
   d. Metformin is contraindicated in clients with late-stage renal impairment; assess renal function before instituting metformin and monitor regularly.
   e. Metformin must be stopped 24 to 48 hours before any procedure with radiographic dye.
3. Progestin:
   a. Medroxyprogesterone acetate (Provera) is used for a withdrawal bleed 5 to 10 mg daily for 10 days every 1 to 2 months. This withdrawal bleeding is advised to protect the endometrium.
   b. Progestin-releasing intrauterine device (IUD)
4. Spironolactone (Aldactone) 100 to 200 mg twice a day is used after a 4- to 6-month oral contraceptive trial as antiandrogen therapy.

TABLE 20.5 ANDROGEN EXCESS SOCIETY SCREENING AND TREATMENT REQUIREMENTS FOR IGT

All clients with PCOS, regardless of BMI, should be screened for IGT using a 2-hour OGTT.
Clients with a normal glucose test should be rescreened at least once every 2 years or earlier if additional risk factors are identified.
Clients with IGT should be screened annually for the development of type 2 DM.
Adolescents with PCOS should be screened for IGT using a 2-hour OGTT every 2 years. If IGT develops, the treatment with metformin should be considered.
The mainstay of treatment with PCOS and IGT is intensive lifestyle modification (diet, exercise, and weight loss).
Screening for depression, anxiety, and eating disorders and appropriate pharmacological/counseling management should be initiated.
Insulin-sensitizing agents should be considered for clients with PCOS and IGT.

BMI, body mass index; DM, diabetes mellitus; IGT, impaired glucose tolerance; OGTT, oral glucose tolerance test; PCOS, polycystic ovary syndrome.

Source: Data from the 2007 Androgen Excess Society Position Statement (Salley, K. E. S., Wickham, E. P., Cheang, K. I., Essah, P. A., Karjane, N. W., & Nestler, J. E. (2007). POSITION STATEMENT: Glucose intolerance in polycystic ovary syndrome—A position statement of the Androgen Excess Society. *The Journal of Clinical Endocrinology & Metabolism, 92*(12), 4546–4556. Retrieved from http://press.endocrine.org/doi/pdf/10.1210/jc.2007-1549); and Polycystic Ovary Syndrome Society position statement (update) for depression, anxiety, quality of life, and eating disorders (2018).

a. Spironolactone is also a good alternative when OCPs are contraindicated. However, spironolactone can be used in combination with OCPs.

b. Alternative methods of birth control should be used when spironolactone is used alone secondary to potential congenital defects such as abnormal development of the male fetus' external genitalia.

c. Monitor potassium level during spironolactone therapy.

5. Eflornithine (Vaniqa) topical may be prescribed to prevent facial hair regrowth.

6. Letrozole is used to induce ovulation. Weight loss should be attempted before starting ovulation induction treatment.

Follow-Up

A. Glucose tolerance needs to be evaluated regularly for type 2 diabetes in women with PCOS (see Table 20.5).

Consultation/Referral

A. Refer to an obstetrician/gynecologist or a reproductive endocrinologist for consultation and management of:
   1. Infertility/pregnancy
   2. Menstrual bleeding that is not controlled despite OCPs

B. An endocrinologist may be an appropriate consultation.

C. Consider a nutritional consultation for weight-loss recommendations.

Bibliography

Androgen Excess and Polycystic Ovarian Syndrome Society. (2019). *Polycystic ovarian syndrome*. Retrieved from http://ae-society.org/sub/resources.php

Azziz, R. (2017, December). Epidemiology and pathogenesis of polycystic ovarian syndrome in adults. *UpToDate*. Retrieved from http://www.uptodate.com

Barbieri, R. L., & Ehrmann, D. A. (2018, November). Treatment of polycystic ovary syndrome in adults. *UpToDate*. Retrieved from http://www.uptodate.com

BMI Calculator. (n.d.-a). *BMI calculator*. Retrieved from http://www.bmi-calculator.net

BMI Calculator. (n.d.-b). *Waist to hip ratio calculator*. Retrieved from http://www.bmi-calculator.net/waist-to-hip-ratio-calculator

Centers for Disease Control and Prevention. (n.d.-a). *Adult BMI calculator: English version*. Retrieved from https://www.cdc.gov/healthyweight/assessing/bmi/adult_bmi/english_bmi_calculator/bmi_calculator.html

Centers for Disease Control and Prevention. (n.d.-b). *BMI percentile calculator for child and teen: English version*. Retrieved from https://nccd.cdc.gov/dnpabmi/calculator.aspx

Dorkras, A., Stener-victorin, E., Yildiz, B., Li, R., Shah, D., Epperson, N., & Teede, H. (2018). Androgen excess—Polycystic ovary syndrome society: Position statement on depression, anxiety, quality of life, and eating disorders in polycystic ovary syndrome. *Fertility Sterility, 109*(5), 888–899. doi:10.1016/j.fertnstert.2018.01.038

Lee, A. (Ed.). *NPPR: Nurse practitioners' prescribing reference*. (2019). New York, NY: Haymarket Media. Retrieved from https://www.empr.com/

Rosenfield, R. L. (2018a, November). Definition, clinical features, and differential diagnosis of polycystic ovary syndrome in adolescents. *UpToDate*. Retrieved from http://www.uptodate.com

Rosenfield, R. L. (2018b, October). Treatment of polycystic ovary syndrome in adolescents. *UpToDate*. Retrieved from http://www.uptodate.com

Salley, K. E. S., Wickham, E. P., Cheang, K. I., Essah, P. A., Karjane, N. W., & Nestler, J. E. (2007). POSITION STATEMENT: Glucose intolerance in polycystic ovary syndrome—A position statement of the Androgen Excess Society. *The Journal of Clinical Endocrinology & Metabolism, 92*(12), 4546–4556. Retrieved from http://press.endocrine.org/doi/pdf/10.1210/jc.2007-1549

Thyroid Disease: Hyperthyroidism

Jill C. Cash and Mellisa A. Hall

Definition

A. Hyperthyroidism is a condition in which thyroid hormone exerts greater than normal responses. Hyperthyroidism may be subclinical and may not be easily recognized or exhibit overt symptoms. The most common hyperthyroid conditions are Graves' disease and toxic multinodular goiter. The USPSTF does not currently recommend screening for thyroid dysfunction in asymptomatic adults who are not pregnant.

Incidence

A. Overall incidence of Graves' disease is 0.5 per 1,000. Graves' disease is responsible for 60% to 80% of cases of thyrotoxicosis.

B. Female gender:
   1. The ratio of 5:1 is higher in women than men.
   2. Older women: 4% to 5% incidence

3. Graves' disease is more common in younger women.
4. Toxic nodular goiter is more common in older women.
C. Children:
   1. Graves' disease in children: 0.02% (1:5,000)
   2. Most often occurs in 11- to 15-year-olds
D. Elderly: Toxic multinodular goiter (Plummer disease) occurs in 15% to 20% of clients with thyrotoxicosis.
E. Symptomatology incidence:
   1. Ophthalmopathy is more common in smokers.
   2. Atrial fibrillation occurs in 10% to 25% of clients and is more common in the elderly.
   3. Autoimmune thyroid diseases have a peak incidence in people aged 20 to 40 years.

Pathogenesis

A. Hyperthyroidism is one form of thyrotoxicosis in which an excess of hormone is excreted by the thyroid gland. The diseases that can cause hyperthyroidism include Graves' disease, toxic multinodular goiter, thyroid cancer, and increased secretion of the TSH. Thyrotoxicosis not related to hyperthyroidism may be subacute thyroiditis, ectopic thyroid tissue, and ingestion of excessive thyroid hormone. Postpartum thyroiditis can precipitate a short-term mild hyperthyroidism, which has an onset at 2 to 6 months postpartum. Severe thyrotoxicosis of any cause is called thyrotoxic crisis or storm.
B. In Graves' disease, the normal feedback mechanisms that regulate hormone secretion are taken over by some abnormal thyroid-stimulating mechanism. Thyroid auto-antibodies of the immunoglobulin G (IgG) class are present in more than 95% of clients with Graves' disease. The hyperfunctioning of the thyroid gland causes suppression of TSH and thyrotropin-releasing hormone (TRH). There are profound increases in iodine uptake and thyroid gland metabolism, which are believed to be the causes of the gland enlargement. The resulting increase in the level of circulating thyroid hormone is responsible for the thyrotoxic symptoms.
C. In the condition called toxic multinodular goiter, the thyroid gland enlarges in response to some bodily need such as puberty; pregnancy; iodine deficiency; and immunologic, viral, and genetic disorders. As TSH levels rise, the gland enlarges; when the condition demanding increased thyroid hormone resolves, TSH levels usually return to normal and the gland slowly assumes its original size.

Predisposing Factors

A. Graves' disease:
   1. Women in the second through fifth decades of life
   2. Familial autoimmune thyroid disease
   3. Concomitant disorders believed to be autoimmune
   4. Increased incidence in clients diagnosed with trisomy 21
   5. Higher incidence in persons who smoke
B. Toxic multinodular goiter:
   1. Older people
   2. Recent exposure to iodine-containing medications (amiodarone and radiocontrast dye)

3. Long-standing simple goiter
4. Conditions such as puberty, pregnancy, iodine deficiency, and immunologic, viral, or genetic disorders

Common Complaints

A. Graves' disease:
   1. Prominence/protrusion of the eye (exophthalmos)
   2. Prominent "stare"
   3. Visual changes:
      a. Diplopia
      b. Photophobia
      c. Eye irritation: gritty feeling or pain
B. Weight loss with no change in diet or an increase in appetite
C. Anorexia (may be prominent in the elderly)
D. Weakness and fatigue
E. Tachycardia
F. Decreased tolerance to heat
G. Thinning scalp hair
H. Fingernail separation from the nail bed
I. Smooth, thin skin
J. Heart palpitations (atrial fibrillation)
K. Bowel symptoms:
   1. Increase in frequency and loose bowel movements (not diarrhea)
   2. Constipation (more frequent in the elderly)
L. Swelling of feet and ankles

Other Signs and Symptoms

A. Goiter: **Approximately 50% of clients will not have an enlargement of the thyroid gland**. Elderly clients are less likely to have a goiter.
B. Periorbital edema
C. Flushing, warm skin
D. Fine hand tremors
E. Dyspnea (especially elderly)
F. Exertional fatigue/exercise intolerance
G. Insomnia
H. Irritability
I. Nervousness
J. Mood swings
K. Inability to concentrate
L. Depression and apathy (elderly)
M. Hyperactivity (children)
N. Decreased menses
O. Impotence and decreased libido in men
P. Gynecomastia
Q. Galactorrhea (TSH-mediated hyperthyroidism)
R. Atrial dysrhythmias (atrial fibrillation), left ventricular dilation (common in elderly)
S. Urinary frequency and nocturia (enuresis is common in children)
T. A combination of these noted symptoms should lead to the assessment of hyperthyroidism.

Subjective Data

A. Identify when symptoms began, duration, and any change or progression.
B. Identify if perceived thyroidmegaly, difficulty swallowing, or change in voice

C. Assess for change in weight over the past 3 months, past 6 months, and last year. Ask the client whether his or her appetite has changed.
D. Explore the client's family history of thyroid problems.
E. Obtain the client's medical history of associated diseases (especially those of autoimmune pathogenesis: pernicious anemia, type 1 diabetes mellitus [T1DM], myasthenia gravis, RA, ulcerative colitis).
F. Review the client's medication history, including amiodarone, interferon alpha, levothyroxine (overdose), expectorants, and health food supplements containing seaweed.
G. Ask the client to identify any changes in bowel habits, loose (nondiarrhea) stools, frequency of bowel movements, or constipation.
H. Ask about moods, changes in concentration, feelings of restlessness, nervousness, anxiety, and change in sleep habits.
I. Assess for any cardiac symptoms, such as palpitations, chest pain, shortness of breath, and decreased tolerance for activities previously done.
J. Ask whether the client has noticed any swelling or puffiness anywhere.
K. Determine whether the client has experienced changes in vision and/or eye irritation.
L. Assess for hand tremors, increase in the moistness and coolness of the skin, flushing, and blushing.
M. Ask the client to identify any menstrual changes or whether the client has had a recent pregnancy, or is in the postpartum period.
N. Review for a recent history of a viral infection.
O. Review recent trauma to the neck (significant trauma can cause thyrotoxicosis).

Physical Examination
A. Check temperature, if indicated, pulse (tachycardia), respirations (dyspnea), BP (systolic hypertension), and weight. Children: plot height/weight on growth curve (accelerated growth is noted).
B. Inspect:
1. Observe overall appearance: Does the client have any difficulty with breathing, including dyspnea, or difficulty swallowing from tracheal obstruction secondary to a large goiter?
2. Note eyelid retraction, lid lag, and exophthalmos. The clinician may see periorbital edema and an elevated upper eyelid, which leads to decreased blinking and a staring quality in Graves' disease.
3. Note tremors that are best demonstrated from outstretched hands.
4. Inspect the skin for temperature and texture.
5. Inspect the fingernails for:
    a. Onycholysis, also known as Plummer's nails (loosening of the nails from the nail beds)
    b. Softening of the nails
6. Inspect scalp hair.
7. Assess Tanner stage in preadolescence/adolescence. Puberty may be delayed.

C. Auscultate:
1. The thyroid for bruits
2. The heart and pulse rate. Clients with subclinical hyperthyroidism frequently present with atrial fibrillation.
3. The carotid arteries for bruits
4. Bowel sounds
D. Palpate:
1. Palpate the neck and thyroid for nodules, thrills, and enlargement. Depending on the etiology of the hyperthyroidism, the thyroid may range from normal to massive (Graves' disease or toxic multinodular goiter). Palpation of the thyroid can induce the gland to release increased hormone; be alert for signs and symptoms of thyroid storm.
2. If the thyroid is tender and painful to palpation, granulomatous thyroiditis may be the etiology of hyperthyroidism.
3. Palpate the heart for thrills.
4. Palpate extremities for edema. Pretibial myxedema is noted in Graves' disease.
E. Neurologic examination:
1. Assess DTRs.
2. Tests for lid lag:
    a. Have the client follow your finger as it moves up and down.
    b. Have the client look down and observe whether sclera can be seen above the iris.
3. Have the client stick out the tongue to observe for presence of tremors.

Diagnostic Tests
A. TSH, free T4, triiodothyronine (T3) (see Table 20.6)
B. Radioactive iodine (131I) uptake (RAIU) if needed. If the client has ophthalmopathy, clinical symptoms of hyperthyroidism, and a diffusely enlarged thyroid gland, the RAIU test is not necessary to confirm Graves' disease. Pregnancy and breastfeeding are absolute contraindications to radionuclide imaging.
C. Sonography provides information about gland size and structure. RAIU is needed if information about thyroid gland functioning is required.
D. Consider additional laboratory testing:
1. CBC: look for possible normochromic, normocytic anemia
2. Serum ferritin (may be high)
E. If T4 and T3 are high, but TSH is normal or high, an MRI of the pituitary should be ordered to look for a pituitary mass.
F. An echocardiogram should be considered when an irregular heart rate and signs of heart failure are noted on examination.

Differential Diagnoses
A. CVD such as CAD and heart failure
B. Gastrointestinal disorders such as irritable bowel syndrome (IBS), ulcerative colitis, and Crohn's disease
C. Cancer: testicular germ cell tumors
D. Neurologic disorder

TABLE 20.6   TEST RESULTS IN HYPERTHYROIDISM

Disorder	TSH	Free T4	T3	RAIU and Thyroid Scan
Overt hyperthyroidism	L	H	H	H
Graves' disease	L	H	H	H
Multinodular goiter	L	H	–	H
T3 thyrotoxicosis (may be caused by antithyroid drug therapy)	L	N or H	H	N or H

H, high; L, low; N, normal, RAIU, radioactive iodine uptake; T3, triiodothyronine; T4, free thyroxine; TSH, thyroid-stimulating hormone.

E. Hydatidiform mole (molar pregnancy)
F. Psychological disorder

Plan

A. General interventions:
1. Carefully assess for complications of hyperthyroidism—cardiac, ophthalmologic, gastrointestinal, musculoskeletal, and psychological—and address each area identified.
2. Clients with tachycardia, palpitations, tremors, anxiety, and eyelid lag can be treated with a beta-adrenergic antagonist for some relief from those symptoms until they become euthyroid.
3. For infiltrative dermopathy over the lower extremities, the use of occlusive wraps on the affected side is recommended.
4. Only 5% of clients with Graves' disease develop severe ophthalmopathy. An initial ophthalmologic examination is recommended as baseline, with follow-up determined by the ophthalmologist.
B. Client teaching:
1. Clients taking propylthiouracil (PTU) or methimazole (MMI) should be instructed to immediately report any side effects, including rash, hives, fever, jaundice, abdominal pain, and clay-colored stools.
2. Less than 1% of clients develop agranulocytosis, but all clients should be instructed to call the provider immediately if a fever, sore throat, or joint ache develops due to their susceptibility to serious infection.
3. Clients receiving radioactive iodine (RAI) should be informed that they most likely need to take life-long hormone replacement after the RAI treatment is completed.
4. Teach safety measures to guard against the possibility of fractures due to bone density loss secondary to hyperthyroidism.
5. Inform clients that an episode of serious depression may follow successful treatment of hyperthyroidism.
6. No special diet is required; however, clients should be told to avoid herbal supplements and sushi that contains seaweed.
C. Pharmaceutical therapy:
1. Antithyroid drugs: The choice of drugs depends on clinician experience, the severity of the disease, and client preference. Provide titration of antithyroid drug dose every 4 weeks until thyroid function normalizes and to ensure the client does not become hypothyroid. Graves' disease may go into remission after treatment for 12 to 18 months and drug therapy can be discontinued.
    a. PTU:
        i. Initial dose 100 to 150 mg by mouth three times daily. Dosage decrease is almost always required at 4 to 8 weeks of start.
        ii. Thyroid storm: 150 to 200 mg orally every 4 to 6 hours
        iii. Not a first-line agent in pediatrics
        iv. Except in thyroid storm, PTU is considered a second-line drug therapy. It is reserved for use in clients who are allergic to or intolerant of MMI and in women who are in the first trimester of pregnancy or planning pregnancy.
    b. MMI (Tapazole):
        i. Adults: 20 to 40 mg/d or in divided twice-a-day dose. Maintenance doses are 2.5 to 15 mg/d.
        ii. Pediatrics: 0.2 mg/kg/d
        iii. MMI is more potent than PTU and has a longer duration of action.
        iv. MMI is not recommended for use in the first trimester of pregnancy.
2. RAI therapy is one of the most common treatments in adults. It is administered orally as a single dose. RAI is contraindicated in pregnancy and lactation.
3. Beta-blockers, such as propranolol (Inderal), are also used for hyperthyroidism until TSH levels are normalized.
4. Atrial fibrillation treatment is directed toward restoring an euthyroid state. Other therapies include the following:
    a. Beta-blockers (unless contraindicated, including chronic obstructive pulmonary disease [COPD] and asthma)
    b. Calcium channel blockers if unable to use beta-blocker
    c. Oral anticoagulation (keeping the international normalized ratio [INR] between 2 and 3)
    d. Antiarrhythmic drugs and cardioversion may be unsuccessful until euthyroid.

D. Medical/surgical management:
1. RAI is a common choice of therapy for adults. It is administered in capsule form or in water.
   a. One dose is usually sufficient; however, a second dose may be given if necessary.
   b. Permanent hypothyroidism requiring lifelong hormone replacement is the only notable complication.
2. A thyroidectomy is seldom used except in limited client conditions.
   a. Pregnancy if women are noncompliant or cannot tolerate thionamides because of allergies or agranulocytosis
   b. Severe hyperthyroidism in children
   c. Clients who refuse RAI therapy
   d. Refractory amiodarone-induced hyperthyroidism
   e. Clients with unstable cardiac conditions that require quick normalization of thyroid function

Follow-Up

A. Depending on the experience of the clinician, a specialist, such as an endocrinologist, best performs treatment and therapy, including RAI and antithyroid medication.
B. Clients receiving PTU or MMI should be seen in the office every 4 to 6 weeks for evaluation and have blood drawn for serum TSH and free T4 measurements until euthyroid state is achieved and maintained.
C. Clients are usually maintained on these drugs for 1 to 2 years, with office visits every 3 months. The drug is then gradually withdrawn; 25% to 90% of clients experience permanent remission.
D. Clients with RAI therapy should be seen in the office to monitor thyroid levels. It is anticipated that most of them will require lifelong hormone replacement medication following treatment.
E. Due to the increased risk of bone loss, perform dual-energy x-ray absorptiometry (DEXA) scans to evaluate for osteopenia/osteoporosis.
F. Consider testing for IGT in untreated clients.

Consultation/Referral

A. Ophthalmology consultation is recommended for clients with ophthalmologic involvement.
B. If surgery is the choice of treatment, refer the client to an endocrinologist and a surgeon.
C. An experienced obstetrician or perinatologist should follow pregnant women.

Individual Considerations

A. Pregnancy:
1. Pregnant clients with mild hyperthyroidism may be followed with treatment.
2. If an antithyroid drug is necessary, PTU is the drug of choice in the first trimester. MMI has been associated with congenital anomalies such as tracheoesophageal fistula and choanal atresia. After the first trimester, mothers may be switched to MMI.
3. Monitor thyroid function every 4 weeks during pregnancy.
4. RAI therapy is contraindicated during pregnancy and breastfeeding.
5. Thyrotoxicosis may improve during pregnancy; however, symptoms may relapse during the postpartum period.
6. Hyperthyroidism in the third trimester may increase the risk of low birth weight.
7. Prolonged high-dose iodine therapy can cause fetal goiter.
8. Ultrasounds should be performed to evaluate fetal hyperthyroidism, such as goiter, poor growth, cardiac failure, and hydrops fetalis.
B. Pediatrics:
1. Low thyroid function at birth is present in approximately half of the neonates whose mother received PTU or MMI during pregnancy.
2. Graves' disease can occur in prepubescent girls. Symptoms can be vague and include hyperactivity or slowness and fatigue.
3. Carefully assess for goiter in children who present with a variety of symptoms otherwise unexplained.
4. PTU should not be used in pediatrics unless there is allergy to, or intolerance of, MMI and other options are not available.
C. Adults:
1. Sympathetic activation (anxiety, hyperactivity, etc.) is seen in adult years more commonly than in the elderly population.
D. Geriatrics:
1. Older patents exhibit only three clinical signs (tachycardia, fatigue, and weight loss), whereas younger clients may exhibit as many as 12 symptoms.
2. Rare signs in this population include atrial fibrillation, hyperactive reflexes, increased sweating, heat intolerance, tremors, nervousness, polydipsia, and increased appetite. Goiter is much less common.
3. Elderly women with hyperthyroidism are at increased risk for accelerated bone loss.

Bibliography

Centers for Disease Control and Prevention, NCHS National Center for Health Statistics. (n.d.). *Clinical growth charts*. Retrieved from https://www.cdc.gov/growthcharts
LaFranchi, S. (2018, July). Clinical manifestations and diagnosis of Graves in children and adolescents. *UpToDate*. Retrieved from http://www.uptodate.com
Lee, A. (Ed.). *NPPR: Nurse practitioners' prescribing reference*. (2019). New York, NY: Haymarket Media. Retrieved from https://www.empr.com/
National Guideline Clearinghouse. (2015, May). *Screening for thyroid dysfunction: U. S. Preventative Services task force recommendation statement*. Retrieved from http://www.guideline.gov/content.aspx?id=49227&search=thyroid+screening
Prescriber's Letter. (2019, March). Consider the new Beer's criteria when prescribing meds for older adults. Retrieved from https://prescriber.therapeuticresearch.com/Content/Articles/PRL/2019/Mar/Consider-the-New-Beers-Criteria-When-Prescribing-Meds-for-Older-Adults
Rubin, D. I. (2018, November). Neurologic manifestations of hyperthyroidism and Graves' disease. *UpToDate*. Retrieved from http://www.uptodate.com

Thyroid Disease: Hypothyroidism

Jill C. Cash and Mellisa A. Hall

Definition

A. Hypothyroidism is a condition in which the body does not produce enough thyroid hormone. In general, hypothyroidism is considered permanent, requiring life-long therapy to restore a euthyroid state. The most common physical finding is a goiter. The most common worldwide cause of hypothyroidism is iodine deficiency, whereas the most common cause in the United States is Hashimoto thyroiditis, an autoimmune thyroid disease.

Incidence

A. Hypothyroidism occurs in 5% of the population.
B. It occurs in women more than men (five to eight times higher).
C. The incidence is higher in Whites (5.1%) and Mexican Americans than in African Americans (1.7%).
D. It may present in up to 15% of people older than 65 years.
E. In adolescents, approximately 6% have acquired hypothyroidism.
F. Approximately 10% of clients with type 1 diabetes will develop chronic thyroiditis.
G. After pregnancy, up to 10% of women develop lymphocytic thyroiditis in the postpartum period (up to 10 months postpartum).
H. Approximately 1:4,000 newborns have congenital hypothyroidism (cretinism).

Pathogenesis

Hypothyroidism is caused by an insufficient production of thyroid hormones by the thyroid gland, either by a primary or a secondary cause.

A. Primary causes include decreased hormone production caused by autoimmune thyroiditis, endemic iodine deficiency, congenital defects, or decreased thyroid activity after treatment for hyperthyroidism.
  1. The most common cause of primary hypothyroidism is chronic autoimmune thyroiditis called Hashimoto's thyroiditis. In this disease, circulating thyroid antibodies and the infiltration of lymphocytes destroy thyroid tissue. Autoimmune thyroiditis may also be a result of an inherited immune defect.
B. Secondary causes are much less common but may include insufficient stimulation from the pituitary or hypothalamus and peripheral resistance to thyroid hormones.
C. Acute thyroidism is a rare cause of hypothyroidism in which the cause is an acute bacterial infection. Subacute thyroiditis, a nonbacterial inflammation of the thyroid, is often preceded by a viral infection. Both of these conditions cause inflammation of the thyroid gland by lymphocytic and leukocytic infiltration into the thyroid tissue, resulting in hypothyroidism.

Predisposing Factors

A. Iodine deficiency
B. Women older than 40 years at highest risk
C. Presence of other autoimmune disorders (diagnosed and previously undiagnosed)
D. Recent acute bacterial or viral infection
E. Treatment with RAI for thyroid gland problems
F. Surgical removal of thyroid gland
G. Exposure to external radiation
H. Evidence of pituitary or hypothalamic disease
I. Postpartum period
J. Type 1 (autoimmune) DM
K. Chromosomal disorders:
  1. Down syndrome
  2. Turner's syndrome
  3. Klinefelter's syndrome
L. Celiac disease
M. Drug-induced:
  1. Amiodarone
  2. Interferon alpha
  3. Thalidomide
  4. Lithium
  5. Stavudine
  6. Dopamine

Common Complaints

A. Weight gain/obesity
B. Fatigue/sluggishness
C. Cold intolerance
D. Constipation
E. Dry and flaky skin
F. Coarseness hair or loss of hair, inability of hair to hold a curl, hair loss at eyebrows, and reduced growth of hair
G. Reduced growth of nails
H. Hoarseness
I. Memory or mental impairment, difficulty concentrating, and slowed speech or thinking
J. Periorbital edema and facial puffiness
K. Irregular or heavy menses and infertility
L. Muscle aching and stiffness
M. Children:
  1. Short stature
  2. Delayed skeletal maturation
  3. Overweight
  4. Delayed puberty
  5. Some adolescents have sexual precocity:
    a. Girls: breast development
    b. Boys: macro-orchidism

Other Signs and Symptoms

A. Asymptomatic if subclinical hypothyroidism and have no overt symptoms
B. Delayed reflexes
C. Elevated BP
D. Hyperlipidemia
E. Jaundice
F. Painful subacute thyroiditis:
  1. Sudden neck pain with sore throat, radiating to jaw and ears, and pain shifting to sides of the neck

2. Late stage: myxedema, thick scaly skin, muscle weakness/joint pain, enlarged tongue, hearing loss, bradycardia, cardiac hypertrophy, pleural effusion, and ascites

G. Pituitary or hypothalamic failure:
   1. Loss of axillary and pubic hair
   2. Cessation of menses
   3. Postural hypotension

H. Exercise intolerance

I. Carpal tunnel syndrome a common occurrence

J. Depression

K. Ataxia

L. Decreased concentration/memory impairment

Subjective Data

A. Note history of recent illness and/or pregnancy.

B. Evaluate the client's medical/surgical history for any treatment of hyperthyroid, including radioactive treatment or thyroidectomy.

C. Review dietary and weight history, how much weight has been gained, and over what period of time.

D. Review any changes in health status or symptoms associated with other body systems (thyroid symptoms usually involve multiple body systems).

E. Review any history of OSA.

F. Assess for pain or swelling of the neck or difficulty swallowing.

G. Inquire as to the client's history of supervoltage x-ray therapy to the neck for nonthyroid cancer or for polio.

H. Identify family history:
   1. Does the client have a first-degree relative with thyroid disease?
   2. Is there a family history of any endocrine problems, including thyroid, T1DM, and/or RA?

I. Review the client's medication history for current medication, OTC medications, vitamins, or herbal supplements.

J. Review the client's menstrual history or history of infertility.

K. Inquire about constipation (new onset or worsening).

Physical Examination

A. Check pulse (bradycardia), respirations, BP (decreased systolic BP and increased diastolic BP), and weight. Plot the height/weight on a growth curve for children.

B. Inspect:
   1. Inspect the skin (dry/flaky) for presence of jaundice.
   2. Inspect the hair (coarse, thin, brittle) and decrease in pubic/axillary hair pattern.
   3. Perform oral examination for evaluation of macroglossia (enlarged tongue).
   4. Inspect the face/eye for periorbital puffiness/edema.
   5. Inspect the neck for the presence of a goiter and surgical scar.
   6. Child: assess Tanner stage of puberty.

C. Auscultate:
   1. The thyroid and carotids
   2. The heart
   3. The lungs
   4. The abdomen for bowel sounds in each quadrant (hypoactive)

D. Palpate:
   1. The neck, thyroid gland, and lymph nodes
   2. The abdomen for presence of abdominal distension, ascites, masses in left lower quadrant, and hepatomegaly
   3. Palpate/evaluate extremities for edema.

E. General observation:
   1. Gait problems, such as ataxia or rigidity, and spasticity of the trunk and proximal extremities
   2. Quality of the client's voice (hoarseness)
   3. Signs of depression, decreased concentration, or memory impairment

F. Musculoskeletal examination: perform a detailed musculoskeletal examination

G. Neurologic examination:
   1. Check visual fields (restricted with hypothyroidism).
   2. Test hearing:
      a. Whisper words and have the client repeat.
      b. Use a ticking watch.
      c. Use a tuning fork:
         i. Weber test: Place vibrating fork on top midline of head (sound hearing equally in both ears).
         ii. Rinne test: Place vibrating tuning fork on mastoid, begin counting, and ask the client to tell you when he or she no longer hears; then quickly reposition 1/2 to 1 inch from the ear and ask the client when he or she no longer hears (hearing should be twice as long as bone conduction).
   3. Check for loss or reduction of DTRs.
   4. Evaluate proximal muscle weakness/strength.
   5. Test for abnormal tandem gait: have the client walk across the room in a heel–toe, heel–toe fashion.
   6. Check for sensory loss:
      a. Evaluate the first three fingers and one half of the fourth finger on testing loss of sensation from carpal tunnel syndrome.
      b. Evaluate sensory loss of the feet/legs (generally symmetrical in a "stocking-glove" distribution).

Diagnostic Tests

A. TSH

B. When a high TSH is noted, repeat the test and add a free T4.

C. T3 resin uptake

D. Thyroid antibodies (see Table 20.7)

E. TSH assay (if TSH assay is elevated, it indicates hypothyroidism)

F. Thyroid scan

G. CBC (anemia)

H. Lipid profile

I. Ultrasound of the neck and thyroid to detect nodules (not a first-line test)

Differential Diagnoses

A. Obesity: Clients with elevated total cholesterol levels or triglyceride levels are often misdiagnosed by assuming that these symptoms are caused by obesity and high-fat diets.

TABLE 20.7   TEST RESULTS IN HYPOTHYROIDISM

Disorder	TSH	Free T4	T3	RAIU and Thyroid Scan	Peroxidase Antibodies
Hypothyroid	H	L	Sometimes L	N or L	n/a
Hashimoto's disease	H or variable	N or L	Not helpful	Variable	Positive
Subacute hypothyroidism	L	H	H or variable	L or absent	Negative/low titers
Silent lymphocytic thyroiditis (usually postpartum)	L when toxic; H when hypothyroid	n/a	L when toxic	Positive	Positive

H, high; L, low; N, normal, RAIU, radioactive iodine uptake; TSH, thyroid-stimulating hormone.

B. Depression
C. Ischemic heart disease
D. Nephrotic syndrome
E. Cirrhosis
F. Side effects/adverse effects of medications
G. Constipation
H. Sleep apnea/sleep disorder
I. Fibromyalgia
J. Infectious mononucleosis

Plan

A. General interventions:

1. The American Thyroid Association clinical practice guideline for detection of both subclinical and symptomatic hypothyroidism recommends that all adults age 35 years and older be screened for hypothyroidism every 5 years to identify thyroid disease in the early stages. However, Medicare does not cover a screening TSH in an asymptomatic client.

2. Clients with underactive thyroids require lifelong treatment with levothyroxine.

3. In clients with subacute thyroiditis, relatively large doses of nonsteroidal anti-inflammatory drugs (NSAIDs) or prednisone may be prescribed.

4. For clients with enlarged thyroid glands, surgery may be recommended if the gland begins obstructing the airway.

5. The treatment of clients with malignant thyroid nodules depends on the type of cancer.

B. Client teaching:

1. Teach the client about the nature and course of the disease, as well as the signs and symptoms. Frequently, clients are relieved that their perceived symptoms are real and that there is treatment. This may also improve client compliance.

2. Teach the client to report any side effects of the levothyroxine and desiccated thyroid medications:

   a. Tachycardia
   b. Palpitations
   c. Chest pain

3. Emphasize the need for lifelong treatment with levothyroxine and the dangers of noncompliance.

4. **Thyroid replacement should be taken on an empty stomach.**

5. The beneficial effects of thyroid replacement occur in about 3 days to 1 week; the client may not feel the clinical effects for several months.

6. When switching brands or using a generic, the serum TSH should be checked in 6 weeks.

C. Pharmaceutical therapy:

1. **Clients requiring therapy with levothyroxine should be treated with the same brand/generic consistently because potency varies between brands and generics.**

   a. Levothyroxine (Synthroid, Levoxyl, Levothroid, Unithroid):

      i. Adult dose is 1.6 mcg/kg/d by mouth administered as a single dose in the morning on an empty stomach.

      ii. Elderly with comorbid CAD or severe COPD should be started at 25 to 50 mcg/d.

      iii. Maintenance dose is 50 to 200 mcg by mouth every morning.

      iv. Pediatric dosing is age and weight dependent.

   b. Desiccated thyroid (Armour thyroid):

      i. Adult initial dosing is 15 to 30 mg/d by mouth and increased by 15 to 30 mg/d every 4 weeks.

      ii. Maintenance dose is 60 to 180 mg/d.

      iii. Pediatric dosing is age and weight dependent.

2. The medication should be titrated to the lowest dosage needed to maintain euthyroidism and a nonelevated serum TSH and a normal or slightly elevated T4.

3. Elderly clients and those with CVD should be started on very low doses (25 mcg/d) of levothyroxine; doses are increased very gradually, over 8 to 12 weeks, as tolerated. Close monitoring for the development of cardiac complications such as angina, arrhythmias, and MI needs to be undertaken.

4. Thyroid hormones should be taken on an empty stomach in the mornings to avoid insomnia.

5. Other drugs that can reduce the effectiveness/affect of the absorption of thyroid hormone are the following:

   a. Cholesterol-reducing drugs

   b. Cholestyramine interferes with absorption in the gut.

   c. Calcium carbonate

   d. Aluminum hydroxide

   e. Sucralfate (Carafate)

   f. If taking one of these drugs and levothyroxine, they should be taken 4 to 6 hours apart.

6. Dietary fiber can interfere with levothyroxine absorption. Coffee reduces the absorption of levothyroxine.

7. Pharmacological treatment of the client with subclinical hypothyroidism is controversial. If goiter is present, treatment may be considered.

Follow-Up

A. Clients who are not treated with medication should be seen every 6 to 12 months for reevaluation.

B. When medication is instituted, monitor laboratory values and client well-being in the office every 4 to 6 weeks.

C. After the dosage is stabilized, the client with an elevated serum TSH level should be seen every 6 to 12 months.

1. Undetectable TSH levels are indicative of overmedication.

2. High TSH levels are indicative of insufficient medication or client noncompliance.

D. After the TSH is normalized, regular annual follow-up visits are required.

E. Order DEXA scan as indicated to screen for bone loss/osteopenia/osteoporosis.

Consultation/Referral

A. Consultation with an endocrinologist is recommended for:

1. Children/teens younger than 18 years

2. Clients unresponsive to therapy

3. Pregnant clients

4. Presence of goiter, nodule, or other structural changes in the thyroid

5. Compression symptoms of dysphagia

6. Any client with myxedema, significant cardiac disease, or involvement or hypothyroidism secondary to pituitary or hypothalamic failure should be managed in consultation with a physician or should be referred to an endocrinologist for continued care.

7. If fine-needle aspiration biopsy is required

Individual Considerations

A. Pregnancy:

1. Monitor TSH levels monthly during the first trimester.

2. Small increases in medication dosage may be required.

3. Some women develop postpartum thyroiditis and hypothyroidism after taking hyperthyroid medication during pregnancy or immediately thereafter.

4. Postpartum: monitor TSH level at 6 weeks' postpartum examination.

5. A common cause of congenital hypothyroidism is maternal and infant iodine deficiency.

6. Monitor TSH to avoid overtreatment in postpartum women because excess thyroid hormone levels increase the risk of osteoporosis.

7. Hypothyroidism in pregnancy is associated with preeclampsia, anemia, postpartum hemorrhage, cardiac ventricular dysfunction, spontaneous abortion, low birth weight, impaired cognitive development, and fetal mortality.

B. Geriatrics:

1. Some elderly clients who are actually hyperthyroid exhibit symptoms of hypothyroidism.

Bibliography

Centers for Disease Control and Prevention, NCHS National Center for Health Statistics. (n.d.). *Clinical growth charts*. Retrieved from https://www.cdc.gov/growthcharts

Grundy, S. M., Bailey, A. L., Beam, C., Birtcher, K. K., Blumenthal, R. S., Braun, L. T., … Yeboah, J. (2018). 2018 Guideline on the management of blood cholesterol. A report of the American College of Cardiology/American Heart Association task force on clinical practice guidelines. *Journal of the American College of Cardiology*. doi:10.1016/j.jacc.2018.11.003

LaFranchi, S. (2018, November). Clinical features and detection of congenital hypothyroidism. *UpToDate*. Retrieved from http://www.uptodate.com

Lee, A. (Ed.). *NPPR: Nurse practitioners' prescribing reference*. (2019). New York, NY: Haymarket Media. Retrieved from https://www.empr.com/

Prescriber's Letter. (2019, March). *Consider the new Beer's criteria when prescribing meds for older adults*. Retrieved from https://prescriber.therapeuticresearch.com/Content/Articles/PRL/2019/Mar/Consider-the-New-Beers-Criteria-When-Prescribing-Meds-for-Older-Adults

Ross, D. S. (2017a, November). Diagnosis and screening for hypothyroidism in non-pregnant adults. *UpToDate*. Retrieved from http://www.uptodate.com

Ross, D. S. (2017b, September). Treatment of primary hypothyroidism in adults. *UpToDate*. Retrieved from http://www.uptodate.com

Ross, D. S. (2018, May). Hypothyroidism during pregnancy: Clinical manifestations, diagnosis, and treatment. *UpToDate*. Retrieved from http://www.uptodate.com

Thyrotoxicosis/Thyroid Storm

Jill C. Cash and Mellisa A. Hall

Definition

A. Severe thyrotoxicosis of any cause is called thyrotoxic crisis or storm.

Incidence

A. It is rare; the incidence varies, depending on the cause of the thyrotoxicosis.

Pathogenesis

A. Thyrotoxic crisis or storm usually develops in clients either undiagnosed as being hyperthyroid or those who are known to be severely hyperthyroid, are being treated insufficiently, and are subjected to excessive stress from other causes. Oversecretion of T3 and T4 is followed by a release of epinephrine. Metabolism is dramatically increased, and the adrenal glands produce excessive corticosteroids, which is a response to stress.

Predisposing Factors

A. Severe, uncontrolled hyperthyroidism
B. Noncompliance with antihyperthyroid medication
C. Inadequate preparation for thyroid surgery

Common Complaints

A. Sudden onset of:
   1. Hyperthermia
   2. Tachycardia (usually atrial tachydysrhythmias)
   3. High-output cardiac failure
   4. Altered sensorium (usually agitation, restlessness, delirium)
   5. Nausea, vomiting, and diarrhea

Subjective Data

A. Elicit information regarding the onset, duration, and nature of symptoms.
B. Determine the presence of cardiac symptoms.
C. Take a complete drug history, including whether or not the client has been taking antithyroid medication as prescribed.
D. Rule out any excessive acute stressors such as infection, pulmonary or cardiac problems, dialysis, plasmapheresis, and/or emotional stressors.
E. Rule out illicit substance abuse.

Physical Examination

A. Check temperature, pulse, respirations, and BP.
B. Inspect:
   1. The skin
C. Auscultate:
   1. The heart and lungs
D. Palpate:
   1. Neck carefully for thyroid nodules and enlargement

Diagnostic Tests

A. Serum T3 and free T4
B. TSH

Differential Diagnoses

A. Thyrotoxic crisis

Plan

A. General interventions:
   1. Closely monitor temperature, pulse, respirations, and BP
   2. Assess the need to hospitalize the client for supportive therapy: intravenous fluids, medication treatment, antipyretics, and/or oxygen.
B. Client teaching:
   1. See "Client Teaching" in the "Hyperthyroidism" section.
C. Pharmaceutical therapy:
   1. See "Pharmaceutical Therapy" in the "Hyperthyroidism" section.

Follow-Up

A. Following resolution of the crisis, see the client in the office every 3 to 4 weeks for evaluation and monitoring of serum TSH and free T4 levels.
B. See "Follow-Up" in the "Hyperthyroidism" section.

Consultation/Referral

A. Refer the client to a physician immediately for possible hospitalization.

Individual Considerations

A. Pregnancy: see "Individual Considerations" in the "Hyperthyroidism" section.

Bibliography

Lee, A. (Ed.). *NPPR: Nurse practitioners' prescribing reference.* (2019). New York, NY: Haymarket Media. Retrieved from https://www.empr.com/

National Guideline Clearinghouse. (2015, May). *Screening for thyroid dysfunction: U. S. Preventative Services task force recommendation statement.* Retrieved from http://www.guideline.gov/content.aspx?id=49227&search=thyroid+screening

Ross, D. S. (2019, January). Thyroid storm. *UpToDate.* Retrieved from http://www.uptodate.com

21 Rheumatological Guidelines

Ankylosing Spondylitis

Jill C. Cash

Definition
A. Ankylosing spondylitis (AS) is a chronic inflammatory joint disease that causes joint pain/swelling, which primarily affects the spine and sacroiliac (SI) joints; however, larger peripheral joints can also be affected.

Incidence
A. AS occurs in approximately 1% to 2% of the general population.
B. Prevalence rates differ between races. AS occurs in approximately 0.04% to 0.06% of non-Caucasians and in approximately 0.1% to 1.4% of Caucasians.

Pathogenesis
A. Inflammation occurs at the entheses (insertion site of the ligaments and tendons of the bone) throughout the body. Primary sites of involvement include the lower back, SI joint, and lower extremities. Inflammatory cells invade the joint and erode the bone and fibrocartilage of the joints. The body responds by trying to repair the tissue and forms fibrous scar tissue. The structure is replaced by the ossified scar tissue, which causes fusion of the joint; in return, flexibility of the joint is lost. The eroded joint tries to repair itself by osteoblast formation in building new bone tissue. This results in the production of new enthesis that deposits itself on top of the existing enthesis. Calcification of the spinal ligaments also occurs and the appearance of the vertebral bodies looks more "square" and distinct. This appearance is referred to as a "bamboo spine."

Predisposing Factors
A. Gender (men > women, 3:1 ratio)
B. Race (Caucasians more prevalent, occurring more in the northern European countries)
C. Age: Onset of symptoms usually occurs during the early 20s. However, diagnosis usually is made several years after the onset of symptoms, more into the late 20- to 30-year range. AS rarely occurs after the age of 50.
D. Family history of AS
E. Thought to have a genetic predisposition: serum HLA-B27 positive. Approximately 90% to 95% of clients with AS have a positive HLA-B27. However, only 5% of clients with a positive HLA-B27 develop any type of spondyloarthropathy.

Common Complaints
A. Chronic back pain that has been gradual with the onset of low back pain symptoms occurring in the early 20s
B. SI joint pain
C. Joint pain (back pain) occurring for more than 3 months, with morning stiffness
D. Low back pain/joint pain that improves with activity, worsens with rest
E. Dactylitis (sausage digits of the fingers/toes)
F. Enthesitis (inflammation/pain at insertion site of the tendon or ligament to the bone)

Other Signs and Symptoms
A. Peripheral joint pain and swelling
B. Decreased range of motion (ROM) in joints/back/neck
C. Extra-articular features such as anterior uveitis or iritis
D. Fatigue
E. Weight loss
F. Shortness of breath (SOB)
G. Psoriasis

Subjective Data
A. Ask the client when back pain/joint pain began. Have symptoms been present for several months/years? At what age did pain initially begin?
B. Is pain intermittent or constant?
C. Does pain improve or worsen with activity? Inflammatory back pain (IBP) improves with activity and worsens with rest.
D. Does client have complaints of other joint pain?
E. Has the client noted any weight gain/loss, fatigue, or fevers?
F. Any history of psoriasis or other skin rashes?
G. Any gastrointestinal (GI) changes or chronic problems such as Crohn's disease, ulcerative colitis, or diarrhea?
H. Any pulmonary problems such as SOB, difficulty breathing, or SOB with activity?

I. Any cardiac changes or problems?

J. Any history of amyloidosis?

Physical Examination

A. Check vital signs, blood pressure (BP), pulse, respirations, and temperature as indicated.

B. Inspect:

1. Assess the cervical spine. Ask the client to stand straight and assess the degree of cervical change. Ask the client to perform flexion, extension, lateral flexion, and rotate the head.

2. Inspect the thoracic and lumbar spine. Note degree of chest expansion of thoracic spine. Assess lumbar spine noting the ROM with flexion/extension. Have the client bend to the right and left sides and note any difference in flexion.

3. Assess gait. If abnormal gait, assess for hip pain/involvement.

4. Inspect hands/feet for sausage digits.

5. Inspect joints in hands/wrists/feet/knees for tender, swollen joints.

C. Auscultate:

1. Heart

2. Lungs

D. Palpate:

1. Examine the SI joints by palpating the SI joint while lying supine and while lying on the side. Have the client flex one knee while lying supine, and externally rotate the hip. Assess for pain at the SI joint area while pressure is applied on the knee.

2. Assess for pain at the entheses site. Assess Achilles tendon and plantar fascia areas where the tendon attaches to the calcaneus.

Diagnostic Tests

A. Serum blood work:

1. HLA-B27 commonly positive

2. Rheumatoid factor (RF) usually negative

3. C-reactive protein (CRP)

4. Erythrocyte sedimentation rate (ESR)

5. Complete blood count (CBC)

6. Comprehensive metabolic panel (CMP)

7. Creatinine kinase

8. Alkaline phosphatase

9. Complement levels (C3, C4)

B. Radiographic studies:

All clients with complaints of chronic low back pain prior to the age of 45 years should have x-rays of the pelvis/SI joints.

1. X-ray of cervical/thoracic/lumbar spine and pelvis:

a. In AS, the spine is noted to have "squaring" of the vertebral bodies.

b. Sclerosis of the SI joint: sacroiliitis grade 2 or above (grade 2 is bilateral sacroiliitis)

2. X-ray of peripheral joints: erosions noted in the larger joints, loss of joint space, sclerosis

3. MRI of SI joints

4. Bone mineral density (BMD) screening: high incidence of osteoporosis noted in clients diagnosed with AS

Differential Diagnoses

A. Reactive arthritis

B. Psoriatic arthritis (PsA)

C. Spondylitis associated with inflammatory bowel disease

D. Rheumatoid arthritis (RA)

Plan

A. General interventions:

1. Treatment for AS includes nonpharmacological and pharmacological interventions.

2. Osteoporosis screening and treatment are recommended for AS clients.

3. Systemic steroids are not routinely prescribed; however, for severe symptoms of pain and swelling, joint injection may be considered.

B. Client teaching:

1. Encourage a healthy, active lifestyle. Activity improves symptoms. Regular exercises are recommended as tolerated. Physical therapy and/or structured exercises recommended most days of the week

2. Medications prescribed should be used on a routine basis.

3. Fall prevention should be reviewed with the client. The home should be modified to prevent falls. Suggestions include installing grab bars in the bathroom tub/shower, removing loose rugs in the house, keeping walkways in the home clear and clutter free.

4. Seat belts should always be worn properly.

5. For persons with severe spinal involvement, contact sports and high-impact exercises/sports should be avoided.

C. Pharmaceutical therapy:

1. Nonsteroidal anti-inflammatory drugs (NSAIDs) are first-line therapy for pain/symptoms produced from AS. All medications should not be used longer than 4 weeks.

a. Ibuprofen 400 mg every 4 to 6 hours as tolerated

b. Naproxyn 500 mg twice a day (bid) as tolerated

c. Celecoxib (Celebrex) 100 to 200 mg daily to bid as tolerated

d. Indomethacin 75 mg one to two times per day

e. Meloxicam 7.5 to 15 mg daily

f. Diclofenac 50 mg every 8 hours

2. Nonopioid analgesic:

a. Acetaminophen 325 to 650 mg every 4 to 6 hours or 1,000 mg three times a day (tid)

3. Tumor necrosis factor alpha antagonists (anti-TNF) medications may be prescribed by a rheumatologist after failed NSAID use.

Follow-Up

A. Clients treated with NSAIDs should have routine follow-up at 2 weeks following initial diagnosis or sooner if not improving with treatment.

B. Clients treated with NSAIDs should be followed every 3 months, with close monitoring of kidney and liver function.

Consultation/Referral

A. Clients diagnosed with AS should be referred to rheumatology for evaluation and treatment.

Individual Considerations

A. Adults:

1. Young adults diagnosed with AS are typically in the 20- to 30-year range. Clients commonly present to the office with complaints of low back pain are treated for noninflammatory chronic back pain. These clients may go years without the proper diagnosis and treatment. Therefore, delayed diagnosis is not uncommon in these clients.

2. All clients with chronic low back pain with the onset prior to 40 years old should be screened for AS.

3. The three criteria commonly present for diagnosing AS are chronic low back pain, x-ray sacroiliitis grade 2 bilaterally or grade 3 unilaterally, and one additional characteristic (such as positive HLA-B27).

4. If x-rays or MRI do not support sacroiliitis, 4 of 11 symptoms must be present for the diagnosis of AS:

   a. IBP

   b. Heel pain (enthesitis)

   c. Dactylitis

   d. Uveitis

   e. Positive family history for spondyloarthritis (SpA)

   f. Inflammatory bowel disease

   g. Alternating buttock pain

   h. Psoriasis

   i. Asymmetric arthritis

   j. Positive response to NSAIDs

   k. Elevated acute phase reactants (ESR or CRP)

5. Standard precautions should be followed for NSAIDs for clients with renal insufficiency and clients taking anticoagulants, systemic glucocorticoids, and other interacting medications.

B. Geriatrics:

1. Not commonly diagnosed in this group of clients

Bibliography

Di Lorenzo, A. L. (2015). HLA-B27 syndromes. *Medscape*. Retrieved from http://emedicine.medscape.com/article/1201027-overview#a1

Yu, D. (2019). Diagnosis and differential diagnosis of axial spondyloarthritis (ankylosing spondylitis and nonradiographic axial spondyloarthritis) in adults. *UpToDate*. Waltham, MA: Wolters Kluwer. Retrieved from https://www.uptodate.com/contents/diagnosis-and-differential-diagnosis-of-axial-spondyloarthritis-ankylosing-spondylitis-and-nonradiographic-axial-spondyloarthritis-in-adults

Fibromyalgia

Jill C. Cash

Definition

Fibromyalgia syndrome is a clinical condition characterized by generalized aching and stiffness, associated with the finding of numerous tender points in characteristic locations.

A. The most current guidelines for diagnosis are presented by the American College of Rheumatology (ACR; Wofle et al., 2010). The criteria for diagnosis include characteristic symptoms of pain at specific trigger point locations that are displayed by the client for the past 3 months when there is no other reason or explanation for the associated pain. According to ACR 2016 revisions, the trigger points of 19 body areas are no longer required for the diagnosis of fibromyalgia; diagnosis is based on the client's significant symptoms.

B. Trigger point locations are found primarily in the back, neck, jaw, shoulders, chest, abdomen, arms, hips, and legs.

C. Somatic symptoms are also assessed for and present with fibromyalgia. Somatic complaints may include cognitive problems, sleeping difficulties, fatigue, headaches, and other associated symptoms. These criteria can be found at the ACR website www.rheumatology.org.

> Areas palpated are considered positive if the client verbalized the area as being "painful" when palpated.

Incidence

A. Fibromyalgia affects females more than males at a ratio of 10:1 and clients with an average age of 47 years; 5% of the population is affected with fibromyalgia. Usual onset is between 20 and 50 years; however, it has also been diagnosed in the young as well as the elderly. Often clients have symptoms for longer than 5 years before finally being diagnosed. The prevalence of fibromyalgia in rheumatology practice is 20%.

Pathogenesis

A. The cause is unclear. Studies of sleep physiology, neurohormonal function, muscular function, and psychological factors support a central mechanism for the disorder linked to depression. Other research suggests a pathophysiologic and psychological disorder.

Predisposing Factors

A. Life stress

B. Depression

C. Female gender

D. Age mid-30s and older

Common Complaints

A. Common complaints are multifocal pain present longer than 3 months; moderate to extreme fatigue; morning stiffness; nonrestorative sleep; pain worsening with stress, exposure to cold, inactivity, or overactivity; sensitivity to touch, light, and sound; cognitive difficulties; and pain associated with changes in barometric pressure.

Other Signs and Symptoms

A. Numbness

B. Swelling

C. Reactive hyperemia of skin

D. Raynaud's phenomenon (RP)

E. Irritable bowel syndrome (IBS) and bladder symptoms

F. Headaches

G. Restless legs syndrome (RLS)

H. Anxiety/depression

Subjective Data

A. Determine onset, duration, and course of complaints

B. Does fatigue interfere with the client's daily activity?

C. Note sleep quality. Does the client feel rested after sleeping?

D. Do exacerbations of discomfort occur with stress, activity, and cold?

E. Has the client experienced stress and/or depression in the past?

F. Does the client have a family history of rheumatoid disease?

G. Has the client ever been diagnosed with chronic fatigue syndrome, Lyme disease, or thyroid disease?

Physical Examination

A. Check temperature if indicated, pulse, and BP

B. Inspect:
1. Observe overall appearance.
2. Observe the nails, skin, mucous membranes, eyes, joints, and spine. If clubbing is noted and tender points are minimal, consider hypertrophic osteoarthropathy.
3. Check joints for swelling, deformities, erythema. If clubbing is noted and tender points are minimal, consider hypertrophic osteoarthropathy.

C. Palpate the muscles as outlined in the aforementioned criteria for classification of fibromyalgia. Note the following when palpating for tender points:
1. Pressure should be insufficient to produce pain in normal clients or at uninvolved sites in affected clients.
2. Pain on digital palpation must be present in at least 11 of 18 tender point sites.
3. "Positive pain reaction" is related to the client stating that palpation causes pain. Tenderness is not to be considered as pain.
4. Painful points must be differentiated from trigger points of myofascial syndrome which produce referred pain on compression.
5. Control areas not expected to be tender in fibromyalgia, such as middle of the forehead and fingertips, should be examined to exclude psychological pain or malingering.

D. Auscultate:
1. Heart
2. Lungs

Diagnostic Tests

A. Laboratory studies are normal with fibromyalgia.

B. Tests to consider for assessing for other conditions include:
1. CBC
2. CRP
3. ESR

C. If the history and physical suggest some type of inflammatory rheumatic condition, also order:
1. Antinuclear antibody (ANA)
2. RF
3. Cyclic citrullinated peptide (CCP)

D. If there are concerns regarding a possible thyroid or muscle condition, also order:
1. Thyroid-stimulating hormone (TSH)
2. Creatinine phosphokinase

E. Assessment for a sleep disorder should include ordering a sleep study.

Differential Diagnoses

A. RA

B. Osteoarthritis (OA)

C. Polymyalgia rheumatica (PMR)

D. AS

E. Myositis

F. Systemic lupus erythematosus

G. Hypothyroidism

H. Chronic fatigue syndrome

I. Obstructive sleep apnea

Plan

A. General interventions:
1. Routine follow-up is recommended. Multiple therapies may be beneficial for controlling symptoms.
2. Stress importance of daily exercises and therapy to control pain.
3. Clients should also be screened for other disorders such as sleep disorders, RLS, and for psychiatric disorders.
4. Support groups are beneficial for clients and families.

B. Client teaching: *See Section III: Client Teaching Guide for this chapter, "Fibromyalgia."* ◀
1. Teach the client that fibromyalgia is a recognizable syndrome that does not progress or cripple and does not warrant further testing. Clients can be assured it is not "all in their head."
   a. Exercise: encourage the client to exercise daily, including stretching programs along with walking, low-impact cardiovascular conditioning such as cycling, and low-impact aerobics. Initially, pain may increase with the first 2 weeks of exercise; then it improves with a routine exercise program.
   b. Pain control: Pain may improve with exercise, hot baths, heating pads, warm weather, and stress reduction.

C. Pharmaceutical therapy:
1. Amitriptyline 10 to 50 mg at bedtime for sleep
2. Cyclobenzaprine 10 to 40 mg daily or other muscle relaxants
3. NSAIDs such as ibuprofen 200 to 600 mg every 4 to 6 hours. Maximum dose is 1.2 g/d.
4. Analgesics such as acetaminophen (Tylenol) as needed
5. Selective serotonin reuptake inhibitors (SSRIs) if depression is present
6. Pregabalin (Lyrica) 75 mg twice a day to 150 mg twice a day; maximum dose of 450 mg/d
7. Duloxetine Hcl (Cymbalta) 30 to 60 mg once a day. Caution about nausea with medication. If nausea

is severe, consider prescribing Zofran 8 mg 30 minutes prior to Cymbalta dose. Advise client that nausea will resolve after 3 to 4 weeks.

8. Milnacipran (Savella) titrated dose 12.5 mg on day 1; 12.5 mg twice a day for 2 days; 25 mg twice a day from days 4 to 7; then 50 mg twice a day (recommended dose). Maximum dose is 100 mg twice a day. Withdraw gradually. Precautions to be carried out of renal impairment

9. Current guidelines suggest guarded use of opioids chronically in nonmalignant pain. Opioids have not been studied in randomized controlled trials and should be considered only after all other medicinal therapies have been exhausted. Tramadol, a centrally acting analgesic with atypical opioid and antidepressant-like activity, is moderately effective in treating fibromyalgia pain.

10. Neurontin (Gabapentin) is approved for use in the treatment of neuropathic pain but not for fibromyalgia. Neurontin 300 mg orally three times a day should be the starting dose, with titrations upward as tolerated.

Follow-Up

A. Schedule regular visits in initial 2 to 4 weeks to evaluate how therapy is helping. Educate the client each visit, and stress positive reinforcement and supervision of treatment regimen. Visits may then be scheduled every 3 months to monitor progress.

Consultation/Referral

A. Consult with a physician if the client has abnormal laboratory results
B. Consult or refer the client to a physician if depression is suspected and current medication therapy is unsuccessful

Individual Considerations

A. Geriatrics:
1. Fibromyalgia is common in the elderly and can be more painful for this population because of other coexisting conditions such as OA.
2. Fibromyalgia prevalence has accelerated for the geriatric population. Studies show that older adults suffering from fibromyalgia are more depressed and less physically active. Treatment options include antidepressants titrated according to Beers guidelines rather than prescribing chronic use of steroids/NSAIDs.
3. Fibromyalgia syndrome is associated with increased risk of falls and fractures. Calcium and vitamin D levels should be monitored. Vitamin D3 recommendation for clients older than 70 years of age is 24,000 IU per month.

Bibliography

Arumugam, V., & MacDermid, J. C. (2019). Appraisal of clinical practice guideline: EULAR revised recommendations for the management of fibromyalgia. *Journal of Physiotherapy (Elsevier)*, 65(2), 112. doi:10.1016/j.jphys.2019.01.003
Centers for Disease Control and Prevention. (2015a). *Fibromyalgia*. Retrieved from www.cdc.gov/arthritis/basics/fibromyalgia.htm
Goldenberg, D. L. (2019). Diagnosing fibromyalgia as a disease, an illness, a state, or a trait? *Arthritis Care & Research*, 71(3), 334–336.
Gota, C. E., Kaouk, S., & Wilke, W. S. (2015). Fibromyalgia and obesity: The association between body mass index and disability, depression, history of abuse, medications, and comorbidities. *Journal of Clinical Rheumatology*, 21(6), 289–295. doi:10.1097/RHU.0000000000000278
Hassan, N., Clarke, L., Minaur, N., & Creamer, P. (2019). Accuracy of fibromyalgia diagnosis in primary care, British society for rheumatology annual conference 2019, April 30-May 02 2019, Birmingham, United Kingdom. *Rheumatology*, 58(Suppl. 3), 1–2. doi:10.1093/rheumatology/kez106.050
Perrot, S. (2019). Fibromyalgia: A misconnection in a multiconnected world? *European Journal of Pain*, 23(5), 866–873.
Wolfe, F., Clauw, D. J., Fitzcharles, M. A., Goldenberg, D. L., Katz, R. S., Mease, P., … Yunus, M. B. (2010). The American college of rheumatology preliminary diagnostic criteria for fibromyalgia and measurement of symptom severity. *Arthritis Care & Research*, 62(5), 600–610. doi:10.1002/acr.20140

Gout

Jill C. Cash

Definition

A. Gout is an acute sudden inflammatory disease of the joint caused by high concentrations of uric acid in the joints and bones.
B. Three stages of gout:
1. Acute gouty arthritis: attack exhibiting severe pain, redness, and swelling of a joint, which may last from days to weeks
2. Intercritical gout: period without flares
3. Chronic/tophaceous gout: the progression of gout that has been inadequately treated, resulting in urate crystal deposits (tophaceous deposits) in the joints that can cause deformity and disability of the joint

Incidence

A. Gout is most common in men from ages 30 to 60 years. Women become increasingly susceptible to gout after menopause. It is estimated that gout occurs in approximately 3% of the adult population in the United States.

Pathogenesis

A. Primary: high levels of uric acid result from either increased production or decreased excretion rates of uric acid.
B. Secondary: hyperuricemia resulting from primary disease processes such as hypertension, renal failure, kidney disorders, and so forth. See the following section, "Predisposing Factors."
C. Medications/toxins can also cause hyperuricemia.

Predisposing Factors

A. Chronic conditions: hyperuricemia, chronic kidney disease, hypertension, diabetes mellitus, ischemic cardiovascular disease, hyperlipidemia, obesity, OA
B. Gender (men older than 30 years, postmenopausal women)
C. Medications that alter uric acid level (diuretics, acetylsalicylic acid, alcohol, nicotinic acid, ethambutol, pyrazinamide)
D. Dietary factors (high intake of beer and meat/fresh seafood products)
E. Family history of gout
F. Lead poison

Common Complaints

A. Redness, swelling, warmth, and/or pain in the joint (usually one joint only)—podagra (big toe). The pain is likely to be the most severe in the first 12 to 24 hours.

B. History of having severe joint pain with inflammation in other joints, followed by pain-free episodes

Other Signs and Symptoms

A. Tophi are seen from several years of untreated gout.

B. Fever may be present in acute stages.

Subjective Data

A. Note when initial symptoms began

B. Review client history of gout

C. Determine what makes the symptoms worse or better

D. List medications/therapies used and the result of the different therapies used

E. Review recent dietary preferences (alcohol, meat, seafood)

Physical Examination

A. Check temperature, pulse, respirations, and BP.

B. Inspect:
1. Inspect the joints.
2. Note the presence of tophi on other joints.

C. Palpate the joints for tenderness, pain, and increase in temperature of skin.

Diagnostic Tests

A. Joint fluid aspiration for urate crystals is the gold standard in diagnosing gout. Inspect fluid with polarized light microscopy to identify uric acid crystals.

B. CBC: white blood cell count elevated

C. ESR: elevated in gout

D. Serum uric acid level: uric acid >6.8 mg/dL. Serum uric acid level may be normal during acute attacks. Perform test at least 2 weeks after acute attack or when flare has resolved.

E. RF titer

F. X-ray or MRI: identify bone cysts/gout tophi

Differential Diagnoses

A. Infectious arthritis

B. RA

C. Hyperparathyroidism

D. Pseudogout (calcium pyrophosphate [CPP] deposition disease) in the knee, wrist, or other joints

E. Bursitis

F. Cellulitis

Plan

A. General interventions:
1. Rest the joint area; no heavy lifting or weight-bearing activity
2. Aspirin products should not be used.

B. Client teaching:
1. *See Section III: Client Teaching Guide for this chapter, "Gout."*
2. Increase fluid intake to at least eight glasses of water daily.

3. Avoid alcohol intake and excessive meat and seafood products that trigger flares.

4. Medication treatment and compliance of taking the prescribed medications can be very effective in preventing the development of the chronic tophaceous gout stage.

5. *Aspirin products should not be used.*

C. Pharmaceutical therapy:
1. Analgesia:
   a. NSAIDs—most effective if started within 48 hours of presenting symptoms
      i. Indocin 50 mg every 8 hours for eight doses, then 25 mg every 8 hours until pain-free for 1 to 2 days. Normal course is 5 to 7 days.
      ii. Naproxen, 750 mg initially, followed by 500 mg every 12 hours
      iii. NSAIDs are contraindicated for clients with the diagnosis of renal insufficiency, heart failure, ulcer disease, NSAID allergy, and anticoagulation therapy.
   b. Colchicine (Colcrys) is most effective if started within 12 to 24 hours of presenting symptoms: 1.2 mg initial dose, followed by 0.6 mg 1 hour later. Continue 0.6 mg one to two times daily until symptoms resolve. Medication may be stopped after the client is free from symptoms after 2 to 3 days. Colchicine may also be used to prevent attacks. Colchicine warnings: be aware of contraindications; caution regarding drug interactions; intolerable side effects of colchicine include nausea, vomiting, and diarrhea. Be cautious with use in clients with kidney/liver impairment.
   c. Corticosteroids may be used for clients who cannot tolerate oral medications. Intra-articular steroid injection of methylprednisolone acetate may be given. Oral steroids may also be prescribed for clients who cannot take NSAIDs or colchicine and who cannot tolerate intra-articular steroid injection. Prednisone is safe. Be aware of rebound effects.
2. For hypersecretion of uric acid, long-term therapy is needed to decrease uric acid production; allopurinol (Zyloprim) is the drug of choice. Starting dose is 100 mg/d and titrated up over several weeks to a maximum of 300 mg/d. The goal is to keep the uric acid level <6.0 mg/dL. Febuxostat (Uloric) is also used to lower blood uric acid levels. The recommended dose is 40 mg/d with or without food; maximum dose is 80 mg/d. Initial laboratory studies include liver enzymes before beginning Uloric. Common side effects include liver problems, nausea, gout flares, joint pain, and rash.
3. For reduced excretion rates of uric acid, consider probenecid (Benemid) 250 mg by mouth twice a day for 1 week, then increase to 500 mg by mouth twice a day. Increased consumption of fluids must be encouraged. Avoid if CrCl is less than 50.

4. Chronic gout: if clients have three or more attacks per year, consider long-term therapy, low dose of NSAIDs, or allopurinol for 2 to 12 months.

5. Alternative medications for intolerance, renal insufficiency, and extensive tophi include oxypurinol, febuxostat, and uricase. Refer to rheumatology specialist.

Follow-Up

A. The client should be contacted within 24 hours for evaluation.

B. Schedule follow-up visit in 1 month to reevaluate status.

C. Monitor serum urate during medication titration every 2 to 5 weeks to target goal of uric acid level <6.0.

D. Chronic gout: obtain yearly uric acid levels; before initiating long-term therapy, obtain baseline blood urea nitrogen (BUN), serum lipid profile, and CBC and periodic liver enzymes.

Consultation/Referral

A. Consult and refer to physician or rheumatologist for aspiration of joint fluid and newer treatment options.

Individual Considerations

A. Adults:

1. Between gout flares, the client is asymptomatic. Compliance with medication treatment to avoid flares is imperative. Without adequate control, gout flares occur more frequently, last for longer periods of time, may affect more joints, as well as may cause client to develop fever during flare.

B. Pregnancy:

1. Colchicine not recommended

C. Pediatrics:

1. Colchicine not recommended

2. If gout is seen in this population, consider underlying primary cause (i.e., inborn error of metabolism).

D. Geriatrics:

1. Reformation in joint areas may be seen in clients who have a history of gout from the uric acid deposits.

2. Complications for chronic gout include nephrolithiasis and chronic urate nephropathy.

3. Avoid Indocin in elderly clients because of the increased risk of adverse effects with other medications when compared with other NSAIDs.

4. NSAIDs are not recommended in the elderly with a history of heart failure, GI ulcers/disease, and renal impairment.

5. Individual considerations must be given in this population regarding GI, cardiac, renal, and liver disease.

6. Glucocorticoids are generally well tolerated in this population and a safer alternative if NSAIDs or colchicine may increase the risks for the client.

7. Allopurinol in elderly clients is safe; however, it can have a negative interaction with warfarin, cyclosporine, chlorpropamide, and thiazide diuretics.

8. Beers criteria recommends avoiding colchicine in the geriatric population with CrCl <30 mL/min secondary to increased risk of bone marrow toxicity, GI complications, and neuromuscular adverse effects.

Bibliography

Becker, M. A. (2016a). *Clinical manifestations and diagnosis of gout*. *UpToDate*. Retrieved from http://www.uptodate.com/contents/clinical-manifestations-and-diagnosis-of-gout

Becker, M. A. (2016b). *Prevention of recurrent gout: Pharmacologic urate-lowering therapy and treatment of tophi*. *UpToDate*. Retrieved from http://www.uptodate.com/contents/prevention-of-recurrent-gout-pharmacologic-urate-lowering-therapy-and-treatment-of-tophi

Becker, M. A. (2019). *Treatment of gout flares*. *UpToDate*. Retrieved from www.uptodate.com/contents/treatment-of-gout-flares

Centers for Disease Control and Prevention. (2019). *Gout*. Retrieved from www.cdc.gov/arthritis/basics/gout.htm

Neogi, T., Jansen, T. L., Dalbeth, N., Fransen, J., Schumacher, H. R., Berendsen, D., … Taylor, W. J. (2015). 2015 Gout classification criteria: An American College of Rheumatology/European League Against Rheumatism collaborative initiative. *Annals of the Rheumatic Diseases*, *74*(10), 1789–1798. doi:10.1136/annrheumdis-2015-208237

Osteoarthritis (OA)

Jill C. Cash

Definition

A. OA, formerly known as degenerative joint disease, is a chronic noninflammatory disease that affects the movable joints. OA is characterized by destruction of the cartilage with resultant decrease in the joint spaces and bony overgrowth. OA is considered to be primary when there are no underlying conditions, and secondary to conditions such as trauma, septic arthritis, inflammatory arthritis, metabolic disorders, or congenital or acquired joint abnormalities.

Incidence

A. It is estimated that up to 12% of the general population between the ages of 25 and 74 years have OA. The incidence clearly increases with age as up to 85% of the general population older than 65 years of age have radiographic changes suggestive of OA.

Pathogenesis

A. Damage to the articular cartilage and subchondral bone may be because of local trauma and results in chondrocyte injury.

B. Chondrocytes release proteolytic enzymes that assist in repair of the cartilage.

C. In OA, the remodeling process of chondrocytes and release of enzymes is impaired and results in a loss of strength and greater trauma and destruction of the subchondral bone. The end result is joint destruction and bony overgrowth most frequently in hands, knees, hips, and spine.

Predisposing Factors

A. Increasing age: among clients older than 55 years

B. Gender: women more commonly affected and exhibit greater disease severity

C. Genetic predisposition; distal interphalangeal (DIP) joint involvement

D. Trauma such as previous fractures, ligamentous injuries, or occupationally related repetitive stress

E. Altered joint anatomy or instability

F. Obesity: Mechanical injury in the knee may increase OA.

G. Secondary inflammation such as infections, inflammatory arthropathies, and metabolic disorders

Common Complaints

A. Unilateral joint pain frequently involving the joints of the hands, neck, lower back, knees, and hips
B. Morning stiffness lasting less than 1 hour

Other Signs and Symptoms

A. Unilateral joint pain involving the DIP and proximal interphalangeal (PIP) joints, first carpometacarpal joint, hips, knees, cervical and lumbar spine, and first metatarsophalangeal joint
B. Mild OA, or early disease, pain that increases with joint use and decreases with rest
C. Severe OA, or late disease, pain that is present with rest

Subjective Data

A. Elicit the client's age at onset of pain.
B. Has the pain gradually gotten worse over the months or years?
C. How long does the pain last in the morning? Does the pain get worse with joint use and better with rest?
D. What joints are involved?
E. Is the joint pain described as "aching?"
F. What does the client take to relieve the pain?
G. Is there any joint deformity, redness, swelling, or warmth?
H. Is there any decrease in ROM of the joint?
I. Is there any family history of OA?

Physical Examination

A. Check pulse and BP.
B. Inspect the joints for enlargement, edema, and erythema.
C. Palpate:
1. Palpate the joints, noting temperature, edema, and tenderness. Joints are cool. Bony enlargement may be present in the PIP (Bouchard's nodes) or DIP joints (Heberden's nodes) and other weight-bearing joints.
2. Palpate extremities. Perform assisted and active ROM exercises. With examination, limited ROM of the joint and/or pain on palpation may be present, along with crepitus.

Diagnostic Tests

A. ESR: OA does not cause an increase of the ESR
B. Chemistry profile
C. CBC
D. RF
E. Routine radiography: confirms disease severity and presence of joint narrowing
F. CT scan or MRI: considered with nerve impingement syndrome (spine) or spinal stenosis

Differential Diagnoses

A. Inflammatory OA
B. RA
C. Gout or pseudogout
D. Septic arthritis
E. Bursitis or tendonitis
F. Systemic lupus erythematosus (SLE)
G. Fracture or trauma

Plan

A. General interventions:
1. Confirm diagnosis:
2. Provide the client with support and education to improve client well-being and reduce discomfort.
3. Physical therapy and/or occupational therapy should be initiated, if indicated.
B. Client teaching:
1. *See Section III: Client Teaching Guide for this chapter, "Osteoarthritis."* ◀
2. Reinforce the importance of joint protection; avoid repetitive stress or trauma.
3. Encourage daily exercises and strengthening.
4. Encourage weight loss if the client is obese. Joint pain can be significantly reduced with weight loss.
C. Pharmaceutical therapy:
1. First-line agents: The goal of treatment is to preserve joint mobility. First-line agents should be used in a stepwise approach.
   a. Acetaminophen up to 1 g four times daily; in early disease, may be given on an as-needed basis
   b. NSAIDs if acetaminophen has failed to control the pain. Use with caution. Consider renal function and risk factors for peptic ulcer disease (PUD) and cardiovascular disease:
      i. Naproxen 220 to 375 mg one to two times daily
      ii. Inflammatory OA: consider naproxen 375 to 500 mg twice a day. Recommend taking this medication for 2 to 4 weeks for maximum effect
      iii. Ibuprofen 200 to 400 mg, three times a day, may also be considered. Doses may be increased at a gradual pace for maximum benefit as tolerated. If one NSAID does not work, consider other NSAIDs.
         1) Cox-2 inhibitors, such as celecoxib (Celebrex), may also be considered. Celebrex 200 mg daily to twice a day as tolerated
         2) Meloxicam (Mobic) 7.5 to 15 mg daily
   c. For high-risk clients, an H_2 receptor blocker may decrease gastritis and be helpful in preventing duodenal ulcers. Consider Arthrotec 50, one tablet three times a day.
   d. Misoprostol may be considered in clients who are at high risk of gastric ulcers. It should not be used by pregnant women. It is considered high risk for fetal death and possible congenital abnormalities.
   e. Topical creams:
      i. Diclofenac gel (Voltaren gel) may be applied to affected area; recommended for clients with severe pain who are not able to tolerate oral NSAIDs
      ii. Capsaicin cream may be applied to the affected area. Capsaicin creams may cause local burning at the site of application for the first several days.

2. Second-line agents, such as intra-articular cortico-steroid injections, may prevent some joint erosion and decrease pain. The same joint should not be injected more than three to four times a year in 3-month intervals. If the joint is injected at this frequency for more than 1 year, alternative options, such as surgery, should be considered. Narcotics may provide relief from more severe OA pain, but they carry a risk of dependence. These should be reserved for clients who do not respond to other treatments and are not surgical candidates. Follow state protocols for scheduled pain medications.

3. The use of glucosamine and chondroitin has not been established and is not recommended for clients. There does not appear to be any risks associated with using glucosamine and chondroitin. If the client does not notice any relief within the first 6 months of use, then recommend discontinuing product.

4. Physical therapy to create an individualized exercise regimen to strengthen muscles, increase ROM, and reduce pain

5. Lubrication injections (Hyalgan or Synvisc) may also be considered. Referral to the rheumatologist should be considered for this treatment.

Follow-Up

A. Follow-up is based on disease severity and therapeutic treatment. If the client is treated with first-line agents, follow up on pain control, nonpharmocological interventions, and possible side effects of medications within 2 to 4 weeks.

Consultation/Referral

A. Referral to an orthopedic surgeon may be considered for moderate to severe pain, as indicated.

Individual Considerations

A. Pregnancy:
  1. NSAIDs should not be used in pregnancy unless clearly indicated. Misoprostol should be used with great caution in women of childbearing age because of its potential for fetal abnormalities and abortive properties.
B. Adults and geriatrics:
  1. Clients on chronic NSAIDs should be monitored closely for toxicity such as renal insufficiency, gastritis, and PUD. Elderly clients and those with preexisting GI disease, diabetes, congestive heart failure, and cirrhosis should be monitored closely.
  2. Topical therapies are preferred for clients over 75 years old due to the increased risk for complications from oral NSAIDs.
  3. Sedentary lifestyle contributes to OA disease and increased, progressive pain. Quality of life can be improved with increasing physical activity.
  4. Avoid long-term splinting and orthotics due to the risk of the client's vulnerability to periarticular muscle weakness and wasting. Splints worn at bedtime can prevent unintentional injury.

Bibliography

Centers for Disease Control and Prevention. (2015c). *Osteoarthritis (OA)*. Retrieved from www.cdc.gov/arthritis/basics/osteoarthritis.htm

Deveza, L. A. (2019). *Overview of the management of osteoarthritis. UpToDate*. Retrieved from https://www.uptodate.com/contents/overview-of-the-management-of-osteoarthritis

Solomon, D. H. (2019). *Overview of selective COX-2 inhibitors. UpToDate*. Retrieved from http://www.uptodate.com/contents/overview-of-selective-cox-2-inhibitors

Osteoporosis/Kyphosis/Fracture

Jill C. Cash

Definition

A. Osteoporosis is a condition of reduced bone mass resulting in bone fragility and fracture. The World Health Organization (WHO) has defined it as "spinal or hip BMD of 2.5 standard deviations or more below the mean for healthy, young women (T-score of –2.5 or below) as measured by dual energy x-ray absorptiometry." BMD is performed on the lumbar spine, hip, and/or forearm (see Figure 21.1).

(A)　　　　　　　　　(B)

FIGURE 21.1 (A) Normal bone matrix. (B) Osteoporotic bone matrix.

B. Clinical diagnosis of osteoporosis can also be defined as having a fragility fracture of the spine, hip, wrist, pelvis, rib, and/or humerus without evidence of a BMD.

C. Osteopenia is defined as low bone mass of the spinal or hip BMD between 1 and 2.5 standard deviations below the mean as evidenced by the T-score (T-score between –1.0 and –2.5).

D. Kyphosis (dowager's hump) is the forward curvature of the thoracic spine. It is estimated that kyphosis occurs in approximately 20% to 40% of clients older than 60 years of age. Kyphosis may occur because of many different causes, including vertebral fractures, muscle weakness, degenerative disk disease, postural changes, and genetic/metabolic changes. Kyphosis is associated with other conditions such as decreased pulmonary function, back pain, increased risk of fracture of the spine, limited mobility, and an increase in mortality.

E. Osteoporotic fracture occurs from a fall while standing at normal height or less, without any type of trauma and/or while performing daily activities. A vertebral compression fracture is the most common type of osteoporotic fracture.

F. Vertebral fractures: There are three primary types of vertebral fractures:
1. Biconcave deformity
2. Wedge fracture
3. Compression fracture

Incidence

A. There are approximately 25 million people in the United States diagnosed with osteoporosis; 80% of those are women. Women are diagnosed with osteoporosis six to eight times more often than men and this is thought to be related to hormone deficiency (estrogen). The peak incidence of fractures in men occurs 10 years later in life than for women, averaging at 70 years of age.

B. Approximately 50% to 60% of 50-year-old women sustain osteoporosis-related fractures during their remaining life. Spinal fractures occur in 25% of White women by age 65 years, causing pain, deformity, and disability. Most common fractures include 25% at distal radius (Colles' fracture), 50% in vertebrae, and 25% in the hip.

C. Approximately 33% of all women and 17% of men suffer a hip fracture before age 90 years, and 20% of those who sustain a fracture die within 3 months of the event.

Pathogenesis

A. Osteoporosis occurs because of bone reabsorption being greater than bone formation.

Predisposing Factors

A. Hypogonadal states, particularly menopause
B. Small body frame, low body weight (<127 lbs)
C. Cigarette smoking
D. Low calcium intake
E. Lack of weight-bearing exercise
F. Family history of hip/pelvic fracture
G. Excessive alcohol intake
H. Asian or Caucasian
I. Advanced age
J. Previous fracture
K. Secondary causes:
1. Hyperparathyroidism
2. Hyperthyroidism
3. Cushing's syndrome
4. Multiple myeloma
5. Thyroid replacement therapy
6. Corticosteroid therapy
7. Renal disease

Common Complaints

A. Loss of height
B. Kyphosis, or dowager's hump
C. Back pain as a result of a compression fracture

Other Signs and Symptoms

A. Cervical lordosis
B. Fracture with little or no trauma
C. Crush fracture of vertebra
D. Pain

Subjective Data

A. Explore history of the following:
1. Loss of height. Ask client to compare current height with height written on the driver's license if height is unknown.
2. Low initial bone mass
3. Early menopause, oophorectomy, postmenopause, or amenorrhea
4. European or Asian family origin
5. Family history of spinal fractures and osteoporosis
6. Sedentary lifestyle with little weight-bearing activity
7. Endocrine disorders
8. Review medications taken in the present and past, including over-the-counter (OTC) and herbal supplements, with attention to medications such as corticosteroids, barbiturates, heparin, and thyroid hormone.
9. Dietary review for low calcium and vitamin D intake
10. Increased alcohol, caffeine, and protein intake
11. Renal disease/dialysis

B. Determine onset, duration, location, and characteristic of back pain if present.

C. Has the client had any recent falls?

Physical Examination

A. Check pulse, BP, height, and weight.
B. Inspect:
1. Compare present height with previous height.
2. Observe presence of dorsal kyphosis.
3. Observe physical abnormalities that interfere with mobility.
C. Palpate the joints and over the back for pain.

Diagnostic Tests

A. Laboratory studies:
1. Women: CMP (calcium, phosphorus, albumin, total protein, creatinine, liver enzymes, alkaline phosphatase, electrolytes), TSH, and 25-hydroxyvitamin D level
2. Men: CMP (calcium, phosphorus, albumin, total protein, creatinine, liver enzymes, alkaline phosphatase, electrolytes), TSH, 25-hydroxyvitamin D level, and testosterone level
3. CBC, ESR, and serum protein electrophoresis to rule out multiple myeloma and leukemia, if concerned

B. BMD or dual-energy x-ray absorptiometry (DEXA) scan:
1. The DEXA scan measures bone density of the lumbar spine and/or hip. Medicare will reimburse for this test to be performed every 2 years. If the spine is compressed or has severe scoliosis, BMD values may not be valid for the lumbar spine. Consider assessing the forearm for radial interpretation.
2. The result of this procedure is read in "T-scores" or "Z-scores." T-scores are evaluated for postmenopausal women and older men. A T-score is a number

given to identify the amount of bone present when compared with other healthy adults. Z-scores are recommended for premenopausal women. A Z-score is a score given to identify the amount of bone present when compared with other people of the same age, gender, and weight.

3. WHO Fracture Risk Assessment Tool (FRAX) was developed to determine the absolute fracture risk of breaking a bone in the next 10 years. This tool may be used with the BMD results to determine who needs to be treated with medication for prevention of fracture when treatment is unclear. FRAX should be used on women who have not previously been treated with antiresorptive therapy when T-scores are between –1.5 and –2.5. The FRAX tool can also be used on clients who have been treated with prior antiresorptive medications if they have been off these medications for more than 2 years. FRAX scoring is not recommended for clients currently being prescribed antiresorptive medications.

C. Radiography: x-ray the lumbar and thoracic spine for suspected vertebral fracture and/or for height loss greater than 2 in. Consider a CT to assess for instability of a wedge fracture. An MRI is recommended to assess for the extent of a compression fracture and/or possible malignancy.

Differential Diagnoses

A. OA
B. Secondary causes:
1. Thyroid disease
2. Glucocorticoid therapy
3. Malabsorption syndromes
4. Renal or collagen disease
5. Vitamin D deficiency
6. Metastatic cancer
7. Multiple myeloma

Plan

A. General interventions: Lifestyle changes should be introduced to the client.
B. Client teaching:
1. Educate the client regarding calcium and vitamin D intake in diet.
  a. Calcium intake:
    i. Men younger than 50 years up to 69 years: 1,000 mg/d
    ii. Men older than 70 years: 1,200 mg/d
    iii. Women younger than or equal to 50 years: 1,000 mg/d
    iv. Women older than 50 years: 1,200 mg/d
    v. Food sources high in calcium include salmon or sardines with bones, low-fat yogurt and skim milk, green vegetables, and cheese
  b. Vitamin D intake:
    i. Men younger than 50 years of age: 400 to 800 IU/d
    ii. Men 51 to 69 years: 800 to 1,000 IU/d
    iii. Men older than 70 years of age: 800 to 1,000 IU/d
    iv. Women younger than 50 years of age: 400 to 800 IU/d
    v. Women 50 years of age and older: 800 to 1,000 IU/d
    vi. Food sources high in vitamin D include vitamin D–fortified milk and cereals, fish liver oils, cod liver oil, mushrooms, herring, catfish, salmon, sardines, egg yolks, cheese, and beef liver.
2. Encourage the client to eliminate alcohol and caffeine from diet.
3. Encourage the client to eliminate cigarette smoking.
4. Prescribe regular moderate exercise, such as 30 minutes of walking at least three times per week. Walking 50 to 60 minutes three times per week provides optimal benefits.
5. Fall prevention: advise the client to avoid medications that may cause drowsiness and precipitate falls. Use extra light at night in the bathroom to help prevent falls. Remove all loose rugs and clutter from the home. Install handrails on steps.
6. Discuss safety issues and fall prevention with the client and family.
C. Pharmaceutical therapy:
1. Calcium supplements

> Calcium supplements may be contraindicated in clients who have a history of renal stones.

  a. Calcium carbonate (Os-Cal) 500 mg is given orally one to three times per day, or Tums 1 tablet orally two to three times a day. See the section "Plan" discussed earlier for recommendations.
2. Vitamin D supplements: See the section "Plan" discussed earlier for recommendations. Clients diagnosed with vitamin D deficiency should ingest an increased dosage according to the deficiency.
3. Bisphosphonates: first-line therapy recommended for postmenopausal women to reduce fracture risk in osteoporosis
  a. Acts by reducing bone resorption and bone loss by preventing osteoclast activity
  b. May be given daily, weekly, or monthly according to individual medication
    i. Alendronate sodium (Fosamax): available in 5, 10, 35, 40, and 70 mg tablets; 70 mg liquid; 70 mg tablet + 2,800 IU vitamin D tablet
    ii. Risedronate (Actonel): available as 5 mg daily, 35 mg weekly, or 150 mg monthly tablets
    iii. Zoledronic (Reclast): 5 mg/100 mL (intravenous [IV]) infusion once yearly as 15-minute infusion. Check serum creatinine and calcium before infusion
  c. Instruct the client to take medication with 6 to 8 ounces of water one-half hour before breakfast

or any medication for the day. Advise standing or sitting upright after taking medication. No food should be ingested for 30 minutes after taking the medication. Precautions should be used for clients who have upper GI side effects.

4. Receptor activator of nuclear factor kappa B ligand (RANKL):

   a. Acts by inhibiting osteoclast formation, decreasing bone resorption, reducing bone fracture, and increasing bone density

      i. Denosumab (Prolia) 60 mg subcutaneous injection once every 6 months. Clients with chronic kidney disease and/or a risk of hypocalcemia should have a serum calcium level checked 10 days after the administration.

      ii. Denosumab is recommended as an alternative initial treatment option for postmenopausal women with osteoporosis and high risk for osteoporotic fracture.

5. Selective estrogen receptor modulator (SERM):

   a. Raloxifene (Evista): 60 mg orally daily

   b. For postmenopausal women who have never had a fragility fracture, raloxifene prevents osteoporosis, is cardio-protective, and appears to decrease estrogen receptor breast cancer by 65% more than 8 years (National Osteoporosis Foundation, n.d. -a,-b). Client may note side effects of increased vasomotor symptoms and increased risk of venous thromboembolism.

6. Calcitonin:

   a. Calcitonin is no longer recommended for treatment for osteoporosis. Studies do not support the beneficial effect on bone health when compared with bisphosphonate and parathyroid hormone (PTH) therapy. Long-term use also has concerns for increased risk of cancer.

7. PTH:

   a. Recombinant human PTH rebuilds bone density and increases strength of bone. Approved for severe osteoporosis for postmenopausal women and men with the diagnosis of osteoporosis for clients with T-score of –3.5 or below without fracture, T-score of –2.5 or below with a fragility fracture, who have failed antiresorptive therapy and are not able to tolerate bisphosphonates. See package insert for contraindications.

   b. Teriparatide (Forteo) 20 mcg prefilled, 28 day pen/syringe; subcutaneous injection daily, taken for a maximum of 2 years. Check calcium and renal function before prescribing. Contraindicated for clients with a history of kidney stones and prior history of radiation therapy. See package insert.

   c. Abaloparatide (Tymlos) 80 mcg subcutaneously once daily, taken for a maximum of 2 years

8. Hormone replacement therapy (HRT)

> Estrogen therapy and estrogen/progesterone therapy are available as tablets or transdermal patches and come in a wide variety of doses. HRT is approved for prevention of bone loss, but not approved for the treatment of osteoporosis.

Follow-Up

A. If the client is on calcium supplements, check urinary calcium excretion two times per year. If it is below 250 mg/d, nephrocalcinosis and the risk of renal stones are decreased.

B. Fracture risk is recommended to be assessed by performing a bone density test for postmenopausal women.

   1. Every 2 years for postmenopausal women not treated with bisphosphonates

   2. Every 3 to 5 years for postmenopausal women treated with bisphosphonates

C. It is recommended that women with high risk of fracture remain on bisphosphonates.

D. It is recommended that women with low to moderate risk of fracture take a "bisphosphonate drug holiday" (discontinuing bisphosphonate therapy) for up to 5 years.

Consultation/Referral

A. If fracture is suspected, consult with a physician.

Individual Consideration

A. Geriatrics:

   1. Assessment and treatment for osteoporosis must be performed routinely to prevent the risk of fracture, which may increase the risk of morbidity and mortality rates in this population.

   2. The mortality rate postfracture for geriatric men with osteoporosis is 18.7% and for geriatric women is 13.9%.

   3. Bisphosphonates are contraindicated for clients with whom have CrCl ≤ 35 to 40 mL/min/1.73.

   4. Delay treatment with bisphosphonate therapy a few months postdental surgery until facial and mandibular bones are healed.

   5. Stress fall prevention when educating geriatric client about osteoporosis.

Bibliography

Curtis, E. M., Moon, R. J., Dennison, E. M., Harvey, N. C., & Cooper, C. (2015). Recent advances in the pathogenesis and treatment of osteoporosis. *Clinical Medicine (London, England), 15*(Suppl. 6), s92–s96. doi:10.7861/clinmedicine.15-6-s92

Eastell, R., Rosen, C. J., Black, D. M., Cheung, A. M., Murad, M. H., & Shoback, D. (2019). Pharmacological management of osteoporosis in postmenopausal women: An endocrine society* clinical practice guideline. *Journal of Clinical Endocrinology & Metabolism, 104*(5), 1–28. doi:10.1210/jc.2019-00221

Farford, B., Balog, J., Jackson, K. D., & Montero, D. (2015). Osteoporosis: What about men? *Journal of Family Practice, 64*(9), 549–552, 542–552.

Kado, D. M. (2019). *Overview of hyperkyphosis in older persons. UpToDate.* Retrieved from http://www.uptodate.com/contents/overview-of-hyper-kyphosis-in-older-persons

Mackey, P. A., & Whitaker, M. D. (2015). Osteoporosis: A therapeutic update. *Journal for Nurse Practitioners*, *11*(10), 1011–1017. doi:10.1016/j.nurpra.2015.08.010

Martin, G. M., Thornhill, T. S., & Katz, J. M. (2019). *Total knee arthroplasty*. *UpToDate*. Retrieved from www.uptodate.com/contents/total-knee-arthroplasty

National Osteoporosis Foundation. (n.d.[a]). *Medications to prevent & treat osteoporosis*. Retrieved from https://www.nof.org/?s=osteoporosis+prevention

National Osteoporosis Foundation. (n.d.[b]). *Prevention: Vitamin D*. Retrieved from https://www.nof.org/?s=osteoporosis+prevention

Robinson, P. G., Campbell, V. B., Murray, A. D., Nicol, A., & Robson, J. (2019). Stress fractures: Diagnosis and management in the primary care setting. *British Journal of General Practice*, *69*(681), 209–300.

Rosen, H. N., & Drezner, M. K. (2019). *Overview of the management of osteoporosis in postmenopausal women*. *UpToDate*. Retrieved from http://www.uptodate.com/

Rosen, H. N., & Walega, D. R. (2019). *Osteoporotic thoracolumbar vertebral compression fractures: Clinical manifestations and treatment*. *UpToDate*. Retrieved from http://www.uptodate.com/contents/osteoporotic-thoracolumbar-vertebral-compression-fractures-clinical-manifestations-and-treatment

Polymyalgia Rheumatica

Jill C. Cash

Definition

A. Polymyalgia rheumatica (PMR) is an inflammatory condition with an insidious or abrupt onset that causes morning muscle stiffness, pain, and decreased ROM, primarily in the hips, shoulders, and neck.

Incidence

A. PMR occurs in all racial groups; however, it is rarely seen in the African American and Latino populations. It is commonly seen in adults older than 50 years, with an increased incidence in the 70- to 80-year-old population. Women are affected two to three times more often than men. PMR is occasionally associated with giant cell arteritis (GCA). Approximately 15% of diagnosed clients with PMR will also have GCA. Approximately half of clients diagnosed with GCA will be diagnosed with PMR.

Pathogenesis

A. The cause of PMR is unknown. Environmental and genetic factors have been shown to play a role in PMR. Studies speculate that environmental triggers, such as viruses, may cause the onset of symptoms. There are common similarities between PMR and GCA.

Predisposing Factors

A. Age (older than 50 years)
B. Gender (women are affected two to three times more often than men)
C. Ethnicity (those of Northern European origin have a higher rate of PMR)

Common Complaints

A. Early morning joint stiffness and pain lasting for approximately 20 to 30 minutes after waking for at least 2 weeks
B. Stiffness and pain commonly occur in the shoulders, hips, and neck.
C. Decreased ROM of joints
D. Muscle pain
E. Weakness of joints and muscles

Other Signs and Symptoms

A. Fever
B. Fatigue
C. Malaise

Potential Complications

A. Difficulty performing daily activities, such as getting up out of a chair, dressing, and bathing
B. Decreased activity
C. Overall a decrease in general health because of limitations

Subjective Data

A. Ask the client if there was an activity that brought about or preceded the episode of joint pain.
B. Has the client had any recent illness or injury?
C. Ask the client to describe the onset, duration, and intensity of pain, noting what particular joints are involved.
D. How long does pain and stiffness last in the morning?
E. Does the client notice a decrease in ROM? Are there activities that the client is not able to perform?
F. Ask the client to list all medications currently being taken, particularly substances not prescribed and OTC products. What medications improve pain?
G. Has the client noticed a problem with sleeping since the symptoms began?

Physical Examination

A. Vital signs: check temperature, pulse, respirations, and BP.
B. Inspect:
    1. Hands, wrists, elbows, shoulders, hips, and neck for erythema and synovitis
C. Auscultate:
    1. Heart
    2. Lungs
D. Palpate:
    1. Palpate joints for swelling and pain. Marked swelling is not usually seen in clients with PMR.
    2. Assess ROM of the shoulders, hips, back, and neck. Perform passive ROM of the shoulders and hips.
    3. Assess trigger points for tenderness, assessing for symptoms of fibromyalgia.
    4. Assess muscle strength of upper and lower extremities and neck.
    5. Assess temporal arteries for signs of inflammation.

Diagnostic Tests

A. CBC—normocytic anemia common
B. ESR—elevation
C. CRP, noncardiac—elevation
D. RF—negative
E. X-rays or MRI of the affected joints

Differential Diagnoses

A. RA

B. GCA

C. Fibromyalgia (symptoms will have been present for years)

Plan

A. General interventions:

    1. Treat the client with steroid therapy to improve symptoms, starting at a dose adequate to resolve symptoms. Treatment includes slowly tapering the steroids over a period of weeks/months to keep the client symptom-free until off of steroids.

B. Client teaching:

    1. *See Section III: Client Teaching Guide for this chapter, "Polymyalgia Rheumatica."*

    2. Educate the client and family that PMR is primarily a self-limiting condition that will improve slowly over time.

    3. Treatment includes several weeks/months of low-dose prednisone therapy, tapering slowly until completion of steroid therapy. Tapering slowly and patience prevents recurrent attacks and rebound flares.

C. Pharmaceutical therapy:

    1. Low-dose prednisone is used to treat the symptoms. Steroids should be given to relieve symptoms (starting dose may be 10 to 20 mg orally [po] daily) and then tapered slowly over the next 6 months. Gradually decreasing the steroid dose by very small increments over time has the best results, minimizing the possibility of relapse.

Follow-Up

A. A follow-up appointment is recommended 2 weeks after the initial appointment.

B. If symptoms are improving with the steroid therapy, a follow-up appointment is recommended every 1 to 2 months until there are not any flares of symptoms and the client has completed the steroid therapy. This treatment may take several months and even up to greater than 1 year.

Individual Considerations

A. Another condition to consider with the symptoms is remitting seronegative symmetrical synovitis with pitting edema. This condition presents with hand and distal extremity swelling, noting marked pitting edema in extremities. It is commonly seen in clients older than 50 years of age with an acute onset of swelling and pain. Symptoms respond quickly to the use of low-dose steroids. Laboratory testing for RA is negative.

B. Clients on long-term steroids should have a BMD performed to evaluate for osteoporosis.

Bibliography

Yurdakul, F. G., Bodur, H., Sivas, F., Başkan, B., Eser, F., & Yilmaz, O. (2015). Clinical features, treatment and monitoring in patients with polymyalgia rheumatica. *Archives of Rheumatology*, *30*(1), 28–33. doi:10.5606/ArchRheumatol.2015.4643

Pseudogout

Jill C. Cash

Definition

A. Pseudogout is an acute inflammatory condition primarily affecting the larger joints in which crystal deposits of CPP dihydrate occur in the connective tissues.

Incidence

A. Acute attacks occur more often in men than in women.

B. Women diagnosed with OA with CPP have a higher incidence of occurrence.

C. Approximately 50% of cases occur in clients older than the age of 84 years, 36% occur during the ages of 75 to 84 years, and 15% occur in those from 65 to 74 years old.

D. Joints affected: The knee is affected approximately 50% of the time; other joints affected include wrists, shoulders, ankles, feet, and elbows.

Pathogenesis

A. Pseudogout occurs from crystal formation in the cartilage that is shed into the synovial joint. Excessive cartilage pyrophosphate production leads to CPP production and CPP crystals are formed and deposited in the joint.

Predisposing Factors

A. Older adults

B. Joint trauma

C. Hospitalization/illness

D. Familial chondrocalcinosis

E. Endocrine/metabolic disorders:

    1. Gout

    2. Hyperparathryroidism

    3. Hemochromatosis

    4. Hypophosphatasia

    5. Hypothyroidism

    6. Hypomagnesemia

    7. Gitelman syndrome

    8. Hemosiderosis

Common Complaints

A. Asymptomatic (may be visible on x-ray)

B. Acute attack of pain and swelling of affected joint, commonly a large joint

C. Erythema

D. Decreased ROM secondary to severe pain; inability to bear weight

Other Signs and Symptoms

A. Fever

B. Pain, swelling, and redness in several joints

Subjective Data

A. Ask the client about the onset, progression, and duration of symptoms.

B. How many joints are affected?

C. Is this the first time this has occurred, or is this a chronic problem?

D. Ask the client to describe the onset of symptoms, in the order of occurrence

E. Has this occurred in other joints?

F. Does the client have a history of RA, OA, or other types of arthritis?

G. Any previous injury to the joint?

H. What has the client used for pain or fever?

Physical Examination

A. Check vital signs, temperature as indicated.

B. Inspect:
1. Inspect the affected joint for erythema, edema, and synovitis.
2. If erythema is present, note location of erythema and evaluate if erythema extends beyond joint area.
3. While examining the joint, note facial grimaces, guarding with examination.
4. If weight-bearing joint is affected, note if the client is able to bear weight.

C. Auscultate:
1. Lungs and heart

D. Palpate:
1. Palpate affected joint, noting pain and swelling in the joint.
2. Assess ROM in joint if possible.

Diagnostic Tests

A. CBC

B. ESR

C. Serum CRP

D. CMP

E. Magnesium level

F. TSH

G. Iron studies (iron, total iron-binding capacity, ferritin level)

H. Joint aspiration for synovial fluid (microscope evaluation for crystals)

I. X-ray of joint: Results may demonstrate linear and punctate calcifications in articular hyaline or fibrocartilage, also known as chondrocalcinosis.

Differential Diagnoses

A. Gout

B. Septic arthritis

C. RA

D. OA

Plan

A. General interventions:
1. Acute attacks should be treated with rest, immobilization, and education.
2. Differentiate between acute and chronic attacks and treatment.
3. Recurrent attacks should have long-term management.

B. Client teaching:
1. For acute attacks, encourage rest and elevation of affected joint.

2. Encourage no weight bearing until symptoms subside. Suggest the use of crutches or cane for assistance.
3. Warm, moist compresses may be used as needed for comfort.
4. As symptoms improve, suggest ROM exercises for affected joint.
5. Once symptoms have improved, weight-bearing activities may resume.
6. Symptoms should continue to improve over the next 7 to 10 days. Full recovery should be expected.

C. Pharmaceutical therapy:
1. For acute attack, with one to two joints affected and no signs of infection:
   a. Large joints (knees/shoulders): joint aspiration and glucocorticoid steroid injection: triamcinolone acetonoid 30 to 40 mg mixed with 1% procaine, 1 to 2 mL. Smaller joints require less steroid.
2. If not meeting the criteria discussed earlier, the next treatment option recommended is the use of NSAIDs:
   a. Naproxen (Naprosyn) 500 mg twice a day with food
   b. Indomethacin (Indocin) 50 mg three times a day with food (not recommended in high-risk clients with heart failure, GI effects, or decreased renal function)
   c. Sulindac 200 mg twice a day with food
3. If NSAIDs are contraindicated, use colchicine 1.2 mg within 24 hours of attack, followed by 0.6 mg 1 hour later, then 0.6 mg bid.
4. If injection and use of NSAIDs are contraindicated, use oral prednisone 30 to 50 mg daily until flare begins to resolve, then taper prednisone over the next 7 to 10 days.
5. Recurrent attacks (more than three attacks in 1 year) should be treated with colchicine. Monitor liver and kidney function. Consult with physician and/or refer to rheumatologist.

Follow-Up

A. The client should return to the office in 48 to 72 hours after diagnosis and treatment.

B. Client follow-up in 1 week is recommended for continued care.

C. If symptoms are not improving or are worsening, client should return to the clinician's office or present to the ED for further evaluation and treatment.

Consultation/Referral

A. Refer all clients who appear to have a septic joint to the ED for evaluation and treatment. Refer to an orthopedic surgeon for consult.

B. Consider referring clients with pseudogout to rheumatology for evaluation and continued care.

Individual Considerations

A. Adults:
1. Most commonly seen in adults older than 60 years
2. Precautions should be used in treating clients with long-term NSAIDs. Clients with active GI ulcers or history of GI disease should avoid NSAID use.

3. Clients on blood thinner medications should avoid the use of NSAIDs.

4. All precautions for the use of NSAIDs in adults should be considered, including chronic kidney disease.

5. Clients diagnosed with diabetes who are prescribed oral or injection steroids should be advised that steroids may increase blood sugar and to monitor blood sugar values at home as indicated.

B. Geriatrics:

1. Most common in the older adult

2. Precaution should be used with using NSAIDs in the older adult

3. Monitor renal function

Bibliography

Sholter, D. E., & Russell, A. S. (2019). *Synovial fluid analysis. UpToDate.* Retrieved from www.uptodate.com/contents/synovial-fluid-analysis

Psoriatic Arthritis

Jill C. Cash

Definition

A. Psoriatic arthritis (PsA) is a systemic inflammatory condition that occurs in the joints that presents with symptoms of joint pain, stiffness, and swelling around the tendons and ligaments. Other symptoms include psoriasis and IBP. PsA is a chronic disease, and when left untreated, it can cause irreversible joint damage.

B. Five different types of PsA:

1. Symmetrical polyarthritis

2. Asymmetric oligoarthritis (fewer than four joints involved)

3. DIP joint involvement

4. Arthritis mutilans (destructive and deforming, causes resorption of the phalanges)

5. Axial arthritis (spondyloarthritis [SpA])

C. The 2006 Classification of Psoriatic Arthritis (CASPAR) was developed to assist in diagnosing clients with PsA. The client must score at least three points from the following list:

1. Skin psoriasis:

   a. Present: 2 points

   b. Previous history of skin changes: 1 point

   c. Family history of psoriasis if client not affected: 1 point

2. Nail lesions (onycholysis, pitting): 1 point

3. Dactylitis (present or past): 1 point

4. RF negative: 1 point

5. X-ray evidence of new bone formation near a joint: 1 point

Incidence

A. Occurs in approximately 1% to 2% of the U.S. population

B. Estimated to occur in approximately 4% to 30% of clients diagnosed with psoriasis

Pathogenesis

A. Individuals are genetically susceptible to PsA. It is thought that the immune system is triggered by something in the environment, which may include infection and/or trauma. The immune system is stimulated, activating T-cells that produce inflammatory cytokines and mediators that attack the joints, causing inflammation, pain, and/or erosions that can potentially destroy the joint. This response occurs in the joint and causes damage to the ligament or tendon attachment area (enthesis), as well as producing bone spurs and changes in the skin and/or nails.

Predisposing Factors

A. Gender: men and women affected equally

B. Commonly seen in adults ranging from 30 to 55 years of age

C. The client has a first-degree relative with psoriasis

D. More common in Caucasians than African American and Native American populations

Common Complaints

A. Pain and stiffness in joints, usually lasting longer than 30 minutes in the morning after wakening

B. Pain and stiffness that usually improves with activity

C. Enthesopathy (pain and inflammation at the ligament or tendon attachment site of the bone, commonly seen on the Achilles tendon, plantar fascia, or tibial tuberosity area)

Other Signs and Symptoms

A. Skin and nail psoriasis, nail pitting

B. Uveitis

Subjective Data

A. Does the client have a history of skin rash, plaques, and so forth? If present, ask the client when psoriasis began. What treatments have been used, including topical, light therapy, oral, and subcutaneous treatments?

B. Does the client complain of photosensitivity?

C. Ask the client to describe joint changes, such as swelling, pain, redness, and so forth. What joints are affected with pain and swelling?

D. Have any treatments used for psoriasis improved joint pain?

E. What medications or treatments are being used for the joint pain and swelling? What is the result of medications/treatments being used?

F. Does the client have a history of back pain? If so, when did symptoms begin? Ask the client to describe his or her back pain. Does pain improve or worsen with physical activity?

G. Does the client have a history of frequent infections or high fevers?

H. Any history of frequent eye infections?

Physical Examination

A. Check vital signs and temperature as indicated.

B. Inspect:

1. Skin for plaques or rash.

2. Nails for pitting.

3. Joints for inflammation, synovitis, and erythema.
4. Eyes for erythema and infection.

C. Auscultate:
1. Heart
2. Lungs

D. Palpate:
1. All joints (hands, wrists, feet, elbows, ankles, knees, and shoulders) for synovitis/pain.
   a. Dactylitis (swelling of the entire finger/toe that appears as a "sausage digit") occurs in approximately 50% of clients diagnosed with PsA.
   b. Enthesopathy is commonly seen in the Achilles tendon, plantar fascia, or tibial tuberosity.
2. Note ROM of all joints.
3. Palpate lumbar/thoracic spine.
4. Palpate sacroiliac joint for tenderness.

Diagnostic Tests

A. ESR: may be elevated or normal
B. CRP: may be elevated or normal
C. CBC
D. RF: commonly negative in these clients. Only 2% to 16% of clients with PsA have a positive RF.
E. X-rays of affected joints

Differential Diagnoses

A. RA
B. AS
C. OA
D. Gout
E. Reactive arthritis

Plan

A. General interventions:
1. Early identification is necessary to prevent irreversible joint damage.

B. Client teaching:
1. Nonpharmacological treatment options include the following:
   a. Exercise on most days of the week. ROM exercises are encouraged for joint stiffness.
   b. Heat application for stiffness and ice to affected joint for swelling may be used.
   c. For extended joint stiffness/pain, recommend physical therapy for assessment and treatment

C. Pharmaceutical therapy:
1. First-line treatment: The European League Against Rheumatism (EULAR) recommends the use of NSAIDs for first-line treatment. Precautions should be given for all clients using NSAIDs (cardiovascular, renal, and GI risks should be considered). NSAIDs are used for mild symptoms.
2. Second-line treatment: Disease-modifying antirheumatic drugs (DMARDs), such as methotrexate (MTX), sulfasalazine, and leflunomide, are used. These medications should be prescribed by a rheumatology specialist.
3. Third-line treatment: biological TNF inhibitors (adalimumab, certolizumab pegol, etanercept, golimumab, and infliximab). These medications should be prescribed by a rheumatology specialist.

Follow-Up

A. Recommend follow-up in 2 weeks if prescribing NSAIDs for treatment of early disease.
B. Recommend follow-up every 3 months if not referred to rheumatology.

Consultation/Referral

A. Clients diagnosed with PsA who are not controlled with NSAIDs or who have evidence of joint changes should be referred to a rheumatology specialist for evaluation and treatment. NSAIDs do not prevent joint damage and prevention of irreversible joint damage is imperative.
B. Clients presenting with uveitis should be referred to an ophthalmologist for evaluation and treatment.
C. Clients diagnosed with severe joint damage should be referred to orthopedics for evaluation and treatment options (surgery).
D. Clients diagnosed with severe skin psoriasis should be referred to dermatology for evaluation and treatment.

Individual Considerations

A. Adults:
1. The use of oral steroids is not recommended for clients with PsA. Oral steroids have not been found to be effective; they also present a high risk of skin psoriasis flare when tapering the steroid dose.
2. Clients diagnosed with PsA are at higher risk for cardiovascular disease and should be screened and monitored annually.
B. Geriatrics:
1. When prescribing NSAIDs, monitor renal, cardiac, and GI systems for adverse events with use

Bibliography

Dewing, K. A. (2015). Management of patients with psoriatic arthritis. *Nurse Practitioner*, *40*(4), 40–46; quiz 46. doi:10.1097/01.NPR .0000461950.23292.18

Raynaud's Phenomenon

Jill C. Cash

Definition

A. Raynaud's phenomenon (RP) is an idiopathic disease in which an exaggerated vascular response occurs in extreme circumstances (heat, cold, and stress). It is manifested by bilateral blanching of the skin that is well demarcated, discomfort in the fingers, then by cyanosis, then erythema after warming the digits.
B. Cold hands and feet are very common complaints. RP involves both cutaneous color change and cool skin temperature. Although the hands are the most common area of attacks, RP also can occur in the toes, ears, nose, face, knees, and nipples.

C. A Raynaud attack typically begins in a single finger and spreads symmetrically; however, the thumb is often spared.

D. RP may be either primary or secondary. Spontaneous remission may occur with primary RP.

E. Criteria for diagnosis of primary RP:
1. Symmetric episodic attacks
2. No evidence of peripheral vascular disease
3. No tissue gangrene, digital pitting, or tissue injury
4. Negative nailfold capillary examination
5. Negative ANA test
6. Normal ESR

F. Indications of secondary RP:
1. Age of onset older than 40 years
2. Painful severe attacks with signs of ulceration/ischemia
3. Ischemic signs/symptoms proximal to the fingers or toes
4. Asymmetric attacks
5. Abnormal laboratory suggesting vascular or autoimmune disorders

Incidence

A. 3% to 20% of women
B. 3% to 14% of men
C. 3% of African Americans
D. Wide global differences from the United States

Pathogenesis

A. Primary RP: occurs alone, without any other disease process. Speculated theories include digital microvascular vasospasm because of increased response of alpha-2-adrenergic receptors and a high sympathetic vascular tone.

B. Secondary RP: Symptoms occur as a secondary manifestation from other diseases or products such as autoimmune disorders (connective tissue disorders, systemic sclerosis, SLE, RA, vasculitis, Sjögren's syndrome, dermatomyositis, polymyositis, etc.), atherosclerotic diseases, hematologic disorders (polycythemia, cryofibrinogenemia, etc.), metabolic/endocrine disorders (diabetes mellitus, pheochromocytoma, myxedema), neoplastic syndromes (lymphoma, leukemia, polycythemia, monoclonal/type 1 cryoglubulinemia), infections (hepatitis B, hepatitis C, mycoplasma infections), environmental exposures/neurologic changes (frostbite, vibratory injuries from use, lead exposure, vinyl chloride exposure, arsenic exposure, organic solvents [xylene, toluene, acetone, chlorinated solvents], carpel tunnel syndrome), and some medications/drugs (cyclosporines, antineoplastics, oral contraceptives, narcotics, ergot alkaloids, bromocriptine, beta-adrenergic blocking agents, and nicotine). Symptoms may be unilateral and may affect only one or two fingers. Secondary RP usually has a poorer morbidity than the primary disease.

Predisposing Factors

A. Primary RP:
1. Female
2. Onset of symptoms after menarche (15–30 years)
3. Smoking
4. Emotional stress

B. Secondary RP:
1. Onset after age 40 years
2. Male gender

C. Family history: multiple family members
D. Frostbite
E. Vascular trauma (distal ulnar artery)
F. Vibration-induced/occupation exposure (jackhammers, pneumatic drills, weed eaters)
G. Medication-associated RP (see Table 21.1)

Common Complaints

A. Paleness of the fingertips after exposure to cold temperatures, followed by redness and discomfort after warming fingers

B. "White attack": sharp, demarcated color of skin pallor
C. "Blue attack": cyanotic skin
D. White or blue attack, usually lasting 15 to 20 minutes
E. Age of onset between 15 and 30 years

Other Signs and Symptoms

A. Paresthesias and numbness
B. Clumsiness of the aching hand/finger
C. Loss of pulp in pads of fingers (severe cases)

Subjective Data

A. Determine the age of onset, time, duration, and course of presenting symptoms.

B. Question the client regarding location and symptoms, noting blanching, followed by erythema and pain after hands are warm.

C. Note frequency of attacks.

D. Review the presence of any other skin alterations that have occurred. Does client also note skin mottling of the arms and legs? Livedo reticularis is a lilac or violet mottling or reticular pattern that occurs during a cold response.

E. Ask the client to identify any events that precipitate occurrences and what makes symptoms worse or better:
1. Air-conditioning
2. Grocery cold/freezer food sections
3. Cold weather
4. Cold water
5. Emotional stress
6. Sudden startling

F. Identify any other symptoms that occur at the same time such as migraine headaches.

G. Review the client's health history for underlying disorders such as hypothyroidism and autoimmune disorders/connective tissue disease.

H. Review current or past occupation (especially those that include the use of vibratory tools).

I. Review current medications, stimulants, herbals, and OTC medications.

TABLE 21.1	DRUGS THAT INDUCE RP	
Amphetamines	Clonidine	Interferon-Alpha
Beta-blockers	Cocaine	Nicotine
Bleomycin	Cyclosporine	Vinblastine
Cisplatin	Ergot	Vinyl chloride

Physical Examination

A. Check pulse, respirations, and BP.

B. Inspect:

1. Dermal examination: note malar/petechial rash, telangiectasias, digital pallor, or erythema. Examine for any ulceration or signs of ischemia.

2. Inspect joints for swelling or redness and overall ischemic changes.

3. Examine several fingernails using a microscope or ophthalmoscope; examine capillaries at nailfold:

   a. Normal: fine red capillaries lined in the same direction

   b. Abnormal: capillaries dilated, tortuous, and irregularly spaced. Avoid using the index finger for evaluation

C. Auscultate:

1. Heart

2. Lungs

D. Palpate:

1. Joints for tenderness and peripheral pulses bilaterally

E. Neurologic examination: sensory function:

1. Sensory discrimination (hot/cold, sharp/dull)

2. Location of sensation (proximal/distal to previous stimuli)

3. Vibratory sensation with tuning fork (distal to proximal joints)

4. Graphesthesia (draw a number or letter in the palm of the hand with a blunt object, such as a pencil, applicator stick, or pen and have the client identify the letter/number)

Diagnostic Tests

A. There is no gold standard diagnostic test.

B. History alone is accepted as diagnostic as no office test application consistently triggers an attack. A history of at least two color changes, pallor, and cyanosis after cold exposure is adequate for the diagnosis of RP. Ask the client to take a picture when symptoms occur and bring it into the office for evaluation.

C. The cold water challenge test is no longer recommended.

D. Tools to assess vascular response (usually not readily available):

1. Nailfold capillaroscopy

2. Videomicroscopy

3. Thermography

4. Angiography

5. Laser Doppler

6. Direct measures of the skin temperature and local blood flow

E. Laboratory tests:

1. ANA

2. ESR

3. Thyroid profile if hypothyroidism is suspected

4. Other tests are used, depending on suspected etiology; testing should be guided by results of history and physical examination.

   a. CBC

   b. Chemistry profile with renal and liver function

   c. Urinalysis

   d. RF

   e. Complement (C3 and C4)

   f. ANA

Differential Diagnoses

A. Scleroderma

B. SLE

C. Occupational trauma

D. Medication induced

E. Peripheral vascular disease

F. Neurovascular processes (diabetes, atherosclerosis, thromboangitis obliterans)

Plan

A. General interventions:

1. If ulcerations are present, monitor for secondary infections. Consider topical/systemic antibiotics if secondary infection. Debridement may be necessary.

2. Biofeedback and relaxation techniques are frequently used for treatment.

B. Client teaching:

1. Stress the importance of not smoking.

2. Keep the body warm:

   a. If in extreme temperatures, wear extra clothing (thermal underwear) to maintain temperature.

   b. Wear mittens instead of gloves to protect hands and keep them warm.

   c. Wear a hat to conserve heat.

3. If possible, stop all medications that could be inducing symptoms. Other drugs that should be avoided include:

   a. Decongestants

   b. Herbs that contain ephedra

   c. Medications used for migraine headaches; for example, serotonin agonists such as sumatriptan, or caffeine plus ergotamine

4. If vibrator injury is present, stop the repetitive activity that induces symptoms. Consider alternative methods of work. If unable to totally stop the activity, decrease time spent using the vibratory equipment.

5. Emotional stress can be a trigger because of the vasoconstriction of the sympathetic nervous system being triggered. Counsel the client regarding controlling the stress in his or her life and treatment (nonpharmacological/pharmacological) options that may be beneficial.

C. Surgical therapy (only recommended for clients resistant to initial therapies):

1. Temporary sympathectomy involving a local chemical block with lidocaine or bupivacaine (without epinephrine) relieves the pain.

2. Chemical and cervical sympathectomy may be used for severe cases with digital ischemia for temporary measures.

3. Vascular reconstruction is an option.

D. Pharmaceutical therapy:

1. Therapy may be required only during the winter months.

2. Long-acting calcium channel blockers are used. Doses may be adjusted every 4 weeks or as tolerated.

Monitor by side effects: headaches, dizziness, flushing tachycardia, and edema:

    a. Nifedipine 30 to 180 mg/d

    b. Amlodipine 5 to 20 mg/d

3. Low-dose aspirin antiplatelet therapy 75 to 81 mg/d may be considered in secondary RP with a history of ischemic ulcers or other thrombotic events.

4. Vasodilators (sildenafil) and endothelin receptor antagonists (bosentan) may be useful in refractory cases with associated digital ulcers/infarcts. However, these medications are not FDA approved for this treatment.

Follow-Up

A. Follow up in 1 month or as needed by client symptoms

Consultation/Referral

A. Consult a physician if signs of ischemia are present and/or if refractory symptoms are present.

B. Refer to a rheumatologist if there is a moderate/high suspicion of secondary RP.

C. Refer for surgical therapies.

Individual Considerations

A. Pediatrics:

    1. RP is commonly seen in children with SLE and scleroderma.

B. Adults:

    1. The onset of RP after age 40 years is commonly associated with an underlying disease.

C. Geriatrics:

    1. Recommend clients wear gloves and socks in extreme cold weather and carry a jacket for sudden temperature changes such as outdoors, restaurants, freezer section of the grocery store, etc.

    Older adults are sensitive to triggers causing vasoconstriction, such as vibratory tools, decongestants, herb/medications, emotional stress, and second-hand smoke.

    2. Due to neuropathy and cognitive decline in this population, monitor for increased risk of digital ischemia and potential ulceration of digits.

Bibliography

Hansen-Dispenza, H. (2015). *Raynaud phenomenon treatment & management. Medscape.* Retrieved from http://emedicine.medscape.com/article/331197-treatment

Jordan, S., Maurer, B., Toniolo, M., Michel, B., & Distler, O. (2015). Performance of the new ACR/EULAR classification criteria for systemic sclerosis in clinical practice. *Rheumatology (Oxford, England), 54*(8), 1454–1458. doi:10.1093/rheumatology/keu530

Miller, M. L., & Viegels, R. A. (2019). *Clinical manifestations of dermatomyositis and polymyositis in adults. UpToDate.* Retrieved from www.uptodate.com/contents/clinical-manifestations-of-dermatomyositis-and-polymyositis-in-adults

Varga, J. (2019). *Diagnosis and differential diagnosis of systemic sclerosis (scleroderma) in adults. UpToDate.* Retrieved from www.uptodate.com/contents/diagnosis-and-differential-diagnosis-of-systemic-sclerosis-scleroderma-in-adults

Varga, J., & Steen, V. (2019). *Pulmonary arterial hypertension in systemic sclerosis (scleroderma): Definition, classification, risk factors, screening and prognosis. UpToDate.* Retrieved from www.uptodate.com/contents/pulmonary-arterial-hypertension-in-systemic-sclerosis-scleroderma-definition-classification-risk-factors-screening-and-prognosis

Rheumatoid Arthritis

Jill C. Cash

Definition

A. Rheumatoid arthritis (RA) is a chronic systemic disease that involves articular inflammation of the joints. The disease is generally insidious, and symmetrical involvement of synovial joints is a characteristic feature. Typically, the interphalangeal joints of the fingers and thumbs are noted; however, other joints involved include the elbows, shoulders, ankles, knees, and toes. Left untreated, the client is at high risk of joint deformity and disability. Treatment goals of RA include remission, preventing functional decline of the client, and halting progression of the disease (see Figure 21.2).

FIGURE 21.2 Ulnar deviation of fingers due to rheumatoid arthritis.

Source: Image courtesy of James Heilman, MD.

B. RA is not limited to the joints; extra-articular features of RA include anemia, pleuropericarditis, neuropathy, myopathy, splenomegaly, Sjögren's syndrome, scleritis, vasculitis, and renal disease. Most clients with extra-articular symptoms also have the classic RA joint symptoms. Clients with RA are at increased risk of development of carpal tunnel syndrome, stroke, an osteoporotic fracture, and renal disease (secondary to drug toxicity).

C. The ACR criteria for RA require that an algorithm be used to assess for criteria to meet the diagnosis for RA. A score of ≥6/10 is recommended for the client to be diagnosed with RA based on the working algorithm. Clients who should be screened for RA include those who have had at least one swollen joint, with the joint swelling not being caused by any other known etiology. Scoring for the algorithm is available at www.rheumatology.org/Portals/0/Files/ACR%202015%20RA%20Guideline.pdf.

D. Classification criteria for screening for RA:

    1. Duration of symptoms for more than 6 weeks

    2. Joint swelling involvement (synovitis)

3. Serology: RF and/or anti-citrullinated peptide/protein antibody (CCP)

4. Acute-phase reactants: CRP and ESR

E. Four stages of RA:

1. Stage 1: no symptoms or signs; normal activity; RF and/or CCP antibody is present.

2. Stage 2: morning stiffness, warmth at joint, normal activities of daily living (ADLs), minimal limitation in joint use; increased T-cells, B-cells, antibody production, and synovial cells are observed.

3. Stage 3: morning stiffness, warmth at joint, and extra-articular manifestations; marked limitation in ADL; increased T-cells, B-cells, antibody production, and synovial cells are observed.

4. Stage 4: same as stage 3 plus proliferating synovial membrane involved, causing injury to the bone, tendons, and cartilage. Client is now incapacitated or confined to a wheelchair.

Incidence

A. It is estimated that RA occurs in approximately 1.5 million adults in the United States. RA occurs at twice the rate in women compared with men. The prevalence of RA is approximately 1.06% of women compared with 0.61% of men.

Pathogenesis

A. The cause is unknown. Articular inflammation results in joint destruction. Antibody formation in the joint area results in inflammation and pain in the joint area.

Predisposing Factors

A. Family history, including 15% prevalence in monozygotic twins

B. Female gender

C. Age 20 to 50 years

D. Recent systemic illness or trauma

Common Complaints

A. Joint pain

B. Morning stiffness in joints for at least 1 hour that has been present for more than 6 weeks

C. Swelling and warmth in at least three joints or more for at least 6 weeks. Common joints affected include the wrists and hands, the metacarpal phalangeal (MCP) joints, and the PIP joints.

Other Signs and Symptoms

A. Fatigue

B. Malaise

C. Subcutaneous nodules

D. Joint deformities:

1. PIP joints: boutonniere deformities

2. Fingers: swan-neck contractures, ulnar deviation

3. Wrists: loss of extension

4. Hips: loss of internal rotation, followed by flexion contractures

5. Knees: suprapatellar pouch distension

6. Elbows: decreased extension, olecranon bursitis

7. Shoulders: limited ROM movement

8. Cervical spine: subluxation rare

9. Temporomandibular joint: pain with biting

E. Depression

F. Low-grade fever

G. Weight loss

H. Myalgia

I. Anemia

J. Carpal tunnel syndrome

Subjective Data

A. Review when joint pains began and identify the joints involved. Is pain and stiffness worse in the morning? How long does it last? Is it symmetrical?

B. Elicit the client's description of pain and a description of how the pain interferes with ADL (walking, climbing stairs, using the toilet, getting up from a chair, opening a jar).

C. Review the family history of RA.

D. Has the client ever had any type of injury to the specific joint area? Rule out recent injuries.

E. Identify what makes the pain worse and alleviating factors. In clients with RA, activity typically alleviates symptoms, which is indicative of inflammation.

F. Review list of medications, including herbal and OTC medications. What therapies have specifically been used, and what were the results?

G. Review the client's history for recent infections.

H. Does the client use any assistive devices, including cane, crutches, walker, wheelchair/power mobility device, kitchen devices/grips, and so forth?

Physical Examination

A. Check temperature, if indicated, pulse, respirations, BP, and weight.

B. General observation:

1. Observe the client getting up and down in the chair.

2. Observe the client walking (may have a tendency to bear weight on heels and hyperextend toes secondary to tenderness to the metatarsophalangeal joints).

3. Observe the client handling objects in his or her hands.

4. Observe for signs of depression.

C. Inspect:

1. Inspect all joints, noting deformities, erythema, and temperature. (Heat and redness are not prominent features of RA.)

2. Evaluate for pitting edema in the hand (may have a "boxing glove" appearance).

3. Inspect for subcutaneous rheumatoid nodules (elbow is the most common site).

4. Evaluate skin for ulcerative lesions (secondary from venous stasis and neutrophilic infiltration), skin atrophy and ecchymoses from glucocorticoids, and petechiae (side effect from medications causing thrombocytopenia).

5. Eye examination:
   a. Episcleritis: acute redness and pain without discharge
   b. Scleritis: deep ocular pain with dark red discoloration
D. Auscultate:
   1. Heart
   2. Lungs (at risk of infectious complications from immunosuppression and pulmonary toxicity from methotrexate [MTX] if currently being treated with medications)
E. Percuss:
   1. Perform a patellar tap to evaluate synovial thickening/effusion of the knee.
F. Palpate:
   1. Lymph nodes
   2. Perform oral examination to palpate the salivary glands (may have lymphocytic infiltration).
   3. All joints to evaluate for tenderness with pressure, pain with movement of the joint, and "bogginess" of the joint (synovial thickening).
   4. Popliteal fossa for evidence of a popliteal (Baker's) cyst.
   5. Examine abdomen for splenomegaly.
G. Musculoskeletal examination:
   1. Assess grip (a reduced grip is a useful parameter in evaluating disease activity and progression). Is the client able to close fingers to make a fist?
   2. Assess the strength of the extremities.
   3. Assess the ROM (active and passive) and flexion.

Diagnostic Tests

A. CBC and platelets
B. ESR
C. CRP
D. RF, quantitative
E. CCP antibody
F. Uric acid level
G. Synovial fluid (optional)
H. Plain film radiography of the hands, wrists, and feet as a baseline and to monitor disease progression

Differential Diagnoses

A. OA
B. PsA
C. Crystalline arthritis (gout and pseudogout)
D. Polyarthritis
E. Reactive arthritis
F. Acute viral/infectious process:
   1. Lyme disease
   2. Hepatitis B
   3. Hepatitis C
   4. Parvovirus B19
G. Sjögren's syndrome: keratoconjunctivitis sicca, splenomegaly, and lymphadenopathy
H. Sarcoidosis
I. Polymyositis

Plan

A. General interventions:
   1. Focus on exercise and joint mobility to maintain functional abilities.
   2. Encourage smoking cessation, especially among females on glucocorticoids because of the risk of increased bone loss/fracture.
B. Client teaching:
   1. Once diagnosed, it is recommended that treatment with medications begins to prevent joint damage. First-line medications include DMARDs. Depending on what medication is used, educate the client regarding benefits, risks, side effects, and precautions for medications. If MTX is used, educate the client that alcohol should be avoided to prevent hepatotoxicity.
   2. Stress the importance of returning for laboratory follow-up while on DMARDs.
   3. Discuss vaccinations, especially pneumonia and influenza vaccines. Emphasize the importance of keeping all vaccinations up to date. Most treatment medications suppress the immune system and increase the risk of infections.
C. Pharmaceutical therapy:
   1. Early disease:
      a. Daily NSAIDs and pain-relieving medications:
         i. Ibuprofen 600 to 800 mg every 6 to 8 hours as needed
         ii. Naproxen 500 mg orally every 12 hours as needed
         iii. Celecoxib (Celebrex) 200 mg by mouth daily
         iv. Acetaminophen (Tylenol) 500 to 1,000 mg orally every 4 to 6 hours as needed
      b. Comorbid conditions, such as a history of heart failure, renal disease, and peptic ulcers, should be considered before starting NSAID therapy.
      c. Be aware of other medications the client is prescribed by other providers and consider possible drug-to-drug interactions. Examples include NSAIDs, antacids, anticoagulants, oral hypoglycemic agents, antihypertensives/diuretics, lithium, MTX, and diphenylhydantoin (Dilantin).
   2. Moderate to severe RA disease:
      a. Oral glucocorticoids: prednisone 5 to 10 mg/d for active joint inflammation. Prednisone may be used up to 6 months, but shorter courses are recommended because of the consequences of long-term steroid use. Steroids should be tapered over a period of a few months and then completely discontinued if possible.
      b. Intra-articular long-acting glucocorticoid injections are used for the reduction of synovitis in inflamed joints.
      c. DMARDs are recommended by AMR if early RA manifestations have been present for

<6 months. Adding DMARDs depends on the number of inflamed joints, severity of inflammation, functional impairment, and the number of poor prognostic signs (bony erosions and extra-articular disease). The benefits, risks, and side effects of all medications should be explained to the client before beginning therapy. Recommended blood work monitoring should also be followed according to the medication recommendations.

    i. MTX is given on a weekly basis starting with 7.5 mg/wk and is increased as tolerated to control symptoms. Titration: increase the dose after 4 weeks at a rate of 2.5 mg/wk to a maximum of 25 mg/wk. MTX should not be given to clients who desire to become or who are pregnant or clients with liver disease.

    ii. Sulfasalazine (Azulfidine) 500 to 1,000 mg is given daily initially.

    iii. Hydroxychloroquine (Plaquenil) 200 to 400 mg is given daily. Plaquenil is an antimalarial medication for which the patient must be closely monitored for eye changes. Before starting clients on hydroxychloroquine, the client must be counseled regarding the possible risks of the medication, including retinal damage that can lead to blindness. A baseline eye examination must be performed, followed by eye examination every 6 months to monitor for retinal changes.

    iv. Leflunomide (Arava) 10 to 20 mg/d. Monitoring blood work every 3 months is recommended.

d. If response is not adequate, biological agents, TNF-alpha inhibitors, and other classes of drugs may be instituted. Because of the associated side effects, rheumatology consult is recommended for treatment of these medications.

    i. Examples of TNF inhibitors:

      1) Infliximab (Remicade) 3 to 10 mg/kg every 4 to 6 weeks; IV infusion

      2) Adalimumab (Humira) 0.8-mL (40 mg) subcutaneous injection into abdomen or thigh every 2 weeks

      3) Etanercept (Enbrel) 50-mg subcutaneous injection into the abdomen or thigh weekly

      4) Golimumab (Simponi) 50-mg subcutaneous injection monthly

      5) Certolizumab pegol (Cimzia) 200-mg subcutaneous injection every other week

    ii. Janus kinase inhibitor:

      1) Tofacitinib citrate (Xeljanz) 5 mg orally twice a day (po bid) or 11 mg po daily

    iii. Interleukin-6 (IL-6) inhibitor:

      1) Tocilizumab (Actemra) 162-mg subcutaneous injection every 1 to 2 weeks or 4 to 8 mg/kg IV infusion every 4 weeks

    iv. T-cell depletion:

      1) Abatacept (Orencia) IV infusion every 4 weeks or subcutaneous injection weekly; dosage based on weight

    v. B-cell depleting therapy:

      1) Rituximab (Rituxan) 1,000-mg IV infusion given at week 0 and week 2, and then repeated approximately every 6 months or as indicated

e. Clients may also use combination therapy. Examples of this include using MTX plus a TNF inhibitor or sulfasalazine, and so forth.

f. Clients receiving treatment with pharmacological agents should be evaluated at routine intervals, every 3 months, regarding their functional status to identify whether treatment therapies are improving the symptoms. There are several functional forms that are available for use. The Stanford Health Assessment Questionnaire (HAQ) is a well-known questionnaire that is recommended for use.

g. Drug monitoring, by performing serum blood work, is also recommended at routine intervals when prescribing pharmacological agents to avoid adverse effects of the medications being prescribed.

Follow-Up

A. Follow-up is guided by medication therapy. Disease activity and response to therapy should be reassessed every 4 to 6 weeks.

B. Certain medications require frequent monitoring. When prescribing MTX, blood work for liver function (ALT, AST), albumin, CBC with differential, platelets, and urinalysis is initially recommended monthly.

C. Assume all clients with RA are at risk of osteoporosis. DEXA scan is used to evaluate bone loss secondary to glucocorticoid-induced osteopenia. Initiate bisphosphonate therapy as indicated for signs of bone loss. Use a low threshold for prescribing bisphosphonates in postmenopausal women with RA.

D. Anti-TNF agents are contraindicated in clients with an active infection and those who are at high risk of reactivation of tuberculosis (TB). A TB skin test is required before administration. Clients with a positive skin test should be treated with prophylactic antituberculosis therapy 1 month before therapy with anti-TNF agents.

E. Clients should receive a baseline ophthalmologic examination before starting Plaquenil, and then follow-up examinations every 6 to 12 months while on therapy.

Consultation/Referral

A. Refer all clients with early inflammatory arthritis to a rheumatologist if RA is the suspected. Early intervention may prevent bone destruction of the joints and improve the long-term outcome for the client.

B. Clients with a history of chronic swelling and pain of the joints should be referred to a rheumatologist.

C. Refer all clients to the rheumatologist, orthopedist, or ED if a septic joint is suspected.

Individual Considerations

A. Pregnancy:
  1. RA activity improves substantially in pregnancy.
     a. Approximately 70% to 80% of clients have symptoms improve during pregnancy.
     b. Approximately 90% of women have a flare in the postpartum period. Flares usually occur within the first 3 months postpartum.
  2. Leflunomide, etanercept, adalimumab, and infliximab are contraindicated in pregnancy and while breastfeeding.
  3. Pregnancy should be avoided with the use of MTX and Arava. Women need to have one normal menstrual cycle following discontinuation of MTX before attempting pregnancy. Men should wait at least 3 months after discontinuing MTX before attempting to conceive.
  4. Therapy during pregnancy should be coordinated with the perinatologist and the rheumatologist.
B. Pediatrics:
  1. In children, consider juvenile-onset RA.
  2. If suspected, consider referral to a pediatric rheumatologist for evaluation and diagnosis.
C. Geriatrics:
  1. Use NSAIDs with caution. Consider the client's age, weight, and chronic conditions when prescribing NSAIDs. NSAIDs are not recommended in clients with renal conditions.
  2. The immune status is compromised in these clients. Close monitoring for infection should occur for clients with upper respiratory infection and mild illnesses.
  3. Clients treated with long-term glucocorticoids should be monitored closely for osteoporosis.

Bibliography

Aletaha, D., Neogi, T., Silman, A. J., Funovits, J., Felson, D. T., Bingham, C. O., … Hawker, G. (2010). 2010 rheumatoid arthritis classification criteria: An American College of Rheumatology/European League Against Rheumatism collaborative initiative. *Arthritis and Rheumatism*, *62*(9), 2569–2581. doi:10.1002/art.27584

American College of Rheumatology (2020). *ACR*-endorsed criteria for rheumatic diseases. Retrieved from http://www.rheumatology.org/Practice-Quality/Clinical-Support/Criteria/ACR-Endorsed-Criteria

Brinkmann, G. H., Norli, E. S., Bøyesen, P., van der Heijde, D., Grøvle, L., Haugen, A. J., … Lie, E. (2017). Role of erosions typical of rheumatoid arthritis in the 2010 ACR/EULAR rheumatoid arthritis classification criteria: Results from a very early arthritis cohort. *Annals of the Rheumatic Diseases*, *76*(11), 1911–1914. doi:10.1136/annrheumdis-2017-211350

Ikdahl, E., Rollefstad, S., Olsen, I. C., Kvien, T. K., Hansen, I. J., Soldal, D. M., … Semb, A. G. (2015). EULAR task force recommendations on annual cardiovascular risk assessment for patients with rheumatoid arthritis: An audit of the success of implementation in a rheumatology outpatient clinic. *BioMed Research International*, 2015, 1–6. doi:10.1155/2015/515280

Marcus, D. M. (2015). *Herbal remedies, supplements & acupuncture for arthritis*. Retrieved from www.rheumatology.org/i-am-a/patient-caregiver/treatments/herbal-remedies-supplements-acupuncture-for-arthritis

Raza, K., Klareskog, L., & Holers, V. M. (2016). Predicting and preventing the development of rheumatoid arthritis. *Rheumatology (Oxford, England)*, *55*(1), 1–3. doi:10.1093/rheumatology/kev261

Schur, P. H., & Moreland, L. W. (2019). *General principles of management of rheumatoid arthritis in adults*. *UpToDate*. Retrieved from http://www.uptodate.com/contents/general-principles-of-management-of-rheumatoid-arthritis-in-adults

Sholter, D. E., & Russell, A. S. (2019). *Synovial fluid analysis*. *UpToDate*. Retrieved from www.uptodate.com/contents/synovial-fluid-analysis

Singh, J. A., Saag, K. G., Bridges, S. L., Akl, E. A., Bannuru, R. R., Sullivan, M. C., … McAlindon, T. (2016). 2015 American College of Rheumatology guideline for the treatment of rheumatoid arthritis. *Arthritis & Rheumatology (Hoboken, NJ)*, *68*(1), 1–26. doi:10.1002/art.39480

Systemic Lupus Erythematosus (SLE)

Jill C. Cash

Definition

A. SLE is a chronic, inflammatory autoimmune disorder. It may affect multiple organ systems. The body's immune system forms antibodies that attack healthy tissues and organs. The clinical course is marked by spontaneous remission and relapses. Severity varies from a mild episodic disorder to a rapidly fulminating fatal disease. The three types of lupus are as follows:
  1. Discoid lupus erythematosus (DLE) affects the skin, causing a rash, lesions, or both.
  2. SLE attacks body organs and systems, such as joints, kidneys, brain, heart, and lungs. SLE is usually more severe than DLE and can be life-threatening.
  3. Drug-induced lupus symptoms usually disappear when medication is discontinued.

Incidence

A. The incidence of SLE in relation to gender, ancestry, and familial history has been repeatedly documented. About 85% of clients with SLE are women; it affects mainly young women after menarche and before menopause. The majority of clients who develop SLE during childhood or after age 50 years are also women. SLE occurs in 1:1,000 Caucasian women and 1:250 African American women. The disorder is concordant in 25% to 75% of identical twins. The risk of developing the disease if a mother has SLE is 1:40 for a daughter and 1:250 for a son. Positive ANA is seen in asymptomatic family members, and the prevalence of other rheumatic diseases is increased among close relatives of clients. There is a high frequency of specific genes in SLE. Ten percent of DLE clients go on to develop SLE.

Pathogenesis

A. The exact cause of SLE is unknown, but clinical manifestations of SLE are secondary to the trapping of antigen–antibody complexes in capillaries of visceral structures, or to autoantibody-mediated destruction of host cells such as thrombocytopenia. SLE is commonly precipitated by recent exposure to illness, infections, UV light, surgery, pregnancy, and stress.

Predisposing Factors

A. Female gender
B. African American, Asian, Hispanic ancestry
C. Childbearing age
D. Positive family history of SLE

E. Drug use:
1. Procainamide
2. Hydralazine
3. Isoniazid

Common Complaints
A. Joint pain: Joint symptoms occur in 90% of clients.
B. Fever
C. Loss of appetite
D. Fatigue
E. Weight loss
F. Oral or nasal ulcers
G. Hair loss
H. Photosensitive skin rash and skin lesions over areas exposed to sunlight
I. Relapsing polychondritis

Other Signs and Symptoms
A. DLE:
1. Rash: erythematosus (round, scaling papules 5 to 10 mm in diameter, appearing as "butterfly" shape across bridge of nose)
2. Rash, commonly on the trunk, extremities, scalp, external ear, and neck
3. Photosensitivity
B. SLE: According to the 1997 Updated ACR Criteria, for diagnosis the client must have four or more of the first 11 of the following criteria:
1. Malar rash
2. Discoid rash
3. Photosensitivity
4. Oral ulcers
5. Arthritis (generally bilateral, symmetric, especially in hands and wrists)
6. Serositis
7. Renal disorder: chronic renal problems as indicated by proteinuria (>0.5 g/d of protein or >3+ protein) or cellular casts
8. Neurologic disorder (seizures or personality changes, psychosis)
9. Hematologic disorder
10. Immunologic disorder
11. ANA; abnormal titer of ANA
12. Other signs and symptoms:
    a. Weight loss
    b. Fatigue
    c. Acute abdominal pain
    d. Alopecia
    e. Tendon involvement
    f. Urinalysis: active urine sediment (blood or protein without urinary tract infection [UTI])
    g. Fever and malaise
    h. Lymphadenopathy
13. Other complications:
Probable SLE: have two or three of the first 11 ACR guidelines criteria along with one other feature.
Possible SLE: Have one of the first 11 ACR guidelines criteria, along with one other feature.
    a. Hashimoto's thyroiditis
    b. Hemolytic anemia

c. Thrombocytopenia purpura
d. Arterial and venous thrombosis in the presence of antiphospholipid antibodies
e. Recurrent pleurisy
f. Pleural effusion, pneumonitis
g. Pulmonary embolism
h. Pericarditis, endocarditis, myocarditis
i. Hypertension
j. Splenomegaly
k. Recurrent miscarriages in the presence of antiphospholipid antibodies
l. Relapsing polychondritis
C. Central nervous system (CNS) problems:
1. Chronic headaches (migraine)
2. Seizures or epilepsy
3. Personality changes, chronic brain syndrome
D. Decreased hemoglobin (Hgb), white blood cells (WBC), and platelets

Subjective Data
A. Determine systemic features and onset, course, and duration of symptoms (see "Other Signs and Symptoms" section).
B. Obtain medication history (see "Predisposing Factors" section).
C. Determine family history of rheumatoid diseases or other autoimmune disorders.
D. Review the client's recent history for possible allergen exposure.

Physical Examination
A. Check temperature, pulse, respirations, and BP.
B. Inspect:
1. Observe general overall appearance and generalized movement of extremities.
2. Conduct dermal examination for color, petechiae, rashes, lesions, and hair loss.
3. Conduct funduscopic examination; note photosensitivity.

Funduscopic examination: Cotton–wool exudates are the most common eye lesion.

---

4. Examine mouth and nose for oral lesions/ulcers.
5. Observe for pericardial lifts and heaves.
6. Inspect joints for subluxation of the MCP joints and swan-neck deformities of the hands.
C. Auscultate:
1. Heart
2. Lungs
3. Abdomen
D. Percuss:
1. The chest, anterior and posterior lung fields, for consolidation
2. The abdomen for splenomegaly
E. Palpate:
1. The back for tactile fremitus; palpate the heart for lifts, heaves, and thrills
2. The neck for thyroid enlargement
3. The neck, axilla, and groin for lymphadenopathy

4. The abdomen for organomegaly, masses, and tenderness; palpate suprapubic area for suprapubic tenderness and assess back for costovertebral angle (CVA) tenderness

F. Musculoskeletal examination:
1. Examine for bone or joint swelling, tenderness, and increased warmth.
2. Check lower extremities for evidence of phlebitis, asymmetrical swelling, calf tenderness, and palpable cord.

G. Neurologic examination: complete neurologic examination with mental state.

Diagnostic Tests

A. CBC with differential

B. Platelets

C. ANA: indirect immunofluorescence assay (IFA) positive. In clients with SLE, the ANA will typically be positive with a high-titer ANA. Note pattern associated with positive ANA. A negative ANA by the IFA method dramatically decreases the risk of SLE.

D. Complement levels (decreased C3 and C4)

E. RF can be positive in clients with SLE.

F. Thyroid profile

G. Anti-DNA antibodies (seen in approximately 30% of clients with renal disease)

H. Antiphospholipid antibodies: lupus anticoagulant immunoglobulin A (IgA), immunoglobulin G (IgG), and immunoglobulin M (IgM) anticardiolipin antibodies; IgA, IgG, and IgM anti-beta-2-glycoprotein

I. ESR

J. Urinalysis (check for hematuria, proteinuria, and cellular casts) and urine culture

K. Collection of 24-hour urine for protein and creatinine clearance

L. Skin biopsy

M. Follow-up Coombs' test: positive

N. Microhemagglutination assay for *Treponema pallidum* antibodies (MHA-TP) to confirm reactive syphilis for positive rapid plasma reagin (RPR). False-positive serologic test for syphilis needs follow-up.

O. Chest x-ray film may show changes.

P. X-ray of joints for nondestructive arthritis

Differential Diagnoses

A. DLE

B. Undifferentiated connective tissue disease

C. Drug-induced lupus

D. RA: Lupus can resemble RA, especially early in the course of SLE. Unlike RA, the arthritis is nonerosive; there is no joint destruction.

E. Vasculitis

F. Scleroderma

G. Chronic active hepatitis

H. Acute drug reactions

I. Polyarteritis

J. Infection

K. Influenza

L. Rosacea

M. Neoplasm

Plan

A. General interventions:
1. After diagnosis, refer the client to a rheumatologist and comanage with a physician

B. Client teaching: *See Section III: Client Teaching Guide for this chapter, "Systemic Lupus Erythematosus."* ◀

C. Pharmaceutical therapy:
1. NSAIDs for arthritis symptoms
2. Prednisone 40 to 60 mg initially for the control of thrombocytopenic purpura, hemolytic anemia, myocarditis, pericarditis, convulsions, and nephritis
3. Always give the lowest dose that controls the condition.
4. Corticosteroids can usually be tapered to low doses, 10 to 15 mg/d, during disease inactivity.
5. Antimalarial drug, hydroxychloroquine sulfate, every day may help treat lupus rashes and joint symptoms that do not respond to NSAIDs. Do not exceed 400 mg/d. *Consult with a rheumatology specialist.*
6. Alternative drug therapy: Immunosuppressive agents, such as cyclophosphamide, chlorambucil, and azathioprine, are used in cases resistant to corticosteroids. The exact role of immunosuppressive agents is controversial.

Follow-Up

A. Very close follow-up by a physician specialist is needed when immunosuppressants are employed.

B. If fever is present on examination, explore cause of fever to rule out infection. Monitor the client for infections, especially with opportunistic organisms.

C. Preventive heart care is important because of the presence of premature atherosclerosis seen in these clients.

D. Up-to-date immunizations

E. Osteoporosis screening

> Infections are the leading cause of death secondary to the depression of WBCs, followed by active SLE, chiefly because of renal or CNS disease.

Consultation/Referral

A. After diagnosis, refer the client to a medical specialist, a rheumatologist

B. Referral to a specialist for a biopsy of the skin or kidney may be necessary to confirm the diagnosis

Individual Considerations

A. Pregnancy:
1. Infertility: 25% of clients have a problem getting pregnant.
2. Clients with SLE experience frequent miscarriages and stillbirths.
3. Clients are considered high risk when consultation and management with a perinatologist are needed.

4. Approximately 33% of clients have an antibody (anticardiolipin) that is associated with early failure of the placenta.

5. Approximately 10% have a related antibody (lupus anticoagulant) that allows early pregnancy, but compromises fetal growth as the placenta fails.

6. It is estimated that 25% of the remaining pregnancies deliver prematurely.

7. Family planning:

a. Barrier methods or intrauterine devices (IUDs) are best and safest.

b. Clients with active SLE should avoid use of birth control pills with estrogen. Consider alternate methods of birth control.

8. Exacerbations of lupus are sometimes caused by pregnancy.

B. Pediatrics:

1. Prematurity is the greatest danger of lupus's effects on the baby.

2. There are no known congenital abnormalities related to lupus.

3. Three percent of all lupus clients have a baby with neonatal lupus. This is a syndrome, not SLE, and it is transient.

C. Geriatrics:

1. Males are affected more than females.

2. Older adults with SLE have an increased incidence of developing cognitive impairment. Early detection of cognitive decline is necessary to assist the client and family to adapt and prevent further decline.

3. Impaired sleep and depression contribute to cognitive decline. These need to be diagnosed and treated to prevent further deterioration and cognitive decline.

Bibliography

Bartels, C. (2015). *Systemic lupus erythematosus. Medscape.* Retrieved from www.emedicine.medscape.com/article/332244-overview

Centers for Disease Control and Prevention. (2019). *Systemic lupus erythematous (SLE or lupus): Prevalence and incidence.* Retrieved from www.cdc.gov/arthritis/basics/lupus.htm

Chasset, F., Francès, C., Barete, S., Amoura, Z., & Arnaud, L. (2015). Influence of smoking on the efficacy of antimalarials in cutaneous lupus: A meta-analysis of the literature. *Journal of the American Academy of Dermatology, 72*(4), 634–639. doi:10.1016/j.jaad.2014.12.025

Jordan, S., Maurer, B., Toniolo, M., Michel, B., & Distler, O. (2015). Performance of the new ACR/EULAR classification criteria for systemic sclerosis in clinical practice. *Rheumatology (Oxford, England), 54*(8), 1454–1458. doi:10.1093/rheumatology/keu530

Montes, R. A., Mocarzel, L. O., Lanzieri, P. G., Lopes, L. M., Carvalho, A., & Almeida, J. R. (2016). Smoking and its association with morbidity in systemic lupus erythematosus evaluated by the systemic lupus international collaborating clinics/American college of rheumatology damage index: Preliminary data and systematic review. *Arthritis & Rheumatology (Hoboken, NJ.), 68*(2), 441–448. doi:10.1002/art.39427

Shur, P. H., & Wallace, D. J. (2019). *Diagnosis and differential diagnosis of systemic lupus erythematosus in adults. UpToDate.* Retrieved from www.uptodate.com/contents/diagnosis-and-differential-diagnosis-of-systemic-lupus-erythematous-in-adults

Tunnicliffe, D. J., Singh-Grewal, D., Kim, S., Craig, J. C., & Tong, A. (2015). Diagnosis, monitoring, and treatment of systemic lupus erythematosus: A systematic review of clinical practice guidelines. *Arthritis Care & Research, 67*(10), 1440–1452. doi:10.1002/acr.22591

Varga, J. (2019). *Diagnosis and differential diagnosis of systemic sclerosis (scleroderma) in adults. UpToDate.* Retrieved from www.uptodate.com/contents/diagnosis-and-differential-diagnosis-of-systemic-sclerosis-scleroderma-in-adults

Varga, J., & Steen, V. (2019). *Pulmonary arterial hypertension in systemic sclerosis (scleroderma): Definition, classification, risk factors, screening and prognosis. UpToDate.* Retrieved from www.uptodate.com/contents/pulmonary-arterial-hypertension-in-systemic-sclerosis-scleroderma-definition-classification-risk-factors-screening-and-prognosis

Temporal Arteritis/Giant Cell Arteritis

Jill C. Cash

Definition

A. Temporal arteritis, also known as giant cell arteritis (GCA), is a vascular illness that can affect the entire body; however, it primarily affects the blood vessels. There is inflammation of the arteries that begins in the aortic arch and branches out to the cranial arteries.

Incidence

A. GCA occurs in approximately 1 in 500 individuals older than 50 years. GCA rarely occurs in individuals younger than 50 years and is more commonly seen during later years (older than 70 years). It can also be seen in clients diagnosed with polymyalgia rheumatica (PMR). Approximately 50% of clients diagnosed with GCA will also have PMR.

Pathogenesis

A. The cause of GCA is unknown. The immune system attacks the body and causes inflammation of the medium and large arteries, which causes thickening of the arterial walls and narrowing of the lumen. When these changes occur, the result is a decrease in blood flow that can potentially cause an occlusion in the artery, leading to ischemia. Arteries commonly involved include the temporal artery, medium and large vessels, and the vessels of the eyes. Blindness is the major acute morbidity with GCA.

Predisposing Factors

A. Age (older than 50 years)
B. Ethnicity (Scandinavian) Northern European descent
C. Gender (women > men)

Common Complaints

A. Abrupt onset of headaches
B. Visual impairment
C. Joint pain (PMR)

Other Signs and Symptoms

A. Fever
B. Anemia
C. Jaw or arm claudication
D. Fatigue
E. Weight loss

Potential Complications

A. Visual loss, blindness
B. Joint pain

Subjective Data

A. Have the client describe the presenting complaints. What makes it better or worse?

B. Ask the client when presenting symptoms began. Discuss the course of new-onset symptoms. Note systemic symptoms such as fever, weight loss, fatigue, headache, vision changes, jaw/arm pain

C. Ask the client to describe pain, for example, crushing, stabbing, or burning

D. Have client rate pain on a scale of 1 to 10, with 1 being the least painful

E. What has the client taken to relieve the pain or symptoms?

F. Has the client noted any visual disturbance or changes? Is vision change constant or does it occur when headache is present? What makes the headache worse? What makes the headache better?

Physical Examination

A. Vital signs: check temperature, pulse, respirations, and BP (take BP in both arms and note discrepancies).

B. Inspect:

1. Inspect overall general appearance. Clients with GCA usually appear chronically ill.

2. Perform funduscopic examination, looking for a pale disk and blurred margins of the disk. Assess pupils equal and reactive to light and accommodation (PERLA), extraocular muscles (EOMs), and visual acuity.

C. Auscultate:

1. Heart for murmurs

2. Carotid, brachial, femoral arteries for bruits

3. Abdomen, noting any bruits

D. Palpate:

1. Pulses (carotid, brachial, radial, pedal, and femoral pulses)

2. Perform ROM of all joints (shoulders, neck, hips, and extremities), noting limitations because of pain and/or swelling.

3. Assess joints for swelling and pain (note symptoms of PMR).

Diagnostic Tests

A. Serum laboratory studies (ESR, CBC, CRP, and CMP)

B. Temporal artery biopsy. Any client suspicious of having temporal arteritis should have a temporal artery biopsy performed. This is the gold standard for diagnosing GCA. Recommended sample size of the artery for biopsy should be ≥4 cm. False-negative biopsy results may be up to 20%.

Differential Diagnoses

A. Vasculitis

B. PMR

Plan

A. General interventions:

1. Educate the client and family regarding the disease process of GCA.

B. Client teaching:

1. Educate the client and family that common symptoms of GCA include headaches, vision change, and jaw/arm joint pain.

2. Teach the client that GCA causes inflammation of the blood vessels in the head and neck, but not the blood vessels in the brain.

3. Advise the client that PMR may also occur in some clients, in which joint pain may be present.

4. Medications commonly used for GCA are steroids. Steroids will improve the inflammation, which in return will improve pain. The steroids are commonly used for the duration of treatment and are tapered down over several months. Steroids are the only medication that has proven to prevent blindness. Any side effects or problems should be reported to the primary provider.

5. A baby aspirin is commonly taken daily.

6. Any vision changes should be immediately reported to the primary provider. Vision loss/blindness is one of the greatest risks of GCA.

C. Pharmaceutical therapy:

1. If GCA is suspected, consult with collaborating physician and begin steroids immediately: prednisone 40 to 60 mg daily. Do not wait for biopsy results. Steroids are used to suppress the manifestations of symptoms and decrease the risk of blindness. Steroids are tapered when symptoms begin to improve, commonly after 1 month or so.

2. Aspirin 81 to 325 mg/d is recommended.

Follow-Up

A. Follow up with physician rheumatologist/surgeon as recommended.

Consultation/Referral

A. Consultation with collaborating physician or surgeon should be obtained regarding any client with the suspicion of having temporal arteritis.

B. Refer all clients to a rheumatologist within 1 week of diagnosis to manage the client with GCA.

C. All clients suspected of having temporal arteritis should be referred to a general surgeon for a temporal artery biopsy within 2 to 3 days after beginning steroids.

D. Refer the client to the ophthalmologist for evaluation and treatment.

Individual Considerations

A. Pediatrics:

1. Vasculitis is rare in children. It is estimated to occur in 12 to 50 per 100,000 children younger than 17 years.

B. Geriatrics:

1. Most commonly seen in older clients. Symptoms may occur after the age of 50 years; however, GCA is most commonly seen in clients older than 70 years.

2. Geriatric clients diagnosed with GCA have a higher risk for stroke. Low-dose ASA (81 mg) should be considered to reduce the risk of visual loss, transient ischemic attack/cerebrovascular accident, and thoracic aortic aneurysm.

Bibliography

Docken, W. P., & Rosenbaum, J. T. (2019). *Clinical manifestations of giant cell (temporal) arteritis*. UpToDate. Retrieved from www.uptodate.com/contents/clinical-manifestations-of-giant-cell-temporal-arteritis

Seetharaman, M. (2015). *Giant cell arteritis (temporal arteritis) workup*. *Medscape*. Retrieved from http://emedicine.medscape.com/article/332483-workup

Vitamin D Deficiency

Jill C. Cash

Definition

A. Vitamin D deficiency is defined as having a serum 25-hydroxyvitamin D (25[OH]D) level lower than 15 ng/mL. Vitamin D insufficiency is defined as having a serum 25-(OH)D level lower than 30 ng/mL. Recommended vitamin D levels range between 30 and 40 ng/mL.

Incidence

A. Vitamin D deficiency is seen in all ages. It is highest in the elderly, institutionalized, and/or hospitalized clients. It is found to be more common in women than in men (83% vs. 48%), the difference most likely being less skin exposure to the sun. There is a higher incidence in the winter months, again because of less sun exposure during the winter months.

Pathogenesis

A. The best source of vitamin D is direct sunlight exposure to the skin. It is also absorbed by ingesting foods that are rich in vitamin D. The liver is responsible for breaking vitamin D down. The liver hydroxylates the vitamin D to storage form, 25[OH]D, which then breaks down into the bioactive form in the kidneys, 1,25-dihydroxyvitamin D (1,25[OH]2D). The 1,25(OH)2D is regulated by the PTH and causes calcium absorption to occur in the intestine, which in turn affects bone metabolism and muscle function. When any part of this cascade is interrupted, the cascade is broken and vitamin D deficiency occurs.

Predisposing Factors

A. Race (darker skin population)
B. Age: elderly population highest risk
C. Long-term institutionalized individuals (nursing home)
D. Obese individuals
E. Decreased sun exposure (individuals who spend very little time outdoors in the sun)
F. People with serious nervous or digestive disorders (chronic kidney disease and malabsorption problems)
G. Medications: Drugs, such as dilantin, phenobarbital, and rifampin, induce hepatic p450 enzymes and accelerate catabolism of vitamin D.

Common Complaints

A. Complaints vary from none to severe.
B. Chronic muscle aches/pain/fatigue/weakness
C. Joint pain and bone pain

Other Signs and Symptoms

A. Fracture of bone
B. Frequent falls and muscle weakness
C. The most severe form of vitamin D deficiency can cause nutritional rickets.

Subjective Data

A. With clients presenting with complaints, assess onset, duration, and course of complaints.
B. Assess daily nutritional habits. Does the client get enough calcium and vitamin D in current diet?
C. Does the client live in a nursing home or an institution? Is the client allowed to spend time outdoors in sunlight? What time of the season/year is it? Is 20 to 30 minutes in the sun without sunscreen reasonable?
D. Is the client currently taking any vitamin supplements? If so, review vitamin and ingredients in that particular vitamin.
E. Review the client history and determine if the client has a chronic condition, malabsorption condition, chronic kidney condition, or medications interfering with absorption. If there is no current diagnosis of a GI problem, inquire regarding food intolerances, stool patterns, constipation, and diarrhea history.
F. Does the client currently take a vitamin D and/or calcium supplement?
G. Has the client had a recent vitamin D level drawn?
H. Inquire regarding the client's fatigue level.
I. Assess for muscle weakness and frequent falls, especially if a pattern of more falls in the winter months is noticed.
J. Has the client been diagnosed with osteoporosis? If so, the client needs to be screened for vitamin D deficiency.

Physical Examination

A. Check pulse and BP.
B. Inspect
   1. Observe the client walk in the room and assess for stability.
   2. Observe the skin color and overall appearance and type of skin texture.
   3. Note any deformities in the spine:
      a. Kyphosis
      b. Bowing of the legs
      c. Waddling of gait
C. Auscultate:
   1. Heart
   2. Lungs
D. Palpate:
   1. Joints or areas of complained tenderness that the client presented with
   2. The abdomen if intestinal absorption problems are suspected and workup is needed

Diagnostic Tests

A. Serum 25(OH)D: normal 30–80 ng/mL
B. PTH: normal 14–72 pg/mL
C. Calcium level: normal 8.5–10.2 mg/dL

Differential Diagnoses

A. Osteoporosis
B. Rickets
C. Cystic fibrosis
D. Malabsorption syndrome
E. Chronic kidney disease

Plan

A. General interventions:

1. For low-risk adults, routine screening for vitamin D deficiency is not recommended. Suggest 600 to 800 IU vitamin D daily.

2. Educate the client regarding the importance of calcium and vitamin D for the body.

3. High-risk adults with suspicion of vitamin D deficiency should be screened. Measurement of serum (OH)D concentration should be done. Vitamin D levels <10 ng/mL are at risk for osteomalacia and should also have serum calcium, phosphorus, alkaline phosphatase, PTH, electrolytes, BUN, creatinine, and tissue transglutaminase antibodies measured to assess for celiac disease.

4. High-risk clients complaining of bone pain should have an x-ray of the bone in which they are having pain.

B. Client teaching:

1. Educate the client about vitamin D deficiency and the importance of getting vitamin D into the diet on a daily basis.

2. Suggest eating foods that are higher in vitamin D in the diet. These foods include fish oil, cod liver oil, salmon, and foods fortified with vitamin D such as milk and cereals.

3. Discuss how inadequate sun exposure can increase the risk of vitamin D deficiency. Recommend 20 to 30 minutes of sunlight during summer months without use of sunscreen, if this is not contraindicated to other chronic conditions.

4. Foods higher in calcium should also be included in the diet on a daily basis.

C. Pharmaceutical therapy:

1. Vitamin D-level recommendations:

a. For vitamin D levels <20 ng/mL: vitamin D_2 or D_3 50,000 IU weekly for 8 weeks and recheck vitamin D level. If still <30 ng/mL at that point, repeat the dose for another 8 weeks and recheck when second course is finished.

b. Vitamin D levels between 20 and 30 ng/mL: vitamin D_3 600 to 800 IU daily

c. Cholecalciferol (vitamin D_3) is preferred to ergocalciferol (vitamin D_2) for supplementation when available.

2. Calcium levels should be maintained with a recommended dietary intake of 1,000 mg/d for ages 19 to 70 years and of 1,200 mg/d for women 51 to 70 years and all adults over 71 years of age.

D. For malabsorption problems, recommend magnesium 250 mg daily supplement. May also refer to a GI specialist for workup

Follow-Up

A. Follow-up should be performed according to recommendations based on laboratory results. Initial laboratory results should be repeated in 8 weeks after initial treatment. As soon as vitamin D levels are stable, repeat lab work routinely to confirm that levels remain within normal range. If levels continue to fall, refer to a specialist.

Consultation/Referral

A. Consult with a physician or refer the client to a gastroenterologist for those who consistently have low vitamin D levels or if malabsorption problems are diagnosed

Individual Considerations

A. Pregnancy:

1. No contraindications for treatment during pregnancy. The same prescribing dose is safe for pregnancy and breastfeeding clients.

B. Pediatrics:

1. The American Academy of Pediatrics recommends infants fed exclusively by breast milk should have vitamin D supplementation.

2. Up to 1 year of age: vitamin D_2 or D_3 1,000 to 2,000 IU/d with calcium supplementation recommended for 6 weeks then followed by 400 IU/d

3. Ages 1 to 18 years: 50,000 IU vitamin D_2 recommended every week for 6 weeks, then 600 to 1,000 IU/d

C. Geriatrics:

1. Vitamin deficiencies are commonly seen in this population.

2. All clients diagnosed with osteoporosis should be assessed for vitamin D deficiency.

3. Clients with a serum 25(OH)D level of <10 are at risk for developing osteomalacia.

4. High doses of vitamin D (60,000 IU D3/month) increases the risk of falls by 15% and fracture risk by 26% due to the side effect of impaired balance with high doses of vitamin D. The recommendation of total vitamin D intake/month for clients older than 70 years of age is 24,000 IU/month.

5. Treatment guidelines for geriatric clients include intake of vitamin D 400 to 800 IU/day and calcium 1,000 to 2,000 mg/day in divided doses.

Bibliography

Ali, Y., Anderson, L. N., Smile, S., Chen, Y., Borkhoff, C. M., Koroshegyi, C., … Borkhoff, C. M. (2019). Prospective cohort study of vitamin D and autism spectrum disorder diagnoses in early childhood. *Autism: The International Journal of Research & Practice, 23*(3), 584–593. doi:10.1177/1362361318756787

Dawson-Hughes, B. (2019). *Vitamin D deficiency in adults: Definition, clinical manifestations, and treatment. UpToDate.* Retrieved from http://www.uptodate.com/contents/vitamin-d-deficiency-in-adults -definition-clinical-manifestations-and-treatment

Hiemstra, T., Lim, K., Thadhani, R., & Manson, J. E. (2019). Vitamin D and atherosclerotic cardiovascular disease. *Journal of Clinical Endocrinology & Metabolism, 104*(9), 4033–4050. doi: 10.1210/jc.2019-00194

Low vit D linked to higher blood glucose levels. (2019). *Clinical Advisor, 22*(4), 12.

National Osteoporosis Foundation. (n.d.). *Prevention: Vitamin D.* Retrieved from https://www.nof.org/?s=osteoporosis+prevention

Sharifi, N., & Amani, R. (2019). Vitamin D supplementation and non-alcoholic fatty liver disease: A critical and systematic review of clinical trials. *Critical Reviews in Food Science & Nutrition, 59*(4), 693–703. doi:10.1080/10408398.2017.1389693

22 Psychiatric Guidelines

Anxiety

Moya Cook and Alyson Wolz

Definition

A. Generalized anxiety disorder (GAD) is a condition exhibited by excessive worry, tension, apprehension, and uneasiness from anticipated danger that is not controlled on most days of the week for at least 6 months. It is the "fight-or-flight" response that is part of the survival instinct. Anxiety is distinguished from fear in that fear is a response to consciously recognized external danger. The source of anxiety is largely unknown or unrecognized.

Normal anxiety allows us to get in touch with developmental learning that is part of our human growth. Anxiety in its chronic form is maladaptive and is considered a psychiatric disorder. Many cases of anxiety disorder in late life are chronic, having persisted from younger years. In its pathologic form, anxiety interferes with developmental learning because it infers significant distress.

When a client presents with anxiety, it is often comorbid with other psychiatric disorders, particularly depression. Anxiety may act as a predispositional factor to early-onset depression (before age 26 years) and to increased frequency of depressive episodes. Clients also present clinically with only anxiety, in one of its many forms, such as GAD, posttraumatic stress disorder (PTSD), obsessive-compulsive disorder (OCD), adjustment disorder with anxious mood, phobic disorder, acute anxiety, or panic disorder, with or without agoraphobia.

Incidence

A. Anxiety disorders are the most common mental illness in the United States, affecting approximately 18% of the adult population. Although highly treatable, only about one-third of individuals suffering from anxiety seek treatment. Anxiety is present in many medical illnesses and must be distinguished to treat it appropriately. GAD and panic disorder are associated with frequent suicide attempts.

Pathogenesis

A. Some degree of familial transmission of GAD, as well as panic disorder, has been noted. Unconscious conflict is thought to be the underlying cause of anxiety, which signals the ego to be careful expressing unacceptable impulses. Behavioral anxiety is considered a conditioned response to a stimulus associated with danger.

Clinically, however, identifying specific anxiogenic stimuli is difficult. The onset of GAD is also thought to be the cumulative effect of several stressful life events. Many studies have found that phobic/anxiety symptoms predated clinical alcoholism by a number of years. t-Aminobutyric acid–benzodiazepine receptor complex, the locus coeruleus–norepinephrine system, and serotonin are three neurotransmitter systems implicated in the biological basis of anxiety. These systems are thought to mediate "normal" anxiety and pathologic anxiety.

Predisposing Factors

A. Young to middle-aged women; onset usually at 20 to 30 years of age
B. Non-White
C. Single
D. Lower socioeconomic status
E. A childhood overanxious disorder
F. Excessive worrying
G. Unresolved unconscious conflict

Common Complaints

A. Inability to control worrying
B. Motor tension
C. Autonomic hyperactivity vigilance
D. Sleep disturbance

Statements concerning self-medication with alcohol to help with sleep may indicate a coexistent alcohol abuse/dependence diagnosis that must be treated concomitantly.

E. Shortness of breath
F. Increased heart rate and respirations

G. Feelings of apprehension

H. Dizziness

I. Abdominal disturbances/nausea

J. Increased perspiration

K. Trembling

Other Signs and Symptoms

A. According to the *Diagnostic and Statistical Manual of Mental Disorders* (5th ed.; *DSM-5*; American Psychiatric Association [APA], 2013), other symptoms include excessive worry out of proportion to the likelihood or impact of the feared events that occurs for a period of 6 months or longer, during which the person has been bothered more days than not by these concerns.

B. At least three of the following six symptoms are present:

1. Muscle tension

2. Restlessness or feeling keyed up or on edge

3. Easy fatigability

4. Difficulty concentrating or "mind going blank" because of anxiety

5. Trouble falling or staying asleep

6. Irritability

C. If another Axis I disorder is present, such as depression, or bipolar affective disorder, the anxiety may be in response to fear of:

1. Being embarrassed in public in the presence of a social phobia

2. Being contaminated in the presence of OCD

3. Gaining weight in the presence of anorexia nervosa

4. Having an illness (as in hypochondriasis or somatization disorder)

D. Impaired social or occupational function. The anxiety, worry, or physical symptoms significantly interfere with the person's normal routine or usual activities or cause marked distress.

Subjective Data

A. Review the onset, course, and duration of symptoms. How often does the anxiety occur (e.g., every day, week, and month)?

B. Review any history of anxiety and age of onset. If treated, how was the previous anxiety treated and what was the success of the treatment?

C. Determine whether there is a history of suicide attempts. Does the client have a current plan or vague ideas of suicide? Ask the client, "Have you ever thought of hurting yourself or others?" If there is any concern regarding suicide/homicide, immediately refer the client to a mental health provider.

D. Review drug history for prescription, over-the-counter (OTC) medications, and recreational/illicit drug use, and the client's use of caffeine, which precipitates anxiety symptoms.

E. Review the client's history of alcohol consumption. Mild or moderate alcohol withdrawal presents primarily with anxiety symptoms. In clients who have developed tolerance to the effects of alcohol or benzodiazepines, abrupt cessation of these agents may produce heightened anxiety over baseline, as well as a risk of seizure.

F. Review the client's history for major stressors. Are these stressors new or chronic? If chronic problems, ask what made the client come in today.

G. Determine how the client has been coping with stress up until today (exercise, medication).

H. Review the client's history of other medical problems.

I. Does anyone else in the family have the same problem? How are they treated?

Physical Examination

A. Check pulse, respirations, blood pressure, and weight.

B. Inspect:

1. Observe general appearance; note grooming, dress, ability to communicate, body movements, nail biting, playing with hair, and inability to sit still.

C. Administer mental examination of choice:

1. *DSM-5* Diagnostic Criteria for GAD available from the APA (2013)

2. Beck Anxiety Scale

D. Physical examination as indicated by somatic complaints

Diagnostic Tests

A. Blood alcohol

B. Thyroid profile

C. Blood glucose

D. Medication level (e.g., theophylline) if applicable

E. Urine drug screen

F. Additional testing related to suspected physical pathology

Differential Diagnoses

A. Substance/medication-induced anxiety disorder

B. Psychiatric syndrome:

1. Mood disorders such as depression or bipolar disorder

2. Psychotic disorders

3. Somatoform disorders (characterized by physical complaints lacking known medical basis or demonstrable physical finding in the presence of psychological factors judged to be etiologic or important in the initiation, exacerbation, or maintenance of the disturbance)

4. Personality disorders

5. Alcoholism and drug abuse/dependence

6. Attention deficit hyperactivity disorder (ADHD)

C. Medical conditions. Anxiety syndromes mimic many medical illnesses, including intracranial tumors, menstrual irregularities, hypothyroidism, hyperparathyroidism and hypoparathyroidism, postconcussion syndrome, psychomotor epilepsy, and Cushing's disease.

1. Consider hypoglycemia if anxiety is chronic

2. Hypothyroidism

3. Hyperthyroidism: Rapid-onset anxiety could be a symptom of hyperthyroidism.

4. Tumor

5. Cushing's disease

Plan

A. General interventions:

1. Treat medical conditions as appropriate.

2. Refer the client for cognitive behavior therapy. Counseling is effective for learning new techniques to help with alleviating symptoms. Cognitive behavior therapy may be effective alone and/or may also be used as adjunct to medication treatment.

3. Encourage the client to perform self-calming techniques at home, such as deep breathing/relaxation techniques and exercise.

▶ B. Client teaching: *See Section III: Client Teaching Guide for this chapter, as appropriate: "Sleep Disorders/Insomnia" and "Alcohol and Drug Dependence."*

C. Pharmaceutical therapy:

1. Selective serotonin reuptake inhibitors (SSRIs) or selective serotonin norepinephrine reuptake inhibitors (SNRIs):

   a. Fluoxetine (Prozac), 5 to 10 mg/d orally initially; usual dose 20 to 80 mg/d. Long half-life; alters metabolism of cytochrome P-450 2D6-cleared agents. Use caution

   b. Paroxetine (Paxil), 10 mg/d orally initially; usual dose 25 to 50 mg/d

   c. Sertraline (Zoloft), 25 to 50 mg/d orally initially; usual dose 50 to 200 mg/d

   d. Escitalopram (Lexapro), 10 mg/d initially; usual dose 10 to 20 mg/d. Caution: use 10 mg for geriatric clients. Use with caution in clients with severe renal impairment

   e. Citalopram (Celexa), 5 to 10 mg/d orally initially; usual dose 20 to 40 mg/d. Caution: risk for QT prolongation, contraindicated in clients with congenital long QT syndrome, and should not exceed 20 mg daily if prescribed to clients also taking CYP2C19 inhibitors (cimetidine, fluconazole, omeprazole)

   f. Venlafaxine (Effexor), 37.5 mg/d orally initially; usual dose 75 to 300 mg/ d

   g. Duloxetine (Cymbalta), 30 mg/d for 1 week, then usual dose 40 to 60 mg/d. Maximum dose is 120 mg/d. Caution: do not use in clients with severe renal impairment, chronic liver disease, or cirrhosis

   h. These medications can take 4 to 6 weeks to take effect.

   i. Warn clients that they should not stop these medications abruptly; they should taper off gradually

2. Nonbenzodiazepine anxiolytic:

   a. Buspirone (Buspar), 7.5 mg twice a day

   b. May increase by 5 mg/d orally every 2 to 3 days

   c. Usual range: 20 to 30 mg orally every day; maximum 60 mg orally every day

   d. Not recommended for children younger than 18 years

   e. Therapeutic effects delayed from 1 to 4 weeks

3. Short-acting benzodiazepines:

   a. Alprazolam (Xanax), 0.25 to 0.5 mg orally two to three times daily

   b. Clonazepam 0.25 to 0.5 mg orally one or two times daily, titrated up to 1 mg two to three times daily as needed

   c. Lorazepam (Ativan), 0.5 to 2 mg, up to 6 mg, orally every day in divided doses. Maximum dose of 10 mg/d in divided doses

      i. In 2016 the Centers for Disease Control and Prevention (CDC) issued new guidelines recommending that clinicians avoid prescribing benzodiazepines concurrently with opioids. Both carry a Food and Drug Administration (FDA) "black box" warning highlighting the danger of using these drugs together.

      ii. Use benzodiazepine for initial short-term stabilization while simultaneously prescribing buspirone because therapeutic effects of buspirone are delayed from 1 to 4 weeks.

      iii. Limit use from several weeks to a few months to prevent dependence.

> Remember to check the state prescription monitoring system when starting therapy with benzodiazepines and periodically thereafter (every 1 to 3 months) to avoid potential drug–drug interactions and abuse.

Follow-Up

A. Follow up in 1 to 2 weeks to assess the client's status.

B. Follow up every 2 to 4 weeks after that to check the client's progress.

C. Assess suicide potential with every office visit.

Consultation/Referral

A. Refer to a psychiatric clinician for complex medication management and psychotherapy after initial assessment.

B. If the client expresses suicidal thoughts, immediately refer to the ED (in-client therapy) or psychiatric specialist for continuing assessment and psychotherapy.

Individual Considerations

A. Pregnancy:

   1. Caution should be used in prescribing medications for anxiety during pregnancy; the benefits must be weighed against the risks.

   2. If the client becomes pregnant while taking these medications, taper the medication dose instead of ceasing abruptly.

B. Pediatrics:

   1. Children with suspected anxiety disorders should be immediately referred to a pediatric psychiatrist.

C. Geriatrics:

   1. Anxiety is often unrecognized and inadequately treated in this population because of concomitant medical illness; overlap with cognitive disorders; and comorbid depression, ageism, and cohort effects.

   2. Start with the lowest dose of medication and increase slowly.

D. Partners:

   1. If available in the community, provide resources for partners, such as the National Alliance on Mental Illness (NAMI).

   2. Psychotherapy for the client and partner is often helpful.

Bibliography

Anxiety and Depression Association of America. (2014). *Facts and statistics.* Retrieved from http://www.adaa.org/about-adaa/press-room/facts-statistics

Centers for Disease Control and Prevention. (2019, August 28). *Guidelines for prescribing opioids for chronic pain.* Retrieved from https://www.cdc.gov/drugoverdose/prescribing/guideline.html

Crum, R. M., Anthony, J. C., Bassett, S. S., & Folstein, M. F. (1993). Population-based norms for the mini-mental state examination by age and educational level. *Journal of the American Medical Association*, *269*(18), 2386–2391. doi:10.1001/jama.1993.03500180078038

Attention Deficit Disorder (ADD)/ Attention Deficit Hyperactivity Disorder (ADHD)

Moya Cook and Alyson Wolz

Definition

A. ADHD is a syndrome that consists of a cluster of behaviors that emerge early in a child's life and persist over time. Excessively high levels of motor activity and problems with attention span, concentration, and/or impulsivity characterize ADHD. Up to 50% of clients with ADHD also have other psychosocial disorders such as oppositional defiant disorder (ODD), depression or bipolar disorder (develops in 25% of children with ADHD), PTSD, or Tourette's syndrome.

B. The diagnostic criteria for ADHD include symptoms of inattention and symptoms of hyperactivity/impulsivity, as published by the APA, in the *DSM-5* (2013). These criteria are available at www.cdc.gov/ncbddd/adhd/diagnosis.html.

Incidence

A. 3% to 5% of all school-aged children and 2.5% in adults

B. Occurs in all races and socioeconomic groups

C. Boys are more likely than girls to have symptoms by a ratio of 2:1.

D. Not uncommon for this disorder to persist into adulthood

E. Approximately 33% of children with learning disabilities also have ADHD.

Pathogenesis

A. Unknown, but several studies suggest a biochemical basis involving deficits in the availability of neurotransmitters to the frontal–orbital circuits of the neurobehavioral regulatory systems of the brain. ADHD may also be inherited.

B. Associated problems with ADHD include academic, social, and emotional problems.

Predisposing Factors

A. A close relative with a mood disorder, anxiety, or ADHD

B. Brain trauma

C. Selective therapeutic regimens, such as intrathecal chemotherapy

D. Recent studies have suggested a possible link to maternal smoking, alcohol abuse, or other toxins during pregnancy.

E. Some perinatal influences have been theorized to be connected to ADHD, including fetal distress, prolonged labor, prematurity, and perinatal asphyxia.

Common Complaints

A. Hyperactivity, impulsivity, and/or inattentiveness

B. Poor school performance

C. Poor peer relationships

Other Signs and Symptoms

A. Inattentive and easily distracted when completing tasks: daydreams, does not finish work, loses things, has difficulty concentrating

B. Impulsive: risk taking, impatient, very emotional

C. Hyperactivity/over activity: speech and motor skills overactive

D. Difficulty with learning, poor performance in school/work

Subjective Data

A. Determine the presenting symptoms and ascertain when symptoms first began.

B. Note duration of symptoms:
1. Have they been present for at least 6 months?
2. Ask regarding specific behaviors as listed in the diagnostic criteria.

C. Review settings in which symptoms are present (home, school, day care).

D. Discuss the child's past medical history.

E. Discuss the child's developmental history; did he or she meet all of the developmental milestones?

F. Review the child's family, social, and school histories.

G. Review all current medications, including any OTC medications and herbals. Specifically review medication history for theophylline, prednisone, and albuterol.

H. Review the child's diet, eating habits, and sleeping habits.

I. Review the child's routines and habits: Stimulation may come from TV, video, and computer viewing.

Physical Examination

A. Check temperature, pulse, respirations, blood pressure, weight, and height.

B. Inspect:
1. Observe overall appearance. Note behavior and interactions with others.
2. Inspect the skin, eyes, ears, nose, and throat.

C. Auscultate:
1. Heart
2. Lungs
3. Abdomen

D. Palpate:
1. Neck
2. Thyroid
3. Chest
4. Abdomen

E. Perform neurologic examination:
1. Hearing/vision evaluation: evaluate constant, involuntary movement of the eyes (nystagmus).
2. Evaluate coordination difficulties/impaired motor skills.
3. Evaluate visual-motor control problems (hand–eye coordination).

Diagnostic Tests

A. Complete blood count (CBC) to rule out iron-deficiency anemia

B. Lead level

C. Thyroid studies to rule out other organic problems

D. CBC with differential (if indicated)

E. Administer the National Institute for Children's Health Quality (NICHQ) Vanderbilt Assessment Scale available at www.nichq.org/~/media/files/resources/nichq vanderbiltassessment-full.ashx. See *DMS-5* criteria for diagnosing the type of ADHD. Criteria are available at www.cdc.gov/ncbddd/adhd/diagnosis.html.

F. Refer for psychological tests to measure IQ, social/ emotional adjustment, and presence of learning disabilities.

G. EEG may be considered.

H. MRI may be considered to rule out organic diagnoses.

Differential Diagnoses

A. ODD

B. Autism spectrum disorder

C. Hyperthyroidism/hypothyroidism

D. Lead poisoning

E. Other behavioral/psychological disorders (pervasive developmental delay, mood disorders, anxiety, or personality disorder)

F. Learning disorders

G. Seizure disorder, nonconvulsive

H. Impaired hearing related to chronic or recurrent otitis media

I. Adverse reactions to medications (theophylline, prednisone, or albuterol)

J. Substance use/abuse disorder (caffeine, alcohol/drugs)

Plan

A. General interventions:

1. Multimodal and multidisciplinary approaches are imperative and include parent education regarding the nature of ADHD. Effective behavioral management, appropriate educational placement and support, and family and/or individual therapy are strongly encouraged.

2. It is important to obtain written reports (which consist of a standardized rating, such as the Connors Tool and/or the Vanderbilt Screening Tool of ADHD) from teachers, parents, and other adults who have regular contact with the child. The Vanderbilt Assessment Scale for Parent and Teacher may be found at https:// www.nichq.org/sites/default/files/resource-file/ NICHQ_Vanderbilt_Assessment_Scales.pdf.

3. The primary care provider, school nurse, school psychologist, and/or parent may function as the case manager to coordinate services.

B. Client teaching:

▶ 1. *See Section III: Client Teaching Guide for this chapter, "ADHD: Tips for Caregivers of a Child With ADHD" and "ADHD: Coping Strategies for Teens and Adults."*

2. Provide ADHD resources for parents, children, teens, and adults.

C. Pharmaceutical therapy:

1. Begin with short-acting stimulants. Advance dose as needed for desired result.

2. Consider adding a long-acting agent to a short-acting agent if needed.

3. Long-acting agent used alone

4. First-line agents: rapid onset with short duration:

a. Methylphenidate (Ritalin, Methylin)

b. Dextroamphetamine (Dexedrine, ProCentra, Zenzedi)

c. Amphetamine–dextroamphetamine (Adderall)

d. Dexmethylphenidate (Focalin)

5. Rapid onset with long duration:

a. Methylphenidate (Concerta, Ritalin LA, Ritalin SR, Daytrana patch, Metadate CD, Metadate ER, Methylin ER, Quillivant XR)

b. Amphetamine–dextroamphetamine (Adderall XR): duration 10 hours

c. Dexmethylphenidate (Focalin XR): duration 12 hours

d. Lisdexamfetamine (Vyvanse): duration 13 to 14 hours

6. Medications to use if substance abuse is a concern:

a. Vyvanse

b. Bupropion

c. Strattera

7. Medications recommended for comorbidity of depression:

a. Bupropion (Wellbutrin, Wellbutrin SR, Wellbutrin XL)

b. Venlafaxine (Effexor, Effexor XR)

8. Medication doses:

a. Methylphenidate (Ritalin) starting dose: 0.3 to 0.6 mg/kg/dose; short half-life (3–6 hours) necessitates two to three doses per day. Children: not recommended for younger than 6 years of age. Greater than or equal to 6 years: 5 mg before breakfast and 5 mg before lunch. Increase dose by 5 to 10 mg weekly; maximum dose 60 mg/d. Adults: 10 to 60 mg in two or three divided doses before meals

b. Methylphenidate HCl (Ritalin LA): swallow whole; do not crush. Not recommended in children younger than 6 years. Children 6 years or older: 20 mg in morning; may increase dose 10 mg weekly; maximum dose 60 mg/d

c. Methylphenidate HCl liquid (Quillivant XR): Children: not recommended for children younger than 6 years of age. Starting dose: 10 to 20 mg orally in morning. Increase the dose weekly by 10 to 20 mg; maximum daily dose 60 mg/d

d. Methylphenidate HCl (Concerta): Children: not recommended for children younger than 6 years; 6 to 12 years: 18 mg/d. Increase dose in 18-mg increments weekly as needed. Maximum is 54 mg daily. Adolescents/adults: 18 mg/d with maximum 72 mg daily; increase by 18-mg increments weekly as needed. Contraindicated with severe anxiety

e. Dexmethylphenidate HCl (Focalin XR): Children: not recommended for children younger than 6 years of age. Starting dose: 5 mg/d in morning; titrate weekly in 5-mg increments. Maximum dose for children: 30 mg daily in morning; for adults: 40 mg daily in morning

f. Lisdexamfetamine dimesylate (Vyvanse): Children 6 to 12 years old: 30 mg daily in a single dose in the morning; may be increased by 10 mg/d. Maximum dose of 70 mg daily in the morning

g. Atomoxetine (Strattera): Not a controlled substance. Weight <70 kg: <0.5 mg/kg/d (maximum 1.4 mg/kg/d); weight >70 kg: 40 mg/d (maximum 100 mg/d). Increase dose after 3 days as needed, then after 2 to 4 weeks for maximum dose; may take a few weeks to see the full effect. Should be taken daily at the same time every day to avoid SNRI effects. FDA-approved indication for adults

h. Side effects of these medications include anorexia, insomnia, stomach pain, growth suppression, and tics. If weight loss occurs, give medication after meals.

i. If psychostimulants are not effective, other medications used include antihistamines, guanfacine (Tenex), clonidine, carbamazepine (Tegretol), divalproex (Depakote), beta-blockers, and antidepressants.

j. Be cautious when prescribing other medications concurrently.

Follow-Up

A. At 1 month, inquire about improvements in each area of life and duration of the medication's actions.

B. Medication dose and/or frequency may need to be altered.

C. Consider adding a third dose if the duration of action is very short and the child needs better afternoon or evening coverage to successfully complete homework or participate in other extracurricular activities.

D. When medication schedule is stable, subsequent visits can be every 3 months.

Consultation/Referral

A. Consult with the psychiatric provider to help coordinate the medications.

B. Consult with the school psychologist if indicated for additional data.

C. Refer the client for individual and/or family therapy if indicated.

Individual Considerations

A. Pediatrics:

1. The overall goal of ADHD therapy is to build the child's sense of competence and performance.

2. Not all behavior issues are ADHD. The diagnosis must be carefully and cautiously established according to the diagnostic criteria of the APA.

3. Individualize medications, preparations, and timing; 80% of children respond positively to stimulants.

4. Instituting routine drug holidays should be done with caution. The child's ability to concentrate and manage behavior at all times is critical. Not instituting drug holidays may prevent a "yo–yo" behavior experience for the client.

5. Use caution when medicating children with a personal or family history of Tourette's syndrome. Tics may worsen in these children.

6. When prescribing psychostimulants to children with seizure disorders who are already on anticonvulsants, closely monitor plasma levels of both medications.

7. Treat the child, not the parents, teachers, day-care personnel, or coaches.

B. Adults:

1. Up to half of the affected children have some symptoms of ADHD that persist into adulthood. Adults tend to outgrow the "hyperactivity" aspect; however, they may still require treatment for the ADD. Teens and adults benefit from specific coping strategies for ADD.

Resources

Attention Deficit Disorder Association: http://www.add.org

CHADD (Children With ADD): CHADD National Office

8181 Professional Place

Suite 150

Landover, MD 20785

Phone: 301-306-7070

Fax: 301-306-7090

http://www.chadd.org

Bibliography

McCarney, S. B., & Bauer, A. B. (1995). *Parent's guide to attention deficit disorders: Intervention strategies for the home* (2nd ed.). Columbia, MO: Hawthorne Educational Services. Retrieved from http://www.hawthorne-ed.com/pages/adhd/ad3.html

National Initiative for Children's Healthcare Quality. (2002A). *NICHQ vanderbilt assessment follow-up: Teacher informant*. Retrieved from http://www.copakids.com/Follow%20Up%20Vanderbilt%20Teacher%20Form.pdf

National Initiative for Children's Healthcare Quality. (2002B). *NICHQ vanderbilt assessment scale—PARENT informant*. Retrieved from www.nichq.org/childrens-health/adhd/resources/vanderbilt-assessment-scales

National Initiative for Children's Healthcare Quality. (2002C). *NICHQ vanderbilt assessment scale—TEACHER informant*. Retrieved from www.nichq.org/childrens-health/adhd/resources/vanderbilt-assessment-scales

National Initiative for Children's Healthcare Quality. (2014). *Scoring instructions for NICHQ vanderbilt assessment scales*. Retrieved from www.aap.org/en-us/Documents/sodbp_vanderbilt_scoringinstructions.pdf

Bipolar Disorder

Alyson Wolz

Definition

A. Bipolar disorder, commonly called manic-depressive disorder, is a psychiatric disorder that causes changes in moods, thoughts, and behaviors. These changes may range from mania (excessive energy, euphoria, racing thoughts, decreased need for sleep, grandiosity, pressured speech, and impulsive behavior) to depression (low energy, sadness, diminished interest and pleasure in most activities, recurrent thoughts of death, changes in sleep patterns, cognitive impairment, and difficulty carrying out daily activities).

B. There are four types of bipolar disorder:

1. Bipolar I disorder: Individual meets the diagnostic criteria for a manic episode, which may have been preceded or followed by a hypomanic or depressive episode.

2. Bipolar II disorder: Individual has a pattern of depressive episodes and hypomanic episodes (no mania). Often symptoms of depression and hypomania, especially agitation, irritability, and verbal impulsivity, are displayed in the same episode (mixed).

3. Cyclothymic disorder: A chronic pattern of hypomanic and depressive symptoms that do not meet the full criteria for hypomania or depressive episodes. Symptoms occur for at least 2 years (1 year in children and adolescents).

4. Unspecified bipolar and related disorder: This category applies to situations in which there are symptoms that are characteristic of bipolar disorder but do not meet the full criteria. There may be insufficient information to make a diagnosis, or underlying medical conditions or substance use contributing to the condition.

Specific criteria for bipolar disorder as published by the APA(*DSM-5*, 2013) are available at the National Institute for Mental Health website: www.nimh.nih.gov/health/topics/bipolar-disorder/index.shtml.

Incidence

A. 5.7 million or 2.6% of adults ages 18 years or older in the United States

B. Median age of onset is 25 years, although can range from childhood to late onset (50s).

C. Occurs in all races and socioeconomic groups

D. Men may present with symptoms of mania earlier than women. Women are more likely to present with symptoms of depression and experience more rapid cycling.

E. Bipolar disorder is the sixth leading cause of disability in the world.

F. Results in 9.2 years reduction in expected life span. One in five individuals diagnosed with bipolar disorder will die by suicide.

Pathogenesis

A. No specific biological markers for bipolar disorder have been identified to date; however, studies indicate a significant genetic component. Individuals with a first-degree relative with bipolar disorder are 7 to 10 times more likely to develop the disorder.

Predisposing Factors

A. A family history of bipolar disorder or schizophrenia

B. Periods of high stress

C. Drug or alcohol abuse

D. Major life changes such as the death of a loved one or a traumatic experience

Common Complaints

A. Frequently seek treatment for depressive episodes

B. Poor work or school performance; unfinished tasks

C. Mood swings, irritability, or anger episodes

D. Social problems

E. Sleep disturbance

Other Signs and Symptoms

A. Mania: Symptoms last at least 1 week and may include inflated self-esteem, grandiosity, decreased need for sleep, talkativeness, racing thoughts, distractibility, increase in goal-directed activity, impulsive behavior (buying sprees, sexual indiscretions, poor business decisions). Symptoms cause marked impairment in functioning and may require hospitalization.

B. Hypomania: Symptoms last at least 4 days. Symptoms are the same as mania, but are not severe enough to cause marked impairment. Person frequently displays irritability and agitation.

C. Depression: Symptoms last for at least 2 weeks. They include depressed mood most of the day; diminished interest in pleasure; changes in weight; sleep disturbance; restlessness or low energy; fatigue; feelings of worthlessness, guilt, and burdensomeness; cognitive changes; and thoughts of death.

D. Clients in primary care settings are more likely to present for symptoms of depression, which may look like a depressive disorder. It is important to rule out bipolar disorder before initiating treatment. Screening tool for bipolar symptoms is as follows:

The Mood Disorder Questionnaire (Hirshfeld et al., 2000) https://www.vraylar.com/content/resources/Mood%20Disorder%20Questionnaire.pdf

Note: During a manic episode, individuals often do not perceive that there is anything wrong and will often refuse treatment or become angry with those who are trying to intervene.

E. Impulse control: Client may present as extremely happy and sociable, but may have rapid mood changes, such as irritability or aggression when wishes are denied, especially if using substances.

F. Suicidal or homicidal thoughts or acts: Any statements made by the client, such as "Life isn't worth living, I wish I were dead, I don't deserve to be alive, I can't deal with this," should be taken seriously. Refer the client to a mental health professional for further assessment and treatment.

Subjective Data

A. Review the onset, duration, and course of presenting symptoms.

B. Review any previous history of depression, mania, or mood disorders.

C. Determine how the previous mood disorder was treated, if applicable.

D. Evaluate the client's suicide potential. Ask: "Have you ever thought of hurting yourself or others?" Does the client have a current suicide plan or vague ideas of suicide? Has the client had any previous history of suicide attempts? If so, evaluate how life-threatening they were.

E. Review the client's medical history.

F. Review the client's drug history for prescription, OTC, and recreational/illicit drug use (how much, how long, how often), and review his or her history of alcohol consumption (how much, how long, how often).

G. Assess client's compliance with prescribed medications.

H. Review the client's history for recent major life changes such as pregnancy, death, divorce, or any loss that may be normal throughout the stages of life. The *client's perception* of the loss is what is important.

I. Review dietary intake since the symptoms began.

J. Establish usual weight, review weight gain/loss, and note in what time span.

K. Review the client's activities of daily living. Does the client get up and dress daily, perform daily hygiene, put on makeup?

L. Review how many hours of sleep and quality of sleep per day.

M. Review the disruption of usual activities: return to work, return to school, exercise. Has the client been engaging in activities outside the norm?

N. Assess mood patterns, rate of cycling, seasonal changes.

O. Review occupational/home exposure to neurodegenerative products.

P. Review any exposures to infectious diseases, including Lyme disease. Does anyone else, such as family, friends, or coworkers, have similar symptoms?

Q. If female, review for symptoms of menopause (sleep disturbances, irregular menses/amenorrhea, hot flashes, vaginal dryness, dyspareunia).

Physical Examination

A. Check pulse, respirations, blood pressure, and weight.

B. Inspect:

1. Observe overall appearance; note grooming, tone of voice, eye contact, conduct of client during communication, and breath (smell of alcohol).

2. Complete neurologic examination with screening tool of choice.

3. Complete dermal examination for signs of substance use (refer to "Substance Use Disorders" section).

C. Auscultate:

1. Heart
2. Lungs
3. Abdomen (as applies to physical complaints)

D. Palpate:

1. Neck and thyroid; note goiter if present.
2. Axilla and groin for lymphadenopathy (infectious etiology)
3. Check the joints for swelling and arthritis and range of motion (ROM; rule out musculoskeletal cause).

E. Neurologic examination:

1. Complete the Mental States Examination (MSE), including appearance, affect/mood, thought content, perception, suicide/self-destruction, homicide/aggression, judgment/insight, and cognition.

Diagnostic Tests

A. CBC to rule out iron-deficiency anemia

B. Urine/serum drug screen

C. Thyroid studies to rule out other organic problems

D. Comprehensive metabolic panel (CMP)

E. Erythrocyte sedimentation rate (ESR)

F. Liver and lipid panel

G. Refer for psychological testing to confirm diagnosis, rule out other mental health disorders, and assess for social/emotional adjustment and for the presence of learning disabilities.

H. EKG

I. EEG may be considered.

J. CT scan or MRI may be considered to rule out organic diagnoses.

Differential Diagnoses

A. Substance-induced mood disorder, including from caffeine, alcohol/illicit drugs

B. Head trauma

C. Hyperthyroidism/hypothyroidism

D. Lead poisoning

E. Other behavioral/psychological disorders (pervasive developmental delay, ODD, seasonal affective disorder (SAD), anxiety disorder, schizoaffective disorder, schizophrenia, and personality disorder)

F. PTSD

G. ADHD/learning disorders (in children)

H. Seizure disorder, nonconvulsive

I. Medical conditions (menopause, neurosyphilis, multiple sclerosis, Lyme's disease)

J. Adverse reactions to medications (theophylline, prednisone, albuterol, Levequin, and antidepressant medications may induce mania)

Plan

A. General interventions:

1. Keep the client safe from self-harm.

2. Treat physical/laboratory findings. Recommend dietary change, iron supplements, and hormone replacement therapy per findings (see related chapters).

B. Client teaching:

1. Encourage the client to take medications as prescribed. Educate the client that some medications may take time to get into the system to work and time should be allowed to see the effects of the medication. Review side effects.

2. Encourage the client to express feelings or worsening of symptoms if this occurs before next appointment. Have the client make a client contract with you that he or she will not cause harm to self or others and if the client begins having these thoughts, the client will contact you or go to the nearest ED.

3. Encourage exercise on a daily basis for 20 to 30 minutes to increase energy and enhance a feeling of well-being.

4. Encourage the client to get at least 7 to 8 hours of sleep each night. If sleep is a problem, address this issue with the client.

5. Avoid caffeine at night and/or watching TV late at night.

6. Encourage the client to seek counseling with a professional counselor. Refer to the appropriate site (psychologist, psychiatrist, group therapy, etc.). Offer local resources to the client.

7. Advise client to participate in activities to enhance interpersonal relationships and build self-esteem. Include family and friends in recommended therapies and advise them to encourage the client to participate in activities to enhance self-esteem.

8. Once the client is feeling better, encourage continued use of medication, activities, and resources.

> Bipolar disorder is a chronic condition requiring long-term, continuous treatment. Untreated, episodes of mania and depression may become more severe and more difficult to treat over time.

C. Pharmaceutical therapy:

Medication choice depends on the current episode: mania/depression.

1. Mood stabilizers:
   a. Divalproex sodium (Depakote, Depakote ER):
      i. Indicated for mania
      ii. Initial dose of 25 mg/kg/d mg daily in divided doses
      iii. Increase as quickly as possible to achieve target plasma concentrations of 50 to 125 mcg/mL.
      iv. Maximum concentration achieved within 14 days
      v. Maximum recommended dose is 60 mg/kg/d.
      vi. Drug–drug interactions: may increase concentrations of clonazepam, diazepam, lamotrigine, and carbamazepine. Aspirin increases Depakote blood levels.
      vii. Labs: check valproic acid level, liver function test (LFT), and CBC after 1 week, then at 1 to 2 months, then every 6 to 12 months thereafter
      viii. Side effects: dizziness, sedation, nausea, tremor, thrombocytopenia, elevated liver enzymes, polycystic ovarian syndrome, and hepatotoxicity (rare)
      ix. Monitoring: serum drug levels during treatment initiation; monitor weight and menstrual history every 3 months for the first year, then annually.
   b. Carbamazepine ER (Equetro):
      i. Indicated for mania and mixed episode
      ii. Initial dose of 200 mg twice daily
      iii. Adjust dose in 200-mg increments.
      iv. Capsules may be taken whole or opened and sprinkled on food.
      v. Do not use with monoamine oxidase inhibitors (MAOIs) or within 14 days of using an MAOI.
      vi. Side effects include dizziness, somnolence, dry mouth, constipation, aplastic anemia, agranulocytosis, rash, toxic epidermal necrolysis (TEN), and Stevens–Johnson syndrome (SJS). Clients of Asian ancestry have a 10-fold greater risk of TEN/SJS.
      vii. Monitoring: serum drug levels during treatment initiation and as clinically indicated. CBC, LFT, electrolytes, blood urea nitrogen (BUN), creatinine monthly for 3 months, then annually
   c. Lithium:
      i. Indicated for mania and maintenance
      ii. **Lithium workup** before initiating the medication: EKG, BUN/creatinine, urinalysis, CMP, and thyroid-stimulating hormone (TSH)
      iii. Initial dose of 300 mg twice daily
      iv. Lithium levels drawn two times per week with dose adjustments in 300 mg increments until target serum levels are reached: target serum levels 0.6 to 1.2 mEq/L. Levels should be drawn 12 hours after last dose.
      v. Lithium toxicity: nausea, vomiting, diarrhea, muscular weakness, lack of coordination, giddiness, and large output of dilute urine; may involve multiple organs and organ systems
      vi. Monitoring: serum drug levels every 3 to 6 months once stable; electrolytes, BUN, creatinine every 3 to 6 months to exclude renal impairment; TSH, calcium, and weight after 6 months, then annually
   d. Lamotrigine (Lamictal):
      i. Indicated for maintenance therapy
      ii. Must titrate slowly due to risk of rash/SJS
      iii. Initial dose:
         1) Weeks 1 and 2: 25 mg daily
         2) Weeks 3 and 4: 50 mg daily
         3) Week 5: 100 mg daily
         4) Week 6: 200 mg daily
         5) Target dose of 200 to 400 mg
      iv. Titration dose adjustments required if client is on Depakote (slower titration) or carbamazepine (faster titration)
      v. Side effects: nausea, insomnia, somnolence, rash, leg cramps, aphasia, and SJS
   e. Topiramate (Topamax):
      i. Off-label use as adjunctive treatment for bipolar disorder
      ii. Side effect: weight loss
2. Atypical antipsychotics:

Potential Side Effects for All Atypical Antipsychotics

- *Extrapyramidal and/or withdrawal symptoms in neonates with third-trimester exposure*
- **Lower seizure threshold**
- *Leukopenia, neutropenia, and agranulocytosis*
- *Metabolic changes including hyperglycemia/diabetes, dyslipidemia, and weight gain*
- *Orthostatic hypotension*
- *Tardive dyskinesia*
- *Cognitive and motor impairment*
- *Increased risk of stroke in elderly clients with dementia-related psychosis; elderly clients with a history of cerebrovascular accident (CVA) treated with antipsychotic medications are at an increased risk of death.*
- *Suicidal thinking*
- *Neuroleptic malignant syndrome (NMS): high fever, stiff muscles, confusion, sweating, changes in pulse, heart rate, and elevated blood pressure*
- Laboratory tests: monitor body mass index (BMI), **waist circumference, hemoglobin A1c (HbA1c), fasting plasma glucose**, and fasting lipid panel at baseline, 3 months, and then annually

a. Aripiprazole (Abilify):

i. Indicated for mania, mixed episodes, and maintenance

ii. Initial dose: 15 mg daily (10–15 mg if using in addition to a mood stabilizer), once daily with or without meals

iii. Available in tablets, orally disintegrating tablets, oral solution, and injectable 9.75 mg/1.3 mL single-dose vial

iv. Maximum recommended dose is 30 mg daily.

v. Drug/drug interactions: known CYP2D6 poor metabolizers, strong CYP2D6, *or* CYP3A4 inhibitors: ½ dose; known CYP2D6 poor metabolizers and strong CYP3A4 inhibitors: ¼ dose

vi. Common side effects: akathesia (restlessness), weight gain, nausea, constipation, headache, dizziness, and stuffy nose.

b. Ziprasidone (Geodon):

i. Indicated as monotherapy for mania and mixed episodes and as an adjunct to lithium or valproate for maintenance

ii. Initial dose for mania: 40 mg twice daily, with increase to 60 to 80 mg twice daily on day 2 of treatment. **Giving oral doses with food increases absorption up to twofold.**

iii. Available in capsules and injectable 20 mg/mL single-dose vial

iv. Maximum recommended dose: 60 to 80 mg twice daily with food

v. Drug/drug interactions: do not give with other medications known to cause QT prolongation.

vi. Side effects: QT prolongation. Do not use in clients with recent heart failure, recent heart attack, or arrhythmias. Other more common side effects include akathesia (restlessness), sleepiness, weight gain, nausea, constipation, headache, dizziness, and stuffy nose. Less common effects include severe cutaneous adverse reactions (SCAR) such as SJS.

c. Risperidone (Risperdal/Risperdal Consta):

i. Indicated as monotherapy for mania and mixed episodes, and as an adjunct to lithium or valproate for maintenance therapy

ii. Dosing:

1) Risperidone: 2 to 3 mg daily with titration in 1 mg increments at intervals of 24 hours or greater. Target dose of 1 to 6 mg daily, max dosing 6 mg/d, once or twice daily with or without meals. Available in tablets, orally disintegrating tablets, and oral solution 1 mg/mL

2) Risperdal Consta: 25 mg intramuscular (IM) q 2 weeks with dose increase in 4-week intervals, max dosing 37.5 to 50 mg IM q 2 weeks. Oral dose of risperidone should be used along with the first injection of Risperdal Consta and continued for 3 weeks. Available in dose strengths of 12.5, 25, 37.5, or 50 mg

3) Drug/drug interactions: CYP2D6 enzyme inducers (carbamazepine) may need to increase dose up to double the client's usual dose. CYP2D6 enzyme inhibitors (paroxetine, fluoxetine): Dose of risperidone should be titrated slowly and dose may need to be decreased.

4) Side effects: dizziness, drooling, nausea, tiredness, weight gain, akathesia, tremor, blurred vision, QT prolongation, and increased prolactin levels. Dose adjustment recommended for clients with severe renal or hepatic impairment. Monitor prolactin levels along with other recommended labs.

d. Asenapine (Saphris): dissolvable:

i. Indicated as monotherapy for mania and mixed episodes, and as an adjunct to lithium or valproate for maintenance therapy

ii. Initial dose: 5 to 10 mg sublingually twice daily

iii. Available in sublingual tablets only

iv. Maximum recommended dose: 10 mg twice daily

v. Drug/drug interactions: Antihypertensive drugs: Saphris may cause hypotension. Paroxetine (CYP2D6 substrate and inhibitor): reduce paroxetine dose by ½ when used in combination with Saphris

vi. Common side effects: orthostatic hypotension, syncope, akathesia (restlessness), weight gain, nausea, constipation, headache, dizziness, and stuffy nose. Contraindicated in clients with severe hepatic impairment

e. Quetiapine (Seroquel/Seroquel XR):

i. Indicated as monotherapy for bipolar mania, mixed, and depressive episodes, and as an adjunct to lithium or valproate for maintenance therapy

ii. Dosing:

1) Quetiapine:

Mania: 50 mg twice daily; dose adjustments in increments of 100 mg daily up to total of 400 mg. Further dose adjustments up to 800 mg/d should be in increments of no greater than 200 mg/d. Target dose: 400 to 800 mg daily. Maximum recommended dose: 800 mg/d

Depression: Administer once daily at bedtime. Initial dose of 50 mg at bedtime; increase to 100 mg on day 2 with further increases of 100 mg daily up to 300 mg/d. Target dose: 300 mg/d. Maximum daily dose: 300 mg

2) Quetiapine extended release: *Bipolar mania/mixed episode:* Initial dose of 300 mg daily in evening without food or with light meal. Target dose: 400 to 600 mg daily. Maximum daily dose: 600 mg. *Bipolar depression:* 50 mg daily in evening without food or with a light meal. Target dose: 300 mg daily. Maximum recommended dose: 300 mg daily

3) Drug/drug interactions: Dose should be increased up to fivefold of the original dose when used in combination with a potent CYP3A4 inducer. Titrate dose based on clinical response and tolerability. Dose should be reduced to one-sixth of the original dose when used in combination with a potent CYP3A4 inhibitor. Quetiapine may cause hypotension, thus enhancing the effects of antihypertensive medications.

4) Side effects: somnolence, dry mouth, dysarthria, increased appetite, weight gain, nausea, constipation, dizziness, stuffy nose, joint pain, QT prolongation, and hypotension

f. Olanzapine (Zyprexa, Zydis):

i. Indicated for mania, mixed episodes, and maintenance monotherapy

ii. Initial dose: 10 to 15 mg once daily with or without meals, with dose adjustments of 5 mg daily

iii. Available in tablets, orally disintegrating tablets, and injectable 10 mg/2.1 mL single-dose vial

iv. Maximum recommended dose: 20 mg daily

v. Drug/drug interactions: Coadministration with diazepam may potentiate orthostatic hypotension. Known CYP1A2 inducers, such as carbamazepine, increase the clearance of olanzapine. Titrate dose based on clinical response and tolerability. When used in combination with CYP1A2 inhibitors, such as fluvoxamine, lower doses of olanzapine should be considered.

vi. Side effects: postural hypotension, akathesia (restlessness), increased appetite, weight gain, somnolence, nausea, constipation, headache, dizziness, stuffy nose, and tremors

g. Olanzapine/fluoxetine combination (Symbyax):

i. Indicated for bipolar depression

ii. Initial dose: 6 mg/25 mg capsule daily in the evening (mg equivalent olanzapine/mg equivalent fluoxetine); dose adjustments as needed and tolerated; target dose within the approved dosing range of 6/25, 6/50, 12/25, 12/50 mg

iii. Maximum recommended dose: 18 mg/75 mg daily in evening

iv. Drug/drug interactions: same as with olanzapine and fluoxetine individually

v. Common side effects: akathesia (restlessness), increased appetite, fatigue, somnolence, peripheral edema, blurred vision, weight gain, nausea, constipation, headache, dizziness, and stuffy nose

h. Chlorpromazine (Thorazine):

i. Indicated for mania/mixed episode

ii. Initial dose: 25 mg orally three times daily with gradual increase until effective dose is reached. Target dose: 400 to 500 mg daily in divided doses

iii. Available in tablets, spansule/sustained release, single and multidose vials for IM injection, and suppositories

iv. Maximum recommended dose: 1,000 mg daily

v. Drug/drug interactions: multiple drug/drug interactions, alpha-blockers, anticholinergic/antispasmodic drugs. Avoid use with other medications that may cause QT prolongation or respiratory depression

vi. Side effects: drowsiness, postural hypotension, akathesia (restlessness), dystonia, tremor, weight gain, nausea, constipation, headache, dizziness, stuffy nose, and QT prolongation

i. Caraprazine (Vraylar):

i. Indicated for mania/mixed episode

ii. Initial dose: 1.5 mg orally daily with or without food. Increase to 3 mg on day two. Due to the long half-life and active metabolites, changes in dose may not be reflected in plasma levels for several weeks. Gradually increase until effective dose is reached. Target dose: 3 mg to 6 mg daily

iii. Available in capsules 1.5 mg, 3 mg, 4.5 mg, and 6 mg

iv. Maximum recommended dose: 6 mg daily

v. Drug/drug interactions: reduce dose of Vraylar if used with strong CYP3A4 inhibitor. Not recommended to use with strong CYP3A4 inducer

vi. Side effects: uncontrolled movements of the body and face, muscle stiffness, vomiting, indigestion, sleepiness, and restlessness

3. Antidepressants:

a. Use of traditional antidepressants to treat bipolar depression is controversial and not FDA approved.

b. Using antidepressants alone to treat bipolar depression is not recommended due to the potential to cause hypomania, mania, and rapid cycling.

c. According to the International Society for Bipolar Disorders (ISBD), antidepressants may be used in combination with another medication, typically a mood stabilizer, when there is a history of a positive response to antidepressants or if the client relapses into a depression after an antidepressant is discontinued.

  d. Do not prescribe an antidepressant during manic or mixed episodes.

4. Electroconvulsive therapy (ECT):

  a. Short-term treatment for severe manic or depressive episodes, especially when suicidal or psychotic symptoms are present, or when medication intervention is ineffective or not well tolerated

  b. ECT is among the safest treatments for severe mood disorders and is effective in up to 75% of clients.

Follow-Up

A. Initially, monitor clients closely to assess for response to treatment, need for medication dose adjustment, side effects, and changes in level of functioning.

B. Monitor for emergence of suicidal thoughts, psychosis, mania, or depression.

C. As appropriate, order lab work to monitor serum blood levels of medications and assess for potential side effects, such as metabolic changes, elevated liver enzymes, decreased kidney functioning, cardiac changes, and blood dyscrasias.

D. After initial stabilization, follow-up appointments should be made every 1 to 3 months.

E. Client teaching related to importance of self-care and medication compliance

Consultation/Referral

A. If the client is experiencing suicidal/homicidal ideations, refer immediately to the nearest ED to be evaluated by a mental health professional for possible emergency admission.

B. Consult with the psychiatric provider to help coordinate care.

C. Refer the client for individual and/or family therapy if indicated.

Individual Considerations

A. Pregnancy:

  1. Some of the medications used to treat bipolar disorder can potentially lower the effectiveness of hormone contraception. Women should be counseled on the use of additional methods of pregnancy prevention.

  2. Medications, such as mood stabilizers, cause an increased risk of birth defects in the first trimester. Women of childbearing age should be counseled on planned pregnancy to allow for medication adjustment and initiation of supportive therapy/close monitoring.

  3. Stopping bipolar medications during pregnancy puts a woman at high risk of relapse during the pregnancy and developing postpartum depression. Some bipolar medications pass through the breast milk. Risk versus benefits of medication use during pregnancy and breastfeeding should be discussed with the client and significant other, if appropriate. Refer to a psychiatric specialist for consultation.

B. Pediatrics:

  1. Bipolar disorder in children/adolescents is difficult to diagnose and does not present with the same clinical picture as adults. Children and adolescents with suspected bipolar disorder should be referred to a pediatric mental health specialist.

C. Partners/family:

  1. Provide educational materials and information on local support resources to partners and family members. The NAMI provides family support groups and online resources in many rural and urban areas. Information may be accessed at www.nami.org.

D. Geriatrics:

  1. Dementia and delirium are common in the elderly. Rule out underlying medical conditions and possible medication-induced mood/cognitive changes.

  2. Caution should be used in the treatment of bipolar mania/mixed symptoms in geriatrics. Atypical antipsychotic medications increase the risk of stroke and death in elderly clients with a history of CVA and dementia-related psychosis.

Bibliography

Depression and Bipolar Support Alliance. (2019). *Peer inspiration*. Retrieved from https://www.dbsalliance.org/support/peer-inspiration/

Hampton, T. (2015). *Epidemiology and pathogenesis of bipolar disorders*. Retrieved from http://www.medpagetoday.com/resource-center/bipolar-resource-center/epidemiology_pathogenesis/a/44242

National Institute of Mental Health. (2016). *Bipolar disorder*. Retrieved from https://www.nimh.nih.gov/health/topics/bipolar-disorder/index.shtml

Depression

Moya Cook and Alyson Wolz

Definition

A. Depression is a mental health disorder that interferes with a person's daily life. Depression may be mild or severe, depending on signs and symptoms expressed, as well as the length of time symptoms are present. Depression affects multiple body systems and may impact one emotionally, cognitively, physically, as well as one's behavior. Symptoms of depression may include difficulty sleeping, depressed mood, inability to function at work, change in appetite, and inability to enjoy activities that bring one pleasure. There are many forms of depression, and treatment varies depending on the specific diagnosis. Types of depression include (a) major depression, single episode, or recurrent (mild, moderate, or severe with or without psychotic features); (b) persistent depressive disorder (dysthymia); (c) premenstrual dysphoric disorder; (d) postpartum depression; (e) SAD; and (f) bipolar disorder. Depression is frequently a concomitant diagnosis with other physical or mental disorders.

Incidence

A. One in 10 adults experiences one or more episodes of depression during his or her lifetime. Depression can occur at any age. The median age of depression occurs between 25 and 32 years of age. The lifetime risk is estimated to be as high as 30%. Women have a twofold to threefold higher rate of reported depression than men. Estimated rates of major depression in the elderly are 3% to 5% for those living in a community dwelling; 15% to 30% for those living in an institutional setting; and 13% for those living in nursing homes.

B. Only 10% to 25% of people with depressive disorders seek treatment. There is a high mortality from suicide if untreated (see "Suicide" section that follows).

C. No single causal factor has been identified. Depressive syndromes are so varied in course and symptomatology that a single cause is unlikely. Several factors appear to contribute, including genetics; neurochemical abnormalities (reductions in adrenergic or serotonergic neurotransmission); electrolyte disturbances; and neuroendocrine abnormalities such as hypothalamic, pituitary, adrenal cortical, thyroid, and gonadal functions. Depression is frequently a concomitant diagnosis with other physical or mental disorders. Personality and psychodynamic factors of depression include low self-esteem, self-criticism, and interpersonal loss. A childhood history of emotional, physical, and/or sexual abuse can also contribute to adult-onset depression.

Predisposing Factors

A. Age (between 25 and 32 years and the elderly)
B. Lack of social support/living alone
C. A history of early parental loss
D. Female gender:
    1. Most common in childbearing years from age 25 to 45 years
    2. Premenstrual
    3. Perimenopausal
    4. Postpartum
E. Family history of depression
F. Frequent exposure to stressful events
G. Nutritional disorders:
    1. Vitamin B_{12} deficiency
    2. Pellagra (niacin deficiency)
H. Personality characteristics that include absence of hardiness factors in response to stress (lack of resilience, flexibility, and optimism)
I. Anger not dealt with and turned in on the self
J. Negative interpretation of one's life experiences
K. Poor physical health
L. Postsurgical diagnosis of cancer
M. Chronic pain
N. Chronic medical problems such as hypothyroidism and hyperthyroidism, Cushing's syndrome, hypercalcemia, hyponatremia, diabetes mellitus, lupus erythematosus, fibromyalgia, rheumatoid disease, and chronic fatigue syndrome
O. Neurologic disorders such as stroke, subdural hematoma, multiple sclerosis, brain tumor, Parkinson's disease, epilepsy, dementia, and Huntington's disease
P. Alcoholism/drug abuse or dependence/withdrawal
Q. Infectious etiology such as mononucleosis and other viral infections, syphilis, HIV, and Lyme disease

R. Side effect of prescription drugs, such as methyldopa, antiarrhythmic, benzodiazepines, barbiturates/central nervous system (CNS) depressants, beta-blockers, cholinergic drugs, corticosteroids, digoxin, H_2-blockers, and reserpine

Common Complaints

A. Lack of interest in pleasurable activities
B. Digestive problems
C. Chronic aches and pains that are not otherwise explained

Other Signs and Symptoms

A. Vegetative:
    1. Changes (increased or decreased) in sleep, appetite, and weight
    2. Changes in appearance: poor grooming and hygiene
    3. Poor eye contact, staring downward, flat affect
    4. Loss of energy
    5. Decreased interest in sex
    6. Psychomotor retardation or agitation
B. Cognitive:
    1. Sense of guilt, worthlessness, low self-esteem
    2. Problems with attention span, concentration or memory, frustration tolerance, negative distortions, mild paranoia, and psychosis
C. Impulse control:
    1. Suicidal or homicidal thoughts or acts. Any statements made by the client, such as "Life isn't worth living, I wish I were dead, I don't deserve to be alive, I can't deal with this," should be taken seriously. Refer the client for counseling and assessment and treatment.
D. Behavioral:
    1. Depressed mood, anxiety, and irritability
    2. Isolation, decreased motivation, fatigability, and anhedonia (unable to derive gratification from pleasurable activities)
E. Physical symptoms:
    1. Digestion problems, nausea, constipation, diarrhea (less common), and dry mouth
    2. Fatigue, but difficulty sleeping
    3. Physical pain, chronic aches, and pains that cannot be explained
    4. Recurrent headaches, backaches, or stomachaches that have no cause
    5. Migrating pain that disappears when depression lifts
    6. Increased muscle tension

Subjective Data

A. Review the onset, duration, and course of presenting symptoms.
B. Review any previous history of depression (such as postpartum depression).
C. Determine how the previous depression was treated.
D. Evaluate the client's suicide potential. Ask: "Have you ever thought of hurting yourself or others?" Does the client have a current suicide plan or vague ideas of

suicide? Has the client had any previous history of suicide attempts? If so, evaluate how life-threatening they were.

E. Review the client's medical history (see "Predisposing Factors" section).

F. Review the client's drug history for prescription, OTC medications, and recreational/illicit drug use (how much, how long, how often), and review his or her history of alcohol consumption (how much, how long, and how often).

G. Review the client's history for recent major life changes such as pregnancy, death, divorce, or any loss that may be normal throughout the stages of life. The *client's perception* of the loss is what is important.

H. Review dietary intake since the symptoms began.

I. Establish usual weight, review weight gain/loss, and note in what time span.

J. Review the client's activities of daily living. Does the client get up and dress daily, perform daily hygiene, put on makeup?

K. Review how many hours of sleep and quality of sleep per day.

L. Review the disruption of usual activities: return to work, return to school, exercise.

M. Review the amount of crying per day, for what length of time (days, weeks).

N. Assess whether the depression is cyclic/seasonal (starts in the fall, ends in the spring).

O. Review occupational/home exposure to lead and lead-based products.

P. Review any exposures to infectious diseases, including Lyme disease (refer to Chapter 16, "Infectious Disease Guidelines" for specific questions). Does anyone else, such as family, friends, or coworkers have similar symptoms?

Q. If female, review for symptoms of menopause (sleep disturbances, irregular menses/amenorrhea, hot flushes, vaginal dryness, dyspareunia).

Physical Examination

A. Check pulse, respirations, blood pressure, and weight.

B. Inspect:

1. Observe overall appearance; note grooming, tone of voice, conduct of client during communication, and breath (smell of alcohol).

2. Complete neurologic examination and Mini-Mental State Examination (MMSE) available for download at https://www.ncbi.nlm.nih.gov/projects/gap/cgi-bin/GetPdf.cgi?id=phd001525.2.

3. Complete dermal examination for signs of substance use (refer to "Substance Use Disorders" section in Chapter 2).

C. Auscultate:

1. Heart
2. Lungs
3. Abdomen

D. Palpate:

1. Neck and thyroid; note goiter
2. Axilla and groin for lymphadenopathy (infectious etiology)
3. Check the joints for swelling and arthritis and ROM; rule out musculoskeletal cause.

Diagnostic Tests

A. CBC with differential

B. Electrolytes, serum calcium, and phosphorus

C. Thyroid profile

D. Liver profile

E. Vitamin D_{25} hydroxy

F. Vitamin B_{12}/folate

G. Lead level

H. Follicle-stimulating hormone/luteinizing hormone (FSH/LH)

I. Viral cultures

J. Blood alcohol

K. Urine drug screen

L. Monospot

M. CT and MRI scans

N. Dexamethasone suppression test

O. Perform MSE with depression rating scale of choice:

1. Beck Depression Inventory Scale (Beck, Ward, Mendelson, Mock, & Erbaugh, 1961): www.beckinstitute.org/get-informed/tools-and-resources/professionals/patient-assessment-tools/

2. Geriatric Depression Scale (GDS): Short version (Yesavage, 1988): https://sagelink.ca/sites/default/files/clinical-resources/5-Item-Geriatric-Depression-Scale-print-form.pdf

Differential Diagnoses

A. Mood disorder due to another medical condition

B. Adjustment disorder with depressed mood

C. Chronic untreated anxiety disorders such as GAD, PTSD, or OCD

D. Personality disorder

E. Schizoaffective disorder

F. SAD:

1. Seasonal pattern: starts in the fall, linked to lack of light exposure

2. Women more than men

3. Age typically in the 20s

G. Alcoholism and drug abuse/dependence

H. Early dementia

I. Endocrine etiologies (see "Predisposing Factors")

J. Infectious etiologies (see "Predisposing Factors")

K. Menopause

L. Side effect of medication (see "Predisposing Factors")

M. Cancer: 50% of clients with tumors, particularly of the brain and lung, and carcinoma of the pancreas develop symptoms of depression before the diagnosis of tumor is made.

N. Heavy metal poisoning

O. Nutritional deficit (see "Predisposing Factors")

Plan

A. General interventions:

1. Keep the client safe from self-harm.

2. Treat physical/laboratory findings. Recommend dietary change, iron supplements, and hormone replacement therapy per findings.

B. Client teaching:

1. Encourage the client to take medications as prescribed. Educate the client that some medications

may take time to get into the system to work and time should be allowed to see the effects of the medication. Review side effects.

2. Encourage client to call provider and return to clinic if feelings or symptoms of depression worsen before next appointment. Have the client make a client contract with you that he or she will not bring harm to self or others and if he or she begins having these thoughts, the client will contact you or go to the nearest ED.

3. Encourage exercise on a daily basis for 20 to 30 minutes to increase energy and enhance a feeling of well-being.

4. Encourage the client to get at least 7 to 8 hours of sleep each night. If sleep is a problem, address this issue with the client.

5. Avoid caffeine at night and/or watching TV late at night.

6. Encourage the client to seek counseling with a professional counselor. Refer to appropriate site (psychologist, psychiatrist, group therapy, etc.). Offer local resources to the client.

7. Advise client to participate in activities to enhance interpersonal relationships and build self-esteem. Include family and friends in recommended therapies and advise them to encourage the client to participate in activities to enhance self-esteem.

8. Once the client is feeling better, encourage continued use of medication, activities, and resources for at least 6 months after the client has started feeling better to prevent relapse.

C. Pharmaceutical therapy: Table 22.1 presents dosage information.

1. Drugs of choice: SSRI antidepressants. Caution should be used when coadministering SSRIs with drugs that have a narrow therapeutic window, such

TABLE 22.1 DOSAGES FOR COMMON ANTIDEPRESSANT DRUGS

Generic (Brand Name)	Adults Aged 18–60 Years	Elderly >60 Years or Renal or Hepatic Clients
Fluoxetine hydrochloride (Prozac) Therapeutic onset occurs in 1–4 weeks. Serum levels peak in 4.5–8.5 hours.	20 mg daily in a.m., dosage increased according to client response May be given bid—in the morning and at noon Maximum dosage 80 mg/d	10–20 mg daily in a.m. with clinical response monitored q 1–2 weeks Gradual dose increases q 6 week until optimal therapeutic response is obtained.
Paroxetine hydrochloride (Paxil) Therapeutic onset occurs in 1–4 weeks. Serum levels peak in 2–8 hours.	10 mg daily in a.m., p.m., or @ HS. May increase 10 mg/d increments at weekly intervals Maximum dosage 50 mg/d	10–20 mg daily in a.m., p.m., or @ HS with clinical response monitored q 1–2 weeks and gradual increase
Sertraline hydrochloride (Zoloft) Therapeutic onset occurs in 2–4 weeks. Serum levels peak in 4.5–8.5 hours.	50 mg daily in a.m. May increase to 100 mg Dosage adjustments should be made at intervals of no less than 1 week. Maximum dosage is 200 mg/d.	25–50 mg daily in a.m. with clinical response monitored q 1–2 weeks and gradual increase
Citalopram hydrobromide (Celexa) Therapeutic onset occurs in 2–4 weeks. Serum levels peak in 4 hours.	20 mg daily in a.m., p.m., or @ HS May increase 10 mg/d increments at weekly intervals Maximum dosage is 40 mg/d (due to potential for QT prolongation at higher doses).	20 mg daily in a.m., p.m., or HS with clinical response monitored q 1–2 weeks and gradual increase
Escitalopram oxalate (Lexapro) Therapeutic onset occurs in 1–2 weeks. Serum levels peak in 5 hours.	10 mg daily in a.m. May increase in 5–10 mg/d increments at weekly intervals Maximum dosage is 20 mg/d.	5 mg daily in a.m. with clinical response monitored q 1–2 weeks and gradual increase
Vortioxetine (Trintellix/Brintellix) Therapeutic onset occurs in 2–4 weeks. Serum levels peak in 7–11 hours.	5–10 mg daily in a.m. or p.m. May increase in 5 mg/d increments at weekly intervals Maximum dosage is 20 mg/d.	10–20 mg daily in a.m., p.m. with clinical response monitored q 1–2 weeks and gradual increase
Vilazodone hydrochloride (Viibryd) Therapeutic onset occurs in 2–4 weeks. Serum levels peak in 4–5 hours.	10 mg daily in a.m. or p.m., with food May increase 10 mg/d increments at weekly intervals Maximum dosage is 40 mg/d.	10–20 mg daily in a.m. or p.m. with food, clinical response monitored q 1–2 weeks and gradual increase
Venlafaxine (Effexor) Therapeutic onset occurs in 1–4 weeks. Serum levels peak in 2 hours. **(Effexor XR)** Therapeutic onset occurs in 2–4 weeks. Serum levels peak in 8 hours.	75 mg daily in divided dose May increase 75 mg/d increments at 4-day intervals Maximum dosage is 375 mg/d in divided doses q 8–12 hr. 37.5–75 mg daily in a.m. or p.m. May increase by 75-mg/d increments at 4-day intervals Maximum dosage is 225 mg daily.	75–225 mg daily in divided doses q 8–12 hr with clinical response monitored q 1–2 weeks and gradual increase 75–225 mg daily dose with clinical response monitored every 1–2 weeks and gradual increase

(continued)

TABLE 22.1   DOSAGES FOR COMMON ANTIDEPRESSANT DRUGS *(continued)*

Generic (Brand Name)	Adults Aged 18–60 Years	Elderly >60 Years or Renal or Hepatic Clients
Desvenlafaxine (Pristiq) Therapeutic onset occurs in 1–2 weeks. Serum levels peak in 7.5 hours.	50 mg daily in a.m. or p.m. May increase to 100 mg after 1–2 weeks, although there is no evidence of increased efficacy over 50 mg dose. Maximum dosage is 100 mg/d.	25–50 mg daily in a.m. or p.m. with clinical response monitored q 1–2 weeks and gradual increase
Duloxetine delayed-release (Cymbalta) Therapeutic onset occurs in 2–4 weeks. Serum levels peak in 6–10 hours.	30 mg daily in a.m. or p.m. with increase to 60 mg after 1 week daily dosing or bid May increase 30-mg/d increments at weekly intervals Maximum dosage is 120 mg/d.	40–120 mg daily in a.m., p.m., single dose, or bid with clinical response monitored q 1–2 weeks and gradual increase
Nortriptyline hydrochloride (Pamelor) Therapeutic onset occurs in 2–4 weeks or longer. Serum levels peak in 7–8.5 hours.	25 mg tid or qid initially, gradually increase to maximum dose 150 mg qd	30–50 mg daily tid or qid or in 1 day's dose
Desipramine hydrochloride (Norpramin) Therapeutic onset occurs in 2–4 weeks or longer. Serum levels peak in 4–6 hours.	100–200 mg po in single or divided dose	25–100 mg daily in divided doses, increase gradually to maximum of 150 mg qd
Amitriptyline (Elavil) Therapeutic onset unknown—thought to take several weeks. Serum levels peak 2–12 hours.	75 mg po in divided doses initially or 50–100 mg HS Dose not to exceed 150 mg/d	10–20 mg po tid and 20 mg HS daily

Paxil works well for clients who have a component of anxiety to their depression. **Monitor prothrombin time for clients taking warfarin, sertraline, and paroxetine.**

bid, twice a day; HS, at bedtime; po, by mouth; q, every; qd, every day; qid, four times a day; tid, three times a day.

as carbamazepine (Tegretol), warfarin, tricyclic antidepressants (TCAs), antiarrhythmics, and some antipsychotic medications (risperidone, haloperidol, and phenothiazine), and other drugs including diazepam (Valium) and MAOIs:

  a. Most antidepressant therapy takes 3 to 4 weeks for onset of action to elicit visible changes.

  b. Never prescribe more than a week's supply or a total of 2 g of a TCA if there is a risk of suicide.

  c. Medication should not be changed until a trial of 6 to 8 weeks has been given to measure the progress.

  d. Before concluding that the antidepressant is ineffective, verify that the client is taking the medication correctly.

  e. First-line therapy in the elderly is SSRIs, which have significantly fewer side effects than the traditional TCAs. Paroxetine and sertraline have short half-lives and can be withdrawn quickly.

  f. Antidepressant therapy should be continued for 6 months to 1 year (up to 5 years if necessary) because of the risk of recurrence of depression.

  g. Taper the medication off instead of abruptly withdrawing.

2. TCAs: avoid administration after acute myocardial infarction. **Men with prostatic hypertrophy do best with a nonsedating TCA that has a mild anticholinergic activity, such as desipramine (Norpramin) or nortriptyline (Pamelor).**

3. Adrenergic modulators: a weak inhibitor of norepinephrine, dopamine, and serotonin reuptake: bupropion hydrochloride (Wellbutrin):

  a. For clients older than 18 years

  b. No dosage established for the elderly

  c. Therapeutic onset in 1 to 3 weeks

  d. Serum level peak within 2 hours

  e. Initially 100 mg twice a day for at least 3 days

  f. If well tolerated, increase to 375 or 400 mg daily.

  g. After 3 days more, 450 mg daily in four divided doses at least 4 hours apart

  h. Maximum single dosing 150 mg, maximum 450 mg daily:

    i. Avoid bedtime dosing.

    ii. Do not give to clients with predisposition to seizures.

    iii. Give reduced dose to clients with renal or hepatic impairment.

4. Dual reuptake inhibitors: block the reabsorption of the norepinephrine and serotonin into the neurons in the CNS. When this occurs, higher levels of norepinephrine and serotonin remain and improve the nerve transmission in the brain, which then improves mood:

a. Venlafaxine hydrochloride (Effexor):

   i. With hepatic impairment, reduce dose by 50%.

   ii. Withdraw gradually over 2 weeks when discontinuing medication.

   iii. Interacts with MAOIs. Do not start venlafaxine within 14 days of discontinuing an MAOI.

b. Duloxetine (Cymbalta) also blocks reuptake of serotonin and norepinephrine:

   i. Avoid use in clients with chronic liver disease or cirrhosis.

   ii. Clients should be warned about stopping the medication abruptly; have them taper down slowly.

   iii. Duloxetine is also helpful in treating the physical pain that accompanies some depression symptoms as well as clients with chronic musculoskeletal pain and fibromyalgia.

5. **MAOIs** should be prescribed only by a psychiatrist.

Follow-Up

A. Follow up in 1 to 2 weeks to assess client's status, drug effectiveness, and adverse reactions.

B. Clients can become suicidal after the depression is treated and they begin to have more energy to act on the suicidal ideation. **Assess suicidality with every office visit.**

C. Follow up every 2 to 4 weeks afterward to check client's progress.

D. Once positive change is seen, the client can be seen monthly.

E. Refer to other applicable medical diagnoses for the follow-up recommendations.

Consultation/Referral

A. If there is any potential for suicidal/homicidal behavior, refer client immediately to a psychiatrist for possible emergency admission.

B. Consult with the psychiatric specialist, or the client may need immediate referral/consult for continuing psychotherapy.

C. Clients who fail to respond to antidepressants after 1 to 2 months of appropriate antidepressant therapy should have a psychiatric consultation.

Individual Considerations

A. Pregnancy:

1. A woman with a history of depression or previous postpartum depression is at a high risk of postpartum depression (recurrent). Caution should be used in prescribing antidepressants during pregnancy. Review the benefits versus risks.

2. Refer to Chapter 13, "Obstetrics Guidelines," for the section, "Postpartum Depression."

B. Pediatrics:

1. Children with depression are more difficult to diagnose and do not necessarily meet adult criteria. The clinical picture can be completely different, that is, acting-out behavior. Children suspected to be depressed should be referred to a child psychiatrist.

C. Adolescence:

1. Teens are at risk for suicide after recent losses from death (especially if one of their friends/family commits suicide). Recent loss includes breaking up with a boyfriend or girlfriend.

2. If a teen has had a depressive episode, he or she may be at a higher risk for suicide if he or she is suddenly happy and things are "just fine." He or she may have decided on a suicide plan and may be experiencing a sense of relief because plans have been made.

D. Partners:

1. If available in the community, provide resources for partners, such as the NAMI (listed in most telephone books).

2. Frequently, partners will take too much responsibility for the depressed client's state of mind and, over time, also become depressed. Relating to other people with depressed partners will assist them in dealing with their significant other's depression.

E. Geriatrics:

1. Dementia masked as "pseudodepression" is common in the elderly. Check for memory impairment and disorientation because delirium can often be mistaken for depression.

2. Elderly clients who are depressed may experience agitation rather than retardation in psychomotor function.

3. White men, aged 80 years, have the highest rate of suicide of any age group in the United States.

4. Look for depression in caretakers of clients with Alzheimer's disease.

> Elderly clients who are suicidal may present with atypical symptoms of depression and may not express their distress directly. Three identified behaviors include impaired ability to communicate, intractable tinnitus, and feelings of helplessness.

Bibliography

American Psychiatric Association. (2013). *Diagnostic and statistical manual of mental disorders* (5th ed.). Arlington, VA: American Psychiatric Publishing.

Anxiety and Depression Association of America. (2014). *Facts and statistics*. Retrieved from http://www.adaa.org/about-adaa/press-room/facts-statistics

Beck, A. T., Ward, C. H., Mendelson, M., Mock, J., & Erbaugh, J. (1961). An inventory for measuring depression. *Archives of General Psychiatry*, 4(6), 561–571. doi:10.1001/archpsyc.1961.01710120031004

Crum, R. M., Anthony, J. C., Bassett, S. S., & Folstein, M. F. (1993). Population-based norms for the mini-mental state examination by age and educational level. *Journal of the American Medical Association*, 269(18), 2386–2391. doi:10.1001/jama.1993.03500180078038

Depression and Bipolar Support Alliance. (2015). *Peer support*. Retrieved from http://www.dbsalliance.org/site/PageServer?pagename=education_statistics_bipolar_disorder

Ng, C. W., How, C. H., & Ng, Y. P. (2017). Managing depression in primary care. *Singapore medical journal*, 58(8), 459–466. doi:10.11622/smedj.2017080

U.S. Preventive Services. (2016). *Depression in adults: Screening*. Retrieved from https://www.uspreventiveservicestaskforce.org/Page/Document/RecommendationStatementFinal/depression-in-adults-screening1

World Health Organization. (2013). *Gender and women's mental health.* Retrieved from http://www.who.int/mental_health/prevention/gender women/en

Yesavage, J. A. (1986). The use of rating depression series in the elderly. In L. W. Poon (Ed.), *Clinical memory assessment of older adults.* Washington, DC: American Psychological Association.

Yesavage, J. A. (1988). Geriatric depression scale. *Psychopharmacology Bulletin, 24*(4), 709–711. Retrieved from https://medworksmedia.com/product-category/psychopharmacology-bulletin/

Failure to Thrive

Moya Cook and Alyson Wolz

Definition

Failure to thrive (FTT) is an abnormality in growth in which an individual fails to gain weight or grow. FTT is a manifestation of an underlying problem, whether the problem be mental, physical, or psychological.

A. Children: In a growing child, a child measuring below the third to fifth percentile on the growth curve, or exhibiting a drop greater than two percentiles on the growth curve in the past several months, is referred to as FTT.

B. Adults: FTT is also seen in adults who have a weight <80% of the ideal average body weight for the adult.

C. Geriatrics: FTT in the geriatric population is defined as a deterioration in functional status disproportional to their disease burden. Signs are decreased appetite, weight loss of >5% of their weight, decreased physical activity, along with dehydration, depression, and compromised immune status.

Incidence

A. Incidence depends on the population; however, it is estimated that FTT is seen in 5% to 10% of low-birth-weight children and children who live in poverty. In the elderly population, it is estimated to occur in 5% to 35% of the elderly population, with nursing home residents having an occurrence rate of 25% to 40%.

Pathogenesis

A. Organic causes for FTT:
 1. Gastrointestinal (reflux, celiac disease, Hirschsprung's disease, and malabsorption)
 2. Cardiopulmonary (cardiac diseases, congestive heart failure)
 3. Pulmonary (asthma, bronchopulmonary dysplasia, cystic fibrosis)
 4. Renal (diabetes insipidus, renal insufficiency, urinary tract infections)
 5. Endocrine (hypothyroidism, adrenal diseases, parathyroid disorders, thyroid disorders, pituitary disorders)
 6. Neurologic (mental retardation, cerebral hemorrhages)
 7. Metabolic disorders (inborn errors of metabolism)
 8. Congenital (congenital syndromes such as fetal alcohol syndrome, chromosomal abnormalities, perinatal infections)
 9. Infectious (gastrointestinal infections, tuberculosis, HIV)
 10. Allergies to certain foods such as lactose, gluten, or proteins

B. Inorganic causes for FTT:
 1. Poor eating habits such as unscheduled meals, or eating in front of television or electronic game systems
 2. Exposure to toxins or parasites
 3. Emotional deprivation as a result of parental withdrawal or absence
 4. Socioeconomic factors that affect nutrition and living conditions
 5. Physical, sexual, and/or emotional abuse
 It is common to see both organic and inorganic problems as causative factors for FTT.

C. Geriatric population:
 1. Feel fuller with less food; this may be an endorphin response that decreases the adaptive relaxation of the fundus of the stomach.
 2. Increased number of cytokines, which contributes to anorexia
 3. Diminished sense of smell or taste
 4. Dysphagia
 5. Medications
 6. Depression, delirium, dementia
 7. Alcohol or substance abuse

Predisposing Factors

A. Children: low birth weight, prematurity

B. Geriatrics: dementia, comorbidities (cancer, chronic infections, malabsorption syndromes, psychiatric disorders), limited mobility, despair

C. Poverty

D. Organic conditions with the major organs noted in the Pathogenesis section

E. Parents with psychosocial disorders

F. Altered family processes

Common Complaints

A. Failure to grow and gain weight

B. Weight loss

> Clients do not always present for this problem. Many clients are diagnosed at a routine examination in the ambulatory setting.

Other Signs and Symptoms

A. No growth in height

B. Loss of subcutaneous fat tissue

C. Muscle atrophy

D. Alopecia

E. Dermatitis

F. Marasmus (severe malnutrition from poor caloric intake over a period of time contributing to growth retardation and muscle wasting)

G. Kwashiorkor (severe malnutrition from protein deficiency with symptoms of edema and liver enlargement with fatty infiltrates)

Subjective Data

A. Obtain detailed history of the client's diet. Note the differences between foods offered and foods eaten. If formula is used, note type, frequency, amount taken each feeding, spits, and so forth.

B. Assess quality of nutrients offered to the client. Consider knowledge deficit of care provider if inadequate.

    1. Children: If breastfeeding, note frequency, duration, milk supply, medications, or foods that would alter breast milk.

    2. Geriatrics: Is client able to chew and swallow food offered? Are supplements being offered?

C. Query regarding financial resources, and, if needed, does the family participate in low-income opportunities (Women, Infant, and Children [WIC], food stamp programs, etc.)?

D. Evaluate whether religious or unusual dietary beliefs/habits contribute to the food preparation, if inadequate.

E. For infants and children, obtain a detailed perinatal history, noting complications with mother or baby.

F. For infants and children, determine whether the formula is being prepared correctly (powder, concentrate, ready-to-feed).

G. Rule out any difficulty in swallowing or retaining ingested food.

H. Note regular bowel/bladder habits.

I. Note any recent illness, chronic or acute.

J. Query regarding lead exposure.

K. Rule out family history of cystic fibrosis or lactose intolerance.

L. Note whether a short/small stature runs in the family history.

M. Geriatrics: evaluate nutritional screening using the Mini Nutritional Assessment.

Physical Examination

A. Check temperature, pulse, respirations, blood pressure, height, and weight.

    1. Measure head circumference in children.

B. Inspect:

    1. Observe overall appearance.

    2. Observe oral pathology; for geriatrics, check for ill-fitting dentures, dental and gum condition.

    3. Note muscle tone, strength, and movement.

    4. Note social interactions among family members.

    5. Note social skills of the client.

    6. Perform Denver Developmental II on children.

Note any changes in growth curve, especially if crossing over percentiles, and if height and weight are not concordant. If premature, adjust for gestational age as appropriate.

C. Auscultate:

    1. Heart

    2. Lungs

D. Percuss:

    1. Abdomen

E. Palpate:

    1. Abdomen

    2. Back

    3. Extremities

Diagnostic Tests

A. CBC, urinalysis, electrolytes

B. Thyroid panel if indicated

C. Lead screen

D. Sweat test if indicated

E. X-rays if appropriate

F. Serum albumin in geriatrics

G. MSE

H. Purified protein derivative (PPD)

I. HIV, rapid plasma reagin (RPR)

J. MRI

Differential Diagnoses

A. Weight loss

B. Depression

C. Impaired physical function

D. Cognitive impairment

E. Depression

F. Malnutrition related to malabsorption (e.g., bariatric surgery)

Plan

A. General interventions:

    1. The plan is based on the cause of FTT. Children with organic etiologies need follow-up regarding the specific problem.

    2. Severe malnutrition requires hospitalization.

    3. Geriatrics: obtain nutritional consult to evaluate the dietary needs for protein, iron, and other nutrients.

B. Client teaching:

    1. Reinforce positive eating habits and encourage dietary meal planning.

    2. Offer nutrition counseling with dietitian.

    3. Educate the client and family about the importance of meeting the dietary requirements for protein, iron, calcium, and other nutrients to prevent weight loss, loss of muscle and bone mass, and to prevent infection and other complications that can stress the body.

C. Pharmaceutical therapy:

    1. High-calorie supplements are recommended for some clients (Polycose, Carnation Instant Breakfast, Pediasure, Ensure).

Weight gain with high-calorie supplements is commonly seen with clients who have psychosocial etiology of FTT.

---

    2. Geriatrics: Short-term aggressive caloric replacement has been shown to be effective in reversing FTT. Severe malnutrition may require hospitalization with total parental nutrition. Medications may be used to increase appetite.

        a. Megestrol 400 or 800 mg daily with meal

        b. Antidepressants such as SSRIs, TCAs, and mirtazapine (Remeron) have been shown to be beneficial to help stimulate appetite and increase weight.

D. Dietary management:

1. Meal suggestions: offer adequate time for meals (20–30 minutes), offer solid food before drinks/juices, and provide a pleasant environment for eating.

2. Encourage all family members to sit down and eat at least one meal a day together. This time will also enhance family social interactions.

3. Provide handout for high-calorie foods (peanut butter, cheese, whole milk, etc.).

4. Consider exercise sessions for geriatrics to stimulate appetite.

5. Encourage clients to attend centers where meals are served as a group or have meals delivered to the home.

6. Encourage small frequent meals with snacks between meals and before bedtime.

Follow-Up

A. Two-week evaluation for weight/height measurements and to evaluate compliance with regimen at home. Routine visits recommended every 2 to 4 weeks to monitor progress

B. Reevaluate client in 1 to 2 months. After 2 months, if no improvement or further loss is noted, refer to a specialist.

Consultation/Referral

A. Consult with a physician if height/weight measurements are noted below the third percentile on a graphic chart.

B. For the majority of clients, a nutrition consultation is needed to assist the parents or food provider in providing adequate resources/calories for the client.

C. Consider social service and visiting nurses for outpatient assistance in the home.

Individual Considerations

A. Pediatrics:

1. The prognosis for inorganic etiologies of children in the first year of life is ominous due to the poor brain growth. These children will be at high risk for developmental delay, poor cognitive and emotional developments, and social/emotional problems.

2. Approximately 10% of children are normally small children by genetic makeup. These children are not diagnosed with FTT. FTT is most commonly seen in children younger than 3 to 5 years.

3. Consider keeping small children on formula past the 12-month age mark if FTT is diagnosed.

4. Early intervention programs should be considered for children.

B. Geriatrics:

1. FTT in the elderly may lead to a decline in physical and mental functions. Aggressive treatment should be employed to improve the nutritional status of these clients.

2. FTT increases the risk of morbidity and mortality.

3. FTT increases the risk of depression and social isolation in the elderly.

Bibliography

Homan, G. (2016). Failure to thrive: a practical guide. *American Family Physician*, *94*(4), 295–299. Retrieved from https://www.aafp.org/afp/2016/0815/p295.html

National Initiative for Children's Healthcare Quality. (2014). *Scoring instructions for NICHQ Vanderbilt assessment scales*. Retrieved from www.aap.org/en-us/Documents/sodbp_vanderbilt_scoringinstructions.pdf

National Institute on Aging. (2016, December 16). *Elder abuse*. Retrieved from https://www.nia.nih.gov/health/elder-abuse

Grief

Moya Cook and Alyson Wolz

Definition

A. Grief is defined as the normal, appropriate emotional response caused by a loss. This feeling of loss is a response caused by a particular event in one's life. It is unique to the individual experiencing it, and there is no general timetable for completing it. Grief is commonly seen following the death of a loved one, but grief also follows other losses (e.g., loss of independence, loss of affection, loss of body parts, loss of comfort caused by pain, or loss of mental soundness from distress). Mourning is defined as the process by which grief is resolved. Mourning is individual and helps in reaching acceptance of a loss.

B. The process through which one resolves grief usually follows a typical course that can be viewed in five stages:

1. Denial: Denial occurs when one refuses to accept the circumstance that has occurred. It is a natural defense mechanism that occurs to protect the body.

2. Anger: Pain, tears, anxiousness, anger, and feelings of guilt may be seen.

3. Bargaining: In this stage, the person tries to negotiate alternatives that will make him or her feel better.

4. Depression: One begins to understand what has happened and may show feelings of sadness and fear.

5. Acceptance: One begins to rebuild one's life and think about the past with pleasure. In this phase, one regains interest in activities and forms new relationships.

C. It is important to distinguish between the normal grief reactions of pathologic grief and major depression. Approximately 10% to 15% of individuals experience a severe grief reaction. Often, depressive symptoms are a pervasive part of the grief response, and a clear delineation of grief versus depression is not always possible.*

Incidence

A. Grief is a universal emotional response. Each year, approximately 5% to 9% of the population lose a close family member or friend. Grief is a normal emotional response that will follow this loss for an individual.

Pathogenesis

A. Grief is a normal emotional response to the loss of a loved one, pain, and/or distress. Abnormal, pathologic grief can occur if the mourner is not encouraged to grieve losses. Normal grief resolution begins to subside at approximately 6 months but may sometimes take longer.

---

* Based on the Grief Cycle model first published in *On Death and Dying,* Elisabeth Kübler-Ross, 1969. Interpretation by Alan Chapman 2006–2009. Retrieved from www.ekrfoundation.org/five-stages-of-grief

Predisposing Factors

A. Sudden or terrible deaths
B. Excessive dependency on the deceased and feelings of ambivalence
C. Traumatic losses earlier in life
D. Social isolation
E. Actual or imagined responsibility for "causing" the death
F. Avoidance of grief and denial of loss
G. Survived a traumatic experience that killed the deceased

Common Complaints

A. Angry feelings at God or medical personnel for not doing more, anger at oneself for not seeing the warning signs, anger at the deceased for not taking better care of himself or herself. Common feelings of being left alone and not making proper financial/legal preparations may also occur.
B. Sleeping all the time or inability to sleep without medication
C. Change in eating habits with significant weight loss or gain
D. Fatigue, lethargy, or lack of motivation
E. Decreased concentration and memory, forgetfulness
F. Increased irritability
G. Unpredictable bouts of crying
H. Fears:
    1. Of being alone or with people
    2. Of leaving the house
    3. Of staying in the house

Other Signs and Symptoms

A. Normal grief:
    1. Protest, disbelief, shock, and denial
    2. Profound sadness and survivor guilt
    3. Multiple somatic symptoms without actual organic disease
    4. Sense of unreality and withdrawal from others
    5. Disruption of normal patterns of conduct, with restlessness and aimlessness
    6. Preoccupation with memories of the deceased, dreams of the deceased, hallucinations, fear of going crazy, and transient psychotic symptoms
    7. Responds to support, displaying an improvement with normal patterns of conduct and reconnecting with others.
B. Complicated or prolonged grief:
    1. Persistence of denial with delayed or absent grief
    2. Depression with impaired self-esteem, suicidal thoughts, and impulses with self-destructive behavior
    3. Actual organic disease and medical illness
    4. Progressive social isolation
    5. Persistent anger and hostility leading to paranoid reactions, especially against those involved in medical care of the deceased, or suppression of any expression of anger and hostility
    6. Continued disruption of normal patterns of conduct, often with a persistent hyperactivity unaccompanied by a sense of loss or grieving
    7. Continued preoccupation with memories of the deceased to the point of searching for reunion (sustained depressive delusions)
    8. Conversion symptoms similar to the symptoms of the deceased
    9. Self-blame
    10. Prolonged grief longer than 6 months is commonly linked to complications and impairment for the next 1 to 2 years.

Subjective Data

A. Review onset, duration, and course of presenting symptoms. Review the mourner's grief symptoms.
B. Obtain an in-depth personal history of the mourner and his or her relationship to the identified loss or with the deceased.

> Understanding the bereaved's history is critical to understanding the individual's loss.

C. Identify anniversary dates pertinent to the mourner's relationship with the deceased/loss.
D. Determine whether the mourner has suicidal ideation (especially with a plan). **Be sure to ask: "Have you ever thought of hurting yourself or others?"**
E. Assess whether the mourner experiences self-blame.
F. Review the mourner's appetite.
G. Establish usual weight, review weight gain/loss, and in what time span.
H. Review the mourner's activities of daily living. Does the mourner get up and dress daily and perform daily hygiene?
I. Review the mourner's sleep quality.
J. Review the mourner's daily routines: return to work, return to school, and exercise.
K. Review the mourner's amount of crying per day, for what length of time (days, weeks).
L. Review the mourner's drug and alcohol consumption since the loss.

> Statements suggesting self-medication with alcohol to facilitate sleep could indicate a coexistent alcohol abuse/dependence diagnosis.

M. Review the mourner's usual medical problems and how the loss/grief has affected these problems.

Physical Examination

A. Check temperature, pulse, respirations, blood pressure, and weight.
B. Inspect:
    1. Observe overall appearance. Note grooming habits, dress, and appearance.
    2. Note social interactions among family members.
    3. Note social skills of the client.
C. Auscultate:
    1. Heart
    2. Lungs

Diagnostic Tests

A. As indicated to rule out other pathology
B. Blood glucose

C. Thyroid studies

D. If depression is suspected, perform Beck's Depression Inventory; see "Depression" section.

Differential Diagnoses

A. Depressive disorder

B. PTSD

C. Somatoform disorders (characterized by physical complaints lacking known medical basis or demonstrable physical findings in the presence of psychological factors)

D. Alcoholism and drug abuse/dependence

Plan

A. General interventions:

1. Evaluate the nature of the grief and any accompanying psychiatric symptoms.

2. Treat physical/laboratory findings as indicated.

3. Encourage the client to eat a healthy diet, exercise daily, and maintain normal sleep habits and activities.

4. Encourage support by family and friends.

5. Offer counseling with professional psychologist or group sessions.

6. Assess for depression at each office visit and treat accordingly.

▶ B. Client teaching: *See Section III: Client Teaching Guide for this chapter, "Grief."*

C. Pharmaceutical therapy: Antidepressants should not be prescribed for acute grief, but reserved for a possible subsequent major depression. Clinical data suggest that SSRIs may assist the client with mobilizing the energy necessary to assist him or her through the grieving process.

> Resist sedation of individuals suffering from acute grief because this tends to delay and prolong the mourning process. Refer to the "Depression" section for pharmaceutical therapy.

1. Drug of choice: sedative to help sleep

a. Sedative anxiolytic hypnotics may be prescribed for **no more than 2 weeks at a time.** Try initially for 1 week to establish a sleep pattern. If insomnia continues, refer the client to a specialist.

b. Temazepam (Restoril) 7.5 to 30 mg at bedtime *or* flurazepam (Dalmane) 15 to 30 mg at bedtime

c. Zolpidem (Ambien) 5 to 10 mg at bedtime (not to be used for more than 1 month)

2. Sedating antihistamines:

a. Hydroxyzine HCl (Atarax) 50 to 100 mg at bedtime

b. Hydroxyzine pamoate (Vistaril) 50 to 100 mg at bedtime **(not to be used for more than 4 months)**

3. Antidepressant with sedating properties:

a. Trazodone HCl (Desyrel) 50 to 100 mg at bedtime

b. Paroxetine (Paxil) 10 to 20 mg given at bedtime

c. Mirtazapine (Remeron) 15 mg every day at bedtime. Increase at 1 to 2 weeks: Usual range is 15 to 45 mg every day at bedtime.

Follow-Up

A. Follow up in 1 week to assess the client's status and symptoms.

B. Then follow up every 2 weeks to assess the client's progress.

C. Assess for depression and suicide at every office visit.

D. Once positive change is seen, the client can be seen monthly.

Consultation/Referral

A. Provide immediate referral/consult for continuing psychotherapy for severe depression and/or suicidal threats.

B. Consult with a prescribing psychiatric provider for evaluation of pharmacologic agents versus referral.

Individual Considerations

A. Pregnancy:

1. Miscarriage, stillbirth, and neonatal death should be considered a major loss and treated as a grief reaction.

2. Grief is also seen in pregnancy termination. The woman who terminates a pregnancy (regardless of gestational age and reason for termination) may exhibit a major response to this loss.

3. Hospitals often provide photographs, footprints, and identification bracelets of deceased baby and connect families with perinatal grief support groups.

4. Use the baby's name when discussing feelings about the loss of a child.

5. Suggest that friends and family not put away the baby clothes and bedroom furniture. The couple should do this as part of their closure process.

B. Pediatrics:

1. Grief in children may be delayed or difficult to identify.

2. Children who suddenly experience behavioral problems not present before the death of a significant person should be immediately referred to a child psychiatrist.

3. Children should not be told the deceased person is "asleep" or died because they were "sick"; this may cause fears of falling asleep and becoming sick themselves.

4. Use proper terms: heart attack, stroke, "Your baby brother had a congenital heart defect." Use the correct terms and draw pictures to help explain.

5. Young children do not understand death is forever and may continue to ask to see the deceased.

C. Adults:

1. Grief responses vary among individuals. Look for behaviors outside the norm.

D. Geriatrics:

1. Grief in the elderly should be closely assessed to rule out medical diagnoses.

E. Partners:

1. Involvement in grief/loss psychotherapy groups is extremely helpful.

Bibliography

Linde, K., Treml, J., Steinig, J., Nagl, M., & Kersting, A. (2017). Grief interventions for people bereaved by suicide: A systematic review. *PLOS ONE, 12*(6), e0179496. doi:10.1371/journal.pone.0179496

Sleep Disorders/Insomnia

Moya Cook and Alyson Wolz

Definition

Insomnia disorders are categorized as situational, persistent, or recurrent.

A. In normal sleepers, transient insomnia occurs in those who have traveled to another time zone (i.e., "jet lag"), are under situational stress, or are sleeping in unfamiliar surroundings. Treatment is not required in these situations because time takes care of the problem. With short-term insomnia, the normal sleeper experiences difficulty sleeping that does not resolve within a few days. This can be the result of stress, such as financial difficulty and/or divorce. These clients may require short-term symptomatic relief of insomnia.

B. Long-term insomnia is persistent and disabling. Studies suggest that 40% to 50% of these insomniacs have an associated psychiatric disorder, especially depression, an associated drug use/abuse/withdrawal problem, or an associated medical disorder.

C. Other types of sleep disorders:

1. Inadequate sleep hygiene: habitual behaviors that harm sleep, such as delaying morning awakening time or napping, use of electronic devices prior to hour of sleep, and interrupted sleep due to notifications on electronic devices

2. Insufficient sleep syndrome: curtailing time in bed in response to social and occupational demands over long periods of time (shift work, circadian rhythm sleep–wake disorder)

3. Adjustment sleep disorder: acute emotional stressors (job loss or hospitalization) resulting in difficulty falling asleep because of tension and anxiety

4. Psychophysiologic insomnia: anticipatory anxiety over the prospect of another night of sleeplessness and the next day of fatigue

5. Narcolepsy: persistent daytime sleepiness with brief naps accompanied by vivid dreams:

   a. Cataplexy or abrupt paralysis or paresis of skeletal muscles following anger, surprise, laughter, or physical exercise

   b. Hypnagogic hallucinations (vivid and often frightening dreams that occur shortly after falling asleep or on awakening)

   c. Sleep paralysis, a transient global paralysis of voluntary muscles that occurs shortly after falling asleep and lasts a few seconds or minutes

   d. Disturbed and restless sleep

Incidence

A. Difficulties with sleep are among the most common complaints of medical clients and affect a large percentage of the population. One third of adults express sleep-related complaints they consider to be serious. Sleep disorders also can affect proper mental functioning (53% of chronic insomniacs complain of memory difficulties). Sleep disorders are also implicated in decreased work efficiency, impaired industrial productivity, and increased risk of traffic accidents. They also seem to enhance the propensity for cardiovascular disease and increase the risk of death. Insomniacs are also at increased risk for the development of depression and anxiety disorders. Clients with obstructive sleep apnea (OSA) syndrome have significant performance impairments on complex motor tasks.

The risk of depression increases with time if insomnia is left untreated.

Pathogenesis

A. Other than situational stress, jet lag, and sleeping in unfamiliar surroundings, difficulty with sleep can be related to psychiatric illness or medical problems. It is most frequently due to chronic depression and/or anxiety. Antisocial and obsessive-compulsive features are also common among these clients. Clients may self-medicate, which produces more insomnia.

Predisposing Factors

A. Alcohol use: initially assists with sleep but produces fragmented sleep

B. Hypnotic medications can produce tolerance, which causes sleep disruption and rebound insomnia with withdrawal from the medication.

C. Substances such as caffeine, nicotine cigarettes, amphetamines, steroids, methylphenidate, hallucinogens, aminophylline, ephedrine, decongestants, bronchodilators, weight loss/diet pills, thyroid preparations, MAOIs, and anticancer agents

D. Women with fibromyalgia syndrome

E. Women experiencing menopausal symptoms

F. Upper respiratory symptoms

G. OSA disorders such as nasal obstruction, large uvula, low-lying soft palate, craniofacial abnormalities, excessive pharyngeal tissue, pharyngeal masses (tumors, cysts), macroglossia, tonsillar hypertrophy, and vocal cord paralysis

H. Obesity

I. Hypothyroidism

J. Acromegaly

K. Chronic pain

L. Urinary frequency possibly due to prostatism, diabetes, diuretics, and infection

Common Complaints

A. Statements regarding impaired sleep pattern:

1. Inability to fall asleep

2. Restless throughout the night

3. Early morning awakening with inability to fall back to sleep

4. Difficulty concentrating during the daytime hours

5. Feels fatigued after 8 hours of sleep, no energy

6. Partner complains of the client's snoring

Other Signs and Symptoms

A. Excessive daytime sleepiness

B. Feels tense, irritable, and agitated

C. Heightened anxiety and aggressiveness (occasionally)

D. Reports of prolonged pauses in respiration during sleep
E. Weight gain
F. Frontal headaches on awakening
G. Difficulty with short-term recall

Subjective Data

A. Review the onset, course, and duration of problems and symptoms.
B. Take a thorough history of the sleep problem, including the 24-hour sleep–wake cycle: sleep–wake habit history, sleep hygiene history, meal and exercise times, ambient noise, and light and temperature.
C. Identify the pattern: trouble falling asleep, trouble staying asleep (frequent awakenings), and early morning awakenings.
D. Inquire about life stresses, drug and alcohol use, and marital and family problems.

> Statements suggesting self-medication with alcohol to facilitate sleep could indicate a coexistent alcohol abuse/dependence diagnosis. In clients who have developed tolerance to alcohol or sleep medications, abrupt cessation of these agents may produce increased insomnia and anxiety.

E. Determine whether the insomnia is simply normal sleep. Some "insomniacs" get ample sleep (pseudoinsomnia) and the problems are psychological.
F. Review the client's smoking and caffeine intake history.
G. Review all medications, including prescribed and OTC medications, recreational drug use, and weight-loss medications.
H. Review the client's medical history: thyroid problems, hypertension, steroid use, diabetes, and cancer.
I. Conduct an interview with the client's bed partner to elicit information about snoring, breathing pauses, and unusual body positions or movements. Is the partner concerned/frightened about the apneic pauses?
J. Review cardiopulmonary dysfunction: orthopnea, paroxysmal nocturnal dyspnea, or nocturnal angina.
K. If female, establish past menses to rule out pregnancy or menopause. Is there regular menses, vaginal dryness, and/or hot flashes?
L. If male, review for signs of prostatism (greater than age 50 years, hesitancy, dribbling, nocturia, frequency, incomplete emptying, and so on). *See Section III: Client Teaching Guide, "Prostatic Hypertrophy/Benign."*

Physical Examination

A. Check pulse, respirations, blood pressure, and weight.
B. Inspect:
   1. Observe general overall appearance; note grooming and behaviors during interview.
   2. Evaluate eyes: pupil dilation/constriction (may indicate recent medication/nonprescription drug use).
   3. Inspect nasal mucosa for erythema, edema, discharge, and nasal patency; look for septal deviation and polyps. Transluminate sinus (if indicated).
   4. Inspect the mouth for erythema, the teeth for uneven surfaces (grinding), and the retropharynx for abnormality.

C. Auscultate:
   1. Heart
   2. Lungs
   3. Abdomen
D. Palpate:
   1. Conduct a neurologic examination.
   2. Palpate the neck and thyroid; note goiter.
   3. Check the joints for swelling, arthritis, and ROM to rule out musculoskeletal cause.
   4. Rectal examination if indicated for men with prostate symptoms.
   5. Perform speculum/bimanual examination if indicated to evaluate menopausal atrophy and bladder complaints.

Diagnostic Tests

A. CBC with differential
B. Electrolytes
C. TSH or full thyroid profile, FSH, LH
D. Prostate-specific antigen (PSA) for men
E. Serum creatinine and BUN
F. Urinalysis: check hematuria
G. Urine culture (if indicated)
H. Glucose tolerance test
I. Urine drug screen
J. Sinus x-rays
K. Urodynamics tests if bladder issues suspected
L. Postvoid residual (catheterization or ultrasound)
M. Nocturnal polysomnography or actigraphy
N. Psychiatric evaluation if indicated

Differential Diagnoses

A. Insomnia/sleep disorder
B. Alcoholism and drug abuse/dependence
C. Major depressive disorder
D. Acute psychosis, mania, and hypomania
E. Medical problems such as chronic pain, anxiety, depression, hyperthyroidism, epilepsy, general paresis, diabetes, benign prostatic hypertrophy, urinary problems related to age/diuretic use, cardiopulmonary dysfunction, and menopause

Plan

A. General interventions:
   1. Identify cause of insomnia
   2. Treat physical/laboratory findings if underlying condition exists. Treat condition according to diagnosis made, that is, hormone replacement therapy, thyroid medications, diabetes, and so forth, as indicated.
B. Client teaching:
   1. Have the client record a 2-week log for sleep–wake habits. A sleep diary is available from the National Sleep Foundation at https://sleepfoundation.org.
   2. Advise the client to avoid alcohol, caffeine, and stimulating agents during the evening hours.
   3. Avoid exercising before going to bed.
   4. Encourage smoking cessation. Avoid smoking in the evening hours. *See Section III: Client Teaching Guide, "Nicotine Dependence."*

5. Encourage regular sleep habit/hygiene. Recommend going to bed the same time every night and waking up the same time every day.
6. Recommend keeping the bedroom cool, quiet, and dark while sleeping.
7. Encourage relaxation exercises before going to bed.
8. If stress/anxiety contributes to sleeping disorder, recommend counseling with psychologist or counselor to identify and deal with issues.
9. *See Section III: Client Teaching Guide for this chapter, "Sleep Disorders/Insomnia."*
C. Pharmaceutical therapy:
1. Eliminate prescription medications (when possible) and OTC products as part of management plan *before writing another prescription.*
2. Only after making the assumption that the insomnia cannot be adequately treated by addressing the underlying medical problem responsible for causing the insomnia should medications for sleep be prescribed.

> Do not prescribe medications for sleep to clients with alcohol/drug or depressive disorders.

3. Use short-term pharmaceutical therapy.
4. Drug of choice: *sedative anxiolytic hypnotics:* try initially for 1 week to establish a sleep pattern:

> If insomnia continues for more than 1 month, refer the client to a sleep specialist.

a. Temazepam (Restoril) 7.5 to 30 mg at bedtime (1–2 weeks)
b. Flurazepam (Dalmane) 15 to 30 mg at bedtime (1–2 weeks)
c. Zolpidem (Ambien) 5 to 10 mg at bedtime (4 weeks maximum)
d. Zolpidem XR (Ambien XR) 6.25 to 12.5 mg at bedtime
e. Eszopiclone (Lunesta) 2 to 3 mg at bedtime; start with 1 mg in the elderly
f. Ramelteon (Rozerem) 8 mg by mouth 30 minutes before bedtime; do not take with meals
g. Suvorexant (Belsomra) 10 to 20 mg by mouth 30 minutes before bedtime

> Anxiolytic agents, such as diazepam (Valium) and alprazolam (Xanax), tend to increase the duration and frequency of sleep apneas and are contraindicated for clients with possible/undiagnosed apnea spells.

5. **Sedating antihistamines are not recommended for use over 4 months.**
a. Hydroxyzine HCl (Atarax) 50 to 100 mg at bedtime
b. Hydroxyzine pamoate (Vistaril) 50 to 100 mg at bedtime

6. Antidepressants with sedating properties:
a. Trazodone HCl (Desyrel) 50 to 100 mg at bedtime
b. Paroxetine (Paxil) 10 to 20 mg at bedtime

Follow-Up
A. Follow up at 1 week to assess the client's status.
B. Then, follow up every 2 weeks to check the client's progress.
C. Once positive change is seen, the client can be seen monthly as needed.
D. Assess the client's potential for suicide with every office visit.
E. If coexisting medication conditions exist, refer to medical diagnosis for follow-up recommendations.

Consultation/Referral
A. Refer to a psychiatric clinician for medication management and psychotherapy after initial assessment if psychiatric differential diagnosis is made.
B. Refer for psychological testing.
C. If insomnia continues for more than 1 month, refer to a physician if the client requires a sedative anxiolytic hypnotic for more than 4 weeks.

Individual Considerations
A. Pregnancy:
1. Sleep difficulties are more prevalent in second and third trimesters of pregnancy because of the growing size of the uterus and difficulty finding comfortable sleeping positions. Treat with comfort measures.
B. Pediatrics:
1. Children normally require about 10 hours of sleep.
2. Children younger than 18 years with sleep problems should be referred to a pediatrician or pediatric psychiatrist, depending on clinical findings.
C. Adults:
1. The "right" amount of sleep results in optimal daytime alertness and a sense of mental efficiency and well-being.
2. Daytime naps often interfere with the quality of night sleep. Encourage eliminating naps during the day.
3. Nocturia and disturbed sleep are the symptoms that cause older men to seek medical help with prostatism.
D. Geriatrics:
1. With aging, it is normal for sleep time to decrease (<7 hours), with a tendency toward sleep fragmentation and an increase in the frequency of awakenings and brief arousals. Explain this to older adults to avoid "worry over sleeplessness."
2. Always assess for depression in elderly clients.
3. Start with the lowest dose of pharmaceutical agents.
4. Chronic pain is a leading cause for sleep disruption in elderly persons with degenerative joint pain.
5. Review elderly clients' medications and dosage for insomnia because of known side effects or as a medication toxicity.

6. Gastroesophageal reflux is commonly seen in geriatric clients at nighttime and causes them to wake up at night. Correcting the reflux with sleeping position, avoiding late night meals and spicy food, prescribing medications (proton pump inhibitors [PPIs]), and making possible weight-loss interventions could improve sleep disturbance in these clients.

7. Clients with end-stage renal disease may have nocturnal leg movement disorders and anemia due to renal failure. Improving the anemia will improve the insomnia and will decrease the leg movements.

E. Partners:

1. Those who find it necessary to sleep in another room because of their partner's snoring should refer the snorer to the primary care physician/advanced practice nurse to rule out an OSA syndrome.

Resource

National Sleep Foundation: www.sleepfoundation.org

Bibliography

National Sleep Foundation. (n.d.). *National Sleep Foundation sleep diary*. Retrieved from https://sleepfoundation.org/search/node/sleep%20diary

Qaseem, A., Kansagara, D., Forciea, M., Cooke, M., & Denberg, T. (2016). Management of chronic insomnia disorder in adults: A clinical practice guideline from the American College of Physicians. *Annals of Internal Medicine, 165*, 125–133. doi:10.7326/M15-2175

Suicide

Moya Cook and Alyson Wolz

Definition

A. Suicide is defined as the intentional destruction of one's own life. It is the most critical consequence of mental illness and occurs in all diagnostic psychiatric categories. Therefore, knowing the risk factors for suicide and eliciting key clinical features that differentiate the truly suicidal client from the attention seeker are of utmost importance. **Symptoms are often missed because they can be very subtle. Because there are important legal, social, and religious implications to suicide, the general healthcare practitioner should not attempt to treat these high-risk clients. This section focuses on identifying the suicidal client for immediate referral to a psychiatrist or psychiatric inpatient facility.**

Incidence

A. Approximately 15% of clients with recurrent depressive illness commit suicide.

B. Approximately 75% of suicides are due to depressive illness (jumps to 90% if other mental illnesses and substance abuse are included).

C. It is estimated that 75% of people who attempt suicide have seen their primary care provider within the 6 weeks prior to the attempt.

D. Suicide is the **10th leading cause of death** in the United States; for young people between the ages of 15 and 24 years it is the second leading cause of death.

The United States averages 13 suicides per 100,000 population annually. Every year more than 38,000 people take their own lives, not including those individuals who die as a result of fatal accidents due to impaired concentration and attention, and death due to illnesses that may be sequelae (e.g., alcohol abuse).

According to the World Health Organization (WHO), by the year 2020, depression will be the number two cause, worldwide, of individuals losing healthy years of their lives. Estimates associate 16,000 suicides in the United States annually with depressive disorder. Fifteen percent of those hospitalized for major depressive disorder attempt suicide. Fifteen percent of clients with severe primary major depressive disorder of at least 1 month's duration eventually commit suicide.

The rate of suicide in young adults has more than doubled since 1950. Midlife suicide rates tend to be highest among White men, although female suicide rates peak in midlife. Males are three to four times more likely to complete suicide, but females are three times more likely to attempt suicide. Whites are twice as likely as non-Whites to commit suicide, although in the 25- to 34-year age group they are equal. Rates for widowed, divorced, or separated individuals are higher than for those who are married. Rates are highest in Protestants, intermediate in Jews, and lowest in Catholics.

Pathogenesis

A. Recent studies confirm that some changes in the noradrenergic system along with reduced serotonin levels are associated with suicide. In recent studies independent of psychiatric diagnoses, one researcher identified a suicidality syndrome consisting of hopelessness, ruminative thinking, social withdrawal, and lack of activity as core symptoms.

B. Familial, genetic, early life-loss experiences, and comorbid alcoholism may be causal factors. In adolescence, depression is the largest single risk factor for suicidal behavior, although family relationship difficulties make a significant independent contribution to this. Environmental stressors in the presence of psychiatric disorders may also be responsible for initiating the impulsive behavior leading to suicide. The risk of suicidal behaviors is higher in those with mental disorders than those with mood disorders.

Predisposing Factors

A. **SAD PERSONAS**

   S = sex
   A = age
   D = depression
   P = previous attempts
   E = ethanol abuse
   R = rational thinking loss
   S = social support loss
   O = organized plan
   N = no spouse
   A = availability of lethal means
   S = sickness

Also, consider gender, race and ethnicity, medications, and other medical conditions.

Common Complaints

A. Overt or indirect suicide talk or threats: "You won't be bothered by me much longer."

> Any mention of dying or ending one's life must be taken seriously.

B. Depressed or anxious mood due to depression

> Every depressed client must be assessed for suicide risk.

C. Significant recent loss such as spouse, job, or self-esteem
D. Unexpected change in behavior, such as making a will, intense talks with friends, and giving away possessions
E. Unexpected change in attitude, such as suddenly cheerful, angry, or withdrawn
F. Atypical symptoms of depression in the elderly, such as impaired ability to communicate, intractable tinnitus, and feelings of helplessness

Other Signs and Symptoms

Indications for hospitalization of suicidal clients:
A. Psychosis
B. Intoxication with drugs or alcohol that cannot be evaluated and treated over a period of time in the ED
C. No change in affect or symptoms despite the intervention of the physician, family, and friends
D. Command hallucinations
E. Lack of access to, or low availability of, outpatient resources
F. Family exhaustion
G. Escalating number of suicide attempts
H. Uncertainty about the risk of suicide
I. Severe psychic anxiety, anxious ruminations, and global insomnia are acute risk factors.

Subjective Data

A. Ascertain the client's intention. Ask why he or she wants to die.
    1. Asking the client about suicide does not give the client any ideas about suicide.
B. Determine whether the client has thought of a suicide plan. The more specific the plan, the more likely the act. A well-worked out, realistic, and potentially lethal plan suggests great risk.
C. Rule out the presence of psychiatric or organic factors such as psychotic depression, thought disorder, or sedative self-medication.
D. Determine whether the precipitating crisis is resolving satisfactorily to the client.
E. Take an "inventory of loss." Determine the losses the client has incurred in the past several months or years.
F. Review the client's plans for the future.
G. Determine whether the client thinks he or she is going to commit suicide.

H. Evaluate whether the client has a caring family or other support systems.

Physical Examination

A. Check pulse, respirations, blood pressure, and weight.
B. Inspect:
    1. Observe overall appearance; note grooming, tone of voice, conduct of client during communication.
    2. Complete dermal examination. Check for physical evidence of suicidal behavior such as wrist lacerations or rope burns around the neck. Look for signs of substance use.
C. Auscultate:
    1. Heart
    2. Lungs
    3. Abdomen (as applies to physical complaints)
D. Palpate:
    1. The neck and thyroid; note goiter
    2. Axilla and groin for lymphadenopathy (infectious etiology)
E. Neurologic examination:
    1. Complete mental status review: Specific concern exists when client displays a flat affect when discussing thoughts or plans for suicide.
    2. Assess for thought disorder: Is the client having command hallucinations telling him or her to harm or kill him- or herself? Is the client having delusions or a strong sense of "burdensomeness," thinking that others will be better off without him or her?
    3. Is the client exhibiting obsession with taking his or her own life?

Diagnostic Tests

A. CBC with differential
B. Electrolytes, serum calcium, and phosphorus
C. Thyroid profile
D. Liver profile
E. BUN, creatinine
F. Blood alcohol
G. Urine drug screen
H. EKG
I. RPR
J. CT and MRI scans
K. Perform the MMSE to rule out dementia/delirium.
L. Perform suicide assessment using an assessment tool such as the Suicide Behavior Questionnaire-Revised (SBQ-R) available at www.integration.samhsa.gov/images/res/SBQ.pdf.

Differential Diagnoses

A. Mood disorder due to another medical condition
B. Adjustment disorder with depressed mood
C. Personality disorder
D. Psychotic disorder
E. Alcoholism and drug abuse/dependence
F. Dementia/delerium
G. Side effect of medication (antidepressants, antipsychotics)

Plan

A. General interventions:

1. If the client is suicidal, refer immediately. Make sure there is someone with the client at all times.

2. If the client came to the office alone, call a family member or friend to accompany the client to the hospital ED or treatment center.

3. If you are fearful the client will try to escape or leave unaccompanied, call an ambulance to escort the client to the hospital ED where commitment papers for involuntary hospital admission can be completed.

> Documentation is critical. Make sure all statements are recorded and the decision-making process followed.

> Be sure to advise the hospital staff of your concerns regarding the client's suicidal status.

B. Client teaching:

1. Educate client and family regarding treatment with medication for depression. Discuss benefits/risks of medication and side effects.

2. Encourage the client to enroll in counseling with a psychologist/therapist to discuss current problems/needs.

3. Determine whether social services needs to be contacted for client to provide support services.

4. Provide local resources for counseling and social services as appropriate.

5. If the client is not hospitalized, make sure that family or friends are aware of the client's status and that he or she has someone to talk to and monitor his or her condition until the next office appointment.

C. Pharmaceutical therapy:

1. See this chapter for sections on "Depression" and/or "Bipolar Disorder" for complete pharmacological interventions for specific mood disorders.

2. Antidepressants such as SSRIs, SNRIs, and anti-anxiety medications can help to reduce symptoms of depression and severe anxiety, which may help the client to feel less suicidal.

3. Clozapine is an FDA-approved medication for reduction of suicidal behavior in clients with schizophrenia.

4. Quetiapine and lithium have been shown to prevent suicide in clients with bipolar depression.

Follow-Up

A. After emergency admission for suicidal ideation or threats, clients should be closely observed, especially in the first year after the serious suicide attempt.

B. With each visit, question the client regarding suicidal ideation or a plan (see "Subjective Data" section for important questions to ask).

Consultation/Referral

A. Consult with the client's psychiatric practitioner. Obtain a release of information from the client.

B. Be sure the client continues to follow up with psychiatric counseling and medication management (see "Depression" section).

Individual Considerations

A. Pregnancy:

1. A woman with a history of depression or previous postpartum depression is at high risk for postpartum depression (recurrent) (see "Postpartum Depression" section in Chapter 13, "Obstetrics Guidelines").

B. Adolescents:

1. Teens are at risk after recent losses from death (especially if one of their friends/family commits suicide). Recent loss includes breaking up with a boyfriend or girlfriend.

2. If a teen has had a depressive episode, he or she may be at a higher risk if he or she suddenly seems happy and things are "just fine." The teen may have decided on a suicide plan and is experiencing a sense of relief because he or she has made plans.

C. Geriatrics:

1. Suicide is the eighth leading cause of death in males older than 65 years.

2. Older persons use the usual means for suicide as well as a slower plan, including not eating, stopping prescription drugs or overmedicating, increasing alcohol intake, and refusing treatment.

3. The elderly population is more susceptible to the adverse effects of medications.

4. Antidepressants should be started at the lowest doses and slowly increased for the elderly. The SSRIs are considered the first line of antidepressant therapy in the elderly population (see "Depression" section in this chapter).

Resource

National Alliance on Mental Illness. (2016). NAMI family support group: https://www.nami.org/Local-NAMI/Programs?classkey=72e2fdaf-2755-404f-a8be-606d4de63fdb

Bibliography

Beck Institute for Cognitive Behavior Therapy. (2013). *Identifying suicide risk*. Retrieved from https://www.beckinstitute.org/identifying-suicide-risk.

Linde, K., Treml, J., Steinig, J., Nagl, M., & Kersting, A. (2017). Grief interventions for people bereaved by suicide: A systematic review. *PLOS ONE, 12*(6), e0179496. doi:10.1371/journal.pone.0179496

Osman, A., Bagge, C., Guitierrez, P., Konick, L., Kooper, B., & Barrios, F. (2001). The suicidal behaviors questionnaire-revised (SBQ-R): Validation with clinical and nonclinical samples. *Assessment, 8*(4), 443–454. doi:10.1177/107319110100800409. Retrieved from http://www.integration.samhsa.gov/images/res/SBQ.pdf

Patterson, W. M., Dohn, H. H., Bird, J., & Patterson, G. A. (1983). Evaluation of suicidal clients: The SAD PERSONS scale. *Psychosomatics, 24*(4), 348–349, 343–345. doi:10.1016/S0033-3182(83)73213-5

Suicide Awareness Voices of Education. (2003–2013). *Suicide facts*. Retrieved from http://www.save.org/about-suicide/suicide-facts

World Health Organization. (2019). *Suicide fact sheet*. Retrieved from https://www.who.int/news-room/fact-sheets/detail/suicide

23 Assessment Guide for Sport Participation

Mariya Tankimovich

Student athletes who plan to participate in sport activities are required by most states to have a preparticipation sports physical examination (American Academy of Family Physicians et al., 2015; Mirabelli, Devine, Singh, & Mendoza, 2015; Roberts et al., 2014). School districts and individual schools customarily provide a form to be completed by healthcare providers for reviewing health history and completing physical examinations. Other organizations, for example, Boy Scouts of America, require participation clearance forms for participation in different activities as well (https://www.scouting.org/health-and-safety/ahmr/). These forms may be found on organization websites. The primary goals of preparticipation examination are (a) to assure that the student is safe to participate in the specified sport; (b) to assess the growth and development of the person, evaluating maturation and size of the athlete; (c) to identify any congenital or new anomalies/conditions that would pose a threat of injury with activity; (d) to assess the preparticipation condition of the athlete that would put the athlete at risk while participating in the sport; and (e) to eliminate any unnecessary barriers that would restrict the student's participation in the identified sport.

Ideally, the examination should be performed several weeks (typically 6 weeks) before season activity. In the event that any conditions need to be addressed, this time frame would allow adequate time for evaluation and resolution, if possible, of the problem before participation in the sport. There is controversy regarding the frequency of these sports examinations; however, many states address this frequency and/or resort to an annual physical examination. The annual examination would suffice for each sport that the athlete is engaged in throughout the academic year.

The physical examination may be performed by the primary care provider or by multiple providers in a multistation setting. Multistation examination settings are frequently arranged by schools. Each station has a specialty provider who assesses a particular part of the body. The evaluation includes blood pressure, pulse, respiration, height, weight, body mass index (BMI), vision, dental and physical examination, musculoskeletal examination, nutrition, flexibility/strength, speed/agility, and balance. A lead primary care provider evaluates the results from each substation and determines the clearance of the athlete. The American Academy of Pediatrics (AAP) has developed four forms to use for completing the athlete history and physical examination.

The sports physical forms are available on the AAP website at https://www.aap.org/en-us/about-the-aap/Councils/Council-on-Sports-Medicine-and-Fitness/Pages/Preparticipation-Physical-Evaluation.aspx.
A. Preparticipation Physical Evaluation History Form
B. Preparticipation Physical Evaluation Physical Examination Form
C. Preparticipation Physical Evaluation Clearance Form
D. Preparticipation Physical Evaluation of the Athlete With Special Needs: Supplemental History

A thorough medical history is imperative to identify potential risk factors for the athlete. A complete review of systems should be discussed with the athlete to identify possible risks. Prior personal conditions/injuries should be reviewed and assessed, such as previous head concussions (Bernhardt, 2015). See "Mild Traumatic Brain Injury" in Chapter 19, Neurologic Guidelines Section for assessment and treatment guidelines. The morbidity rate increases with repetitive head concussions and new guidelines are emerging regarding assessment and clearance for athletes with a history of head concussions.

Dizziness or syncope episodes should be evaluated. There are many causes for these symptoms; however, cardiac conditions can present with these symptoms and an in-depth cardiac evaluation should be performed (Sharma, Merghani, & Gati, 2015). There are conflicting recommendations on routine cardiac screening for all athletes because of the poor sensitivity and high false-positive rates of the EKG. At this time, the American Heart Association recommends a screening history and physical examination, unless further screening is warranted. A thorough family history should also be obtained. An athlete with a family history of conditions such as exercise-related deaths or heart attacks before the age of 50 years should be further evaluated.

Previous injuries, illnesses, fractures, or other trauma should be evaluated for complete resolution and healing.

Prior history of heat illness poses a higher risk for recurrence. Prior surgery or other procedures need to be assessed to document that the athlete has been released by the surgeon and there is no risk involved with participation in the sport.

Flexibility and endurance should also be evaluated and are commonly performed by sport trainers. There are several techniques available to assess flexibility and endurance. Flexibility may be assessed by having the athlete perform range of motion of extremities and comparing the left side to the right side. A goniometer is an instrument that is useful to measure the motion of specific joints. Active and passive range of motion can be used to assess the joints. Normal degrees of range of motion of particular joints can be found at http://highered.mheducation.com.

Lower extremity range of motion can be assessed by a "sit-and-reach" test. Examples of the "sit-and-reach" and other methods of evaluation can be found on the Top End Sports website (Wood, 2008) at www.topendsports.com/testing/tests/sit-and-reach.htm.

Endurance can be evaluated by having the athlete perform a timed test, such as measuring the distance run in a 12-minute period. Routine blood work is not recommended at this time.

Clearance for sport participation is determined once the history and examination are completed. There are different levels of clearance depending on the sport. AAP has developed two classifications of participation, depending on the level of contact in each sport. The athlete may be cleared for all sports without restriction or may be cleared for all sports without restriction with further evaluation or treatment for the particular condition diagnosed at the time of examination. An example of the latter is an athlete with a history of well-controlled exercise-induced asthma. Clearance may be denied at the time of examination and the athlete given further recommendations.

Common conditions in which the athlete may be disqualified for clearance to participate in the sport include dizziness with exercise, asthma history, musculoskeletal abnormality, heart murmur, visual impairment, elevation in blood pressure, and/or BMI outside of normal parameters.

Athletes with concerns regarding their medical history or examination and unsure of how clearance status is determined can review the AAP guidelines for clearance for sports participation, which is available for purchase as an eBook at https://shop.aap.org/preparticipation-physical-evaluation-4th-edition-ebook/.

The time spent with the athlete during the physical examination also provides an opportunity to discuss prevalent risk behaviors and issues he or she may be experiencing at that time. In addition, this is an ideal time to review preventive health strategies to help the athlete achieve his or her optimal health and participate at his or her fullest ability. Topics to consider discussing include:

A. Preventive care: Use of proper gear and safety equipment for each particular sport, such as mouth guards, goggles, proper fitting head gear/helmets, and so forth, are important for the athlete to prevent injury and enhance his or her best performance.

B. Injury prevention: Correct techniques of stretching, warming up, and cooling down should be encouraged during every practice and sport. Stretching properly can prevent musculoskeletal injuries.

C. Chronic conditions: Use of proper medications for chronic conditions, such as asthma, is imperative to prevent complications. Proper use of the rescue inhaler before exercise should be reinforced. Proper administration of the inhaler should also be reviewed. See Chapter 9, Respiratory Guidelines, "Asthma" for assessment and treatment. *See Client Teaching Guides in Section III, "Asthma: Action Plan and Peak Flow Monitoring"* and *"Asthma: How to Use a Metered-Dose Inhaler"* for educational material.

D. Substance abuse: Education about abstinence regarding substance abuse (drugs, alcohol, and tobacco). See Chapter 2, Public Health Guidelines, "Substance Use Disorders" for screening questions and treatment. Discuss the detrimental effects of each substance on the body and the way studies show that athletes who use these substances have decreased performance. Long-term risks, such as dependence, cancer, and death, should also be discussed.

E. Depression: Screening for depression should be incorporated into the examination. See Chapter 22, Psychiatric Guidelines, "Depression" for screening questions and treatment.

F. Domestic violence: assess for domestic violence by observing bruising, scars, cigarette burns, and so forth. See the section "Children" under "Violence" in Chapter 2, Public Health Guidelines for assessment and treatment guidelines.

G. Bullying: Bullying takes different forms and roles (the perpetrator or the victim). Assist the family in ending inappropriate behavior by offering counseling services and interventions to end the problem (Pigozi & Bartoli, 2016).

H. Nutrition: Eating disorders are commonly seen in student athlete population. See the Section "Nutrition" in Chapter 1, Health Maintenance Guidelines, for assessment and education for the athlete's nutrition. Discuss and stress the importance of hydration during the sporting event to prevent dehydration and explain the ways dehydration can affect the body and performance.

Bibliography

American Academy of Family Physicians, American Academy of Pediatrics, American College of Sports Medicine, American Medical Society for Sports Medicine. (2015). *Preparticipation physical evaluation* (4th ed.). Elk Grove Village, IL: American Academy of Pediatrics.

Bernhardt, D. T. (2015). Concussion. *Medscape*. Retrieved from www.medscape.com

Boy Scouts of America. (2019). *Annual health and medical record*. Retrieved from www.scouting.org/health-and-safety/ahmr/

Mirabelli, M. H., Devine, M. J., Singh, J., & Mendoza, M. (2015). The preparticipation sports evaluation. *American Family Physician, 92*(5), 371–376.

Pigozi, P. L., & Jones Bartoli, A. (2016). School nurses' experiences in dealing with bullying situations among students. *Journal of School Nursing:*

The Official Publication of the National Association of School Nurses, *32*(3), 177–185.

Roberts, W. O., Löllgen, H., Matheson, G. O., Royalty, A. B., Meeuwisse, W. H., Levine, B., … Pigozzi, F. (2014). Advancing the preparticipation physical evaluation: An ACSM and FIMS joint consensus statement. *Clinical Journal of Sport Medicine: Official Journal of the Canadian Academy of Sport Medicine, 24*(6), 442–447.

Sharma, S., Merghani, A., & Gati, S. (2015). Cardiac screening of young athletes prior to participation in sports: Difficulties in detecting the fatally flawed among the fabulously fit. *JAMA Internal Medicine, 175*(1), 125–127.

Wood, R. (2008). *Sit and reach test.* Top End Sports website. Retrieved from www.topendsports.com/testing/tests/sit-and-reach.htm

II

PROCEDURES

Canalith Repositioning (Epley) Procedure for Vertigo

Cheryl A. Glass

Description

A. Benign paroxysmal positional vertigo (BPPV) occurs with changing position and rapid head movement causes imbalance, disorientation, and nausea. Vertigo develops when there is a disturbance of the crystals that are normally evenly distributed in the fluid-filled semicircular canal and they become clumped together. Often the imbalance can be corrected by performing canalith repositioning (Epley maneuver) to redistribute the crystals in the vestibule.

Indications

A. BPPV

Contraindications

A. **Testing should never be done in the case of head injury or suspected or confirmed cervical spine injury/ dysfunction, severe kyphoscoliosis, a history of unstable carotid disease, or recent retinal detachment.**

Equipment Required

A. Examination table
B. Stool at the head of the table for the practitioner

Procedure

A. Explain the procedure (see Figure II.1).
B. Have the client sit on the examination table (position 1):
   1. Reposition the client to sitting in the center of the table.
   2. The edge at the head of the table should be at the client's shoulder height (head will hang off the table).
   3. Your position will be at the head of the examination table, and you will use the stool for comfort while holding the client's head with your hand.
C. Rapidly lay the client down (position 2).
   1. The client's head should be hanging over the table in a slightly downward tilt, supported by both of your hands.
   2. The client should be instructed to keep his or her eyes open and try to focus on a stationary object on

Particles in semicircular canal

FIGURE II.1 Epley procedure for vertigo.

Source: From the *Merck Manual Consumer Version* (known as the Merck Manual in the United States and Canada and the MSD Manual in the rest of the world), edited by Robert Porter. Copyright 2016 by Merck Sharp & Dohme Corp., a subsidiary of Merck & Co, Inc, Kenilworth, NJ. Retrieved from http://www .merckmanuals.com/consumer.

the wall throughout the positions on his or her back and sides.

3. The client's head is turned to the same side as the affected ear with the provider supporting the head.

   a. If the client has vertigo affecting both inner ears, turn the client's head to the dominantly affected side.

   b. As an alternative to just turning the head, the client may quickly turn and lie down on the affected side while you support the head with both of your hands.

4. After a few minutes, the client will be ready to be repositioned as evidenced by his or her lack of nystagmus (rhythmic side-to-side eye movement) and confirmation that the dizziness has stabilized.

D. Turn the client's head in the opposite direction while you continue to support the head (position 3). Again, the head should be in a slightly downward tilt.

1. If the client was using the side-lying position, have him or her turn to his or her back.

2. Have the client continue to keep the eyes open and focus on a stationary object on the wall.

3. Again, the time lapse to repositioning is evidenced by the lack of nystagmus and subjective confirmation that the dizziness has stabilized or abated.

E. Ask the client to roll from his or her back to the opposite side (or from the back to the opposition side; position 4). The client's head should be parallel to the floor.

F. With the client side-lying (position 5), have him or her quickly turn only his or her face to the floor, while you are supporting the head.

G. After the client verbalizes that the dizziness has abated from side-lying (position 5):

1. The client is to swing the legs to the edge of the table and quickly sit up.

2. He or she will continue to feel vertigo at this point.

H. Assist the client off the examination table.

I. The client should be instructed to be in a sitting position or with the head no farther back than a 45-degree angle for the next 24 hours.

J. The Epley does not immediately stop the vertigo. The client may begin to feel better within a few days.

K. If the Epley procedure needs to be repeated, allow 1 week between attempts.

Cervical Evaluation During Pregnancy: Bimanual Examination

Cheryl A. Glass

Description

A. The bimanual examination is a digital evaluation of the cervix with the index and middle fingers of the examiner's hand.

Indications

A. To assess cervical dilation, effacement, presentation of the fetus, and position and station of fetal presenting part

B. The cervix may be assigned a Bishop score to evaluate cervical change and to determine difficulty/ease with induction of labor. There is an inherent subjective difference among examiners; however, the Bishop score can be used to evaluate preterm labor cervical changes over time (see Table II.1).

Precautions

A. **Bimanual examination should never be performed when there is suspicion of or history of documented placenta previa. Vaginal bleeding in second or third trimester of pregnancy should be treated as placenta previa until this is ruled out.**

B. **Suspicion of ruptured membranes with preterm contractions: first perform sterile speculum examination to assess for rupture. Then, if membranes are intact, proceed with bimanual examination.**

C. If membranes are ruptured in the absence of active labor, avoid bimanual examination until frequent, painful uterine contractions are present.

Equipment Required

A. Gloves (nonsterile if membranes are intact; sterile if suspicion of or documented ruptured membranes)

B. Water-soluble lubricant (sterile lubricant required if membranes are ruptured)

C. Examination table or bed

Procedure

A. Stand at the foot of the examination table or sit near the foot of the bed and face the client.

B. Place the client in the lithotomy position, or have the client draw knees up and allow knees to drop to opposite sides.

C. Suggest relaxation techniques to reduce discomfort. If the client is in active labor, the cervix will be tender.

D. Place lubricant on the index and middle fingers of the examining hand.

E. Inform the client of each step before performance. Touch inner thigh first, then touch posterior portion of introitus and introduce gloved fingers into the vagina. Encourage the client to relax pelvic muscles (a deep breath will often encourage relaxation).

F. Palpate the cervix and lower uterine segment evaluating (see Figure II.2):

Score	0	1	2	3
Dilation	0	1–2	3–4	5–6
Percentage effacement	0%–30%	40%–50%	60%–70%	80% or more
Station	–3	–2	–1 to 0	+1 to +2
Consistency	Firm	Medium	Soft	–
Position	Posterior	Mid	Anterior	–

TABLE II.1   BISHOP SCORING

Total score: 0 to 5 = difficult induction; ≥6 = easy induction.

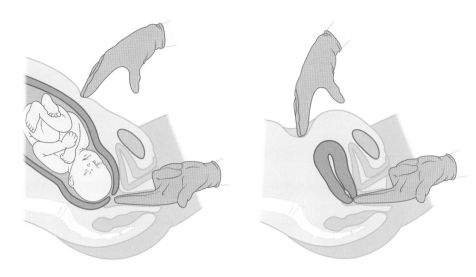

FIGURE II.2 Bimanual examination.

1. Dilatation
2. Effacement
3. Station
4. Consistency (softness)
5. Anterior versus midposition versus posterior placement of the cervix
6. In cases of preterm uterine contractions, it is helpful to assess the development of the lower uterine segment. A well-developed lower uterine segment (even in the absence of cervical dilation or effacement) is often a sign of preterm labor.

7. Note fetal presentation and station of the presenting part. Use ischial spines as landmarks to determine fetal descent through the pelvis.
8. If the fetus is sufficiently descended into the pelvis, determine the position of the presenting part.
9. If present, note bag of amniotic membranes. A bulging bag, known as a "forebag," may be present, even in the presence of documented ruptured membranes.
G. Following the examination, note if blood or vaginal discharge is on gloves.

Clock-Draw Test

Cheryl A. Glass

Description

The clock-draw test (CDT) is a quick screening tool assessing visuospatial and praxis abilities (may reflect both attention and executive dysfunction). The tool can be used by itself or as a complement to other screening tests. The test is a component of the Mini-Cog and also the "7-Minute Neurocognitive Screening Battery." It can be administered repeatedly over time to evaluate deterioration of function. The CDT evaluates:

A. Orientation
B. Conceptualization of time
C. Visual spatial organization
D. Visual memory
E. Auditory comprehension
F. Numeric knowledge
G. Concentration
H. Frustration tolerance

Indications

A. Evaluation of dementia
B. Evaluation of delirium
C. Evaluation of neurologic insult:
   1. Head trauma
   2. Stroke
   3. Alcohol and drug use
D. Evaluation of psychiatric illness:
   1. Schizophrenia
   2. Psychotic state

Administering the CDT

A. A number of variations can be used in administering the CDT.

The CDT is not a timed test. There is no limitation to administration time, although the test generally takes 1 to 2 minutes. However, in the Mini-Cog test, if the clock is not completed within 3 minutes, the client should proceed with word recall.

General Information

A. Provide the client with an 8.5 by 11 inches blank sheet of paper and a pencil with a predrawn clock and pencil.
B. Instructions can be repeated if necessary.
C. Clients may use their nondominant hand.
D. The ages for CDT testing are for adults 18 to 64 and the elderly (age 65+ years).

Setup

A. Equipment required includes a sheet of paper with a predrawn clock, a pen, and a chair or table for ease of drawing.
B. A clock should not be visible to the client during the CDT.

Client Instructions

The following instructions are given:
A. If using a blank page, instruct the client to:
   1. Draw a clock face.

   2. Place all of the numbers on the clock.
   3. Draw hands pointing to 10 minutes after 11.
B. If using a page with a predrawn clock, instruct the client to:
   1. Copy the clock on the top of the page onto the lower part of the same sheet of paper.

Scoring

Scoring consists of the evaluation of errors and/or distortions. There are several variations on scoring the CDT. The quickest scoring involves dividing the clock into four quadrants and counting the numbers in the correct quadrant. More complex assessment evaluates up to 20 traits or categorizes errors.

A. The placement of the arms of the clock is the most abstract feature and is useful in evaluating the early dementing process.
B. A normal clock suggests that multiple functions are intact and contributes to the assessment of the client's ability to continue independently. This is a "normal" clock draw:

C. A grossly abnormal clock is an indicator of potential problems that require attention (see the following figures):

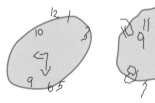

D. There are several scoring systems for evaluating the CDT results. The most basic involves awarding 1 point for each of the following:
   1 point for the clock circle
   1 point for the numbers placed in the correct position
   1 point for the clockface numbers placed in their proper order around and inside the clockface
   1 point for the presence of the two clock hands
   1 point for the correct time as instructed
A normal score is 4 or 5 points.
Refusal to draw a clock is scored as abnormal.
Note: The next page may be used for serial testing.

Name: _____   Date: _____

Copy this clock.

Cystometry

Cheryl A. Glass

Description

A. Cystometry testing is an office procedure to determine bladder capacity, how full the bladder gets when the urge to urinate begins, postvoid residual (PVR), any fluid leak with stress maneuvers, or inhibited bladder capacity. Cystometry measures the intravesical bladder pressure during bladder filling. Often, cystometry is performed in conjunction with uroflowmetry.

Indications

A. Clients presenting with complaints of urinary incontinence, stress incontinence (leaking), overactive bladder (OAB), and urinary retention (inability to empty bladder) are candidates for cystometry testing.

Before the Procedure

A. A thorough urologic/gynecologic history should be taken and a physical examination should be performed, including a digital rectal examination.

Precautions

A. Rule out the presence of a urinary tract infection as a cause of the incontinence prior to cystometry testing.
B. Use universal precautions. This is a sterile procedure and is contraindicated when infection or inflammation is present.
C. Risks of the procedure:
   1. Discomfort
   2. Bleeding
   3. Infection
   4. Autonomic dysreflexia (AD) from bladder instrumentation and bladder distension:
      a. Flushing
      b. Hypertension
      c. Reflex bradycardia
      d. Severe headache

Equipment Required

A. Sterile straight catheter (12–14 French catheter)
B. Catheter insertion kit
C. 60-mL sterile syringe
D. 1,000 mL sterile water (CO_2, saline, or contrast medium may also be used)
E. Sterile measurement container
F. Urine collection device
G. A vaginal or rectal pressure catheter or insertion of a second catheter with a manometer to measure pressures
H. Light source for catheterization
I. Gown and drape for the client

Procedure

A. Explain the procedure.
B. Obtain consent (if required).
C. Ask about any latex or Betadine allergies.
D. Throughout the procedure, ask the client to speak to his or her sensation of the feeling of the bladder filling, any discomfort, when the urge to void, and bladder fullness. Sensations noted by the client are subject to the rate of bladder filling and temperature of the fluid.
E. During the initial physical examination, have the client bear down and/or cough to evaluate urinary incontinence.
F. Have the client void, measure the urine, and collect the specimen for urinalysis:
   1. The measurement of the urine flow rate also screens abnormalities of micturition.
      a. A simple way to measure the flow rate is to time the duration of urination and measure the volume voided. A woman usually voids in a continuous flow rate until the bladder is empty. Intermittent flow patterns indicate dysfunction with voiding.
   2. The evaluation of urine speed and flow rate may be measured by uroflowmetry equipment using a special toilet with a computer to record the flow rates.
G. Catheterize, using sterile technique:
   1. Measure urine drained from the catheter inserted post voiding; this amount is the PVR.
      a. Normal: less than 100 mL PVR
      b. Abnormal: more than 100 mL PVR
      c. Differential diagnostic evaluation: overflow incontinence secondary to retention
H. Attach the 60-mL syringe to the catheter.
   1. Observe whether there was any difficulty passing the catheter.
      a. Normal findings: catheter passes with ease
      b. Abnormal findings: catheter difficult or impossible to pass
      c. Differential diagnostic evaluation: overflow incontinence possibly due to obstruction
I. Place the rectal or vaginal catheter to measure intra-abdominal pressure and involuntary/voluntary detrusor contractions.
J. Using gravity, fill the bladder slowly through the catheter/syringe with sterile water (saline or contrast medium).
   1. Avoid instilling the sterile water too quickly; instill approximately 30 to 50 mL amounts at a time.
   2. Measure the amount of water instilled when the client has the urge to void, different degrees of filling, and pain during filling.
      a. Normal: bladder capacity usually at 300 mL when urge is sensed
      b. Abnormal: urge at less than 200 mL
      c. Differential diagnostic evaluation: urge incontinence due to small capacity
   3. Continue to fill, noting if there is any fluctuation of the sterile water in the syringe during filling.
      a. Normal: Contractions or fluctuations occur around 200 to 250 mL from bladder into syringe (detrusor muscle contraction).

b. Abnormal: fluid moving into the syringe

c. Differential diagnostic evaluation: urge incontinence related to bladder spasm

4. The rectal/vaginal probe measures detrusor activity/overactivity and notes phasic pressure increases associated with symptoms of urgency or urge incontinence, indicating detrusor overactivity.

5. During the procedure, ask the client to cough or bear down to help elicit involuntary bladder contractions. The Valsalva maneuver or cough assesses the sphincter competence.

6. The instillation of sterile water should be stopped when the client reports a full bladder. Measure the bladder capacity; that is, the client reports a perception that voiding can no longer be delayed.

7. If the client has not reported a full bladder before the instillation of 600 mL, the test should be discontinued.

8. The urodynamic test is done until the point of leakage.

    a. Have the client cough or strain; observe for leaking, clamp catheter

    b. Normal: normal capacity 400 mL, no leaking with cough

    c. Abnormal: urge before 400 mL, or leaking with pressure

    d. Differential diagnostic evaluation: urge incontinence due to small capacity and/or stress incontinence due to leakage with pressure

    e. Coughing and straining during the procedure are also done to evaluate bladder pressure changes. The manometer also measures the pressure inside the bladder when leakage occurs.

9. Remove the catheter after the bladder is filled to capacity (strong urge to void); have the client cough.

    a. Normal: no leakage

    b. Abnormal: leakage of fluid

    c. Differential diagnostic evaluation: stress incontinence associated with weak pelvic muscles

10. Have the client void; measure output, compare with amount instilled.

    a. Normal: return with a maximum of 100 mL retained (PVR)

    b. Abnormal: greater than 100 mL retained after voiding

    c. Postprocedure, while the client is emptying the bladder, the manometer measures the bladder pressure and flow rate. After bladder has emptied, remove the vaginal/rectal probe.

    d. Differential diagnostic evaluation: overflow incontinence either from obstruction or an atonic bladder

K. Discuss treatment options, including pharmaceutical therapy and/or consultation with the urologist.

L. Give postprocedure instructions and discuss when to report problems.

1. Expect some discomfort; it should lessen over time.

2. Blood during urination may be expected after the procedure. The amount of blood lessens over time and with urination.

3. Drinking additional fluids (noncaffeinated and noncarbonated beverages) will increase urination and ease discomfort and passage of blood.

4. An antibiotic may be prescribed (per protocol).

5. Anti-inflammatories, such as ibuprofen, may be discussed.

6. Have the client report:

    a. Chills and fever

    b. Any abdominal pain

    c. Continued bloody urine 1 day post procedure

Foreign Body Removal From the Nose

Cheryl A. Glass

Description

A. This technique is for removing a nasal foreign body (NFB) that is anterior to the pharynx and can be visualized with a nasal speculum.

Indications

A. Clients with retained NFB often present with unilateral, foul rhinorrhea, nosebleeds, or the request for foreign-body removal. NFB is most commonly seen toddlers.

Precautions

A. Try to identify the type of object: organic or inorganic.
   1. Organic foreign objects include food items (e.g., peas and beans), sponges, or rubber
   2. Inorganic foreign objects include a rock, pearl, battery, or small toy parts
B. If you cannot identify the object, do not irrigate the nares before removal.
   1. Vegetable matter will swell if hydrated, so remove it in a dry environment when possible.
   2. Small "button" batteries from toys are common and should not be irrigated due to the destruction from the low-volt current and potential spread of alkaline content.
C. When the object is too far into the nasal turbinate/cavity or when in doubt, do not attempt the procedure and refer to an otolaryngologist.
   1. The procedure may need to be done under sedation.
   2. The object may need to be removed in a surgical setting utilizing sedation.

Equipment Required

A. Proper lighting (headlight or head mirror)
B. Nasal speculum
C. Topical anesthetic for use before procedure (topical 1% lidocaine with 0.5% phenylephrine)
D. Fogarty suction and several suction tips
E. Other equipment should be available depending on the type of foreign body: wire loop or curette, alligator or Hartman forceps, bayonet forceps, right-angle hooks, a Foley catheter, and Fogarty suction.

Procedure

A. Determine the type of object in the nostril during history taking in order to determine the best approach for removal.
B. Explain the procedure to the client.

C. Obtain the client's consent for removal.
D. To best visualize the nasal cavity, have the client lie down or sit erect with the head slightly tilted back.
E. Visualize the nostril with the nasal speculum (insert speculum into nares with handles horizontal).
F. If tissue edema is present in the nares, you may use a topical anesthetic with vasoconstrictor to the affected nares to help prevent bleeding.
G. If the client is willing, have him or her dislodge the foreign body with forceful nose blowing while occluding the unaffected nostril and keeping the mouth closed.
   1. The client should be supine or with a slight elevation of the head with assistance to stabilize the client's head.
H. If forceful blowing is not successful, attempt to remove the foreign object using the most appropriate instrument or technique (wire loop or curette, alligator or Hartman forceps, bayonet forceps, right-angle hooks and suctioning). The choice of instrument for removal is dependent on the type of object, location, and how well the client is able to cooperate during the procedure.
   1. Use of a catheter involves lubricating the tip, inserting catheter past the foreign body, and inflating the balloon with approximately 2 mL of air or water.
   2. Gentle withdrawal will pull the foreign object out.
   3. Use of cyanoacrylate glue involves placing a drop of the adhesive on the wooden tip of a cotton-tipped applicator, touching the foreign body with the wooden tip, and gently pulling the object out of the nares.
   4. Simple external pressure should be applied to prevent bleeding.

Evaluation/Results of Procedure

A. **Evaluate the other nares and ear if one foreign object is found.**
B. Bleeding is common after the removal of a foreign object. Pressure should be applied to stop the bleeding.
C. Follow up in 2 days to evaluate the mucosa.
D. Consult a physician if you are unable to dislodge or remove the object.
E. Button batteries require prompt removal and inspection due to alkaline-induced liquefactive necrosis to the mucosa.

Hernia Reduction (Inguinal/Groin)

Cheryl A. Glass

Description
A. A hernia reduction may be done by a manual technique used for external replacement of the bowel (occasionally omentum) from the hernia back into the abdomen/groin.

Indications
A. Herniation of bowel contents occurs secondary to pregnancy, straining, hard physical labor, or congenital defect.

Precautions
A. ***Do not try to reduce a strangulated hernia. This hernia type is a surgical emergency and should be referred immediately to a surgeon for evaluation and treatment. Reduction of a strangulated hernia can cause gangrenous bowel to enter the peritoneal cavity. Strangulation symptoms include tenderness, discoloration, edema, fever, and signs of bowel obstruction.***
B. Sedation and analgesia may be necessary to decrease guarding and abdominal muscular constriction.

Equipment Required
A. Gown/drape for the client
B. Nonsterile gloves
C. Ice or cold compress

Procedure
A. After doing a complete assessment, explain the reduction procedure to the client, discussing each step just before performing it.
B. Obtain consent if required by protocol.
C. Ask the client to void.
D. Apply ice or cold compress to the hernia for several minutes to reduce swelling and allow for easier reduction.
E. Apply the gloves.
F. Have the client lie in a 20-degree Trendelenburg position to allow gravity to help retract the herniated tissue into the pelvis.
G. After the client has had the ice pack, been positioned in the Trendelenburg position, and had light sedation and analgesia for up to 30 minutes, the hernia may self-reduce because of the reduction of edema, force of gravity, and relaxation of muscles.
H. Ask the client to take deep, slow, relaxing breaths. Hernia reduction should cause minimal discomfort.
   1. *Males*: gently invaginate the scrotal skin and replace the herniated contents back through the external/internal inguinal or femoral rings by slowly applying pressure distal to the hernia while guiding the proximal portion. Use two hands to assist in the guidance through the defect and simultaneously add gentle pressure.
   2. *Females*: gently invaginate the herniated bowel contents back through the external/internal inguinal or femoral rings by slowly applying pressure distal to the hernia while guiding the proximal portion. Use two hands to assist in the guidance through the defect and simultaneously add gentle pressure.
I. Hernias should be easily reducible. Do not force any contents back into the abdominal wall defect. Too much distal pressure causes the hernia to balloon around the fascial opening.
J. After the reduction, ask the client to cough and strain to evaluate successful reduction prior to discharge.

Evaluation/Results of Procedure
A. Consult a physician if unable to reduce the hernia. The hernia may be strangulated.
B. Have the client return in 1 week for reexamination or sooner if needed.
C. Tell the client not to strain with bowel movements, lift heavy objects, or exercise strenuously.
D. Review symptoms of obstruction or strangulation of entrapped bowel: pain, nausea, and vomiting. At discharge, educate the client to seek immediate medical attention for strangulated bowel.
E. Recurrent hernias and congenital defects eventually require surgical repair.
F. Hernias secondary to pregnancy may not require surgery.

Intrauterine Device Insertion

Cheryl A. Glass and Rhonda Arthur

> Note: Only trained healthcare providers who carefully reviewed the selected device's manufacturer's package insert for indications and use as well as specific insertion instructions should place intrauterine devices (IUDs).

Description

A. The long-acting reversible contraceptive (LARC) is a method of contraception that is inserted into the uterine cavity.

1. Copper T 380 A (ParaGard):
   a. T-shaped bound in fine copper wire
   b. **Approved for 10 years**
   c. Clear or white knotted double string
2. Levonorgestrel-releasing intrauterine system (LNG-IUS):
   a. Levonorgestrel (Mirena®):
      i. T-shaped polyethylene frame with levonorgestrel (LNG) reservoir coating
      ii. 52 mg—initial release rate of LNG is 20 mcg/d; this rate is reduced by about 50% after 5 years. Mirena must be removed or replaced after 5 years.
      iii. Dark monofilament strings
      iv. **Approved for 5 years**
   b. Kyleena:
      i. T-shaped polyethylene frame with LNG reservoir coating
      ii. 19.5 mg—release rate of LNG is 17.5 mcg/day after 24 days and declines to 7.4 mcg/d after 5 years. Kyleena must be removed or replaced after 5 years.
      iii. White monofilament strings
      iv. **Approved for 5 years**
   c. Skylar:
      i. T-shaped polyethylene frame with LNG reservoir coating
      ii. 13.5 mg—release rate of LNG is 14 mcg/d after 24 days and declines to 5 mcg/d after 3 years. Skylar must be removed or replaced after 3 years.
      iii. White monofilament strings
      iv. **Approved for 3 years**
   d. Liletta:
      i. T-shaped polyethylene frame with LNG reservoir coating
      ii. 52 mg—release rate of LNG is 19.5 mcg/d initially and declines progressive to approximately 17.0 mcg/d at 1 year, 14.8 mcg/d at 2 years, 12.9 mcg/d at 3 years, and 11.3 mcg/d at 4 years after insertion. Liletta can be removed at any time but must be removed by the end of the fourth year.
      iii. Blue monofilament strings
      iv. **Approved for 5 years**

Indications

A. To provide a long-acting method (3–10 years) of contraception
B. The LNG IUDs are therapeutic with severe dysmenorrhea and severe menorrhagia.

Precautions

A. Pregnancy must be ruled out before insertion.
B. Use universal precautions. Insertion is a sterile procedure and is contraindicated when infection or inflammation is present.
C. Risks at the time of insertion include the following:
   1. Uterine perforation
   2. Discomfort
   3. Bleeding
   4. Infection
   5. Autonomic dystreflexia (AD) from IUD insertion:
      a. Flushing
      b. Hypertension
      c. Reflex bradycardia
      d. Severe headache
D. Ask about any latex or Betadine allergies.
E. Small amounts of progestins pass into breast milk with LNG IUDs.
F. To minimize the risk of expulsion, it is advisable to insert an IUD when the woman is *not* on her menstrual cycle.
G. **An existing IUD should be removed during the menstrual cycle.**
H. Consent(s) is required by the manufacturer and by individual institutional protocols. The client should know the type of IUD device inserted and when it should be replaced.

Contraindications

A. Women who have a history of sexually transmitted disease and/or currently have more than one sexual partner may not be good candidates for IUD use.
B. Uterine anomaly
C. Cervical stenosis (unable to pass a uterine sound)
D. Active pelvic infection (recent, acute, or subacute)
E. Purulent cervicitis
F. History of ectopic pregnancy (strong relative risk)
G. Abnormal Papanicolau (Pap) smear/endometrial hyperplasia/cervical intraepithelial neoplasia (CIN)/cancer (review last recent Pap results); uterine or cervical neoplasm
H. Concern for future fertility
I. Allergy to copper (ParaGard) or allergy to component of LNG IUDs as applies
J. Valvular heart disease

> Insertion of an IUD may theoretically increase the woman's susceptibility to subacute bacterial endocarditis (SBE). No current evidence supports this. Optional therapy: Some clinicians require antibiotics for valvular coverage. High-risk clients may receive intravenous (IV) ampicillin and gentamicin, and moderate-risk clients may receive oral amoxicillin 2 g before insertion or removal.

K. Acute liver disease

L. Known or suspected breast carcinoma

Equipment Required

A. IUD

B. Speculum

C. Iodine solution

D. Tenaculum

E. Uterine sound

F. Scissors

G. Sterile gloves (two pairs)

H. Urine pregnancy test kit

I. Atropine 0.5 mg should be available at the time of insertion for severe AD response.

> Backup staff should be available for complications such as vasovagal response and perforation of uterus.

Procedure

A. Perform a urine pregnancy test.

B. Perform a baseline blood pressure and pulse.

C. Obtain the client's consent after full history and review of last Pap smear; discuss alternative methods, pros and cons of each method, procedure, side effects, and complications of IUD insertion and device.

D. With the client draped in the lithotomy position, perform a bimanual examination to determine uterine position and size

E. Apply sterile gloves.

F. Cleanse the vagina and cervix with antiseptic solution.

G. Use the tenaculum to grasp the anterior lip of the cervix approximately 1.5 to 2.0 cm from the os:

1. Atropine should be readily available for severe vasovagal response.

2. Lidocaine (Xylocaine) gel or benzocaine (Hurricane spray) can be used to decrease discomfort with the application and use of the tenaculum.

H. Insert the uterine sound into the cervix/uterus slowly and gently.

1. Moisture mark on the sound will indicate the depth of insertion for the IUD. (Depth less than 6 cm is contraindication.)

I. Change sterile gloves.

J. Load the IUD as directed by manufacturer.

K. Set indicator for depth of insertion as guided by the uterine sound.

L. While maintaining gentle traction with the tenaculum, insert the IUD gently to the predetermined mark on the guide sheath.

1. Spasm of the internal cervical os may occur and will resolve by waiting a few minutes.

M. Gently push the IUD through the guide into the fundal position. Excessive pain or bleeding is often a sign of perforation. Consult a physician immediately (most common perforation sites: fundus, body of uterus, and cervical wall).

N. Remove the guide sheath.

O. Remove the tenaculum.

P. Cut the IUD strings to approximately 1-inch length past the cervix.

Q. Remove the speculum.

R. Check the client's blood pressure and pulse to rule out vasovagal potential.

S. Recommend a prostaglandin inhibitor if cramping occurs/persists (Motrin 400 mg by mouth four times a day).

T. Prophylactic antibiotics may be used for SBE prophylaxis. Amoxicillin is used unless there is an amoxicillin/penicillin allergy, then erythromycin or clindamycin may be prescribed. Amoxicillin 3.0 g by mouth 1 hour before the procedure, then 1.5 g by mouth 6 hours later.

1. Erythromycin (EES) 800 mg by mouth 2 hours before the procedure, then 400 mg by mouth 6 hours later.

2. Clindamycin 300 mg by mouth 1 hour before the procedure, then 150 mg 6 hours later.

U. Instruct the client regarding string location and periodic checks. The client should not have vaginal intercourse or use a tampon for 7 days (decreases infection).

Evaluation/Results of Procedure

A. See the client after first menses to check for expulsion.

B. If the client has missed two or more periods, perform a beta human chorionic gonadotropin (HCG) test.

1. Rule out ectopic pregnancy.

2. Explore the canal for IUD.

3. Consider ultrasound to rule out pregnancy/expulsion.

4. Consider flat plate of abdomen.

5. Consult a physician.

C. Yearly evaluation with Pap smear/annual checkup

D. Consider hemoglobin for reports of heavy bleeding with ParaGard:

1. If hemoglobin (Hgb) is less than 9, remove the IUD, provide an alternative method of contraception, and prescribe iron supplement for 2 months.

2. Repeat Hgb in 1 month.

IUD Removal Procedure

A. Remove only during menses (cervix is more dilated).

B. Apply gentle, steady traction; remove slowly.

C. **Consider uterine embedding if unable to remove and need for consultation.**

Client should call the office for:

A. A missed period

B. Abdominal pain (severe)

C. Temperature 100.4°F not associated with other problems (sinus infection, urinary tract infection [UTI])

D. Foul vaginal odor/discharge, especially if bloody or greenish color

E. Heavy bleeding with clots

Neurologic Examination

Cheryl A. Glass

Description

A. Performance of the neurologic examination is a diagnostic component of many physical examinations. Examination of all cranial nerves is not necessary for every client. The neurologic examination should be performed based on client-focused presenting complaints. The purpose of this support tool is to review the cranial nerves and the equipment needed for a neurologic examination.

A neurologic examination identifies dysfunction and assists in accurate diagnosis (see Table II.2).

Components of the Neurologic Examination

A. Thorough history
B. Assessment of mental status
C. Assessment of cranial nerve function

TABLE II.2   CRANIAL NERVE FUNCTION

Cranial Nerve Number	Cranial Nerve	Functional Test
I	Olfactory	Smell reception and interpretation: assess patency of one nostril at a time. Occlude one nostril, have person close eyes, ask person to sniff item on hand, such as vanilla or cinnamon, and report name of substance
II	Optic	Vision: assess acuity and visual fields using Snellen chart
III	Oculomotor	Motor: eye/lid movement up, pupil constriction, visual accommodation. Ask client to look at the object far away, then place the object in close proximity, noting pupillary constriction at near object. Holding finger in front of face, move finger closer to the nose, noting convergence of eyes when moving closer to nose
IV	Trochlear	Eye movement up/down: using penlight, ask client to follow penlight with eyes, without moving head. Move penlight upward, downward, sideways, and diagonally
V	Trigeminal	Chewing, jaw opening and clenching, facial sensation: palpate temporal and masseter muscles as person clenches teeth closed, resisting examiner's attempt to open jaw. Corneal, forehead, eyes, nose/mouth mucosa, teeth, tongue, and ears: ask person to close eyes. (a) Using light sensation, brush cotton ball across forehead to see whether client feels sensation. (b) Using blunt/sharp object, assess deep sensation alternating blunt/sharp object on skin for sensation
VI	Abducens	Lateral gaze/eye movement: holding penlight in front of person's eyes, ask person to follow the movements of penlight with eyes without moving head, while examiner performs testing for the six cardinal fields of gaze
VII	Facial	Corneal reflex, facial expression, taste to the lateral two thirds of tongue, and sensation to pharynx, parasympathetic secretion of tears and saliva: look for facial symmetry. Ask the person to smile, frown, close eyes tightly while resisting attempt by examiner to open eyes. Show all teeth, close mouth, and puff cheeks out. Note symmetry of cheeks
VIII	Acoustic (vestibulocochlear)	Hearing and equilibrium: assess hearing by whispered voice, or ticking watch. May use tuning fork for Weber and Rinne tests. Ask client to walk across room and return, noting gait stability
IX	Glosso-medulla or glossopharyngeal	Gag reflex, cough, swallow, taste on posterior third of tongue, parasympathetic secretion of salivary glands, and carotid reflex: using tongue blade, depress tongue, ask the person to say "Ahh." Watch soft palate and uvula rise midline, tonsils move medially. Gag reflex may be elicited by depressing back of tongue with tongue depressor.
X	Vagus	Laryngeal muscles: muscles of phonation, swallowing, sensation behind ear and part of external canal, parasympathetic secretion of digestive enzymes/peristalsis, as well as involuntary action of heart and lungs. Ask the client to swallow and speak, noting hoarseness in voice if present representing vocal cord abnormality
XI	Spinal accessory	Head and shoulder movement: have client shrug shoulders against resistance from examiner
XII	Hypoglossal	Tongue movement/muscles, swallowing, and sound articulation: ask the person to stick tongue out and move tongue from side to side

Source: Adapted from Seidel, H., Ball, J. W., Dains, J. E., & Benedict, G. W. (1991). *Mosby's guide to physical examination* (2nd ed.). New York, NY: Mosby.

D. Assessment of motor function
E. Assessment of sensory function
F. Assessment of gait
G. Assessment of reflexes

Equipment Required
A. Multiple mental examinations are available. The clock-draw test (CDT) and the Mini-Mental Examination are two examples.
B. Penlight/ophthalmoscope: light source

C. Ophthalmoscope
D. Snellen chart/Rosenbaum pocket card
E. Items to taste (salt, sugar)
F. Items to smell (vanilla, cinnamon)
G. Tongue depressor
H. Tuning fork
I. Ticking watch/clock
J. Cotton or soft tissue
K. Pin or other sharp object
L. Reflex hammer

Nonstress Test

Cheryl A. Glass

Description

A. The nonstress test (NST) is a noninvasive test to assess fetal well-being. A fetus with an intact central nervous system with adequate oxygenation will demonstrate transient fetal heart rate (FHR) accelerations in response to fetal movement. Results of the NST must be evaluated with consideration of gestational age. It is not uncommon for a neurologically intact fetus between the ages of 26 and 28 weeks' gestation to have a nonreactive NST.

Indications

A. Clients at risk of adverse perinatal outcome:
1. Maternal indications:
   a. Hypertension
   b. Maternal cardiac disease
   c. Diabetes (including gestational diabetes)
   d. Renal disease
   e. Hyperthyroidism
   f. Collagen vascular disease
   g. Sickle cell disease
   h. Previous stillbirth
2. Fetal indications:
   a. Intrauterine growth restriction (IUGR)
   b. Postdates (greater than 41 weeks)
   c. Decreased fetal movement

B. Frequency of testing: One must consider prognosis for neonatal survival and severity of maternal disease. In general, most high-risk pregnant women should begin testing by 32 to 34 weeks estimated gestational age (EGA). In case of multiple or severe high-risk conditions, testing may begin at 26 to 28 weeks. Frequency may be weekly or biweekly. If clinical deterioration is noted, reducing the testing interval is prudent.

Precautions

A. A reactive NST is reassuring. However, the significance of abnormal results is less clear. Loss of FHR reactivity may be benign, or it may be a sign of the metabolic consequences of hypoxemia.

Equipment Required

A. Electronic FHR monitor (EFM)
B. Reclining chair or bed/stretcher
C. Sphygmomanometer
D. Vibroacoustic stimulator (protocol dependent)

Procedure

A. Place the client in the semi-Fowler's position in a recliner or on a stretcher. Optimal positioning includes the client tilted to the left or right side to avoid vena caval compression. The client is preferably nonfasting and has not recently smoked.
B. Measure the client's blood pressure.
C. Apply EFM on the maternal abdomen.
D. Record FHR for 20 to 40 minutes. Ask the mother to record fetal movements with a marker button, if available.

However, all accelerations may be counted as they probably have the same significance whether or not they occur in response to the fetal movement felt by the mother.
E. Interpret FHR tracing as reactive or nonreactive (see the following).
F. If the fetus is suspected to be in a sleep state, a vibroacoustic stimulation device may be applied (protocol dependent). The vibroacoustic stimulator is placed on the maternal abdomen and used for a 1- to 5-second stimulation in an attempt to awaken the fetus. If no fetal response occurs, the stimulus may be repeated up to three times for progressively longer duration of up to 3 seconds.

Evaluation/Results of Procedure

A. Reactive NST: baseline FHR 110 to 160 beats per minute (bpm) with two or more accelerations of greater than or equal to 15 bpm amplitude that last at least 15 seconds or more, within a 20-minute period (**Note: Before 32 weeks of gestation, accelerations are defined as two accelerations or more greater than 10 bpm amplitude that last at least longer than 10 seconds over a 20-minute period.**) If these criteria are met before 20 minutes, the test may be declared reactive. The FHR tracing may be continued for at least 40 minutes to account for the typical fetal sleep–wake cycle.
B. Nonreactive NST: The aforementioned criteria are not met within the 40-minute time frame.

Treatment

A. If the NST is a reactive, reassuring test, continue obstetrical prenatal care. Further testing is required for maternal and fetal indications as previously noted.
B. Causes of a nonreactive NST includes fetal immaturity, fetal sleep, maternal smoking, fetal neurologic or cardiac anomalies, or maternal ingestion of drug.

Consultation/Referral

A. Further evaluation is mandatory for a nonreactive NST (variable, late, or prolonged decelerations) noted during testing. Consult with a physician. Depending on the situation, the client could be given juice or sent to eat and return later for a repeat NST. She may undergo a modified NST, which includes single vibroacoustic stimulation applied to the maternal abdomen plus the assessment of amniotic fluid and/or biophysical profile (BPP). Doppler velocimetry may also be used for additional evaluation in the setting of fetal growth restriction. Management decisions are guided by the results of the additional evaluation and clinical situation. The client may also be sent to the hospital for another NST, modified NST, BPP, or a contraction stress test (CST).

The CST should only be performed in a setting where immediate delivery could occur if indicated for fetal distress.

Oral Airway Insertion

Cheryl A. Glass

Description

A. An oropharyngeal airway is a semicircular device used to hold the tongue away from the posterior wall of the pharynx. To insert this device, the mouth and pharynx should first be cleared of secretions, blood, or vomit, using a suction tip catheter (if available).

Indications

A. Oral airway insertion can be used to help control the airway and to suction, ventilate, and provide oxygenation of the unconscious client.

Precautions

A. **Oral airways should be inserted only if the client is unconscious, unresponsive, and has no gag reflex.** If the client is conscious, airway insertion may stimulate vomiting and laryngospasm.

B. It is important to measure for the correct size of the oral airway. If the airway is too long, it could press the epiglottis against the entrance of the larynx and produce a complete airway obstruction.

C. If the airway is not inserted properly, it can push the tongue posteriorly and worsen an upper airway obstruction.

D. If the tongue and/or lips are between the teeth, trauma will result.

Equipment Required

A. An oropharyngeal airway (selection/measurement of the airway size is measured from the earlobe to the corner of the mouth)

B. A tongue blade

C. Gloves

D. A suction tip and canister (if available)

Procedure

A. Place head/neck in the correct position (see Figure II.3).

B. The best way to insert an oral airway is to turn it backward (upside down) as it enters the mouth.

C. As the airway transverses the oral cavity and approaches the posterior wall of the pharynx, rotate it into the proper position.

FIGURE II.3   Insertion of an oral airway.

D. Open the client's mouth using a cross-finger technique. An alternate method is to move the tongue out of the way with a tongue blade before insertion of the airway.

E. The end flared flange of the airway should rest on the client's lips.

F. Suction if necessary.

G. If the client vomits, the airway should be removed. The mouth and airway should be cleared and the oral airway reinserted only if the client remains unconscious and has no gag reflex.

Evaluation/Results of Procedure

A. The airway is in the proper position and of the proper size when you hear clear breath sounds on auscultation of the lungs during ventilation.

B. Resuscitation will be necessary to ventilate if there is no spontaneous breathing.

Pap Smear and Maturation Index Procedure

Cheryl A. Glass and Rhonda Arthur

Description

A. A Papanicolaou (Pap) smear is a cytologic *screen* that is performed to detect the presence of cancerous and pre-cancerous lesions of the uterine cervix. The procedure involves procuring a sample of both the ectocervix and endocervix. The maturation index (endocrine assessment) is a tool to evaluate decreased estrogenization of the vagina. Both liquid-based and conventional methods for collecting cervical cytology are acceptable.

Indications

A. Human papillomavirus (HPV) increases the risk for cancer, including cervical, vulvar, vaginal, penile, and anal cancer as well as cancer of the oropharynx. Since cervical cancer is believed to be caused by sexually transmissible HPV infections, women who have not had sexual exposures are likely at low risk. Women aged older than 21 years who have not engaged in sexual intercourse may not need a Pap test depending on circumstances. The decision should be made at the discretion of the women and her physician. Women who have had sex with women are still at risk of cervical cancer.

B. Persistent infection of the uterine cervix with high-risk types of human papillomavirus (hrHPV) is required for the development of invasive cervical cancer. Infection with hrHPV is common, especially with sexually active young women; most infections are transient and spontaneously clear without clear clinical consequences. The American Cancer Society, the American Society for Colposcopy and Cervical Pathology, and the American Society for Clinical Pathology clinical guidelines recommend screening strategies with cytology or cotesting (cytology in combination with hrHPV) by age-specific guideline. The American College of Obstetricians and Gynecologists (ACOG) recommends screening for women ages 21 to 65 with cytology alone, and HPV cotesting by age-specific guideline. The 2018 U.S. Preventive Services Task Force (USPSTF) recommendation statement for cervical cancer for women ages 21 to 65 years recommends screening for cervical cancer with cervical cytology alone and hrHPV testing alone dependent on the woman's age. See Table II.3 for cervical cancer screening recommendations for average-risk women. Women who are infected with HIV, who are otherwise immunocompromised (e.g., solid organ transplants), women previously treated for cervical intraepithelial neoplasia 2 (CIN2) or cervical intraepithelial neoplasia 3 (CIN3) or cancer, and women exposed to diethylstilbestrol (DES) before birth need more frequent screening.

Precautions

A. Ask the woman not to douche, use any antifungals or spermicides, or have intercourse the night before the procedure so that there will be nothing to interfere with obtaining a good sample.

B. Practitioners should be aware that some women experience discomfort during the Pap smear procedure and should be sensitive to this possibility.

C. In order to procure an adequate Pap smear, care must be taken to obtain a sample from the entire squamocolumnar junction of the cervical portio. (The squamocolumnar junction is more prominent in teens and women on oral contraceptives.)

D. Blood may obscure an adequate cytology interpretation. It is advisable, therefore, to obtain the endocervical sample following the ectocervical sample. Bleeding from the endocervix is common, particularly if a cytobrush is used. A cytobrush is recommended for sampling the endocervix as more cells are retrieved using this tool as compared to a Q-tip.

Equipment Required

A. Speculum (size appropriate for teen/woman)
B. Warm water for lubrication (excessive K-Y jelly may interfere with the smear and reading)
C. Spatula (wooden or plastic)
D. Q-tip or cytobrush
E. Glass slide (two if maturation index)
F. Container for slide(s)
G. Cytology fixative

Procedure (Conventional Method)

A. With the client draped in a lithotomy position, insert the lightly lubricated speculum and visualize the cervix.

B. With the spatula, sample the entire (360-degree sweep) squamocolumnar junction using gentle pressure applied directly to this area (if visualized). The goal of the technique is to scrape exfoliated cells or those cells held loosely on the surface of the cervix. Vigorous scraping that abrades the cervix yields tissue that is virtually uninterpretable in the cytology smear.

C. Insert the cytobrush or Q-tip until the brush or cotton swab is no longer visible. It is not necessary to insert further to obtain an adequate sample. A fiber-tipped swab should be introduced in the canal and rotated clockwise several times to obtain cells. A cotton-tipped swab should first be moistened with saline to prevent cells from adhering to the cotton; a synthetic fiber swab is nonabsorbent and can be used without moistening. Pap smears taken with a brush have been found superior in containing endocervical cells.

D. Wipe the sample from the spatula and roll and twist the brush of the cytobrush or the Q-tip on the glass slide as quickly as possible. The cytobrush sample can be rolled through the spatula sample. It is not necessary to separate these two areas or obtain two slides.

E. Spray the slide with cytology fixative held at a distance of approximately 12 inches to avoid "blasting" the cells from the slide. If held too far away, inadequate spray reaches the slide and drying distortion could result.

1. Allow the slide to dry before covering in transport container.

2. To obtain a cytology specimen from the vaginal cuff (posthysterectomy), use a spatula (rounded end) to scrape the upper lateral third of the vaginal wall. Spread on a slide and fix the slide with cytology fixative.

3. Vaginal pool specimens for a maturation index are often recommended in perimenopausal women; sampling is done by scraping the posterior fornix with the spatula. Spread on a separate slide from the Pap smear and fix the slide.

Procedure (Liquid-Based Cytology)

A. With the client draped in a lithotomy position, insert the lightly lubricated speculum and visualize the cervix

B. With the spatula, sample the entire (360-degree sweep) squamocolumnar junction using gentle pressure applied directly to this area (if visualized). The goal of the technique is to scrape exfoliated cells or those cells held loosely on the surface of the cervix. Rinse the spatula as quickly as possible in the solution by swirling vigorously 10 times and discard the spatula.

C. Insert the cytobrush until only the bottom-most fibers are visible. Rotate slowly one half-turn in one direction (do not overrotate). Rinse the brush quickly by rotating the brush against the container wall and swirling. Place the cap on the specimen container and label properly (see Figure II.4).

D. Alternatively, you may use the broom device instead of the cytobrush. If so, insert the central bristles of the broom device into the endocervical canal (deep enough for the short bristles to contact the ectocervix) and rotate clockwise

FIGURE II.4 Pap smear cytology brush.

five times. Rinse the broom by quickly pushing against the bottom of the specimen container and swirling 10 times.

Evaluation/Results of Procedure

A. A Pap smear may be classified as "inadequate" if no endocervical cells are present for interpretation (unless the client has had a hysterectomy).

B. Pap smear adequacy may be compromised if the slide is allowed to air dry before spraying with cytology fixative.

C. A Pap smear reading may be compromised due to the presence of blood, lubricant, or certain vaginal infections creating an increase in vaginal discharge.

D. See Pap Smear Interpretation and American Society for Colposcopy and Cervical Pathology Consensus guidelines on the management of women with abnormal cervical cancer screening tests algorithms on the Internet at www.asccp.org/asccp-guidelines.

TABLE II.3 CERVICAL CANCER SCREENING GUIDELINES FOR *AVERAGE-RISK* WOMEN

Recommending Body	ACS, ASCCP, and ASCP 2012 Guidelines	USPSTF 2018 Guidelines	ACOG 2016
Statement about annual screening	Women of any age should not be screened annually by any screening method.	Cervical cancer screening visits are an opportunity to discuss other health problems and preventative measures.	• Clients should be counseled that annual well-woman visits are recommended even if bimanual pelvic exam with cervical cancer screening is not performed at each visit. The components of the examination may vary depending on the client's age, risk factors, and physician preference. • The visit is valuable in promoting prevention practices, recognizing risk factor for disease, identifying medical problems, administration of immunizations based on age and risk factors, and establishing clinician–client relationship.
Women aged <21 years	Recommends no screening, regardless of the age of sexual initiation or other risk factors	Recommends no screening for women <21	Recommends no screening for women <21, regardless of the age of sexual initiation and other behavior-related risk factors

(*continued*)

TABLE II.3	CERVICAL CANCER SCREENING GUIDELINES FOR *AVERAGE-RISK* WOMEN (*continued*)		
Recommending Body	**ACS, ASCCP, and ASCP 2012 Guidelines**	**USPSTF 2018 Guidelines**	**ACOG 2016**
Women aged 21–29 years • Cytology (conventional or liquid based) alone **OR** • HPV cotest (cytology and HPV test administered together)	• Cervical cytology every 3 years is recommended. • HPV cotesting should not be used for women <30.	Cervical cytology alone **every 3 years** is recommended.	• Cervical cytology **every 3 years** is recommended. • Liquid-based and conventional methods of cervical cytology collection are acceptable for screening. • HPV cotesting is not recommended in women <30 years.
Women aged 30–65 years • Cytology (conventional or liquid-based) alone **OR** • hrHPV cotest (cytology and HPV test administered together)	Pap test and hrHPV cotesting **every 5 years**	• Cervical cytology alone **every 3 years** **OR alternatively** • hrHPV testing alone **every 5 years** • For women age 30–65, cotesting is no long recommended.	• Cervical cytology test alone **every 3 years** is acceptable. • **Pap test + hrHPV cotesting every 5 years** (*preferred over cytology alone every 3 years*)
When to stop screening for average-risk women	• Women >65 years with adequate screening history and who have had a total hysterectomy for benign indications do not need further screening.	• For women >65 years, no screening is recommended for women who have had adequate prior screening and are not otherwise at high risk for cervical cancer.	• For women >65 years, no screening is recommend if no history of cervical changes **AND** either three negative Pap test results in a row or two negative cotest results in a row within the past 10 years, with the most recent test performed within the past 5 years.
Primary hrHPV testing alone	2015—ASCCP and SGO issued interim guide recommendation for the use of HPV test for primary testing	For average- risk women aged 30–65, hrHPV testing **every 5** years is an alternative to cytology alone **ever 3 years.**	hrHPV primary screening is considered an acceptable alternative per the ASCCP and SGO interim guidance.
Screening post-hysterectomy	• Women who have had a total hysterectomy (removal of the uterus and cervix) should stop screening. • Women who have had a supra-cervical hysterectomy (cervix intact) should continue screening according to guidelines.	No screening is recommended for women who have had a hysterectomy with removal of the cervix and do not have a history of high-grade precancerous lesions (i.e., cervical intraepithelial neoplasia grade 2 or 3) or cervical cancer.	• For women who have had a total hysterectomy with removal of the uterus and cervix and no history of cervical cancer or cervical change, screening with routine cytology screening and HPV testing should be discontinued and not restarted for any reason. • For women who had a hysterectomy in which the cervix was removed **AND** have a history of cervical cancer or moderate to severe cervical changes, the recommendation is to continue screening for 20 years after surgery.
Screening among those immunized against HPV 16, 18	Women at any age with a history of HPV vaccination should be screened according to the age-specific recommendation for the general population.	The possibility that vaccination might reduce the need for screening with cytology or hrHPV testing has not been established; therefore, women who have been vaccinated should be screened as recommended until further evidence accrues.	Women who have been vaccinated against HPV still need to be screened according to the same guidelines for the age-specific recommendation.

ACOG, American College of Obstetricians and Gynecologists; ACS, American Cancer Society; ASCCP, American Society for Colposcopy and Cervical Pathology; ASCP, American Society for Clinical Pathology; HPV, human papillomavirus; hrHPV testing, high-risk HPV testing; SGO, Society of Gynecologic Oncology; USPSTF, U.S. Preventive Services Task Force.

Pregnancy: Estimating Date of Delivery

Cheryl A. Glass

The first 12 weeks of pregnancy are vital as the fetal organ systems are developing.

Early Diagnosis of Pregnancy

A. Allows counseling about potential risks to the developing fetus

B. Enables the woman contemplating elective abortion to consider her options

C. Affords diagnosis/intervention in an ectopic pregnancy

D. Fosters early entry into prenatal care, which in turn may provide early identification of pregnancy complications

Obtain Menstrual History

A. Obtain sexual history.

B. Obtain fertility history:

1. Length of cycles
2. Regularity of cycles. Regularity of menstruation is influenced by:
   a. Recent previous pregnancy and cycles that have not yet reestablished themselves
   b. Breastfeeding
   c. Oral contraceptive pills
   d. Intramuscular contraceptive
   e. Subdermal implant contraceptive
   f. Intrauterine device (IUD) contraceptive
   g. Polycystic ovarian syndrome (PCOS)
   h. Comorbid medical conditions

C. Is this a planned pregnancy? If so, how long did it take to conceive?

D. Has the client been pregnant before? If so, what was the outcome of each pregnancy (miscarriage, stillbirth, live birth), the delivery method, and fetal and/or pregnancy complications for each pregnancy?

Initial Assessment/Diagnosis of Pregnancy

A. Is the exact date of the last menstrual period (LMP) known, using the first day of the last period?

B. Was the LMP a normal period? If not, when was the most recent normal period?

C. Is there a known isolated sexual incident that could pinpoint a possible conception date?

D. Does the client know when conception may have occurred?

Pregnancy Testing

Testing includes analysis of maternal blood or urine for the presence of human chorionic gonadotropin (HCG), a hormone produced by the trophoblastic cells of the developing placenta. **Positive testing is not diagnostic of a normal intrauterine pregnancy.**

A. Maternal blood: HCG

1. Most accurate
2. Earliest to become positive

3. Negative test should be repeated in 2 weeks with suspected pregnancy.

B. Urine:

1. More commonly used
2. Accurate 4 to 7 days following conception
3. Available over the counter
4. First-void morning specimen is best (most concentrated)
5. Negative test should be repeated in 1 week to ensure that the first test was not done too early to detect urine HCG. HCG production decreases after 60 to 70 days, and thereafter declines below the sensitivity of some tests.

Presumptive Signs of Pregnancy

A. Amenorrhea

B. Has experienced pregnancy before and feels pregnant now

C. Nausea/vomiting: Nausea is not limited to "morning sickness."

D. Fatigue

E. Breast tenderness

F. Urinary frequency

G. Enlarging abdomen

H. Unexplained weight gain

I. Constipation

Probable Signs of Pregnancy

A. Positive Chadwick's sign: purplish coloration of vagina and cervix; may be seen on speculum examination

B. Positive Hegar's sign: softening of the lower uterine segment; may be palpated on bimanual examination

C. Uterine enlargement:

1. 8 weeks' gestation = two times nonpregnant size
2. 10 weeks' gestation = three times nonpregnant size
3. 12 weeks' gestation = four times nonpregnant size; uterine fundus (size of orange) palpable at symphysis pubis
4. 16 weeks' gestation = uterine fundus midway between symphysis pubis and umbilicus (size of grapefruit)
5. 20 weeks' gestation = uterine fundus at umbilicus (size of large honeydew melon)

D. Increased skin pigmentation (face [chloasma], nipples, abdomen [linea nigra])

E. Striae gravidarum: "stretch marks"

Positive Diagnostic Signs

A. Fetal heart tones (FHTs):

1. 10 to 12 weeks with ultrasonic Doppler (fetal Doppler)
2. If unable to hear FHTs with Doppler at 12 weeks (by size and dates), have the client return at 14 weeks.

3. If unable to hear FHTs at 14 weeks' gestation, repeat visit; the client needs ultrasound examination to confirm fetal viability. Consult with physician if abnormal ultrasound results.

B. Fetal movements palpated by the mother or health-care provider

C. Ultrasound examination:

1. Gestational sac visualized by 4 to 4.5 weeks
2. Yolk sac by 5 to 5.5 weeks
3. Fetal cardiac activity should be visualized by 6 to 6.5 weeks when the embryo measures greater than 7 mm.
4. Embryo should be visualized when the gestational sac measures greater than 25 mm.

Estimated Date of Delivery/Estimated Date of Confinement

A. 280 days (40 weeks) after LMP

B. 266 days (38 weeks) from last ovulation (in a 28-day cycle)

C. **Naegele's rule** for establishing estimated date of confinement (EDC): first day of the LMP plus 7 days minus 3 months plus 1 year = EDC

D. Gestational calculator (in the form of a wheel) may be used to determine EDC. *Gestational wheels are based on a 28-day cycle.*

E. An online gestational calculator is located at www.perinatology.com/calculators/Due-Date.htm

Prostatic Massage Technique: Two-Glass Test

Cheryl A. Glass

Description
A. Obtaining prostatic fluid by prostate massage using the two-glass test known as the Nickel premassage and postmassage test. The Meares–Stamey four-glass test is considered too time-consuming and is rarely used by urologists.

Indications
A. Expressed prostatic secretion (EPS) is used to distinguish chronic prostatitis from acute prostatitis or urinary tract infection.

Precautions
A. Do not perform test in clients with acute prostatitis (swollen, tender, boggy prostate) as it may cause septicemia.

Equipment Required
A. Clean-catch specimen cups (two)
B. Labels (two) marked:
   1. Premassage
   2. Postmassage
C. Sterilized towelette

Procedure
A. Collection of a clean-catch midstream urine specimen for male clients. The client should retract the foreskin (if applies) and cleanse the glans penis with a sterilized towelette in order to avoid contamination.
B. The client should collect a midstream flow of urine by starting the flow of urination, then catch at least 10 mL urine specimen in the first clean-catch specimen cup marked "premassage." The client should be instructed to then stop the flow of urine.
C. The client is asked to lean over the examining table for a digital rectal examination. With a lubricated index finger, gently enter the rectum. The prostate should be massaged by stroking it from the periphery toward the midline several times on each side (similar to a windshield wiper).
D. Following the massage, ask the client to provide more urine in the second clean-catch specimen cup labeled "post massage."
E. Send both the premassage and postmassage urine specimens for urine cultures

Treatment
A. See Table II.4.

TABLE II.4   EVALUATION AND RESULTS OF PROSTATIC SECRETIONS

Diagnosis	Microscopic Evaluation	Treatment
Urethritis	WBC, bacteria in VB_1; in no other specimens	<40 years, probably STI; Rx ceftriaxone 250 mg in a single dose PLUS azithromycin 1 g PO in a single dose
		>40 years, probably coliform bacteria nongonococcal urethritis; Rx: azithromycin 1 g PO in a single dose OR doxycycline 100 mg BID × 7 days
Cystitis	WBC, RBCs, bacteria in VB_2	**First-line therapy**: trimethoprim-sulfamethoxazole PO BID × 7–10 days **Second-line therapy**: quinolones: ciprofloxacin 500 mg BID for 3 days **Alternative therapy**: amoxicillin-clavulanate 875/125 mg BID × 7 days OR **amoxicillin**-clavulanate 500/125 mg TID × 7 days
Acute prostatitis	WBC, bacteria in VB_2 and/or EPS, VB_3	**First-line therapy**: quinolones: Ciprofloxacin 500 mg BID for 4 weeks, OR Ofloxacin 400 mg BID × 4–6 weeks, OR Levofloxacin 500–750 mg daily × 4 weeks **Second-line therapy**: trimethoprim-sulfamethoxazole DS BID × 14 days
		May need hospitalization for IV antibiotics
Chronic prostatitis	Bacteria in EPS and/or VB_3, but not in VB_1 or VB_2	Trimethoprim-sulfamethoxazole BID for 3–4 months PO OR Ciprofloxacin BID 500 mg BID for 3–4 months OR Tetracyclines: doxycycline 100 mg BID × 4 weeks

BID, twice a day; EPS, expressed prostatic secretion; IV, intravenous; PO, per os; RBC, red blood cell; Rx, prescription; STI, sexually transmitted infection; TID, three times a day; VB_1, voided bladder 1, represents the urethra; VB_2, voided bladder 2, represents the bladder; VB_3, voided bladder 3, represents the prostate; WBC, white blood cells.

Rectal Prolapse Reduction

Cheryl A. Glass

Description

There are three types of rectal prolapse:

A. *Internal*: Client complains of a protrusion, but no protrusion is noted on examination.

B. *Partial*: Anus is inverted; rectal mucosa protrudes 1 to 3 cm out of rectal sphincter.

C. *Complete*: All layers of rectum have intussuscepted through the anus (rare in adults; most often seen in children and the elderly).

Indications

A. Diagnosis of rectal prolapse is made by inspection. Several populations are at risk for rectal prolapse, including infants, multiparous women, and the elderly. Other factors associated with rectal prolapse include malnutrition, severe constipation, severe chronic diarrhea, obstetrical injuries, rectal intercourse, and multiple sclerosis, as well as neuromuscular diseases.

Hemorrhoids, mucosal prolapse, polyps, and cancer must be ruled out. Conditions associated with rectal prolapse include cystic fibrosis, ulcerative colitis, intussusception, and Hirschsprung's disease.

Precautions

If a manual reduction fails, an emergent surgical referral should be done.

A. Refer clients with complete prolapse to a physician for evaluation and treatment. After a rectal prolapse reduction by proctoscope, follow-up testing by a barium enema, endoscopy, manometry, defocography, or MRI is indicated.

B. Surgery may also be indicated, depending on the degree of prolapse, recurrence, and risk of strangulation. **Children need further assessment for sexual abuse and cystic fibrosis.**

C. Clients with a history of surgery for rectal prolapse should be evaluated and assessed for hemorrhage, bowel obstruction, pelvic abscess, fecal impaction, and recurrent prolapse.

D. Instruct the client on a high-residue diet and adequate fluid intake to prevent constipation. Instruct the client to avoid straining to induce a bowel movement.

Equipment Required

A. Sterile gauze
B. Normal saline
C. Anoscope
D. Water-soluble lubricant
E. Gloves
F. Chux pads and tissue
G. Light source
H. Examination table

Procedure

A. Explain the procedure to the client and discuss all the steps just before performing. Explain that during the procedure relaxation of the anal sphincter is the key.

B. Obtain the client's consent

C. Ask the client to void. (Urinary stress incontinence is common during the procedure.)

D. Apply gloves.

E. As the procedure is being done, give the client and/or caregiver instructions on how reduction is done in the event of another prolapse:

  1. Provide the client with gloves and lubricant for future need.

  2. Prolapses may also reduce spontaneously without any manual reduction.

F. Have the client lie in the left lateral position and give extra tissues for urinary incontinence.

G. Ask the client to strain (perform Valsalva's maneuver). This action allows the practitioner to fully evaluate the prolapse through the anal sphincter. If straining does not produce the prolapse, have the client squat and/or sit on the toilet to strain.

H. With a good light source, do a detailed visual examination to rule out hemorrhoids versus a complete/partial prolapse:

  1. Thrombosed hemorrhoids appear as blue, shiny masses.

  2. A normal hemorrhoid appears as a painless, flaccid skin tag.

  3. Anoscope reveals internal hemorrhoids as bright red to purplish bulges.

  4. Rectal prolapse looks like a pink doughnut or rosette; a complete prolapse involving the muscular wall is larger, red, and has circular folds.

I. After visual inspection/evaluation, reposition the client into a knee–chest position. This allows the bowel to be pulled back into the anus.

J. If, after changing positions, the prolapse does not reduce with gravity, place a saline-soaked 4-by-4 gauze over the prolapse to prevent drying.

K. Gentle pressure with the saline gauze should be applied distally to slide the distal end of the prolapse/protusion into the lumen and through the anal sphincter.

L. A rectal prolapse that is large and/or difficult may be reduced by an application of sugar, used as an osmotic agent, to reduce swelling.

M. Using a lubricated gloved hand, perform a rectal examination to evaluate sphincter tone at rest and with some straining. This rectal examination should be painless. Pain raises suspicion for other pathology, such as incarceration or an unrelated lesion.

N. Apply lubricant to anoscope and slowly insert it anteriorly into the rectum. Remove inner cannula of anoscope, and slowly withdraw it to evaluate and identify any lesions. It is rare to see a polyp or carcinoma. Usually, erythema and edema will be noted.

Evaluation/Results of Procedure

A. If reduction of rectal prolapse occurs with minimal discomfort, have the client return in 1 week to assess sphincter function.

B. If unable to reduce prolapse, send the client for *immediate* evaluation by a physician. Keep prolapse covered with saline-soaked gauze during transport.

C. If prolapse was partial or complete, refer the client to a physician after reduction.

D. Further evaluation may include a sigmoidoscopy, barium enema, or biopsy.

E. Presence of pain may indicate an incarceration with impending strangulation and requires *immediate* referral.

F. All clients need to follow a high-fiber diet and have instructions on avoiding straining. Stool softeners, laxatives, and enemas may need to be used to prevent constipation. To reduce the recurrence of prolapse, pelvic floor exercises (Kegel) that strengthen the pelvic floor muscles may be used.

Sprain Evaluation

Cheryl A. Glass

Evaluate each leg, comparing the injured with the uninjured and examining for signs of edema, deformity, tenderness, range of motion, strength, and discoloration. A neurovascular assessment should be performed for any limb injury. Palpate the dorsalis pedis and the posterior tibial arterial pulses and test for sensation.

Knee

A. Lachman test

The Lachman test is used to diagnose injury to the anterior cruciate ligaments (ACL) and posterior cruciate ligaments (PCL). This procedure is considered the gold standard for the evaluation of anterior cruciate and posterior cruciate knee ligament damage:

1. Explain the procedure.
2. Ask the client to lie down on his or her back (supine).
3. The injured knee is flexed 15 to 30 degrees.
4. Lachman's anterior: stabilize the client's femur with one hand and then pull the tibia anteriorly with the other hand.
5. Lachman's posterior: perform the same procedure except repeatedly push the tibia posteriorly.
6. Positive Lachman test interpretation:
    a. Pain with normal anterior translation: ACL sprain
    b. Pain with increased anterior translation (more than 2 mm of the tibia): ACL rupture
    c. Pain with normal posterior: PCL sprain
    d. Pain with increased posterior: PCL rupture

B. Active posterior drawer test

The active posterior drawer test is a method of diagnosing PCL injury:

1. Explain the procedure.
2. Ask the client to be seated with knees flexed 90 degrees.
3. Instruct the client to isometrically contract the hamstring while the examiner stabilizes the foot and palpate the knee joint line.
4. The test is positive if there is posterior sublaxation of the tibial plateau: posterior knee instability.

C. McMurray test

The McMurray test is a **clinical** rotation test for evaluating the knee joint for tears in the meniscus of the knee:

1. Explain the procedure.
2. Ask the client to lie down on his or her back (supine) or side-lying.

3. The affected leg, right or left, should have hip flexed 90 degrees.
4. The injured knee is flexed 90 degrees.
5. Hold the foot in one hand and place the fingers of the other hand on the joint line.
6. Evaluate the client's pain level when palpating the joint when the knee is flexed.
7. Apply valgus force by holding the femur steady and slowly move the lower leg laterally while still applying the valgus stress.
8. Next flex the knee to 135 degrees and switch to varus stress.
9. Finally, extend the knee in the varus position.
10. If the test is positive, a crepitus sensation with movement (meniscus click or pop) can be felt, as well as knee joint line pain or "locking of the knee," which is characteristic of an anterior cruciate ligament tear or relocation.

Ankle

A. Anterior drawer test

The anterior drawer test is an examination for lateral ankle sprain, mechanical instability, or hypermobility:

1. Explain the procedure.
2. Perform this test on the uninjured ankle first, then repeat on the injured ankle.
3. The client should be seated with knees flexed 90 degrees. Ask the client to position the affected foot in the plantar flexion position (foot slightly at rest).
4. Grasp the lower portion of the uninjured leg for bracing. Use one hand at the shin and attempt to draw the heel anteriorly (forward) with your other hand.
5. Repeat the test on the injured ankle.
6. Anterior drawer test is positive for an ankle sprain if the talus at the injured point slides 4 mm or more than the same bone in the other joint.
7. A dimple appears in the area in the anterior talofibular ligament (ATFL) on anterior translation. This dimple sign indicates compromise of the ligament.

B. Prone anterior drawer test (also tests for ligamentous instability):

1. Explain the procedure.
2. Perform this test on the uninjured ankle first, and then repeat on the injured ankle.
3. To perform the prone anterior drawer test, the client must lie prone with his or her feet extending over the end of the examination table. The heel is pushed steadily forward with one hand.
4. The test is positive if there is excessive anterior movement and dimpling of the skin on both sides of the Achilles tendon.

C. Talar tilt test

The talar tilt test (inversion stress maneuver) evaluates injury to the lateral ligaments of the ankle:

1. Explain the procedure.

2. Perform this test on the uninjured ankle first, and then repeat on the injured ankle.

3. The client should be supine or on his or her side, with the foot relaxed.

4. To perform the talar test, grasp the lower heel with one hand while adducting or inverting the foot with your other hand.

5. The degree of tilt ranges from 0 to 23 degrees. The test is positive if the tilt is 5 to 10 degrees greater around the injured joint.

Tick Removal

Cheryl A. Glass

Description

A. Ticks are vectors for Lyme disease, deer tick fever, and Rocky Mountain spotted fever. Ticks should be removed as soon as possible since they pass bacteria that cause the fevers and rashes.

Indications

A. There are several populations at risk of tick-borne transmission diseases, including participants in any outdoor recreational activity; those in contact with heavy brushy areas, such as hunters, campers, and landscapers; and persons in contact with dogs, deer, rodents, and other animals with ticks.

Equipment Required

A. Fine-tip tweezers
B. Antiseptic or rubbing alcohol
C. Gloves: nonsterile may be used.
D. Office setting: scalpel if the tick head remains embedded

Procedure

A. Use gloves.
B. To remove the tick, care should be taken to avoid squeezing the body of the tick:
   1. Tick should be grasped with fine-tip tweezers close to the skin.
   2. Remove by gently pulling the tick upward straight out without using any twisting motions (see Figure II.5).
   3. Do not crush the tick during removal.
C. Examine to ensure the entire head and body removed. If the head is embedded, a small incision may be required for its removal.
D. Cleanse the skin with antiseptic or rubbing alcohol.
E. Save the tick for identification. Write the client's name, date of removal, and date of the tick bite on a piece of paper. Place the paper and the tick in a resealable bag and place it in the freezer.
F. If your office protocol does not require saving the tick for identification, dispose by placing the tick in alcohol, then put it a sealed bag/container and dispose.

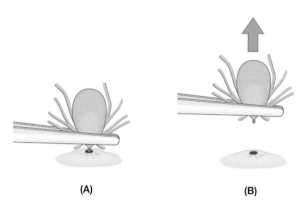

(A)   **(B)**

FIGURE II.5 Tick Removal. (a) Grasp the tick's body as close to the skin as possible using a fine-tip tweezers. Avoid squeezing the body. (b) Remove by pulling the tick straight upward without using twisting motions.

Source: Centers for Disease Control and Prevention. Retrieved from https://www.cdc.gov/ticks/index.html.

Evaluation/Results of Procedure

A. Examine the rest of the body for other ticks.
B. Try to determine the length of time the tick was on the skin.
C. Assess for symptoms of Lyme disease, deer tick fever, and Rocky Mountain spotted fever.
D. Consider serum laboratory studies, medications, and consultants as applicable. See Chapter 16: "Infectious Disease Guidelines," "Lyme Disease," and "Rocky Mountain Spotted Fever" for assessment, diagnosis, and treatment guidelines.

Trichloroacetic Acid/Podophyllin Therapy

Cheryl A. Glass and Rhonda Arthur

Description

A. Trichloroacetic acid (TCA) and podophyllin are substances used to eliminate exophytic warts on the external genitalia and perianal area.

Indications

A. External genitalia and perianal warts

Precautions

A. Podophyllin use is contraindicated in pregnancy.

B. Either substance should be applied sparingly to avoid contact with unaffected skin.

Equipment Required

A. Examining table with stirrups for positioning the female client in the lithotomy position

B. Light source for examining the genitalia and perianal area

C. Gown/drape for the client

D. Gloves: Nonsterile glove may be used.

E. Cotton-tipped applicators

F. Petroleum jelly

G. Sodium bicarbonate (baking soda) or powder with talc

H. Plastic medicine cups

I. TCA 80% to 90% *OR*

J. Podophyllin 10% to 25% in compound tincture of benzoin

Procedure

A. Assist the female client to the lithotomy position; assist the male client to a sitting or supine position on the examination table.

B. Inspect the external genitalia and perianal areas for exophytic warts.

C. Pour small amount (0.5–1.0 mL) of solution (TCA or podophyllin) to be used in a plastic medicine cup.

D. Use the cotton-tipped applicator to apply petroleum jelly on unaffected skin surrounding areas identified for therapy.

E. Use the wooden end of the cotton-tipped applicator to apply a small amount of solution (TCA or podophyllin) to warts.

F. If TCA is used, apply sodium bicarbonate or powder with talc to absorb unreacted acid.

    1. The client should not sit or stand and dress until the treatment has dried.

G. If podophyllin is used, the area should air dry before the client dresses.

    1. Instruct the client to thoroughly wash off the solution in 1 to 4 hours.

H. Repeat weekly if necessary. If warts persist after six applications, consider other therapeutic methods.

I. Advise the client that mild to moderate pain or local irritation may occur after treatment.

Wet Mount/Cervical Cultures Procedure

Cheryl A. Glass

Description

A. The wet mount procedure is a technique used to identify vulvovaginitis commonly caused by trichomoniasis, bacterial vaginosis, and vulvovaginal candidiasis. Any client complaining of vaginal discharge, irritation, vaginal pain, and/or a vaginal odor should have a wet mount performed to aid in identifying the organism to assist in the diagnosis.

Indications

A. Vaginal discharge
B. Vulvar/vaginal irritation or pain
C. Vaginal discharge with an odor
D. Prior to the examination: take a thorough history before the physical examination to determine whether other testing needs to be performed.
E. Presenting complaints (refer to Table II.5 for a comparison of bacterial vaginosis, candidiasis, and trichomoniasis):
　　1. Bacterial vaginosis: thin off-white "grayish" discharge, as well as a musty "fishy" amine odor. The odor increases after intercourse.
　　2. Vulvovaginal candidiasis: thick white "cottage cheese" discharge with no odor observed, as well as pruritus and some dysuria
　　3. Trichomoniasis (parasite *Trichomonas vaginalis*): copious frothy yellow-gray to green-colored malodorous vaginal discharge, pruritus, and vaginal irritation. *The client may also be asymptomatic.*

Precautions

A. Use universal precautions when obtaining specimens.
B. All specimens need to be disposed of as biohazard waste.

Equipment Required

A. Examining table with stirrups for positioning the client in the lithotomy position
B. Light source for examining the cervix
C. Gown/drape for the client
D. Gloves, two pairs (nonsterile)
E. Speculum: several different types and sizes of speculums on hand for appropriate sizing, visualization, and comfort
F. Condoms available if needed
G. Q-tip/cotton-tipped applicators
H. Gen-Probe or other collecting tubes for *Neisseria gonorrhoeae* and *Chlamydia* specimens
I. Small test tube/plastic collection tube
J. Normal saline (NS) and 10% potassium hydroxide (KOH)
K. Glass slides (two): one marked "KOH" and one marked "NS"
L. Cover slips for slides (two)
M. Nitrazine pH test tape
N. Microscope with 10× and 40× objectives

Procedure

A. After the client has voided and changed into a gown, assist the client into the lithotomy position.
B. Apply gloves.
C. Prepare the test tube/specimen tube with 1 mL of NS. Prepare slides (one marked "KOH" and the other marked "NS"); apply one drop of each solution to a clean slide and set aside.
D. Inspect the perineum for lesions, erythema, fissures, condyloma, and lacerations:
　　1. Bacterial vaginosis: usually normal-appearing tissue

TABLE II.5	VAGINITIS DIFFERENTIATION			
	Normal	**Bacterial Vaginosis**	**Candidiasis**	**Trichomoniasis**
Symptom presentation		Odor, discharge, itch	Itch, discomfort, dysuria, thick discharge	Itch, discharge, Merken 70% asymptomatic
Vaginal discharge	Clear to white	Homogeneous, adherent, thin, milky white; malodorous "foul fishy" smell	Thick, clumpy, white "cottage cheese"	Frothy, gray or yellow-green; malodorous
Clinical findings			Inflammation and erythema	Cervical petechiae, "strawberry cervix"
Vaginal pH	3.8–4.2	>4.5	Usually ≤4.5	>4.5
KOH "whiff" test	Negative	Positive	Negative	Often positive
NaCl wet mount	Lacto-bacilli	Clue cells (≥20%), no/few WBCs	Few to many WBCs	Motile flagellated protozoa, many WBCs
KOH wet mount			Pseudohyphae or spores if non-*albicans* species	

KOH, potassium hydroxide; NaCl, sodium chloride; WBCs, white blood cells.

2. Vulvovaginal candidiasis: vulvar and vaginal erythema, edema, and fissures

3. Vulvar and vaginal edema and erythema

E. Gently insert the speculum into the vagina. Do not use lubricant as this may interfere with the quality of the specimen; use warm water for lubrication.

F. While inserting the speculum, visualize the vaginal vault, walls, and cervix. Note any irregularities, such as lesions, masses, and lacerations.

G. If the lateral sidewalls collapse and decrease visualization of the cervix, withdraw the speculum. Apply a condom to the speculum and cut the condom tip. Reinsert the condom-covered speculum to visualize the cervix.

H. Observe for vaginal discharge, noting the amount, color, consistency, and odor:

1. Bacterial vaginosis: discolored discharge with odor, homogeneous discharge that adheres to the vaginal walls

2. Vulvovaginal candidiasis: thick white discharge that adheres to the vaginal walls

3. Frothy, purulent discharge and a "strawberry" cervix

I. Collect a sample of discharge with the two Q-tips:

1. Place one Q-tip into a prefilled test tube/specimen tube and make the slide later OR

2. Collect a sample of discharge with the Q-tip and roll the Q-tip into the NS-prepared slide, then cover with a cover slip.

3. *Next* roll the Q-tip into the KOH-prepared slide.

4. Note any "musty/fishy" amine odor before placing the cover slip on the slide. (Whiff test is positive if amine odor is noted.)

J. Using the second Q-tip, roll the Q-tip over a strip of nitrazine test tape to evaluate pH.

K. Using the Gen-Probe, insert the tip onto the cervical os and rotate the tip in the os several times to obtain an adequate specimen (sample for a minimum of about 30 seconds).

L. Withdraw the Gen-Probe applicator and place in the appropriate specimen container.

M. Gently remove the speculum and perform a bimanual examination, assessing for cervical motion tenderness and pain.

N. After completing this examination, take the specimens to the lab area for evaluation (while the client is dressing).

O. Prepare slides (if steps I.1–I.4 not followed):

1. Slide 1: place one drop of NS on the slide; roll the Q-tip and apply cover slip.

2. Slide 2: place one drop of KOH on the slide and roll the Q-tip; note any "musty/fishy" amine odor from the slide before placing the cover slide.

P. Observe the NS slide first under the microscope. Start on low power, 10×, and adjust the focus until the specimen is clearly seen under the microscope.

Q. Observe the entire field and note the number of squamous cells.

R. Switch to the high-powered field, 40×, making sure the light source and the visual focus are adequate

S. Observe the slide for:

1. Vaginal squamous epithelial cells: appear flat, with clear edges. Red blood cells (RBCs), sperm, and polymorphonuclear neutrophils (PMNs) may also be identified (see Figure II.6).

2. Clue cells: epithelial cells with irregular borders and a granular appearance; may see the presence of coccobacilli bacteria (not present on slide; see Figure II.7)

3. Bacteria

4. *Lactobacilli*: appear as rods (see Figure II.8)

5. White blood cells (WBCs): Note, a large number of WBCs is not normal.

6. Trichomonads: appear as ovoid mobile organisms that dart around on the slide (see Figures II.9 and II.10)

7. *Candida*: appear as branching pseudohyphae or budding yeast (best seen under the KOH slide; see Figure II.11)

Treatment

A. Refer to specific chapters for treatment recommendations and medication dosages.

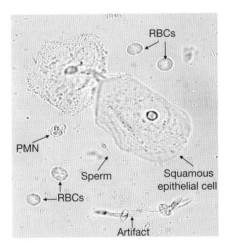

FIGURE II.6 Epithelial cells.

PMN, polymorphonuclear neutrophils; RBC, red blood cell.

Source: Used with permission from the University of Washington STD Prevention Training Center.

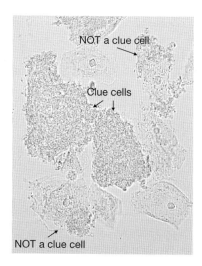

FIGURE II.7 Clue cells.

Source: Used with permission from the University of Washington STD Prevention Training Center.

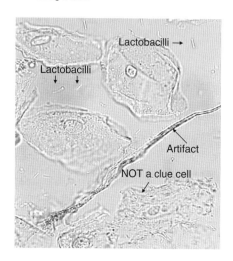

FIGURE II.8 Lactobacilli.

Source: Used with permission from the University of Washington STD Prevention Training Center.

FIGURE II.9 *Trichomonas vaginalis*.

Source: Used with permission from the University of Washington STD Prevention Training Center.

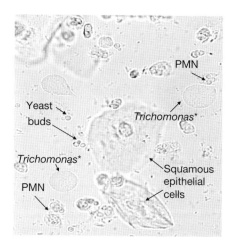

FIGURE II.10 *Trichomonas* (1,000×).

PMN, polymorphonuclear neutrophils.

Note: Organism is enlarged.

Source: Used with permission from the University of Washington STD Prevention Training Center.

FIGURE II.11 Budding yeast cells, pseudohyphae, and septate hyphae and spores.

PMN, polymorphonuclear neutrophils.

Source: Used with permission from the University of Washington STD Prevention Training Center.

Bibliography

Allergan. (2018, October). *Liletta highlights of prescribing information.* Retrieved from https://www.allergan.com/assets/pdf/liletta_pi

American Cancer Society. (2018, December 28). *Cervical cancer prevention and early detection.* Retrieved from https://www.cancer.org/cancer/cer-vical-cancer/prevention-and-early-detection/cervical-cancer-screening-guidelines.html

American College of Obstetricians and Gynecologists. (2009, July, reaffirmed 2015). ACOG practice bulletin no. 106: Intrapartum fetal heart rate monitoring: Nomenclature interpretation, and general management principles. *Obstetrics and Gynecology, 114,* 192–202. doi:10.1097/AOG.0b013e3181aef106

American College of Obstetricians and Gynecologists. (2010, November, reaffirmed 2015). ACOG practice bulletin no. 116: Management of intrapartum fetal heart tracing. *Obstetrics and Gynecology, 116,* 1232–1240. doi:10.1097/AOG.0b013e3182004fa9

American College of Obstetricians and Gynecologists. (2014, July, reaffirmed 2019). Practice bulletin no. 145: Antepartum fetal surveillance. *Obstetrics and Gynecology, 124,* 182–192. doi:10.1097/01.AOG.0000451759.90082.7b

American National Red Cross. (2011). *Airway adjuncts.* Retrieved from https://www.redcross.org/images/MEDIA_CustomProductCatalog/m4240191_AirwayAdjunctsFactandSkill.pdf

American Urological Association. (2012). *Adult urodynamics: AUA/SUFU guideline.* Retrieved from www.auanet.org/education/adult-urodynam-ics.cfm

Bayer. (2017, June). *Mirena: Highlights of prescribing information.* Retrieved from https://labeling.bayerhealthcare.com/html/products/pi/Mirena_PI.pdf

Bayer. (2018a, March). *Kyleena: Highlights of prescribing information.* Retrieved from http://labeling.bayerhealthcare.com/html/products/pi/Kyleena_PI.pdf

Bayer. (2018b, March). *Skyla: Highlights of prescribing information.* Retrieved from http://labeling.bayerhealthcare.com/html/products/pi/Skyla_PI.pdf

Bhattacharyya, N., Grubbels, S. P., Schwartz, S. R., Edlow, J. A., El-Kashlan, H., Fife, T., ... Corrigan, M. D. (2017, March 1). Clinical practice guideline: Benign paroxysmal positional vertigo (Update). *Otolaryngology–Head and Neck Surgery, 156*(3S), S1–S47. doi:10.1177/0194599816689667

Blumenfeld, H. (n.d.). *Neuroanatomy through clinical cases: Extraocular movements (CN III, IV, VI).* Retrieved from http://www.neuroexam.com/content.php?p=20

Castro, D., & Freeman, L. A. (2019, January 19). Oropharyngeal airway. *StatPearls [Internet].* Retrieved from https://www.ncbi.nlm.nih.gov/books/NBK470198/

Cheuck, L. (2017, April 17). *Diagnostic prostatic massage technique.* Medscape. Retrieved from http://emedicine.medscape.com/article/1948091-technique#2aab6b3b2

Collins, C. W., Winters, J. C., American Urological Association, & Society of Urodynamics Female Pelvic Medicine and Urogenital Reconstruction. (2014). AUA/SUFU adult urodynamics guideline: A clinical review. *Urologic Clinics of North America, 41*(3), 353–362, vii. doi:10.1016/jucl.2104.04.011

Cooper Surgical. (2018, January). *Paragard intrauterine copper contraceptive prescribing information.* Retrieved from https://hcp.paragard.com/wp-content/uploads/sites/2/2018/09/ParaGard-PI.pdf

Da Costa Andrade, S., Chianca da Silva, F., dos Santos Oliveira, S., Souza Leite, K., Ferreira da Costa, T., & Lacet Zaccara, A. A. (2014). Microbiological agents of vulvovaginitis identified by Pap smear. *Journal of Nursing UFPE/Revista De Enfermagem UFPE, 8*(2), 338–345. doi:10.5205/reuol.4688-38583-1-RV.0802201414

Davis, R., Jones, J. S., Barocas, D. A., Castle, E. P., Lang, E. K., Leveillee, R. J., ... Weitzel, W. (2012 and validity confirmed 2016). *Diagnosis, evaluation, and follow-up of asymptomatic microhematuria (AMH) in adults: AUA guideline.* Retrieved from https://www.auanet.org/guidelines/asymptomatic-microhematuria-(amh)-guideline

Dickey, R. P. (2014). *Managing contraceptive pill patients* (15th ed.). Fort Collins, CO: EMIS Medical Publishing.

Dubey, P. K. (2016). Another method for the removal of spherical nasal foreign bodies in pediatric patients. *Journal of Emergency Medicine, 50*(1), 125–126. doi:10.1016/j.jemermed.2015.01.043

Family Practice Notebook.com. Orthopedics Book. (n.d.a). *Ankle anterior drawer test.* Retrieved from http://www.fpnotebook.com/Ortho/Exam/AnklAntrDrwrTst.htm

Family Practice Notebook.com. Orthopedics Book. (n.d.b). *McMurray test.* Retrieved from http://www.fpnotebook.com/Ortho/Exam/McmryTst.htm

Family Practice Notebook.com. Orthopedics Book. (n.d.c) *Talar tilt.* Retrieved from http://www.fpnotebook.com/Ortho/Exam/TlrTlt.htm

Fetzer, S. (2015, July). Advance practice nursing guide to the neurological exam. [Review of the book *Advanced Practice Nursing Guide to the Neurological Exam,* by Alexandra Armitage.] *New Hampshire Nursing News, 39*(3), 14. Retrieved from https://www.nursingald.com/publications/1206

Fisher, J. I. (2017, July). *Nasal foreign bodies.* Medscape. Retrieved from https://emedicine.medscape.com/article/763767-overview

Fundakowski, C. E., Moon, S., & Torres, L. (2013). The snare technique: A novel atraumatic method for the removal of difficult nasal foreign bodies. *Journal of Emergency Medicine, 44*(1), 104–106. doi:10.1016/j.jemermed.2012.07.070

Heerema, E. (2019, March 16). *How the clock-drawing test screens for dementia.* Retrieved from https://www.verywellhealth.com/the-clock-drawing-test-98619

Hubbard, E. J., Santini, V., Blankevoort, C. G., Volkers, K. M., Barrup, M. S., Byerly, L., ... Stern, R. A. (2008, May). Clock drawing performance in cognitively normal elderly. *Archives of Clinical Neuropsychology, 23*(3), 295–327. doi:10.1016/j.acn.2007.12.003

Interstitial Cystitis Association. (2015, May 20). *Urodyamics: What, when, why.* Retrieved from https://www.ichelp.org/diagnosis-treatment/diagnosis-of-ic/urodynamics-what-when-why/

Jørgensen, K., Kristensen, M. K., Waldemar, G., & Vogel, A. (2015). The six-item clock drawing test—Reliability and validity in mild Alzheimer's disease. *Neuropsychology, Development, and Cognition, Section B: Aging, Neuropsychology and Cognition, 22*(3), 301–311. doi:10.1080/13825585.2014.932325

Krapf, J. M. (2018, January 19). *Vulvovaginitis.* Retrieved from https://emedicine.medscape.com/article/2188931-overview

Krause, R. S. (2017, May 9). *Reduction of rectal prolapse.* Medscape. Retrieved from http://emedicine.medscape.com/article/80982-overview

Lab Tests Online. (2018, July 23). *Vaginitis and vaginosis.* Retrieved from https://labtestsonline.org/conditions/vaginitis-and-vaginosis

Lustig, L. R. (2018, October). Benign paroxysmal positional vertigo: BPPV. The Merck manual professional version. In R. Porter (Ed.), *Merck manual: Professional version.* Kenilworth, NJ: Merck & Co. Retrieved from https://www.merckmanuals.com/professional/ear,-nose,-and-throat-disorders/inner-ear-disorders/benign-paroxysmal-positional-vertigo

Massad, L.S., Einstein, M. H., Huh, W. K., Katki, H. A., Kinney, W. K., Schiffman, M., ... Lawson, H. W. (2013, April). 2012 updated consensus guidelines for the management of abnormal cervical cancer screening test and cancer precursors. *Journal of Lower Genital Tract Disease, 17,* S1–S27. doi:10.1097/LGT.0b013e318287d329

McMurray's test. (2016). *MediSavvy.* Retrieved from https://medisavvy.com/mcmurrays-test

Miller, D. (2019). Intrapartum fetal heart rate assessment. *UpToDate.* Waltham, MA: Wolters Kluwer. Retrieved from https://www.uptodate.com/contents/intrapartum-fetal-heart-rate-assessment?search=Antepartum%20fetal%20heart%20rate%20assessment&source=search_result&selectedTitle=1-140&usage_type=default&display_rank=1

Miller, M. (2014, August 1). Recurrent vulvovaginitis: Tips for treating a common condition. *Contemporary OB/GYN, 59*(8), 22–27. Retrieved from https://www.contemporaryobgyn.net/vaginal-infection/recurrent-vulvovaginitis-tips-treating-common-condition

Moses, S. (2014a, February 23). *McMurray test.* Family practice notebook. Retrieved from https://fpnotebook.com/ortho/Exam/McmryTst.htm

Moses, S. (2014b, September 8). *Ankle anterior drawer test.* Family practice notebook. Retrieved from https://fpnotebook.com/Ortho/Exam/AnklAntrDrwrTst.htm

Moses, S. (2014c, September 8). *Talar tilt.* Family practice notebook. Retrieved from https://fpnotebook.com/Ortho/Exam/TlrTlt.htm

Murray, T. A., Kelly, N. R., & Jenkins, S. (2002). The complete neurological examination: What every nurse should know. *Advance for Nurse Practitioners, 10,* 24–28.

National Kidney and Urologic Diseases Information Clearinghouse. (2014, January). *Urodynamic testing* (NIH Publication No. 12–5106). Retrieved from https://www.niddk.nih.gov/health-information/diagnostic-tests/urodynamic-testing

Peters, R., Beckett, N., Pereira, L., Poulter, R., Pinto, E., Ma, S., … Bulpitt, C. (2015). The clock drawing test, mortality, incident cardiovascular events, and dementia. *International Journal of Geriatric Psychiatry, 30*(4), 416–421. doi:10.1002/gps.4153

Ricci, M., Pigliautile, M., D'Ambrosio, V., Ercolani, S., Bianchini, C., Ruggiero, C., … Mecocci, P. (2016). The clock drawing test as a screening tool in mild cognitive impairment and very mild dementia: A new brief method of scoring and normative data in the elderly. *Neurological Sciences, 37*(6), 867–873. doi:10.1007/s10072-016-2480-6

Sand, P. K. (2008). Diagnostic procedures in the evaluation of female urinary incontinence and voiding dysfunction. In S. Arulkumaran (Ed.), *The global library of women's medicine*. Carlisle, United Kingdom: The Foundation for The Global Library of Women's Medicine. Retrieved from www.glowm.com/section_view/heading/DiagnosticProceduresintheEvaluationofFemaleUrinaryIncontinenceandVoidingDysfunction/item/55. Update currently under review due 2019.

Saslow, D., Solomon, D., Lawson, H. W., Killackey, M., Kulasingam, S., Cain, J., … Myers, E. R. (2012). American Cancer Society, American Society for Colposcopy and Cervical Pathology, and American Society for Clinical Pathology screening guidelines for the prevention and early detection of cervical cancer. *CA: A Cancer Journal for Clinicians, 63*(3), 147–172. Retrieved from https://onlinelibrary.wiley.com/doi/epdf/10.3322/caac.21139

Seidel, H. M., Ball, J. W., Dains, J. E., & Benedict, G. W. (1991). *Mosby's guide to physical examination* (2nd ed.). New York, NY: Mosby Year-Book.

Shah, A. R. (2018, September 14). *Hernia reduction technique*. Medscape. Retrieved from https://emedicine.medscape.com/article/149608-technique#showal

Shirley Ryan Abilitylab. (n.d.) *Clock drawing test*. Retrieved from https://www.sralab.org/rehabilitation-measures/clock-drawing-test

Winters, J. C., Dmochowski, R. R., Goldman, H. B., Herndon, C. D. A., Kobashi, K. C., Kraus, S. R., … Wein, A. J. (2012, December). Urodynamic studies in adults: AUA/SUFU guideline. *The Journal of Urology, 188*(Suppl. 6), 2464–2472. doi:10.1016/j.juro.2012.09.081

Young, C. C. (2019, January 14). *Ankle sprain*. Medscape. Retrieved from https://emedicine.medscape.com/article/1907229-overview

Zasler, N. D. (2015). Validity assessment and the neurological physical examination. *NeuroRehabilitation, 36*(4), 401–413. doi:10.3233/NRE-151229

III CLIENT TEACHING GUIDES

- Head Injury: Mild
- Hemorrhoids
- Herpes Simplex Virus
- Herpes Zoster or Shingles
- HIV/AIDS: Resources for Clients
- Human Papillomavirus
- Infant Nutrition
- Influenza (Flu)
- Insect Bites and Stings
- Insulin Therapy During Pregnancy
- Iron-Deficiency Anemia (Pregnancy)
- Irritable Bowel Syndrome
- Jaundice and Hepatitis
- Kidney Disease: Chronic
- Knee Exercises
- Lactose Intolerance And Malabsorption
- Lice (Pediculosis)
- Lichen Planus
- Lyme Disease and Removal of a Tick
- Lymphedema
- Mastitis
- Menopause
- Mononucleosis
- Myasthenia Gravis
- Nicotine Dependence
- Nosebleeds
- Oral Thrush in Children
- Osteoarthritis
- Osteoporosis
- Otitis Media With Effusion
- Parkinson's Disease Management
- Pelvic Inflammatory Disease
- Peripheral Arterial Disease
- Pharyngitis
- Pityriasis Rosea
- Pneumonia, Viral: Adult
- Pneumonia, Viral: Child
- Polymyalgia Rheumatica
- Postpartum: Breast Engorgement and Sore Nipples
- Premenstrual Syndrome
- Preterm Labor

- Prostatic Hypertrophy/Benign
- Prostatitis
- Pseudogout
- Psoriasis
- Respiratory Syncytial Virus
- RICE Therapy and Exercise Therapy
- Ringworm (Tinea)
- Rocky Mountain Spotted Fever and Removal of a Tick
- Roundworms And Pinworms
- Scabies
- Seborrheic Dermatitis
- Shortness of Breath
- Sinusitis
- Skin Care Assessment
- Sleep Apnea
- Sleep Disorders/Insomnia
- Superficial Thrombophlebitis
- Syphilis
- Systemic Lupus Erythematosus
- Testicular Self-Examination
- Tinea Versicolor
- Tinnitus
- Toxoplasmosis
- Transient Ischemic Attack
- Trichomoniasis
- Ulcer
- Urinary Incontinence: Women
- Urinary Tract Infection (Acute Cystitis)
- Urinary Tract Infection During Pregnancy: Pyelonephritis
- Vaginal Bleeding: First Trimester
- Vaginal Bleeding: Second and Third Trimesters
- Vaginal Yeast Infection
- Warts
- Wound Care: Lower Extremity Ulcers
- Wound Care: Pressure Ulcers
- Wound Care: Wounds
- Wound Infection: Episiotomy and Cesarean Section
- Xerosis (Winter Itch)
- Zika Virus Infection

ABDOMINAL PAIN: ADULTS

PROBLEM

Problems relating to abdominal organs may range from simple gas to appendicitis. Acute pain is pain that has started recently; recurrent pain is present on three or more separate occasions over at least a 3-month period.

It is important that you call the healthcare provider if you have pain that lasts 3 hours or longer, have fever, vomiting, or pain that is unusually sharp or intense.

CAUSE

Pain may result from inflammation, ischemia (poor blood supply), distension, constipation, or obstruction. Gastroenteritis is the most common cause of acute pain, and chronic stool retention (constipation) is the most common cause of chronic pain. Urinary tract infections (UTIs) can also cause abdominal pain.
A. Males: Torsion of the testicles or a strangulated inguinal hernia may cause abdominal pain
B. Females: If you have missed a period or suspect you are pregnant, tell your healthcare provider; ectopic pregnancies are a medical emergency

PREVENTION/CARE

The following suggestions can prevent abdominal pain from constipation:
A. Go to the bathroom as soon as you have the urge to have a bowel movement (BM)
B. Establish a regular toilet time such as after breakfast; 15 to 20 minutes after breakfast provides a good time, because spontaneous colonic motility is greatest during that period.

TREATMENT PLAN

Do not take laxatives, enemas, drugs, food, or liquids (including water) until consulting your healthcare provider for suspected abdominal pain and the following:
A. Increased or odd-looking vomit or stools
B. Hard, swollen abdomen
C. Lump in scrotum, groin, or lower abdomen
D. Missed period or suspected pregnancy

Activity: Engage in activity as tolerated. Abdominal pain with nausea and vomiting, with fever, or pain that lasts more than 3 hours and makes you stop doing daily activities should be reported.

Diet: Eat regular foods as tolerated. Do not eat food or drink liquids until you see a healthcare provider if you have pain with nausea and vomiting, with fever, or pain that lasts longer than 3 hours.

Medications:

You Have Been Prescribed: _____

You Need to Take: _____

You Need to Notify the Office If You Have:
A. Any change in first symptoms that brought you to the office
B. Fever higher than _____ degrees

C. Other: _____

Phone: _____

ABDOMINAL PAIN: CHILDREN

PROBLEM

Pain in your child's "tummy" may range from simple gas to appendicitis. It is important to call the healthcare provider if your child has abdominal pain that lasts 3 hours or longer, has a fever, vomiting, or pain that is unusually sharp or intense. Signs that your child has abdominal pain include lying down and drawing his or her knees into the stomach; crying when you try to touch his or her stomach; or pointing to an area, such as the navel, when crying.

CAUSE

Pain may result from inflammation, distension, constipation, or obstruction. A gastrointestinal (GI) stomach bug (gastroenteritis) is the most common cause of acute pain. Chronic pain happens if your child holds in BMs, which causes constipation. UTIs can cause abdominal pain, and often the child with a bladder infection does complain of burning on urination and having to go to the bathroom more often.

PREVENTION/CARE

There is no way to prevent stomach pain, but the following can prevent abdominal pain from constipation:
A. Tell your child to go to the bathroom as soon as he or she feels the urge to go
B. If possible, set up a regular toilet time such as 15 to 20 minutes after breakfast or after school

TREATMENT PLAN

Do not give laxatives, enemas, drugs, herbal products, food, or liquids (including water) until consulting your healthcare provider for suspected abdominal pain and the following:
A. Unusual cry, especially loud crying
B. Increased or odd-looking BMs or vomiting
C. Hard, swollen abdomen
D. Lump in scrotum, groin, or lower abdomen (tummy)
E. If you notice pain symptoms, especially if when the child bends his or her legs, draws the knees to his or her chest, and/or points to his or her navel

Activity: Allow activity as tolerated. Children may not be able to tell you in words what is wrong with them. Children tell you they are in pain with a change in the pitch of their crying and by making faces (grimacing). For example:
A. Refusing to eat or breastfeed
B. Drawing knees to tummy when you touch the stomach
Diet: Do not give baby food or liquids until you see a healthcare provider if you notice a change in the pitch of your baby's crying, facial grimacing, refusal to suck, or your child draws the knees up to his or her stomach, especially after being touched.
Medications:

You Have Been Prescribed: _____

You Need to Take: _____

You Need to Notify the Office If You Notice That Your Child Has:
A. Any change in first symptoms that brought you to the office
B. Fever higher than _____ degrees

C. Other: _____

Phone: _____

ACNE ROSACEA

PROBLEM

Acne rosacea is a skin condition that affects primarily the nose and face, causing redness, flushing, pimples, and bumps. The blood vessels may be more prominent on the face, causing the skin to appear reddened.

CAUSE

The cause is not known. It is thought to be caused by the blood vessels in the face being too active, causing flushing and redness of the skin.

PREVENTION/CARE

A. Avoid rubbing or massaging the face, which can irritate the skin.
B. Avoid alcoholic beverages.
C. Avoid using harsh soaps/creams on face, including cosmetics that irritate the skin.
D. Wash face with a mild soap, such as Cetaphil or Purpose soap daily. Other suggested daily cleansers are sulfa-based cleanser (Rosanil) or benzoyl peroxide cleanser.
E. Protect the skin when outdoors by wearing protective clothing, hats, and so on, to cover the face. Use a sunscreen with a sun protection formula (SPF) 30 or a zinc-based ointment, such as zinc oxide, on the skin for protection.
F. You may be prescribed an antibiotic by mouth or an antibiotic cream/gel to place on the skin. Use medications as prescribed by your provider
G. Avoid using steroid creams on your face unless prescribed by your provider.
H. If your skin condition begins to affect your eyes, you need to notify your provider immediately. Do not apply any medications or creams on your eyes unless prescribed by your provider.

TREATMENT PLAN

A. Use antibiotics/medications as prescribed by your provider.
B. Wash face with mild cleanser daily.

Activity: As tolerated. No limitations in physical activity.
Diet:
A. Drink plenty of fluids daily.
B. Avoid alcoholic beverages.
Medications:

You or Your Child Has Been Prescribed: _____

You Need to Take: _____

You Need to Notify the Office If:
A. You have a reaction to any of the medications or cleansers prescribed.
B. Rash appears on your eyes or other new places.
C. Symptoms worsen, or new signs or symptoms present before your next follow-up appointment.

D. Other: _____

Phone: _____

RESOURCE

www.rosacea.org

ACNE VULGARIS

PROBLEM

Acne vulgaris refers to blackheads, whiteheads, or red nodules noted on the face, back, chest, and arms.

CAUSE

Accumulation of cells and bacteria clogs the pores and stimulates an inflammatory response, which results in papule or pustule (pimple or blackhead) formation.

PREVENTION/CARE

A. Wash area with mild soap (Purpose or Basis soap) no more than two times per day.
B. Avoid oil-based makeup and creams. Use matte-finished makeup or pore minimizer.
C. Use facial cleansers and moisturizers such as Cetaphil and Moisturel. These prevent the skin from drying out. Benzoyl peroxide 5% lotion or gel may be used at bedtime to help open pores and kill bacteria.
D. To prevent scarring, do not pick lesions.
E. Avoid excessive sun exposure. Use oil-free sunscreen with SPF 15 or greater.
F. Do not get frustrated if lesions return. Do not stop medications without the direction of your provider.
G. Stress can influence outbreaks of lesions. Follow a routine exercise program, practice stress management tactics, and take other measures that decrease stress levels in your daily routine.

TREATMENT PLAN

Activity: As tolerated. Physical activity encouraged
Diet: Eat a well-balanced diet. Drink 8 to 10 glasses of water a day to help keep your skin well hydrated. Cocoa and chocolate do not have an effect on the development of acne vulgaris.
Medications: Antibiotics may need to be prescribed.

You Have Been Prescribed: _____

You Need to Take: _____

You Need to Notify the Office If:
A. You have a reaction to any of the medications prescribed.
B. You are unable to tolerate the prescribed medications.

Phone: _____

ACUTE OTITIS EXTERNA (SWIMMER'S EAR)

PROBLEM

Your practitioner has diagnosed a condition known as acute otitis externa, sometimes also referred to as "swimmer's ear." This is a common condition characterized by itching in the ear, sometimes followed by severe ear pain, swelling, and drainage of the ear canal. Difficulty hearing may also occur. The eardrum is rarely affected.

CAUSE

Acute otitis externa occurs from irritation to the external canal of the ear. The most common causes for otitis externa are long exposure to water in the ear canal after frequent swimming and self-cleaning of the earwax. It may involve either a bacterial or a fungal infection.

PREVENTION/CARE

The following measures may prevent future problems with otitis externa:
A. Clean the outer ear only as needed. Do NOT attempt to clean in internal ear canal. Do not use cotton-tipped swabs or any other device to clean down into the ear canal. Usually, wax is just pushed deeper into the canal with this method, and the canal may be traumatized by the instrument used.
B. For swimmers or others susceptible to frequent recurrences of otitis externa, it may be helpful to dry the ear canals with a blow dryer on a low setting after exposure to water. Also, isopropyl alcohol (rubbing alcohol), may be instill into the ear canal after showering, bathing, or swimming. Do not instill rubbing alcohol into the ear if the ear is already infected or if there is a hole in the ear drum.

TREATMENT PLAN

For the most common bacterial infections associated with otitis externa, antibiotic/steroid eardrops are usually prescribed. In addition, the ear should be kept dry until it is healed. This means no swimming until symptoms are totally resolved. To bathe or shower, first coat cotton balls with petroleum jelly and use them to plug ears.

Activity: The only activity restrictions are those involving submersion in water. Bathing and hair washing are permitted as described previously.
Diet: No changes are required in your diet.
Medications:
A. Prescription eardrops are used to treat otitis externa.
B. The drops should be applied down the ear canal's opening.
C. In severe cases, oral antibiotics may be given.

You Have Been Prescribed: _____

You Need to Instill _____ **Drops into the Affected Ear** _____ **Times Per Day.**

You Need to Notify the Office or Go to the Emergency Department If You:
A. Have symptoms that have not cleared up in 3 days
B. Have a fever over 100°F
C. Have severe ear pain or new symptoms present
D. Are unable to instill ear drops into the ear due to swelling of the ear canal

E. Other: _____

Phone: _____

ACUTE OTITIS MEDIA

PROBLEM

Acute otitis media inflammation of the space between the eardrum and the inner ear is characterized by the rapid onset of ear pain and possible hearing loss.

CAUSE

Usually caused by bacteria or viruses

PREVENTION/CARE

A. Wash your child's hands often. Always wash hands before eating and after playing, especially when playing with other children.
B. **Do not smoke. Children should not be exposed to secondhand smoke. Secondhand smoke increases the risk of ear infections in children.**
C. Avoid exposure to other children/people as much as possible, especially during the first year of life. Exposure to others increases the risk of contracting a virus that may lead to getting a cold. Many ear infections occur after having a cold or upper respiratory infection.
D. If your child is bottle-fed, do not "prop" the bottle. Always hold your baby when bottle feeding.
E. Do not allow your child to have a bottle at bedtime.
F. Wean your child from the bottle by his or her first birthday.
G. Breastfeeding your baby for the first 6 to 12 months of life is highly recommended. Breastfeeding reduces the risk of ear infections because breast milk contains antibodies that fight against ear infections.
H. Childhood immunizations are encouraged to be given at the recommended ages. Some immunizations, such as the flu vaccine and pneumococcal vaccine, may protect your child from getting ear infections.

TREATMENT PLAN

Follow up with a healthcare provider as instructed to avoid complications of otitis media or permanent hearing loss.

Activity: Your child may not play as much when he or she is sick. Activity is encouraged as tolerated.
Diet: Your child may not eat well when he or she is sick. No change in diet is recommended. Encourage fluids for hydration.
Medications:
A. Children's Tylenol and/or ibuprofen may be used for fever or pain.
B. **Do not use aspirin for children**
C. Antibiotics may be prescribed. Give as prescribed.

You Have Been Prescribed: _____

You Need to Take: _____

Your child needs to finish all the antibiotics, even though he or she may start to feel better.

You Need to Notify the Office If You Have:
A. Continued fever or no improvement in symptoms in 48 hours
B. A child who acts as if he or she has a stiff neck, headache, or other new symptoms
C. Continual crying or not being able to console your child
D. Rash while taking medicine

E. Other: _____

Phone: _____

ADDISON'S DISEASE

PROBLEM

Addison's disease has many symptoms, including weakness and fatigue, fainting or dizziness, poor appetite, weight loss, nausea, vomiting, diarrhea, abdominal discomfort, skin discoloration, and low blood pressure, as well as cravings for salty foods.

CAUSE

Addison's disease is most commonly caused by your body's unusual ability to attack its own tissues, called autoimmunity. This results in inadequate amounts of cortisol and/or aldosterone produced by the adrenal glands.

TREATMENT PLAN/CARE

A. Wear your identification band stating that you have Addison's disease and that lists treatment, as well as your healthcare provider's name and phone number.
B. Increased medication dosage will be required during any significant illness, especially with vomiting and/or diarrhea, before dental extractions, and before major surgical procedures. **These issues need to be discussed with your healthcare provider so you will know the correct dosage of medication to take.**
C. Have injectable cortisol available for emergencies when you are unconscious or otherwise unable to take pills.

Activity: As tolerated, avoid overexertion
Diet: High-sodium, low-potassium, high-protein diet
Medications:

You Have Been Prescribed: _____

You Need to Take: _____

You Need to Notify the Office If:
A. You have a reaction to your medications.
B. You cannot tolerate the prescribed medications.
C. You are having dental procedures or surgery to discuss adjusting your medicines.
D. You are sick with nausea and vomiting to discuss adjusting your medicines or coming into the office.

E. Other: _____

Phone: _____

RESOURCES

National Adrenal Diseases Foundation (NADF): www.nadf.us
You can build your own identification bracelets or neck chains from American Medical ID: www.americanmedical-id.com

ADHD: COPING STRATEGIES FOR TEENS AND ADULTS

PROBLEM

Attention deficit hyperactivity disorder (ADHD) is a common mental health problem in which a person has difficulty paying attention, has a short attention span, and frequently gets in trouble because of behavior issues. The client may show signs of hyperactivity, difficulty with concentrating, reacting without thinking first, and may also have anger issues.

CAUSE

The cause of ADHD is unknown. However, it may be hereditary.

TREATMENT PLAN/PREVENTION CARE

A. Identify coping skills. Identify what things help you to control your behavior and prevent outbursts.
B. Counseling and therapy are commonly encouraged to help you learn new coping skills to help with your problem. Make sure you keep all appointments with your counselor/therapist.
C. Make sure to clarify all assignments and tasks.
D. Keep simple lists of your chores for the day.
E. Attach reminder notes to logical items; for example, put a self-adhesive note on your bathroom mirror to remind yourself to do something.
F. Organize your things in a logical way. For example, put your medication bottle with your toothbrush so you will be sure to take it in the morning.
G. Establish a daily routine and stick to it
H. Keep your environment as quiet and peaceful as possible. Seek out work and study sites that are quiet and peaceful
I. Be good to yourself: eat well, get enough rest, and exercise.
J. Take your medications as prescribed. If you feel that your medication is not improving your behavior, notify your parent and/or care provider so this can be evaluated.

RESOURCES

Children and Adults With Attention Deficit Hyperactivity Disorder (CHADD): www.chadd.org
The National Attention Deficit Disorder Association: www.add.org
National Resource Center for ADHD: www.help4adhd.org

ADHD: TIPS FOR CAREGIVERS OF A CHILD WITH ADHD

A child with ADHD may not respond to your direction and discipline as easily as other children. Here are a few ways you can organize your home and your child to try to help him or her.

A. Accept your child's limitations. Understand that his or her activity and inattention are intrinsic. Be as tolerant, low key, and client as you can possibly be.

B. Provide an outlet for the release of excess energy, such as active games, especially outdoors or in open spaces.

C. Keep your home well organized. Have routines for the usual activities for the day. This will help your child to anticipate activities. Eliminate extraneous noise and clutter, such as having the TV on or piling your kitchen table high with newspapers.

D. Be sure your child gets plenty of rest and good nutrition.

E. Avoid formal gatherings or other places where you and your child will have added stress to behave well.

F. Establish discipline that is firm, reliable, and nonphysical.

G. Stretch your child's attention span by quietly and regularly reading to or playing with him or her. Praise whenever possible.

H. Medications may be very helpful. *Often* they will allow your child to attend to his or her schoolwork; school performance and experience may be much improved.

I. Be active with your child's school. *You* are his or her most interested advocate.

J. Make sure that his or her school placement and program are appropriate. Enlist the support of the school nurse, school psychologist, or principal if needed.

K. Most important, enjoy your child as much as possible. Try to take breaks whenever possible.

ADOLESCENT NUTRITION

A. Adolescents need a well-balanced diet. However, requirements vary depending on the build and gender of the adolescent.

B. Adolescents go through a growing spurt and require extra nutrients during this time:
1. Girls have a growth spurt generally between 10 and 14 years of age.
2. Boys have a growth spurt generally between 12 and 15 years of age.

C. To help prevent obesity, it is important to set a good example:
1. Limit junk foods.
2. Limit sugary sodas.
3. Limit fast food.
4. Serve regular portions, not "super-sized"
5. Teens need snacks between meals.
6. Buy fresh vegetables and fruits for snacking.
7. Many teens do not get enough vitamins from their regular diet and may need a vitamin supplement.

D. Enhance your diet with foods that are a good source of calcium and vitamin D:
1. Dairy products are an excellent source of calcium and support the bones, making them healthy and stronger. Strong bones decrease the risk of the development of osteoporosis.
2. Dairy products also provide potassium and maintain and support a healthy blood pressure.
3. Dairy products fortified with vitamin D are also recommended to support bone health.

E. Choosing foods that are lower in saturated fats and cholesterol will also help to keep cholesterol levels low and decrease the risk of developing high cholesterol and heart disease.

F. Since body image is important to teens, making good decisions for weight control and participating in daily exercises will help reduce the risk of obesity.

Note: If you are concerned about your child's eating habits, eating too much, "binging," or not eating enough to control his or her weight, "anorexia," you need to notify our office.

G. A use resource is the U.S. Department of Agriculture Food Pyramid: www.ChooseMyPlate.gov

SUGGESTED NUMBER OF SERVINGS OF FOOD GROUPS PER DAY	
Food Group	**Number of Servings Per Day**
Milk/dairy	3
Meat	2–3
Fruits	3–4
Vegetables	4–5
Grains (breads and cereal)	**9–11**

ALCOHOL AND DRUG DEPENDENCE

PROBLEM

Dependence on alcohol or drugs is a disease with signs and symptoms and a progressive course that requires treatment, just like diabetes or cancer.

CAUSE

Factors that contribute to dependence on alcohol and drugs may include inherited traits, the environment, occupation, socioeconomic status, family and upbringing, personality, life stress, and emotional stress. These factors vary among individuals, but no one factor can account entirely for the risk.

PREVENTION/CARE

The only way to prevent alcohol and/or drug abuse and dependence is not to start. Warning signs for needing help are not always dramatic. The following questions can help identify dependence.

A. **Are you or someone you know experiencing any of the following:**
   1. Steadily drinking or using more at a time or more often?
   2. Setting limits on how much, how often, when, or where you will drink or use other drugs and repeatedly violating your limits?
   3. Keeping a large supply on hand or becoming concerned when you run low?
   4. Drinking or using other drugs before going to activities where they won't be available (e.g., class or work)?
   5. Drinking or using other drugs alone? Drinking or using other drugs every day?
   6. Spending more money than you can afford on alcohol or other drugs?
   7. Doing or saying things when you are under the influence that you regret later or do not remember?
   8. Lying to friends and family about your drinking or other drug use?
   9. Becoming accident prone when you are under the influence (spilling, dropping, or breaking things)?
   10. Regularly hung over the morning after drinking?
   11. Worrying about your drinking or other drug use?
   12. Having work or school problems, such as tardiness or absenteeism?
   13. Reducing contact with friends, or experiencing increasing problems with important relationships?
   14. Used naloxone for overdose/hospitalization?
B. **If you answered "yes" to any of these questions, it suggests your drinking or drug use may be a problem.**

TREATMENT PLAN

A. There are no "quick cures" for alcohol and drug dependence, but early intervention is important because it helps avoid the harmful effects of long-term alcohol or other drug use.
B. Your healthcare provider will be suggesting a plan of action for you to consider. You are strongly encouraged to follow the recommendations.
C. Do not hang around your drinking/drug-using friends. Instead, go to new areas, play new sports, and develop new hobbies.
D. Talk to your provider about seeking professional rehab treatment. No single treatment is right for everyone. Your provider will assist in the location of treatment centers.
E. Ask about a support group in your area. Individual and group supports are the most common treatments.
F. Your friends and family may ask about having/using naloxone for opioid to reverse an overdose. Some states require a prescription and others have pharmacies that do not require a prescription. Discuss availability and how to use naloxone.

Activity: Daily exercise is helpful in alleviating the craving for alcohol and drugs. Walking daily and increasing your tolerance for distance are recommended.

Diet:
A. Avoid caffeine and nicotine, if possible.
B. Try to eat three meals a day and three snacks.
C. You may be given vitamin supplements to help restore the vitamins and minerals that have been depleted as a result of your alcohol or drug dependence.

(*continued*)

ALCOHOL AND DRUG DEPENDENCE   *(continued)*

Medications: Usually, medications are not prescribed because they may make the problem worse. If you are prescribed any medications, take them exactly as directed by your healthcare provider.

You Have Been Prescribed: _____

Vitamins/Minerals: _____

You Need to Take: _____

You Need to Notify the Office If You Have:
A. Severe craving and the urge to use alcohol or drugs
B. Any thoughts of hurting yourself or others
C. Impulsive feelings, like you might do something you will later regret
D. You or your family wants to discuss naloxone

Phone: _____

RESOURCES

Adult Children of Alcoholics: 562-595-7830; https://www.adultchildren.org

Al-Anon Family: 888-4AL-ANON; www.al-anon.alateen.org

Alcohol Help Line 24 hours a day, 7 days a week: 800-345-3552; www.adcare.com

American Council for Drug Education: 800-488-3784 (DRUG); www.health.gov/nhic

Cocaine Anonymous: 310-559-5833; www.ca.org. Online meetings are available at https://ca.org/meetings/online-meetings/

Cocaine Hotline 24 hours a day, 7 days a week: 888-633-3239; http://drughelpline.org/cocaine-hotline/

Co-Dependents Anonymous (CoDA®): 888-444-2359; http://www.coda.org

Families Anonymous: 800-736-9805: familiesanonymous.org

Marijuana Anonymous World Services: 800-766-6779; http://www.marijuana- anonymous.org

Mothers Against Drunk Driving (MADD) 24 hours a day, 7 days a week: 877.MADD.HELP; www.madd.org

National Suicide Prevention Lifeline: 1-800-273-TALK (8255)-free and confidential support for people in distress, 24/7

The Phoenix House: Drug Addiction, Alcohol Abuse Treatment & Rehab: 1-888-671-9392; https://www.phoenix house.org/

Veteran's Crisis Line: 1-800-273-TALK (8255)

Women for Sobriety: 215-536-8026; www.womenforsobriety.org. Online support is available.

ALLERGIC RHINITIS

PROBLEM

Allergic rhinitis is a chronic or recurrent condition. Common symptoms are nasal congestion, sneezing, and clear nasal discharge. It is not contagious; therefore, you cannot catch it from anyone, and you cannot spread it to others.

CAUSE

You are having an allergic response after being exposed to small airborne particles called allergens (substances that provoke an allergic reaction).

PREVENTION/CARE

A. The best prevention is to avoid things you know you are allergic to, for example: pollens and molds; pet dander; dust mites; and insects (cockroaches).
B. Target to make bedroom as "allergy-free" by removing carpets, rugs, and window drapes; wash sheets weekly using hot water; mop floors weekly; remove books and stuffed animals; and use pillow and mattress covers.
C. Do not blow your nose too frequently or too hard. This will irritate the nasal tissue. It may also cause your eardrum to perforate (tear). Blow through both nostrils at the same time to equalize the pressure.
D. Use tissues when you blow your nose. Dispose of them and then wash your hands. If no tissue is available, do the "elbow sneeze" into the bend of your arm (away from your open hands). Always wash your hands.

TREATMENT PLAN

A. Use a high-efficiency particulate air (HEPA) filter to reduce exposure to dust mites.
B. Keep humidity level between 30% and 50% to reduce exposure to dust mites and molds.
C. Dust your house often, using a cloth and cleaner or polish to keep dust from flying.
D. Allergy testing may need to be done if you have had allergies for a long time. Ask your healthcare provider about a consultation with an allergist.

Activity: There are no activity restrictions. However, you may want to exercise indoors during the spring, summer, and fall when pollen counts are high.
Diet: Eat well-balanced meals. Drink at least 6 to 8 glasses of water a day.
Medications: Common medications used include antihistamines, decongestants, and nasal sprays.
Antihistamines: Some antihistamines may cause drowsiness. Use with caution. You may consider using a different antihistamine during the day that does not cause drowsiness or take the antihistamine at night before bed.
Decongestants: Decongestants may increase blood pressure and may also interact with other medications. Please consult with your provider before using these medications.
Nasal Sprays: Nasal saline spray is safe to use in the nose several times a day. Nasal steroid spray is treatment of choice for chronic management of nasal allergies. Nasal decongestant sprays may be used for a short period of time. Do not use longer than 3 days to prevent causing rebound side effects from this medication. Consult with your provider if using a nasal decongestant spray.

You Have Been Prescribed: _____

You Need to Take: _____

You Need to Notify the Office If:
A. You experience trouble breathing or catching your breath.
B. You have asthma; call if your symptoms are worse.
C. Your symptoms are worse after using the medications for three complete days or if they do not improve after 4 to 6 weeks of using the allergy medications.

D. Other: _____

Phone: _____

CLIENT TEACHING GUIDE

AMENORRHEA

PROBLEM

For any number of reasons, you have stopped ovulating (putting out an egg each month), and you have stopped having menstrual periods. This is a very common issue women experience.

It is not immediately dangerous for you. However, it is not good to have long stretches of time without having a period because the inner lining of your uterus is still being stimulated by estrogen, which causes the lining to become full and thick. Having a period every month (or using certain contraception types) keeps the lining thin. Over a long period of time, a constantly thickened lining that continues to have estrogen stimulation could produce abnormal cells that can become cancerous.

CAUSE

Sometimes the cause can be found and other times it is unknown. Amenorrhea is often associated with low thyroid activity, excessive exercise such as that of an athlete or dancer, or excessive weight loss. Another common cause is polycystic ovarian syndrome (PCOS).

PREVENTION/CARE

There is no specific prevention. However, if you notice a decreased frequency of menstrual periods, or absence of menstrual periods, when you increase your exercise, you may need to decrease the intensity of exercise. Maintaining weight in a normal (rather than under or overweight range) can help to avoid amenorrhea due to very low body mass index (BMI). If you lose too much weight, you could stop having periods.

TREATMENT PLAN

Progesterone may be prescribed to induce shedding of the lining.

Activity: Decrease intensity of exercise if your periods stop after undertaking a strenuous exercise routine. Take at least 2 days off each week, and decrease the amount of time during each exercise session.

Sexual Activity: You may have a return of fertility without warning. If pregnancy is undesired, be sure to use an effective birth control prevention method to prevent unintended pregnancy.

Diet: Increase calories and try to put on 5 pounds if the amenorrhea occurs shortly after weight loss.

Medications: Your healthcare provider will prescribe progesterone to replace what your ovaries are not making at the present time.

You Have Been Prescribed: _____

You Need to Take: _____

You Need to Notify the Office If:
A. You have any new symptoms.
B. You have problems taking your medication.
C. You think you might be pregnant.

D. Other: _____

Phone: _____

ANKLE EXERCISES

A. Education:
1. Exercise in your bare feet or in stocking feet.
2. Count slowly (1,001, 1,002, etc.) when you must hold a position and count.
3. Do each exercise 10 times the first day and increase the repetitions by 5 each following day until you reach a maximum of 30, unless otherwise instructed.
4. Repeat prescribed exercises three times a day.
5. Exercise slowly and get the greatest stretch possible.
6. Stop any exercise that causes new, unusual, or intense pain.
7. You need to perform daily stretching exercises and toning to speed your recovery.
8. It takes months to adequately heal these types of injuries; therefore, do not be discouraged that it takes time for your ankle to heal.
9. Sports to avoid: stop-and-go activity, basketball, running, and impact aerobics
10. You may need to wear a Velcro-secured ankle brace or high-top tennis shoes for support.

B. Toe and foot bend (floor):
1. Sit on the floor or bed with legs out straight.
2. Bend the injured foot back toward the head and curl toes.
3. Then point the injured foot away and bend the toes back.

C. Toe rise and foot slide (chair):
1. Sit in a chair with knees bent at a right angle and feet flat on the floor.
2. Raise all toes on the injured foot and slide the foot back 3 to 4 inches.
3. Relax.
4. Continue the sliding and toe raising until the heel can no longer be kept on the floor.

D. Toe and foot bends (chair):
1. Sit in a chair with knees bent at a right angle and feet flat on the floor
2. Slide the foot on the injured side forward as far as possible while keeping the toes and heel in contact with the floor.
3. From the straight-leg position, bend the foot toward the head as far as possible.
4. Lower your foot back onto the floor.
5. Bend the foot back and forth from the straight-leg position.

E. Heel-cord stretch
1. Stand straight and face a wall with feet together, arms straight out, and palms flat against the wall.
2. Lean toward the wall, bending the elbows, to stretch the cords above the heels.
3. Continue leaning to a count of 5 and then straighten up again.

F. Inner-tube stretch:
1. Sit with feet dangling side by side at a right angle to your legs.
2. Tie stretch bands around your feet until they are snug.
3. Keeping ankles together, move the toes as far apart as possible.
4. Hold the stretch for a count of 5.

G. Inner-tube stretch:
1. Sit with feet dangling.
2. Cross your feet at the ankles.
3. Tie bands snugly around feet.
4. Move toes as far apart as possible.
5. Hold the stretch for a count of 5.

APHTHOUS STOMATITIS

PROBLEM

Aphthous stomatitis describes tender ulcers in the mouth that recur.

CAUSE

The cause is unknown. Possible causes include diet (lack of iron, zinc, or B vitamins), menstrual or hormonal changes, and viruses.

PREVENTION/CARE

A. Preventing ulcers in the mouth can be difficult when the cause is unknown. Some suggestions of prevention include the following:
   1. Avoiding trauma/injury to the inside of your mouth (biting cheek, etc.)
   2. Avoiding toothpastes and mouth rinses that include sodium lauryl sulfate
   3. Avoiding certain foods that tend to trigger the onset of an ulcer (spicy foods, nuts, cheese, coffee, acidic food, etc.)
   4. Maintaining a healthy diet in vitamin B12, folate, iron, and/or zinc
   5. Avoiding stress

TREATMENT PLAN

A. Use an over-the-counter gel such as Anbesol or Orajel four times daily.
B. You may be prescribed a mouthwash made of diphenhydramine (Benadryl), Maalox, and lidocaine or fluocinonide gel to "swish" in your mouth two to four times daily.

Activity: No restrictions are required.
Diet:
A. Avoiding spicy, salty, or hot foods may help.
B. Using a straw when drinking may decrease pain.
C. Cold foods may be easier to tolerate.
D. Avoid hard or sharp food.
E. Use a soft toothbrush.
Medications:

You Have Been Prescribed: _____

You Need to Take: _____

You Need to Notify the Office If You Have:
A. Worse symptoms than seen at the office visit today
B. Ulcers that do not heal in approximately 1 to 2 weeks

C. Other: _____

Phone: _____

ASTHMA

PROBLEM

Asthma is a chronic condition with wheezing, coughing, breathlessness, and chest tightness.

CAUSE

The most common cause is inflammation that results from exercise or exposure to environmental irritants, allergens, furry animals, cockroaches, dust mites, pollens and molds, cold air, or viral respiratory infections.

PREVENTION/CARE

Those with asthma are encouraged to get the flu vaccine every year.

You may be able to prevent frequent recurrences of asthma by following these asthma trigger avoidance strategies:

A. *Dust mite allergens:* Wash bedding weekly in hot water and dry it in a hot dryer. Encase pillows and mattresses in airtight covers. Remove carpets, especially from your bedroom. Avoid use of fabric-covered furniture, especially for sleeping.

B. *Cockroach allergens:* Clean your house thoroughly. Use poison bait or traps. Do not leave food or garbage exposed.

C. *Animal fur allergens:* Avoid keeping house pets, or at least do not allow them in sleeping areas.

D. *Smoke allergens:* Avoid all of the following: smoking, contact with tobacco smoke, smoke from wood-burning stoves or fireplaces, and unvented stoves or heaters

E. *Outdoor pollens and molds:* Keep windows closed when pollen or mold counts are high.

F. *Indoor mold:* Reduce dampness in your home by using a dehumidifier. Clean damp areas often. Remove carpets that are laid on concrete.

G. *Other irritants:* Avoid perfumes, cleaning agents, and sprays.

TREATMENT PLAN

See the Client Teaching Guides "Asthma: Action Plan and Peak Flow Monitoring" and "Asthma: How to Use a Metered-Dose Inhaler."

Activity:

A. If cold air causes symptoms, wear a scarf over your mouth and nose when you go outside during the winter.

B. Avoid vigorous exercise if this causes asthma symptoms. Learn to recognize activities that trigger your breathing problems.

C. Make an asthma action plan to follow. Copy the plan and place it on the refrigerator door, take a copy of your action plan to school, and give each coach a copy of your asthma action plan.

D. Color code your inhalers with tape or markers, for example, use green tape for quick-relief inhalers, and blue tape for long-acting inhalers.

Diet: There are no diet restrictions unless you have found a food that causes an allergic reaction resulting in trouble with breathing.

Medications: Cough medicines should not be used for asthma symptoms.

You Have Been Prescribed: _____

You Need to Take: _____

You Need to Notify the Office If You Have:

A. A peak flow reading below 60% of your personal best number that does not return to the yellow or green zone after taking your medication

B. Other: _____

Phone: _____

ASTHMA: ACTION PLAN AND PEAK FLOW MONITORING

A peak flow meter is a device that measures how well air moves out of your lungs. This measurement is referred to as your "peak expiratory flow," or PEF.

HOW TO USE A PEAK FLOW METER

A. Place the indicator at the bottom of the numbered scale.
B. Stand up.
C. Take a deep breath, filling your lungs as deeply as possible.
D. Place the mouthpiece in your mouth and close your lips around it. Do not put your tongue inside the hole.
E. Blow into the mouthpiece as hard and fast as you can. It is important to give this your best effort.
F. Write down the number on the indicator. If you cough or make a mistake, do not record that number—do it over again.
G. Repeat steps A through F two more times.
H. Write down the highest number of the three attempts. This is your PEF.

CALCULATING YOUR PERSONAL BEST PEAK FLOW NUMBER

This number is the highest peak flow number you can achieve over a 2- to 3-week period when your asthma is under good control (when you do not have any symptoms). To find this number, take peak flow readings:
A. Twice daily for 2 to 3 weeks
B. When you wake up and between noon and 2 p.m.
C. Before and after taking your quick-relief medication
D. Or as directed by your healthcare provider

THE PEAK FLOW ZONE SYSTEM

Once you have determined your personal best peak flow number, your healthcare provider can give you the numbers that let you know what medications to take based on your PEF. The numbers are set up like a traffic light system (red, yellow, and green).

Green Zone (80%–100% of your personal best number): Signals *good control.* No asthma symptoms are present, and you should take your medication as usual.

Yellow Zone (50%–80% of your personal best number): Signals *caution.* You may be having an episode of asthma that requires an increase in your medications.

Red Zone (below 50% of your personal best number): Signals a *medical alert.* You must use your "fast" inhaler to help open up your airways right away and call your healthcare provider immediately if your peak flow number does not return to the yellow or green zone and stay there.

Use the following "Asthma Action Plan," which specifies what medications you should take when you are in each zone and also use the self-assessment diary provided in the table.

ASTHMA ACTION PLAN

A. My personal best PEF is _____
B. When I am in the *green zone*, PEF above _____, I should continue to take my regularly scheduled asthma medications. They are:
    1. _____
    2. _____
    3. _____
C. When I am in the **yellow zone**, PEF between _____ and _____, I should add the following to my regularly scheduled medications:
    1. _____
    2. _____
    3. _____

(continued)

ASTHMA: ACTION PLAN AND PEAK FLOW MONITORING   (*continued*)

ASTHMA DIARY SELF-ASSESSMENT

Symptom Codes: Rate Your Symptoms 1 (Mild), 2 (Moderate), or 3 (Severe)							
My Personal Best PEF Is _____							
Date	PEAK FLOW ZONES *Green* = Good Control *Yellow* = Caution *Red* = Emergency			Symptoms (Use Codes) W = Wheeze C = Cough S = Shortness of Breath	Quick-Relief Medication (Include the Number of Times Needed for Relief)	Anti- Inflammatory Medication	Additional Medications or Activity
Monday	A.M.	P.M.	ZONE				

PEF, peak expiratory flow.

D. When I am in the ***red zone,*** PEF below _____, I should immediately take the following rescue medication and contact my healthcare provider:
   1. Rescue Medication: _____
E. Other Directions: _____

_____

_____

ASTHMA: HOW TO USE A METERED-DOSE INHALER

USING AN INHALER

To receive the proper dose from your inhaler, you must use good technique. Your healthcare practitioner may provide you with a drug-free practice inhaler. Practice the following steps until you are comfortable administering your inhalant:

A. Shake the inhaler well immediately before each use.
B. Using a spacer helps to deliver more medication.
C. Remove the cap from the mouthpiece. Hold the inhaler upright. Make sure the medication canister is firmly inserted into the plastic holder (actuator).
D. The first time you use your new inhaler (or if it has been 1 month or longer since the last use), test spray four times into the air.
E. Breathe out through your mouth to the end of a normal breath.
F. Position the mouthpiece about 1 to 2 inches in front of your open mouth. Or you may close your lips in a tight seal around the mouthpiece.
G. Open your mouth widely (unless you are using the closed-lip method) and position your head in a neutral position.
H. While breathing in slowly and deeply, firmly depress the container once.
I. Continue breathing in slowly until your lungs are full.
J. Once you have breathed in fully, hold your breath for 10 seconds or as long as you can.
K. If you need a second puff of the same medication, wait a minimum of 1 minute before repeating steps A through J. If you are using a different inhaler for the second puff, wait at least 5 minutes before using the second inhaler.

OTHER TIPS

A. If you are taking a steroid inhalant, rinse your mouth and throat with water after each dose.
B. When you are short of breath, use your bronchodilator ("rescue medicine") first; then wait about 5 minutes before using your steroid inhaler. The rescue inhaler opens your airways so more of the steroid medication reaches your lungs.
C. Keep the inhaler clean. Once a week, remove the medication canister from the actuator and wash the actuator in warm, soapy water. Rinse and allow to air dry. Replace the medication canister in the holder and recap the mouthpiece.
D. Always check the expiration date on your inhaler and make sure to refill your prescription before the medication expires.
E. Color code your inhalers with tape or markers; for example, use green tape for quick-relief inhalers, and blue tape for long-acting inhalers.

ATHEROSCLEROSIS AND HYPERLIPIDEMIA

PROBLEM

Hyperlipidemia (excess lipids in the blood) is often called "hardening of the arteries." The excess lipids increase your risk of developing heart disease and heart attacks.

CAUSE

Elevated blood cholesterol levels lead to plaque formation in the walls of the major arteries in the body. The higher the level of low-density lipoprotein (LDL), or "bad" cholesterol, the greater the chance of getting heart disease. On the other hand, the higher the level of high-density lipoprotein (HDL), or "good" cholesterol, the lower the risk of heart disease.

PREVENTION

Lowering your risk of heart disease involves the following:
A. Diet changes to lower your bad cholesterol (LDL) and raise your good cholesterol (HDL)
B. Lose weight. Start with losing 5 to 10 lb.
C. Start or increase your physical activity. Walking is a good exercise to start getting active.
D. Other ways to modify your risk factors:
   1. Stop smoking.
   2. Control your blood pressure.
   3. If you are a diabetic, control your blood sugar level.

TREATMENT PLAN

Activity:
A. Regular exercise, such as walking vigorously for 30 minutes three times a week, increases your good cholesterol levels, lowers blood sugar, and promotes weight loss.

Diet: Follow the dietary approaches to stop hypertension (DASH) and low-fat/low-cholesterol diet:
A. Decrease total fat calories and cholesterol.
B. Decrease total saturated fats and replace with monounsaturated fats such as canola oil, olive oil, and margarine.
C. Increase fiber with oatmeal, bran, or fiber supplements.
D. Increase daily intake of fruits and vegetables.
E. Try garlic, soy protein, and vitamin C to help lower LDL cholesterol.

Medications: You may be prescribed a medicine to lower your cholesterol. You will need to come into the doctor's office to have your blood drawn to monitor your liver and cholesterol levels.

You Have Been Prescribed: _____

You Need to Take: _____

You Need to Notify the Office If You Have:
A. Chest pain
B. Shortness of breath or trouble breathing while exercising
C. Abdominal pain
D. Muscle pain or weakness

E. Other: _____

Phone: _____

ATRIAL FIBRILLATION

PROBLEM

Atrial fibrillation is the condition that causes the upper chambers of the heart (the atria) to beat faster and irregularly (also called fibrillation). The upper chambers of the heart do not beat at the same time as the lower chambers (the ventricles). When atrial fibrillation occurs, blood clots can form in the heart and then travel to the brain, causing a stroke.

CAUSE

Atrial fibrillation is caused by a malfunction of the heart's pacemaker. Many things can cause the heart's pacemaker to malfunction, including excessive alcohol intake, emotional stress, physical stress, recent heart surgery, medication side effects, and a long list of medical conditions. These medical conditions include coronary artery disease, leaky heart valves, high blood pressure, heart failure, heart attack, thyroid disease, infections, inflammation around the heart, sleep apnea, obesity, and lung diseases such as chronic obstructive pulmonary disease, bronchitis, asthma, and emphysema.

PREVENTION/CARE

A. Stop smoking. Discuss smoking cessation with your healthcare provider.
B. Reduce or eliminate intake of alcohol and caffeine.
C. Lose weight. Discuss losing weight with your healthcare provider.
D. Make a list of your current medical conditions and current medications. Keep an updated copy in your wallet.
E. When traveling:
    1. Always travel with enough of your medication to last through your vacation plus an additional 3 days.

TREATMENT PLAN

A. Take your medications as ordered by your healthcare provider.
B. Effectively manage all other medical conditions, paying special attention to cholesterol, blood pressure, thyroid disease, sleep apnea, and any lung diseases.
C. Follow up with your primary healthcare provider and/or cardiologist on a regularly scheduled basis.

Activity:
A. Get regular exercise, after discussing the type and frequency of exercise that is safe for you with your healthcare provider.

Diet:
A. Eat a balanced, low-fat, and low-salt diet in addition to dietary guidelines suggested by your healthcare provider.
B. If you are taking the blood thinner Coumadin, you will be given a list of foods that are high in vitamin K. These foods can interfere with how the blood thinner works. Please discuss these foods further with your healthcare provider.

Medications:

You Have Been Prescribed: _____

You Need to Take: _____

You Need to Notify the Office If:
A. You have any of the following symptoms:
    1. Palpitations or a fluttering in your chest
    2. Chest pain
    3. Weakness or extreme tiredness
    4. Shortness of breath at rest or with activity
    5. Dizziness
    6. Disorientation
    7. Confusion
    8. Passing out or losing consciousness
    9. Severe headache

(*continued*)

ATRIAL FIBRILLATION   (*continued*)

    10. Frequent urination or a compelling urge to urinate

    11. Anxiety or panic symptoms

B. Vomiting or other illness causes you to miss more than one dose of your medications.

C. Other: _____

Phone: _____

RESOURCES

American Heart Association: www.heart.org

National Heart, Lung, and Blood Institute: www.nhlbi.nih.gov

ATROPHIC VAGINITIS

PROBLEM

You have been diagnosed with atrophic vaginitis. This means that the lining of your vagina is thinner, less pliable, and less lubricated. This condition leaves the lining more prone to tears and abrasions. This is a natural part of aging, and it is also very common with teens as they begin menstruating and with breastfeeding women.

CAUSE

Atrophic vaginitis is caused by an alteration in estrogen either from premature ovarian failure, delayed puberty, breast-feeding, or naturally occurring menopause.

PREVENTION/CARE

A. This is a physical problem, *not* an emotional problem.
   1. If you are a preadolescent girl, the symptoms will decrease as puberty approaches.
   2. If you are breastfeeding, your symptoms will resolve after weaning the baby.
   3. If you are menopausal, or have premature ovarian failure, your symptoms will improve after starting a hormone replacement pill or using a hormonal vaginal cream.
B. You also can help your symptoms by doing the following:
   1. Avoid perfumed hygiene sprays, talcs, and deodorant soaps in the perineal area.
   2. Wear cotton crotched underwear, preferably white (free of dye).
   3. Sleep without wearing underwear.
   4. Use a water-soluble, nonglycerine-containing vaginal lubricant with sexual intercourse, such as Good Clean Love or Slippery Stuff. **Do not use Vaseline.** Vaseline can contribute to infections.
   5. Regular sexual activity/masturbation facilitates the natural production of lubricating secretions of your body.
   6. Kegel exercise (using the muscles that start and stop the flow of the urine stream) improves the muscle tone and elasticity of the vagina.
   7. The female-superior "on top" or side-lying position for sexual intercourse gives you the ability to control the depth of thrusting with the penis, and this may make sex more comfortable.
   8. Plain yogurt douches or acidophilus tablets by mouth, or inserted into your vagina, can help maintain the vaginal pH to prevent vaginitis,

TREATMENT PLAN

A. Vitamin E oil may be used for vaginal dryness.
B. Use water-soluble, non-glycerine-containing vaginal lubricants for intercourse.
C. You may be prescribed an estrogen cream or hormone replacements for menopause.
D. If you still have your uterus, hormones need to be balanced with estrogen and progesterone to prevent the lining of the uterus from overgrowing. Follow your hormone therapy instructions.
E. You still need regular cervical cancer screening (Pap, and HPV test if indicated by age) even if you do not have a period.

Activity: Increase foreplay for increased lubrication. Try the previous suggestions on sexual positions for greater comfort and control.
Diet: As tolerated
Medication:

You Have Been Prescribed: _____

You Need to Take It/Use It: _____

(*continued*)

ATROPHIC VAGINITIS   (*continued*)

You Need to Notify the Office If You Have:

A. No relief of symptoms after following the aforementioned instructions

B. No relief of symptoms after beginning the hormonal replacements

C. Vaginal bleeding after intercourse

D. A change in your symptoms

E. Other: _____

Phone: _____

BACK STRETCHES

You have been approved to do back-stretching exercises to help with your low back pain. Follow the instructions, starting slowly to build your strength.

EQUIPMENT

Use a mat or a towel on the floor for extra padding and comfort.

A. In the lying position:
   1. Lie on your back with knees bent. Cross your arms over your chest.
   2. Raise your head and shoulders and curl your trunk upward, no more than 6 inches.
   3. Keep the small of your back pressed against the mat.
   4. Exhale during the curl up.
   5. Hold _____ seconds; do _____ repetitions _____ times a day (see Figure III.1).

B. In the standing position:
   1. Stand with your back against the wall.
   2. Place your feet shoulder width apart and 18 inches from the wall.
   3. Slowly slide down the wall until you are in the "chair" position.
   4. Hold for 10 seconds and relax, then slide back up the wall to a standing position.
   5. Do _____ repetitions _____ times a day (see Figure III.2).

C. In the lying position:
   1. Bring your right knee slowly to your chest, holding it in place with your hands on your knee.
   2. Relax the buttock and your back muscles.
   3. Hold _____ seconds, then relax with your right knee down.
   4. Repeat with your left knee.
   5. Now that you have stretched both legs, pull both of your knees up, holding them in place with your hands on your knees.
   6. You will be curled in the fetal position.
   7. Hold _____ seconds, then relax with your knees down.
   8. Do _____ repetitions, _____ times per day (see Figure III.3)

FIGURE III.1   Lie on a mat or towel. Raise head and shoulders as demonstrated.

(*continued*)

BACK STRETCHES (*continued*)

FIGURE III.2   Place your feet shoulder width apart. Slide down against the wall to the "chair" position.

FIGURE III.3   Pull your left knee toward your chest to stretch; repeat with your right knee as demonstrated.

D. In the lying position:
1. Lie on your back with your knees bent
2. Tighten your abdominal muscles and squeeze. As you squeeze the buttock muscles, flatten your back toward the mat/towel Relax.
3. Tighten your buttock muscles and lift your abdomen or "tummy" toward your knees while arching your back. Relax.
4. Hold _____ seconds; do _____ repetitions _____ times a day (see Figure III.4).

BACK STRETCHES (*continued*)

FIGURE III.4   Lie with knees bent, flatten your back, and then lift your tummy toward knees with back arched.

BACTERIAL PNEUMONIA: ADULT

PROBLEM

Pneumonia is a lung infection that causes fluid to collect in the air sacs. You may have a fever, cough, or trouble breathing.

CAUSE

Respiratory bacteria or viruses cause pneumonia.

PREVENTION/CARE

People older than 65 years and younger people with severe lung disease may receive a vaccine to prevent pneumococcal pneumonia.

The flu vaccine is recommended to be taken every year.

TREATMENT PLAN

A. Use a cool-mist humidifier. Clean the humidifier daily.
B. Do not smoke and avoid smoke-filled rooms.
C. Cover your mouth when you cough and cover your nose when you sneeze.
D. Use tissues when you blow your nose. Throw away tissues as soon as they are used. If no tissue is available, do the "elbow sneeze" into the bend of your arm.
E. Wash your hands frequently with soap and water.

Activity: Rest during the early phase of the illness.
Diet: Eat a nutritious diet. Drink 8 to 10 glasses of water a day.
Medications:
A. Do not use cough suppressants if your cough produces sputum. Use them only for a dry, nonproductive cough.
B. Acetaminophen (Tylenol) may be used for fever or body aches.
C. Antibiotics are given for pneumonia that is caused by bacteria. Take your medication as directed.
D. Finish all of your antibiotics even though you may feel better.

You Have Been Prescribed: _____

You Need to Take: _____

You Need to Notify the Office If You Have:
A. Increased difficulty breathing
B. Fever after 48 hours on an antibiotic
C. Blood in your sputum
D. Worsening discomfort or fatigue

E. Other: _____

Phone: _____

BACTERIAL PNEUMONIA: CHILD

PROBLEM

Bacterial pneumonia is a lung infection that causes fluid to collect in the air sacs. Your child may have a fever, cough, or trouble breathing.

CAUSE

Respiratory bacteria cause pneumonia.

PREVENTION/CARE

A. Keep your children away from people with respiratory illnesses.
B. The flu vaccine is recommended every year.

TREATMENT PLAN

A. Encourage fluids.
B. Use a vaporizer or humidifier to increase humidity in your child's room. Clean the humidifier or vaporizer daily.
C. Keep your child away from cigarette smoke.
D. Teach your child to cover his or her mouth when coughing and to cover his or her nose when sneezing.
E. Use tissues when your child blows his or her nose. Throw away all tissues as soon as they are used. If there are no tissues available, teach your child to do the "elbow sneeze" into the bend of the arm.
F. Use good handwashing with soap and water.

Activity: Have your child rest at first (during the acute phase). Children may return to school after 24 hours of antibiotic therapy and when they have no fever for 24 hours.

Diet: There are no diet restrictions with pneumonia. Your child may not be very hungry when he or she is feeling very sick. Encourage the child to drink liquids or suck on ice pops.

Medications:
A. Your child should take all of the antibiotics prescribed as directed.
B. It is very important for your child to finish the antibiotic, even though he or she may feel well.
C. Acetaminophen (Tylenol) may be given for fever. ***Children 18 years or younger should not be given aspirin.***
D. Do not give your child cough medicine; it is important that he or she can cough to break up any mucus. **The American College of Chest Physicians clinical guidelines recommend that cough suppressants and over-the-counter cough medications *not* be given to young children. Cough and cold medicines should *not* be given to children younger than 6 years.**

You Have Been Prescribed: _____

You Need to Take: _____

You Need to Notify the Office Immediately If:
A. Your child's breathing becomes faster, more labored or difficult.
B. Retractions (tugging between ribs) become worse.
C. Your child's lips become blue.
D. Grunting sounds occur when breathing out.
E. Your child starts acting very sick.

F. Other: _____

You Need to Notify the Office Within 24 Hours If:
A. Your child is unable to sleep.
B. Your child is not drinking enough.
C. Fever lasts longer than 48 hours on antibiotics.
D. You feel your child is getting worse.

E. Other: _____

Phone: _____

BACTERIAL VAGINOSIS

PROBLEM

You have been diagnosed with a vaginal infection, also known as bacterial vaginosis (BV). This is the most common infection in women. The discharge is thin, white or gray-white, and has a "fishy" odor. The odor, and any vaginal irritation or itching, tends to increase after sexual intercourse, but it is not considered a sexually transmitted infection. Recurrence is common.

YOU CAN BE TREATED IN PREGNANCY

BV has been associated with premature rupture of the membranes in pregnancy and preterm labor.

CAUSE

BV is caused by an alteration in the normal flora of the vagina. There are many contributing pathogens and factors, including the routine use of douches, antibiotic use, menses, and pregnancy.

PREVENTION/CARE

A. Wear cotton panties, or at least panties with a cotton crotch. White panties are best (no dyes).
B. Try to avoid wearing restrictive clothing that limits air flow to the area, such as tight jeans.
C. Sleep without wearing underwear.
D. Avoid the use of bubble bath, feminine deodorant sprays, and perfumed sanitary products (sanitary pads, tampons, and toilet paper).
E. Use good hygiene:
    1. Wipe with toilet tissue from front to back after urinating and bowel movements.
    2. Wipe from front to back using clean towels with each bath or shower.
    3. Change your tampons and pads often during your period.
F. Routine douching destroys the normal vaginal flora. Avoid douching unless you are prescribed a medicated douche.

TREATMENT PLAN

A. Try the prevention tips to decrease the recurrence of BV.
B. You may be given a prescription for pills or vaginal creams.
C. Do not use a tampon with vaginal creams because it will absorb the medication.
D. Clindamycin is an oil-based, medicated cream used to treat BV. It can weaken latex condoms for at least 72 hours after stopping the therapy.
E. All treatments (medications and douches) may be used during your period.
F. Metronidazole (Flagyl) oral tablets may be prescribed. The side effects include a sharp, unpleasant metallic taste in the mouth, furry tongue, and some urinary tract symptoms. Please remind your provider if you have a history of seizures or if you are on any blood-thinning drug.

Other Methods of Treatment

A. Vinegar and water douches: 1 tablespoon of white vinegar in 1 pint of water. Douche one to two times a week.
B. *Lactobacillus acidophilus* culture four to six tablets daily
C. Insertion of a tampon soaked in hydrogen peroxide in the vagina for three minutes, three nights in a row

Activity: As tolerated
Diet: When taking the medicine metronidazole (Flagyl), you must **avoid alcohol during the entire week you are taking the medicine and for 48 hours after your last dose. If you are taking the medicine tinidazole (Tindamax), you should avoid alcohol while taking and for 72 hours after completing.** The combination of the medicine and alcohol may cause nausea, vomiting, stomach upset, and a headache.

*(**continued**)*

BACTERIAL VAGINOSIS *(continued)*

Medications:

You Have Been Prescribed: _____

You Need to Take: _____

You Need to Notify the Office If:
A. You vomited your medication.
B. Your vaginal odor and discharge are not relieved after the medications.
C. You continue to have repeated infections after following the instructions.

D. Other: _____

Phone: _____

BASAL BODY TEMPERATURE MEASUREMENT

DEFINITION

Basal body temperature (BBT) assessment is done to determine if and when a woman ovulates. It may be used to achieve or prevent pregnancy. During the follicular phase of the normal menstrual cycle (the first 2 weeks), one follicle and the oocyte it contains mature. The normal body temperature during the follicular phase when estrogen dominates ranges from 97.2°F to 97.6°F.

At midcycle, when progesterone dominates, the ovum is extruded from the ovary and may be fertilized any time from 12 to 24 hours later. Ovulation manifests as an increase in BBT from 0.6° to 1°F above your baseline temperature. Some women have a dip in temperature just before the day of ovulation and then their temperature may rise.

CHECKING YOUR BBT

A. A BBT thermometer must be used. They are easily accessible in the contraceptive section of any pharmacy. If using any other type besides a basal body thermometer, such as a digital thermometer, it must be able to measure to 0.10° due to the slight changes that will be measured.

B. Record your temperature on the temperature chart provided in the thermometer packet or by a healthcare provider. The chart can be easily copied for as many months as needed.

C. Keeping your BBT calendar:
1. Day 1 of the cycle is the first day of menstruation/bleeding.
2. Mark the days of bleeding and other discharge, especially mucus, on the calendar.
3. Mark any days that you are sick, stay up late, or sleep less than 6 hours because this will interfere with your temperature.
4. Mark the days that you have sexual intercourse.
5. Mark your medications on your BBT calendar.

D. Each morning, prior to arising or any activity, place the thermometer under the tongue, leaving it in for 1 minute. Take your temperature consistently at the same time every morning.

E. A temperature elevation that is 0.2°F or greater from your past 6 days of temperature (and that stays elevated) indicates an ovulatory pattern.
1. This is the time when you are more likely to get pregnant.
   a. If pregnancy is desired, the standard recommendation is that sexual intercourse should begin 2 days before ovulation is expected and occur every 2 days thereafter until 2 to 4 days have passed following the rise in body temperature. Having sex only once daily, and every other day beginning 2 days prior to ovulation allows the sperm count to regenerate to adequacy. Too frequent intercourse can actually decrease the chance of conception.
   b. If pregnancy is not desired, avoid sexual intercourse.

F. The record should be kept for 2 to 6 months minimum.

CHECKING YOUR CERVICAL MUCUS

Your cervical mucus ranges from thick and tacky feeling to thin and slippery, the consistency of egg whites. The type of mucus you have also signals the time of ovulation.

A. Your mucus can be checked daily by inserting one finger in your vagina to check the cervix.
1. Wash your hands.
2. Sit on the toilet and gently insert your finger to feel the cervix.
3. The cervix feels firm, like the end of your nose.
4. Check the thickness of the mucus and note it on your BBT chart.

B. After you have your period, the cervical mucus is thick and tacky. It is more difficult to get pregnant when the mucus is thick.

C. As ovulation approaches, you will notice the mucus getting thinner.

D. When the mucus is the consistency feeling of egg whites, that signals ovulation and you are the most fertile.
1. This is the time to have sexual intercourse/avoid intercourse.
2. Continue until you see your BBT rise.
3. You will notice the cervical mucus getting thicker.

CLIENT TEACHING GUIDE

BELL'S PALSY

PROBLEM

Bell's palsy is a disorder that can occur at any age, but most frequently occurs between the ages of 20 and 60 years. The disorder affects the muscles associated with expression on one side of the face, including the muscles that allow smiling, closing of the eyes, and raising of the eyebrows.

The exact cause of Bell's palsy remains unknown. Possible causes may include viral infections, a type of inflammatory process, or possibly an autoimmune disease.

Prevention/Care

A. Bell's palsy is usually treated with a steroid, such as prednisone.

B. Pain is usually managed with acetaminophen (Tylenol) or another over-the-counter pain medication; for example, nonprescription anti-inflammatory medications (NSAIDs) such as ibuprofen or naproxen.

C. Sometimes it is helpful to use gentle massage or electrical stimulation of the nerve to help with the pain.

D. Applying heat or cold packs for 15 to 20 minutes three to four times a day may also help with pain. When applying ice packs, do not directly apply ice to the skin and be cautious on skin to avoid frostbite to the area.

E. Protection of the eye is very important if there is loss of lid function. Eye drops and lubricating ointment may be recommended along with taping the affected eye while sleeping.

F. Wearing eyeglasses, sunglasses, or goggles is also recommended to protect the eye.

G. Physical therapy may also be helpful with recovering function in the muscles that are weak.

H. Symptoms usually resolve within 3 or 4 weeks to a few months. Occasionally, clients have symptoms lasting longer than this. If symptoms change or worsen, notify your healthcare provider immediately.

TREATMENT PLAN

Activity: Engage in activities as tolerated. Use caution when performing activities requiring visual demands such as depth perception (driving, walking, etc.).

Diet: Eat a regular diet as tolerated.

Medications:

You Have Been Prescribed: _____

You Need to Take: _____

You Need to Notify the Office If You Have:

A. No relief of symptoms in 4 weeks

B. New symptoms, such as headaches, visual changes, or other problems such as trouble walking

C. Other: _____

Phone: _____

BIPOLAR DISORDER

PROBLEM

Bipolar disorder, formerly called manic-depressive disorder, causes extreme mood changes, ranging from mania or hypomania (emotional "highs") to depression ("lows"). Mania may cause feelings of extreme happiness and increased energy. Sometimes mania causes people to behave in ways that are outside their normal behaviors such as spending too much money, arguing, or making impulsive decisions. Depression can cause feelings of sadness, low energy, low motivation, sleep disturbance, and suicidal thoughts.

CAUSE

The exact cause of bipolar disorder is unknown, but may have to do with physical changes or an imbalance in naturally occurring chemicals in the brain. Bipolar disorder is common in people who have a first-degree relative with the condition.

TREATMENT PLAN

Bipolar disorder is a long-term condition and is sometimes disruptive to daily living. By following a treatment plan and working closely with a mental health professional, mood swings can be managed. The process of finding the right medication may take some trial and error and it can take several weeks for medications to take full effect. Medication doses may need to be adjusted as symptoms change.

A. **Take your medications as prescribed**. Even when you are feeling better, do not stop or change your medication without consulting with your provider.

B. **Keep your appointments with your provider.** You are the most important member of your treatment team. It is important for you to visit regularly to your medical provider to discuss your progress, keep your prescriptions current, and to check your lab work when needed. It may be helpful to take along a support person to help you remember questions, instructions, and treatment information. Be honest with your providers about how you feel and worries you may have.

C. **See a therapist or a counselor.** Your medical provider will work with you in managing your medications and your general health needs. A counselor or therapist will meet with you on a regular basis to help you learn about bipolar disorder and to work on effective ways to manage symptoms, cope with stressful situations, and make lifestyle changes that will improve your mental and physical health.

D. **Manage stress.** Stress can make you feel more anxious, worried, irritable, moody, and can get in the way of a good night's sleep. Take time to relax, get creative, spend time with friends/family, take a few deep breaths several times a day, focus on the "positives" in your life, and ask for help when you need it.

E. **Avoid drug and alcohol use.** Drugs and alcohol can alter your mood and interfere with prescribed medications.

F. **Practice good sleep habits.** Let your provider know about any changes in your sleep pattern. Problems with sleeping too much, or too little, can be an early warning sign for mania and/or depression.

Activity: Exercise regularly. Exercise naturally improves mood and gives an overall sense of well-being. Taking a brisk walk for 20 to 30 minutes on most days can help to relieve stress, improve your mood, help you feel better physically, and help to maintain a healthy weight. Check with your provider before starting any exercise program.

Diet: Eat well. Eating foods that are high in fats, sugars, salt, and carbohydrates can cause weight gain and make you feel more tired and sluggish. Eat plenty of fresh fruit and vegetables and try to avoid fried foods, soda, sweet tea, candies, and baked goods.

Medications:

You Have Been Prescribed: _____

Labs Ordered:

(*continued*)

BIPOLAR DISORDER *(continued)*

You Need to Notify the Office If You Have:

A. Thoughts of harming yourself or someone else. If you are having suicidal thoughts, call 911 or have someone take you to the nearest ED.

B. No improvement, or worsening of your symptoms, even though you are taking your medications as directed

C. Physical symptoms that may be side effects from prescribed medications

D. Any new symptoms that you are concerned about

E. Other: _____

Phone: _____

Your next scheduled appointment: _____

BRONCHIOLITIS: CHILD

PROBLEM

Bronchiolitis is a lung infection that causes difficulty breathing (respiratory distress), wheezing, coughing, and fever.

CAUSE

Respiratory viruses, usually respiratory syncytial virus (RSV), cause bronchiolitis. The symptoms generally last approximately 7 to 10 days. Bronchitis usually occurs in fall, winter, and early spring.

PREVENTION/CARE

A. Isolate young infants from people with respiratory illnesses.
B. Avoid large crowds.
C. Wash your hands with soap and water frequently if you are caring for your child.
D. Wash toys and surfaces that your child touches.
E. The flu vaccine should be given to children every year.

TREATMENT PLAN

A. Use a cool-mist humidifier in your child's bedroom and clean the humidifier frequently. If a humidifier is not available, you and your child may stay in a steamy bathroom for 20 minutes two to three times a day.
B. Use warm water and a bulb syringe to clear your baby's stuffy nose.
C. Children should not be exposed to secondhand smoke.
D. Teach your child to cover his or her mouth when he or she coughs and to cover his or her nose when he or she sneezes
E. Use tissues when your child blows his or her nose. Throw away tissues as soon as they are used.
F. Wash your child's hands with soap and water after coughing and sneezing into a tissue. If a tissue is not available, teach your child to "elbow sneeze" into the bend of his or her arm.

Activity: Children need rest during the early stages of the illness.
Diet:
A. Offer fluids, such as juice and water. Try ice pops if the child does not feel like drinking. Dilute juice for younger infants.
B. Your child may not be hungry but try to get him or her to eat small, frequent feedings.
Medications:
   Antibiotics are not prescribed for viral infections, but your child may be given medicines for other symptoms.
   The American College of Chest Physicians clinical practice guidelines recommend that cough suppressants and over-the-counter cough medications *not* be given to young children. Cough and cold medicines should *not* be given to children younger than 6 years of age.

You Have Been Prescribed: _____

You Need to Take: _____

You Need to Notify the Office Immediately If:
A. Your child's temperature is 101°F or greater.
B. Breathing becomes labored or difficult or is faster than 60 times a minute.
C. Wheezing becomes severe.
D. Retractions (tugging between ribs) become worse.
E. Your child stops breathing or passes out.
F. Lips become bluish.
G. Your child starts acting very sick or is difficult to arouse.

H. Other: _____

(*continued*)

BRONCHIOLITIS: CHILD (*continued*)

You Need to Notify the Office Within 24 Hours If:
A. Your child is unable to sleep or would not drink enough fluids.
B. Your child has symptoms of an earache such as tugging at his or her ears.
C. Your child has yellowish to green nasal discharge.
D. Fever greater than 100°F lasts more than 72 hours.
E. You feel your child is getting worse.

F. Other: _____

Phone: _____

BRONCHITIS, ACUTE

PROBLEM

Acute bronchitis is a lung infection followed by a productive cough.

CAUSE

Respiratory viruses cause bronchitis.

PREVENTION/CARE

A. Avoid exposure to other people with respiratory illnesses.
B. Do not smoke and avoid secondhand smoke and other smoke-filled environments.
C. Avoid air pollutants, such as wood smoke, solvents, and cleaners.
D. Cover your nose and mouth when you sneeze or cough.
E. Use tissues when you blow your nose. Throw away all tissues as soon as they are used. If no tissue is available, do the "elbow sneeze" into the bend of your arm.
F. Use good handwashing techniques with soap and water.
G. You are encouraged to take the flu vaccine every year.

TREATMENT PLAN

A. Humidity and mist may be helpful.
B. Always clean the humidifier daily to prevent bacteria from growing.
C. Twenty minutes several times a day in a steamy bathroom may provide relief.

Activity: Rest is important when you have been diagnosed with bronchitis; then increase activity as tolerated when the fever subsides. Children may attend school or day care without any problems after their fever subsides.
Diet: Eat a nutritious diet. Drink 8 to 10 glasses of water daily.
Medications:
A. Acetaminophen (Tylenol) may be used to relieve discomfort.
B. For a nonproductive cough, take cough suppressants if recommended. You may be prescribed a cough medicine or be told the best kind to buy in the drugstore. **The American College of Chest Physicians clinical practice guidelines recommend that cough suppressants and over-the-counter cough medications should *not* be given to young children. Cough and cold medicines should *not* be given to children younger than 6 years of age.**
C. Because a virus almost always causes acute bronchitis, **antibiotics will rarely be needed to get better.**

You Have Been Prescribed: _____

You Need to Take: _____

You Need to Notify the Office If You Have:
A. No improvement after 48 hours
B. Worsening symptoms
C. High fever, chills, chest tightness or pain, shortness of breath
D. Symptoms that last longer than 3 weeks

E. Other: _____

Phone: _____

BRONCHITIS, CHRONIC

PROBLEM

Chronic bronchitis is an upper respiratory infection followed by a productive cough. To be diagnosed with chronic bronchitis, you should have had the symptoms for 3 months for 2 years in a row.

CAUSE

Both viral and bacterial infections cause chronic bronchitis.

PREVENTION/CARE

A. Avoid exposure to others with respiratory illnesses.
B. Do not smoke and avoid secondhand smoke and smoke-filled environments.
C. Avoid other air pollutants, such as wood smoke, solvents, and cleaners.
D. Use good handwashing techniques.
E. Use tissues for the mucus coughed up. Dispose of the tissues after use.
F. Cover your mouth when you cough. If you do not have a tissue, the "elbow sneeze" into the bend of your arm will prevent you from spreading your illness.
G. Although the flu vaccine does not prevent bronchitis, a yearly flu vaccine is recommended.
H. A pneumonia vaccine is recommended for people older than 65 years of age and for younger people with chronic respiratory conditions.

TREATMENT PLAN

A. Humidity and mist may be helpful.
B. Always clean the humidifier daily to prevent bacterial growth.
C. Twenty minutes several times a day in a steamy bathroom may provide relief.

Activity: Rest during the early stage of the illness, then increase activity as tolerated when the fever subsides. It is not uncommon to feel tired for several weeks.
Diet: Eat a nutritious diet. Drink 8 to 10 glasses of water daily.
Medications:
A. Acetaminophen (Tylenol) may be used to relieve fever and discomfort.
B. You may be prescribed an inhaler to help your breathing.
C. You may be prescribed steroids to help with the inflammation of your lungs. The steroids may be given by an inhaler or as a pill.
D. It is very important that you use the inhaler properly so that the medicine can go into your lungs. A teaching sheet on how to use an inhaler is available.
E. You may also be prescribed an antibiotic for a bacterial infection. Take all of your antibiotics, even if you feel better.
F. You may be prescribed a cough suppressant to take at night to help you rest. However, coughing up the mucus is very important to clear out your "wind pipes."

You Have Been Prescribed: _____

You Need to Take: _____

You Need to Notify the Office If You Have:
A. No improvement after 48 hours
B. Worsening symptoms
C. High fever, chills, chest tightness or pain, shortness of breath
D. Symptoms that last longer than 3 weeks after taking all of your antibiotics

E. Other: _____

Phone: _____

CELIAC DISEASE

PROBLEM

Celiac disease is a condition where a protein called gluten can damage the lining of the small bowel. Gluten is found in wheat, rye, or barley. People with celiac disease can experience diarrhea, abdominal discomfort, bloating, weight loss, and nutritional deficiencies.

CAUSE

The exact cause of celiac disease is not clear. Environmental and genetic factors contribute to this condition. Small intestine is responsible for absorbing nutrients. When there is a damage to the small intestine, the absorption of the nutrients is affected, which causes malabsorption.

PREVENTION/CARE

A. Maintain a gluten-free diet. Avoid foods containing wheat, rye, or barley.
B. Consult a dietitian regarding the foods to avoid and the foods to add for nutritional balance.
C. Discuss the need for vitamin and nutritional supplementation with your healthcare provider.
D. Keep all your follow-up appointments with your healthcare provider.

TREATMENT PLAN

A. Eat a strict gluten-free diet.
B. Take vitamin and nutritional supplements as directed by your provider.
C. Untreated celiac disease can increase the risk of certain GI cancer. Eating a gluten-free diet reduces this risk.

Medications: There are no medications to treat celiac disease. Your physician may prescribe vitamin and nutritional supplements as needed for any deficiencies.

You Have Been Prescribed: _____

You Need to Take: _____

You Need to Notify the Office If You Have:
A. Severe abdominal pain
B. Diarrhea causing dehydration

C. Other: _____

RESOURCE

Kelli, C.P., & Dennis, M. (2018, Oct 8). Patient education: Celiac disease in adults (Beyond the Basics). *UpToDate*. Retrieved from https://www.uptodate.com/contents/celiac-disease-in-adults-beyond-the-basics#H21

CERUMEN IMPACTION (EARWAX)

PROBLEM

A buildup of earwax in the external ear canal that may cause itching, pain, dizziness, ear ringing, and/or temporary hearing loss

CAUSE

Earwax production is a normal, healthy process of the gland of the ear. Earwax is produced to protect the ear from infection and trauma. The wax is continuously being produced and removed from the ear via its own mechanism. However, at times, an overproduction of wax may build up and remain in the external ear canal. With age, the normal mechanisms of the ear for removing earwax are decreased. This is called cerumen impaction. Use of cotton swabs to remove earwax can push wax further into the ear and cause problems deeper into the ear canal.

PREVENTION/CARE

Do not use cotton swabs, paper clips, or other objects to clean your ears. These can damage the ear canal and lead to an external ear infection.

TREATMENT PLAN

A. It is generally safe to clean the external ears with a wet washcloth. The external ear that is visible is the only part of the ear that should be cleaned.
B. In general, it is preferable to allow your healthcare provider or your otolaryngologist to clean your ears.

Activity: As tolerated
Diet: As tolerated

Medications: _____

You Have Been Prescribed: _____

You Need to Take: _____

You Need to Notify the Office If:
A. You are unable to hear.
B. You have colored drainage or fluid draining from your ears.
C. You run a fever.
D. You have dizziness.

E. Other: _____

Phone: _____

CERVICITIS

PROBLEM

You are being treated for cervicitis. The cervix is the lower section of the uterus that opens into the vagina. Cervicitis is an inflammation of the cervix.

CAUSE

Certain germs, such as *Chlamydia trachomatis* or *Neisseria gonorrhea*, may cause cervicitis; however, in many cases no specific bacteria or virus may be identified. In these cases, inflammation may be due to douching, chemical irritants, or altered vaginal flora. In many cases, no cause may be found.

Your healthcare provider will perform a physical evaluation, including pelvic examination, and obtain certain tests to diagnose the cause of cervicitis. If a sexually transmitted organism is found, you and your partner will need to be treated.

PREVENTION/CARE

In cases in which cervicitis is caused by sexually transmitted organisms, use of condoms may prevent infection.

Do not douche or use any other chemically irritating products.

TREATMENT PLAN

A. You may be prescribed an antibiotic by your healthcare provider.
B. Depending on the cause of cervicitis, your sexual partner(s) may also need medical evaluation and treatment.

Activity: Avoid sexual activity until treatment is completed.
Medications:

You Have Been Prescribed: _____

You Need to Take: _____

You need to finish all of your antibiotics even though you may feel good.

You Need to Notify the Office If:
A. You are not able to take your medicine.
B. You have other new symptoms.

C. Other: _____

Phone: _____

CHICKENPOX (VARICELLA)

PROBLEM

Chickenpox is a virus in which a rash occurs, appearing like red, small bumps that usually occur in crops on the body. The virus can affect all ages, but usually affects children and older adults. If you have chickenpox, it may come back later as shingles.

CAUSE

Varicella-zoster virus is a herpes virus that is highly contagious. It is spread by direct person-to-person contact and sometimes by airborne means from respiratory secretions.

PREVENTION/CARE

A. Avoid contact with anyone with chickenpox.
B. If infected, stay in strict isolation until lesions are all crusted over.
C. Sores ("lesions") should be covered by clothing or a dressing until they have crusted. **Covering sores prevents spreading and helps prevent scarring.**
D. Practice good handwashing any time you touch the sores.

TREATMENT PLAN

A. Stay away from other people. Remain in strict isolation.
B. Children may return to day care or school only after all sores have dried and crusted.
C. Care for skin with daily cool-water bathing or soaks.
D. Keep fingernails short and clean; try to prevent scratching.
E. Using a cornstarch bath, baking soda, or oatmeal (Aveeno) or topical lotions, such as calamine, to help with itching.
F. Change your bed sheets and clothes often.
G. **Aspirin should never be used for a fever; it may contribute to the development of Reye's syndrome when given to children during a viral illness.**

Activity: Bed rest is not necessary. Quiet-play activity in a cool room or outside in the shade during nice weather is permitted. Keep all ill children away from others and away from school and day care until all blisters have crusted and there are no new ones.

Diet: No special foods are needed.

Medications: Acetaminophen may be administered for fever. Your child may have a medication prescribed for itching.

You Have Been Prescribed: _____

You Need to Take: _____

You Need to Notify the Office If You Have or Your Child Has:
A. Symptoms of chickenpox
B. Lethargy, headache, sensitivity to bright light
C. Fever over 101°F
D. Chickenpox sores that contain pus or otherwise appear infected
E. A cough that occurs during a chickenpox infection

F. Other: _____

Phone: _____

CHILDHOOD NUTRITION

TODDLERS

Appetite often decreases during the toddler years. Parents should monitor the child's nutrition by weekly intake instead of daily intake. Just like adults, children's appetites change, leaving them hungrier at certain times than others.

Toddlers love to be busy. Therefore, if mealtime tends to be a struggle, after the child tells you he or she is finished with the meal, let the child get up and move around, but continue to offer bites of the meal between the child's activities.

Toddlers also do best with finger foods, which are easy to pick up and eat. Finger-food snacks, such as crackers, carrots, and celery, are great choices. Snacks between meals are important for children. Fresh fruit and vegetables are excellent snacks. Try to limit the amount of sweets and fats the child consumes. Obesity can be a nutritional concern, especially in the early childhood stages. As a parent, set a good example and eat healthy foods and snacks. Toddlers and children learn by watching and eating the same foods that they see their parents and siblings eat.

FAMILY TEACHING TIPS FOR FEEDING TODDLERS

A. Serve small portions and provide a second serving when the first has been eaten. Just 1 or 2 tablespoons are an adequate serving for the toddler. Too much food on the dish may overwhelm the child.
B. There is no *one* food essential to health. Allow substitution for a disliked food. Food jags in which toddlers prefer one food for days on end are common and not harmful. If the child refuses a particular food, such as milk, use appropriate substitutes such as pudding, cheese, yogurt, and cottage cheese. Avoid a battle of wills at mealtime.
C. Toddlers like simply prepared foods, served warm or cool, *not* hot or cold.
D. Provide a social atmosphere at mealtimes; allow the toddler to eat with others in the family. Toddlers learn by imitating the acceptance or rejection of foods by other family members.
E. Toddlers prefer foods they can pick up with their fingers; however, they should be allowed to use a spoon or fork when they want to try.
F. Try to plan regular mealtimes with small nutritious snacks planned between meals. Do not attach too much importance to food by urging the child to choose what to eat.
G. Dawdling at mealtime is common with this age group and can be ignored unless it stretches on to unreasonable lengths or becomes a play for power. Mealtime for the toddler should not exceed 20 minutes. Calmly remove food without comment.
H. Do not make desserts a reward for good eating habits. It gives unfair value to the dessert and makes vegetables or other foods seem less desirable.
I. Offer regularly planned nutritious snacks, such as milk, crackers, and peanut butter, cheese cubes, and pieces of fruit. Plan snacks midway between meals and at bedtime.
J. Remember that the total amount eaten each day is more important than the amount eaten at a specific meal.
K. Useful resources for parents and children are available at www.ChooseMyPlate.gov. This site provides daily food plans, interactive games, and teaching tools for adults and children regarding nutritional guidelines and recommendations for a healthy lifestyle.

CLIENT TEACHING GUIDE

CHLAMYDIA

PROBLEM

Chlamydia is a sexually transmitted infection. Often, no problems are present, but you may notice a yellowish discharge from the penis or vagina, burning during urination, frequent and urgent urination, or pelvic pain.

Untreated chlamydia in females may lead to a condition called pelvic inflammatory disease (PID). PID is a leading cause of infertility, increased ectopic pregnancies, and chronic pelvic pain in women.

CAUSE

Chlamydia is caused by a bacterium called *Chlamydia trachomatis*. This bacterium is spread through sexual contact and may infect the eyes, throat, vagina, penis, or rectum.

PREVENTION/CARE

A. Limit sexual partners.
B. Have routine screening tests for chlamydia prior to beginning a new sexual relationship.
C. Use condoms with sexual activity.

TREATMENT PLAN

Abstain from sexual activity until you and your partner(s) have completed your prescribed medication. Your healthcare provider is required to report this disease to the public health department. The health department may contact you.

Diet: As desired

Medications: Chlamydia can be cured by the prescribed antibiotics.

You Have Been Prescribed: _____

You Need to Take: _____

You need to take all of your antibiotics. It is very important that you keep your follow-up appointment with your provider in 3 months: Your appointment has been scheduled for: _____

You Need to Notify the Office If:
A. You are unable to take your antibiotics because of nausea, vomiting, or a reaction.

B. Other: _____

Phone: _____

CHOLECYSTITIS

PROBLEM

Cholecystitis is the inflammation of the gallbladder. Your gallbladder is situated in the right upper side of your abdomen, beneath your liver. Clients with cholecystitis can experience pain in the right upper or middle of the abdomen, and the pain might spread to your right shoulder or back. Other symptoms may be nausea, vomiting, and/or fever.

CAUSE

Most commonly, gallstones that form inside the gall bladder are the cause of cholecystitis. Other causes include infections, decreased blood flow to gall bladder, bile duct problems, and tumors.

PREVENTION/CARE

A. Maintain a healthy body weight. This decreases chance of formation of gall stones.
B. Chose a healthy diet.
C. Lose weight slowly. Rapid weight loss can increase the risk of gall stones.
D. Exercise regularly, 30 minutes, 5 days per week.

TREATMENT PLAN

A. You may need to get admitted to the hospital if your symptoms are severe.
B. Surgery—gall bladder may need to be removed depending on the severity of your symptoms.
C. Procedure. Your doctor may perform procedure to remove any stones that block the bile duct.

Medications:
A. Pain medications to help control the pain
B. Antibiotics to fight infection
C. Bile acid pills can break down certain types of gall stones. However, it may take several years for these stones to disappear with this treatment.

You Have Been Prescribed: _____

You Need to Take: _____

You Need to Notify the Office If You Have:
A. Severe abdominal pain
B. Fever

C. Other: _____

RESOURCE

Zakko, S.F. (2018, Feb 21). Patient education: Gallstones (Beyond the Basics). *UpToDate*. Retrieved from https://www.uptodate.com/contents/gallstones-beyond-the-basics

CHRONIC OBSTRUCTIVE PULMONARY DISEASE

PROBLEM

Chronic obstructive pulmonary disease (COPD) is a chronic, progressive, debilitating disease of the lungs that does not have a cure. Most people with COPD have a combination of emphysema and chronic bronchitis. Persons with COPD usually have some of the following symptoms: cough (usually productive), shortness of breath at rest or with exertion, wheezing, decreased energy level, and weight loss.

CAUSE

COPD is most commonly associated with cigarette smoking and long-term exposure to pulmonary irritants in the environment (e.g., coal dust). Repeated respiratory infections may also contribute to the development of COPD.

PREVENTION/CARE

A. Avoid smoking and exposure to secondhand smoke.
B. Avoid exposure to environmental irritants, including pollution, household cleaning products, and smoke from fires.

TREATMENT PLAN

A. Stopping smoking is one of the most important treatments. Talk to your healthcare provider about support for stopping.
B. Reduce your exposure to lung irritants and extremely hot and cold air temperatures.
C. Begin an exercise program with your healthcare provider's approval. Walking is a good aerobic exercise. Begin with a pace that is tolerable and easy to maintain; then increase the duration and intensity of the exercise as tolerated. Stop if you experience shortness of breath or chest pain. A realistic goal may be to walk 5 to 10 minutes a day, eventually increasing to 30 to 40 minutes a day.
D. Receive the influenza vaccine every fall. The pneumococcal vaccine is recommended every 5 years and may be given at the same time as the influenza vaccine.
E. Use a spacer/holding chamber to help you inhale all of your medicine. Spacers help you place more of your medicine in your lungs instead of at the back of your throat and mouth. Keep your spacer clean.
F. Use slow, deep breathing or pursed-lip breathing when you are short of breath. Breathe out like you are blowing out a candle.
G. Ask your healthcare provider if you are a candidate for low-flow oxygen treatment when shortness of breath occurs at night and causes insomnia and restlessness.

Activity: Group activities together such as planning shopping with going to the post office. Schedule rest periods throughout the day. Exercise programs should help increase activity tolerance.

Diet: Good nutrition is important. Six small, high-calorie meals a day are suggested. Avoid excessive intake of carbohydrates, especially simple carbohydrates like candy, soda, and potato chips. Milk and milk products do not increase the production of mucus. Ask your healthcare provider to refer you to a dietitian if nutritional problems persist.

Medications:

You Have Been Prescribed: _____

You Need to Take: _____

You Need to Notify the Office If:
A. Your mucus changes color, or increases in amount, or the consistency becomes thicker.
B. After you start your medication, call if your wheezing or shortness of breath is getting worse.
C. You have trouble walking or talking due to your shortness of breath.

D. Other: _____

Phone: _____

CLIENT TEACHING GUIDE

CHRONIC PAIN

RESOURCES

Many client resources on pain are available at your local library, bookstores, and on the Internet. Look for a local support group in your area to join and learn how other people are coping with your same condition.

An excellent resource for clients, families, and physicians is *How to Cope With Chronic Pain*, by Nelson Hendler, MD (Cool Hand Communications, 1993).

There are many pain organizations available to assist clients. Clients may wish to visit these websites for further information:

American Academy of Pain Medicine: painmed.org

American Chronic Pain Association: www.theacpa.org

Arthritis Foundation: www.arthritis.org

National Fibromyalgia Association: www.fmaware.org

United States Pain Foundation: https://uspainfoundation.org

International Association for the Study of Pain—patient resources: www.iasp-pain.org/PatientResources?navItem Number=678

CHRONIC VENOUS INSUFFICIENCY

PROBLEM

Chronic venous insufficiency (CVI) is a condition in which blood has difficulty flowing back to the heart from the arms or legs. This usually occurs when the valves along the inside of the veins are damaged and allow blood to flow backward. The pooling of blood leads to swelling, pain, a heavy feeling, darkening of the skin, and infections. Without treatment, CVI can lead to blood clots and serious infections that could lead to amputation.

CAUSE

Many things may increase the chance of having CVI. Some, like gender, age, or how tall you are, cannot be changed. Others can be changed; these include prolonged standing or sitting and excessive weight.

PREVENTION/CARE

A. Avoid standing or sitting for long periods.
B. If overweight or obese, lose weight. Discuss what you can do to lose weight with your healthcare provider.

TREATMENT PLAN

A. Take your medications as ordered by your healthcare provider.
B. Wear compression stockings. Put them on before getting out of bed in the morning. Take them off just before going to bed at night.
C. Raise the affected arm or leg whenever lying down to reduce pain and swelling.
D. Avoid standing or sitting for long periods of time.
E. Follow up with your primary healthcare provider on a regularly scheduled basis.

Activity:
A. Get regular exercise. Discuss what type and frequency of exercise is safe for you with your healthcare provider.
B. Exercise leg muscles by pumping ankles when sitting. Rocking in a rocking chair is another option.

Diet:
A. Discuss the type of diet that best suits your needs with your healthcare provider: diabetic diet, low-fat diet, low-cholesterol diet, and/or low-sodium diet.

Medications:

You Have Been Prescribed: _____

You Need to Take: _____

You Need to Notify the Office If You Have:
A. Fever greater than 101°F
B. Increased redness, pain, tenderness to touch, swelling, and/or warmth
C. Sudden shortness of breath
D. Chest pain
E. New wound or sore on the affected arm or leg
F. If you are taking a blood-thinning medication and have any of these symptoms:
    1. Vomit that is bright red or dark and looks like coffee grounds
    2. Bright-red blood in your stools or black, tarry stools
    3. Severe headache
    4. Sudden weakness in an arm or leg
    5. Memory loss or confusion

(continued)

CHRONIC VENOUS INSUFFICIENCY   (*continued*)

6. Sudden change in vision
7. Trouble speaking or understanding others

G. Other: _____

Phone: _____

RESOURCE

Vascular Disease Foundation: vasculardisease.org/flyers/chronic-venous-insufficiency-flyer.pdf

COLIC: WAYS TO SOOTHE A FUSSY BABY

PROBLEM

Your baby has been diagnosed with colic if the following symptoms are noticed: repeated episodes of excessive crying that cannot be explained; crying may range from fussiness to screaming; and crying that follows a pattern:

A. It occurs at the same time of the day, usually late afternoon or evening.

B. The crying episodes last a total of more than 3 hours per day and infants are difficult to soothe.

C. It usually begins at 3 weeks of age and lasts through 3 to 4 months of age.

D. The baby's stomach may rumble, and then the baby may draw up his or her legs as if in pain.

E. No specific cause or disease can be found.

CAUSE

The cause of colic is unknown.

PREVENTION/CARE

There are no specific preventive measures. Remove any causes that can be identified.

TREATMENT PLAN

A. Record time when colic episodes occur. Soothe and comfort your baby before the "attack."

B. Do not feed your baby every time he or she cries. Look for a reason, such as a gas bubble, cramped position, too much heat or cold, soiled diaper, or a desire to be cuddled.

C. Make sure your baby is not overfed or underfed (see "Diet" section that follows). During an attack of gas, hold your baby securely, and gently massage his or her lower abdomen. Rocking may be soothing.

D. Feed your baby with the head up, such as sitting up, and use frequent burping.

E. Using a collapsible bag/bottle may help to reduce air-swallowing

F. Do not give your baby any herbal products without a healthcare provider's approval.

Activity:

A. Overstimulation may cause infant upset. A quiet environment or being left alone in the crib to work off excess tension may be necessary.

B. Allow your baby to cry if you are certain that everything is all right. Colic is distressing, but not harmful.

C. Take time away from your infant to rest and recoup.

D. Try the following remedies:
   1. Rhythmic rocking, use swings
   2. Car rides
   3. Walking the baby in a stroller
   4. Running vacuum or vaporizer for calming noise
   5. Giving your baby a pacifier for sucking
   6. Swaddling and cuddling to soothe the baby
   7. Playing music to quiet the baby

E. If you are breastfeeding, review all of your medications and any herbal products that you are taking with your healthcare provider.

Diet:

A. Your baby should be taking at least _____ ounces of _____ formula at each feeding. Interrupt bottle feedings halfway through the feeding and burp the baby. Burp your baby at the end of the feeding, too.

B. If breastfeeding, do not switch to formula unless you have discussed it with a healthcare provider. Interrupt breastfeeding every 5 minutes to burp. If breastfeeding, you should avoid eating the following foods: chocolate, cabbage, beans, pizza, or spicy foods.

(*continued*)

COLIC: WAYS TO SOOTHE A FUSSY BABY   *(continued)*

C. Allow at least 20 minutes to feed your baby. Hold your baby while he or she is feeding; do not prop the baby with a bottle for feeding.

D. Do not try a home remedy, such as feeding homegrown mint teas, to your baby.

You Need to Notify the Office If:

A. The baby has a rectal temperature of 100. 4°F or higher.

B. You fear you are about to lose emotional control or afraid that someone has shaken the baby.

C. Your baby is taking a prescription drug and new unexplained symptoms develop; the drug may produce side effects.

D. You notice a change in your baby's eating patterns, or he or she has vomiting, diarrhea, or constipation.

E. You notice a change in your baby's pattern of behavior: He or she refuses to suck, has a high-pitched cry, draws the legs up when you touch the tummy, or your baby is limp with no activity.

F. Crying could be the result of an injury or fall.

G. Other: _____

Phone: _____

RESOURCE

Turner, T.L., & Palamountain, S. (2019, Jan 22). Patient education: Colic (excessive crying) in infants (Beyond the Basics). UpToDate. Retrieved from https://www.uptodate.com/contents/colic-excessive-crying-in-infants-beyond-the-basics

COMMON COLD

PROBLEM

The common cold is swelling of the mucous membranes of the respiratory tract. Most people complain of feeling tired and have a runny or stopped-up nose, a sore throat, hoarseness, and watery and/or red eyes. You may have a low-grade fever or no fever at all.

CAUSE

A virus usually causes the common cold.

PREVENTION/CARE

A. Colds are spread from one person to another through hand-to-hand contact and contact with air droplets from sneezing, coughing, and talking.
B. Practice good handwashing techniques with soap and water or hand sanitizers.
C. Do not drink from the same glass as others.
D. Cover your mouth and nose when you sneeze or cough.
E. Use tissues when you blow your nose. Dispose of them and then wash your hands. If no tissue is available, do the "elbow sneeze" into the bend of your arm (away from your open hands). Always wash your hands afterward.
F. The flu vaccine is recommended every year.

TREATMENT PLAN

A. Using a humidifier for your bedroom or inhaling steam helps keep the mucous membranes of your nose from drying.
B. Use a rubber suction bulb to clear nasal congestion in babies.
C. Discuss using saline nose drops.
D. Secondary infections of the respiratory tract (sinuses, lungs) may occur. If these do occur, then antibiotic therapy may be needed.
E. Zinc preparations are not recommended for an acute cough due to the common cold.

Activity: There are no activity restrictions. Frequent rest periods or naps can help with fatigue.
Diet: Eat well-balanced meals and snacks. Drink extra liquids (10–12 glasses a day). Warm fluids, such as tea and soups, can increase the rate of mucus flow and provide some symptom relief.
Medications: The American College of Chest Physicians clinical practice guidelines recommend that cough suppressants and other over-the-counter cough medications *not* be given to young children. Cough and cold medicines should *not* be given to children younger than 6 years.
A. Antibiotics are not prescribed for a cold, but they may be prescribed for a secondary infection.
B. All cold medications are available over the counter. Take as directed.

You Have Been Prescribed: _____

You Need to Take: _____

You Need to Notify the Office If:
A. Your child is listless or hard to wake up, refuses a bottle or would not drink liquids, does not want to play, has a fever, or has other symptoms such as shortness of breath.
B. You experience pain that is getting worse in your ears, sinuses, throat, neck, or chest.
C. You have green or yellow nasal drainage.
D. Your temperature is higher than 100.4°F.
E. You are a diabetic and your blood sugars are elevated, or you notice ketones in your urine while you are sick.

F. Other: _____

Phone: _____

CONJUNCTIVITIS

PROBLEM

You have an infection of the eye, or conjunctivitis, that causes redness, itching, drainage from the eye, and crusting on the eyelids.

CAUSE

Bacteria, viruses, or allergies can cause eye infections.

PREVENTION/CARE

A. Wash your hands frequently.
B. Avoid persons with conjunctivitis (pink eye).
C. Avoid known allergens.

TREATMENT PLAN

A. All types:
　　1. Wash your hands frequently, especially after touching the eyes, to avoid spread.
　　2. Use cool compresses on the eyes as needed.
　　3. Wash crusting eyelids with baby shampoo daily.
　　4. Wipe the eyes from the inner to outer corners.
B. *Bacterial*: Bacterial conjunctivitis is contagious until 24 hours after beginning medication.
C. *Viral*: Viral conjunctivitis is contagious for 48 to 72 hours, but it may last up to 2 weeks.

Activity: As tolerated
Diet: As tolerated
Medications: No medications are prescribed for viral infections. You will be given instructions on how to use eyedrops or eye ointment.

You Have Been Prescribed: _____

You Need to Take: _____

You Need to Notify the Office If You Have:
A. A reaction to your medication
B. Trouble seeing
C. New symptoms

D. Other: _____

Phone: _____

CONSTIPATION RELIEF

PROBLEM

Constipation is an infrequent and difficult passing of hard stools and the sensation of not emptying or having to strain.

CAUSES

There are many reasons why you have constipation. You may have just one or a combination of these common causes:
A. Not drinking enough liquids
B. Eating a low-fiber diet
C. Sedentary lifestyle, lack of exercise
D. Ignoring the urge to go to the bathroom
E. Side effects of medicine taken, including blood pressure (BP) medications, antidepressants, pain medications and antacids, or overusing laxatives
F. Depression
G. Other medical conditions

PREVENTION/CARE

A. Go to the bathroom as soon as you have the urge to have a BM; do not wait.
B. Establish a regular toilet time such as after breakfast; 15 to 20 minutes after breakfast is a good time because spontaneous colonic motility is greatest during that period.
C. Use a footrest during elimination to provide support and decrease straining.
D. Do not rely on laxatives; use prune juice as a natural substitute.
E. Stimulate the intestine by drinking hot or cold water or prune juice before meals.
F. Decrease the intake of sweets, which increases bacterial growth in the intestine and can lead to gas.
G. Stop taking enemas and nonessential drugs and herbals.

TREATMENT PLAN

A. Follow the suggested prevention tips.
B. Change to a high-fiber diet.
C. Get daily exercise.

Activity: Daily exercise, such as walking, helps to maintain healthy bowel patterns.
Diet:
A. Eat a high-fiber diet.
B. Restrict cheese: It causes constipation.
C. Drink at least eight glasses of water each day.
D. Avoid refined cereals and breads, pastries, and sugar.
E. Coffee, tea, and alcohol decrease water to the colon. Limit your intake to two of these drinks per day.
Medications: You may be prescribed a stool softener or a laxative for short-term use only. You may be prescribed a bulk-forming agent to take on a regular basis to increase the bulk of your stool.

You Have Been Prescribed: _____

You Need to Take: _____

You Need to Notify the Office If:
A. Constipation continues in spite of the self-care instructions, including diet and exercise.
B. You notice a change in your BMs. Changes in bowel patterns may be an early sign of cancer.
C. You develop fever or severe abdominal pain with your constipation.

(*continued*)

CONSTIPATION RELIEF   *(continued)*

D. If there are any concerning features such as blood on the toilet paper or stool, weight loss, fever, and weakness

E. Other: _____

Phone: _____

RESOURCE

Wald, A. (2018, Sep 18). Patient education: Constipation in adults (Beyond the Basics. UpToDate. Retrieved from https://www.uptodate.com/contents/constipation-in-adults-beyond-the-basics

CONTRACEPTION: HOW TO TAKE BIRTH CONTROL PILLS (FOR A 28-DAY CYCLE)

You have been prescribed an oral contraceptive, also known as a *birth control pill*. Most birth control pills contain a combination of synthetic estrogen and progesterone.

A. Birth control pills suppress ovulation.

B. They make the lining of the uterus unreceptive for an egg to implant and grow. Birth control pills also alter the cervical mucus, making it thicker and harder for sperm to penetrate.

C. A birth control pill does not prevent any sexually transmitted infection or HIV. A condom must still be used to protect yourself from the HIV virus or other infections.

D. You will be asked to return to the office in 3 months after starting birth control pills to check your blood pressure and to check for other side effects of the pill.

E. If your blood pressure is normal and you are not having any other problems taking the pills, your prescription for birth-control pills may be written for 1 year.

F. At the end of that time, you will need another physical examination and possibly a Pap and HPV test, depending on your age. Your prescription can be refilled annually at your preventative care exam appointment.

You Have Been Prescribed:

A. This prescription is a combination pill of estrogen and progestin.

1. Your packet contains 28 pills. Notice that your pills are different colors. **You must take them in the order that they come in the packet.** There are 21 "active" pills, and the last 7 are "inactive or sugar pills" to keep you in the habit of taking a pill every day.

2. You must take a pill **every day** at approximately the same time. Develop the habit of taking the pill with brushing your teeth, for example.

3. You can start your pill pack on any day of the month. Take the pill marked "1," "start here," or "Sunday."

4. You take a pill every day for 21 days; when you start the last 7 pills, you will have a period or "withdrawal bleed."

5. Your period may not start for 1 to 2 days into the last week of pills; this is normal. You generally have a shorter, lighter period on birth control pills.

6. When you start your period, it is time to refill your prescription for your next month of pills.

7. If you are new to the pill, and begin taking it within the first 5 days of your menstrual period, you do not need to use any backup method for protection. If you begin taking it on any other day of your cycle, you need to use a backup method for 7 days.

8. **Missed pills instructions:**

    a. If you miss one pill: take it as soon as you remember, then get back on your regular schedule (you can take two pills in 1 day).

    b. If you miss two pills: take two pills as soon as you remember, then two pills the next day. Continue on with one pill daily as you would normally. There is a possibility you could become pregnant that cycle so you should use a **backup method of birth control** such as a condom until you finish that packet of pills. You may have spotting if you miss two pills. This is normal.

    c. If one or more birth control pills are missed, no backup method of contraception is used.

You Need to Notify the Office If You:

A. Vomit your birth control pills

B. Have a severe or migraine-like headache

C. Are depressed

D. Have pain in your legs, especially if your calf hurts when walking or flexing your foot

E. Break your leg and need to have a cast

F. Think you are pregnant

G. Have blurred vision, loss of vision, or spots before your eyes

H. Feel chest pain or shortness of breath

I. Feel severe abdominal pain

J. Have swelling of the fingers, hands, ankles, or face

K. Other: _____

Phone: _____

COUGH

PROBLEM

Coughing is an important defense mechanism your body uses to clear your airways of mucus and inhaled particles.

CAUSE

A cough is often associated with other respiratory symptoms and may be a sign of infection. Coughing is often related to environmental or chemical irritants such as smoking.

PREVENTION/CARE

A. Coughing cannot be prevented, but you do have some voluntary control over it.
B. Occasionally, medications can cause a cough. It is important to review all medications with your healthcare provider.
C. The flu vaccine is recommended each year; however, the flu vaccine does not prevent a cough.

TREATMENT PLAN

A. **The American College of Chest Physicians clinical practice guidelines recommend that cough suppressants and other over-the-counter cough medications *not* be given to young children. Cough and cold medicines should *not* be given to children younger than 6 years.**
B. Stop smoking, including exposure to secondhand smoke. At the minimum, maintain a smoke-free bedroom.
C. Using a room humidifier may be helpful. Keep your humidifier clean—it can grow bacteria.
D. Change heating and air-conditioning filters often to decrease environmental irritants.
E. Coughing for several minutes may tire you, so you may need extra rest.

Activity: No activity restrictions
Diet: Drink at least 10 to 15 glasses of liquids a day.
Medications: The American College of Physicians clinical practice guidelines recommend that cough suppressants and over-the-counter cough medications *not* be given to children younger than 6 years.

You Have Been Prescribed: _____

You Need to Take: _____

You Need to Notify the Office If:
A. You have difficulty breathing.
B. Your child makes noises with coughing, such as wheezing, singsong sounds, or crowing sounds.
C. You cough up blood.
D. You develop other symptoms besides coughing, such as green sinus drainage and/or a sore throat.
E. You cannot sleep because of coughing.
F. You develop a fever over 101°F.

G. Other: _____

Phone: _____

CROHN'S DISEASE

PROBLEM

Crohn's disease (CD) is an inflammatory disorder of the GI tract that produces ulceration and decreased absorption of nutrients through intestine. CD is chronic, relapsing, and incurable. The symptoms are abdominal pain, diarrhea, fatigue, and weight loss, and medications can help to keep the disease and symptoms under control.

CAUSE

The exact cause is unknown, but it can result from inflammation as the body's immune system that normally fights the infection attacks digestive tract.

TREATMENT PLAN

A. Adequate nutrition is critical to the promotion of healing.
B. Vitamin, mineral, and folic acid supplementation is necessary for proper healing and to avoid secondary complications such as bone disease and low blood counts.
C. To relieve pain, apply a heating pad or warm compress to your abdomen.
D. Check your BMs daily for signs of bleeding.
E. Surgery may be required to help control symptoms.
F. There may be a support group near where you live. The Crohn's and Colitis Foundation website has an area to find a support group at www.ccfa.org/living-with-crohns-colitis/find-a-support-group.
G. Take your medicine as your healthcare provider ordered to help prevent an attack.

Activity: During acute attacks, rest in bed or in a chair. Get up only to go to the bathroom, bathe, or eat. Between attacks, resume normal activities, as tolerated.
Diet:
A. When you have diarrhea, increase the fiber content of your diet.
B. Restricting milk products may stop the diarrhea. Stop using milk products for a short time; then try them again in a few weeks.
C. Decreasing the amount of fat and gluten in your diet may help.
D. Ensure, Sustacal, and Isocal have been found to improve symptoms.
E. Severe relapse may require you stop eating or drinking called a partial bowel rest. Contact the office for instruction
Medications: There are different medications that are used to treat CD. Your medical healthcare provider prescribes your medication depending on the severity of your disease and the part of your intestine that is affected. You may also be prescribed vitamins and minerals, medicine to control pain and relieve diarrhea, and a steroid for a limited time to reduce the inflammation. Do not stop taking the steroid abruptly. Your healthcare provider can tell you how to taper the dose over several days. Take all your medications as prescribed.

You Have Been Prescribed the Following Vitamins and Minerals: _____

You Need to Take: _____

You Have Been Prescribed the Following to Relieve Diarrhea: _____

You Need to Take: _____

You Have Been Prescribed the Following Steroids: _____

You Need to Take: _____

Other medications to treat CD include pills, intravenous infusions, and injectable medications to control the severity of symptoms. Your healthcare provider will discuss these with you and the need for close follow-up monitoring.

You Have Been Prescribed: _____

You Need to Take: _____

You Need to Return to the Office for Blood Work: _____

(continued)

CROHN'S DISEASE   (*continued*)

You Need to Notify the Office If You Have:
A. Black, tarry stools or blood in the stool
B. A swollen abdomen
C. A temperature of 101.0°F or higher

D. Other: _____

Phone: _____

RESOURCES

Crohn's and Colitis Foundation of America:
386 Park Avenue South, 17th Floor
New York, NY 10013
800-932-2423
info@ccfa.org
www.ccfa.org

Peppercorn, M, A., & Kane, S.V. (2018, May 18). Patient education: Crohn disease (Beyond the Basics. UpToDate.
Retrieved from https://www.uptodate.com/contents/crohn-disease-beyond-the-basics

CLIENT TEACHING GUIDE

CROUP, VIRAL

PROBLEM

Croup is a childhood illness of the respiratory system involving the voice box, vocal cords, windpipe, and bronchial tubes. Children become hoarse and have a barking cough, which usually gets worse at night. There may be a sore throat, fever, and a harsh sound with each inward breath (stridor). Infants may be irritable, sleepy, and have a poor appetite.

CAUSE

Croup is usually caused by a virus. Occasionally, it is caused by a bacterial infection.

PREVENTION/CARE

A. Isolate the child from others who are ill with respiratory symptoms.
B. The virus is most contagious during the first few days of fever.
C. Although the flu vaccine does not prevent croup, the vaccine is recommended every year.

TREATMENT PLAN

A. Cool mist has not been shown to be effective with croup.
B. Avoid hot steam because it may cause scalding.
C. Cool night air is often helpful, so open the window or take the child outdoors.
D. Croup tents are not generally recommended unless no alternative therapy is available.
E. Do not expose children to tobacco smoke and other irritants.
F. Count the child's breathing, and look for breathing problems, flaring of nostrils, or retractions (pulling in of chest wall while breathing).

Activity: Let your child rest. Handle your child as little as possible. Your child may return to day care or school when his or her temperature is normal and he or she feels better. A lingering cough is no reason to keep the child home.

Diet: Your child may have decreased appetite during the early part of the illness. It is more important to give plenty of fluids, such as juice and water.

Medications:

The American College of Chest Physicians clinical practice guidelines recommend that cough suppressants and over-the-counter cough medications *not* be given to young children. **Cough and cold medicines should *not* be given to children younger than 6 years.**

Antibiotics do not help viral croup. Your child may be prescribed other medications.

You Have Been Prescribed: _____

You Need to Take: _____

You Need to Notify the Office Immediately If:
A. Your child's breathing becomes difficult or fast, or his lips become blue.
B. Your child has difficulty swallowing or begins to drool.
C. Retractions develop.
D. Your child cannot sleep.
E. Mist from the vaporizer or bathroom does not help.
F. You feel your child is getting worse.

G. Other: _____

You Need to Notify the Office Within 24 Hours If:
A. The cough becomes worse.
B. More than three episodes of labored breathing occur.
C. Your child is not drinking enough fluids.
D. Fever is greater than 104°F.

E. Other: _____

Phone: _____

CUSHING'S SYNDROME

PROBLEM

Cushing's syndrome has many symptoms, including weight gain, obesity, moon-shaped face, excessive hair growth, easy bruising, thin skin, muscle weakness, decreased or no menstrual periods, increased blood pressure, osteoporosis, and impaired wound healing.

CAUSE

Cushing's syndrome is caused by excessive cortisol production.

TREATMENT/CARE

A. Take medications precisely as directed.
B. Avoid excessive alcohol.
C. You may be instructed to purchase a medic alert bracelet or necklace for any emergencies. This can be used to list your treatment and healthcare provider's name and phone number.

Activity: Exercise is encouraged.
Diet: Low-sodium, high-potassium, high-calcium diet
Medications:

You Have Been Prescribed: _____

You Need to Take: _____

You Need to Notify the Office If You:
A. Have a reaction to the medications
B. Cannot tolerate the prescribed medicines

C. Other: _____

Phone: _____

RESOURCES

NADF: www.nadf.us
You can build your own identification bracelets or neck chains from American Medical ID: www.americanmedical-id.com

DEEP VEIN THROMBOSIS

PROBLEM

You have inflammation or a blood clot in one of the veins in your body. Phlebitis is inflammation, and thrombosis means you have a blood clot. Symptoms include:

A. Pain
B. Fever
C. Swelling
D. Tenderness in the affected leg or arm
E. The vein may feel somewhat "hard" to touch.

CAUSE

Blood clots form because of bed rest, surgery, a heart attack, a severe illness, and birth control pills. A blood clot can also form after breaking a hip or leg, pregnancy, cancer, and some medications.

TREATMENT PLAN/CARE

A. If you have phlebitis, you may be given an anti-inflammatory medicine.
B. Some clients need to go to the hospital and get intravenous (IV) medicine to break up the clot.
C. You may be given blood thinners either as a pill or by self-injection.
D. Be sure to take all of the medicine as directed to help with the blood clot.
E. Do not smoke: This worsens your condition.
F. If you currently take any hormones, such as birth control pills, your healthcare provider may talk to you about stopping them.
G. Manage all other medical conditions, especially high blood pressure, diabetes, and high cholesterol, and try to lose any extra weight.
H. Follow up with your primary healthcare provider and/or cardiologist on a regularly scheduled basis.

Activity:
A. Get out of bed as soon as possible after surgery.
B. While in bed, perform range-of-motion exercises with your legs.
C. Exercise leg muscles by pumping your ankles when sitting.
D. Do not sit with your legs crossed.
E. Avoid standing or sitting for long periods of time.
F. Do not wear tight clothing such as knee-high hosiery.
G. Wear special supportive hosiery called compression stockings. Put them on before getting out of bed in the morning and take them off before going to bed at night.
H. When traveling:
   1. Try to take rest breaks on a regular basis.
   2. Continue to do the ankle-pumping exercise when in the car or on the plane.
   3. Wear loose-fitting clothes that are comfortable.
   4. Avoid drinking alcohol.
   5. Drink plenty of fluids unless you are instructed not to do so by your healthcare provider.
   6. Ask your healthcare provider if you should wear compression stockings.
I. Wear a medic alert bracelet if you are put on blood thinners.
J. You will notice that you bruise easier while on your blood thinner.
K. You may need to come back to the office to have your labs drawn.

Diet:
A. Discuss the type of diet that best suits your needs: diabetic diet, low-fat diet, low-cholesterol diet, and/or low-sodium diet.
B. If you are taking the blood thinner Coumadin, you will be given a list of foods that are high in vitamin K. These foods can interfere with how the blood thinner works. Please discuss these foods further with your healthcare provider.
C. Avoid alcohol.

*(**continued**)*

DEEP VEIN THROMBOSIS (*continued*)

Medications: If you currently take birth control pills, ask your healthcare provider if you should stop taking them. You may be prescribed a blood thinner by injection or pills. Take this medicine even if you feel better.

You Have Been Prescribed: _____

You Need to Take: _____

You Need to Notify the Office If You Have:
A. Increased swelling, pain, or warmth in your leg or arm with the deep vein thrombosis (DVT)
B. Fever
C. Sudden shortness of breath
D. Chest pain
E. If you are on a blood-thinner medicine, call for signs of bleeding, including:
   1. Nosebleed that will not stop with pressure
   2. Coughing up blood
   3. Vomiting that is bright red or dark that looks like coffee grounds or grape jelly
   4. Blood in your bowel movements that looks black or tarry in color
   5. Heavy periods
   6. Severe headache
   7. Sudden weakness in an arm or leg
   8. Sudden change in vision
   9. Trouble speaking or understanding others
  10. Memory loss or confusion
F. Any new symptoms not present at your last office visit

Phone: _____

You can build your own identification bracelets or neck chains from American Medical ID: www.americanmedical -id.com

RESOURCES

Patient Education Center—Thromboembolism (DVT and Pulmonary Embolism): patienteducationcenter.org/articles/ thromboembolism-deep-vein-thrombosis-and-pulmonary-embolism
Vascular Disease Foundation: vasculardisease.org/about-vascular-disease/2011-05-05-02-02-59/deep-vein-thrombosis-dvt

CLIENT TEACHING GUIDE

DEMENTIA

PROBLEM

Dementia is mental impairment due to a variety of disorders.

CAUSE

Dementia is caused by degeneration and loss of the gray matter from the brain; common causes of Alzheimer's disease are inadequate blood supply to the brain, alcoholism, chronic infections, inherited conditions, brain injury, or brain tumors.

PREVENTION/CARE

Early medical treatment is required for reversible causes of dementia. Prevention includes protection from head injury, eating a balanced diet, preventing alcoholism, avoiding drug abuse, and preventing atherosclerosis.

TREATMENT PLAN

A. Minimize changes in daily routines.
B. Provide simple memory reminders such as notes, calendars, and clocks.
C. Encourage social contacts.
D. Caregivers should treat the individual with respect.
E. Provide a safe environment.
   1. General home safety review:
      a. Wear shoes that fit your feet well and have solid, nonskid soles.
      b. Wear shoes instead of slippers and wear shoes instead of going barefoot.
      c. Remove scatter rugs or use nonslip rugs. Fix any loose and torn carpeting.
      d. Remove clutter and clear a path instead of having to walk around furniture
      e. Add lighting by using nightlights and higher-watt light bulbs.
      f. Install handrails on both sides of the stairs inside and outside the home.
      g. Fix loose or uneven steps.
      h. Lock closets.
      i. Lock up matches and firearms.
   2. Bathroom safety review:
      a. Add grab bars on the inside and outside of the shower.
      b. Add at least one grab bar located at the toilet.
      c. Add a nonslip bath mat in your tub or shower.
      d. Use a nonslip mat to set on getting out of the tub or shower.
      e. Use a raised toilet seat.
      f. Consider the need for a bedside commode.
   3. Bedroom safety review:
      a. Place a lamp close to the bed so that you do not have to reach it from the edge of the bed.
      b. Use a nightlight.
      c. Use a comforter and blankets instead of long bedspreads that touch the floor.
   4. Kitchen safety review
      a. Install stove cutoff switch.
      b. Date leftovers and check expiration dates on refrigerated and pantry items.
F. Encourage "thinking" games such as puzzles, word games, and reading.
G. Provide frequent gentle reorientation to surroundings.

(*continued*)

DEMENTIA *(continued)*

Activity: Client may engage in as much activity as possible with *supervision* and *direction*.

Diet: Eat a well-balanced diet low in saturated fat.

Medications: A variety of medications are available to treat symptoms including memory, sleep, and depression.

You Have Been Prescribed: _____

You Need to Take: _____

You Need to Notify the Office If:

A. The symptoms/behaviors are getting worse.

B. You are unable to tolerate the medications because of side effects.

C. You need help with social services.

D. Other: _____

Phone: _____

RESOURCE

Alzheimer's Association: www.alz.org

The Alzheimer's Association's website includes information on locating the closest support group; search by zip code: https://www.alz.org

24/7 Helpline 1-800-272-3900

DERMATITIS

PROBLEM

Inflammation of the skin that occurs from contact with an irritant substance (poison ivy, soaps, etc.)

CAUSE

Skin contact with irritating agent

PREVENTION

A. Avoid aggravating agents.
B. Learn to recognize all plants (poison ivy, poison oak, etc.).
C. Flare-ups are common.
D. Avoid all known stimuli (poison ivy, soaps, etc.).
E. Do not wear tight, restrictive clothing.
F. When around irritating substances, wear gloves for protection.
G. For poison ivy:
    1. Wash all clothes, shoes, pets, or other substances that may have come in contact with the poison ivy oil.

TREATMENT PLAN

Activity: As tolerated. Take cool baths as needed for itching. Oatmeal baths (Aveeno bath) help soothe the itching.
Diet: Regular diet
Medications: Take Benadryl as needed for itching. Use calamine lotion as needed. Steroid creams may also be prescribed if reaction is severe. Steroid dose packs may be needed if you are not getting better.

You Have Been Prescribed: _____

You Need to Take: _____

You Need to Notify the Office If You Have:
A. Worsening symptoms
B. Sores on your face, eyes, or ears
C. More redness, swelling, pain, or drainage
D. Secondary bacterial infection
E. Fever

F. Other: _____

Phone: _____

DIABETES

PROBLEM

You have been diagnosed as having diabetes. Diabetes does not go away; you have to manage it every day. It is a condition in which your body cannot use the glucose from food properly. Some signs that your blood sugar is too high and too low are listed here.

A. *Hyperglycemia* (high blood sugar) signs/symptoms: fruity breath odor, abnormal breathing pattern, rapid, weak pulse, confusion, or stupor

B. *Hypoglycemia* (low blood sugar) signs/symptoms: hunger, weakness, sweating, headache, shaking, rapid heartbeat, paleness, fainting, seizures, or coma

CAUSE

Your body has an organ close to the stomach called a pancreas. Your pancreas is not making enough insulin, or your body is not using the insulin it is making properly.

TREATMENT/CARE

A. Lifestyle changes—exercise, stop smoking, follow your diet, and lose some weight—are necessary to control your diabetes:
   1. Stop smoking. Smoking doubles your risk of developing heart or blood vessel disease.
   2. Weight loss of even 5 to 10 pounds could help control your diabetes.
   3. You need to wear an identification tag that tells others you have diabetes in case of an emergency.

B. Foot care is very important:
   1. Check feet every day.
   2. Wash with mild soap and lukewarm water.
   3. Apply lotion.
   4. File or clip nails after washing and drying.
   5. Do not tear skin around calluses.
   6. Wear clean socks daily.
   7. Wear well-fitted shoes at all times: no bare feet. You may not be able to feel or detect damage.
   8. Avoid crossing your legs.
   9. Take shoes off at every office visit.

C. Blood glucose monitoring: You will be instructed on how to check your blood sugar at home.
   Goals of Glycemia Control:
   1. Fasting blood sugar: 80 to 120 mg/dL
   2. 2-Hour postprandial glucose: Less than 180 mg/dL
   3. Bedtime glucose: 100 to 140 mg/dL
   4. Hemoglobin A_{1c}: Less than 7%

D. For low blood sugar you need to follow the 15:15 rule:
   1. After having low blood sugar, you need to check your blood every 4 hours for the next 24 hours.
   2. 15:15 rule: eat 15 g of carbohydrates and wait 15 minutes. Choose one to follow:
      a. Take three glucose tablets.
      b. Drink 1/2 cup orange juice.
      c. Drink 1/2 cup apple juice.
      d. Drink 1/3 cup grape juice.
      e. Drink 6 oz of regular coke.
   3. If your blood sugar drops less than 59, then you need to follow the 15:15 rule, (drinking juice or taking glucose tablets), and then follow that intake with 1/2 cup of milk, and a starch, and 1 ounce of protein.

(*continued*)

DIABETES *(continued)*

4. **If you have severe low blood sugar, you could pass out and go into a coma. You need to have glucagon for emergencies.**
   a. Glucagon is not glucose, but it helps the liver raise your blood glucose.
   b. Glucagon is a prescription drug and is given by injection; it usually works within 15 minutes.
   c. If you do not respond with the first shot of glucagon, your family needs to call 911.
   d. A second dose of glucagon should be given by your family if you do not awaken in 15 minutes.
   e. After receiving glucagon and you respond, you need to eat a snack.

REGULAR CARE

A. You will need to come to the office at regular times to have your diabetes checked and make sure you do not have any complications. Your provider will follow national standards of care, including:
   1. Order a dilated eye examination every year.
   2. Check your blood pressure and keep it less than 140/80.
   3. Check your cholesterol at least once a year.
   4. Do a special foot examination at least once a year. Wear shoes in your home to protect your feet, and look at the bottom of your feet for injuries every day.
   5. Check your HgbA$_{1c}$ every 3 months to see if your blood sugar is under control.
   6. Check your urine for protein/kidney problems.
   7. Update your flu vaccine every year.
   8. Update your pneumonia vaccines based on the CDC's recommendations.
   9. Update other vaccines you may need as an adult (shingles, tetanus, etc.).

SICK DAY RULES

You will also need a special plan in the event you are sick or have a special occasion.
A. Test blood sugar more often up to every 2 to 4 hours.
B. Increase your fluids, even if you do not feel like drinking.
C. Follow a meal plan if you can.
D. Call your healthcare provider if your blood sugar is less than 70 or greater than 240 for two readings in a row that cannot be explained; if you are unable to retain food/fluids; and if you are spilling ketones.
E. Check your ketones if your blood sugar is greater than 240. If your ketones are negative, keep testing if your blood sugar stays up.
F. Continue to take your usual insulin dose.
G. **Do not take Glucophage (metformin) if you are dehydrated.**

Activity:
A. Exercise is very important in controlling your diabetes. It not only improves blood sugar by helping your insulin to work, but it also reduces your risk of heart attack and stroke and helps with losing weight.
B. Talk with your healthcare provider before starting an exercise plan. If you are currently doing some form of exercise, please continue; however, avoid any strenuous exercise.
C. Moderate exercise (walking, cycling, and swimming) is the best exercise. Your goal will be to develop a consistent exercise activity three to four times a week for 20 to 45 minutes. Drink plenty of fluids before and after you exercise to prevent dehydration.
D. Exercise causes a decrease in your blood sugar for up to 24 hours. Do not exercise if your fasting blood sugar is greater than 250 or your sugar at any time is over 300. Exercise is not recommended if you have ketones (burning fat instead of sugar).

DIET:

A. You will be seeing a dietitian to develop a nutritional plan that is suited for you.
B. Consistency with meal times and amounts and food from all the six major food groups is important.

(continued)

DIABETES *(continued)*

C. Even though we stress carbohydrate counting, diabetes has abnormalities in carbohydrate, fat, and protein metabolism that cause hyperglycemia.

D. Dietary control includes control of fats such as cholesterol and saturated fat to help control blood lipid levels and prevent cardiovascular disease.

E. Eat a balanced diet, eat at regular times, and try not to skip meals; eat about the same amount of food at meal/snack times.

F. Use portion control, decrease the fats that you eat, and decrease fast simple sugars.

G. Decrease your alcohol consumption.

Medications:

A. You may need a combination of medications or insulin to help control your blood sugar to prevent complications.

B. If you use insulin injections or the insulin pump, the best place to give it is your stomach.

C. The American Diabetes Association recommends that you take an angiotensin-converting enzyme (ACE) inhibitor (blood pressure medicine) to help protect your kidneys.

D. You may be told to take an aspirin every day (if you are not allergic).

You Have Been Prescribed: _____

You Need to Take: _____

You Have Been Prescribed: _____

You Need to Take: _____

You Have Been Prescribed: _____

You Need to Take: _____

You Need to Notify the Office If:

A. You are sick and unable to keep foods/fluids down (vomiting) or have severe diarrhea.

B. You intend to take over-the-counter medications because they could react with your diabetes medication.

C. You are using Glucophage (metformin) and are going to have x-rays using any dyes. You must stop your medicine.

D. Other: _____

Phone: _____

Remember to carry an ID and carbohydrate source. Glucagon should be available for severe low blood glucose due to risk of aspiration and/or inability to swallow.

RESOURCES

American Diabetes Association (ADA): www.diabetes.org

You can build your own identification bracelets or neck chains from American Medical ID: www.americanmedical-id. com

DIARRHEA

PROBLEM

Diarrhea is a condition that causes loose, watery stools. Diarrhea is a symptom, not a disease. If you are a diabetic and have more than 1 day of diarrhea, please contact the office.

CAUSE

There are many causes of diarrhea, including infections caused by virus, bacteria, and even parasites. Diarrhea can also be caused by infection resulting from eating or drinking contaminated food or water.

PREVENTION/CARE

A. Avoid raw seafood and undercooked foods. Cut away any damaged or bruised areas on fruits and vegetables before eating.
B. Store food in the refrigerator within 1 hour of cooking to prevent the growth of bacteria. Store fruits and vegetables away from raw meat, chicken, and seafood.
C. Avoid buffet or picnic foods left out for several hours and food served by street vendors.
D. Wash your hands well before and after preparing foods, after going to the bathroom, and after handling diapers.
E. When traveling:
   1. Avoid local water supplies (including ice) when they are in question: drink bottled water instead.
   2. Do not eat fresh vegetables that may have been washed in contaminated water.
   3. If possible, travel with antiseptic hand lotion and wipes.
F. When hiking or camping, do not drink from streams, springs, or untested wells. Boil all water used for drinking or cooking.
G. Do not allow people with diarrhea to handle food.
H. Do not buy turtles, iguanas, or reptiles for pets: They carry *Salmonella*.
I. Thoroughly cook eggs. Do not eat raw eggs or foods containing raw eggs, such as cookie dough. Store fruits and vegetables away from raw meat, chicken, and seafood.
J. Cook chicken, beef, and pork until the meat does not have any pink color.
K. Call your day-care center if your child has diarrhea, especially if he or she has fever. Keep your child away from child-care centers if the diarrhea is too much for a diaper or if he or she is unable to get to the toilet.

TREATMENT PLAN

A. Diarrhea usually goes away in 24 to 48 hours.
B. Keep drinking liquids.
C. If you think a prescription drug is causing diarrhea, consult with the doctor before stopping the medication.
D. Clean toys and hard surfaces with soap and water. Chlorine-based disinfectants inactivate rotavirus and may help prevent the spread in child-care centers.

Activity: Decrease activities until diarrhea stops.
Diet:
A. If diarrhea is accompanied by nausea, suck ice chips.
B. Drink clear liquids frequently, such as 7-Up, Gatorade, ginger ale, broth, or gelatin, until diarrhea stops.
C. Use popsicles for added liquid.
D. After symptoms disappear, eat soft foods, such as cooked cereal, rice, baked potatoes, and yogurt, for 1 to 2 days.
E. Resume your normal diet in 2 to 3 days after the diarrhea stops.
F. Avoid fruits, alcohol, and highly seasoned foods for several more days.
Medications:

You or Your Child Has Been Prescribed the Following Antidiarrheal Medication: _____

You or Your Child Need to Take: _____

(*continued*)

DIARRHEA (*continued*)

You Need to Notify the Office If:

A. You or your child has diarrhea lasting more than 2 days or has chronic diarrhea.

B. You or your child has mucus, blood, or worms in the stool.

C. You or your child has a fever of 101.0°F or higher.

D. You or your child has severe pain in the stomach or in the rectum.

E. You or your child has dehydration symptoms, including dry mouth, wrinkled skin, excessive thirst, or little or no urine.

F. Your child:

　　1. Becomes listless, refuses to eat, or cries loudly and persistently, even when picked up

　　2. Has abnormal growth and development

G. Other: _____

Phone: _____

RESOURCE

LaRoque, R., & Harris, J.B. (2018, March 17). Patient education: Acute diarrhea in adults (Beyond the basics). *UpToDate*. Retrieved from https://www.uptodate.com/contents/acute-diarrhea-in-adults-beyond-the-basics

CLIENT TEACHING GUIDE

DYSMENORRHEA (PAINFUL MENSTRUAL CRAMPS OR PERIODS)

PROBLEM

Painful menstrual cramps, or dysmenorrhea, can cause occasional diarrhea, nausea or vomiting, and headache with menstrual periods.

CAUSE

A substance called prostaglandin causes most painful menstrual cramps. This substance is released in the uterus and causes the uterus to contract. Most menstrual cramps are normal and are not a sign of anything wrong. However, menstrual cramps may cause you to feel bad enough that you are unable to go to school or work. If that is the case, your healthcare provider can suggest medication to decrease the painful periods.

TREATMENT PLAN/CARE

A. Your healthcare provider may suggest a medicine such as a prostaglandin inhibitor. This medication helps decrease or eliminate the most likely substance that is causing the cramping of your uterus. The medication most often suggested is ibuprofen (Motrin IB, Advil, Nuprin, or others). Another medication is naproxen (Aleve).
   1. These are available at your local drug store, grocery store, or convenience store.
   2. Take any of these with a snack or meal to protect your stomach lining and prevent nausea.
   3. If you usually have very painful menstrual cramps, begin your medication as soon as your period begins or even the day before your period. This helps stop the production of prostaglandin.
B. If your cramps are not better using over-the-counter medications, your healthcare provider may write a prescription for a stronger medicine.
C. Many women take oral contraceptive pills to relieve menstrual cramps. A prescription is necessary. Notify your care provider if you are a cigarette smoker as smoking may increase your chance of side effects with oral contraceptives.
D. Some women find that exercise, such as walking, helps ease the cramps.
E. Another idea is a warm bath, shower, or a warm heating pad placed on your abdomen.
F. General health practices such as regular exercise, yoga, routine sleep habits, and regular sexual activity are beneficial.

Activity: Try to continue your usual activity. Try taking a walk, swimming, or doing yoga. Try a warm bath or shower.
Diet: Eat your normal diet. Red raspberry leaf tea may be helpful as a uterine toner.
Medication:

You Have Been Prescribed: _____

You Need to Take: _____

You Need to Notify the Office If You Have:
A. Any questions concerning your condition
B. Problems taking the medicine
C. No relief when taking the medicine, and other measures do not help
D. Any signs of infection, such as fever, chills, bad-smelling vaginal discharge, or burning sensation when you urinate

E. Other: _____

Phone: _____

DYSPAREUNIA (PAIN WITH INTERCOURSE)

PROBLEM

As many as 60% of women complain of pain with sexual intercourse, also known as dyspareunia. Pain may occur with insertion of and/or with deep penetration of the penis into the vagina.

CAUSE

There are physical causes, such as episiotomy scars, a short vagina, and infections; musculoskeletal causes such as disc problems; hormonal causes such as the lack of estrogen in menopause; and poor communication with partners and lack of foreplay.

PREVENTION AND TREATMENT PLANS

A. Inadequate lubrication:
1. More prolonged foreplay increases natural vaginal lubrication.
2. Use a water-soluble glycerine-free lubricant such as Slippery Stuff or Good Clean Love.
3. Do not use Vaseline as a lubricant.
4. Do not use contraceptive creams for lubrication; they often cause dryness (dehydration) and may worsen soreness.
B. Pain on insertion of penis:
1. Try different positions that give you more control.
2. Guide the penis for insertion.
3. If menopausal, you may be prescribed estrogen cream to use on an intermittent basis.
C. Pain with deep penetration:
1. Use a side-lying position during intercourse; this may be more comfortable so that deep penetration is limited.
2. You may need to be referred to a gynecologist for further treatment and/or surgery if you have any masses or scar tissue noted on a physical examination.
D. If you have or suspect an infection:
1. Inform your provider that you may have an infection.
2. A culture will be done.
3. Antibiotics will be prescribed for you and possibly your partner(s).
4. Refrain from sexual intercourse until all medications are gone (unless otherwise instructed).
5. If you have a Bartholin's duct cyst, it will be drained and you will be treated with antibiotics.
E. If you have a very narrow vaginal opening, you may be referred to a gynecologist for vaginal dilation.
F. Spasm of the muscles upon touching the vaginal area may be treated with medication, relaxation techniques, and Kegel exercises.
G. You and your partner may be referred to a clinician specializing in sexual health.

Medication:

You Have Been Prescribed: _____

You Need to Take/Use It: _____

You Need to Notify the Office If You Have:
A. No relief of your symptoms after your prescribed treatment

B. Other: _____

Phone: _____

CLIENT TEACHING GUIDE

ECZEMA

PROBLEM

Red, itching, scaling, and thickening of skin occurs in patches. You may have papules (bumps) with vesicles (clear fluid) that can be found especially on the hands, scalp, face, back of the neck, or skin creases of elbows and knees.

CAUSE

The cause is unknown. If it is an allergic reaction, it may be caused by foods such as eggs, wheat, milk, or seafood; wool clothing; skin lotions and ointments; soaps; detergents; cleansers; plants; tanning agents used for shoe leather; dyes; and topical medications. The risk for developing eczema increases with stress, medical history of other allergic conditions, clothing made of synthetic fabric (which traps perspiration), and weather extremes (cold, hot).

PREVENTION/CARE

A. Avoid risk factors.
B. Wear rubber gloves for household cleaning tasks.
C. Wear loose, cotton clothing to help absorb perspiration.
D. Keep fingernails short and wear soft gloves during sleep.
E. Scratching worsens eczema.
F. Bathe less frequently to avoid excessive skin dryness.
G. Use special nonfat soaps (Purpose or Basis soap) and tepid water.
H. Do not use soap on inflamed areas.
I. Lubricate the skin after bathing; avoid lubricants with alcohol in the ingredients.
J. Recommended creams include Eucerin, Keri Lotion, and Lubriderm. Steroid creams may be prescribed.
K. Avoid extreme temperature changes.
L. Avoid anything that has previously worsened the condition.

TREATMENT PLAN

Activity: No restrictions
Diet: You may be told to try a special diet. Eliminate any foods known to cause flare-ups.
Medications:

You Have Been Prescribed: _____

You Need to Take: _____

You Need to Notify the Office If:
A. You have a reaction to any of the medications prescribed.
B. You cannot take the medications.
C. New symptoms develop.

Phone: _____

EMERGENCY CONTRACEPTION—LEVONOGESTREL

You have indicated that you want to use an emergency contraception (EC) method. **There are several levonorgestrel emergency contraceptive pills with different brand names available** over the counter without prescription.

TREATMENT PLAN

A. You must start levonorgestrel-based EC within 72 hours.

B. It is best to start within the first 12 to 24 hours.

C. Your healthcare provider can give you clear instructions, though the packaging information on the over-the-counter products is very clear.

D. The sooner you begin EC, the more effective it will be.

E. The levonorgestrel EC prevents pregnancy because the hormones cause the mucus in the cervix to thicken and the lining of the uterus and tubes to change.

F. You may not ovulate, but if you do ovulate, the chance of fertilization is decreased because of the mechanism of action of the EC.

G. EC in the form of hormonal pills will *neither* interrupt *nor* harm an already established pregnancy.

H. Nausea is a common side effect.

I. Your healthcare provider will tell you what medication to buy, or give you a prescription for medicine to keep you from being sick to your stomach.

J. Take this medicine at least 1 hour before you take the hormone pills.

K. Other common side effects include breast tenderness, headache, or dizziness. These side effects go away in a day or two.

L. You should have a menstrual period a week or so after you take the pills.

M. If you have not had a period by 3 weeks, call the office

N. It is unlikely that you would get pregnant, but if you do and choose to have a baby, the EC is *not* associated with any increased chance of birth defects.

O. Be sure to discuss reliable methods of birth control that are best suited for you.

Medication:

You Have Been Prescribed the Following EC Medication: _____

You Have Been Prescribed the Following Nausea Medication: _____

You Need to Call Us If You Have Any Questions or Problems.

You Need to Notify the Office If You Have:

A. Serious side effects of medicine

B. Severe chest pain

C. Severe abdominal pain

D. Headache

E. Vision changes

F. Shortness of breath

G. No period for 3 weeks

H. Other: _____

Phone: _____

EMERGENCY CONTRACEPTION—ULIPRISTAL ACETATE

You have indicated that you want to use an EC method. **You have been prescribed ulipristal acetate.**

TREATMENT PLAN

A. You must start ulipristal acetate within 120 hours of unprotected intercourse.
B. Your healthcare provider will give you clear instructions.
C. The sooner you begin EC, the more effective it will be.
D. This method of EC prevents pregnancy by delaying ovulation.
E. Common side effects are headache and nausea.
F. Notify your healthcare provider if vomiting occurs within 3 hours of taking.
G. You should have a menstrual period 1 to 3 weeks after you take the pills.
H. If your period is delayed by more than 1 week, call the office.
I. Do not take if you are breastfeeding or pregnant.
J. Do not take repeated doses in the same menstrual cycle.
K. This EC may decrease the effectiveness of hormonal contraceptives. Use a barrier backup method (condoms) for 14 days after taking this EC.
L. Do not use as routine contraception. Talk to your healthcare provider about birth control options that are best suited to you.
M. Seek medical attention if you experience lower abdominal pain 3 to 5 weeks after taking.

Medication:

You Have Been Prescribed the Following EC Medication: _____

You Need to Call Us If You Have Any Questions or Problems.

You Need to Notify the Office If You Have:
A. Serious side effects of medicine
B. Severe chest pain
C. Severe abdominal pain
D. Headache
E. Vision changes
F. Shortness of breath
G. Menses delayed more than 1 week of expected date

H. Other: _____

Phone: _____

CLIENT TEACHING GUIDE

EMPHYSEMA

PROBLEM

Emphysema is a chronic lung disease that is incurable. Emphysema can only be managed; the goal of treatment is to improve the activities of daily living and the quality of life by preventing symptoms and by preserving optimal lung function.

CAUSE

Cigarette smoking increases the risk of COPD (another name for several lung diseases) by about 30 times. Environmental irritants have also been linked with chronic lung diseases.

PREVENTION/CARE

Emphysema cannot be prevented once lung changes have taken place.

TREATMENT PLAN

A. **Stop smoking—it causes more lung irritation, mucus/sputum production, and coughing. It is never too late to quit smoking.**
B. Eliminate other lung irritants, such as wood smoke; secondhand smoke; hair spray; and paint, bleach, and other chemicals found at home. Avoid sweeping and dusting. Stay indoors when air pollution or pollen counts are high.
C. Pulmonary rehabilitation may be ordered. Exercising is a very important component of pulmonary rehabilitation as well as learning breathing techniques.
D. Report respiratory infections to your healthcare provider as soon as possible.
E. Get a flu shot every year.
F. Get a vaccination for pneumonia: once as an adult before 65 years old; then 2 more doses at 65 years and older.
G. Use postural drainage: lean over the side of the bed, rest your elbows on a pillow placed on the floor, and cough as someone gently pounds on your back.
H. Stay indoors during extremely hot or cold weather. If you must be outside in the cold, cover your nose and face. Use an air conditioner in hot weather.
I. Avoid people who have respiratory illnesses; also avoid crowds and poorly ventilated areas.
J. Oxygen therapy may be ordered if you have trouble breathing.
K. Use community resources such as Meals on Wheels, handicap tag, or parking stickers.
L. You may be asked to talk to a social worker.

Activity:
A. Pace yourself to avoid shortness of breath.
B. Follow a daily exercise plan. Start with three to four times a day, each lasting 5 to 15 minutes. Start at half-speed and build up.
C. Sexual dysfunction can occur because of lack of physical energy and trouble breathing. Find other ways to show affection such as kissing, hugging, or massage.

Diet:
A. If you do not have congestive heart failure, drink 3 L of fluids a day—equal to one and a half large soda bottles.
B. Avoid dairy products; they increase mucus/sputum production.
C. Eat five to six small meals a day. Big meals feel like pressure on your stomach and lungs.
D. Avoid foods that cause gas and stomach discomfort.
E. Use oxygen during meals, if necessary; take your time eating, rest between bites, and avoid hard-to-chew foods, because eating may tire you. Rest before and after eating if you have shortness of breath.
F. Eat a high-protein diet with a good balance of vitamins and minerals.
G. Avoid excessively hot or cold foods and drinks that may start an irritating cough.
H. Eat high-potassium foods such as bananas, dried fruit, orange and grape juice, milk, peaches, potatoes, tomatoes, and cantaloupe. Symptoms of low potassium include weakness, leg cramps, and tingling fingers.

(*continued*)

EMPHYSEMA *(continued)*

Medications:

You Have Been Prescribed: _____

You Need to Take: _____

Use of a spacer/chamber device improves aerosol delivery to your lungs and reduces side effects.

You Need to Notify the Office If:
A. You have trouble breathing.
B. You develop an infection (signs are fever, change in sputum, sinus drainage).
C. Your inhaler does not help your symptoms.
D. Your symptoms do not improve within 48 hours of starting medication.

E. Other: _____

Phone: _____

ENDOMETRITIS

PROBLEM

You have an infection of the inside of the uterus.

CAUSE

One or more types of bacteria that invade damaged tissue following giving birth could cause endometritis. The bacteria may be from the vagina, the bowel, or the environment.

PREVENTION/CARE

A. Use careful perineal care:
    1. Wipe from front to back after voiding.
    2. Remove pad from front to back.
    3. Change pad at least every 4 hours.
    4. Use your squeeze bottle filled with warm water to cleanse after each time you urinate or have a bowel movement.
    5. Use good handwashing after changing your pads and the baby's diaper.

TREATMENT PLAN

A. You need to be treated with antibiotic therapy.
B. Take your temperature three times a day for the first 3 days on the antibiotics.
C. Take Tylenol or ibuprofen as needed for fever or discomfort.

Activity: It is very important for you to increase rest with an infection. Try to get a nap when the baby is sleeping. You may continue to breastfeed on most antibiotic therapies; your provider will let you know if you are prescribed something that is not compatible with breastfeeding. If you do not breastfeed while you are feeling bad, pump your breast milk to keep up your milk supply.
Diet: Eat well-balanced meals. Drink at least 10 to 12 glasses of liquid a day.
Medications: Continue your prenatal vitamins. Take all of your antibiotics, even if you start feeling better.

You Have Been Prescribed: _____

You Need to Take: _____

You Need to Notify the Office If You Have:
A. Temperature 100.4°F or greater
B. Foul-smelling vaginal bleeding
C. Increase in pain or tenderness in uterus

D. Other: _____

Phone: _____

EPIDIDYMITIS

PROBLEM

Epididymitis is infection of the gland that carries sperm.

CAUSE

The infection may be a urinary tract infection (UTI) or may be from a sexually transmitted disease (STD), such as gonorrhea or chlamydia.

PREVENTION/CARE

A. Prevent UTIs with good hygiene:
   1. Clean under foreskin if uncircumcised.
   2. Wash your hands after each time you go to the bathroom (both urine and bowel movements [BM]).
B. Limit your sexual partners and use a condom to prevent all types of infection.

TREATMENT PLAN

A. Antibiotics are used to kill bacteria that cause infection.
B. Try one of the following comfort measures:
   1. Intermittent cold compresses for acute swelling and pain relief
   2. Local heat or warm bath after the initial discomfort
C. Use an athletic supporter or elevate the scrotum on a small rolled washcloth.
D. Your sexual partner(s) need(s) to be treated for STD.

Activity:
A. Rest; do not engage in strenuous activity or heavy lifting.
B. Avoid sex until you finish the antibiotics.

Diet: Avoid foods that irritate the bladder: caffeine, alcohol, and spicy foods.

Medications:
A. Antibiotics are used to kill bacteria causing infection.
B. Take all of the antibiotics prescribed for you; do not stop taking drugs after symptoms are gone.
C. Do not share your antibiotics with your sex partner(s); a full prescription of antibiotics is needed for each of you to get better.
D. Take pain medications or anti-inflammatory drugs, such as acetaminophen (Tylenol) or ibuprofen, as needed.

You Have Been Prescribed the Following Antibiotics: _____

You Need to Take: _____

Finish all of the antibiotics, even if you feel better.

You Have Been Prescribed the Following for Pain: _____

You Need to Take: _____

You Need to Notify the Office If:
A. You have a great increase in pain or swelling after going home.
B. You have worsening symptoms after starting the antibiotics.
C. You have fever greater than 101.0°F.
D. You get very constipated.

E. Other: _____

Phone: _____

ERYTHEMA MULTIFORME

PROBLEM

An acute inflammatory disorder of the skin and mucous membranes, erythema multiforme, is usually self-limited and benign. A severe form is known as Stevens–Johnson syndrome or erythema multiforme majus, and the less severe form is referred to as erythema multiforme minus.

CAUSE

The cause is unknown in 50% of the cases. Erythema multiforme has been associated with viral infections, particularly the herpes simplex virus; bacterial and protozoan infections; an immunologic reaction of the skin; medications (sulfonamides, penicillins, anticonvulsants, salicylates, barbiturates), with reactions occurring up to 7 to 14 days after using the medication; pregnancy; premenstrual hormone changes; malignancy; or radiation therapy. Risk increases with previous history of erythema multiforme.

PREVENTION/CARE

A. Avoid suspected causes.
B. Seek prompt treatment of any illness or infection.
C. Prevent herpes simplex virus outbreaks by avoiding sun exposure and reducing stress.
D. Seek treatment immediately if at any time symptoms seem to be worsening or increasing.
E. Discontinue any implicated medication.
F. Apply wet dressings or soaks, with Burow's solution, or apply lotions to soothe the skin.
G. Bathe in lukewarm to cool water three times a day for 30 minutes.
H. Monitor yourself for any eye involvement and report it to your healthcare provider immediately.
I. If mouth sores are present, use good oral hygiene (brush two to three times a day using a soft brush) and rinse frequently with cool water.
J. Hospitalization may be required if there is extensive skin involvement.

TREATMENT PLAN

Activity: As tolerated by the extent of the symptoms. Restrict yourself to bed rest if fever is present.
Diet: Usually no special diet is necessary; although if mouth sores are present, a soft or liquid diet may be better tolerated. Increase fluid intake above the general 8 to 10 glasses per day.
Medications: May be prescribed to control symptoms and pain

You Have Been Prescribed: _____

You Need to Take: _____

You Need to Notify the Office If:
A. You have an adverse reaction to or cannot tolerate any of the prescribed medications.
B. Symptoms worsen during treatment, or the rash does not clear in 3 weeks (usual course: rash evolves over 1–2 weeks, usually clears in 2–3 weeks, but may take 5–6 weeks).
C. New or unexplained symptoms develop.
D. You have any questions or concerns.

Phone: _____

EXERCISE

You have been evaluated and cleared for an exercise program. Your maximum target heart rate during exercise based on your age and physical fitness is _____ beats per minute.

 Your goal is to exercise at least three times a week (nonconsecutive days). Your target heart rate should be sustained for 20 to 30 minutes for maximal cardiovascular effect.

A. **Your exercise plan should include four components of activity:**
 1. Warm-up
     a. The warm-up phase prepares the body to increase the blood flow to the heart and decreases muscle tension. **The warm-up phase should last 10 to 20 minutes** and may include such exercises as head rotations, arm and shoulder circles, waist circles or bends, and side leg raises.
 2. Stretching
     a. Stretching prepares the major muscles for exercise. Slow stretching and holding repetitions help to prevent injury. Examples of stretching: sitting hamstring leg stretches and holds, and arm stretches
 3. Aerobic activity
     a. The aerobic phase of exercise should be continuous. **Your target heart rate should be maintained for 20 to 30 minutes for cardiovascular benefit.** Examples of aerobic activity: brisk walking, running, or swimming
 4. Cooldown phase
     a. **A cooldown period for 5 to 10 minutes finishes your exercise.** This gradual cooldown allows the body temperature to cool and slowly decreases the heart rate, preventing dizziness, fatigue, and nausea. Examples of cooldown exercise: walking and cooldown stretches
B. **Exercise should be discontinued if the following symptoms develop:**
 1. Marked increase in shortness of breath (inability to talk while exercising)
 2. Chest pain, including left arm and jaw pain
 3. Irregular heartbeat
 4. Nausea or vomiting
 5. Faintness or light-headedness
 6. Injury to muscle or joints (sprains, tears)
 7. Prolonged fatigue
 8. Muscle weakness

Seek immediate medical attention if you experience chest pain. If your shortness of breath or irregular heartbeat does not subside within 1 to 2 minutes of rest, seek help. Return to your healthcare provider for an evaluation before further exercise after you experience any other symptoms.

C. **Exercise can be easily incorporated into daily activities in other ways:**
 1. Use the stairs instead of the elevator.
 2. Park away from buildings to add extra walking distance.
 3. Use the walking path and carry golf clubs instead of using golf carts.
 4. Play outdoor games of catch, kickball, or hopscotch instead of indoor activities.
 5. Push-mow your yard instead of riding or hiring others for lawn care.
 6. Take an evening walk in your neighborhood or use the local mall for all-weather exercise.
 7. Shovel snow from the sidewalk instead of using a snow blower.
 8. Sweep the porch patio instead of using a leaf blower.
 9. Rake leaves for composting.
 10. Rent or buy an exercise video on yoga, Tai Chi, or aerobics instead of a movie.
 11. Turn on your radio and dance.
 12. Walk your dog for 20 to 30 minutes at a time.

EYE MEDICATION ADMINISTRATION

PROBLEM

You have been prescribed a medication for your eye(s). It is very important that you know the correct way to use your eye medication.

CAUSE

You have been diagnosed with:_____

PREVENTION/CARE

The health of your eyes is important.
A. Use good handwashing and try not to rub your eyes with your fingers.
B. Clean your contacts regularly with contact cleaning solution. Do not put your contacts in your mouth to moisten.
C. Wear sunglasses in bright sunshine.
D. Use eye goggles when working and playing sports to ensure extra protection.
E. Replace your eye makeup often. Mascara, eye shadow, and eyeliner grow bacteria. Do not share makeup.

TREATMENT PLAN

A. Correct use of your medication is important.
B. **You may or may not require an eyepatch or shield.**

How to Apply Eye Ointment
A. Always wash your hands before placing medication in your eyes.
B. Gently pull down the lower eyelid.
C. Make a small pocket between the eyeball and the eyelid.
D. If you have someone helping to put your eye ointment in the lower-lid pocket, look up and away while he or she puts in the medicine.
E. Do not let the tube of medicine touch the eye or eyelid.
F. Squeeze a thin ribbon of the medication into the pocket of the eyelid.
G. Start at the inner fold of the eye going from the nose to the outer eye.
H. Let go of the eyelid and blink to spread the medication.

How to Instill Eye Drops
A. Always wash your hands before placing medication in your eyes.
B. Gently pull down the lower eyelid.
C. Make a small pocket between the eyelid and the eyeball.
D. If you have someone helping to put your eye drops in the lower lid pocket, look up and away while he or she puts in the medicine.
E. **Do not let the bottle of medication touch the eye or eyelid.**
F. Squeeze the prescribed number of drops of the medicine into the pocket of the eyelid.
G. Let go of the eyelid and blink (or tell the client to blink) to spread the medication.

Activity: No restrictions are required unless you require eye surgery; then you will be given specific instructions about the amount of activity allowed.
Diet: No restrictions
Medications:

You Have Been Prescribed: _____

You Need to Take: _____

(**continued**)

EYE MEDICATION ADMINISTRATION   *(continued)*

You Need to Notify the Office If:

A. You are unable to put in the medication yourself or get help from others.

B. You are not better 24 to 48 hours after starting the medication.

C. Your vision is worse after using the medication.

D. You have an allergic reaction to the medicine.

E. Other: _____

Phone: _____

FEBRILE SEIZURES (CHILD)

PROBLEM

Convulsions or seizures may occur with an illness accompanied by a fever.

CAUSE

The cause of seizures with a febrile illness is not certain. Some families have seizures with fever that run in the family.

PREVENTION/CARE

A. Contact the office when your child gets sick with a fever:
   1. You may be instructed to give Tylenol or Motrin by your healthcare provider to help comfort your child. These medications do not prevent febrile seizures. *Aspirin should not be given to your child.*
   2. Be sure that your child gets plenty of fluids and rest.
   3. You do not need to take your child's temperature on a strict schedule if he or she is not getting/feeling worse. For children ages 0 to 5 years, the rectum and mouth areas are *not routinely* used to measure fever.
   4. Do not use the thermometers with mercury in the glass, and many states have banned them from medical use due to toxic risks. Use electronic/digital, infrared/tympanic, or chemical dot thermometers. The mouth, rectum, forehead (chemical dots), ears, or armpit are common areas for taking temperatures in children, depending on the age of the child. Always hold the thermometer while taking your child's temperature.
B. Care during a seizure:
   1. Make sure that your child is breathing without difficulty.
   2. Lay your child down on a safe surface and position the head to the side so that he or she does not spit up and get vomit into his or her lungs.
   3. Try not to restrain your child but protect him or her from hurting himself or herself.
   4. Do not try to open his or her mouth or put your fingers in their mouth.
   5. Do not try to give your child any medications during a seizure.
   6. Seizures from fever generally last less than 5 minutes.
   7. If the seizure lasts longer than 5 to 7 minutes, or if your child is not breathing or looks blue, call 911 for an ambulance.
   8. After the seizure, your child may be sleepy. This is normal, and it is okay to let him or her rest.

Activity: When your child is not sick, there should be no restrictions on normal activity. When your child has a fever, try to keep him or her quiet and avoid strenuous play activity. Follow your child's day-care/school policy about when to return after having a fever/illness

Diet: There is no special diet for a child with a fever; a regular diet is fine. Although your child has a fever, offer fluids to make sure he or she gets plenty of fluids, including formula and breast milk. Use juices or water, and, if directed, use Pedialyte. If your child is old enough, try ice pops for extra fluids.

Medications: You may be directed to use Tylenol or Motrin for your child's fever. These medications do not *prevent* febrile seizures.

Your Child Has Been Prescribed: _____

Take the Medications on This Schedule: _____

You Need to Notify the Office If:
A. Your child continues to have a high fever.
B. Your child is unable to keep fluids down due to nausea, vomiting, or diarrhea.

C. Other: _____

Phone: _____

If your child develops seizures lasting longer than 5 to 7 minutes or is having trouble breathing, *CALL 911*.

FIBROCYSTIC BREAST CHANGES AND BREAST PAIN

PROBLEM

You are being treated for breast pain or breast lumpiness that result from changes that are painful, but not cancerous. You have probably had an extensive examination by your healthcare provider, perhaps a mammogram, sonogram, and/or a breast biopsy.

CAUSE

The cause is unknown. It is probably related to estrogen changes that occur with menstrual periods.

PREVENTION/CARE

None known

TREATMENT PLAN

Be fitted for a well-fitting bra. This helps to eliminate breast movement as a source of pain. Try ice packs on your breasts for 20 minutes every few hours. Some women find that heat on the breast can also relieve discomfort.

Activity: There are no activity restrictions. When exercising, wear a good, supportive bra.

Diet: Decrease the amount of salt in your diet (near your period) to decrease water retention if you have swelling of your breasts near your period. Some women have reported decreased breast pain with reduced caffeine and nicotine intake.

Medications: Several medications have been found to relieve breast pain from fibrocystic breast changes. Ask your healthcare provider which is best for you.

Complementary: Recent research has shown that flaxseed may reduce cyclic pain (flaxseed 25 mg a day). Evening primrose oil (EPO) 1-3 g daily in divided doses may relieve discomfort. Vitamin E, B6, and A supplementation may also be helpful, as well as iodine 3,000 mcg daily. Violet iodine is an over-the-counter formulation for the treatment of fibrocystic breast pain.

You Have Been Prescribed: _____

You Need to Take: _____

You Need to Call Us If You Have Any Questions or Problems.

Phone: _____

FIBROMYALGIA

PROBLEM

You have inflammation or pain in the muscles and connective tissues, usually noted in the low back, shoulders, neck, chest, arms, hips, and thighs. This pain is chronic, and you may also have excessive fatigue and stiffness, difficulty with sleeping, and possibly other symptoms of anxiety, stress, and/or depression.

CAUSE

The cause is unknown. Fibromyalgia has been linked to anxiety, depression, stress, infections, and viruses.

TREATMENT PLAN/CARE

A. Get regular exercise.
B. Get adequate amounts of sleep.
C. For symptoms of discomfort, you may try applying heat to the areas of pain, such as hot showers, heating pad, and whirlpools.
D. Gentle massages by a massage therapist may help with comfort.
E. Try to eliminate the daily stress in your life.
F. Consider alternatives to relieving stress such as biofeedback, relaxation techniques, and yoga.
G. Notify your healthcare provider if you are having symptoms of anxiety or depression that need addressing and possible treatment with medications.

Activity: Regular exercise is recommended. Exercise at least 30 minutes, for three to five times a week, if possible. Even 5 minutes is better than no exercise. Establish a regular sleep time. Adequate and sound sleeping may decrease symptoms. You may require naps during the day.

Diet: Eat a nutritious regular diet. Increase your intake of fruits and vegetables. Avoid foods, caffeine, and alcohol that interfere with your normal sleep.

Medications: There are medications to help with your fibromyalgia. You may be prescribed one of these by your healthcare provider. Examples include duloxetine (Cymbalta), milnacipran (Savella), or pregabalin (Lyrica).

You may also need to treat other symptoms accordingly:

1. Pain: address with nonsteroidal anti-inflammatory drugs (NSAIDs) such as ibuprofen or naproxen
2. Sleep disorder: address this with your healthcare provider for treatment.
3. Anxiety/stress/depression: address this with your healthcare provider.

You Have Been Prescribed: _____

You Need to Take: _____

You Need to Notify the Office If You Have:
A. New or unexplained symptoms that have developed
B. Fever higher than 100°F

C. Other: _____

Phone: _____

RESOURCE

The National Fibromyalgia Association: www.fmaware.org

FOLLICULITIS

PROBLEM

A bacterial (or fungal) infection of the hair follicle, folliculitis is seen when a pustule develops, commonly on the arms, legs, scalp, and face (beard).

CAUSES

A. Bacterial: infection commonly caused by *Staphylococcus* bacteria
B. Fungal: may be caused by yeast infection

PREVENTION

A. Keep skin clean and dry.
B. Avoid warm, moist conditions.
C. Healing generally occurs 10 to 14 days after proper treatment with medications.
D. Practice good handwashing technique, using antibacterial soaps.
E. Use clean razors daily.
F. Throw old razors away.
G. Do not share razors.
H. Shampoo scalp daily.
I. Folliculitis usually resolves within 4 to 6 weeks after proper treatment.

TREATMENT PLAN

Activity: As tolerated
Diet: Regular diet
Medications: Topical and/or oral antibiotics as prescribed

You Have Been Prescribed: _____

You Need to Take: _____

You Need to Notify the Office If:
A. You notice lesions worsening or spreading, despite adequate medication treatment.
B. You have a fever higher than 101°F.
C. Your condition is not getting better.
D. You have a reaction to your medication.

E. Other _____

Phone: _____

GASTROESOPHAGEAL REFLUX DISEASE (GERD)

PROBLEM

Relaxation of the lower esophageal (stomach) sphincter causes reflux of gastric acid or a feeling of "heartburn" and "acid brash."

CAUSE

Heartburn occurs when acidic stomach contents come back into the esophagus. Improper diet, spicy foods, alcohol, smoking, pregnancy, obesity, certain medications, and nervous tension are all causes of gastroesophageal reflux disease (GERD).

PREVENTION/CARE

A. Avoid smoking.
B. Avoid things that increase abdominal pressure:
 1. Wearing tight clothes and belts
 2. Lying down or bending over for 3 hours after eating, which is when there can be a lot of reflux
 3. Coughing
 4. Straining
C. Avoid medications, such as aspirin or ibuprofen, that may irritate your stomach.
D. Avoid alcohol.
E. Avoid large meals.

TREATMENT PLAN

A. Weight loss is advised to relieve symptoms.
B. Stop smoking.
C. You may be instructed to elevate the head of your bed on 6-inch blocks, or sleep on a wedge bolster pillow.
D. Review all of your medications, over-the-counter (OTC) medications, and herbal products with your healthcare provider to help identify any side effects that may cause your symptoms.
E. Take your medications at the correct times.

Activity: Postpone vigorous exercise until your stomach is likely to be empty, about 2 hours after eating.
Diet:
A. Eat a lower fat, bland diet.
B. Eat four to six small meals a day instead of three larger meals.
C. Do not eat 2 to 3 hours before bedtime.
D. Avoid chocolate, garlic, onions, citrus fruits, coffee (including decaffeinated), alcohol, highly seasoned foods, and carbonated beverages.
E. Eat slowly.
Medications: Sit or stand when taking solid medications (pills or capsules). Follow the drug with at least one cup of liquid. When OTC antacids do not make your symptoms better, please notify the office for medications that decrease gastric acid secretions. You may require lifelong therapy.

You Have Been Prescribed: _____

You Need to Take: _____

You Need to Notify the Office If You Have:
A. No relief from antacids or second medication, so that the next step of medication therapy may be prescribed
B. New symptoms, such as blood in vomit

C. Other: _____

Phone: _____

GESTATIONAL DIABETES

PROBLEM

Gestational diabetes only develops during pregnancy because of the new hormones being produced. The hormonal influence makes you "insulin resistant," meaning you still produce insulin, but the hormones prevent it from working effectively.

Your blood sugar needs to be controlled so that the amount of sugar going to your baby is controlled, too. High blood sugar causes a big baby at delivery, increases your risk of a cesarean birth, causes the baby to have low blood sugar after delivery, increases jaundice, and causes other problems for the baby such as lung problems. It can also cause your baby to be overweight in childhood and increases the risk of developing diabetes.

CAUSE

You are producing new hormones that cause insulin resistance. The likelihood of having gestational diabetes increases with other factors, such as the mother's age, and it is more common in certain groups, such as Latin Americans and American Indians.

PREVENTION/CARE

Good control of your diet, exercise, and the possible use of medication and/or possibly insulin will help you to control your blood sugar during your pregnancy.

TREATMENT PLAN

A. You are asked to keep a record of your blood glucose values:
   1. You will be shown how to test your blood.
   2. You need to test your blood four times a day: first thing in the morning, before or after lunch, before or after dinner, and possibly at bedtime, depending on if your diabetes is controlled by diet or by medication.
   3. You will be given specific instructions for before or after meals.
   4. Phone in your blood sugar values every week. Your insulin may be changed weekly.
   5. The goal of your fasting blood sugar before breakfast is 60 to 90 mg/dL.
   6. Your blood sugar goal before meals and 2 hours after meals is less than 120 mg/dL.
B. You need to test your urine for ketones every day:
   1. You will be shown how to test your urine.
   2. You need to test for ketones if you are unable to eat or if you have diarrhea.
   3. You need to test for ketones if you feel like you have a urinary tract infection (UTI), sinus infection, or any kind of infection.
   4. You need to test for ketones if your blood sugar is higher than 150 mg/dL.
   5. You must follow the diet given to you by the dietitian. If you have questions or do not understand what you should be eating, contact your dietitian.

Activity: Exercise lowers blood sugar—gestational diabetes control involves regular exercise. You need to walk at least 20 to 30 minutes a day. Try your local mall for a climate-controlled place to walk. Your heart rate should not get above 140 beats per minute.

Diet: You are placed on a _____ calorie diet. The number of calories needs to be spread out over three meals and three snacks:
1. Breakfast, midmorning snack, lunch, midafternoon snack, dinner, and a snack at bedtime
2. The time you eat is as important as what you eat. Try to keep on a regular schedule.

Medications: Depending on your blood sugar, you may require medication to control it. You will be instructed on how to take the medicine. If you are started on insulin, you will require extra testing for the rest of your pregnancy.

GONORRHEA

PROBLEM

Gonorrhea is a sexually transmitted infection. You may have the following symptoms: burning during urination, yellowish discharge from the penis or vagina, heavier menstrual periods, or pelvic pain.

Untreated gonorrhea in females can lead to a condition called PID. PID is a leading cause of infertility, increased ectopic pregnancies, and chronic pelvic pain in women.

CAUSE

Gonorrhea is caused by an organism called *Neisseria gonorrhoeae.* This organism is spread through sexual contact and may infect the eyes, throat, vagina, penis, or rectum.

PREVENTION/CARE

A. Limit sexual partners.
B. Have routine screening tests for gonorrhea prior to beginning a new sexual relationship.
C. Use condoms when having intercourse.

TREATMENT PLAN

Your healthcare provider is required to report this disease to the public health department. The health department may contact you. **Abstain from sexual activity until you and your partner(s) have completed your prescribed medications.**
Diet: There is no special diet that needs to be followed.
Medications: Gonorrhea can be cured by the prescribed antibiotics.

You Have Been Prescribed: _____

You Need to Take: _____

It is very important that you keep your follow-up appointment that has been scheduled for you on: _____

All of the antibiotics need to be taken.

You Need to Notify the Office If:
A. You have any new symptoms.
B. You are unable to take all of the antibiotics due to nausea or vomiting or a reaction.

C. Other: _____

Phone: _____

CLIENT TEACHING GUIDE

GOUT

PROBLEM

Gout is caused by high uric acid deposits in the joints, which produce pain and swelling at the joint. Gout commonly occurs in the big toe; however, other joints may be affected, too. Other signs/symptoms include red, hot, and swollen joints, which may be tender to the touch. Gout also produces tophi, which are uric acid crystals that have formed under the skin, such as the edge of the ear, elbow, fingers, and toes, and near the Achilles tendon.

Gout is the result of too much uric acid production or not enough uric acid excretion from the kidney.

PREVENTION/CARE

A. The goal is to prevent recurrences of the attacks.
B. Acute attacks: You may apply warm or cool compresses to the affected areas for comfort.
C. Avoid weight-bearing objects on the affected joint.
D. Take your medication as prescribed.

Activity: When you have an attack, resting the joint is the best treatment. Drinking large amounts of water will keep your urine diluted to help prevent kidney stones.

Diet:

A. Drink 10 to 12 glasses of water a day. Avoid dehydration.
B. Refrain from alcohol (beer, wine, liquor). These will worsen your symptoms or trigger a new attack.
C. If overweight, you need to begin a weight-loss program appropriate for you.
D. Avoid crash diets. These will also precipitate an acute attack.
E. Foods to avoid: purine-rich foods such as sardines, anchovies, red meat and organ meats (liver, kidney), dried beans, shrimp, and sweet bread

Medications to avoid: salicylates (aspirin). This drug can interfere with the kidney trying to get rid of the high uric acid levels.

You may be prescribed medications for pain such as NSAIDs (ibuprofen or naproxen), steroids, pain relievers (acetaminophen), or colchicine.

You Have Been Prescribed: _____

You Need to Take: _____

You Need to Notify the Office If You Have:

A. Acute attacks
B. Fever higher than 101°F
C. Rash
D. Swelling of extremities
E. Vomiting/diarrhea
F. Signs/symptoms not improving within 3 to 4 days after starting therapy
G. Any adverse effects from your medication

H. Other: _____

Phone: _____

GRIEF

PROBLEM

Normal grief resolution may take from 6 months up to as long as 2 years.

CAUSES

Grief can follow the death of a loved one, but grief also follows other losses such as a loss of independence, loss of affection, or loss of body parts after an accident.

TREATMENT PLAN

It is important that you talk about your loss and how it affects you. The more you are able to talk about your feelings related to the loss you are experiencing, the more you will be able to work through your feelings.

You may be encouraged to seek supportive therapy in the form of divorce groups, loss groups, or groups dealing specifically with death and dying.

Activity: Moderate exercise, such as daily walking, is encouraged. Vigorous, prolonged exercise, however, may precipitate anxiety attacks.

Diet: Avoid caffeinated beverages, including coffee, tea, and carbonated colas that do not specify "decaffeinated." Try to eat healthy food and avoid overeating or skipping meals.

Medications: Medications for loss and grief are usually avoided at first because the use of drugs can prolong the time it takes to work through your grief. However, your healthcare provider will discuss medications in more depth. If you are having signs of depression or think you may need treatment with medication, contact your healthcare provider.

You Have Been Prescribed: _____

You Need to Take: _____

Do not stop antidepressants quickly. Talk to your healthcare provider if you want to discontinue them.

You Need to Notify the Office If:
A. You feel like you cannot stop crying.
B. You are not eating and are losing weight.
C. You feel like you have no one to turn to and talk about your feelings.
D. You have difficulty sleeping after several weeks.
E. You have thoughts of hurting yourself or others.
F. You do not think you are getting better on the prescribed medication.

G. Other: _____

Phone: _____

Local Support Group: _____

RESOURCES

Arnold, J. H., & Gemma, P. B. (1994). *A child dies: A portrait of family grief* (2nd ed.). Charles Press.

Fritsch, J., & Ilse, S. (1992). *The anguish of loss*. Wintergreen Press.

Ilse, S. (2008). *Empty arms: Coping with miscarriage, stillbirth, and infant death*. Wintergreen Press.

Smith, H. I. (2011). *A Decembered grief: Living with loss while others are celebrating*. Kansas City, MO: Beacon Hill Press of Kansas City. (Original work published 1999)

Zonnebelt-Smeenge, S., & De Vries R. C. (2001). *Empty chair: Handling grief on holidays and special occasions*. Baker Books.

HEAD INJURY: MILD

PROBLEM

Mild head injury includes any bump, jolt, or blow to the head that affects normal brain function, possibly causing confusion or a loss of consciousness.

WHAT TO EXPECT AFTER A HEAD INJURY

After a head injury, it is not unusual to have fatigue, headaches, irritability, dizziness, problems with sleep, trouble keeping your balance, or difficulty working in school or at your job. It is important to **_gradually_** increase your level of activity at home, school, and work. Take time to rest and schedule breaks whenever you feel physically or mentally tired. Usually, these symptoms or problems will lessen within a week and you will continue to improve over the next 3 months. Sometimes it may take longer to recover from a head injury. If you are still having symptoms or problems after 3 months, contact your primary care provider for additional treatment and advice.

GUIDELINES FOR CARE AT HOME

Activity:
A. Have someone stay with you for the next 24 hours to be sure your head injury does not worsen.
B. Limit physical activity, especially sports, heavy exercise, and heavy lifting, and limit other activities that require you to concentrate or focus.
C. Slowly increase your activity. Pace yourself and stop to rest whenever you are mentally or physically tired.
D. Do not drive or operate heavy machinery during the next 24 hours.
E. You must have approval from your primary care provider before returning to work or school.
F. Coaches or trainers must be notified of any head injury.

Diet: Do not eat or drink if you feel sick to your stomach. When you feel better, you can eat or drink anything, except alcohol. You must not drink any alcoholic beverages until your primary care provider tells you it is safe to do so.

Medications: You should not take any medications, including the ones you take every day, until your primary care provider tells you it is safe to continue your medications.

INSTRUCTIONS FOR CAREGIVERS: OBSERVATION AFTER HEAD INJURY

Check the client for signs and symptoms of worsening head injury during the first 24 hours after discharge. If he or she is sleeping through mealtimes or not awakening to go to the bathroom, awaken him or her for testing.

HOW TO TEST THE CLIENT

A. Test orientation: Ask the client to tell you his or her name, where he or she is, the current month/day/year, and to tell you what your name is.
B. Test the client's strength: Ask the client to squeeze one or two of your fingers as hard as he or she can, checking both hands at the same time, and compare them. Also have the client lift one leg at a time off the bed and hold it up for a few seconds.
C. Have the client open both eyes at the same time and check his or her pupils to make sure they are the same size. (The pupil is the black round part in the center of the eye.)
D. If you are uncertain about these test results, repeat them in 5 minutes to be sure of what you see. _Call the primary care provider or go to the ED if you cannot tell what is normal or if the client's head injury worsens._

WARNING SIGNS

Call the primary care provider's office immediately or take the client to the ED if you notice any of the following:
A. The client cannot be easily awakened or sleeps constantly in between activities or tests for no apparent reason.
B. The client cannot answer orientation questions correctly or becomes confused.

(*continued*)

HEAD INJURY: MILD   (*continued*)

C. The client has new or increasing weakness in any arm or leg, or has trouble standing or walking.

D. The client becomes very restless, agitated, is acting unusual, or has any other change in behavior.

E. One pupil in an eye is larger than the other.

F. You cannot understand what the client is saying, or the client cannot understand what you have said.

G. The client complains of a severe or worsening headache.

H. The client continues to complain of nausea or begins vomiting.

I. The client has a fever over 100.9° F.

J. The client has a convulsion, or seizure, or passes out.

K. The client has clear or blood-tinged fluid leaking from the nose or ear.

If any of the previous situations occur or if you have any questions/concerns regarding any of the tests, please call the primary care provider immediately or bring the client to the ED or clinic right away.

Phone: _____

CLIENT TEACHING GUIDE

HEMORRHOIDS

PROBLEM

A hemorrhoid is an enlarged or swollen vein in the anus and rectum. You can have hemorrhoids for years but not known you have them until bleeding occurs. They may cause rectal pain, itching, or a sensation that you have not emptied completely after a BM. Hemorrhoids are often found after painless rectal bleeding with a BM. Hemorrhoids are very common.

CAUSE

Repeated pressure in the anal or rectal veins causes hemorrhoids. They are commonly seen with obesity, pregnancy, constipation, inactive lifestyle, and liver disease.

PREVENTION/CARE

A. Avoid heavy lifting.
B. Try to prevent constipation or straining.
C. Eat a high-fiber diet.
D. Drink 8 to 10 glasses of water a day.
E. Lose weight if you are overweight.
F. Exercise regularly.

TREATMENT PLAN

A. Spend less time sitting on the toilet to reduce pressure in the veins around the anus.
B. Pat with toilet paper instead of rubbing.
C. Take sitz baths or soak in a warm bathtub three or four times a day for comfort.
D. Apply cold packs or witch hazel (Tucks) compresses for symptom relief.
E. Take a stool softener two to three times a day to prevent straining with BMs.
F. A hemorrhoid treatment, such as ligation, freezing, or surgery, may need to be done for severe cases.

Activity: No restrictions are required. Bowel function improves with good physical activity.
Medications: Hemorrhoid cream or suppository containing hydrocortisone may help to relieve pain, inflammation, and itching associated with hemorrhoids. Many of these medications are available OTC.

You Have Been Prescribed the Following Stool Softener: _____

You Need to Take: _____

You Have Been Prescribed the Following Local Cream: _____

You Need to Apply: _____

You Need to Notify the Office If You Have:
A. A hard lump that develops where a hemorrhoid has been
B. Hemorrhoids that cause severe pain that is not relieved by the aforementioned treatment
C. Excessive rectal bleeding: More than a trace or streak on the toilet paper or BM. **Rectal bleeding may be an early sign of cancer.**

D. Other: _____

Phone: _____

HERPES SIMPLEX VIRUS

PROBLEM

You may experience oral or genital bumps or lesions (often painful), burning, itching, sensation of pressure, painful urination, painful lymph nodes (bumps along underwear line), or flu-like symptoms (fever, headache, muscle aches, tired feeling).

CAUSES

A. The herpes simplex virus (HSV) is spread by direct contact with the secretions of someone who has the virus.
B. Viruses cannot be cured, but the problems or symptoms caused by them can often be managed with medication.
C. It is possible for someone to have HSV and have no symptoms. The first outbreak after contact with an infected individual usually occurs within 2 to 10 days, but it may take up to 3 weeks.
D. More severe symptoms are experienced with the first outbreak of HSV. The symptoms usually peak 4 to 5 days after the onset of infection and resolve after 2 to 3 weeks without medication.
E. Medication may decrease the severity and duration of the symptoms. Recurrent outbreaks usually last 5 to 7 days.
F. The virus may be spread even when symptoms are not present. This is known as viral shedding. Medication may also decrease the time of viral shedding.
G. Often, individuals with HSV experience itching, burning, or a feeling of pressure at the site 24 to 48 hours before an outbreak. This is known as a prodrome.
H. Sexual activity should be avoided during this time because the viral shedding is occurring, which means the infection may be spread more easily.

TREATMENT PLAN

A. Avoid sexual activity when lesions are present or when you feel the prodrome.
B. Use condoms with sexual activity.
C. Limit sexual partners.
D. Do not use any creams, lotions, or powders on lesions unless instructed to do so by your healthcare provider.
E. If urination is painful, pour water over the genital area while urinating.
F. Dry affected area thoroughly.
G. If you are pregnant at any time, notify your provider of your diagnosis of herpes to allow the provider to treat you accordingly prior to delivery to prevent spreading the herpes infection to your baby.

Activity: Stress is a trigger for an outbreak. Exercise may help with keeping your stress level down.
Diet: There is no special diet.
Medications: Antiviral medications are used to suppress the virus. They do not cure it but decrease the intensity of viral outbreaks.

You Have Been Prescribed: _____

You Need to Take: _____

You Need to Notify the Office If:
A. You are unable to empty your bladder when you have an outbreak.

B. Other: _____

Phone: _____

HERPES ZOSTER OR SHINGLES

PROBLEM

Shingles is a reactivation of the viral infection of childhood known as chickenpox. **The virus is contagious for those who have not had chickenpox.**

CAUSE

Varicella-zoster virus stimulates and produces a blister-type rash, commonly seen on the chest and trunk area. The rash is commonly confined to one side of the body.

PREVENTION

There are 2 vaccines available for prevention of shingles. The Centers for Disease Control and Prevention (CDC) recommends the Recombinant Zoster Vaccine (RZV, Shingrix) as the preferred vaccine for anyone age 50 years and older; however, Zostavax is also still available if there is a shortage of the preferred vaccine. Shingrix is a 2-dose vaccine, given 2 months apart. Zostavax is a one-time vaccine.

TREATMENT PLAN

A. The shingles vaccine cannot be given if you have a rash/shingles breakout.
B. The shingles rash usually lasts 2 to 3 weeks; however, symptoms may persist beyond this period.
C. The goal is to relieve the itching.
D. Apply warm soaks of Burow's solution (generic 5% aluminum subacetate) three times a day to lesions.
E. Notify family and friends of active virus. Advise anyone who has had contact with you that you have shingles, especially pregnant women and those who have never had chickenpox.

Activity: Avoid touching the shingles. Wash your hands. Your partners should not touch the area, especially when blisters are present. Use separate bath towels.

Diet: There is no special diet for shingles.

Medications: Oral and topical medications may be prescribed to soothe the itching. Take acetaminophen (Tylenol) as needed for comfort. Antiviral medications are available to help slow down the virus if started within 48 to 72 hours after the initial outbreak. You may be prescribed medications to help with the painful sensations (neuralgia).

You Have Been Prescribed: _____

You Need to Take: _____

You Need to Notify the Office If You Have:
A. Severe pain at lesion sites
B. Any new symptoms relating to the shingles, such as excruciating pain, headaches, numbness, tingling sensation, or other symptoms
C. Any questions regarding the shingles

Phone: _____

HIV/AIDS: RESOURCES FOR CLIENTS

AIDS HEALTHCARE Foundation
http://www.aidshealth.org

A Positive Life
Features real people telling their stories
http://www.apositivelife.com

Centers for Disease Control and Prevention (CDC)
1. Provides general information on HIV
http://www.cdc.gov/hiv/default.htm
2. Provides information on the basics: living with HIV
https://www.cdc.gov/hiv/basics/livingwithhiv/index.html

HIVandHepatitis.com
Provides the latest information about coinfection with hepatitis B and hepatitis C
http://www.hivandhepatitis.com

National Association of People With AIDS
POZ AIDS Services Directory is a comprehensive guide to HIV care and services
http://directory.poz.com/napwa

Project Inform (includes Spanish resources)
Provides multiple topics, including the latest treatment options
www.projectinform.org

The AIDS InfoNet
http://www.aidsinfonet.org

The Body
The most-visited Internet site about HIV
http://www.thebody.com

The Well Project
Designed for HIV-positive women
www.thewellproject.org

Treat HIV
Provides information about your treatment options
http://www.treathiv.com

HUMAN PAPILLOMAVIRUS

PROBLEM

Human papillomavirus (HPV), also known as condyloma, or genital or venereal warts, is a sexually transmitted infection.

A. You may experience "bumps" or lesions on genitals or the perianal area. They may be raised and rough appearing or flat and smooth. They are often wart-like in appearance.

B. Lesions may appear singly or in clusters and may be small or large. They are usually soft, painless, and pale pink to grayish in color, and they may itch.

C. **It is very important to get regular Pap smears.**

D. There are several treatment options that your healthcare provider will discuss.

CAUSE

HPV is acquired by having genital contact or intercourse with someone who has the infection.

PREVENTION/TREATMENT PLAN

There is no cure for HPV, but the following may decrease the spread of HPV:

A. Do not have genital contact or intercourse without a condom when the lesions are present. Some people who have the infection never have symptoms (bumps or warts). It is possible to spread the infection even when no symptoms are present.

B. Limit sexual partners and openly discuss the need to use a condom.

C. Examine new partners for bumps or warts.

D. Ask your provider about receiving the Gardasil vaccine for preventing the HPV virus. It is available for males and females ranging from 9 to 45 years of age.

Medications:

You Have Been Prescribed: _____

You Need to Take: _____

You Need to Notify the Office If:

A. You have any new symptoms.

B. It is time for your Pap smear.

C. Other: _____

Phone: _____

INFANT NUTRITION

BREASTFEEDING

Breast milk is the best choice for feeding infants. Mothers are encouraged to breastfeed for at least 6 to 12 months. However, if you are unable to breastfeed for this length of time, breastfeeding for the first few weeks is highly beneficial to the newborn. If breastfeeding, you should consult with your practitioner prior to taking any medications.

Advantages of Breastfeeding
A. It allows increased contact with your baby.
B. Breast milk is digested more easily by infants than baby formula.
C. Breast milk causes fewer spit ups and stomach problems than formula.
D. There is no preparation; it is ready to feed anytime; it is always in the correct temperature.
E. It is inexpensive.
F. Babies who are breastfed have fewer allergies in childhood.
G. Antibodies in the mother's breast milk protect the newborn against infections.
H. It prevents overfeeding. Breastfed babies usually feed "on demand."

General Guidelines for Breastfeeding
A. You should breastfeed your baby when he or she is hungry. It is recommended to breastfeed your baby every 2 to 4 hours, which is approximately 8 to 12 times in a 24-hour period, during the first few days of life.
B. Babies may go through a "growth spurt" on day 3 or 4 after birth. Your baby may want to feed more frequently, every 1 to 2 hours during growth spurts.
C. After the baby is 1 to 2 weeks old, he or she will develop a routine pattern of eating every 2 to 4 hours during waking hours and possibly every 4 to 5 hours at nighttime.
D. Length of time feeding your baby at each feeding should last until the baby is full. Signs of fullness from your baby may include turning away from the breast, no longer feeding, or falling asleep.
E. It is not recommended to feed your baby water or formula in addition to breastfeeding. Some women may choose to occasionally add a supplement with formula. A soy-based formula is usually tolerated best by the baby.
F. The diet of a breastfeeding mother requires increased nutrition: 500 kilocalories above the normal diet and increased fluids are recommended.
  1. Mother's diet should exclude caffeine, chocolate, cabbage, beans, and other gas-forming foods. Alcohol and tobacco should also be avoided.
G. **Fluoride**
  1. When your child is fed solely breast milk, you should consider adding a vitamin and fluoride supplement.
  2. Fluoride supplementation may also be needed for babies who live in an area where the water is low in fluoride.
  3. Fluoride is important for prevention of dental caries.
  4. Even though your baby does not have any teeth, he or she still needs fluoride for building the developing teeth.
  5. Consult with your practitioner regarding this supplementation.
H. All medications and supplements should be avoided by the mother when breastfeeding. If these medications are necessary, please check with your healthcare provider to make sure the medication or supplement is safe while breastfeeding.

BOTTLE FEEDING

If breastfeeding is not an option, nutritional formulas are available. Ask your practitioner which is best suited for your baby.
A. It is best to have 6 to 8 bottles and 6 to 10 nipples prepared.
B. Formula may be purchased in powder, concentrate, or ready-to-feed forms.
C. Please read the can and be aware of the proper mixing method for each type of formula.
D. When feeding your baby, make sure the nipple is full of milk to avoid getting excess air in the baby's stomach.
E. You should never prop bottles on blankets or other objects when feeding your baby.

(*continued*)

CLIENT TEACHING GUIDE

INFANT NUTRITION (*continued*)

ROUTINE SCHEDULE OF FEEDING

A. Newborn
   1. Give a newborn baby 1 to 2 oz of formula every 3 to 4 hours
   2. Increase formula by 1 oz as tolerated by the baby
   3. Give similar amounts at each feeding. The approximate total amount of formula your baby should take per day is determined by his or her weight (see table).
   4. If your baby seems dissatisfied with feedings, you may add 1/2 to 1 more ounce of formula. Be careful not to add more than this at a time, because overfeeding may cause the baby to have a "bellyache" or diarrhea.
   5. By 4 months of age, babies usually take 32 oz of formula per day. At this time, solid foods (e.g., baby cereal) are introduced.

SOLIDS

A. Solid foods are generally introduced to the baby at approximately 4 months.
   1. You may introduce new solid baby food every 3 to 5 days as tolerated by your baby.
   2. It is necessary to use this 3- to 5-day span between foods in case your baby is allergic or does not tolerate a specific food.
   3. If you have waited after trying a new food, you will be able to determine which food your baby was not able to tolerate.
B. Begin with rice infant cereal mixed with breast milk or formula.
C. Begin with 1 tablespoon. You may increase the amount to 2 to 5 tablespoons one to two times a day as tolerated by the baby.
D. Next, introduce fruits followed later by vegetables, increasing the amount as tolerated:
   1. If your baby does not like one vegetable, wait a few weeks to try to introduce it again.
   2. Some babies may be very finicky regarding the texture of solid food. Do not give up! One day the baby may accept the foods he or she used to spit out because of taste or texture.
E. Meats are usually the last food introduced and many babies do not like the texture; however, you should continue to offer them.
F. Juices are usually introduced last, at approximately 6 months.

COW'S MILK

A. It is not recommended to feed cow's milk to a baby during the first year of life.
B. Cow's milk may be introduced after your baby turns 1 year old.

HONEY

Honey is not recommended during a baby's first year of life because of the risk of infant botulism.

NUTRITIONAL INFORMATION

Beechnut Nutrition: 800-BEECH NUT or 1-800-233-2468 or www.beechnut.com
La Leche League Helpline: 800-LALECHE or 1-800-525-3243 or www.llli.org

TOTAL FORMULA NEEDS PER INFANT WEIGHT	
Infant Weight (Pounds)	**Total Infant Formula Per Day (Ounces Per Day in Divided Feedings)**
7	19
8	21
9	24
10	27
11	30

INFLUENZA (FLU)

PROBLEM

Influenza (flu) is an acute, self-limiting, febrile illness of the respiratory tract. You are contagious for 24 to 48 hours before feeling symptoms, and you are contagious up to 7 days after symptoms begin. Coughing and sneezing spread the flu.

CAUSE

There are many flu viruses. Stress, excessive fatigue, poor nutrition, recent illness, crowded places, and immunosuppression from drugs or illness lower your resistance to these viruses.

PREVENTION/CARE

A. Although the flu vaccine neither prevents nor causes the flu. The flu vaccine is recommended for almost everyone.
B. The flu vaccine should be taken yearly (in the fall) if you are at high risk:
1. Healthcare worker
2. Immunocompromised (transplant clients, HIV-positive clients, etc.)
3. Pregnant (after the first trimester)
4. Elderly (older than 65 years)
5. A child with severe asthma
C. Avoid unnecessary contact with sick persons, including in crowded areas.
D. To keep the flu from spreading:
1. Cover your mouth when coughing or sneezing.
2. Use tissues when you blow your nose. Dispose of them and then wash your hands.
3. If no tissue is available, do the "elbow sneeze" into the bend of your arm (away from your open hands).
4. Do not share drinking glasses.
5. Wash your hands with soap and water or use hand sanitizer.

TREATMENT PLAN

A. Rest.
B. Drink lots of fluids.
C. Run a cool-mist vaporizer.
D. Take tepid sponge baths in warm water to prevent chilling and shivering.
E. Gargle with warm salt water for a sore throat.
F. Use warm compresses or a heating pad on low for aching muscles.

Activity: Stay in bed for at least 24 hours after your fever is gone.
Diet: You may not be hungry, but you do not need to be on a special diet for the flu. Drink plenty of liquids (at least 10 glasses a day).

MEDICATIONS:

A. **Antibiotics do not help the flu because it is a virus.**
B. Do not use aspirin for a child because of the risk of Reye's syndrome.
C. Special medications shorten the flu. They must be started within 2 days of contracting the flu.

You Have Been Prescribed for Your Fever: _____

You Need to Take: _____

You Have Been Prescribed for Your Respiratory Symptoms: _____

You Need to Take: _____

(*continued*)

INFLUENZA (FLU)   *(continued)*

The American College of Chest Physicians Clinical Practice Guidelines recommend that cough suppressants and over-the-counter (OTC) cough medicine not be given to young children. Cough medicine should not be given to children younger than 4 years of age.

You Have Been Prescribed for Your Respiratory (Cough Suppressant) Symptoms: _____

You Need to Take: _____

You Need to Notify the Office If You Have:
A. Thick, green nasal drainage
B. Ear pain
C. Increase in fever or cough
D. Shortness of breath (SOB) or chest pain
E. Blood in your sputum
F. Neck pain or stiffness
G. New or unexplained symptoms

H. Other: _____

Phone: _____

INSECT BITES AND STINGS

PROBLEM

Skin changes and insect bites or stings that cause other reactions.

A. **Seek immediate help if you or a family member has any symptoms of allergic reaction or anaphylaxis, either immediately after the bite or in 8 to 12 hours after the bite.**

B. You may need to call 911 or your local emergency response service.

C. If you have had a previous life-threatening allergic reaction, carry an anaphylaxis kit for emergency treatment.

    1. *Local skin reactions* include red bumps on the skin that usually appear within minutes after the bite or sting, but may not appear for 6 to 12 hours. Itching and discomfort may occur at the site.

    2. *Systemic (body) reactions* include nausea or vomiting; headache, fever, dizziness, or light-headedness; swelling; or convulsions.

    3. *Allergic reactions* include itchy eyes, facial flushing, dry cough, wheezing, or chest or throat constriction or tightness.

CAUSE

Bites or stings can be caused by mosquitoes, fleas, chiggers, bedbugs, ants, spiders, bees, scorpions, and other insects. Risk increases with exposure to areas with heavy insect infestation, warm weather in spring and summer, lack of protective measures, use of perfumes or colognes, and previous sensitization.

PREVENTION/CARE

A. **Institute first-aid measures and activate emergency services if severe, life-threatening reactions occur.**

B. Avoid risk factors.

C. Wear protective clothing.

D. Use insect repellents with diethyltoluamide (DEET), avoiding the head, face, eyes, and mouth, especially with children.

E. Products containing DEET are not recommended for children under the age of 2 years.

Specific Insect Care

A. For all stingers: Remove stinger.

B. Bee, wasp, yellow jacket, or hornet stings: Rub a paste of meat tenderizer and water into the site.

C. Ant bites: Rub bite with ammonia, and repeat as often as necessary.

D. Spider and scorpion bites: Capture the arachnid if possible and seek medical attention.

E. Mites: Apply a petroleum product (Vaseline) until the insect withdraws from the skin.

F. Ticks: Remove the tick by following the instructions in Section II: Procedures "Tick Removal."

General Care for All Bites

A. Clean wound with soap and water.

B. Apply ice pack (no ice directly on skin; use towel or cloth to protect skin).

C. Elevate and rest the affected body part.

D. Immerse affected part or apply warm-water soaks to site. However, if site itches, cool water feels best.

E. For minor discomfort, you may use nonprescription oral antihistamines (Benadryl) or topical steroid preparations (hydrocortisone cream).

F. Use only low-potency topical steroid products without fluorine on the face and groin area.

G. You may be prescribed more potent, prescription medications.

TREATMENT PLAN

Activity: No restrictions

Diet: Eat a regular diet. Maintain adequate hydration with 8 to 10 glasses of water per day.

Medications: You may be prescribed an EpiPen to use for future major reactions. You need to keep this with you at all times.

(*continued*)

INSECT BITES AND STINGS   (*continued*)

You Have Been Prescribed: _____

You Need to Take: _____

You Need to Notify the Office If:

A. Self-care treatment does not relieve symptoms or if no improvement is noticed after 2 to 3 days.

B. A bitten area becomes red, swollen, warm, and tender to the touch; these symptoms indicate infection.

C. You have a temperature higher than or equal to 101°F.

D. You have a reaction or cannot tolerate any of the prescribed medications.

Phone: _____

INSULIN THERAPY DURING PREGNANCY

You Have Been Prescribed Insulin Therapy:

A. Your insulin needs may change weekly because of the change in your hormones (you become more insulin resistant as your pregnancy progresses).

B. Insulin therapy is safe for your baby. Insulin does not cross the placenta like the sugar does.

C. The insulin lowers your blood sugar and therefore controls the amount of sugar that goes to your baby.

D. You may have been prescribed Humulin insulin, which works very much like your own body's insulin.

E. Some of the insulin therapies have a mix of short-term regular (clear) insulin with intermediate-acting (cloudy) insulin.

   1. You will be instructed in how to mix and give yourself your insulin.

   2. The first key to insulin therapy is to be able to recognize signs of too much and too little insulin. A chart is included to post on your refrigerator (see the following table).

   3. The second key is to let people know you are on insulin.

   4. You need a Medical Alert bracelet or necklace as well as information to put in your car and billfold.

   5. The third key is to have your baby and yourself evaluated more often when on insulin therapy.

      a. You need to be seen twice a week from 32 weeks' gestation to delivery, or as recommended by your healthcare provider.

      b. You will have extra testing to make sure the baby is doing well and to make sure you are doing well, too.

F. You need to check your blood sugars four times a day. Your blood sugar target is _____

   1. Fasting _____

   2. Before lunch _____

   3. Before dinner _____

   4. Before going to bed _____

G. You will be instructed to check your urine for ketones when you are sick or if you have high blood sugar

Activity: It is important to continue to exercise.

Diet: Eat a good, healthy diet. You will be instructed on how many calories to eat. Eat six smaller meals a day; with insulin, it is important to eat snacks.

SIGNS OF HIGH AND LOW BLOOD SUGAR

Blood Sugar	What to Watch for	What to Do	Causes
HYPOGLYCEMIA Low blood sugar	Excessive sweating Feeling faint Feeling shaky Headache Impaired vision Hunger Irritable feelings Personality change Trouble awakening	**Call the healthcare provider immediately if your blood sugar is _____** Take glucose tablets or eat Do not take your insulin Do not try to force any food or liquids by mouth if client is not conscious	**Too much insulin** Not eating on time or enough food Unusual amounts of exercise
HYPERGLYCEMIA High blood sugar	Increased thirst Need to urinate more often Large amounts of sugar in your blood or urine Ketones in your urine Weakness and generalized aches Heavy, labored breathing with a fruity breath Nausea and vomiting	Test your blood sugar **Call your provider immediately if your blood sugar is _____** Test your urine for ketones Drink extra water if able to swallow	**Too little insulin** Eating more foods and foods not on your diet Infections and fever Stress

*(**continued**)*

INSULIN THERAPY DURING PREGNANCY (*continued*)

You Need to Notify the Office If:

A. You have moderate ketones in your urine.

B. You are unable to eat or you have loose diarrhea stool.

C. You have insulin reactions (blood sugar is below 50 mg/dL or you feel the symptoms of low blood sugar).

D. You have blood sugars higher than 175 mg/dL for two readings.

E. You have any signs of infection.

F. You have a decrease in fetal movement or do not feel your baby moving.

G. Other: _____

Phone: _____

IRON-DEFICIENCY ANEMIA (PREGNANCY)

PROBLEM

You have a "low blood count" called iron-deficiency anemia. Iron is needed for red blood formation.

CAUSE

This is caused by a deficiency of iron in your diet, and it is very common.

PREVENTION/CARE

Anemia may be prevented by increasing iron in your diet and by taking extra iron tablets.

TREATMENT PLAN

A. You need to increase iron-rich food in your diet.
B. You will be prescribed an iron supplement.
C. Antacids for indigestion and dairy products interfere with iron absorption. Do not take your iron supplements with milk or just before or after taking an antacid.
D. You may be eligible for the Women, Infants, and Children (WIC) program, which provides supplemental foods for pregnant women and young children. Ask your healthcare provider for information about WIC availability in your community.

Activity: You may feel more tired than usual because of anemia. You may need to rest more than usual; however, try to continue your current exercise routine as tolerated. Alternative exercise includes walking 20 minutes a day or swimming.
Diet: You need to increase the amount of iron in your diet. Generally, the redder the meat and the greener the vegetable, the richer it is as a source of iron. You also need to make sure you have adequate intake of vitamin C (this helps increase the absorption of iron into your body). Vitamin C is found in fresh, dark-green vegetables and citrus fruits. Drink 8 to 10 glasses of liquids every day.
Medications:

You Have Been Prescribed: _____

You Need to Take: _____

Special Instructions About Iron Supplements:
A. Take the iron medication as prescribed; higher doses are not better. You may need to take the medication for a longer time. High doses of iron can be toxic to children and adults.
B. Your body only absorbs a small portion of the iron pills you take.
C. You may notice green or black bowel movements. This is normal.
D. It is best to take the iron pills on an empty stomach.
E. Try taking your iron pill with a glass of orange juice. The vitamin C in the juice helps the iron be absorbed better.
F. You may have nausea or vomiting when you take iron pills, especially during early pregnancy. If this happens, try taking the pill with food. It is better to take your iron with food than to skip your pill altogether.
G. If you are not able to tolerate the iron in the morning, try taking it in the middle of the afternoon or at bedtime.
H. You may become constipated while taking iron pills. Increase your intake of fruits, vegetables, and water to avoid constipation.
You Need to Notify the Office If You:
A. Have nausea and vomiting while taking the iron supplement even after following the special instructions
B. Become extremely constipated even after increasing the fiber and liquids in your diet

C. Other: _____

Phone: _____

IRRITABLE BOWEL SYNDROME

PROBLEM

Irritable bowel syndrome (IBS) is a chronic condition of the GI system that causes abdominal pain and change in bowel habits. You may have diarrhea, you may have constipation, or you may have problems with alternating constipation and diarrhea.

CAUSE

IBS is **not contagious,** inherited, or cancerous. It has no known direct cause, but it flares with severe stress and may also be triggered by eating.

PREVENTION/CARE

A. Try to reduce stress or modify your response to it. Keep a stress diary to avoid stress triggers.
B. Good food habits also help.
C. No specific food has been identified as responsible for all IBS symptoms. Keep a food diary to identify and avoid your food triggers.

TREATMENT PLAN

A. Quit smoking: nicotine may contribute to the problem.
B. Apply a warm heat compress to your abdomen for comfort.

Activity: Exercise, such as walking 20 minutes a day, improves bowel function and helps reduce stress. Other stress-reduction techniques include self-hypnosis and biofeedback.

Diet:
A. Eat a high-fiber diet. Fiber is good for both diarrhea and constipation.
B. Avoid sorbitol-containing (sugar-free) candies and gum as well as lactose-containing milk products to see if this eases your diarrhea symptoms.
C. Do not eat or drink anything that aggravates your symptoms such as the following:
   1. Coffee may be a major food trigger.
   2. Avoid spicy and gas-producing foods.
   3. Avoid large meals, but eat regularly.
   4. Limit alcohol.

Medications: Your provider may prescribe medications to help relieve symptoms of IBS. These medications do not cure the condition. The choice of the medications depends on the nature and severity of your symptoms.

You Have Been Prescribed: _____

You Need to Take: _____

You Need to Notify the Office If You Have:
A. Fever
B. Black or tarry-looking BMs
C. Vomiting
D. Unexplained weight loss of 5 pounds or more
E. Symptoms that do not improve despite changes in diet, exercise, and medication

F. Other: _____

Phone: _____

JAUNDICE AND HEPATITIS

PROBLEM

Jaundice is a yellow tinge of the skin or mucous membranes that line the mouth and other body cavities. Jaundice is a symptom, not a disease. It occurs when the blood contains too much bilirubin—a yellow pigment found in bile, which is a fluid secreted by the liver.

When the liver is damaged, bilirubin builds up in the body and skin, turning the skin yellow and itchy. Other symptoms that occur with jaundice are dark urine, light-colored BMs, fatigue, fever, chills, appetite loss, nausea, and vomiting.

Hepatitis is the inflammation of the liver. There are several causes of hepatitis. Viral infections such as Hepatitis A, B, C, D, or E are the most common causes of hepatitis. Other causes include certain medications, alcohol, and an autoimmune condition or a disorder that affects your immunity.

CAUSE

Jaundice usually comes from a liver disorder such as cirrhosis, hepatitis, or a disease of the gallbladder or pancreas. However, it can also be a symptom of other disorders such as anemia or severe heart failure. Sometimes jaundice results from taking a drug that damages the liver.

PREVENTION/CARE

Although hepatitis is considered contagious, you do not need to be confined to your home. However, to help prevent the spread of hepatitis:
A. There are vaccinations for hepatitis A and for hepatitis B. There is no vaccination for hepatitis C. The hepatitis B vaccination is recommended for all infants. It is recommended that babies get the first hepatitis B shot before leaving the hospital.
B. Do not prepare or handle food for others until cleared by your healthcare provider.
C. Wash your hands well after using the toilet and changing diapers.
D. If you have hepatitis A, B, or C avoid intimate sexual contact until cleared by your healthcare provider. Discuss safe sex practices with your healthcare provider.
E. If you have hepatitis B or C, do not share razors, toothbrushes, and other personal items.
F. Never donate blood after a hepatitis B or C infection.
G. Your family and sexual partners may need an injection of immune globulin or a vaccination, depending on the type of hepatitis you have.
H. School exposure to hepatitis A does not generally pose a risk to others.
I. Risk of hepatitis B transmission in day-care centers appears to be extremely rare.
J. If you become pregnant, inform your provider if you are positive for hepatitis or at risk for getting hepatitis. Hepatitis can be transmitted from the mother to the baby during the birth process.

TREATMENT PLAN

Treatment for jaundice includes the following:
A. Use good hygiene with bathing, using the bathroom, and handwashing.
B. Apply anti-itch lotions such as calamine.
C. Rest, drink plenty of fluids and eat healthy diet.
D. Review all of the medications, OTC medications, and herbal products that you are taking. Your medications may need to be stopped or have their dose strength changed. Never start any new medications or supplements without consulting your provider.
E. Surgery may be required to remove a gallstone or to have a procedure called lithotripsy to crush it, if a stone blocking the bile duct is causing jaundice.
F. If you have hepatitis, you may need to be referred to a specialist.
G. The public health department will be notified by your healthcare provider for acute hepatitis.
H. Your healthcare provider may discuss the need for a liver biopsy.

(*continued*)

JAUNDICE AND HEPATITIS   (*continued*)

I. Your healthcare provider may discuss treatment to help treat a virus that is causing hepatitis. It is important that you keep all your follow-up appointments with your provider.

J. Avoid alcohol

Activity: Plan rest periods throughout the day. Avoid strenuous exercise. Gradually resume activities and mild exercise during the time you are getting better. You may get extra teaching about ways to protect yourself and others while having sex to prevent giving hepatitis to your partners.

Diet: Eat small, frequent, low-fat, high-calorie meals. You may be instructed to limit protein during acute phases of some types of hepatitis. Sit down to eat to decrease pressure on your liver. Drink 8 to 10 glasses of liquids a day.

Medications: There are several medications to treat hepatitis. Treatment depends on the type of hepatitis. It is important that you take all your medications as prescribed by your healthcare provider.

You Have Been Prescribed: _____

You Need to Take: _____

You Have Been Prescribed: _____

You Need to Take: _____

You Need to Notify the Office If You Have:

A. Mild confusion

B. Personality changes

C. Worsening symptoms

D. Tremors

E. Other: _____

Phone: _____

RESOURCES

Centers for Disease Control and Prevention: www.cdc.gov/hepatitis

Hepatitis B information is available from the Hepatitis B Foundation: www.hepb.org

Hepatitis C information is available from the American Liver Foundation: www.liverfoundation.org

KIDNEY DISEASE: CHRONIC

PROBLEM

Chronic kidney disease (CKD) means that the kidney is having trouble performing its normal function to maintain health.

Functions of a Normal Kidney

The kidney has several functions:

A. Removal and absorption of fluids to maintain balance
B. Filtration of blood to remove waste products
C. Regulation of blood pressure (BP)
D. Hormone regulation for blood production in the bone marrow
E. Regulation of hormones and minerals
F. Maintenance of healthy bones

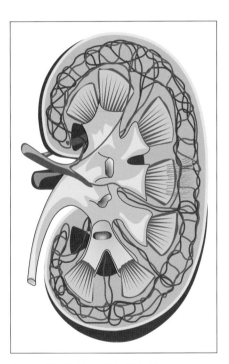

Source: Adapted from Piotr Michal Jaworski.

CAUSE

CKD has multiple causes.

A. Diabetes is the leading cause of CKD in the United States.
B. Hypertension is the second leading cause of CKD in the United States.
C. Other causes of CKD:
    1. Glomerulonephritis
    2. Genetics (inherited) disease: Polycystic kidney disease and Alport's syndrome
    3. Congenital diseases
    4. Autoimmune disease
    5. UTIs
    6. Drugs (legal and illegal) and toxic substances

(*continued*)

KIDNEY DISEASE: CHRONIC (*continued*)

DETECTION

CKD can be detected by:
A. Blood tests: Blood urea nitrogen (BUN) and creatinine
B. Urinalysis (protein in urine and creatinine clearance)
C. Other (ultrasound, immunoassays, CT scan, biopsies, etc.)
D. Glomerular filtration rate (GFR)
    1. Normal rate: 90 or higher without protein in the urine
    2. Gets lower with age
    3. An indicator on the function of the kidney
    4. Used to determine CKD stages
    5. Is lower as the kidney function worsens

STAGES OF CKD

Stage I (with protein in the urine)	GFR: 90 or higher
Stage II (mild)	60–89
Stage III (moderate)	30–59
Stage IV (severe)	15–29
Stage V (kidney failure)	14 or less

GFR, glomerular filtration rate.

SYMPTOMS OF CKD

Symptoms can vary.
A. Usually unnoticed
B. More noticeable symptoms as CKD worsens (usually around Stage III)
C. It can include:
    1. Nausea
    2. Fatigue/weakness, no energy
    3. Decreased or lack of appetite
    4. Weight loss or rapid weight gain
    5. Shortness of breath, which may worsen with activity or at rest (when awakening in the morning)
    6. Swelling of the legs and feet, around the eyes
    7. Cloudy mind or difficulty concentrating
    8. Muscle cramps
    9. Frequent nighttime urination
    10. Difficulty sleeping or staying asleep

PROBLEMS CAUSED BY CKD

CKD can cause multiple problems.
A. Heart, including heart failure and blood vessel dysfunction:
    1. High BP
    2. Cholesterol abnormalities
    3. Heart attack
    4. Stroke
B. Poor nutritional status
C. Weak and unhealthy bones
D. Anemia
E. Water retention
F. Progression to kidney failure

(*continued*)

KIDNEY DISEASE: CHRONIC (*continued*)

LIFESTYLE CHANGES TO PREVENT PROGRESSION OF CKD

Ways you may slow down the progression of CKD and cope with other effects of CKD:

A. Take charge and be proactive:
   1. Be familiar with the healthcare team.
   2. Provide information on beliefs and practices relating to health.
   3. Inform the healthcare team about herbs and other alternative medicine being used.
   4. Be involved in the treatment plan.

B. Diet:
   1. Meet with a registered dietitian.
   2. Eat a well-balanced meal.
   3. Some dietary restrictions may be necessary based on kidney function and stages of CKD.
   4. Follow dietary instructions regarding protein, fats, sodium, and minerals.
      a. Dietary intake of protein is usually restricted to 0.8 to 1.0 g/kg per day.
      b. Dietary sodium should be restricted to no more than 2 g daily.
      c. Potassium should be restricted to 40 to 70 meq/d.
      d. Calories should be restricted to 35 kcal/kg/d; if the body weight is greater than 120% of normal weight or the client is older than 60 years of age, a lower amount may be prescribed.
      e. Fat intake should be about 30% to 40% of total daily caloric intake.
      f. Phosphorus should be restricted to 600 to 800 mg/d.
      g. Calcium should be restricted to 1,400 to 1,600 mg/d.
      h. Magnesium should be restricted to 200 to 300 mg/d.
      i. Carbohydrates: The recommended normal intake is 225 to 358 g/d.

C. Exercise:
   1. Moderate exercise is recommended for at least 30 minutes, five times a week.
   2. The benefits of exercise:
      a. Lowers BP
      b. Improves cholesterol
      c. Lowers hemoglobin A1c (HgA1c) in diabetes
      d. Strengthens bones
      e. Leads to weight loss
      f. Improves signs/symptoms of depression
      g. Boosts the immune system
      h. Reduces stress
      i. Provides an overall better feeling

D. Target heart and blood vessels:
   1. Control BP; goal is less than 130/80 mmHg.
   2. Lower your low-density lipoprotein.
   3. Weight loss.
   4. Lower HgA1c level with the goal of less than 6.9% if you have diabetes.
      a. Exercise.
      b. Diet: No restriction, low-saturated-fat, low-carbohydrate diet.
      c. Smoking cessation is essential.
      d. Reduce or eliminate alcohol intake.
      e. Medications may be necessary for the following:
         i. Hypertension: BP medications.
         ii. Hyperlipidemia: Cholesterol medications.
         iii. Diabetes: Medications to control the blood sugar.

E. Target bones:
   1. Be familiar with your lab results (vitamin D level, calcium level, phosphorus level).
   2. Supplements: Vitamin D, calcium supplements, and phosphate binders may be necessary.

(*continued*)

KIDNEY DISEASE: CHRONIC   *(continued)*

3. Low phosphorous diet may be necessary.
4. Exercise: Weight-bearing exercise will help strengthen bones (walking, dancing, lifting weights, etc.).

F. Target anemia:
1. Goal of the hemoglobin should be 11 g/dL or better.
2. Diet rich in iron
3. Medication may be necessary (depends on the type of anemia):
   a. Erythropoeitin-stimulating agents
   b. Vitamin B12
   c. Folic acid
   d. Iron

G. Target water retention:
1. Limit salt intake.
2. Diet (avoid processed foods/fast foods).
3. Medications may be needed (diuretics).

FOODS HIGH IN PHOSPHORUS

Below is a list of foods with the estimated amount of phosphorus in each food. Limit portions (consultation with registered dietitian is recommended).

Biscuits (mix) 1 (1 oz): 133 mg	Cheese (1 oz): 161 mg
Chocolate 1 bar (2 oz): 137 mg	Cola 1 can (12 oz): 60 mg
Cream soups (1 cup): 151 mg	Dried beans and peas (1 cup cooked): 206 mg
Hot dogs and sausage (2 each): 162/220 mg	Ice cream (1 cup): 157 mg
Liver and organ meats (3.5 oz): 400 mg	Macaroni and cheese (1 oz): 265 mg
Pancake mix 3 (4-inch pancakes): 368 mg	Peanut butter (3 tbsp): 172 mg
Pizza (1 slice): 259 mg	Pork and beans (1 cup): 266 mg
Yogurt (8 fl. oz) and pudding (1/2 cup): 292/280 mg	

POTASSIUM-FRIENDLY FOODS

Limit portion to half cup unless noted otherwise (consultation with registered dietitian is recommended).

Fruits	
Apple (1 small)	Canned pear
Cherries	Grapes (15 small)
Juices (apple, cranberry, grape, lemon, nectar, pear, peach, and pineapple)	Lemon (1/2)
Peach (1/2 cup canned or 1 small fresh)	Pineapple
Plum (1/2 cup canned or 1 medium)	Raspberries (blueberries, blackberries, and cranberries)
Strawberries	Watermelon (1 cup)
Vegetables	
Cabbage	Carrots (1/2 cup cooked or 1 small raw)
Celery (1 stalk)	Corn (1/2 canned or ear)
Cucumbers	Eggplant
Green (or wax) beans	Green peas
Lettuce (1 cup)	Onion
Radishes	Squash (Crookneck, Summer, and zucchini)

(continued)

KIDNEY DISEASE: CHRONIC (*continued*)

RESOURCES

A. BC Renal Agency: www.bcrenalagency.ca
   1. Shopping guide for kidney health: http://www.bcrenalagency.ca/sites/default/files/documents/files/Shopping_Guide_For_Kidney_Health_WEB_Dec_11.pdf
B. National Kidney Foundation: www.kidney.org
   1. Kidney Kitchen recipes: https://www.kidney.org/search-results?solr-keywords=kidney+recipes
C. American Diabetes Association: www.diabetes.org
   1. Food and Fitness: www.diabetes.org/food-and-fitness/?loc=GlobalNavFF

KNEE EXERCISES

CARE FOR YOUR KNEE

Please follow the type of exercises recommended for your knee. You may begin straight-leg raises after the pain resolves. Continue to wear your brace with activities as directed. It may take months for your knee to completely heal. You may gradually resume normal activity as directed by your provider. If you are not sure what activities you may perform, ask your provider before performing the activity.

A. Quad sets:
 1. Exercise may be done while standing, sitting, or lying down.
 2. Straighten knee with intensity.
 3. Hold for 10 counts, then relax.
 4. Repeat the exercise three to four times per day.
 5. If a cast or splint is in place, straighten the knee until the front of the thigh and the cast pinch together.
 6. If the knee is bent, keep the foot planted and use the floor to push against.

B. Co-contractions:
 1. Similar to quads, but the difference is to tighten the entire thigh while straightening the knee.
 2. Hold for 10 counts, then relax.
 3. Repeat the exercise approximately three to four times a day.

C. Hamstring sets:
 1. Pull the leg back against the other foot, floor, or cast.
 2. Hold approximately 10 counts, then relax.
 3. Perform these sets three to four times a day.

D. Heel lifts:
 1. Lie on back with support under the knee.
 2. Lift the heel while resting the knee on support.
 3. Make the knee as straight as possible.
 4. Hold for 10 counts, then relax.
 5. Do not use weights.
 6. Perform these exercises three to four times a day.

E. Straight-leg raises:
 1. Straighten the knee.
 2. Lift and pause for 5 to 10 counts, then relax.
 3. Lower leg and relax, then repeat.
 4. Do three to five sets, three to four times a day. Rest between each set.
 5. Start with _____ pounds of ankle weight and work up to _____ pounds.
 6. Gradually increase weight used.

F. Hip flexors:
 1. While sitting, lift the knee toward the chest.
 2. Hold for 10 counts, then relax.
 3. Lower the leg and relax. Repeat.
 4. Do 10 times, three to four times a day.
 5. Start with _____ pounds of weight and work up gradually to _____ pounds.
 6. The weights should be on the knee or ankle.

G. Hamstring stretches:
 1. While seated on a sturdy table with the foot of your injured leg resting on the floor, lean forward with chin directed toward the toes.
 2. Hold for at least 10 counts, then relax.
 3. The knee should be straight from your hips.
 4. **Do not do this exercise with bouncing or violent movements.**
 5. Do _____ minutes, _____ times a day.

LACTOSE INTOLERANCE AND MALABSORPTION

PROBLEM

You have been diagnosed as having difficulty digesting milk (lactose) products or having problems with absorption. Lactose intolerance can cause gas, bloating, abdominal cramps, diarrhea, and nausea or vomiting. You may be able to eat small portions without problems or be unable to tolerate any foods containing lactose.

CAUSE

Lactose is the sugar present in milk and body makes an enzyme to break down lactose. In people with lactose intolerance, body does not make enough of the enzyme or the enzyme does not work well. Lactose intolerance is very common; it occurs when the body is not able to appropriately digest this milk sugar content and results in diarrhea.

PREVENTION/CARE

Follow a lactose-free or lactose-controlled diet.

TREATMENT PLAN

Activity: No restrictions are required. Resume normal activities as soon as diarrhea symptoms improve. You may be sent to see a registered dietitian to assist in your dietary plan.

Diet:
A. Limit or stop eating foods that contain milk, lactose, whey, or casein.
B. Lactose-controlled diets allow up to 1 cup of milk per day for cooking or drinking, if you can tolerate it.
C. If you cannot tolerate any lactose, choose lactose-free foods with lactate, lactic acid, lactalbumin, whey protein, sodium caseinate, casein hydrolysates, and calcium compounds. Read labels carefully.
D. You may also choose kosher foods marked "pareve" or "parve," which do not contain lactose. Read labels carefully.
E. A low-fat diet is important if you have fat malabsorption.
F. To help with diarrhea caused by malabsorption, avoid more than one serving a day of caffeine-containing drinks.
G. Beverages with high sugar content, such as soft drinks and fruit juices, may increase diarrhea. Juices and fruits with high amounts of fructose include apples, pears, sweet cherries, prunes, and dates.
H. Sorbitol-containing candies and gums may cause diarrhea.

Medications: You may need the enzyme lactase to help you digest your food. You may need vitamins and minerals if you are having problems with malabsorption/diarrhea.

You Have Been Prescribed: _____

You Need to Take: _____

You Need to Notify the Office If You Have:
A. Severe abdominal pain
B. Diarrhea causing dehydration

C. Other: _____

Phone: _____

LICE (PEDICULOSIS)

PROBLEM

A parasite called a louse has been found on your body or hair. Lice tend to live on the scalp, eyebrows, or genital area, or in warm, moist areas of your skin. You may notice you have intense itching, swelling, or reddened areas of the skin, and sometimes even enlarged lymph glands.

CAUSE

The lice bite the skin, which causes the intense itching. Lice and their eggs (called nits) may be difficult to see on the skin and shafts of hair. Lice look like small, 2- to 3-mm, tan-colored bugs. The eggs are tiny white eggs that stick to the hair shaft.

PREVENTION

You can prevent repeated episodes of lice if you bathe daily; avoid crowded living conditions; change the bed linens frequently; do not share hats, combs, brushes, or other belongings. When your children or other family members have been in contact with others diagnosed with lice, check family members closely for lice and treat as appropriate.

TREATMENT PLAN

A. Use medicated shampoo as directed.
B. Machine wash all linens, stuffed animals, or any other items with which the lice may have come in contact.
C. Wash clothes in hot, soapy water.
D. Dry all linens in a hot dryer for at least 30 minutes.
E. Items that cannot be washed must be taken to the dry cleaner or wrapped and sealed in a plastic bag for 14 days.
F. Boil all hair accessories and clean well.
G. Do not share hats and combs.
H. Spray all furniture with appropriate products that kill all nits and lice.
I. Vacuum.

Activity: There is no activity restriction.
Diet: There is no special diet.
Medications:
A. Food and Drug Administration (FDA)-approved over-the-counter products:
1. Pyrethrins combined with piperonyl butoxide—brand names: Rid, Triple X, A-200, Pronto, R & C. Approved for children 2 years and older. Avoid if allergic to ragweed or chrysanthemums.
B. FDA approved for 2 months and older. Permethrin lotion 1%—brand name: Nix. Repeat application on day 9 of initial dose.

You Have Been Prescribed: _____

A. Treat as directed on the bottle.
B. After shampooing as directed, make sure to remove each single nit from each shaft of hair. Any nits left in the hair will hatch and start the cycle over again. Comb any dead or remaining live lice out of the hair with a fine-tooth comb.
C. Repeat in 24 hours, then again in 1 week.
D. Do not use a shampoo/conditioner or conditioner before use of the lice medications. Do not wash the hair for 1 to 2 days after lice medication treatment.

You Need to Notify the Office If You Have: _____

A. Any questions regarding the removal of the nits and lice, or if you need any assistance. If other family members need to be evaluated, please let us know. If secondary infection occurs, please call the office.
B. Precautions: Do not overuse medications or combine different head lice medications. Use only as directed. These medications are insecticides and can be dangerous if used incorrectly.

Phone: _____

LICHEN PLANUS

PROBLEM

A chronic skin eruption, lichen planus, is not cancerous or contagious. It frequently appears as small, slightly raised, itchy, purplish bumps with a whitish surface. Sudden hair loss from the head may occur. Lichen planus may involve the skin of the legs, trunk, arms, wrists, scalp, or penis; the lining of the mouth or vagina; and the nail beds of the toenails and fingernails.

CAUSE

The cause is unknown, but it may be caused by a virus. In a few cases, this may be an adverse reaction to certain drugs. The risk of developing lichen planus increases with stress, fatigue, or exposure to drugs or chemicals.

PREVENTION/CARE

Currently, there are no known preventive measures.
A. The goal of treatment is to relieve symptoms.
B. Use cool water soaks to relieve itching.
C. Reduce stress; this may help to prevent recurrences. Learn relaxation techniques or obtain counseling, if necessary.
D. Speak with your healthcare provider if you suspect a drug to be the cause.

TREATMENT PLAN

Activity: No restrictions
Diet: Eat a well-balanced diet; drink 8 to 10 glasses of water every day.
Medications:

You Have Been Prescribed: _____

You Need to Take: _____

You Need to Notify the Office If:
A. You have a reaction to any of the prescribed medications.
B. You are unable to tolerate the prescribed medications.
C. Hair loss or nail destruction occurs.
D. New lesions appear as old lesions resolve.

E. Other: _____

Phone: _____

LYME DISEASE AND REMOVAL OF A TICK

PROBLEM

Ticks are vectors for Lyme disease and Rocky Mountain spotted fever. You have been diagnosed with Lyme disease.

CAUSE

Lyme disease is caused by a spirochete from ticks.

PREVENTION/CARE

A. Avoid areas with large deer populations.
B. Wear light-colored clothes to make ticks easier to spot. Wear long sleeves and tuck pants into the socks to form a barrier.
C. Stick to hiking trails. Avoid contact with overgrown foliage. Ticks prefer dense woods with thick growth of shrubs and small trees as well as areas along the edge of the woods.
D. Check for ticks after each outdoor activity, especially in hairy regions of the body and beltline, where ticks often attach. Check for ticks before bathing, especially at the back of the neck, knees, and ears.
E. Remove ticks promptly.
F. Inspect pets daily and remove ticks when present.
G. Some manufacturers currently offer permethrin-treated clothing that is effective for up to 20 washings. **This clothing is not recommended for children.**
H. Use tick repellent with diethyltoluamide (DEET; except for small children younger than 2 years). As an alternative, picaridin and oil of eucalyptus preparations have been approved for use as repellents by the U.S. Environmental Protection Agency (EPA).

Precautions When Removing Ticks

A. Do not hold a lighted match or cigarette to the tick. Do not apply gasoline, kerosene, or oil to the tick's body.
B. Avoid squeezing the body of the tick.
C. Grasp the tick with a fine-tip tweezer close to the skin. Remove by gently pulling the tick upward straight out without using any twisting motions (see Figures III.5 and III.6).
D. In the home, if fingers are used to remove ticks, they should be protected with facial tissue or gloves and washed after removal of the tick.
E. Do not crush the tick during removal.
F. **Save the tick for identification in case you become ill. Write the date of the tick bite on paper and place the paper and the tick in a resealable baggie and place it in the freezer.**

TREATMENT PLAN

A. Antibiotics are effective against Lyme disease.
B. If you are prescribed doxycycline, avoid exposure to the sun because a rash may develop.

Activity: As tolerated.
Diet: Eat a regular diet.

MEDICATIONS:

A. Acetaminophen may be taken for body aches and any fever.
B. You may be given antibiotics for infection.

You Have Been Prescribed: _____

(continued)

LYME DISEASE AND REMOVAL OF A TICK (*continued*)

FIGURE III.5 Grasp the tick's body as close to the skin as possible using a fine-tip tweezer. Avoid squeezing the tick's body.

FIGURE III.6 Remove by pulling the tick straight upward without using twisting motions.

Source: Tick Removal (n.d.) Centers for Disease Control and Prevention. Retrieved from https://www.cdc.gov/ticks/removing_a_tick.html

You Need to Take: _____

Take all of your antibiotics even if you feel better.

You Need to Notify the Office If You Have:
1. No signs of improvement with antibiotic therapy
2. Other: _____

Phone: _____

RESOURCE

CDC Understanding Tick Bites and Lyme Disease: https://www.cdc.gov/lyme/resources/toolkit/factsheets/Hooks_Ticks-and-Lyme-Disease-508.pdf

CLIENT TEACHING GUIDE

LYMPHEDEMA

PROBLEM

Lymphedema is the backup of fluid in the lymphatic system into an arm or leg. The fluid causes severe swelling, which restricts movement and can lead to infection and, in rare cases, a form of cancer called lymphangiosarcoma.

CAUSE

Many factors can cause lymphedema. These include a diagnosis of cancer treated with radiation, surgical removal of lymph nodes, infection, and disorders from birth that affect the structure of the lymph system.

PREVENTION/CARE

A. Protect your arm or leg while recovering from cancer treatment.
   1. Avoid heavy lifting, if it involves an arm.
   2. Avoid strenuous exercise.
   3. Avoid heat on your arm or leg.
   4. Avoid tight clothing.

TREATMENT PLAN

A. Raise the affected arm or leg whenever lying down to reduce pain and swelling.
B. Wear compression stockings. Put them on before getting out of bed in the morning. Take them off just before going to bed at night.
C. Apply lotion every day to the affected area.
D. Check the affected area every day and report any skin changes to your healthcare provider, especially any cracks or cuts.
E. Follow up with your primary healthcare provider and other specialty providers on a regularly scheduled basis.

Activity:
A. Get regular exercise. Discuss with your healthcare provider what type and frequency of exercise is safe for you.
B. Exercise leg muscles by pumping ankles when sitting. Rocking in a rocking chair is another option.

Diet:
A. Discuss with your healthcare provider the type of diet that best suits your needs: Diabetic diet, low-fat diet, low-cholesterol diet, and/or low-sodium diet

Medications:

You Have Been Prescribed: _____

You Need to Take: _____

You Need to Notify the Office If You Have:
A. Fever greater than 101°F
B. Increased redness, pain, tenderness to touch, and/or warmth in affected arm or leg
C. New pain, swelling, or warmth in an arm or leg

D. Other: _____

Phone: _____

RESOURCES

National Cancer Institute: cancer.gov/cancertopics/pdq/supportivecare/lymphedema/healthprofessional/page2
National Lymphedema Network: lymphnet.org

MASTITIS

PROBLEM

You have an infection in your breast tissue, not your breast milk.

CAUSE

The most common organism causing mastitis is *Staphylococcus aureus*. The immediate source of the organism is almost always the nursing infant's nose and mouth. Mastitis often develops in the presence of breast injury, such as cracked nipples.

PREVENTION/CARE

A. Prevent injury to the breast:
   1. Avoid overdistension of the breasts; feed infant or use the breast pump frequently (every 2–4 hours).
   2. Avoid clogged milk ducts by applying moist heat to the breasts and massaging the clogged duct while nursing.
   3. Avoid cracking of nipples by proper positioning of the infant's mouth on the nipple during feeding. The baby's mouth should cover the entire areola (dark brown part of the nipple area).
   4. Read the Client Teaching Guide, "Breast Engorgement and Sore Nipples" in this section.
B. Personal hygiene measures:
   1. Avoid soap on the nipples; cleanse nipples with warm water only.
   2. Avoid decrusting the nipple of dried colostrum or milk.
   3. After a feeding, squeeze out a few drops of colostrum/milk and massage that into the nipple and areola. This "Mother Nature's breast cream", with its fat, protein, and antibody content, will help to heal any superficial cracking. Purified lanolin cream is a secondary alternative, after breastmilk, for sore, cracked nipples. It can be applied after nursing. If lanolin is purified, there is no need to remove it prior to the next feeding.
   4. Use good handwashing techniques before handling the breast and before and after breastfeeding.

TREATMENT PLAN

A. Complete course of antibiotics. Be aware that antibiotics increase risk for a vaginal yeast infection.
B. Continue breastfeeding even on the antibiotics.
C. Apply warm soaks to your breast (see the Client Teaching Guide, "Postpartum Breast Engorgement and Sore Nipples" in this section). Breast massage may be needed, too.
D. Use Tylenol or ibuprofen for pain (see the Client Teaching Guide, "Postpartum Breast Engorgement and Sore Nipples" in this section).

Activity: Increased rest is recommended. Try to lie down for a nap when the baby goes to sleep.
Diet: There are no dietary restrictions; continue your regular diet and avoid gas-producing foods that may upset your baby's tummy (cabbage, broccoli, onions, peppers, garlic, chocolate, beans, spicy foods). Increase fluid intake with elevated temperature. Drink at least 10 to 12 glasses of liquid a day. Use caffeine in moderation (eliminate if possible).
Medications: Continue your prenatal vitamins while breastfeeding.

You Have Been Prescribed: _____

You Need to Take: _____

Take all of your antibiotics even if you feel better.

You Have Been Prescribed: Dicloxacillin 500 mg to take four times daily.

You Need to Notify the Office If:
A. You have a fever that does not decrease within 2 days and resolve within 4 days of taking the antibiotics.
B. You have pain that is not controlled with acetaminophen or ibuprofen.
C. Your baby develops thrush. Notify your baby's healthcare provider for medication.

D. Other: _____

Phone: _____

CLIENT TEACHING GUIDE

MENOPAUSE

DEFINITION

Menopause is the cessation of menses (stopping of menstrual periods) for 12 consecutive months and is generally experienced in women between 45 and 55 years of age; however, for some women menopause may be earlier or later.

A. Menopause before the age of 40 years is considered premature.

B. Induced menopause is the abrupt cessation of menses related to chemical or surgical interventions (as is the case with some types of chemotherapy).

Perimenopause is the time preceding menopause and may last several years. The average age of onset is usually in a woman's 40s, but may occur earlier. Symptoms occur during this time period because of fluctuations in hormone levels. Owing to fluctuations in ovarian function, **pregnancy may still occur, and contraception is still necessary if pregnancy is not desired.**

CAUSE

Menopause can be natural or induced. Natural menopause is a normal function of aging. Surgical or chemical intervention can result in induced menopause.

SYMPTOMS

Symptom occurrence and severity vary from very mild to moderate or severe. Symptoms may include:

A. Hot flashes

B. Night sweats

C. Insomnia

D. Vaginal dryness

E. Mood lability

TREATMENT PLAN

Your care provider will work with you to develop a plan of treatment that is based on your individual symptom pattern. Inform your care provider if you have:

A. Acute liver disease

B. Cerebral vascular or coronary artery disease, myocardial infarction (MI), or stroke

C. History of or active thrombophlebitis or thromboembolic disorders

D. History of uterine or ovarian cancer

E. Known or suspected cancer of the breast

F. Known or suspected estrogen-dependent neoplasm

G. Pregnancy

H. Undiagnosed, abnormal vaginal bleeding

Activity:

A. Regular physical exercise can be beneficial for weight reduction and symptom control.

B. Dress in layers to accommodate hot flashes.

C. Regular sexual intercourse is encouraged and you may find glycerine-free, water-soluble vaginal lubricants (Good Clean Live, Slippery Stuff, Replens) helpful for vaginal dryness.

D. Be sure to use a method of **birth control** to prevent undesired pregnancy if you have had a period within 1 year.

Diet: You need to eat a well-balanced diet (three meals). Supplement your diet to achieve calcium 1,000 to 1,200 mg/d and vitamin D 600 IU/d from age 1 year until age 70 years and then 800 IU/d for 71 years and older. Alcohol, caffeine, and spicy foods may trigger hot flashes.

Medication:

You Have Been Prescribed: _____

You Need to Take/Use It: _____

(*continued*)

MENOPAUSE *(continued)*

You Need to Notify the Office If:

A. You experience unexpected vaginal bleeding.

B. Your symptoms interfere with your ability to function.

C. You are on hormone replacement therapy and you experience calf pain, chest pain, or shortness of breath; cough up blood; or have severe headaches, visual disturbances, breast pain, abdominal pain, or yellowing of the skin.

D. Other: _____

Phone: _____

MONONUCLEOSIS

PROBLEM

Mononucleosis (mono) is an acute, infectious, viral disease. Mono causes fever, sore throat, and swollen lymph glands.

CAUSE

Epstein–Barr virus causes mono and is spread to other persons by kissing, sharing food, and coughing without covering your mouth.

PREVENTION/CARE

A. Avoid contact with persons diagnosed with mono.
B. Cover your mouth and nose when you cough or sneeze to prevent the spread of infection.
C. Use tissues to blow your nose and throw them away immediately.
D. If you do not have a tissue, use the "elbow sneeze" using the bend of your arm.
E. Wash your hands or use hand sanitizer.

TREATMENT PLAN

There is no specific cure. Gargle with warm salt water for a sore throat.

Activity:
A. Mono makes you very tired; rest in bed, then gradually return to normal activity.
B. You should not do any physical activity, especially contact sports (football, soccer, basketball, etc.), unless you have been cleared by your healthcare provider.

Diet: Eat a high-calorie diet. Drink plenty of liquids (at least 8 glasses a day).

Medications:
A. Acetaminophen may be taken for body aches.
B. You may be given antibiotics for infection, if indicated.

You Have Been Prescribed: _____

You Need to Take: _____

Take all of your antibiotics even if you feel better.

You Need to Notify the Office If You Have:
A. Fever more than 102°F
B. Severe pain in the upper left abdomen (rupture of the spleen is a medical emergency)
C. Swallowing or breathing difficulty from a severe throat inflammation
D. A rash may follow the use of antibiotics.

E. Other: _____

Phone: _____

MYASTHENIA GRAVIS

PROBLEM

Myasthenia gravis or MG is a chronic disorder in which the body's immune system mistakenly attacks and destroys proteins that help muscles respond to nerve impulses. This causes people to have muscle weakness that is worse with use and better with rest.

Eye muscles and muscles that help with chewing, swallowing, and talking tend to be affected the most. MG can be treated but not cured.

People with myasthenia generally have to take medicine for the rest of their lives to control the disorder. Surgery to remove their thymus gland may be necessary.

TREATMENT PLAN/CARE

A. Wear a medic alert tag and keep a list of medicines and the dosing schedule, with you at all times along with the name and telephone number of your neurologist in case of emergency.
B. Dentists and any other healthcare providers should know that you have MG because many medicines can make your MG worse. Some examples of medicines that can be problems for people with MG are birth control pills, some antibiotics, and some local anesthetics.
C. *Never* start a new medicine without talking to your neurologist first, even if you took it in the past without having problems.
D. Any time you feel worse, particularly if you are having trouble with chewing and swallowing, you should contact your neurologist and plan to go to the hospital, because MG could possibly affect your breathing. You should have a plan for emergencies that includes how you will get to a hospital, child-care arrangements, and how to contact your neurologist.
E. An annual flu shot is recommended because infections can make MG worse.
F. Emotional upset and stress also can make MG worse. Your healthcare provider can supply you with information on handling stress effectively or assist in referring you to a counselor.
G. Surgery can make MG worse, so it should, when possible, be planned with your neurologist. Some changes in your medication schedules in the weeks before the surgery can make problems less likely.
H. Your healthcare provider may recommend a procedure similar to donating blood called plasmapheresis. This procedure is performed to remove the antibodies that make the disease process worse. Blood is removed from a vein, the antibodies are removed, and then the blood is donated back to you in another vein. This procedure may be offered to you many times because the effects are not permanent.

Activity: It is best to plan your activities to take advantage of the peak effects of your medicine and to avoid getting overtired.

Diet: A diet high in potassium-rich foods has been found by some to be helpful because low body potassium is associated with muscle weakness. Bananas, oranges, cantaloupe, prunes, and raisins are high in potassium. Vegetables that are high in potassium include peas, beans, cooked broccoli, spinach, and zucchini. Fish is also high in potassium: tuna, cod, trout, and halibut.

Medications: You may be prescribed steroids or medications that improve muscle strength.

You Have Been Prescribed: _____

You Need to Take: _____

You Need to Notify the Office If:
A. You have worsening or new symptoms.
B. You are unable to tolerate your medicines due to side effects.

(continued)

CLIENT TEACHING GUIDE

MYASTHENIA GRAVIS (*continued*)

C. Other: _____

Phone: _____

RESOURCES

Myasthenia Gravis Foundation of America, Inc.: https://www.myasthenia.org

You can build your own identification bracelets or neck chains from American Medical ID: https://www.americanmedical-id.com

NICOTINE DEPENDENCE

PROBLEM

Cigarette smoking is one of the most **preventable causes of death and disability in the United States.** Other forms of nicotine, such as chewing tobacco and pipe tobacco, hookahs, e-cigarettes can be just as harmful. Risks of lip, tongue, mouth, and throat cancer are associated with use of nicotine. Smoking may cause bleeding in pregnancy and may be responsible for the baby not growing well. It is well documented that infants and children who are exposed to long-term smoke inhalation are at increased risk of **sudden infant death syndrome** and frequent **ear infections and chronic illnesses.**

Nicotine is addictive and so stopping smoking is difficult.

CAUSE

Seeing your parents smoke and using tobacco may be one of the reasons that caused you to start using tobacco. Peer pressure is a big reason why you may have started smoking as a teenager.

REASONS TO QUIT

A. Quitting tobacco will add years to your life.
B. You will have healthier lungs, which will decrease your risk of developing cancer and having a heart attack or stroke.
C. You will also have more energy and feel better physically and mentally.
D. Smoking cessation will also decrease the secondhand smoke exposure around your family and friends, which will also make them healthier too.
E. Secondhand smoke causes asthma attacks and other health problems.
F. Some insurance plans are more expensive if you smoke.
G. You will save a lot of money by not buying cigarettes and e-cigarettes.
H. Do not quit for yourself: Quit for someone you love.
I. You will have fewer wrinkles.

TREATMENT PLAN

A. Set a quit date within 2 to 4 weeks and get information/treatment from your provider.
B. Throw away all cigarettes, matches, lighters, and ashtrays in your home, car, and workplace.
C. Make smoking very inconvenient.
D. Ask your family/friends for support and encouragement to help you stop.
E. Stay in nonsmoking environments and avoid friends/family members who smoke.
F. If you get the urge to smoke, take deep cleansing breaths and try to occupy your time with something else, like chewing gum.
G. Leave the table and change your routine to avoid old triggers such as smoking with your coffee after meals.
H. Reward yourself often for staying smoke free.
I. It is not unusual that you will go back to smoking; it is difficult to quit. Smoking even one less cigarette counts.
J. It may take several times to finally quit for good.

Activity:
A. Exercise daily to help alleviate the craving for nicotine.
B. Avoid caffeine if possible.
C. Chew gum or suck on hard candy when you crave a cigarette.
D. Eat celery sticks or carrots in place of smoking a cigarette.
E. Drink a lot of water and other fluids to keep hydrated.

(*continued*)

NICOTINE DEPENDENCE   (*continued*)

Medications:

A. Discuss options available with your healthcare provider to help you quit.

B. Medications are available to help you quit.

C. The nicotine patch, inhaler, and gum are available and may be right for you. Discuss these options with your healthcare provider because they are good steps to quitting.

D. Nonnicotine therapy such as Chantix and Zyban are also used to help quit smoking.

E. Many of the stop-smoking medicines may be covered by your insurance.

You Have Been Prescribed: _____

You Need to Take: _____

You Need to Notify the Office If You Have:

1. Severe craving and the urge to smoke or chew tobacco even on medicines
2. Feelings of impulsiveness, like you might do something you will later regret
3. Started smoking again after you have stepped down while using the nicotine patch
4. Other: _____

Phone: _____

RESOURCES

The American Cancer Society has some good tips on quitting smoking: www.cancer.org

The American Lung Association also has good guides to help stop smoking: www.lung.org

Drug-Free Workplace: 1-800-WORKPLACE (967-5752); https://www.samhsa.gov/workplace/resources/drug-free-helpline

Nicotine Anonymous 877-879-6422; http://www.nicotine-anonymous.org

CLIENT TEACHING GUIDE

NOSEBLEEDS

PROBLEM

Most nosebleeds stop on their own within 15 to 20 minutes.
If you have trouble breathing, chest pain, or feel woozy with a nosebleed, *call 911*.

CAUSES

Nosebleeds may be caused by several problems:
A. Trauma from nose picking or forcefully blowing the nose
B. Frequent colds.
C. Allergies or exposure to irritants.
D. Drugs, including over-the-counter medications such as aspirin and Pepto-Bismol, or street drugs such as snorted cocaine.
E. Breathing dry air all the time.

PREVENTION/CARE

A. Avoid picking your nose. Keep fingernails trimmed short.
B. Do not blow your nose too frequently or too hard (this may also cause eardrum tearing).
C. Blow your nose through both nostrils at the same time to equalize pressure.
D. Use a humidifier in your home.
E. Keep the inside of your nose moist and promote healing with a nasal saline spray or gel.
F. Avoid smoking and secondhand smoke.

TREATMENT PLAN

A. If you experience a nosebleed, take these steps:
　1. Sit up and lean forward.
　2. Pinch the soft area toward the bottom of your nose below the bone, hold for 15 minutes (5 minutes in children).
　3. If the bleeding continues, spray Afrin into your nostril.
　4. If the bleeding still continues, lightly soak a cotton ball with Afrin, insert it into your nose, and pinch for 15 minutes.
　5. If the bleeding continues, seek medical care.
　6. If the bleeding stops, use nasal saline spray and gel to keep the area moist and promote healing. Avoid picking your nose or hard nose-blowing.
B. Gently blowing your nose also decreases or stops a nosebleed.

Activity: Avoid or limit the following activities for 3 to 5 days after a nosebleed:
A. Heavy lifting
B. Straining
C. Bending over from the waist
D. Very hot showers
Diet: Avoid hot, spicy foods for 3 to 5 days after a nosebleed.
Medications: Avoid medications that increase bleeding, such as aspirin and Pepto-Bismol.

You Have Been Prescribed: _____

You Need to Take: _____

You Need to Notify the Office If:
A. Bleeding does not stop with pressure or nasal spray applied to the bleeding site.
B. You keep having nosebleeds (more than two in a week or four in a month).

C. Other: _____

Phone: _____

ORAL THRUSH IN CHILDREN

PROBLEM

Oral thrush is a white patch that coats the inside of the mouth and tongue. It mainly affects bottle-fed infants, although breastfed infants and debilitated older children may also be affected.

CAUSE

Thrush is caused by a yeast called *Candida* that grows rapidly on the lining of the mouth in areas abraded by prolonged sucking. It may also occur after a course of antibiotic medication.

PREVENTION/CARE

A. Do not use large pacifiers and nipples.
B. Boil bottle nipples and pacifiers.
C. Cleanse your nipples well after breastfeeding.

TREATMENT PLAN

A. Try to remove any large plaques with a moistened cotton-tipped applicator or gauze pad.
B. Cleanse the infant's mouth before giving medication.
C. Place the medication in the front of the mouth on each side.
D. Rub it directly on the plaques with a cotton swab.
E. Feed the infant temporarily with a cup and spoon.
F. Give a pacifier only at bedtime.

Diet: Decrease sucking time until thrush clears up.
Medications: Nystatin is an oral medication used to treat thrush. Nystatin 1 mL four times a day after meals or 30 minutes before feeding. Patches should improve within 2 to 3 days of using the medication.

You Have Been Prescribed: _____

You Need to Take: _____

You Need to Notify the Office If:
A. The child refuses to eat or drink.
B. Symptoms do not improve or thrush lasts longer than 10 days.
C. Unexplained fever occurs.
D. Secondary infection occurs in the mouth (pain, tenderness, sores).

E. Other: _____

Phone: _____

OSTEOARTHRITIS

PROBLEM

Osteoarthritis (OA) is a very common disorder that affects the weight-bearing and movable joints. OA damages the cartilage tissue in the joint. The cartilage provides the cushion around the joint. If the cartilage becomes damaged, it will become inflamed and irritated and start to thin. When this occurs, there is less cushion between the bones, and you will experience more pain and swelling. The joints most commonly involved are the finger and toe joints, knees, hips, and spine.

CAUSE

There are many different causes of OA. A previous injury to the joint, repeated stress to the joint (like a bricklayer's hands), genetics, age, obesity, and other diseases (such as diabetes or infections) may cause OA.

TREATMENT PLAN

A. The goal of treatment is to prevent further joint damage.
B. Learn as much as you can about this disorder and ask your healthcare provider several questions.
C. Heat and massage may increase joint movement and decrease pain.
D. Physical or occupational therapy may be needed.
E. Heat or ice packs may be used for localized relief.

Activity:
1. Range-of-motion (ROM) exercises increase the movement of the joint.
2. Careful exercise may also strengthen the muscles around the joint.
3. Ask your provider to advise the best type of exercise for you.
4. Yoga and acupuncture have been shown to help relieve pain and stiffness.
5. Joint protection: Do not overuse a joint.
6. If you work with your hands and have OA of the fingers, take frequent rest periods. This applies to all the other joints as well.

Diet: Low-fat, low-cholesterol diet may be suggested. Losing weight may help if you have OA of the knees, hips, or spine.

Medications: Your healthcare provider may recommend that you take acetaminophen or an anti-inflammatory drug. This should help relieve the pain and stiffness. Special creams also sometimes help joint pain. In cases of severe OA, your healthcare provider may recommend an injection to the joint or surgery. *Remember* to take only the medicines prescribed for you.

You Have Been Prescribed: _____

You Need to Take: _____

You Need to Notify the Office If You Have:
A. Increased pain despite medication
B. Fever higher than 100.4°F
C. Abdominal pain or discomfort after taking medicine

Phone: _____

RESOURCE

Arthritis Foundation
800-283-7800
www.arthritis.org

OSTEOPOROSIS

PROBLEM

Osteoporosis is a condition in which the bone loses its normal density, mass, and strength, which makes it weak and more vulnerable to fracture (break).

CAUSE

The weakening of the bone can be caused by several factors. Some of these risk factors include:
A. Inadequate amounts of calcium, protein, and vitamin D in the diet
B. Decreased exercise
C. Some chronic diseases such as thyroid disease, diabetes, and heart failure
D. Cancer
E. Smoking
F. Low estrogen levels (menopause)
G. Excessive alcohol intake
H. Advancing age
I. Being a Caucasian or Asian woman
J. Long-term use of certain medications such as steroids, thyroid medications, seizure medications, and some cancer treatment medications

PREVENTION/CARE

A. Be sure to get adequate calcium intake daily (1,500 mg/d) and vitamin D intake (600–2,000 IU/d). Ask your healthcare provider for the appropriate dose of calcium and vitamin D for you.
B. Food sources of calcium are best absorbed.
C. Calcium and vitamin D supplements may also be needed to meet the daily recommendation.
D. Get daily weight-bearing exercise such as walking, jogging, or running. Avoid high-impact exercises.

TREATMENT PLAN

A. If osteoporosis is suspected, your provider may order a bone density study of your bones. Goals are to prevent the disease from occurring.
B. If you have been diagnosed with osteoporosis, you need to prevent the disease from progressing and take measures to prevent all bone fractures.
C. Use caution when walking on wet, slippery surfaces.
D. Avoid risk of falls by making your home safe. Avoid throw rugs on floors and remove small items that are easily tripped over. Use caution when pets are around to prevent falling over your pet.

Activity:
A. Physical activity is vital to maintain and prevent further bone loss.
B. Weight-bearing activity, such as walking or running, is the best activity.
C. Avoid high-impact sports and activities, such as jumping, and high-impact aerobics to prevent fracturing the bones
D. Avoid any risk of falls.
E. Use walking devices, such as a cane or walker, if needed.
F. Bathtubs should have nonskid protection.

Diet:
A. Eat a regular well-balanced diet. Increase food sources rich in calcium, protein, and vitamin D.
B. Sources of vitamin D include milk, some fish (salmon), and drinks and cereals with added vitamin D and minerals.
C. You can also get vitamin D from spending 20 to 30 minutes in the summer sunlight, exposing your skin to the sun without wearing sunscreen for this length of time.
D. Sources of calcium include dairy products, green leafy vegetables (broccoli), almonds, tofu, and drinks fortified with calcium such as orange juice and soy milk.
E. If you are overweight, a low-fat, low-cholesterol diet is suggested to lose weight.

(*continued*)

CLIENT TEACHING GUIDE

OSTEOPOROSIS *(continued)*

Medications:

A. You may be prescribed nonprescription medications like acetaminophen (Tylenol) as needed for pain.

B. Supplements: Calcium, vitamin D, and hormone replacement for women who are menopausal.

C. If prescribed bisphosphonate, take medication with a full glass of water.

D. Wait approximately 30 to 60 minutes before reclining or consuming other medications, beverages, or food to lower the risk of regurgitation or a burning sensation.

You Have Been Prescribed: _____

You Need to Take: _____

You Need to Notify the Office If You Have:

A. Been experiencing any pain; you need to have your provider assess this pain

B. Other: _____

Phone: _____

RESOURCES

National Osteoporosis Foundation: www.nof.org
National Women's Health Information Center: https://www.womenshealth.gov

OTITIS MEDIA WITH EFFUSION

PROBLEM

There is inflammation of the middle ear with effusion, which is the presence of fluid in the middle ear without infection.

CAUSE

The middle ear fluid can remain behind the tympanic membrane after a middle ear infection (acute otitis media) has been treated. The Eustachian tube can be blocked, preventing proper ventilation of the middle ear. Symptoms may include difficulty hearing and a feeling of fullness and/or pain in the ear.

TREATMENT PLAN

A. Determine if there is difficulty with hearing.
B. Make accommodations for the hearing loss, such as sitting in the front of the classroom at school; speaking clearly and loudly. Reduce or eliminate external noises while having a conversation.
C. If the buildup of fluid in the middle ear lasts for longer than 3 months, a hearing evaluation should be completed. A referral to an ear specialist may be required for further care.
D. Follow up with a healthcare provider as instructed to avoid complications and/or permanent hearing loss.

Activity: There is no activity restriction.
Diet: There is no special diet.
Medications: Middle ear fluid often resolves without treatment within 3 months. Nasal spray steroids and nasal spray antihistamines are sometimes prescribed and can improve the time that is taken for resolution of the middle ear fluid. These medications should be taken exactly as has directed.

You Have Been Prescribed: _____

You Need to Take: _____

You Need to Notify the Office if You Have:
A. Fever
B. Decreased appetite
C. Decreased activity level
D. Ear pain
E. Noticed a change in hearing loss or speech development
F. Any other new symptoms that occur

G. Other: _____

Phone: _____

PARKINSON'S DISEASE MANAGEMENT

PROBLEM

Parkinson's disease (PD) is a problem with the central nervous system that causes progressive muscle rigidity and tremors. The ability to move your muscles becomes difficult and you may also notice difficulty with walking and swallowing. Common symptoms you may experience include movements of your muscles slowing down, tremor at rest, and rigidity (feeling stiff and finding it hard to start moving). You may have trouble with your balance, making you feel like you are going to fall down. Other symptoms may also include difficulty speaking, swallowing, drooling, changes in mood, and sleep patterns.

CAUSE

The brain is not able to produce or use the correct amount of a chemical, called dopamine, required by the body, and therefore the nervous system reacts by producing a loss in control of your muscles and movements.

TREATMENT PLAN/CARE

A. There is no cure for PD. However, medications may relieve a lot of your symptoms. Your healthcare provider will share the medications that are available to you.
B. You might be very sensitive to heat. During hot weather, stay outside only for very short periods of time, stay inside during the hottest part of the day, and increase your fluid intake.
C. Balance problems are common and increase the risk of falls. Some ways to avoid injury are not to have loose rugs or other floor coverings; install grab bars around the tub and toilet; ensure a sturdy rail on stairs and adequate lighting so you can see where you are going; use straight-backed, firm chairs with arms.
D. Tremors increase the risk of accidents. Use sturdy plastic cups instead of glasses, use an electric razor to shave, and be cautious with sharp objects and power tools.
E. For clothes, Velcro fasteners, zippers, and snaps are easier to fasten than buttons. Loose clothing is also easier to put on and take off.
F. To avoid sleep problems, stay busy during the day and avoid naps. Discuss any problems you have with your neurologist; sometimes changes in your medication schedule can help.
G. If you have speech problems, work on ways to make your needs known. Practice speech exercises or consider speech therapy with a speech therapist.
H. Stay active in your daily work, hobbies, and other daily activities you enjoy.
I. If you are having signs of anxiety, depression, sleep problems, or other symptoms, please discuss these with your provider. These symptoms are common and can be addressed and treated with other medications.

Activity: Regular exercise helps maintain muscle flexibility and may reduce medication needs. Exercises to improve facial, jaw, and tongue movement are encouraged.
Diet: There is no special diet for PD.
A. If you are having difficulty with swallowing, let your provider know. Take your time eating meals. Sit upright. Thick liquids are easier to swallow than thin liquids.
B. Plan medication schedules so that you are functioning well at meal times. Be sure you allow plenty of time to finish your meal.
C. Your diet should include plenty of fluids and adequate fiber to prevent or manage constipation. Have bran cereal in the morning and eat five or more servings of fruits and vegetables throughout the day. Bananas are low in fiber and should be avoided.
D. If you need help planning your meals, your healthcare provider can suggest a dietitian with whom you can talk about food choices.
E. Alcoholic beverages are discouraged as alcohol can interfere with the effectiveness of your medications.

(*continued*)

PARKINSON'S DISEASE MANAGEMENT (*continued*)

Medications:

A. The medicines you are taking can improve your ability to carry out everyday activities, but they cannot totally eliminate your symptoms. It is important that you know why you are taking each medication as well as the possible side effects of each.

B. Check with your neurologist before starting any new medicine to be sure it does not interact with your Parkinson's medicines. Even vitamins can be a problem, so take only those recommended by your neurologist.

C. If you are having trouble swallowing your medications, call your healthcare provider or pharmacist before breaking or crushing medications. Some medications cannot be broken in half or crushed because of the coating or releasing too much medication at once. Some of your medications may come in syrup form.

D. Keep with you a list of your medicines, including the amounts you take and your schedule for taking them.

You Have Been Prescribed: _____

You Need to Take: _____

You Need to Notify the Office If:

A. You are unable to swallow your medications.

B. You have a reaction to your medication.

C. You are unable to tolerate your medication because of side effects.

D. Your symptoms become worse.

E. Other: _____

Phone: _____

RESOURCES

National Parkinson Foundation: https://www.parkinson.org/

Michael J. Fox Foundation for Parkinson's Research: https://www.michaeljfox.org/

Parkinson's Disease Foundation, 24-hour HELPLINE: 1-800-473-4636; https://www.parkinson.org/Living-with-Parkinsons/Resources-and-Support/Helpline

PELVIC INFLAMMATORY DISEASE

PROBLEM

You have been diagnosed as having pelvic inflammatory disease, also known as PID. This inflammation can involve the uterus, fallopian tubes, ovaries, broad ligament, and/or the pelvic vascular system or pelvic connective tissue.

CAUSE

Organisms that go up from the vagina and cervix into the uterus cause PID. The two most common organisms cultured from clients with PID are *C. trachomatis* and *N. gonorrhoeae*. Your period increases the ability of gonococcal invasion into the upper genital tract. Infection and inflammation spread throughout the endometrium to the fallopian tubes. From there, it extends to the ovaries and peritoneal, or abdominal, cavity.

PREVENTION/CARE

A. Condoms and a spermicidal foam or cream with nonoxynol 9 are very protective against PID.
B. Condoms must be used with *every* act of sexual intercourse.
C. Vaginal douching may lead to an increased risk for PID.
   1. Routine douching is *not recommended;* it wipes out the normal vaginal flora.
D. The more sex partners you have, the greater the chances are of contracting sexually transmitted infections.

TREATMENT PLAN

A. Your partner(s) need(s) to be evaluated and treated with antibiotic therapy, too.
B. Sexual abstinence:
   1. **You should not have sexual intercourse until all of your symptoms are gone and your partner(s) has (have) completed antibiotic therapy.**
   2. If you do have sexual intercourse, you should use condoms consistently.
C. Rescreen:
   1. You should be rescreened for sexually transmitted infections 6 months after treatment ends, or sooner if exposure.

Activity: Limit yourself to light activity for 3 to 4 days, and then pursue activity as tolerated.
Diet:
A. You need to drink at least 10 to 12 glasses of liquid every day.
B. You need to eat a well-balanced diet (three meals).
C. You need to eat high-protein snacks such as peanut butter sandwiches and milk.
D. If you have been prescribed Flagyl (metronidazole), you must avoid all alcohol ingestion while taking and for at least 48 hours after the last dose or you will experience severe nausea and vomiting. If you are taking the medicine tinidazole (Tindamax), you should avoid alcohol for 72 hours after completing.
Medications:
A. You will be prescribed *two or more* antibiotics; it is extremely important to **take all of the antibiotics.**
B. You may take acetaminophen (Tylenol) for fever.
C. You may be prescribed some pain medication.

You Have Been Prescribed: _____

You Need to Take: _____

Take all of your antibiotics, even if you feel better.

Your Second Prescribed Antibiotic Is: _____

You Need to Take: _____

(*continued*)

PELVIC INFLAMMATORY DISEASE (*continued*)

You need to take all of both antibiotics, even if you feel better.

You Have Been Prescribed the Following for Your Pain: _____

You Need to Take: _____

You Need to Notify the Office If:

A. Your fever does not respond to acetaminophen (Tylenol).

B. Your symptoms worsen, even while taking both antibiotics.

C. You vomit or cannot tolerate your antibiotics.

D. Other: _____

Phone: _____

Next Appointment: Date _____ **Time** _____

PERIPHERAL ARTERIAL DISEASE

PROBLEM

Peripheral arterial disease is a condition in which fatty deposits build up on the inside of vessels that carry blood to the hands and feet. This makes it difficult for blood to travel to hands and feet, which causes pain with activity and when resting. If these blockages increase in size, the pain will also worsen and infections can occur that could lead to amputation.

CAUSE

Many things cause these fatty deposits to build up inside arteries. Some, like age, gender, and genetics, cannot be changed. Others can be changed; these include smoking, diabetes, high cholesterol, high blood pressure, and excessive weight.

PREVENTION/CARE

A. Stop smoking.
B. To prevent injury that could progress into an infection, do the following:
  1. Wear well-fitting shoes that protect your feet.
  2. Look and feel inside your shoes before putting them on.
  3. Look at your feet daily for any signs of injury or infection.
  4. Dry feet well after bathing, including between toes.
  5. Do not trim your own toenails or shave off calluses. A healthcare provider should do this for you to prevent infection.
  6. Do not use a heating pad or hot water on your hands or feet to keep warm. Wear gloves or socks instead.

TREATMENT PLAN

A. Take your medications as ordered by your healthcare provider.
B. Effectively manage all other medical conditions, paying special attention to cholesterol, blood pressure, diabetes, and obesity.
C. Follow up with your primary healthcare provider and/or cardiologist on a regularly scheduled basis.

Activity:
A. Get regular exercise, after discussing with your healthcare provider the type and frequency of exercise that is safe for you.
Diet:
A. Discuss the type of diet that best suits your needs: Diabetic diet, low-fat diet, low-cholesterol diet, and/or low-sodium diet.
B. Follow the dietary guidelines suggested by your healthcare provider.
Medications:

You Have Been Prescribed: _____

You Need to Take: _____

You Need to Notify the Office If You Have:
A. Any of the following symptoms:
  1. Worsening pain in your arm or leg
  2. Fever of 101.5°F or greater
  3. Any temperature change in a hand or foot
  4. Any change in feeling of a hand or foot
  5. Any change in the color of a hand or foot
  6. Difficulty walking

(*continued*)

PERIPHERAL ARTERIAL DISEASE *(continued)*

7. Vomiting or other illness that causes you to miss more than one dose of your medications

8. Other: _____

Phone: _____

RESOURCE

Cardiovascular Cell Therapy Research Network NIH: https://sph.uth.edu/research/centers/ccct/cctrn/patient-education-center/peripheral-artery-disease.htm

PHARYNGITIS

PROBLEM

Pharyngitis (sore throat) is a condition that occurs when the throat becomes inflamed.

CAUSE

The inflammation can be due to a virus, a bacterial infection, or a fungus. Other noninfectious causes include postnasal drip, allergies, mouth breathing, and trauma.

PREVENTION/CARE

A. Avoid sick people and crowds. Stay at home if you are sick.
B. Cover your mouth when coughing.
C. Do not share a drinking glass, kiss, or have close contact with anyone who has an upper respiratory infection.

TREATMENT PLAN

A. Hot tea, soup, and throat lozenges soothe your throat.
B. Use disposable tissues when sneezing. Use tissues when you blow your nose. If no tissue is available, do the "elbow sneeze" into the bend of your arm (away from your open hands). Dispose of tissues and then wash your hands.
C. Avoid smoking and secondhand smoke.

Activity: If you have strep throat, do not return to school or work until you have completed a full 24 hours of antibiotic. Rest or nap as often as possible while you are sick.

Diet: Eat a healthy diet. If swallowing is difficult, eat soft foods such as ice cream, Jell-O, pudding, and soup. Avoid salt and spicy foods. Increase your fluid intake to 10 to 12 glasses a day.

Medications: You will be prescribed antibiotics if you have a bacterial infection. If your sore throat is due to a virus, antibiotics would not help. Do not share your prescription medications with other family members who are also sick. They need a full prescription, too. Many other medications are available over the counter, such as throat lozenges, cough suppressants, and so forth.

You Have Been Prescribed: _____

You Need to Take: _____

If you are prescribed antibiotics, complete all of the doses.

You Need to Notify the Office If:
A. You have difficulty breathing because of the sore throat or enlarged tonsils.
B. Your symptoms are worse after 24 hours of antibiotics.
C. You are unable to keep down your antibiotic because of vomiting.
D. Your sick child refuses to eat or drink.
E. You develop a rash or itch after starting the antibiotic.
F. You are a diabetic and your blood glucose is high, or you have ketones in your urine.

G. Other: _____

Phone: _____

PITYRIASIS ROSEA

PROBLEM

Pityriasis rosea is a very common condition characterized by a rash that may or may not itch. You may have noticed a large, scaly patch before breaking out with the more generalized rash. **It is not known to be contagious, and you do not need to isolate yourself.**

CAUSE

The cause of pityriasis rosea is unknown.

PREVENTION/CARE

Because the cause of pityriasis rosea is unknown, there are no recommended preventive measures.

TREATMENT PLAN

Good hygiene and avoidance of scratching are recommended to prevent a secondary infection.

Activity: It is not necessary for you to limit your activity. Sunlight exposure to skin for short periods of time daily for five consecutive days will decrease itching and improve the rash. Care should be taken not to burn skin with short-term exposure to the sun.

Diet: No changes are required in your diet.

Medications: You may be prescribed an antihistamine medication to take by mouth and topical steroid creams to apply to the rash itself. If the itching is severe, oral steroids may be prescribed.

You Have Been Prescribed: _____

You Need to Take: _____

You Need to Notify the Office If You Have:

A. Any new symptoms

B. Any reaction to your medication

Phone: _____

PNEUMONIA, VIRAL: ADULT

PROBLEM

Viral pneumonia is an infection of the lung that causes fluid in the air sacs. You may have fever, cough, or difficulty breathing.

CAUSE

Respiratory viruses cause viral pneumonia and bacteria.

PREVENTION/CARE

A. Avoid contact with people with respiratory illnesses
B. Although the flu vaccine does not prevent pneumonia, a yearly flu shot is recommended
C. The pneumonia vaccine helps prevent pneumonia caused by bacteria. If you are older than 65 years or have other chronic respiratory illness, the pneumonia vaccine is recommended.

TREATMENT PLAN

A. Use a cool-mist humidifier and clean it daily.
B. Take deep breaths and cough frequently to clear secretions from lungs.
C. Avoid smoking and exposure to secondhand smoke.
D. Practice good handwashing techniques or use hand sanitizers.

Activity: Rest frequently during the early phase of the illness. Fatigue may continue for up to 6 weeks.
Diet: Eat a nutritious diet. Drink 8 to 10 glasses of water a day.
Medications:
A. Take acetaminophen (Tylenol) for fever, discomfort, and headache.
B. Do not take cough suppressants. It is important for you to cough and get up any mucus.
C. Antibiotics are not given for a viral infection. If you have a bacterial infection, then you may be put on an antibiotic.

You Have Been Prescribed: _____

You Need to Take: _____

You Need to Notify the Office If You Have:
A. Increased difficulty breathing
B. Fever greater than 101°F or fever that persists after 48 hours of antibiotics
C. Worsening discomfort
D. Shortness of breath
E. Blood in sputum
F. Nausea, vomiting, or diarrhea

G. Other: _____

Phone: _____

PNEUMONIA, VIRAL: CHILD

PROBLEM

Viral pneumonia is an infection of the lung that causes fluid to collect in the air sacs. Your child may have fever, cough, or difficulty breathing.

CAUSE

Respiratory viruses cause viral pneumonia.

PREVENTION/CARE

A. Isolate young infants from people with respiratory illnesses.
B. Although the flu vaccine will not prevent viral pneumonia, children should get an influenza vaccine every year.

TREATMENT PLAN

A. Encourage fluids.
B. Use a vaporizer to increase humidity in the child's room.
C. Keep the child away from cigarette smoke.

Activity: Have your child rest during the acute phase. Your child may return to school or day care when he or she is free from fever for 24 hours.

Diet: There is no special diet for viral pneumonia. Follow a regular diet. Increase fluids.

Medications:
A. You may give your child acetaminophen (Tylenol) for fever.
B. Children should never be given aspirin due to the increased risk of Reye's syndrome.
C. **Do not give cough suppressants. The American College of Chest Physicians clinical practice guidelines recommend that cough suppressants and over-the-counter cough medications should *not* be given to young children. Cough medicines should *not* be given to any child younger than 6 years of age.**
D. Antibiotics are not used for viral infections. Your child may be given an antibiotic if he or she has any infection other than the viral pneumonia.

Your Child Has Been Prescribed: _____

Your Child Needs to Take: _____

You Need to Notify the Office Immediately If:
A. Your child's breathing becomes more labored or difficult, or his or her lips become blue.
B. Retractions (tugging between ribs) become worse.
C. Grunting sounds occur when the child breathes out.
D. Your child starts acting very sick.

E. Other: _____

You Need to Notify the Office Within 24 Hours If:
A. Your child is unable to sleep.
B. Your child is not drinking enough.
C. Fever is over 101°F or persists after 48 hours on antibiotics.
D. Your child is getting worse.

E. Other: _____

Phone: _____

POLYMYALGIA RHEUMATICA

PROBLEM

Polymyalgia rheumatica (PMR) is a common disorder experienced by adults older than the age of 50 years in which complaints involve overall joint stiffness and pain. Common complaints include feeling fine one day and the following day having overall joint pain, with difficulty getting out of bed or standing up from a chair. Symptoms may occur gradually over a period of several days or weeks, or may occur abruptly overnight. Symptoms are usually worse in the morning hours. The joints most commonly affected are the upper arms, shoulders, thighs, hips, and neck.

CAUSE

A. The cause of PMR is unknown.
B. Some theories maintain that PMR may be triggered by an infection; however, research does not identify any specific infection.

PREVENTION/CARE

There is no known way to prevent the onset of PMR.

TREATMENT PLAN

A. You may be treated with low-dose steroid by mouth daily. Prednisone is a common medication used to treat this disorder. Stiffness and joint pain may quickly improve with the use of oral steroids. If improvement with steroids does not occur within 2 weeks of treatment, you should notify your provider.
B. Once improvement is noted, your provider will begin to lower the steroid dose gradually over time. This may take several weeks to months.
C. Do not change or taper your steroid dose on your own. Your provider will advise you on the tapering dose when appropriate.

Activity:
A. Once stiffness and pain have improved, you may resume normal activities. Exercise is encouraged on most days of the week.

Diet:
A. There is not any special diet to follow for this disorder.
B. Blood sugar: Side effects of the prednisone may include increased blood sugar. If you have concerns regarding your blood sugar values, or if you are diabetic, you need to discuss proper management and monitoring of your blood sugar while taking steroids.

Medications:
A. Oral steroids (prednisone) are commonly prescribed over a period. Discuss proper dosages and tapering of this medication with your provider.

You Have Been Prescribed: _____

You Need to Take: _____

You Need to Notify the Office If You Have:
A. Any new symptoms such as headache, jaw pain, or vision changes
B. Side effects from the prednisone or other medications prescribed
C. Increase in pain, or weakness while using prednisone
D. Any other concerns

Phone: _____

RESOURCES

Arthritis Foundation: www.arthritis.org
National Institute of Arthritis and Musculoskeletal and Skin Diseases Information Clearinghouse: www.niams.nih.gov/Health_Info/Polymyalgia/default.asp

POSTPARTUM: BREAST ENGORGEMENT AND SORE NIPPLES

PROBLEM

Engorgement causes swollen, tender breasts, which may have palpable nodular areas.

CAUSE

Engorgement may develop because of inadequate suckling by your baby.

PREVENTION/CARE

A. At first, nurse your baby every 2 to 3 hours.
B. Make sure your baby latches onto the areola (darkened area around the nipple) as much as possible. The baby suckling on the tip of the nipple does not provide the stimulation necessary to let down the milk and can make your nipples sore and cracked.
C. If your baby is not well attached to the breast, detach the baby and make sure he or she opens his or her mouth wide to accommodate most of the areola.
D. Wear a supportive nursing bra (avoid underwire bras as they can exert pressure on certain areas of the breast and cause milk stasis, which is a good medium for bacterial growth and infection); make sure that your bra does not squeeze your breasts too tightly.
E. Make sure that the baby is properly attached to the nipple; this helps to avoid cracking of nipples that can predispose you to an infection of the breast called *mastitis.*
F. After the baby feeds, express some milk and apply it to the areola to keep the nipple hydrated and to avoid cracking.
G. Purified lanolin can also be very helpful for sore nipples and can prevent further cracking and infection. Apply routinely after each breastfeeding session for the first several days of nursing and longer if tender or cracked nipples occur. If the lanolin is purified, there is no need to wash it off before feedings.

TREATMENT PLAN

A. Engorgement:
    1. Treatment of engorgement includes the application of heat, breast massage, and expression of milk for comfort only.
    2. A warm moist washcloth or a warm shower before massaging the breast decreases discomfort.
    3. Massage the breast by making several gentle but firm stroking movements with the fingertips along the swollen ducts, moving toward the nipple. This should be done around the entire breast.
    4. After massaging, milk should be expressed or pumped until the breast softens enough for the baby to latch well. The baby should then be allowed to nurse from both breasts.
    5. The best strategy for engorgement is frequent breastfeeding (at least every half an hour to 2 hours until engorgement resolves).
B. Sore nipples:
    1. Sore nipples are usually caused by the improper positioning of the baby on the nipple.
    2. Ensure your baby is grasping the areola when sucking and not just the nipple.
    3. Continuous suction pressure at the same spot of the nipple can be painful.
    4. Change the position of the baby to change the "latching on" position of your baby's mouth.
    5. If nipples become sore or cracked, start feeding on the less-affected breast first.
    6. Apply purified lanolin to nipples after each feeding.
    7. Prevent mastitis with the following personal hygiene measures:
        a. Avoid using soap on nipples.
        b. Avoid decrusting the nipples of dried colostrum or milk.
        c. Change breast pads frequently.
        d. Wash hands before handling your breast and before breastfeeding.

(*continued*)

POSTPARTUM: BREAST ENGORGEMENT AND SORE NIPPLES *(continued)*

Activity: As tolerated, extra rest is recommended after delivery.

Diet:

A. Breastfeeding mothers need extra liquids for milk production.

B. Drink 10 to 12 glasses of liquid a day.

C. Use caffeine in moderation (eliminate if possible).

D. Continue your regular diet and add about 500 extra calories per day.

E. Avoid gas-producing foods that may upset your baby's stomach.

Medications: Continue your prenatal vitamins while breastfeeding.

You Have Been Prescribed: Acetaminophen 500 mg or ibuprofen 600 mg every 3 to 4 hours for discomfort.

You Need to Notify the Office If You Have:

A. Temperature of 100.4°F or higher

B. Pain that is not controlled with Tylenol or ibuprofen

C. Flu-like symptoms (fever, chills, malaise)

D. Red streaks on breast

E. Headache with the aforementioned symptoms

F. Other: _____

Phone: _____

PREMENSTRUAL SYNDROME

DEFINITION

Premenstrual syndrome (PMS) is a common problem experienced by women in their reproductive years. You may have some or all of the following symptoms:

A. Cravings for food, particularly chocolate and salty foods
B. Irritability
C. Feelings of depression; crying spells
D. Bloated stomach
E. Weight gain and water retention
F. Difficulty concentrating
G. Tiredness
H. Feelings of faintness
I. Sometimes clumsiness
J. Sore breasts

CAUSE

Although the cause is really not known, PMS is a response of your body to the changes in female hormones during the last half of your menstrual cycle.

PREVENTION/CARE

All of your symptoms probably cannot be prevented, but some of them may be made less severe.

TREATMENT PLAN

A. Keep track of your symptoms for at least 3 months so that your healthcare provider can determine if the symptoms always happen in the last half of your cycle.
B. Eat six small meals each day. Eat breakfast, have a morning snack like fruit or a glass of milk, eat lunch, have an afternoon snack, eat supper, and then have another evening snack. This helps keep your blood sugar even, avoiding periods of low blood sugar.
C. Minimize the amount of candy, desserts, and other sugars. They may be associated with episodes of low blood sugar. Complex carbohydrates, such as pasta, potatoes, fresh fruit, rice, and bread, break down more slowly than sweets and keep your blood sugar steadier.
D. Minimize the amount of salty foods such as chips, fast-food, and pickles you eat during the symptomatic phase. They can contribute to bloating.
E. Minimize caffeine intake in soda, coffee, and chocolate. Caffeine makes you irritable and nervous.
F. Exercise daily. Exercise increases chemicals in your brain that help with your mood.
G. Join a PMS group so that you can get support from other women who have similar symptoms. You may get ideas of how other women handle PMS, and you can share your ideas, too.
H. If you smoke, try to cut down or quit.
I. Get a good night's rest and take naps during the day if possible.
J. Try stress-reduction classes or yoga. Local community organizations usually have classes available.

Medications: There are a number of medications available that your healthcare provider may suggest for you.

You Have Been Prescribed: _____

You Need to Take: _____

You Have Also Been Prescribed: _____

You Need to Take: _____

(*continued*)

PREMENSTRUAL SYNDROME   (*continued*)

You Need to Notify the Office If:

A. You have questions or concerns.

B. You feel that things are not improving.

C. Other: _____

Phone: _____

PRETERM LABOR

PROBLEM

Premature contractions and early labor put your baby at risk of premature delivery. Babies born too soon are at risk of breathing problems, bleeding into their brain, infection, and bowel problems, to name a few. Early recognition is the key to stopping premature labor and delivery.

CAUSE

There are several predisposing factors for preterm labor, including previous premature delivery, smoking, incompetent cervix, multiple gestation (twins or triplets), and infection. In most cases, the cause of preterm labor is unknown.

PREVENTION/CARE

You can decrease your risk of preterm labor by living a healthy lifestyle with a balanced diet, proper fluid consumption, and no smoking. Please review any previous preterm labor symptoms with your healthcare provider. Early recognition is a key to success.

TREATMENT PLAN

Treatment depends on the clinical picture. In general, you should remember:
A. Drink at least 8 to 10 glasses of liquid a day; dehydration can increase contractions.
B. Empty your bladder every 2 to 3 hours.
C. Report any bladder infection symptoms, such as burning with urination, to your healthcare provider.
D. Avoid breast stimulation (including showers where the water stream is on your breasts); this can stimulate contractions.
E. Rest frequently. Rest means lying down on either side, not on your back.
F. Contractions and cramping happen more often in the evening and nighttime after activity during the day.
G. Do not have intercourse or sexual stimulation without asking your nurse practitioner, certified nurse-midwife, or doctor. If intercourse is okay, use a condom to decrease infection.
H. Try to arrange for help with housework and child care to help you maintain your bed-rest schedule.
I. Take medications to stop contractions as directed.

Activity: Activity at home is based on how strong your preterm labor has been. You should follow the following activity guidelines:

Level 1: As Tolerated
A. Avoid heavy lifting above 20 lb.

Level 2: Modified Bed Rest
A. You may be out of bed for breakfast.
B. Rest for 2 hours in the morning with only moderate activity until lunch.
C. Rest for 2 hours with only moderate activity until dinner.
D. Go to bed by 8 p.m.
   Moderate activity consists of short periods of cooking and light housework (dusting and sweeping).

Level 3: Strict Bed Rest
A. You may be out of the bed only to go to the bathroom or to move to the couch.
B. You may take a shower, use the toilet, brush your teeth, then return immediately to bed.
C. You should not engage in lifting, bending, housework, or lengthy cooking.
D. You should not have sexual intercourse.
E. Perform range-of-motion (ROM) exercises as directed by your practitioner to avoid muscle weakness and blood clots in your legs. Example: Make small circles with your feet, and bend and straighten your legs.

Level 4: Hospitalization

Diet: Diet as tolerated, or follow your prescribed diet. Drink 8 to 10 glasses of water each day. Avoid beverages with caffeine. Eat fresh vegetables, fruits, and bran cereal to avoid becoming constipated.
Medications: Continue taking your prenatal vitamin every day.

(*continued*)

PRETERM LABOR *(continued)*

You Have Been Prescribed: _____

You Need to Take: _____

You Need to Notify the Office If You Have:
A. Contractions or cramping more frequent than four in 1 hour
B. A gush of fluid or blood from your vagina (it is normal to have spotting after vaginal examination or intercourse)
C. Pelvic pressure or low, dull backache
D. Noticed that your baby is not moving as much as usual: Less than 10 fetal movements in 2 hours after drinking and resting on your side
E. Chest pain or difficulty breathing

F. Other: _____

Phone: _____

PROSTATIC HYPERTROPHY/BENIGN

PROBLEM

Enlargement of the prostate causes the feeling of urge to urinate. Symptoms include having to go to the bathroom more often, especially at night; trouble starting or stopping your urine; decreased stream; and feeling that you do not empty.

CAUSE

The cause is not known, but it may be because of change in hormones with age.

PREVENTION/CARE

None

TREATMENT PLAN

Treatment depends on how bad the symptoms are. Medications can help, but an operation to fix the obstruction may be needed. Empty your bladder on a schedule every 2 to 3 hours to prevent overfilling of the bladder.

Activity: There are no restrictions. You may need to plan schedules with access to bathrooms in mind.

Diet: Avoid spicy foods that irritate the bladder. Caffeine and alcohol act as diuretics and increase your need to urinate.

Medications:

A. Medications that help relieve the blockage may block hormones or relax the muscles that control urination.

B. Antibiotics are used if there is also an infection in your bladder or prostate.

C. Do not take over-the-counter (OTC) medications like cold medications, decongestants, antihistamines (for allergies), and diarrhea medicines; they make symptoms worse.

D. Always read labels to check for the advice: "Do not take if you have prostate enlargement."

E. Avoid drinking liquids before bedtime or before going out.

F. Double void to empty your bladder more completely.

You Have Been Prescribed: _____

You Need to Take: _____

You Need to Notify the Office If: _____

A. You cannot urinate.

B. Your symptoms worsen.

C. You have a fever.

D. Other: _____

Phone: _____

PROSTATITIS

PROBLEM

Prostatitis is infection and/or inflammation of the prostate. Symptoms can be problems with urinating, increased frequency or painful urination, fever, or chills. You may have pain in the scrotum and buttocks and blood in the urine or semen. Prostatitis can be treated and does not cause impotence.

CAUSE

An infection may be caused by bacteria from the bladder or reflux of urine, or it may have started from a rectal infection.

PREVENTION/CARE

A. Prevent prostate infection with good hygiene:
   1. Clean under foreskin if uncircumcised and wash your hands after each time you go to the bathroom (urine and BM)
   2. Limit your sexual partners and use a condom to prevent all types of infection
   3. Urinate when you have the urge. Do not hold your urine for a long period.
B. Staying sexually active with ejaculation may decrease the incidence.

TREATMENT PLAN

A. You may have to be in the hospital for severe infections.
B. At home, try the following comfort measures:
   1. Use a sitz bath or sit in warm bath water or a whirlpool three times a day to provide some relief.
   2. You may feel more comfortable when you empty your bladder in a warm water bath when your pelvic muscles relax.
C. Your sexual partner(s) may need to be evaluated and treated too (ask your healthcare provider).

Activity: Rest; do not engage in strenuous physical activity or heavy lifting.
Diet: Increase fluid intake. *Fluid Exception:* **Decrease caffeine and alcohol, which can irritate the urethra.**
Medications: Antibiotics cure the infection by killing bacteria. You need to continue taking these drugs until the infection is completely cured (usually about 1 month). You need to take all the antibiotics even if your symptoms are gone.

You Have Been Prescribed the Following Antibiotics: _____

You Need to Take: _____

Finish all of the antibiotics even if you feel better.
Pain medications combined with anti-inflammatory drugs to decrease pain are usually taken for 3 to 7 days. Take acetaminophen (Tylenol) to bring down fever.

You Have Been Prescribed the Following for Pain: _____

You Need to Take: _____

You Have Been Prescribed the Following for Fever: _____

You Need to Take: _____

You Need to Notify the Office If You Have:
A. Symptoms that get worse or do not improve during treatment
B. Symptoms that recur after treatment
C. Fever higher than 101.0°F

D. Other: _____

Phone: _____

(*continued*)

CLIENT TEACHING GUIDE

PROSTATITIS *(continued)*

RESOURCES

American Urological Association Foundation: www.UrologyHealth.org
National Kidney and Urologic Disease Information Clearinghouse: www.kidney.niddk.nih.gov
Prostatitis Foundation: www.prostatitis.org
Urology Care Foundation: https://www.urologyhealth.org; Hotline Toll Free 1-800-828-7866

PSEUDOGOUT

PROBLEM

Pseudogout, also known as calcium pyrophosphate deposition disease (CPPD), is a type of disorder that causes acute joint pain and swelling, primarily in the shoulder and knees. It can also occur in smaller joints, such as the ankles, feet, elbows, wrists, and hands.

CAUSE

Pseudogout is caused from calcium crystals building up in the joint, causing inflammation and pain. Having pseudogout can increase your risk of OA. OA is a common type of arthritis seen in older adults that can cause joint pain, stiffness, and sometimes swelling in the joints.

PREVENTION/CARE

There is not anything you can do to prevent this disease from occurring. However, if you are having three or more attacks per year, notify your practitioner. There are medications that can be prescribed to help prevent future attacks.

TREATMENT PLAN

Treatment depends on how many joints are affected. If you have one or two joints affected, your provider may drain the fluid from the joint and inject steroids into the joint, which will reduce the pain. If you have several joints affected, you will probably be given oral medications such as NSAIDs. These medications (indomethacin, naproxen, ibuprofen, etc.) will help with the swelling and pain. If you cannot take these medications because of other illnesses, please make sure your provider is aware of this. There are other medications available if you are not able to take these medications.

Activity: For acute attack, rest and elevation of the affected joint is recommended. If you are having difficulty with bearing weight on the joint, make sure your provider is aware of this; you need to stay off the joint.
Diet: No special diet is recommended.
Medications:
A. NSAIDs:
B. Steroids:

You Have Been Prescribed the Following Medication: _____

You Need to Take: _____

You Have Been Prescribed the Following for Discomfort: _____

You Need to Take: _____

You Need to Notify the Office If You Have:
A. No improvement in 1 to 2 days after being seen by your provider
B. Redness, increase in swelling, and/or pain in the affected joint
C. Redness, swelling, or pain in another new joint
D. Fever or new onset of other symptoms
E. Unable to tolerate medications prescribed by your provider today

F. Other: _____

Phone: _____

CLIENT TEACHING GUIDE

PSORIASIS

PROBLEM

Psoriasis is a chronic, scaly, thickened skin disorder with frequent remissions and recurrences. The skin of the scalp, elbows, knees, chest, back, arms, legs, toenails, fingernails, and fold between the buttocks may be involved.

CAUSE

The cause of psoriasis is unknown.

PREVENTION/CARE

A. There is no known prevention, but symptoms can be controlled.
B. Moving to a warmer climate might be beneficial. Severity increases with cold.
C. Maintain good skin hygiene with daily baths or showers.
D. Avoid harsh soaps.
E. Avoid skin injury, including harsh scrubbing, which can trigger new outbreaks.
F. Avoid skin dryness.
G. To reduce scaling, use nonprescription, waterless cleansers, and hair preparations containing coal tar (Zetar, T/Gel, Pentrax), emollients (Eucerin Plus lotion or cream, Lubriderm, Moisture Plus, Moisturel), or products containing cortisone (often prescription strength).
H. Expose the skin to moderate amounts of sunlight as often as possible. Avoid long periods in the sun to prevent sunburn.
I. Oatmeal baths may loosen scales. Use 1 cup of oatmeal to a tub of warm water.
J. Stress may increase outbreaks of psoriasis. Consider counseling to assist in lifestyle changes, coping, or any psychological problems caused by psoriasis.

TREATMENT PLAN

Activity: There are no activity restrictions.
Diet: Eat a well-balanced diet. You may be instructed to try a gluten-free diet. Drink 8 to 10 glasses of water per day. Avoid alcohol in your diet.
Medications: You may be prescribed the following types of medications:
A. Creams to rub on the skin:
    1. Ointments containing coal tar. These may stain clothing.
    2. Salicylic acid cream, anthralin cream, or vitamin D-like cream (calcipotriene)
    3. Topical cortisone creams may also be used for short periods of time.
B. Psoralen plus UV light (PUVA; combination of a medication and exposure to UV A light)
C. Combination of tar baths with UV B light
D. Antihistamines to relieve itching

You Have Been Prescribed: _____

You Need to Take: _____

You Need to Notify the Office If:
A. You have an adverse reaction to or cannot tolerate any of the prescribed medications.
B. Symptoms recur after treatment. Notify your healthcare provider if, during an outbreak, pustules erupt on the skin and/or are accompanied by fever, muscle aches, and fatigue.
C. New, unexplained symptoms develop.

D. Other: _____

Phone: _____

For severe cases, you may be referred to a dermatologist (specialist for skin disorders).

RESOURCE

National Psoriasis Foundation, Suite 200, 6415 SW Canyon, Ct. Portland, OR 97221, Phone: 800-723-9166, www .psoriasis.org

RESPIRATORY SYNCYTIAL VIRUS

PROBLEM

RSV causes respiratory distress, wheezing, coughing, and fever.

CAUSE

RSV is a common respiratory virus that affects infants and children in fall, winter, and early spring.

PREVENTION/CARE

A. Isolate young infants from people with respiratory illnesses.
B. Wash hands frequently if you are a caregiver.
C. Wash toys and surfaces the child touches.
D. Although the flu vaccine does not prevent RSV, a flu vaccine is recommended every year.

TREATMENT PLAN

A. Do not smoke around the child

Activity: The child needs rest during the early stages of the illness.
Diet: Continue to breastfeed. Offer fluids, such as juice and water, frequently. Dilute juice for younger infants. Offer small, frequent feedings.
Medications:
A. Antibiotics do not help with viruses
B. There is a special vaccination for RSV, but your child must meet special requirements that are recommended by the American Academy of Pediatricians
C. **The American College of Chest Physicians clinical practice guidelines recommend that cough suppressants and over-the-counter cold medicines *not* be given to young children. Cough and cold medicines should *not* be given to children younger than 6 years of age.**
D. Your child may be given other medications to control other symptoms

You Have Been Prescribed: _____

You Need to Take: _____

You Need to Call 911 or Call the Office Immediately If:
A. Your child's breathing gets labored, difficult, or faster than 60 times a minute.
B. Your child's lips become bluish, or he or she stops breathing or passes out.
C. Wheezing becomes severe.
D. Retractions (tugging between ribs) become worse.
E. Your child starts acting very sick and lethargic.

F. Other: _____

YOU NEED TO NOTIFY THE OFFICE WITHIN 24 HOURS IF:

A. Your child is unable to sleep.
B. Your child will not drink enough fluids.
C. Your child has any suggestion of an earache, a yellow nasal discharge, or a fever over 100°F for more than 72 hours.
D. You feel your child is getting worse.

E. Other: _____

Phone: _____

RICE THERAPY AND EXERCISE THERAPY

RICE therapies are used for muscle injuries. RICE stands for rest, ice, compression, and elevation.

REST

A. Take it easy; eliminate abuse; reduce regular exercise or activities of daily living as needed but do not eliminate them.
B. Change activity or components of activity; for example, change running to walking.
C. Stop sports; restrict squatting, kneeling, and repetitious bending.
D. Limit weight bearing; immobilize with crutches for partial weight bearing.

ICE

A. Use cold in the acute phase of the injury (first 72 hours) to reduce pain and swelling.
B. Use cold in the form of ice in a plastic bag or even use frozen peas in a bag.
C. Apply cold four to eight times a day for 20 minutes at a time, with 45 to 60 minutes between applications.

COMPRESSION

A. Use elastic bandages, dry or wet, or open basket-weave tape.
B. Avoid trying to provide support with elastic bandages; a brace, overlap taping, or a cast may be needed.

ELEVATION

A. Elevate the joint above the level of the heart to reduce swelling.
B. Apply cold compresses while the joint is elevated.

EXERCISE THERAPY

A. Begin exercise therapy after the initial 48-hour period if pain and swelling begin to resolve.
B. Do gentle range-of-motion exercises several times a day within limits of pain for 7 to 10 days after knee ligament strain.
C. Exercise after 6 minutes of icing to take advantage of the cold's numbing effect.
D. Start with nonresistive, nonweight-bearing exercises.
E. Use exercises that improve range of motion and strength.
F. Maintain fitness of the extremity.

RINGWORM (TINEA)

PROBLEM

Ringworm is a fungal infection of the skin, which can be found on any part of the body. A worm does not cause ringworm; it gets the name because of the round ring shape that is red on the outside and normal on the inside. It is not uncommon to get more than one time. Other tinea fungal infections are:
A. Tinea pedis (athlete's foot)
B. Tinea cruris (jock itch)
C. Tinea capitis (ringworm on the head)

CAUSE

The fungus is transmitted by direct contact. It can be transmitted from objects, shoes, locker rooms, animals, and people.

PREVENTION

A. Use good hygiene, including not sharing hairbrushes and combs.
B. Keep skin cool and dry.
C. Wear shoes in locker rooms and around pools.
D. Wear loose-fitting clothing.
E. Treat pets' skin problems adequately. Ringworm is often blamed on cats, but it can come from almost any animal, including horses, rabbits, dogs, and pigs.
F. Infections of fingernails and toenails may require prescription medications.

TREATMENT PLAN

Activity: As tolerated. Some contact sports may increase contracting tinea (football and wrestling).
Diet: There is no special diet.
Medications:

You Have Been Prescribed: _____

You Need to Take: _____

You Need to Notify the Office If:
A. Your symptoms get worse.

B. Other: _____

Phone: _____

ROCKY MOUNTAIN SPOTTED FEVER AND REMOVAL OF A TICK

PROBLEM

Ticks are vectors for Lyme disease and Rocky Mountain spotted fever. You have been diagnosed with Rocky Mountain spotted fever.

CAUSE

Rocky Mountain spotted fever is caused by a bacterium from ticks.

PREVENTION/CARE

A. Avoid areas with large deer populations.
B. Wear light-colored clothes to make ticks easier to spot. Wear long sleeves and tuck pants into the socks to form a barrier.
C. Stick to hiking trails. Avoid contact with overgrown foliage. Ticks prefer dense woods with thick growth of shrubs and small trees as well as areas along the edge of the woods.
D. Check for ticks after each outdoor activity, especially in hairy regions of the body and beltline, where ticks often attach. Check for ticks before bathing, especially at the back of the neck, knees, and ears.
E. Remove ticks promptly.
F. Inspect pets daily and remove ticks when present.
G. Some manufacturers currently offer permethrin-treated clothing that is effective for up to 20 washings. This clothing is not recommended for children.
H. Antibiotic therapy to prevent Rocky Mountain spotted fever is not recommended for tick exposure. Instead, tell your healthcare provider if any symptoms, especially fever and headache, occur in the following 14 days.
I. Use tick repellent with diethyltoluamide (DEET; except for small children younger than 2 years). As an alternative, picaridin and oil of eucalyptus preparations have been approved for use as repellents by the EPA.

Precautions When Removing Ticks

A. Do not hold a lighted match or cigarette to the tick. Do not apply gasoline, kerosene, or oil to the tick's body.
B. Avoid squeezing the body of the tick.
C. Grasp the tick with a fine-tip tweezer close to the skin. Remove by gently pulling the tick upward straight out without using any twisting motions (see Figure III.7).
D. In the home, if fingers are used to remove ticks, they should be protected with facial tissue or gloves and washed after removal of the tick.
E. Do not crush the tick during removal.
F. **Save the tick for identification in case you become ill. Write the date of the tick bite on paper and place the paper and the tick in a resealable baggie and place it in the freezer.**

TREATMENT PLAN

Activity: Regular activity as tolerated. Tepid sponge baths may be taken for fever.
Diet: Eat a regular diet. Drink 8 to 10 glasses of water daily.
Medications:
A. Acetaminophen (Tylenol) may be taken for body aches.
B. You may be given antibiotics for a secondary infection if needed.

(*continued*)

ROCKY MOUNTAIN SPOTTED FEVER AND REMOVAL OF A TICK (*continued*)

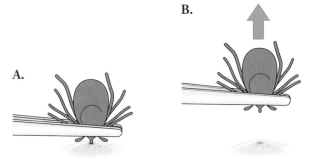

FIGURE III.7 A. Grasp the tick's body as close to the skin as possible using a fine-tip tweezer. Avoid squeezing the tick's body. B. Remove by pulling the tick straight upward without using twisting motions.

You Have Been Prescribed: _____

You Need to Take: _____

Take all of your antibiotics even if you feel better.

You Need to Notify the Office If You Have:
A. No improvement while on antibiotic therapy
B. Decreased urinary output, or dryness of your skin or mouth

C. Other: _____

Phone: _____

ROUNDWORMS AND PINWORMS

PROBLEM

Roundworms and pinworms are intestinal parasites. Roundworms look like earthworms; pinworms are small, white, and threadlike. Both types of worms thrive in the intestinal tract and are very common in children. They can spread to other family members, so the entire family needs to be treated.

CAUSE

Pinworms live in the human rectum or colon and come out during the night onto the skin around the anus. Pinworms are transmitted from person to person by direct transfer of infective eggs to the mouth, or by indirect transfer through clothing, bedding, food, or other items contaminated with the eggs. Nighttime itching is one of the main symptoms of pinworms.

Roundworm eggs enter the human body by drinking contaminated water or eating contaminated food or by transfer from contaminated unwashed hands.

PREVENTION/CARE

The following measures help prevent the spread of worms:
A. Remove sources of infection by treating the infected person and family members.
B. Household measures:
   1. Wash (132°F) or boil soiled bed sheets, nightclothes, underwear, towels, and washcloths used by infected persons.
   2. Soak fabrics that cannot be boiled in an ammonia solution: One cup of household ammonia to 5 gallons of cold water
   3. After treatment, scrub toilet seats, bathroom floors, and fixtures. Vacuum rugs, and clean table tops, curtains, sofas, and chairs carefully.
C. Practice good personal hygiene. Wash hands before handling foods and eating, and after using the toilet. Wash the anus and genitals with warm water and soap at least twice a day. Rinse well and then wash your hands.
D. Take a morning bath to remove most eggs. Other people should not take a bath in the same water.
E. Keep fingers away from the mouth. Cut nails and discourage nail biting and scratching the bare anal area.
F. Clean fingernails before meals and after BMs.
G. Reduce overcrowding when possible.
H. For roundworms: Have pets treated, and avoid stray animals.

TREATMENT PLAN

Parasitic infection is easily treated with medication. All family members need to be treated.

Activity: Resume normal activities after treatment is complete and symptoms improve.
Diet: No special foods are needed.
Medication: There are medications available to treat round worm and pin worm infections. Your provider may want people who live with you to take medications to prevent its spread.

You Have Been Prescribed: _____

You Need to Take: _____

You Need to Notify the Office If You Have:
A. Reappearance of worms after treatment
B. New or unexplained symptoms. Drugs used in treatment may produce side effects.

C. Other: _____

Phone: _____

SCABIES

PROBLEM

Scabies is a common condition characterized by severe itching. You may have noticed small burrows between your fingers and in other locations, or you may have some redness and skin irritation that is aggravated by scratching.

CAUSE

Scabies is caused by an infestation of the skin by a mite. You contract scabies by coming in close contact with an individual who has the condition.

PREVENTION/CARE

You can prevent reinfection of scabies by following these measures:
A. Make sure all close contacts, sexual partners, family, and household contacts are treated.
B. All bedding and clothing that have in contact with the infected skin should be machine washed and machine dried on the highest heat cycle.
C. Any clothing or bedding that cannot be laundered in the way previously mentioned should be placed in a plastic bag that is securely tied for at least a week. The mites cannot live this long away from human skin.
D. Coats, furniture, rugs, floors, and walls do not require any special cleaning or treatment.

TREATMENT PLAN

A. Most clients with scabies are successfully treated with only one overnight application of a cream known as a scabicide.
B. You should let your practitioner know if you are pregnant or breastfeeding.
C. You may itch for up to a week even with successful treatment.
D. If you still have symptoms after 2 weeks, you should see your practitioner, who will determine if you need a second treatment.

Activity: Affected children in day care or school can return the day after treatment is completed.
Diet: There is no special diet.
Medications: The most common medications used to treat scabies include:
A. Permethrin (Elimite cream), which is applied to all body areas from the neck down and washed off in 8 to 14 hours
B. Lindane (Kwell cream), which is applied to all skin surfaces from the neck down and washed off in 8 to 12 hours
C. You may be told to use Benadryl 25 to 50 mg if needed for itching.
D. Do not use near your eyes.

You Have Been Prescribed: _____

You Need to Take: _____

You Need to Notify the Office If:
A. You have new symptoms.
B. You have a reaction to the medication.

C. Other: _____

Phone: _____

SEBORRHEIC DERMATITIS

PROBLEM

Seborrheic dermatitis is a skin condition characterized by greasy or dry, white, flaking scales over reddish patches on the skin. The scales anchor to the hair shafts and may itch, but they are usually painless unless complicated by infection.

CAUSE

The cause is unknown. The risk of seborrheic dermatitis increases with stress; hot and humid or cold and dry weather; infrequent shampoos; oily skin; and other skin disorders such as rosacea, acne, or psoriasis; obesity; Parkinson's disease; use of lotions that contain alcohol; and HIV/AIDS.

PREVENTION/CARE

A. There are no specific preventive measures.
B. The goal of care is to minimize the severity or frequency of symptoms:
   1. Shampoo vigorously and as often as once a day. The type of shampoo is not as important as the way you scrub your scalp. To loosen scales, scrub with your fingernails while shampooing, and scrub at least 5 minutes.
   2. If you suffer from minor dandruff, you may use nonprescription dandruff shampoos with selenium sulfide (Selsun Blue, Exsel) or zinc pyrithione (Zincon) and lubricating skin lotion.
   3. For severe problems, shampoos that contain coal tar or scalp creams that contain cortisone may be prescribed. **Do not use coal tar products on infants or children without specific physician prescription.**
   4. To apply medication to the scalp, part the hair a few strands at a time, and rub the ointment or lotion vigorously into the scalp.
   5. Topical steroids may be prescribed for other affected parts of the skin.
   6. Be sure to dry skin folds thoroughly after bathing.
   7. Wear loose, ventilating clothing. Avoid constant cap wearing.

TREATMENT PLAN

Activity: No restrictions. Outdoor activities in the summer may help alleviate symptoms.
Diet: Eat a well-balanced diet. Drink 8 to 10 glasses of water per day. Avoid foods that seem to worsen your condition.
Medications:

You Have Been Prescribed: _____

You Need to Take: _____

You Need to Notify the Office If:
A. You have an adverse reaction to any of the prescribed medications.
B. You are unable to tolerate any of the medications.
C. You have any secondary infection in affected area.

D. Other: _____

Phone: _____

SHORTNESS OF BREATH

PROBLEM

You have been diagnosed with shortness of breath. Shortness of breath may be due to different reasons, or a combination of reasons. The symptom can come on suddenly or develop slowly, over several months. Some common reasons for shortness of breath are listed subsequently.

CAUSES

A. Being overweight or out of shape
B. Heart or lung disorders
C. Asthma
D. Infections of the upper or lower respiratory systems
E. Pregnancy
F. Nervousness/excessive stress
G. Allergies

PREVENTION/CARE

A. There is no way to prevent shortness of breath that is due to an underlying cause. It can be treated, however, by dealing the underlying disorder.
B. One way to help discover the cause of your shortness of breath is to keep a "diary" of what makes the symptoms worse, and how often it happens.

TREATMENT PLAN

A. You should see your healthcare provider to have your shortness of breath evaluated.
B. Based on the reason for your shortness of breath, a more active lifestyle may be recommended.
C. Everyone's shortness of breath is different and discovering the cause of your symptoms is important to determine your treatment.

Activity:
A. Your recommended activity level is based on the cause of your shortness of breath.
Diet: There is no special diet for shortness of breath; furthermore certain foods make the symptoms worse.
Medications:
The medicines used to treat shortness of breath are chosen based on the underlying reason for the symptom.

You Need to Call the Office Immediately If:
A. Your shortness of breath comes on suddenly or has worsened.

B. Other: _____

Phone: _____

RESOURCES

COPD Foundation: https://www.copdfoundation.org
National Emphysema Foundation: www.emphysemafoundation.org
Breathlessness from the American Thoracic Society: https://www.thoracic.org/patients/patient-resources/resources/breathlessness.pdf

SINUSITIS

PROBLEM

Sinusitis (sinus infection) is classified as an acute, subacute, or chronic condition. In acute sinusitis, the sinus inflammation is resolved after treatment. In subacute sinusitis, there are persistent symptoms despite treatment. In chronic sinusitis, episodes of prolonged inflammation continue longer than 3 months despite treatment.

CAUSE

Sinusitis occurs when the mucous lining in your sinus cavities becomes inflamed because of a virus, bacteria, or allergen. This can also occur after a cold or tooth abscess.

PREVENTION/CARE

A. If you have a tooth abscess, see your dentist and finish all your antibiotics.
B. Do not blow your nose too frequently or too hard. This will irritate the nasal tissue. It may also cause your eardrum to perforate (tear). Blow through both nostrils at the same time to equalize pressure.
C. To prevent spreading germs to others, cover your mouth when you cough:
   1. Use tissues when you blow your nose. Dispose of them and then wash your hands.
   2. If no tissue is available, do the "elbow sneeze" into the bend of your arm (away from your open hands).
D. Always wash your hands after coughing or using tissues.

TREATMENT PLAN

A. Avoid smoking and secondhand smoke.
B. Use steam inhalation to liquefy secretions.
C. Use a room humidifier. Keep your humidifier clean—it can grow bacteria.

Activity: There are no activity restrictions; however, diving, swimming, and flying may increase the occurrence of symptoms or make them worse. Make sure to get plenty of rest each day.
Diet: Eat a healthy diet. Drink at least 8 to 10 glasses of water every day.
Medications: Take all of your prescribed medications (antibiotics and/or steroids), even if you feel better.
Over-the-Counter Medications:
A. **Pain relievers:** Ibuprofen (Advil) or acetaminophen (Tylenol) as needed for facial pain
B. **Antihistamines:** Some antihistamines may cause drowsiness. Use with caution. You may consider using a different antihistamine during the day that does not cause drowsiness or take the medication before bed.
C. **Decongestants:** Decongestants may increase blood pressure and may also interact with other medications. Please consult with your provider before using these medications.
D. **Nasal sprays:** Nasal saline spray is safe to use in the nose several times a day. Nasal decongestant sprays may be used for a short period of time. Do not use longer than 3 days to prevent causing rebound side effects from this medication. Consult with your provider if you are using a nasal decongestant spray.

You Have Been Prescribed: _____

You Need to Take: _____

You Need to Call the Office If:
A. Your eyelids begin to swell or droop, or you experience decreased or double vision.
B. You have stiffness in your neck or increased fever.
C. You have asthma, and you are getting worse.
D. You begin vomiting and are unable to keep down your antibiotic.
E. You are a diabetic and your blood sugars are elevated, or you notice ketones in your urine.
F. You have confusion or difficulty thinking clearly.

G. Other: _____

Phone: _____

SKIN CARE ASSESSMENT

PROBLEM

Skin cancer is the most common type of cancer. In 2006, the Centers for Disease Control and Prevention (CDC) noted that the rate of skin cancer varies by the state where you live. A state map is located on the Internet at www.cdc.gov/cancer/skin/statistics/state.htm.

CAUSE

Skin cancer is frequently caused by damage from the UV rays of the sun. Some people are at a higher risk of developing skin cancer. These risk factors include:
A. Fair complexion
B. Advanced age with sun-damaged skin
C. A history of severe sunburn
D. A history of spending long hours outdoors
E. Having a history of x-ray procedures for skin conditions
F. Genetic susceptibility

PREVENTION/CARE

A. Protect yourself and prevent sun exposure to your skin by staying out of the harmful rays as much as possible, especially between the hours of 11:00 a.m. and 2:30 p.m. This time frame accounts for approximately 70% of the harmful UV radiation.
B. If you are exposed to the sun, wear a sunscreen product with an SPF of 15 or greater at all times.
C. Wear hats that screen your face and neck, as well as your ears.
D. Clothing is available with sun-protective materials. Regular long shirts and long pants also help to protect your skin.
E. Sit in the shade to rest.
F. Do not use a tanning booth.

Steps to Take to Prevent Yourself From Being a Victim of Skin Cancer
A. Examine your skin monthly:
  1. Use a good light source and a mirror to see areas of your skin not clearly visible.
  2. Examine your entire body closely.
  3. Pay particular attention to areas that are frequently exposed to the sun, especially your face, lips, eyes, neck, scalp, and ears.
  4. Monthly screening allows you to familiarize yourself with birthmarks and moles. Note the size, shape, and color of these marks. Note any changes in these marks, using the "ABCDE" method:
    a. *Asymmetry:* The shape of the mark should be noted. Any change in shape or irregularity of the mark needs to be evaluated by your healthcare provider.
    b. *Border:* Look carefully at the border of the mark. If the border edge is ragged, notched, and not smooth, your healthcare provider needs to evaluate it.
    c. *Color:* Note the color of moles. If you notice any change in color, or if you notice the mole to have several colors (brown, black, tan, red, etc.), you need to alert your healthcare provider.
    d. *Diameter:* Measure the size of the mark and document it. Any change in size, especially if it is greater than 6 mm, should be brought to the attention of your healthcare provider.
    e. *Elevation:* Note elevation of the lesion, change in size, and any evolving changes of the lesion. You need to alert your healthcare provider if changes occur.
  5. You should also evaluate lesions on your skin for any type of change. If the lesions begin bleeding or hurting, or change in texture or in any other way, your healthcare provider needs to evaluate the change.
  6. Be alerted to any skin ulcers that do not heal within 1 month. Also, any new moles or lesions need to be evaluated by your healthcare provider for proper diagnosis of the type of lesion.

(*continued*)

SKIN CARE ASSESSMENT   (*continued*)

TREATMENT PLAN

Activity: As tolerated, but protect yourself from sun exposure.

Diet: There is no special diet that will stop skin cancer.

Medications: There are no medications that prevent skin cancer.

You Need to Notify the Office If You Have:

A. Any of the skin changes mentioned previously that need to be evaluated by your healthcare provider

Phone: _____

SLEEP APNEA

PROBLEM

You have been diagnosed with sleep apnea. During your sleep your tongue and throat relax, causing less air to go down into your lungs. When you sleep and snore you have short periods when you stop breathing and may wake up gasping for breath. Your bed partner may shake you awake because of your loud snoring or may notice that you have stopped breathing. The sleep apnea makes you very tired, leading you to take daytime naps.

CAUSES

A. Being overweight and having a "thick neck" can cause sleep apnea.
B. As you get older you are more likely to have sleep apnea.
C. After menopause, women may start having sleep apnea.
D. If you have not had your tonsils removed, they may be part of the problem as your tongue and throat relax.
E. Alcohol and some medicines cause sleep apnea.
F. Allergies may also cause some sleep apnea.

PREVENTION/CARE

A. There is no way to prevent sleep apnea once you have it.
B. One way to help your sleep apnea is to lose weight.

TREATMENT PLAN

A. Review all of your medicines and any herbal products with your healthcare provider.
B. You may be told to sleep with your head up on two pillows, use a tennis ball under your pillow, or even sleep with a backpack under your pillow. This raises your head up higher and prevents your tongue from making your wind pipe smaller.
C. You may also need a mouthpiece to help your tongue from relaxing when you sleep. Your dentist will need to help you find the best one.
D. You may be sent to a lung specialist to help with your treatment.
E. You may be told you need to have a sleep study to check out and measure how often you stop breathing at night.
F. After your sleep study, your lung specialist may order you to have a sleep machine called continuous positive airway pressure (CPAP) or biphasic positive airway pressure (BiPAP).
   1. The sleep machine uses nose tubing, a nasal mask, or a full face mask.
   2. The machine is small and portable.
   3. Your CPAP machine can be taken through the airport.
   4. You will have a supplier who will send you more tubing and breathing tubes/masks on a regular schedule.

Activity:
A. You will continuously need to sleep with your head higher , use the mouth piece, or use the sleep machine to keep from having sleep apnea.
B. Exercise; losing even a small amount of weight will help with sleep apnea.
C. Stop smoking.
D. Avoid alcohol, especially near your bedtime.
Diet: There is no special diet for sleep apnea, but losing weight helps.

(*continued*)

SLEEP APNEA *(continued)*

Medications:

There are no medicines for sleep apnea.

You Need to Notify the Office If:

A. Your bed partner complains that your snoring or sleep apnea has worsened.

B. You want to make an appointment to discuss having a sleep study.

C. Other: _____

Phone: _____

RESOURCE

National Sleep Foundation: www.sleepfoundation.org

SLEEP DISORDERS/INSOMNIA

PROBLEM

Continued loss of sleep over a long period (several days to weeks) can produce a decrease in daytime awareness and functioning, as well as work and driving impairment.

CAUSE

Most sleep difficulties are related to situational problems and are best treated without medications. Medical illness may also predispose you to a sleeping disorder.

PREVENTION/CARE

A. Practice good "sleep hygiene." Here are a few tips:
   1. Try to get to bed at the same time every night (even on weekends).
   2. Plan for 8 hours of sleep.
   3. Maintain the same waking time every morning (even on weekends).
   4. Reserve the bedroom for sleeping. Do not do your work/homework in the bed. Do not watch TV in the bedroom, unless you sit in a chair. Do not read in bed.
   5. Put your children in their own beds/bedrooms.
   6. Try a small bedtime snack.
   7. Do not drink any liquids for at least 1 hour before going to bed. This helps prevent getting up to go to the bathroom during the night.
   8. Review all of your prescription medications, over-the-counter (OTC) drugs, and herbal products with your healthcare provider to evaluate if the drugs are making you stay awake.
   9. Avoid alcohol and tobacco.
B. If you do not get a restful night of sleep, awaken yourself snoring, or your partner complains of your snoring, gasping, or stopping breathing, you may need to have a sleep study.

TREATMENT PLAN

A. Develop a "sleeping ritual": Wear your favorite pajamas and use your favorite pillows.
B. Keep the room dark and quiet. Try not to use a nightlight.
C. Run a small fan for background noise.
D. Arise promptly in the morning.
E. Avoid sleeping medication if possible.
F. Try some relaxation exercises, like yoga, self-hypnosis, or meditation. There are many books on these subjects that will assist you in developing good sleep hygiene. (Try your local library or bookstore.)
G. Keep a sleep diary to help identify the causes of your inability to sleep.
H. Discuss snoring and your partner's concerns about your breathing and the need for a sleep study.

Activity: Regular exercise during the day helps. (Do not exercise vigorously 1 hour before your bedtime—this could keep you awake.)

Relaxation techniques, such as progressive relaxation, biofeedback, self-hypnosis, and meditation, are helpful when done before bedtime. Avoid vigorous mental activities late in the evening.

Diet:
A. Avoid caffeinated drinks, including coffee, tea, and soda.
B. Avoid large meals in the evening.
C. Eat a nutritious balanced diet.
D. Limit your liquids to early evening. Do not drink water after 8 p.m.

(*continued*)

SLEEP DISORDERS/INSOMNIA *(continued)*

Medications: Discuss the need for *short-term* medications to help you sleep.

You Have Been Prescribed: _____

You Need to Take: _____

You Need to Notify the Office If You Have:

A. No relief of your symptoms and you are following the previous recommendations
B. No relief of your symptoms and you are taking your medications as directed
C. Feelings of depression or thoughts of hurting yourself or others
D. Noticeable physical symptoms that were not mentioned in your office visit or any new symptoms that you are concerned about

E. Other _____

Phone: _____

RESOURCES

National Institutes of Health: www.health.nih.gov/topic/SleepDisorders
National Sleep Foundation: www.sleepfoundation.org

SUPERFICIAL THROMBOPHLEBITIS

PROBLEM

Superficial thrombophlebitis occurs when a vein is irritated or injured. The portion of the vein that is affected can develop a blood clot or become infected, causing redness, swelling, and pain. If untreated, the infection and/or blood clot can progress into a life-threatening condition like sepsis, DVT, or pulmonary embolism.

CAUSE

Many things can cause irritation and injury to veins. These include a recent IV line placed during a hospital stay, infection, some medications, and pregnancy. Some risk factors cannot be changed, like genetics, while others can be changed, including inactivity and excessive weight.

PREVENTION/CARE

A. Avoid standing or sitting for long periods of time.
B. If you smoke, stop or reduce the amount you smoke.
C. If overweight or obese, lose weight. Discuss what you can do to lose weight with your healthcare provider.

TREATMENT PLAN

A. Take your medications as ordered by your healthcare provider.
B. Raise the affected arm or leg whenever lying down to reduce pain and swelling.
C. Warm compresses to the affected area may reduce pain.
D. Wear compression stockings. Put them on before getting out of bed in the morning. Take them off just before going to bed at night.
E. Avoid standing or sitting for long periods of time.
F. Follow up with your primary healthcare provider on a regularly scheduled basis.

Activity:
A. Get regular exercise. Discuss with your healthcare provider what type and frequency of exercise is safe for you.
B. Exercise leg muscles by pumping ankles when sitting. Rocking in a rocking chair is another option.

Diet:
A. Discuss with your healthcare provider the type of diet that best suits your needs: Diabetic diet, low-fat diet, low-cholesterol diet, and/or low-sodium diet

Medications:

You Have Been Prescribed: _____

You Need to Take: _____

You Need to Notify the Office If You Have:
A. Fever greater than 101°F
B. Sudden shortness of breath
C. Chest pain
D. New pain, swelling, or warmth in an arm or leg
E. If you are taking a blood-thinning medication and have any of these symptoms:
    1. Vomit that is bright red or dark and looks like coffee grounds
    2. Bright-red blood in your stools or black, tarry stools
    3. Severe headache
    4. Sudden weakness in an arm or leg
    5. Memory loss or confusion

(continued)

SUPERFICIAL THROMBOPHLEBITIS (*continued*)

6. Sudden change in vision
7. Trouble speaking or understanding others

F. Other: _____

Phone: _____

RESOURCES

Mayo Clinic—Thrombophlebitis: mayoclinic.com/health/thrombophlebitis/DS00223

SYPHILIS

PROBLEM

You may have round or oval painless lesions, most commonly in the genital region, but they may occur anywhere on the body where transmission occurred.

A. You may experience a rash covering your body, including palms of hands and soles of feet.

B. **Flu-like symptoms** include fever; headache; sore throat; swollen, tender lymph nodes; and decreased appetite.

CAUSE

Syphilis is contracted by genital or oral contact with someone who has the infection. The infection is spread when lesions are present.

PREVENTION/CARE

A. Use condoms.

B. Limit sexual partners.

C. Screen new sexual partners by asking about any known infections.

TREATMENT PLAN

Do not engage in sexual activity while lesions are present. Notify all partners of the need for treatment. Keep follow-up appointments to determine if treatment has been effective.

Diet: There is no special diet.

Medications: Penicillin is the drug of choice for treating syphilis. Other antibiotics can be used if you are allergic to penicillin. Within 24 hours of receiving antibiotic treatment, you may experience a fever or headache. Aspirin, acetaminophen (Tylenol), or ibuprofen may be taken if these symptoms occur.

You Have Been Prescribed: _____

You Need to Take: _____

You need to finish all of your antibiotics.

You Need to Notify the Office If You Have:

A. Any new symptoms

B. Any reaction to your antibiotics

C. Any other concerns about syphilis

Phone: _____

SYSTEMIC LUPUS ERYTHEMATOSUS

PROBLEM

You have been diagnosed with a condition called systemic lupus erythematosus (SLE) or lupus. Lupus is a chronic, inflammatory, autoimmune disorder. There is currently no cure for lupus; however, it can be managed and can go into remission or a dormant state. Rashes, hair loss, arthritis-like joint pain, and fatigue are very common problems with lupus.

CAUSE

Lupus causes your body to attack its own cells. The exact cause is unknown. Lupus tends to run in families, but it is not contagious.

PREVENTION/CARE

There is no known prevention measure, but long-term management is possible.

TREATMENT PLAN

A. Avoid sun exposure:
  1. Many lupus clients' eyes are sensitive to light; wear sunglasses, and avoid direct exposure.
  2. Light exposure can make your rash worse.
  3. Apply a protective lotion or sunscreen to your skin while outside.
  4. Wear long sleeves and use hats.
B. You may be given steroids for your skin rashes or lesions.
C. Avoid exposure to drugs and chemicals.
D. Review all of your medications and over-the-counter (OTC) drugs with your healthcare provider.
E. Avoid hair sprays and hair-coloring agents.
F. Mouth ulcers may occur with lupus:
  1. Avoid hot or spicy foods that might cause irritation to ulcers.
  2. Use good oral hygiene:
    a. Get regular dental examinations.
    b. Floss your teeth daily.
    c. Brush your teeth at least twice a day.
G. Rest and drugs called NSAIDs are used for minor joint pain.
H. It is very important for you to have your eyes examined **twice** a year to monitor any changes.
I. Talk to your healthcare provider if you are planning a pregnancy.

Activity: You may get tired more easily; plan rest periods. However, you should still get some exercise as tolerated. Many people gain some weight from steroids.
Diet: Eat a regular diet as tolerated; you do not need any special foods.
Medications:

You Have Been Prescribed the Following Steroid: _____

You Need to Take: _____

A. Do not stop taking your steroid abruptly.
B. **Steroid medication should be tapered off (decreased until you are off of it)**
You Need to Notify the Office If:
A. You are unable to tolerate your medication.
B. You have any sign of infections, sinusitis, bronchitis, flu, or urinary tract infections (UTIs).
C. You are getting worse or do not feel better.

(continued)

SYSTEMIC LUPUS ERYTHEMATOSUS   *(continued)*

D. You are planning a pregnancy or think you are pregnant

E. Other: _____

Phone: _____

RESOURCES

Lupus Foundation of America: 800-558-0121 or www.lupus.org
Lupus Research Institute: www.lupusresearchinstitute.org; 212-812-9881 e-mail: lupus@lupusny.org

TESTICULAR SELF-EXAMINATION

The testicular self-examination is easy to do and does not take very much time to perform. Checking every month is a good way to become familiar with this area of your body and will help detect testicular cancer.

Set a date for the same day every month. An easy way to remember is choosing the first day of the month, or the last day of the month, or your birth date. The best time to check your testicles is during or after a hot bath or shower. (Heat makes the testicles relax.)

Tumors can be felt. Boys and men from 15 to 35 years are at the highest risk because of hormonal activity.

PROCEDURE

A. If possible, do the self-examination in front of a mirror after a hot bath or shower.
B. Check for any swelling of the skin.
C. Support each testicle with one hand and examine it with the other hand.
D. Use both hands to feel the entire scrotal bag.
   1. With one hand, lift your penis, and check your sac with the other hand. Feel any change in shape or size.
   2. Look for red veins or veins that are bigger than they used to be.
   3. The left side may hang slightly lower than the right (this is normal).
E. Check each testicle.
   1. Place your left thumb on the front of your left testicle and your index and middle fingers behind it.
   2. Gently but firmly roll the testicle between your thumb and fingers.
   3. Then use your right hand to examine the right testicle the same way.
   4. The testicles should feel smooth, rubbery, oval shaped, and slightly tender. They should move freely.
   5. Locate the epididymis and spermatic cord. The epididymis is the irregular, cord-like structure on the top and the back of the testicle.
      a. Gently squeeze the spermatic cord above your left testicle between your thumb and the first two fingers of your left hand.
      b. Check for lumps and masses along the entire length of the cords.
      c. Repeat on the right side, using your right hand.
F. Call your healthcare provider if you notice:
   1. Any lumps, even small pea-sized ones
   2. Any masses, like a bag of worms
   3. A dull ache in the lower abdomen or in the groin
   4. A feeling of heaviness in the scrotum
   5. A significant loss of size in one of the testicles
   6. Pain or discomfort in a testicle or in the scrotum
   7. Any other changes since the last time you felt yourself for your examination
G. Your healthcare provider may refer you to a urologist for further evaluation.

TINEA VERSICOLOR

PROBLEM

A yeast infection of the skin, tinea versicolor, may cause color changes of the skin, commonly on the chest, back, shoulders, arms, and trunk. During the summer, these spots usually appear pale and do not tan. During the winter, the spots may appear pinker or darker than the normal skin color.

CAUSE

Tinea versicolor is caused by an increased production of yeast on the skin, which is influenced by warm, moist conditions. It is common to have recurring episodes.

PREVENTION/TREATMENT PLAN

A. Air dry skin as much as possible.
B. Apply medication as directed.
C. Patches on skin (color changes) may take several weeks to resolve.
D. Monthly treatments may help prevent recurrences

Activity: There are no activity restrictions with tinea versicolor.

Diet: There is no special diet.

Medications:

A. Apply Selsun Blue shampoo or other medication as directed.
B. Most medications may be washed off from skin 30 minutes after application.
C. Selsun Blue shampoo may be used daily on affected skin for 2 weeks.
D. Keep shampoo out of the eyes and genital area.
E. Leave it on skin for about 20 minutes and then rinse it off.

You Have Been Prescribed: _____

You Need to Take: _____

You Need to Notify the Office If You:

A. Do not see improvement, despite proper treatment
B. Develop new symptoms

C. Other: _____

Phone: _____

CLIENT TEACHING GUIDE

TINNITUS

PROBLEM

Tinnitus is the perception of sound heard in the ear and/or head with no external source. It may be in one or both ears.

CAUSE

Tinnitus is poorly understood, and the cause is not known. It probably originates in the brain, and not the ear. There is a strong association between tinnitus, stress, anxiety, and depression.

TREATMENT PLAN

A. A hearing evaluation will be performed to determine if there is hearing loss
B. A CT or MRI may be performed to rule out rare worrisome causes of the tinnitus
C. There are some medications that are used to help decrease the "ringing, buzzing" noise that you are hearing. Ask your healthcare provider about these medications.
D. Rest, exercise, and mindfulness meditation are encouraged to reduce stress, depression, and anxiety

Activity: There is no activity restriction.
Diet: Some foods may make the tinnitus worsen. Therefore, reducing the amount of sodium, nicotine, alcohol, and caffeine (tea, coffee, soft drinks) is encouraged.
Medications: Consider avoidance of aspirin. Aspirin may aggravate the severity of tinnitus.

You Have Been Prescribed: _____

You Need to Take: _____

You Need to Notify the Office if You Have:
A. Fever
B. Ear pain
C. Noticed a change in hearing loss or speech development
D. Any other new symptoms that occur

E. Other: _____

Phone: _____

TOXOPLASMOSIS

PROBLEM

Toxoplasmosis is an infection acquired through contact with infected cat feces or from eating raw or undercooked meat.

CAUSE

Toxoplasmosis is caused by a parasite. Cats are the primary host, and humans are the intermediate host. **You do not need to destroy your cat.**

PREVENTION/CARE

A. Avoid uncooked eggs and unpasteurized milk.
B. Wash hands after handling raw meat.
C. Meat should be thoroughly cooked at 152°F or higher, or frozen for 24 hours in a household freezer before eating (smoked meats and meats cured in brine are considered safe). Avoid tasting meat while cooking.
D. Wash fruits and vegetables before eating.
E. Wash all kitchen surfaces that come into contact with uncooked meats.
F. Avoid drinking unfiltered water in any setting.
G. Use care in gardening where cats have access.
H. Wear gloves for gardening and landscaping.
I. Wear gloves for handling kitty litter, and wash hands after contact with cats. **Change kitty litter daily.**
J. Keep outdoor sandboxes covered.
K. Domestic cats can be protected from infection by feeding them commercially prepared cat food and preventing them from eating undercooked kitchen scraps and hunting wild rodents.
L. If you are not pregnant and have toxoplasmosis, you should not get pregnant for at least 6 months.

TREATMENT PLAN

A. If you are pregnant, you may be referred to a specialist.
B. If you have AIDS, you will be referred to a specialist.

Activity: There is no activity restriction for toxoplasmosis.
Diet: There is no special diet for toxoplasmosis. Avoid uncooked eggs and unpasteurized milk. Meat should be thoroughly cooked.
Medications: Depending on your risk, you may be prescribed one or two medications. You may be required to take the medication for several weeks.

You Have Been Prescribed: _____

You Need to Take: _____

You Need to Notify the Office If You Have:
A. Headache, dull and constant, with no relief from acetaminophen (Tylenol)
B. Abnormal speech
C. Seizures
D. Loss of visual acuity
E. Poor concentration, forgetfulness
F. Personality changes

G. Other: _____

Phone: _____

TRANSIENT ISCHEMIC ATTACK

PROBLEM/CAUSE

A transient ischemic attack (TIA) is a temporary loss of brain function due to a decrease of blood flow to the brain. It is considered a mini stroke. The symptoms may last only a few minutes, but the risk for a stroke is increased over the next week.

RISK FACTORS FOR TIAs

A. High blood pressure
B. Irregular heartbeat (atrial fibrillation)
C. Smoking
D. High cholesterol
E. Being overweight
F. Diabetes
G. Obstructive sleep apnea

WARNING SIGNS OF A TIA

A. Weakness or numbness of face, arm, or leg on one side of the body
B. Trouble talking or understanding others when they talk
C. Changes in eyesight such as dimness, double vision, or loss of vision
D. Dizziness, unsteadiness, or sudden falls
E. Sudden severe headaches
F. If you experience any of these signs, seek medical attention (call 911) immediately.

PREVENTION/CARE

A. A full workup is necessary to decide why you are having TIAs.
B. You may be referred to a neurologist—a doctor who specializes in medical problems involving the brain.
C. Special tests or surgery may be done to evaluate your heart and blood vessels. Cardiac procedures may be performed to insert a stent into the artery or remove a blockage from the artery. Other treatment depends on your test results.
D. Treatment starts with modifying your risk factors. Weight loss, eating a healthy diet, lowering your cholesterol, and eliminating alcohol in your diet are encouraged. If you are a diabetic, you must keep your diabetes under control to lower your risk.
E. Do not smoke or use any tobacco products or electronic cigarettes.
F. Aspirin is commonly prescribed after a TIA. You may be prescribed a blood thinner. Some blood thinners require regular laboratory testing. Discuss treatment with your healthcare provider.

If you are taking a blood thinner, get a medic alert bracelet/necklace, or carry a card in your wallet and car in case you are in an accident. Medic alert jewelry can be purchased at local drug stores, and there are multiple websites for ordering a medic alert identification. You can build your own identification bracelets or neck chains from American Medical ID: https://www.americanmedical-id.com.

Activity: You need to exercise at least 30 minutes daily three to four times a week. Please make sure you have been released by your healthcare provider to begin exercising.
Diet: Eat a low-fat, low-cholesterol, and low-sodium diet.
Medications:

You Have Been Prescribed: _____

You Need to Take: _____

Phone: _____

RESOURCES

American Heart Association: https://www.heart.org
National Stroke Association: https://www.stroke.org/

TRICHOMONIASIS

PROBLEM

You may experience increased vaginal discharge that is yellow-green or watery gray in color. It may have a foul odor. You may also have vaginal itching or irritation, burning during urination, discomfort during sexual intercourse, spotting or bleeding during or after sexual intercourse, or abdominal discomfort.

CAUSE

Trichomonas vaginalis is acquired by having sex with someone who has the infection.

PREVENTION/CARE

A. Use condom with each act of intercourse.
B. Limit the number of sexual partners.
C. Screen new sexual partners.

TREATMENT PLAN

Do not have sexual activity until you and your partner have both completed your medications. There are no limitations in other physical activity.

Diet: Do not drink alcohol during the use of medication and for 3 days after taking the last dose of your medicine. Alcohol use while taking this medication may result in nausea, vomiting, and severe upset stomach. You may have a metallic taste from the medicine that may slightly alter the taste of food. No other limitations in diet are required.
Medications: Metronidazole (Flagyl) is used to treat the infection.

You Have Been Prescribed: _____

You Need to Take: _____

Finish all of the medication.

You Need to Notify the Office If:
A. You are unable to tolerate the medicine.
B. Any new symptoms develop.

C. Other: _____

Phone: _____

ULCER

PROBLEM

An ulcer is a sore in the lining of the stomach or intestine that occurs in areas exposed to acid and pepsin. People with ulcer may experience upper abdominal pain, heart burn, nausea, vomiting, and blood in the stools. Complications include bleeding ulcer, perforation, and obstruction. These complications can be life threatening.

CAUSE

Although the exact cause of ulcer formation is not completely understood, the process appears to involve excess acid. A type of bacteria called *Helicobacter pylori* and certain medications have been suggested as causing ulcers.

PREVENTION/CARE

Modify your lifestyle to include health practices that prevent recurrences of ulcer pain and bleeding.

TREATMENT PLAN

A. If aspirin or a nonsteroidal anti-inflammatory drug (NSAID) causes the ulcer, eliminate the drug. If you need the drug for other health problems, discuss other options with your healthcare provider. You may need to stop the medicine or take a lower dose.
B. Avoid caffeine, colas, alcohol, and chocolate because they may increase acid production.
C. Stop smoking: It slows the ulcer's healing and increases its chance of coming back.
D. Be sure to tell healthcare providers about your history of ulcer and GI pain if you need new prescriptions or are sent to the hospital.
E. Review all of your medications, OTC medications, and herbal products for possible causes or ulcer irritants.

Activity: Exercise daily, plan rest periods, avoid fatigue, and learn to cope with or avoid stressful situations.
Diet:
A. Eat a well-balanced diet with high-fiber content.
B. Eat meals at regular intervals. Frequent small feedings are unnecessary. Avoid bedtime snacks.
C. Eliminate foods that cause pain or distress; otherwise, your diet is usually not restricted. Examples of foods that cause worse pain are:
   1. Peppermint
   2. Spicy food
   3. Alcohol
D. Avoid extremely hot or cold food or fluids, chew thoroughly, and eat slowly while relaxed for better digestion.

Medications:
A. Acid blockers and medicines called proton pump inhibitors (PPIs) reduce stomach acid.
B. You may need to take antibiotics to fight *H. pylori* infection.
C. Other medications may be prescribed to coat the ulcer area. Antacids can be taken during the ulcer treatment, but should not be used 1 hour before or 2 hours after the ulcer treatment medications because antacids can interfere with absorption.
D. Take the entire prescription: Do not stop when you feel better.
E. If you have been prescribed metronidazole (Flagyl) or clarithromycin, you may notice a metallic taste in your mouth
F. Alcohol (including wine) should be avoided when taking Flagyl. The interaction can cause skin flushing, headache, nausea, and vomiting.
G. If you are prescribed bismuth, you may notice black BMs.

You Have Been Prescribed: _____

You Need to Take: _____

(*continued*)

ULCER   *(continued)*

You Need to Notify the Office If You Have:

A. Worsening symptoms while taking your medication

B. Vomiting that is bloody or looks like coffee grounds

C. Tar-colored or "grape jelly" BMs. If this occurs, bring a stool sample to the office.

D. Diarrhea and/or severe pain despite treatment

E. Unusual weakness or paleness

F. Other: _____

Phone: _____

URINARY INCONTINENCE: WOMEN

PROBLEM

Urinary incontinence is the condition in which you are unable to hold your urine.

CAUSE

The cause depends on the type of incontinence you have.

PREVENTION/CARE

Exercise regularly and practice pelvic floor exercises, commonly called Kegel exercises. Do not become constipated so you do not strain to have a BM. Stop smoking. If you have a cough, you may need to see your healthcare provider to help treat it.

TREATMENT PLAN

Treatment depends on the cause and type of incontinence. Fill out the bladder diary to help figure out what kind of problem you have (see the following table).

A. Pelvic floor exercises should be done every morning, afternoon, and evening; repeat the exercise five times for each set, gradually increase to 10 times each set. To perform these exercises:
   1. Start by doing your pelvic muscle exercises lying down. When your muscles get stronger, do your exercises while sitting or standing.
   2. Do not tighten your tummy, leg, or butt muscles: Just squeeze the muscles you use to start and stop the flow of urine.
   3. Do not hold your breath or practice while you are on the toilet urinating.
   4. Pull in pelvic muscles and hold it tight for a count of 5.
   5. Repeat five times.
   6. Work up to doing 3 sets of 10 repeats.
   7. Kegel exercises take just a few minutes a day, and most women notice an improvement after a few weeks of daily exercise.
B. Empty your bladder frequently. As soon as you feel the urge to urinate, go to the bathroom.
C. You may be taught relaxation techniques to control the feeling of having to go quickly.
D. Fill out your bladder diary and return it to your healthcare provider.

Activity: Try to get daily exercise. Use absorbent undergarments until your bladder leaking is under control.
Diet: Eat a well-balanced diet. If you are overweight, consider a weight-loss program. Avoid drinking lots of liquids, especially caffeinated beverages and alcohol.
Medications: What you take depends on the type of bladder leakage you have.

You Have Been Prescribed: _____

You Need to Take: _____

You Need to Notify the Office If You Have: _____

Phone: _____

RESOURCES

American Urogynecologic Society: www.augs.org
American Urological Association: www.UrologyHealth.org
National Association for Continence: www.nafc.org
Simon Foundation for Continence: https://simonfoundation.org

(*continued*)

URINARY INCONTINENCE: WOMEN   (*continued*)

BLADDER CONTROL DIARY

Your Daily Bladder Diary
This diary will help you and your healthcare team figure out the causes of your bladder control trouble. The "sample" line shows you how to use the diary. Use this sheet as a master for making copies that you can use as a bladder diary for as many days as you need.
Your name: _____
Date: _____

Time	Drinks		Trips to the Bathroom		Accidental Leaks	Did You Feel a Strong Urge to Go?	What Were You Doing at the Time?
	What kind?	*How much?*	*How many times?*	*How much urine? (circle one)*	*How much? (circle one)*	Circle one	*Sneezing, exercising, having sex, lifting, etc.*
Sample	Coffee	2 cups	✓ ✓	⊙ ○ ○ sm med lg	○ ⊙ ○ sm med lg	Yes (No)	Running
6–7 a.m.				○ ○ ○	○ ○ ○	Yes No	
7–8 a.m.				○ ○ ○	○ ○ ○	Yes No	
8–9 a.m.				○ ○ ○	○ ○ ○	Yes No	
9–10 a.m.				○ ○ ○	○ ○ ○	Yes No	
10–11 a.m.				○ ○ ○	○ ○ ○	Yes No	
11–12 noon				○ ○ ○	○ ○ ○	Yes No	
12–1 p.m.				○ ○ ○	○ ○ ○	Yes No	
1–2 p.m.				○ ○ ○	○ ○ ○	Yes No	
2–3 p.m.				○ ○ ○	○ ○ ○	Yes No	
3–4 p.m.				○ ○ ○	○ ○ ○	Yes No	
4–5 p.m.				○ ○ ○	○ ○ ○	Yes No	
5–6 p.m.				○ ○ ○	○ ○ ○	Yes No	
6–7 p.m.				○ ○ ○	○ ○ ○	Yes No	
7–8 p.m.				○ ○ ○	○ ○ ○	Yes No	
8–9 p.m.				○ ○ ○	○ ○ ○	Yes No	
9–10 p.m.				○ ○ ○	○ ○ ○	Yes No	
10–11 p.m.				○ ○ ○	○ ○ ○	Yes No	
11–12 midnight				○ ○ ○	○ ○ ○	Yes No	
12–1 a.m.				○ ○ ○	○ ○ ○	Yes No	
1–2 a.m.				○ ○ ○	○ ○ ○	Yes No	

(*continued*)

URINARY INCONTINENCE: WOMEN *(continued)*

BLADDER CONTROL DIARY *(continued)*

Time	Drinks		Trips to the Bathroom		Accidental Leaks	Did You Feel a Strong Urge to Go?	What Were You Doing at the Time?
	What kind?	*How much?*	*How many times?*	*How much urine? (circle one)*	*How much? (circle one)*	*Circle one*	*Sneezing, exercising, having sex, lifting, etc.*
2–3 a.m.				◯ ◯ ◯	◯ ◯ ◯	Yes No	
3–4 a.m.				◯ ◯ ◯	◯ ◯ ◯	Yes No	
4–5 a.m.				◯ ◯ ◯	◯ ◯ ◯	Yes No	
5–6 a.m.				◯ ◯ ◯	◯ ◯ ◯	Yes No	

I used _____ pads today. I used _____ diapers today (write number).

Questions to ask my healthcare team: _____

_____

_____

_____

_____

Let's Talk About Bladder Control for Women is a public health awareness campaign conducted by the National Kidney and Urologic Diseases Information Clearinghouse (NKUDIC), an information dissemination service of the National Institute of Diabetes and Digestive and Kidney Diseases (NIDDK), National Institutes of Health.

Source: National Kidney and Urologic Diseases Information Clearinghouse, National Institutes of Health (NKUDIC, NIH). Retrieved from kidney.niddk.nih.gov/kudiseases/pubs/bcw_ez/insertB.htm

URINARY TRACT INFECTION (ACUTE CYSTITIS)

PROBLEM

You have a bladder infection. The symptoms include painful, frequent urination, and pain over the bladder. Your symptoms may be mild, moderate, or painful.

CAUSE

Bacteria is the cause for the bladder infection. A bladder infection is more common in women and in men who have prostate problems.

PREVENTION/CARE

A. Empty your bladder often:
　1. As soon as you feel the urge to go, empty your bladder at that time. Do not hold your urine.
　2. You may need to urinate on a schedule during the day, at least every 2 to 3 hours.
B. Wash your hands after going to the bathroom (both urine and BM).
C. Good hygiene for females:
　1. Wipe front to back every time you empty your bladder and especially after BM.
　2. Take showers instead of baths; do not take bubble baths.
　3. Empty your bladder before and after sex.
　4. Avoid feminine hygiene sprays and douches.
D. Wear cotton underwear. Do not wear tight underwear and clothes. Take off your underwear at night while sleeping.

TREATMENT PLAN

Treatment depends on how bad (severity) the infection is. Antibiotics are used to kill bacteria that cause infections. The most important thing is to finish all of your medications even if you feel better.

Activity: Rest; avoid strenuous activity. Avoid sexual activity until you finish the antibiotics.

Diet:
A. Increase fluids; drink at least one large glass of liquid every hour.
B. Avoid foods that irritate the bladder: Caffeine, alcohol, and spicy foods.
C. Drink cranberry juice to help fight bladder infections. If you do not like plain cranberry juice, mix it with another juice such as orange juice.

Medications:
A. Antibiotics kill bacteria that cause infection. Make sure you take all of your medications, not just until you feel better.
B. Take acetaminophen (Tylenol) for fever.
C. You may be prescribed a medication to prevent bladder spasms and pain while urinating. This changes the color of your urine to orange or blue.

You Have Been Prescribed the Following Antibiotics: _____

You Need to Take: _____

Take all of your antibiotics, even if you feel better.

You Have Been Prescribed the Following for Discomfort: _____

You Need to Take: _____

(*continued*)

URINARY TRACT INFECTION (ACUTE CYSTITIS)   *(continued)*

You Need to Notify the Office If You Have:

A. Worsening symptoms or symptoms not improving during treatment

B. Fever higher than 100.4°F

C. Blood in your urine

D. Symptoms that come back after you finish all of your medications: painful urination, back pain, fever, chills, or nausea

E. Other: _____

Phone: _____

URINARY TRACT INFECTION DURING PREGNANCY: PYELONEPHRITIS

PROBLEM

You have been diagnosed with an infection of the kidney (where urine is made). Bladder infections can spread to the kidney.

CAUSE

Bacteria from the bladder can move up to the kidney and cause a kidney infection. Other causes are blockage in the urine system or having a catheter, or tube, in the bladder.

PREVENTION/CARE

A. Urinate frequently. Do not hold urine for a long period.
B. Empty your bladder as soon as you feel it is filling.
C. Urinate before and after sexual intercourse.
D. After urinating, always wipe from front to back with toilet tissue.
E. Do not wear tight underwear or pants that can cause increased moistness and warmth in the perineal area.
F. Cotton panties are the best.
G. Wash your hands every time after going to the bathroom.
H. Do not use the same tissue that you blow your nose with to wipe after emptying your bladder: This spreads infection.

TREATMENT PLAN

Antibiotics kill the bacteria that cause infection.

Activity: Rest; do not engage in strenuous physical activity.
Diet: Increase fluids; drink at least one large glass of water every hour while you are awake. Drink cranberry juice to help fight and prevent urinary tract infections (UTIs). If you do not like the taste of cranberry juice, mix cranberry juice with another juice like grape juice.
Medications: You will be prescribed antibiotics to kill the bacteria causing infection. The drugs may be changed if your urine culture results show different bacteria. You may need mild pain relievers if you have a lot of back pain. Medications, such as Tylenol, may be used to bring down fever. You may be prescribed a medicine to stop bladder spasm and pain.

You Have Been Prescribed the Following Antibiotics: _____

You Need to Take: _____

Finish all of your antibiotics even if you feel better.

You Have Been Prescribed the Following for Bladder Spasms: _____

You Need to Take: _____

This medicine will make your urine turn a different color.

You Need to Notify the Office If You Have:
A. Symptoms that worsen or do not get better during treatment
B. New symptoms that develop during treatment
C. Symptoms that return after treatment when you finish all of your antibiotics
D. Difficulty taking your medication (you break out or vomit)

E. Other: _____

Phone: _____

VAGINAL BLEEDING: FIRST TRIMESTER

PROBLEM

Vaginal bleeding may occur in the first trimester of pregnancy. The amount of bleeding may range from spotting to a complete miscarriage.

CAUSE

Bleeding may occur for a variety of reasons, including smoking, trauma, abnormal fetus, or other problems.

PREVENTION/CARE

In most cases, the cause of vaginal bleeding may not be prevented. If bleeding is light, it may lessen or stop. You need to avoid sexual intercourse, tampons, and douches. If you smoke, it is highly recommended that you cut down and stop smoking.

TREATMENT PLAN

Treatment depends on the cause or suspected cause of your bleeding.

Activity:
A. Many women experience less bleeding and cramping while on limited activities or bed rest. Unfortunately, activity restriction does not prevent miscarriage.
B. Avoid sexual intercourse until at least 2 weeks after the bleeding has stopped, or until your provider tells you.
C. If bed rest is prescribed, perform simple ROM activities as directed by the practitioner. Examples are foot circles and moving legs in bed.
D. Do not use tampons during this period. Use pads so that you can evaluate how much you are bleeding.
   1. **Scant amount:** Blood only on tissue when wiped or less than 1-inch stain on Peri-Pad
   2. **Light amount:** Less than 4-inch stain on Peri-Pad
   3. **Moderate amount:** Less than 6-inch stain on Peri-Pad
   4. **Heavy amount:** Saturated Peri-Pad within 1 hour

Diet: As tolerated. If you are on bed rest, eat fresh vegetables, fruits, and bran cereal to avoid becoming constipated.

Medications: You may not be prescribed any medications.

You Need to Notify the Office If:
A. You develop a fever with your bleeding.
B. You have a gush of blood from your vagina that is more than a period.
C. You pass blood clots or tissue from your vagina.
D. Your vaginal bleeding has a foul odor.
E. You experience abdominal pain or uterine cramping not relieved by taking acetaminophen.

F. Other: _____

Phone: _____

VAGINAL BLEEDING: SECOND AND THIRD TRIMESTERS

PROBLEM

Vaginal bleeding may occur during the second and third trimesters of pregnancy (more than 12 weeks). The bleeding may range from spotting of blood on your panties to bleeding like a menstrual period.

CAUSE

A small amount of bloody mucous discharge or spotting may occur for about 1 day following a pelvic examination or sexual intercourse. This is normal if it is not associated with cramping or contractions.

Other causes of vaginal bleeding may be related to the location of the placenta (placenta previa) or premature separation (abruption) of the placenta from your womb. Placental abruption can be associated with cocaine use, cigarette smoking, and trauma (injuries from car wrecks or physical violence).

PREVENTION/CARE

There is no known way to prevent most types of vaginal bleeding. If you have been diagnosed with placenta previa, you may be able to prevent bleeding by avoiding sexual intercourse and maintaining bed rest.

There is no known method of preventing placenta previa. Smoking has been associated with placental abruption and placenta previa. You should not smoke or at least you should try to cut down and stop smoking during pregnancy. When you stop smoking, it is also good for your baby's health after delivery.

TREATMENT PLAN

A. Treatment depends on the cause of your vaginal bleeding. You may be placed on bed rest.
B. Stop smoking. Ask your provider for a handout on tips to stop smoking.
C. You may need to be on a rest schedule.
D. You may need to stop working.
E. You need to arrange help for child care, grocery shopping, and housework.

Activity: The checked activity restriction(s) are prescribed by the provider.

Level 1: As tolerated, avoid heavy lifting above 20 lb.

Level 2: Modified bed rest.
You may be out of bed for breakfast; rest (lying down) for 2 hours in the morning with moderate activity until lunch; rest for 2 hours with moderate activity until dinner.
Go to bed by 8 p.m.
Moderate activity consists of short periods of cooking and light housework.

Level 3: Strict bed rest.
You may be out of the bed only to go to the bathroom or to move to the couch.
You may take a shower, use the toilet, and brush your teeth, but then return immediately to bed.
No sexual intercourse
Perform ROM exercises as directed by your practitioner.

Diet: Eat fresh vegetables, fruits, and bran cereal to avoid becoming constipated on bed rest. Drinking extra liquids (especially water) also helps to prevent constipation.
Medications: Continue taking your prenatal vitamins every day.
You Need to Notify the Office If You Have:
A. Contractions or cramps, eight in 1 hour or four in 20 minutes
B. Bloody, mucous discharge not associated with recent sexual intercourse or a pelvic examination
C. Bright-red or dark-red vaginal spotting
D. Bleeding like a period

(*continued*)

VAGINAL BLEEDING: SECOND AND THIRD TRIMESTERS (*continued*)

E. A gush of fluid or blood from your vagina
F. Sharp, knifelike pain in your abdomen that does not go away
G. Pelvic pressure or low backache not relieved with emptying your bladder and resting on one side
H. Noticed decreased movement of the baby

I. Other: _____

Phone: _____

VAGINAL YEAST INFECTION

PROBLEM

You have been diagnosed with a vaginal yeast infection. This is an infection or inflammation of the vagina that is caused by a fungus known as yeast (*Monilia* or *Candida albicans*).

CAUSE

Yeast cells (Monilia) are normally present on the skin in healthy people. These cells may be found in the vagina or rectal area. However, due to a disturbance in the body's hormones and pH, an overproduction of these cells has occurred and has caused an infection. Several factors can cause this disturbance, which include menstrual periods, pregnancy, diabetes, antibiotics or other medications, increased dietary intake of sugars and alcohol, and an increase in moisture and warmth in the vaginal or rectal area by wearing tight, restrictive clothing.

PREVENTION/CARE

A. Keep the vaginal and rectal areas clean and dry.
B. Avoid tight, restrictive clothing such as tight jeans and underwear.
C. Wear cotton panties, or at least cotton crotched panties, that allow air to circulate. White underwear is best (no dyes). For sleep it is best not to wear underwear.
D. Avoid douching because this changes the normal flora and pH of the vagina, which can contribute to causing yeast infections.
E. Change damp swimwear or exercise clothing shortly after the activity. *Candida* thrive in warm, moist environments.

TREATMENT PLAN

If self-treated with over-the-counter medications, and symptoms do not resolve, you should be examined by a clinician to verify that the vaginitis is due to *Candida*.

Activity: There is no reason to alter usual activity.
Diet: Drink plenty of water and other liquids. Avoid alcohol and excessive sugars. Increase the intake of yogurt with live active cultures in your diet.
Medications: Antifungal medications may be prescribed for you.
1. Over-the-counter medications may include Monistat vaginal suppositories and cream. This is also known as miconazole nitrate, which you may find in the drug store at a much lower price and which can be just as effective.
2. You must use the full days of the over-the-counter medication. If you stop too early, the yeast can regrow.
    If you have also been diagnosed with a bacterial infection of the vagina, other medications may also be prescribed. If your provider has prescribed Flagyl (metronidazole), **please do not drink any alcohol while taking this medication and for the next 2 days following this medication. If your provider has prescribed tinidazole, alcohol should be avoided for 3 days. The combination of this medication and alcohol can make you very sick.**

You Have Been Prescribed: _____

You Need to Take: _____

You Need to Notify the Office If:
A. Over-the-counter medications do not help your symptoms.
B. You develop other symptoms.

C. Other: _____

Phone: _____

WARTS

PROBLEM

A wart is a raised, rough growth projecting from the skin, which can be contagious.

CAUSE

Warts are caused by a viral infection that stimulates the cells of the skin to multiply rapidly, which results in an outward growth.

PREVENTION/TREATMENT PLAN

A. Wash hands well
B. Avoid scratching or picking warts. Warts bleed easily.
C. Some warts go away spontaneously after time without any treatment.
D. Medications may be prescribed.

To Enhance Destruction

A. Soak the wart in warm water 10 to 15 minutes a day.
B. After soaking, use an emery board to file the wart down.
C. Apply over-the-counter medication as prescribed (Compound W) to the site.
D. Duct tape may be applied over the wart. Perform these steps every night until resolved.
E. Warts may reappear at the same spot or in other areas.
F. Cryotherapy "freezing" is another treatment option. Discuss this with your healthcare provider.

Activity: There are no activity restrictions for warts.
Diet: There are no special diets for warts.
Medications:

You Have Been Prescribed: _____

You Need to Take: _____

You Need to Notify the Office If:
A. You develop an infection at the site of the wart.

B. Other: _____

Phone: _____

WOUND CARE: LOWER EXTREMITY ULCERS

PROBLEM

An ulcer on the body that lies on the lower extremities

CAUSE

Edema, trauma, ischemia, venous insufficiency

PREVENTION/CARE

A. Keep the area clean and free of foreign debris.
B. Dressing changes: _____
C. You may be prescribed antibiotics; if so, take all antibiotics until they are completely gone.

TREATMENT PLAN

Activity: Do not apply direct pressure to the site of the ulcer. You may be prescribed to elevate your lower extremities.
Diet: Eat a well-balanced diet. Increase protein intake.
Medications:

You Have Been Prescribed: _____

You Need to Take: _____

You Need to Notify the Office If You Have:
A. A reaction or cannot tolerate any of the prescribed medications
B. A fever and a general ill feeling
C. Any new or unexplained symptoms related to the ulcer
  1. Increase in size
  2. New odor
  3. Increased drainage
  4. Change in color of the drainage
  5. Increased pain at the site
D. Any questions or concerns

Phone: _____

WOUND CARE: PRESSURE ULCERS

PROBLEM

An ulcer on the body that lies over a bony surface

CAUSE

Prolonged periods of pressure to the area of ulcer causing a breakdown of skin integrity

PREVENTION/CARE

A. Keep the area clean and free of foreign debris.
B. You may be prescribed dressing changes.
   1. Remove dressing.
   2. Clean the ulcer with normal saline.
   3. Apply prescribed medication (see the following).
   4. Cover with dry dressing, change as ordered.
C. You may be prescribed antibiotics; if so, take all antibiotics until they are completely gone.

TREATMENT PLAN

Activity: Do not apply direct pressure to the site of the ulcer.
Diet: Eat a well-balanced diet. Drink 8 to 10 glasses of water per day. Increase protein intake.
Medications:

You Have Been Prescribed: _____

You Need to Take: _____

You Need to Notify the Office If You Have:
A. A reaction or cannot tolerate any of the prescribed medications
B. A fever and a general ill feeling
C. Any new or unexplained symptoms:
   1. Increase in size
   2. New odor
   3. Increased drainage
   4. Change in color of the drainage
   5. Increased pain at the site
D. Any questions or concerns

Phone: _____

WOUND CARE: WOUNDS

PROBLEM

A wound is a break in the external surface of the body.

CAUSE

Wounds are often due to an accidental or intentional injury. Wound infection is usually caused by bacterial contamination of the site.

PREVENTION/CARE

A. Prevent accidental or intentional injury.
B. Immediately after injury, cleanse the wound well with soap and water.
C. Remove all dirt and foreign material.
D. You may be prescribed antibiotics; if so, take all antibiotics until they are completely gone.
E. You may need a tetanus shot.

TREATMENT PLAN

Activity: No restrictions. If infection is present, you may need to increase rest.
Diet: Eat a well-balanced diet. Drink 8 to 10 glasses of water per day.
Medications:

You Have Been Prescribed: _____

You Need to Take: _____

You Need to Notify the Office If You Have:
A. A reaction or cannot tolerate any of the prescribed medications
B. A fever and a general ill feeling
C. A wound/infection that seems to worsen
D. Any new or unexplained symptoms
E. Any questions or concerns

Phone: _____

WOUND INFECTION: EPISIOTOMY AND CESAREAN SECTION

PROBLEM

You have an infection of your episiotomy site or cesarean section incision.

CAUSE

The cause is one or more types of bacteria that invaded the tissue following your delivery. The bacteria may be from the vagina, the bowel, or the environment.

TREATMENT PLAN

A. Take your temperature if you have fever and chills.
B. Episiotomy:
  1. Wash hands before and after changing your sanitary pads and your baby's diaper.
  2. Wipe or pat dry from front to back after every urination or bowel movement (BM).
  3. Apply and remove perineal pad from front to back.
  4. Change perineal pad at least every 4 hours and after each void or BM.
  5. Use a squeeze bottle: Position the nozzle between the legs, empty the entire bottle over the perineum, blot dry with toilet paper, and avoid contamination from the anal area.
  6. Use a blow dryer on the lowest setting to "air dry" your stitches.
  7. Wash the perineum with mild soap and warm water at least once daily.
C. Cesarean section incision:
  1. Wash hands before and after dressing change and wound care.
  2. Follow all of the aforementioned directions (except 6) for your bleeding, too.
  3. After showering, gently pat dry your abdomen.
  4. If the wound is draining, cover it with a clean dressing and call the office for instructions. Otherwise, leave it open to air.
  5. Cleanse the incision with hydrogen peroxide and cotton swab. Do not clean the same area more than once with the same swab.
  6. If your incision opens, notify your practitioner for further instructions.

Activity: Increased rest is recommended; try to lie down for a nap when the baby goes to sleep.
Diet: There are no dietary restrictions; eat well-balanced meals. Increase your fluid intake with an infection. Drink at least 10 to 12 glasses of liquid a day.
Medications: Continue your prenatal vitamins. You may take acetaminophen 1 to 2 tablets every 4 to 6 hours for your fever and/or discomfort.

You Have Been Prescribed the Following Antibiotics: _____

You Need to Take: _____

Take all of your antibiotics, even if you feel better, unless you have an adverse reaction to them. Then call the office.

You Need to Notify the Office If You Have:
A. Temperature that rises significantly or reaches 101°F
B. Foul-smelling drainage from the incision or episiotomy site
C. Increased pain or tenderness
D. Separation of wound or incision

E. Other: _____

Phone: _____

XEROSIS (WINTER ITCH)

PROBLEM

Xerosis is severely chapped skin that becomes cracked, fissured, and inflamed. It can appear on skin anywhere on the body, but it is seen most commonly on the legs.

CAUSE

Xerosis is caused by insufficient oil on the skin's surface, which allows water to evaporate through the skin. Oil in the skin decreases with aging, excessive bathing, and excessive rubbing of the skin. An environment with low humidity also promotes dryness of the skin.

PREVENTION/CARE

A. Reduce water loss from the skin:
  1. Decrease the frequency and duration of baths or showers; use tepid water.
  2. Use soap sparingly.
  3. Avoid detergent soaps.
  4. Pat skin dry rather than rubbing.
  5. Apply skin lubricants (Lac-Hydrin, Eucerin, etc.) to dry skin before chapped areas become inflamed.
  6. Use ultrasonic, cool-mist humidifiers if the air is very dry.
  7. Clean the humidifier daily.
  8. Oil (such as Nivea) in the bath water may be helpful.
  9. Apply lubricants after bathing when possible to trap additional moisture before evaporation occurs.
B. Apply hand cream four to eight times a day to hands and twice daily on the trunk and extremities.

TREATMENT PLAN

Activity: No restrictions. Avoid long-term exposure to drying environments.
Diet: Eat a well-balanced diet; drink 8 to 10 glasses of water per day.
Medications:

You Have Been Prescribed: _____

You Need to Take: _____

You Need to Notify the Office If You Have:
A. Severely chapped skin, and self-care does not relieve the symptoms in 1 week
B. Chapped skin that becomes inflamed or if you see any oozing
C. Any questions or concerns

Phone: _____

ZIKA VIRUS INFECTION

PROBLEM

The Zika virus is a virus that is transmitted to humans by infected mosquitoes. Symptoms of the virus include low-grade fever, hand and/or foot joint pain, skin rash, headache, and/or eye discomfort or pain. The virus can spread to other humans by sexual contact with someone who is infected with the virus. A pregnant woman infected with the virus can spread the virus to her unborn baby.

CAUSE

The disease is caused by a bite from a mosquito infected with the Zika virus.

PREVENTION/CARE

Avoid traveling to countries with known cases of the Zika virus. The outbreak of this virus has been documented in Central and South America, Mexico, the Caribbean, and the Pacific Islands. It has also been documented in the United States territories of Puerto Rico, the U.S. Virgin Islands, and American Samoa.

There have been reported cases in the United States; however, the people diagnosed with the Zika virus had previously traveled to countries in which mosquitoes carry the virus.

TREATMENT PLAN

A. There is no medication or vaccination approved to treat the Zika virus.
B. Prevention of the virus is the most important thing one can do to protect from getting the virus. Avoid traveling to areas in which the Zika virus is transmitted by mosquitoes.
C. Medications, such as acetaminophen (Tylenol), may be given to improve symptoms if present such as headaches, fever, joint pain, eye pain, and muscle weakness.
D. It is thought that the Zika virus can cause another condition called Guillain–Barré syndrome, in which symptoms of severe muscle weakness can occur and even lead to paralysis. Notify your healthcare provider if you have any of these symptoms.

ACTIVITY:

Avoid sexual contact with any person thought to have the Zika virus.
A. Women:
   1. If you have traveled to any of the countries at risk of the Zika virus you should use condoms with sexual activity or do not have sex for at least **8 WEEKS** after your symptoms start.
   2. If you have traveled to any of the countries at risk of the Zika virus and you **DO NOT** have any symptoms, you should use condoms with sexual activity or do not have sex for at least **8 WEEKS** after returning.
   3. Avoid becoming pregnant while traveling to high-risk areas and avoid becoming pregnant up to **8 weeks** after travel.
B. Men:
   1. If you have traveled to any of the countries at risk of the Zika virus and you **HAVE** any of the above symptoms, you should use condoms with sexual activity or do not have sex for at least **6 MONTHS** after your symptoms started.
   2. If you have traveled to any of the countries at risk of the Zika virus and you **DO NOT** have any symptoms, you should use condoms with sexual activity or do not have sex for at least **8 WEEKS** after returning.
   3. If you have traveled to any of the countries at risk of the Zika virus and your **PARTNER IS PREGNANT** you should use condoms with sexual activity, or do not have sex, for the rest of your partner's pregnancy.
C. Precautions to use if you travel to a country with the Zika virus:
   1. Stay indoors. Mosquitoes infected with the Zika virus usually bite during the daytime, but precautions should also be taken for evening and nighttime hours.
   2. If screens in windows are not available, use a bed net to cover you while sleeping.

(*continued*)

ZIKA VIRUS INFECTION *(continued)*

3. Small children in strollers should also be covered with netting for protection.
4. Wear loose clothing to cover most of your body (light-colored clothing, long sleeves and pants, hat) to avoid mosquito bites.
5. Spray clothing with an insect repellant that contains permethrin when going outdoors.
6. Apply insect repellant that contains diethyltoluamide (DEET) or a chemical called *picaridin* to skin. Precautions should be used when using the insect repellant DEET on young children.
7. Insect repellent with DEET should not be used on children younger than 2 years old.
8. Apply insect repellent after sunscreen.
9. Avoid bodies of standing water such as pools, lakes, ponds, and so forth. Empty any containers with standing water such as buckets, plants, and so on.

DIET:

No special diet will prevent or improve the virus. You need to drink plenty of fluids to stay well hydrated.

Medications:

A. Acetaminophen (Tylenol) may be used for fever, body pain, and joint pain.
B. Avoid aspirin and nonsteroidal anti-inflammatory drugs (NSAIDs; ibuprofen, naproxen) because of the risks of bleeding if other conditions are present.
C. Children younger than 18 years should not use aspirin because of the risk of Reye's syndrome.

You Have Been Prescribed: _____

You Need to Take: _____

You Need to Notify the Office If:

A. Muscle weakness occurs. Guillain–Barré syndrome is a condition that is thought to be triggered by the Zika virus. Symptoms include muscle weakness and can lead to paralysis of the muscles and even death.
B. High fever increased joint pain, severe headache, confusion, or any other new symptoms present

C. Other: _____

Phone: _____

RESOURCE

CDC Zika Basics and How to Protect Yourself: https://www.cdc.gov/zika/pdfs/fs-zika-basics.pdf

APPENDICES

A Normal Laboratory Values

Normal laboratory values are presented here. However, ranges of laboratory value differ from laboratory to laboratory. They differ because of age and gender. Different values are presented; all normal values are listed under the Females column. Values for males and children are the same unless otherwise noted. Legend: 10^6 = 1,000,000; 10^3 = 1,000.

NORMAL LABORATORY VALUES

	Females	Males	Children
Complete Blood Count			
Red blood cells (RBCs)	3.8–5.1 10^6/μL	4.2–5.6 10^6/μL	3.5–5.0 10^6/μL
Hemoglobin (Hgb) ↑ Polycythemia, dehydration, ↓ blood loss, severe anemia, low production, or death of blood cell	11–16 g/dL	14–18 g/dL	10–14 g/dL Newborn 15–25 g/dL
Hematocrit (Hct) ↓ Anemia, massive blood loss, ↑ dehydration or hemoconcentration with shock	34%–47%	39%–54%	30%–42%
Mean corpuscular volume (MCV) RBC size: Normocytic, microcytic, macrocytic	78–98 fL		
Mean corpuscular hemoglobin (MCH) RBC color: Normochromic, hypochromic	27–35 pg		
Mean corpuscular hemoglobin concentration (MCHC)	31–37 g/dL or %		
Reticulocyte count Measures the number of new RBCs produced by the bone marrow	0.5–1.5%		
White Blood Cells (WBCs)			
↑ Bacterial infections, infectious diseases (mononucleosis), ↓ stress, tissue death, leukemia, cancer, hemorrhage	3.8–11.0 million/mm	3.8–11.0 10^3/mm³	5.0–10.0 10^3/mm³
Differential			
Segmented neutrophils ↑ stress, trauma, inflammatory disorders, ↓ viral infections, severe bacterial infections, aplastic anemia	50%–81%		
Band neutrophils	2–8 x 10^9/L		
Lymphocytes ↑ chronic bacterial infection, viral infections, ↓ leukemia, AIDS, lupus erythematosus	14%–44%		
Monocytes ↑ chronic inflammatory disorders, viral infections, chronic conditions, ↓ steroid therapy	2%–6%		
Eosinophils ↑ allergies, parasite infections, leukemia	1%–5%		
Basophils ↑ leukemia ↓ allergic reactions, stress, hyperthyroidism	0%–1.0%		
Serum iron concentration of iron bound to transferrin	60–160 mcg/dL	80–180 mcg/dL	
Total iron-binding capacity (TIBC) Amount of iron transferrin can bind	45–85 umol/L		

(*continued*)

NORMAL LABORATORY VALUES (*continued*)

	Females	Males	Children
Erythrocyte sedimentation rate (ESR)	Women <50	Males <50	
↑ Pregnancy, inflammatory conditions, ↓ sickle cell anemia	<20 mm/hr Women >50 <30 mm/hr	<15 mm/hr Males >50 <20 mm/hr	
BUN/Creatinine-Renal Function Tests			
Blood urea nitrogen (BUN)	6–23 mg/dL	0.2–0.6 mg/dL	
Creatinine (Cr)	0.6–1.5 mg/dL	3.5–7.7 mg/dL	
Creatine	0.6–1.0 mg/dL		
Uric acid	2.5–6.6 mg/dL		
Thyroid Studies			
Thyroid-stimulating hormone (TSH)	0.5–5 mIU/L		
T3 ↑ pregnancy and oral contraceptive use	0.7–1.5 ng/dL		
Thyroxine (T4) ↑ hyperthyroidism, ↓ hypothyroidism	10–20 pmol/L		
Aminotransferases			
↑ Liver damage and medications	4–35 U/L	7–46 U/L	
Alanine transaminase (ALT)	5–30 U/L	7–21 U/L	
Aspartate aminotransferase (AST)	5–30 U/L		
Bilirubin (Measures Bile Salt Conjugation and Excretion)			
Direct bilirubin	0.0–0.4 mg/dL		
Indirect bilirubin	Total bilirubin minus direct bilirubin		
Total bilirubin	2–20 umol/L 3.0 mg/dL indicates hepatic disease, jaundice is visible		

Glucose
Fasting 65–100 mg/dL
2-hr postprandial 65–140 mg/dL
Serum albumin (measures protein synthesis)
3.5–5.0 g/dL
↑ Dehydration, inflammatory illness, liver insufficiency, malnutrition, and cancer
Lipid profile—adults
Fasting cholesterol: Less than 200 mg/dL indicates low risk for coronary heart disease (CHD)
200–239 mg/dL: Borderline risk for CHD
>240 mg/dL: High risk for CHD
Triglycerides
<149 mg/dL: Low risk for CHD
150–199 mg/dL: Borderline risk for CHD
>200 mg/dL: High risk for CHD
High-density-lipoprotein (HDL): >40 mg/dL, desirable levels higher than 50 mg/dL
Low-density-lipoprotein (LDL): <100 mg/dL
100–159 mg/dL: Borderline CHD
>160 mg/dL: High risk for CHD
Triglycerides
Ages 0–9 years: <75 mg/dL; ages 10–19 years: <90 mg/dL
Ages 0–9 years: 75–99 mg/dL; ages 10–19 years: 90–129 mg/dL borderline risk for CHD
Ages 0–9 years: >100 mg/dL; ages 10–19 years: >130 mg/dL high risk for CHD
HDL: >45 mg/dL
40–45 mg/dL: Borderline risk for CHD
<40 mg/dL: High risk for CHD
LDL: <110 mg/dL
110–129 mg/dL: Borderline risk for CHD
>130 mg/dL: High risk for CHD

(*continued*)

NORMAL LABORATORY VALUES (*continued*)

	Females	Males	Children

Coagulation
Prothrombin time (PT): 10–14 sec
Partial thromboplastin time (PTT): 32–45 sec
Fibrinogen: 160–450 mg/dL
Bleeding time: 3–7 min
Thrombin time: 11–15 sec
Platelets: 140,000–450,000/mL
↓ Thrombocytopenia, acute leukemia/aplastic anemia during chemotherapy, interferon, infections, and drug reactions
↑ Myeloproliferative disease, cancer, and rheumatoid arthritis (RA)
International normalized ratio (INR): 0.8–1.2

Sickle cell disease
Sickle cell hemoglobin (HgbS): Normal, none present
Homozygous HgbS: Sickle cell disease
Heterozygous HgbS: Sickle cell trait
Hg electrophoresis: Determines Hg types and percentages

Hepatitis B
Hepatitis B surface antigen: Negative
Positive: Acute or chronic infection, further liver function tests needed
Hepatitis B surface antibody: Positive indicates immunity to infection (previous infection or hepatitis B vaccine)

Serum alkaline phosphatase (ALP; marks liver disease)
30–120 IU/L
Pregnancy value 30–200 IU/L
↑ Bile stones, biliary and pancreatic cancer, viral hepatitis, cirrhosis, Paget's disease, osteomalacia, bone metastasis

Urinalysis
Color: Pale yellow/straw to amber
Clarity: Clear
Specific gravity: 1.001–1.035
pH: Normal 4.6–8.0 (acidic)
Glucose: Absent
Ketones: Absent
Protein: Negative

Urine dipstick U/A
Nitrites: Negative (positive = bacteria, infection)
Leukocytes oxidase: Negative (positive = WBCs)

Arterial blood gas values
pH: 7.3–7.45
$PaCO_2$: 35–45 mmHg
HCO_3: 22–26 mEq/L
O_2 saturation: 96%–100%
PaO_2: 85–100 mmHg
Base excess (BE): −2 to +2 mmol/L

Venous blood gas values
pH: 7.31–7.41
$PaCO_2$: 41–51 mmHg
HCO_3: 22–29 mEq/L
O_2 saturation: 60%–85%
PaO_2: 30–40 mmHg
BE: 0 to +4 mmol/L

HIV
ELISA: Negative
ELISA: Positive: Repeat; if second ELISA positive. Perform Western blot
Western blot negative: No evidence of HIV
Western blot positive: Evidence of HIV

Rubella
Titer: >1:10 immune
Titer: <1:8 nonimmune administer Rubella vaccine

Female hormone levels

	Follicle-Stimulating Hormone (FSH)	Luteinizing Hormone (LH)	Progesterone	Prolactin
Follicular phase	2–25 mIU/mL	5–30 mIU/mL	0.2–6.0 mIU/mL	<23 ng/mL
Midcycle phase	10–90 mIU/mL	75–150 mIU/mL	6–30 mIU/mL	<28 ng/mL
Luteal phase	2–25 mIU/mL	3–40 mIU/mL	5.7–28.1 mIU/mL	5–40 ng/mL
Postmenopausal	40–350 mIU/mL	30–200 mIU/mL	0–0.2 mIU/mL	<12 ng/mL

B

Diet Recommendations

Bland Diet

Cheryl A. Glass and Jill C. Cash

You have been prescribed a bland diet. This diet provides adequate nutrition along with the treatment of gastrointestinal (GI) problems such as ulcerative conditions or inflammatory problems of the stomach and intestines. It is intended to decrease irritation in the lining of the stomach and intestines.

Food Tips

Foods to Avoid
Garlic, onions, alcohol, fatty foods, fried foods, chocolate, cocoa, coffee (even decaffeinated), dried fruits, citrus fruit and juices (orange, pineapple, and grapefruit), tomato products, peppermint, whole-grain breads and cereals, prespiced foods such as processed lunch meats and ham, pepper, and chili powder. Avoid pepper, chili powder, and cocoa spices.

General Instructions
A. Eat at least three small meals a day.
B. Avoid alcohol and beer.
C. Avoid caffeinated drinks/colas.
D. Avoid fried, greasy foods.
E. Bake or broil your foods.
F. Trim the fat from meats before cooking.
G. Bake, broil, mash, or cream potatoes.
H. Avoid raw fruits and vegetables, such as corn on the cob, and other gas-forming vegetables such as cabbage, dried beans, and peas.
I. Avoid rich desserts.
J. Avoid bedtime snacks—they may increase acid production and cause discomfort at night.
K. Avoid eating 2 hours before you go to bed.
L. Ask your healthcare provider if nutritional supplements are necessary.

Approved Foods by Food Group
A. Dairy products:
1. Whole milk
2. Low-fat or 2% milk
3. Skim milk
4. Evaporated milk
5. Buttermilk
6. Cottage cheese
7. Yogurt
8. Cheese

B. Meat:
1. Beef
2. Veal
3. Fresh pork
4. Turkey
5. Chicken
6. Fish (canned or fresh)
7. Liver
8. Egg (as a meat substitute)

C. Breads/grains:
1. Enriched breads (plain toast)
2. Oats
3. Cereal
4. Tortillas
5. English muffins
6. Saltine crackers
7. Pasta (all types)

D. Fruits/vegetables:
1. All vegetables
2. All fruits and juices (except citrus)

E. Desserts:
1. Custard
2. Pudding
3. Sherbet
4. Ice cream (except peppermint and chocolate)
5. Gelatin
6. Angel food cake
7. Pound cake
8. Sugar cookies
9. Jams and jellies
10. Honey

F. Drinks:
1. Decaffeinated tea
2. Juices (except citrus)
3. Caffeine-free sodas

G. Spices:
1. Salt
2. Thyme
3. Sage
4. Cinnamon
5. Paprika
6. Apple cider vinegar

7. Prepared mustard
8. Lemon and lime juices

DASH Diet: Dietary Approaches to Stop Hypertension

Cheryl A. Glass and Jill C. Cash

The Dietary Approaches to Stop Hypertension (DASH) diet is based on a combination of different types of foods and is recommended to help control high blood pressure (BP). It is a food plan that is based on foods that are low in cholesterol and high in dietary fiber, potassium, calcium, and magnesium; it is moderately high in protein. DASH eating has a reduction in lean red meats, added sugar, and sugar-containing sodas. The DASH diet's dairy food portions make the diet high in calcium and vitamin D. Overall, Americans, especially African Americans, are deficient in vitamin D.

The DASH diet, along with weight loss and exercise, is used to control other health problems such as type 2 diabetes and heart disease. If your ethnic background is Hawaiian, American Indian, Eskimo, Hispanic, or African American, you are at higher risk for high BP. Following a DASH eating plan will also help lower the bad cholesterol, or low-density lipoprotein (LDL), which can reduce heart disease.

A major way the DASH diet helps lower BP is to limit the amount of salt (sodium). The recommendations are limiting sodium to 2,300 mg a day or less. If you have high BP, you may be limited to 1,500 mg or less a day. One teaspoon of salt contains 2,000 mg of sodium.

Foods high in sodium make you retain extra fluid. If you notice that your hands are swelling (rings are tight) or your feet and legs swell (sock rings or shoes feel tight), you are getting too much salt. Fluid retention is bad if you have heart failure. This diet is rich in potassium, which can help you get rid of the extra sodium and decrease the fluid retention.

Sea salt, even though it may contain less sodium, is not low enough in sodium to use as a substitute for regular salt. Salt substitutes contain potassium chloride; this can cause more fluid retention. Potassium chloride salt substitutes may also interfere with your BP medications, so check with your healthcare provider before using them.

Tips for Reducing Sodium

A. Slowly cut back on your salty foods and begin to use healthier products. Take the saltshaker off the table.
B. Eat fresh foods.
   1. Avoid prepackaged foods.
   2. Eat fresh vegetables instead of canned vegetables. If you use canned vegetables, choose the low-sodium option and/or rinse the vegetables.
C. Read food labels.
   1. Sodium is in almost all processed foods, including milk.
   2. Focus on the amount of sodium per food serving.
   3. Do not forget to read labels on soda and sports drink bottles.

4. Choose your favorite food brand with low-salt or low-sodium labels on the package instead of the same product with more salt.
D. Avoid salty snacks and foods, including:
   1. Crackers, chips, and pretzels
   2. Cheeses
   3. Olives, pickles, pickled okra, and other foods
   4. Processed foods, including jerky, hot dogs, bacon, deli meats, canned fish, and canned meats, contain a large amount of sodium
E. Limit using soy sauce, seasoned salts, and meat tenderizers.
F. Many seasonings, including ketchup and sauces, contain a lot of sodium. Substitute with other flavors such as fresh herbs (e.g., rosemary, thyme, oregano, cilantro, and basil). Use garlic powder, lemon and lime juice, and crushed red peppers, as well as ginger.
G. Try making your own salt-free herb blend to use on your foods. Ingredients that can add flavor without adding salt include:
   1. Peppers such as cayenne, black pepper, and lemon pepper
   2. Dried herbs such as thyme
   3. Garlic powder
   4. Paprika
   5. Celery seed
H. Helpful websites for salt-free herb blend, products, and recipes are:
   1. Salt-free seasoning recipes:
      a. busycooks.about.com
      b. https://www.tasteofhome.com/recipes/salt-free-seasoning-mix/
   2. Websites with low-salt recipes:
      a. http://homecooking.about.com/library/archive/blhelp13.htm
      b. McCormick: www.mccormick.com
      c. Mrs. Dash: www.mrsdash.com

Tips on Eating the DASH Way

A. Start small. Make gradual changes in your eating habits, such as eating smaller portions (see Tables B.1 and B.2).
B. Center your meal around carbohydrates such as pasta, rice, beans, or vegetables.
C. Treat meat as only part of a whole meal instead of the main focus of the meal.
D. Use fruits or low-fat, low-calorie foods such as sugar-free gelatin for desserts and snacks.
E. Choose "whole" grains in breads and cereals.
F. Choose to eat vegetables without butter or sauce.
G. Choose lean cuts of meat. Use fresh poultry, for example, skinless turkey and chicken.
H. Choose ready-to-eat breakfast cereals that are lower in sodium.
I. Eat fruits for dessert. Use fruits that are canned in their own juice.
J. Add fruit to plain yogurt.
K. To increase eating vegetables, stir-fry with 2 oz of chicken and use 1½ cups of raw vegetables.
L. Snack on vegetables, bread sticks, graham crackers, or unbuttered/unsalted popcorn.

TABLE B.1 DASH DIET SERVING PORTION SIZES

Food	Portion Size	Food	Portion Size
1 baked potato	Fist	1 cup of popcorn (unbuttered)	Baseball
1 cup of flaked cereal	Baseball	½ cup of fresh fruit	½ Baseball
1½ oz cheese	4 Dice	½ cup of pasta, rice, or potato	½ Baseball
1 tbsp of margarine	1 Die	½ cup of ice cream	½ Baseball
¼ cup of raisins	Egg	3 oz of meat, includes fish, meat, and chicken	Deck of cards
¼ cup almonds	Golf ball	1 pancake	CD
2 tbsp peanut butter	Ping-Pong ball	1 piece of cornbread	Bar of soap
1 cup of salad	Baseball	3 oz of grilled or baked fish	Checkbook

Source: Adapted from National Heart, Lung, and Blood Institute. (2013). *Serving sizes and portions*. Retrieved from http://www.nhlbi.nih.gov/health/educational/wecan/eat-right/distortion.htm

TABLE B.2 DASH DIET DAILY SERVINGS

Food Group	Daily Servings	Serving Sizes	Examples and Notes	Significance of Each Food Group to the DASH Diet Pattern
Grains and grain product	6–8	1 slice bread ½ cup dry cereal ½ cup cooked rice, pasta, or cereal	Whole-wheat bread, English muffin, pita bread, bagel, cereals, grits, oatmeal, couscous	Major sources of energy and fiber
Vegetables	4–5	1 cup raw leafy vegetables ½ cup cooked vegetables 6 oz vegetable juice	Tomatoes, potatoes, carrots, peas, squash, broccoli, turnip greens, collards, kale, spinach, artichokes, beans, sweet potatoes	Rich sources of potassium, magnesium, and fiber
Fruits	4–5	6 oz fruit juice 1 medium fruit ¼ cup dried fruit ¼ cup fresh, frozen, or canned fruit	Apricots, bananas, dates, grapes, oranges, orange juice, grapefruit, grapefruit juice, mangoes, melons, peaches, pineapples, prunes, raisins, strawberries, tangerines	Important sources of potassium, magnesium, and fiber
Low-fat or fat-free milk and dairy foods	2–3	1 cup milk 1 cup yogurt 1.5 oz cheese	Skim or 1% milk, skim or low-fat buttermilk, nonfat or low-fat yogurt, part-skim mozzarella cheese, nonfat cheese	Major sources of calcium and protein
Lean meats, poultry, and fish	6 or less	1 oz cooked meats, poultry, or fish 1 egg	Select only lean; trim away visible fat; broil, roast, or boil instead of frying; remove skin from poultry	Rich sources of protein and magnesium
Nuts, seeds, and legumes	4–5 per week	1½ oz of nuts ½ oz or 2 tbsp seeds 2 tbsp of peanut butter ½ cup cooled legumes	Almonds, filberts, mixed nuts, peanuts, walnuts, sunflower seeds, kidney beans, lentils	Rich sources of energy, magnesium, potassium, protein, and fiber
Sweets and added sugars	5 or less per week	1 tbsp sugar 1 tbsp jelly or jam ½ cup sorbet or gelatin 1 cup lemonade	Fruit-flavored gelatin, fruit punch, hard candy, jelly, maple syrup, sugar	Sweets should be low in fat

DASH, dietary approaches to stop hypertension.

Source: Adapted from National Heart, Lung, and Blood Institute. (n.d.-a). *DASH Eating Plan*. Retrieved from https://www.nhlbi.nih.gov/health-topics/dash-eating-plan

M. Drink water or club soda.

N. Table B.3 lists the number of servings suggested and Table B.4 offers an example of the caloric adjustment for 2,000 calories a day using the DASH diet.

Resources

DASH Diet Calorie Adjustments for 1,200, 1,600, 2,000, and 2,400 calorie diets: http://dashdiet.org/images/calories.pdf

The DASH Diet Eating Plan: https://www.nhlbi.nih.gov/health-topics/dash-eating-plan

DASH Diet Recipes: https://www.mayoclinic.org/healthy-lifestyle/recipes/dash-diet-recipes/rcs-20077146

DASH for Health: www.dashforhealth.com/index.php

TABLE B.3   TOTAL NUMBER OF SERVINGS IN 2,000 CALORIES PER DAY DASH DIET

Food Group	Servings
Grains	6–8
Vegetables	4–5
Fruits	4–5
Fat-free or low-fat milk and dairy foods	2–3
Lean meats, poultry, and fish	2 (6 oz)
Nuts, seeds, and legumes	1 (4–5/wk)
Fats and oils	2–3
Sweets and added sugars	1 (<5/wk)

TABLE B.4   DASH EXAMPLE MENU (2,000 CALORIES)

Food	Amount	Servings Provided
Breakfast		
Orange juice	6 oz	1 fruit
1% low-fat milk	8 oz (1 cup)	1 dairy
Corn flakes (with 1 tbsp sugar)	1 cup	2 grains
Banana	1 medium	1 fruit
Whole-wheat bread (with 1 tbsp jelly)	1 slice	1 grain
Soft margarine	1 tsp	1 fat
Lunch		
Chicken salad	¾ cup	1 poultry
Pita bread	½ large	1 grain
Raw vegetable medley:	3–4 sticks each	1 vegetable
Carrot and celery sticks	2	1 dairy
Radishes	2 leaves	1 dairy
Loose-leaf lettuce	1.5 slice (1.5 oz)	1 fruit
Part-skim mozzarella cheese	8 oz (1 cup)	
1% low-fat milk	½ cup	
Fruit cocktail in light syrup		
Dinner		
Herbed baked cod	3 oz	1 fish
Scallion rice	1 cup	2 grains
Steamed broccoli	½ cup	1 vegetable
Stewed tomatoes	½ cup	1 vegetable
Spinach salad:	½ cup	1 vegetable
Raw spinach	2	½ fat
Cherry tomatoes	2 slices	1 grain
Cucumber	1 tbsp	1 fat
Light Italian salad dressing	1 small	1 fruit
Whole wheat dinner roll	1 tsp	
Soft margarine	½ cup	
Melon balls		
Snacks		
Dried apricots	1 oz (¼ cup)	1 fruit
Mini-pretzels	1 oz (¾ cup)	1 grain
Mixed nuts	1.5 oz (½ cup)	1 nuts
Diet ginger ale	12 oz	0

Fermentable Oligosaccharides, Disaccharides, Monosaccharides, and Polyols (FODMAP) Diet

Jill C. Cash

Irritable bowel syndrome (IBS) symptoms might be better following a strict low-fermentable oligosaccharides, disaccharides, monosaccharides, and polyols (FODMAP) diet and then reintroducing foods one at a time. You have been recommended to follow a change in your diet by decreasing carbohydrates such as fructose, fructans, lactose, and others called FODMAPs. FODMAPs are also found in certain grains, vegetables, fruits, and dairy product.

General Instructions

A. Keep a food diary of what you are eating and how you feel.

B. When your IBS symptoms are getting better, reintroduce one food at a time to see if it makes your IBS symptoms come back or get worse:

   1. After you feel that the new food does not cause increased IBS symptoms, try a second food.

   2. Foods that make your IBS symptoms worse should be continued to be avoided.

Low FODMAP Foods (Good to Eat)

- Vegetables (bean sprouts, kale, tomato, zucchini, spinach, eggplant, and carrots)
- Legumes (eggs, nuts, seeds, and tofu)
- Fruits (higher glucose than fructose) Eat only 1 serving per meal, 3 ounces (bananas, blueberries, pineapple, strawberries, oranges, mandarins, and kiwi)
- Meats, poultry, and meat substitutes
- Fish and seafood
- Cereals, grains, breads, biscuits, pasta, nuts, and cakes (brown rice, oats, polenta, quinoa, and tapioca)
- Condiments, dips, sweets, sweeteners, and spreads (glucose, maple syrup, sugar, artificial sweeteners including aspartame, saccharin, and stevia)
- Dairy foods and eggs (Cheddar cheese, feta cheese, Parmesan cheese, cream, and lactose-free milk)
- Beverages (black tea, coffee, gin, green tea, vodka, water, and white tea)

High FODMAP Foods (Avoid Eating These Foods)

- Wheat (main ingredient in food), barley, and rye
- Garlic
- Onions
- Fruits (higher in fructose than glucose, including apples, apricots, peaches, pears, watermelon, plums, nectarines, mangoes, and cherries)
- Vegetables (asparagus, brussels sprouts, artichokes, leeks, mushrooms, snow peas, and cauliflower)
- Legumes (baked beans, black-eyed peas, butter beans, kidney beans, lentils, soybeans, and split peas)
- Sweeteners (agave nectar, high-fructose corn syrup, honey, and sugar free gum/mints)
- Dairy (cottage cheese, cream cheese, milk, ricotta, and yogurt)
- Beverages (chai tea, chamomile tea, coconut water, dessert wine, and rum)

Foods to Avoid While Taking Warfarin (Coumadin, Jantoven)

Cheryl A. Glass and Jill C. Cash

Warfarin is a medication that thins the blood to prevent blood clots. Some nutrients and foods can interfere with warfarin and make the warfarin less effective or not work as well. Therefore, it is important to closely monitor the foods that you eat daily to make sure your medication is working for you the same way every day. One nutrient that causes this problem is vitamin K. Vitamin K interferes with the warfarin and can cause problems with thinning the blood. Therefore, it is important to avoid foods and nutrients that would cause this problem. It is suggested to eat foods that contain the same amount of vitamin K every day. This will help to prevent problems with thinning your blood.

The recommended intake of vitamin K for the adult man is 120 mcg and for adult women is 90 mcg.

The following is a list of foods that have a **MODERATE to HIGH level of vitamin K and should be avoided**:

1. Broccoli (cooked)
2. Brussels sprouts
3. Chard
4. Collard greens
5. Green tea
6. Kale
7. Mustard greens
8. Parsley
9. Spinach
10. Turnip greens

Some drinks can also interfere with warfarin and **should be avoided**. These drinks include:

1. Cranberry juice
2. Alcohol

Foods that have a **LOWER level of vitamin K** and are safer to eat in moderate portions include:

1. Asparagus
2. Avocado
3. Blackberries/blueberries
4. Cabbage
5. Carrots
6. Cauliflower
7. Cucumbers
8. Lettuce, iceberg, and romaine
9. Peas
10. Peppers
11. Potatoes
12. Prunes
13. Squash (summer and winter)
14. Sweet potatoes
15. Tomatoes
16. Tuna

Medications (prescribed and over-the-counter [OTC] medications, multivitamins, supplements, and herbal supplements) may also interfere with warfarin and should only be taken after discussing the medication, vitamin, or supplement with your healthcare provider for safety.

If you have questions about certain foods or medications, you need to discuss this with your healthcare provider.

Foods Rich in Vitamin K

If you are taking a blood thinner, you should be aware that certain foods are high in vitamin K

Vitamin K can interfere with how blood thinners work

You do not necessarily have to stop eating these foods, just be consistent and maintain your regular eating habits

Please discuss these foods further with your healthcare provider

These vitamin K–rich foods include the following:

1. Broccoli
2. Brussels sprouts
3. Collard greens
4. Endive
5. Kale
6. Mustard greens
7. Parsley
8. Swiss chard
9. Spinach
10. Turnip greens

Foods that are low in vitamin K:

1. Asparagus
2. Avocado
3. Blackberries
4. Blueberries
5. Cabbage
6. Cranberry juice
7. Green tea

8. Lettuce (iceberg and leafy)
9. Liver
10. Peas
11. Prunes
12. Tuna

Gluten-Free Diet

Cheryl A. Glass and Jill C. Cash

Gluten-Free Diet Tips

The symptoms from celiac disease are triggered from glutens in your diet. Three cereals that contain gluten are wheat, rye, and barley. Glutens are also present in other products, such as food additives, so it is very important to read all the ingredients on food labels (see Table B.5).

Dietary Recommendation for Celiac Disease

A. You may also be told to follow a lactose-free diet for a short time to help your symptoms.

B. Most bread sold in the grocery aisle is not allowed on a gluten-free eating plan.

C. All vegetables and fruits are gluten-free. However, frozen and canned fruits and vegetables may contain an additive with gluten.

D. Although you should not enjoy beer, wine is still on the menu when you go to dinner.

E. Specialty bakeries are able to make gluten-free cakes for special occasions. Plain hard candy, marshmallows, and other candies are usually gluten-free.

F. Caution should be taken when ordering any breaded foods such as chicken nuggets or breaded fish.

G. Deli meats may also contain gluten.

H. Gluten-free foods are often not fortified with vitamins and minerals. It is recommended to take a daily multivitamin.

TABLE B.5   EXAMPLES OF FOODS THAT ARE ALLOWED AND AVOIDED ON A GLUTEN-FREE DIET

Allowed	Avoid
Fresh fruits and vegetables without any processing or additives	Wheat, wheat berry, wheat bran, wheat germ, wheat grass, whole wheat berries
Meat	Flours, bread flour
Soy, soybean, tofu	Bulgur (bulgur wheat, bulgur nuts)
Brown rice	Rye
Enriched rice/instant rice/wild rice	Barley
Buckwheat	Barley malt/barley extract
Millet	Oats, oat bran, oat fiber
Sorghum	Cereals
Alfalfa	Matzo
Almond	Beer, ale, porter, stout
Canola	Farina
Chickpea	Croutons
Corn, corn flour, cornmeal	Bran
Brown rice flour	Tabbouleh
Tapioca	Soy sauce

Resources

Celiac Disease Foundation: www.celiac.org
www.celiac.com
https://www.chex.com/recipes/gluten-freecaramel-chex-mix/
www.BettyCrocker.com/glutenfree
Gluten-Free Recipes: https://www.allrecipes.com/recipes/
741/healthy-recipes/gluten-free/?internalSource=hubcard
&referringContentType=Search&clickId=cardslot%201

High-Fiber Diet

Cheryl A. Glass and Jill C. Cash

Fiber is a plant cell-wall component that is not broken down by the digestive system. An old term for fiber is roughage because it absorbs fluid and moves waste faster through the intestines in a bulky mass. The Food and Drug Administration (FDA) defines as high fiber those products that contain 20% of the daily fiber value. High-fiber diets are used to help prevent constipation as well as diarrhea. Fiber has been used to help several medical conditions such as diabetes, diverticulosis, IBS, and high cholesterol, as well as weight loss. If you have a chronic health condition, check with your healthcare provider about starting any new dietary change.

Fiber provides a full feeling that can help with spacing meals further apart (3–4 hours). Fiber recommendations change with your age (see Table B.6).

Tips for Increasing Fiber in Your Diet

A. Read the Nutrition Facts food label for fiber content per food serving.
  1. Cereals that provide 5 g of fiber per serving give you 20% of your daily fiber.
  2. Look for "whole grain" on the label. Just because bread is brown does not mean it is whole grain.
B. Increase fiber in your diet gradually to prevent gas. Adding too much fiber too quickly may give you abdominal pain, bloating, and constipation. Increase your fiber over several weeks so that it gives time for you to adjust.
C. As you increase fiber, it is also important to increase the amount of fluids you drink up to six to eight glasses a day, including tea, milk, fruit juices, coffee, and even soft drinks. The extra fluids that you drink along with the extra fiber makes you feel fuller, which can help control snacking.
D. Keep a food diary and review it periodically to decide on other diet adjustments that need to be made.
E. Several fiber supplements are available OTC to help you get your daily recommendation of fiber.

Good Food Sources of Fiber

A. Bran: Add 1 teaspoon of whole-grain bran to food three times a day, or take an OTC fiber supplement, such as psyllium (Metamucil), as directed.
B. Whole-grain cereals and breads: Eat oat, bran, multigrain, light, wheat, or rye breads rather than pure white bread or breads that list eggs as a major ingredient. Grains are not only a good source of fiber but also contain vitamins and minerals. Folic acid has been added to breads and cereals to help reduce neural tube defects.
C. Fresh or frozen fruits and vegetables: Citrus fruits are especially good sources of fiber. Eat raw or minimally cooked vegetables, especially squash, cabbage, lettuce and other greens, and beans. Leave the skin on fruits and vegetables; eating the whole fruit is better than drinking the juice. Whole tomatoes offer more fiber than peeling the skin off. The more colorful the fruit and vegetable (dark green, reds, blue, yellow), the better; they provide a good source of antioxidants that are good for the heart and the prevention of some cancers. Apples are a good source of both fiber and water.
D. Legumes (pods): Peas and beans are a good source of fiber. Add chickpeas and kidney beans to salads for extra fiber and flavor. Add baked beans as a delicious side item to your meal.
E. Coffee is another source of fiber.
F. Nuts are an excellent source of fiber. They are considered nutrient-dense and are a good source of vitamins and folic acid. Sprinkle sunflower seeds on a salad to add flavor and fiber. The amount of nuts eaten should be limited to 1 to 2 oz because they are also high in calories.
G. If you have diverticulosis: Avoid foods with seeds or indigestible material that may block the neck of a diverticulum such as nuts, corn, popcorn, cucumbers, tomatoes, figs, strawberries, and caraway seeds.

Lactose-Intolerance Diet

Cheryl A. Glass and Jill C. Cash

Lactose is the sugar present in milk. Lactose intolerance is very common; it occurs when the body is not able to appropriately digest this milk sugar content and the result is diarrhea. You have been diagnosed as having difficulty digesting milk (lactose) products or you have problems with malabsorption. Lactose intolerance can cause gas,

TABLE B.6	FIBER RECOMMENDATIONS BY AGE	
Group/Gender	Age (Years)	Fiber Recommendations (g of Fiber Each Day)
Children	1–3	19
Children	4–8	25
Boys	9–13	31
Boys	14–18	38
Girls	9–13	26
Girls	14–18	26
Men	Younger than 50	38
Women	Younger than 50	25
Men	Older than 50	30
Women	Older than 50	21

Source: Adapted from American Heart Association. (2016). *Fiber and children's diets*. Retrieved from https://www.heart.org/HEARTORG/HealthyLiving/HealthyEating/Fiber-and-Childrens-Diets_UCM_305981_Article.jsp

TABLE B.7   RECOMMENDED FOODS FOR LACTOSE INTOLERANCE

Foods	Recommended	Not Recommended
Milk	Soybean milk, milk treated with lactase, nondairy creamers, whipped topping; up to 1 cup/d of buttermilk, yogurt, sweet acidophilus milk, or whole, low-fat, or skim milk	Milk products in excess of 1 cup/d, malted milk, milkshakes, hot chocolate, cocoa
Meat and protein foods	All meats, fish, poultry, eggs, peanut butter, tofu, or hard, aged, and processed cheese, if tolerated	Sandwich meat, hot dogs that contain lactose, cottage cheese, any meat prepared with milk products
Vegetables	All fresh, frozen, canned, buttered, and/or breaded vegetables	Any vegetable prepared with milk or milk products in excess of allowance (1 cup)
Fruits	All fresh, frozen, or canned fruits	Any fruits processed with lactose
Breads, cereal, and starchy food	White, wheat, rye, or other yeast breads, crackers, macaroni, spaghetti, popcorn, dry or cooked cereals	Commercial bread products (French toast, bread mixes, pancakes, biscuits), cakes/cookies containing milk or milk products
Fats and oils	Butter/margarine, salad dressing, mayonnaise, all oils, nondairy creamers, bacon	Sour cream, salad dressings with milk products in excess of 1 cup allowance
Soups	Vegetable and meat soups, broth, and bouillon	Dried soups, creamed soups made with milk
Desserts	Plain and fruit-flavored gelatins, sherbet, fruit pies, cakes, pudding, pastries, angel food cake, sponge cake	Ice cream, ice milk, cream pie, puddings, custards, cakes, and pastries with milk (unless count as day's allowance)
Beverages	Coffee, tea, soft drinks, fruit juices, carbonated and mineral waters	Beverages with milk over the 1 cup allowance
Miscellaneous condiments	Catsup, mustard, soy sauce, vinegar, steak sauce, Worcestershire sauce, chili sauce	None
Seasonings	Salt, pepper, spices, herbs, and seasonings	None
Sweets	Sugar, jelly, honey, molasses, preserves, marmalade, syrups, hard candy, baker's cocoa, carob powder, artificial sweeteners	Cream or chocolate candies containing milk or milk products (unless count as day's allowance), caramels, toffee, and butterscotch

bloating, abdominal cramps, diarrhea, and nausea or vomiting. You may be able to eat small portions without problems, or you may be unable to tolerate any foods containing lactose (see Table B.7).

Tips for Following a Lactose-Intolerance Diet

A. Limit or omit foods that contain milk, lactose, whey, or casein.

B. Lactose-controlled diets allow up to 1 cup of milk per day for cooking or drinking, if you can tolerate it.

C. Read labels carefully. If you cannot tolerate any lactose, choose lactose-free foods with lactate, lactic acid, lactalbumin, whey protein, sodium caseinate, casein hydrolysates, and calcium compounds.

D. You may also choose kosher foods marked "pareve" or "parve," which do not contain lactose. Read labels carefully.

E. A low-fat diet is important if you have fat malabsorption.

F. To help with diarrhea because of malabsorption, avoid more than one serving a day of caffeine-containing drinks

G. Beverages with high sugar content, such as soft drinks and fruit juices, may increase diarrhea. Juices and fruits with high amounts of fructose include apples, pears, sweet cherries, prunes, and dates.

H. "Sugarless" sorbitol-containing candies and gums may cause diarrhea.

Low-Fat/Low-Cholesterol Diet

Cheryl A. Glass and Jill C. Cash

The connection between fat in the diet and heart attack is cholesterol. Cholesterol is a fatlike substance produced by your liver and also found in many foods. Too much cholesterol causes heart attacks by clogging the arteries that deliver blood to your heart.

Exercising and following a low-fat/low-cholesterol diet can help control your blood cholesterol and reduce your risk of heart attack.

Tips

A. Read food labels. Use the ingredient list on labels to identify products containing saturated fat. High-fat ingredients may have many names. Remember: Foods can say "no cholesterol" and still be high in saturated vegetable fat and calories.

B. Train yourself to think "low fat" in your food and cooking methods:
   1. Bake
   2. Broil
   3. Grill
   4. Stir-fry

C. Eat less-fried food, fast food, and baked products.

D. Eat more fruits and vegetables.

E. Organize your shopping around low-fat foods.

F. Add flavor to foods by using herbs and spices instead of butter and sauces.

G. Choose coleslaw, sliced tomatoes, or a dill pickle instead of fries and chips.

Foods to Avoid or Limit

A. Proteins/meats:
  1. Shrimp
  2. Fried meats, fish, or poultry
  3. Fatty ground meat
  4. Prime or heavily marbled meats
  5. Bacon, sausage, high-fat deli meats, and cheeses
  6. Liver and organ meats

B. Breads/cereals:
  1. High-fat baked foods, such as Danish, croissants, and doughnuts
  2. Fried rice, crispy chow mein noodles
  3. Granola bars with coconut or coconut oil
  4. Chips, cheese, or butter crackers
  5. High-fat cookies and cakes

C. Fruits and vegetables:
  1. Coconut
  2. Fried vegetables such as onion rings and breaded fried pickles, mushrooms, and okra
  3. Cream, cheese, or butter sauces on vegetables

D. Milk/dairy products:
  1. Whole or 2% milk
  2. Cream, half-and-half, nondairy creamers
  3. Ice cream, whipped cream, nondairy whipped toppings
  4. Whole-milk yogurt, sour cream
  5. Cheeses: Cheddar, American, Swiss, cream cheese, Brie, Muenster

E. Very high-fat foods:
  1. Butter or margarine made with partially hydrogenated oils
  2. Lard, meat fat, and coconut or palm oils
  3. Salad dressings made with sour cream or cheese
  4. Chocolate
  5. Beef tallow
  6. Hydrogenated or partially hydrogenated vegetable shortening
  7. Cream
  8. Cocoa butter

Foods That Are Allowed

A. Proteins/meats:
  1. Fish and shellfish
  2. Chicken and turkey cooked without the skin
  3. Ground turkey
  4. Eggs: Limited to two yolks per week
  5. Dried beans, lentils, tofu
  6. Small amounts of meat and seafood

B. Breads/cereals:
  1. Plain bread and English muffins and bagels
  2. Plain pasta, rice
  3. Cereals, oatmeal

  4. Pretzels, air-popped popcorn, rice cakes, Melba toast
  5. Low-fat baked goods: Angel food cake, graham crackers, fruit cookies, and gingersnaps

C. Fruits and vegetables:
  1. Eat several servings per day of high-nutrition, low-fat fruits and vegetables
  2. Prepare vegetables by steaming, broiling, baking, or stir-frying

D. Milk/dairy products:
  1. Skim or 1% milk
  2. Low-fat milk, evaporated milk, nonfat dry milk powder
  3. Frozen yogurt, ice milk, sherbet, sorbet
  4. Low-fat yogurt
  5. Low-fat cheeses: 1% cottage cheese, skim-milk ricotta, mozzarella, and American cheeses

E. Allowed high-fat foods:
  1. Margarine made with liquid safflower, corn, or sunflower oils
  2. Olive, canola, or peanut oils
  3. Nut snacks in moderation (high fat and calories)
  4. Salad dressings made with saturated oils

Nausea and Vomiting Diet Suggestions (Children and Adults)

Cheryl A. Glass and Jill C. Cash

For simple nausea and vomiting with an upset stomach, follow these steps:

Step 1: Replace Lost Fluids

A. Rest your stomach for 1 to 2 hours.

B. Infants and small children: Pedialyte or Ricelyte are recommended because children become dehydrated quickly.

C. Infants: Resume breast- or bottle-feeding as soon as possible.

D. Young children: Give very small sips every 10 to 20 minutes until they keep the fluid down.

E. Older children: Give Gatorade or Pedialyte.

F. Older child and adults:
  1. After vomiting stops, take sips of clear liquids at room temperature, such as flat ginger ale, flat cola, or gelatin.
  2. Suck on lollipops or Popsicles.
  3. Gradually increase the amount of liquids. If 4 hours pass without vomiting, progress to Step 2.

Step 2: Dry Diet

The foods in this diet do not meet all daily food requirements and should be used only for a short period before adding foods or advancing to Step 3.

A. Cheerios

B. Crackers

C. Cornflakes

D. Graham crackers

E. Rice Krispies

F. Vanilla wafers

G. Toast

H. Dinner rolls

Step 3: More Advanced Carbohydrates

A. Oatmeal

B. Grits, unseasoned

C. Rice, unseasoned

D. Mashed potatoes

E. Baked potato

F. Noodles

G. Peanut butter

H. Pudding

Step 4: Bland Foods With Limited Odors

After you are able to eat dry and more complex carbohydrates, a trial of bland foods may be tried. Foods with little or no odors are more easily tolerated after experiencing nausea and vomiting (see Table B.8).

BRAT Diet

You may be told to use a BRAT diet. This is a combination of foods that make up a bland diet and help with nausea and vomiting: Bananas, rice, applesauce, and toast as tolerated.

TABLE B.8   BLAND FOODS WITH LIMITED ODORS

Apple Juice	Canned Pears	Ice Cream
Apple sauce	Chicken noodle soup	Iced tea
Baked chicken	Cottage cheese	Low-fat milk
Baked turkey	Fresh apple	Sherbet
Canned peaches	Fresh banana	½ turkey sandwich

Vitamin D and Calcium Handout

Cheryl A. Glass and Jill C. Cash

VITAMIN D–ENRICHED FOODS

Food Source	Serving Size	Food International Units (IU)
Fish liver oils, cod liver oil	15 mL	1,360
Mushrooms	3 oz	2,700
Fortified milk	8 oz	100
Herring	3 oz	1,383
Catfish	3 oz	425
Mackerel (cooked)	3.5 oz	345
Salmon (cooked)	3.5 oz	360
Sardines (canned in oil, drained)	1.75 oz	250
Fortified orange juice	8 oz	100
Fortified cereal	1 serving	100
Fortified cheese	3 oz	100

CALCIUM-RICH FOODS

Food Source	Serving Size	Food International Units (IU)
Yogurt	1 cup	448
Orange juice	1 cup	350
Fat-free milk	1 cup	316
Shrimp	3 oz	275
Salmon	3 oz	182

(*continued*)

CALCIUM-RICH FOODS

Food Source	Serving Size	Food International Units (IU)
Instant oatmeal	1 packet	165
Tofu	½ cup	130
Broccoli	1 cup	94
Dried beans, cooked	½ cup	50
Cheddar cheese	1½ oz	306
Turnip greens	1 cup	197
Cereal bars, snack bars (fortified)	1 bar	200

Sunlight exposure to the skin is also recommended for approximately 20 to 30 minutes without sunscreen. Sun exposure provides an adequate source of vitamin D. Care should be taken not to burn skin.

1. Vitamin D recommendations:

   a. Men and women age younger than 50: 400 to 800 IU/d

   b. Men and women 50 years and older: 800 to 1,000 IU/d

2. Calcium recommendations:

   a. Women 50 and younger: 1,000 mg/d; women age 51 years and older: 1,200 mg/d

   b. Men age younger than 70: 1,000 mg/d; men 70 years and older: 1,200 mg/d

3. Vitamin D assists with calcium absorption into the bones.

4. Research indicates that caffeine interferes with calcium absorption and lowers bone density. Carbonated beverages appear to be worse than coffee.

5. Vitamin D and calcium deficiency contribute to bone loss, and thus, osteoporosis.

Bibliography

American Dietetic Association Reports. (2014). Position of the academy of nutrition and dietetics: nutrition guidance for healthy children ages 2 to 11 years. *Journal of the Academy of Nutrition and Dietetics, 114*(8), 1257–1276. doi:10.1016/j.jand.2014.06.001

American Heart Association. (2016). *Fiber and children's diets*. Retrieved from https://www.heart.org/HEARTORG/HealthyLiving/HealthyEating/Fiber-and-Childrens-Diets_UCM_305981_Article.jsp

Banks, D. (n.d.). Salt: Too much of a good thing. In *University of Illinois extension: Thrifty living*. Retrieved from http://urbanext.illinois.edu/thriftyliving/tl-salt.html

Gluten Intolerance Group. (2018). *Diabetes and celiac disease*. Retrieved from: https://gluten.org/resources/health-wellness/diabetes-and-celiac-disease/

National Heart, Lung, and Blood Institute. (n.d.-a). *DASH Eating Plan*. Retrieved from https://www.nhlbi.nih.gov/health-topics/dash-eating-plan

National Heart, Lung, and Blood Institute. (n.d.-b). *Tips for reducing sodium in your diet*. Retrieved from www.nhlbi.nih.gov/hbp/prevent/sodium/tips.htm

National Heart, Lung, and Blood Institute. (n.d.-c). *Tips on how to make healthier meals*. Retrieved from www.nhlbi.nih.gov/hbp/prevent/h_eating/tips.htm

National Heart, Lung, and Blood Institute. (2013). *Serving sizes and portions*. Retrieved from http://www.nhlbi.nih.gov/health/educational/wecan/eat-right/distortion.htm

National Heart, Lung, and Blood Institute. (2015). *In brief: Your guide to lowering your blood pressure with DASH*. Retrieved from http://www.nhlbi.nih.gov/files/docs/public/heart/dash_brief.pdf

National Institute of Diabetes and Digestive and Kidney Diseases. (2015). *Lactose intolerance*. Retrieved from https://www.niddk.nih.gov/health-information/health-topics/digestive-diseases/lactose-intolerance/Pages/facts.aspx

National Osteoporosis Foundation. (n.d.). *Calcium and vitamin D: What you need to know*. Retrieved from www.nof.org/articles/10

U.S Department of Agriculture, Agricultural Research Service, Nutrient Data Laboratory. (2014). *USDA national nutrient database for standard reference, release 27*. Retrieved from http://www.ars.usda.gov/nutrientdata. Appendix 13: Food Sources of Dietary Fiber. ªSource. Retrieved from https://health.gov/dietaryguidelines/2015/guidelines/appendix-13/

Tanner's Sexual Maturity Stages

	Sexual Maturity Stages in Females	Sexual Maturity Stages in Males
Stage	**Breasts**	**Penis, Testes, and Scrotum**
1	Preadolescent: Only papilla is elevated above the level of the chest wall	Preadolescent: All are the size and proportion seen in early childhood (testes 1 cm)
2	Breast budding: Breast and papilla elevated as small mound; increased diameter of areola	Slight enlargement, with alteration in color (more reddened) and texture of scrotum (testes 2.0–3.2 cm)
3	Continued breast and areola enlargement; no contour separation	Further growth and enlargement (testes 3.3–4.0 cm)
4	Areola and papilla form secondary mound	Penis significantly enlarged in length and circumference; further development of glands; enlargement of testes and scrotum with darkening of scrotal skin (testes 4.1–4.9 cm)
5	Mature: Nipple projects; areola is part of general breast contour	Genitalia of adult size (testes 5.0 cm)
Stage	**Pubic Hair**	**Pubic Hair**
1	Preadolescent: None or vellus hair in pubis area	Preadolescent: None or vellus hair in pubis area
2	Sparse, straight, lightly pigmented along medial border of labia	Sparse, straight, lightly pigmented at base of penis
3	Darker, coarser, curlier, and in increased amount	Darker, coarser, curlier, and in increased amount
4	Abundant, but has not spread to medial surface of thighs	Abundant, but less quantity than adult type
5	Adult feminine, inverse triangle, spread to medial surface of thighs	Adult distribution, spread to medial surface of thighs

Source: Used with permission from the Child Growth Foundation. Tanner's Sexual Maturity Stages. Retrieved from http://www.childgrowthfoundation.org

D Teeth

DECIDUOUS (BABY)

A, B: Incisors, 6 to 9 months
C: Cuspid (eyetooth), 16 months
D: First molar; 14 months
E: Second molar; 26 months

When they are lost:

A: 6 to 8 years
B: 7 to 9 years
C: 9 to 13 years
D: 8 to 12 years
E: 8 to 12 years
6*: Sixth-year molar*, first permanent tooth

Expected number of teeth up to 24
months = age of child in months −4
(e.g., 18-month-old should have 14 teeth)

PERMANENT

1, 2: Incisors, 7 to 9 years
3: Cuspid (eyetooth), 11 to 13 years
4: First bicuspid, 9 to 11 years
5: Second bicuspid, 10 to 12 years
6: Sixth-year molar, first permanent tooth
7: Second molar, 12 to 14 years
8: Third molar (wisdom), 16 to 20 years

Index